a LANGE medica

MW00753008

CURRENT
Diagnosis & Treatment:
Family Medicine

FOURTH EDITION

Jeannette E. South-Paul, MD, FAAFP
Andrew W. Mathieson UPMC Professor and Chair
Department of Family Medicine
University of Pittsburgh School of Medicine
Pittsburgh, Pennsylvania

Samuel C. Matheny, MD, MPH, FAAFP
Professor and Nicholas J. Pisacano, MD, Chair of Family Medicine
Department of Family and Community Medicine
Assistant Provost for Global Health Initiatives
University of Kentucky College of Medicine
Lexington, Kentucky

Evelyn L. Lewis, MD, MA, FAAFP
Deputy Director
W. Montague Cobb/NMA Health Institute
Washington DC
Adjunct Associate Professor
Department of Family Medicine and Community Health
Rutgers, Robert Wood Johnson Medical School
Piscataway, New Jersey

Mc
Graw
Hill
Education

New York   Chicago   San Francisco   Athens   London   Madrid   Mexico City   Milan
New Delhi   Singapore   Sydney   Toronto

ISBN 978-0-07-182745-4
MHID 0-07-182745-5
ISSN 1548-2189

Notice

Medicine is an ever-changing science. As new research and clinical experience broaden our knowledge, changes in treatment and drug therapy are required. The authors and the publisher of this work have checked with sources believed to be reliable in their efforts to provide information that is complete and generally in accord with the standards accepted at the time of publication. However, in view of the possibility of human error or changes in medical sciences, neither the authors nor the publisher nor any other party who has been involved in the preparation or publication of this work warrants that the information contained herein is in every respect accurate or complete, and they disclaim all responsibility for any errors or omissions or for the results obtained from use of the information contained in this work. Readers are encouraged to confirm the information contained herein with other sources. For example and in particular, readers are advised to check the product information sheet included in the package of each drug they plan to administer to be certain that the information contained in this work is accurate and that changes have not been made in the recommended dose or in the contraindications for administration. This recommendation is of particular importance in connection with new or infrequently used drugs.

This book was set in Minion Pro by Cenveo® Publisher Services.
The editor was Harriet Lebowitz.
The production supervisor was Catherine H. Saggese.
Project management was provided by Anubhooti Saxena, Cenveo Publisher Services.
RR Donnelley was printer and binder.

This book is printed on acid-free paper.

McGraw-Hill Education books are available at special quantity discounts to use as premiums and sales promotions, or for use in corporate training programs. To contact a representative please visit the Contact Us pages at www.mhprofessional.com.

*We would like to dedicate this book
to all family physicians who deliver care in austere environments,
especially our colleagues in uniform, and the families that support them.*

*Jeannette E. South-Paul, MD, FAAFP
Samuel C. Matheny, MD, MPH, FAAFP
Evelyn L. Lewis, MD, MA, FAAFP*

Contents

Section IV. Geriatrics

Section V. Therapeutics, Genetics, & Prevention

Section VI. Psychosocial Disorders

Authors

Pamela Allweiss, MD, MSPH
Community Faculty
Department of Family and Community Medicine
University of Kentucky College of Medicine
Lexington, Kentucky
pallweiss@windstream.net
Endocrine Disorders

Robert Arnold, MD
Leo H Criep Professor of Medicine
Section of Palliative Care and Medical Ethics
University of Pittsburgh
Pittsburgh, Pennsylvania
Hospice & Palliative Medicine

Cindy M. Barter, MD, MPH, IBCLC, CTTS, FAAFP
Residency Faculty
Hunterdon Family Medicine Residency Program
Flemington, New Jersey
cindy@thebarters.net
Abdominal Pain

Kevin Bernstein, MD, MMS, LT, MC, USN
Chief Resident
Naval Hospital
Pensacola, Florida
Kevin.bernstein@med.navy.mil
Hypertension

Samidha Bhat, MD
Family Medicine Resident
University of Pittsburgh Medical Center
McKeesport Family Medicine Resdiency Program
McKeesport, Pennsylvania
samidha.bhat@gmail.com
Breastfeeding & Infant Nutrition

Daphne P. Bicket, MD, MLS
UPMC McKeesport Family Medicine Residency Program
McKeesport, Pennsylvania
bicketdp@upmc.edu
Common Geriatric Problems

W. Scott Black, MD
Associate Professor
Department of Family and Community Medicine
Lexington, Kentucky
wsblac0@uky.edu
Common Upper & Lower Extremity Fractures

Susan C. Brunsell, MD
Medical Director
Executive Medicine Clinic
Walter Reed National Military Medical Center
Assistant Professor of Family Medicine
Uniformed Services University of the Health Sciences
Bethesda, Maryland
Susan.c.brunsell.civ@mail.mil
Contraception

Kim A. Bullock, MD, FAAFP
Director
Community Health Division
Director
HRSA Fellowships
Assistant Director
Service Learning
Associate Clinical Professor
Department of Family Medicine
Georgetown Medical School
Washington DC
kimabullock@hotmail.com
Cultural and Linguistic Competence

Christopher W. Bunt, MD, FAAFP
Assistant Professor
Family Medicine
Uniformed Services University
Major
USAF
Bethesda, Maryland
christopher.bunt@usuhs.edu
Physical Activity in Adolescents

Deepa Burman, MD, D.ABSM
Family Medicine Faculty
Director of Sleep Clinic and Resident Scholarly Activity
UPMC McKeesport
McKeesport, Pennsylvania
burmand@upmc.edu
Travel Medicine

Robert J. Carr, MD
Medical Director
Primary Care of Southbury, Southbury
Connecticut
Danbury Office of Physician Services
Danbury, Connecticut
robber.carr@charter.net
Urinary Incontinence

Elizabeth Cassidy, PharmD, BCPS
UPMC St. Margaret
Pharmacy Residency Program
Pittsburgh, Pennsylvania
forsbergea@upmc.edu
Pharmacotherapy Principles for the Family Physician

C. Randall Clinch, DO, MS
Associate Professor
Department of Family & Community Medicine
Wake Forest University School of Medicine
Winston-Salem, North Carolina
crclinch@wfubmc.edu
Evaluation & Management of Headache

Tracey D. Conti, MD
Assistant Professor Department of Family Medicine
University of Pittsburgh School of Medicine
Program Director
UPMC McKeesport Family Medicine Residency
McKeesport, Pennsylvania
Vice Chair UPMC McKeesport Department of Family
    Medicine
contitd@upmc.edu
Breastfeeding & Infant Nutrition

Barry Coutinho, MD
Clinical Assistant Professor Family Medicine
University of Pittsburgh School of Medicine
Faculty
Family Medicine Residency
UPMC Shadyside Hospital
Pediatric Dermatology
Pittsburgh, Pennsylvania
coutinhobv@upmc.edu
Skin Diseases in Infants & Children

Lora Cox-Vance, MD
Clinical Assistant Professor
Department of Family Medicine
UPMC, Director, Geriatric Fellowship
UPMC St. Margaret Hospital
Pittsburgh, Pennsylvania
coxla@upmc.edu
Healthy Aging & Geriatric Assessment
Health Maintenance for Adults

Amy Crawford-Faucher, MD, FAAFP
Clinical Assistant Professor Family Medicine and Psychiatry
University of Pittsburgh Medical Center
Pittsburgh, Pennsylvania
crawfordfauchera@upmc.edu
Adolescent Sexuality
Interpersonal Violence

K. Michael Cummings, PhD, MPH
Chair, Department of Health Behavior
Roswell Park Cancer Institute
Buffalo, New York
Michael.cummings@roswellpark.org
Tobacco Cessation

Anja Dabelić, MD
Department Head
Family Medicine
Family Medicine Residency Program Faculty
Naval Hospital
Pensacola, Florida
Anja.Dabelic@med.navy.mil
Respiratory Problems

Niladri Das, MD, UPMC
Faculty
UPMC St. Margaret Family Medicine Residency Program
Pittsburgh, Pennsylvania
dasn@upmc.edu
Tickborne Disease

Essam Demian, MD, FRCOG
Clinical Assistant Professor
Department of Family Medicine
University of Pittsburgh School of Medicine
Pittsburgh, Pennsylvania
demiane@upmc.edu
Preconception Care

James C. Dewar, MD
Assistant Professor
Department of Family Medicine
University of Pittsburgh School of Medicine
Pittsburgh, Pennsylvania
Vice Chair for Education
Department of Family Medicine
Dewarjc2@upmc.edu
Common Acute Infections in Children
Failure to Thrive

Stephanie B. Dewar, MD
Associate Professor of Pediatrics
University of Pittsburgh School of Medicine
Pediatric Residency Program
Director Children's Hospital of Pittsburgh of UPMC
Pittsburgh, Pennsylvania
dewarstephanie@upmc.edu
Common Acute Infections in Children
Failure to Thrive

Jeanne M. Doperak, DO
Assistant Professor of Sports Medicine
University of Pittsburgh Department of Orthopedics
UPMC St. Margaret Primary Care Sports Medicine
    Fellowship Director
Team Physician
University of Pittsburgh
Pittsburgh, Pennsylvania
Doperakjm@upmc.edu
Acute Musculoskeletal Complaints

Laura Dunne, MD, CAQSM, FAAFP
Head
Women's Center for Sports Medicine OAA
OAA Orthopaedic Specialists
Allentown, Pennsylvania
lauradunne@aol.com
Abdominal Pain

William G. Elder, PhD
Professor
Department of Family and Community Medicine
University of Kentucky Chandler Medical Center
Lexington, Kentucky
welder@email.uky.edu
Personality Disorders
Somatic Symptom Disorder (Previously Somatoform Disorder),
    Factitious Disorder, & Malingering

Patricia Evans, MD, MA
Assistant Professor
Department of Family Medicine
Georgetown University
Washington DC
Fort Lincoln Family Medicine Center
evansp@georgetown.edu
Vaginal Bleeding

Lawrence S. Fields, MD
University of Louisville
Louisville, Kentucky
University of Kentucky
Lexington, Kentucky
larrysfields@yahoo.com
The Patient-Centered Medical Home

Ronald M. Glick, MD
Assistant Professor of Psychiatry
Physical Medicine and Rehabilitation and Family Medicine
Center for Integrative Medicine
UPMC
Pittsburgh, Pennsylvania
glickrm@upmc.edu
Chronic Pain Management

Wanda C. Gonsalves, MD
Professor and Vice Chair
Department of Family Medicine and Community Medicine
University of Kentucky Chandler Medical Center
Lexington, Kentucky
wcgons0@uky.edu
Oral Health

Darci L. Graves, MPP, MA, MA
Former Instructor and Research Assistant
Office of Medical Education and Research
University of Missouri–Kansas City School of Medicine
Kansas City, Missouri
darci@beyondthegoldenrule.org
Cultural and Linguistic Competence

Mary P. Guerrera, MD, FAAFP, DABIHM
Professor and Director of Integrative Medicine
Department of Family Medicine
University of Connecticut Health Center
Farmington, Connecticut
guerrera@uchc.edu
Complementary & Alternative Medicine

Garry W. K. Ho, MD, CAQSM
Assistant Program Director
Virginia Commonwealth University (VCU)
Fairfax Family Practice Sports Medicine Fellowship
Assistant Professor
Department of Family Medicine
VCU School of Medicine
Medical Director
Fairfax County Public School System Athletic Training
    Program
Fairfax, Virginia
gho@ffpcs.com
Neck Pain

W. Allen Hogge, MD, MA
Milton Lawrence McCall Professor and Chair
Department of Obstetrics, Gynecology, and Reproductive
    Sciences
University of Pittsburgh/Magee–Womens Hospital
whogge@mail.magee.edu
Genetics for Family Physicians

Robert G. Hosey, MD
Professor
Department of Family and Community Medicine
Department of Orthopaedic Surgery and Sports Medicine
Director
Primary Care Sports Medicine Fellowship
University of Kentucky
Lexington, Kentucky
rhosey@email.uky.edu
Common Upper & Lower Extremity Fractures

Thomas M. Howard, MD, FASCM
Program Director
Virginia Commonwealth University (VCU)
Fairfax Family Practice Sports Medicine Fellowship
Associate Professor
Department of Family Medicine
VCU School of Medicine
Fairfax, Virginia
Thmd2020@gmail.com
Neck Pain

Lovie J. Jackson-Foster, PhD, MSW
Assistant Professor
School of Social Work
University of Pittsburgh
Pittsburgh, Pennsylvania
ljj10@pitt.edu
Interpersonal Violence

Carla Jardim, MD
Lead Physician
Delaware Valley Family Health Center
Family Medicine Residency
Hunterdon Medical Center
jardim.carla@hunterdonhealthcare.org
Abdominal Pain

Jennie Broders Jarrett, PharmD, BCPS
Director
Inpatient Pharmacotherapy Education
Clinical Pharmacist/Faculty Member
UPMC St. Margaret
Family Medicine Residency Program
Pittsburgh, Pennsylvania
brodersjk@upmc.edu
Pharmacotherapy Principles for the Family Physician

Martin G. Johns, MD
Associate Residency Director
UPMC McKeesport Family Medicine Residency
McKeesport
Pennsylvania
johnsmg@upmc.edu
Prenatal Care

Bruce E. Johnson, MD
Professor of Medicine
Assistant Dean for Faculty Affairs
Virginia Tech Carilion School of Medicine
Roanoke, Virginia
bejohnson@carilion.com
Arthritis: Osteoarthritis, Gout, & Rheumatoid Arthritis

Joshua R. Johnson, MD, CAQSM
Knoxville Orthopedic Clinic
Knoxville, Tennessee
Common Upper & Lower Extremity Fractures

Wayne B. Jonas, MD
President and CEO
Samueli Institute
Associate Professor
Family Medicine
Uniformed Services University of the Health Sciences
Alexandria, Virginia
wjonas@siib.org
Complementary & Alternative Medicine

Peter J. Katsufrakis, MD, MBA
Vice President
Assessment Programs
National Board of Medical Examiners
Philadelphia, Pennsylvania
pkatsufrakis@nbme.org
Sexually Transmitted Diseases

Michael King, MD
Assistant Professor and Residency Program Director
Department of Family and Community Medicine
College of Medicine
University of Kentucky
Lexington, Kentucky
mrking02@uky.edu
Heart Failure

Joe E. Kingery, DO, CPE
Assistant Professor and Medical Director
Department of Family and Community Medicine
University of Kentucky
Hazard, Kentucky
Joe.kingery@uky.edu
Urinary Tract Infections

Mark A. Knox, MD
Faculty
Hawaii Island Family Medicine Residency Program
Hilo, Hawaii
Clinical Associate Professor
John A. Burns School of Medicine
Department of Family Medicine and Community Health
University of Hawaii
mknox@hhsc.org
Skin Diseases in Infants & Children

N. Randall Kolb, MD
Clinical Associate Professor of Family Medicine
University of Pittsburgh School of Medicine
Program Director
UPMC Shadyside Family Medicine Residency
Pittsburgh, Pennsylvania
kolbnr@upmc.edu
Tuberculosis

Ronald J. Koshes, MD, DFAPA
Private Practice
Washington DC
ronkoshes@aol.com
Combat-Related Posttraumatic Stress Disorder & Traumatic Brain Injury

Matthew D. Krasowski, MD, PhD
Clinical Associate Professor
Director of Clinical Laboratories
Department of Pathology
University of Iowa Hospitals and Clinics
Iowa City, Iowa
mkrasows@healthcare.uiowa.edu
Pharmacogenomics

LTC Mary V. Krueger, DO
PACOM Scholar
Dwight D. Eisenhower School for National Security and Resource Strategy
National Defense University
Fort McNair
Washington DC
mary.v.krueger.mil@mail.mil
Menstrual Disorders

Archana Kudrimoti, MD (MBBS) MPH
Assistant Professor
Clerkship Director
Department of Family and Community Medicine
Lexington, Kentucky
akudr2@email.uky.edu
Hearing & Vision Impairment in the Elderly

Paul R. Larson, MD, MS, DTMH
Director
Global Health Education
UPMC St. Margaret Family Medicine Residency Program
Clinical Assistant Professor
Department of Family Medicine
University of Pittsburgh School of Medicine
Pittsburgh, Pennsylvania
larsonpr@upmc.edu
Health Maintenance for Adults

Evelyn L. Lewis, MD, MA, FAAFP
Adjunct Associate Professor
Department of Family Medicine and Medical and Clinical Psychology
Uniformed Services University, Bethesda, MD
Chief Medical Officer, The Steptoe Group
Deputy Director
W. Montague Cobb/NMA Health Institute
Washington DC
Adjunct Associate Professor
Department of Family Medicine and Community Health
Rutgers, Robert Wood Johnson Medical School
Piscataway, New Jersey
elewismd2504@gmail.com
Eating Disorders
Health & Healthcare Disparities
Combat-Related Posttraumatic Stress Disorder & Traumatic Brain Injury

Kristin Long, MD
General Surgery Resident, PGY-5
University of Kentucky
Department of General Surgery
Lexington, Kentucky
kristin.long@uky.edu
Hepatobiliary Disorders

Charles W. Mackett III, MD, FAAFP
Senior Vice President and Chief Medical Officer
Indian River Medical Center
Vero Beach, Florida
Clinical Associate Professor
University of Pittsburgh School of Medicine
Pittsburgh, Pennsylvania
charles.mackett@irmc.cc
Adult Sexual Dysfunction

Kiame J. Mahaniah, MD
Assistant Professor
Family Medicine Department
Tufts University School of Medicine
Tufts University
Boston, Massachusetts
Associate Residency Director
Greater Lawrence Family Medicine Residency
Lawrence, Massachusetts
K_mahaniah@hotmail.com
Anemia

Martin C. Mahoney, MD, PhD, FAAFP
Associate Professor
Department of Family Medicine
School of Medicine & Biomedical Sciences
State University of New York (SUNY) at Buffalo
Buffalo, New York
Associate Professor
Department of Health Behavior
Roswell Park Cancer Institute
Buffalo, New York
martin.mahoney@roswellpark.org
Neonatal Hyperbilirubinemia
Tobacco Cessation

Robin Maier, MD, MA
Assistant Professor of Family Medicine
Department of Family Medicine
Director of Medical Student Education
Clerkship Director
University of Pittsburgh School of Medicine
Pittsburgh, Pennsylvania
maierrm@upmc.edu
Sexually Transmitted Diseases

Robert Mallin, MD
Dean of Medical Education
American University of Antigua (AUA)
Coolidge, Antigua
rmallin@auamed.net
Substance Use Disorders

Dawn A. Marcus, MD*
Professor
Department of Anesthesiology
University of Pittsburgh Medical Center
Pittsburgh, Pennsylvania
Chronic Pain Management

William H. Markle, MD, FAAFP, DTM&H
Clinical Associate Professor Family Medicine
University of Pittsburgh School of Medicine
UPMC McKeesport
McKeesport, Pennsylvania
marklew@upmc.edu
Travel Medicine

Samuel C. Matheny, MD, MPH, FAAFP
Professor and Nicholas J. Pisacano, MD, Chair of Family
Department of Family and Community Medicine
Assistant Provost for Global Health Initiatives
University of Kentucky College of Medicine
Lexington, Kentucky
matheny@email.uky.edu
Hepatobiliary Disorders

Philip J. Michels, PhD
Michels Psychological Services
PA (Philadelphia) Columbia, South Carolina
michelsfour@hotmail.com
Anxiety Disorders

Donald B. Middleton, MD
Professor
Department of Family Medicine
University of Pittsburgh School of Medicine
Vice President, Family Medicine Residency Education
UPMC St. Margaret
Pittsburgh, Pennsylvania
middletondb@upmc.edu
Well- Child Care
Routine Childhood Vaccines
Seizures

Francis G. O'Connor, MD, MPH, COL, MC, USA
Associate Professor, Chair
Department of Military and Emergency Medicine
Uniformed Services University of the Health Sciences
Bethesda, Maryland
francis.oconnor@usuhs.edu
Low Back Pain in Primary Care

Maureen O'Hara Padden, MD, MPH, FAAFP, CAPT, MC, USN (FS)
Executive Officer
Naval Hospital Pensacola
Pensacola, Florida
maureen.padden@med.navy.mil or scarlettmo@aol.com
Hypertension

Mamta Patel, MD
Resident
University of Pittsburgh Medical Center
McKeesport, Pennsylvania
patel_mamta@yahoo.com
Breastfeeding & Infant Nutrition

Oscar O. Perez Jr., DO, FAAFP
Assistant Professor
Associate Residency Director
Department of Family and Community Medicine
University of Kentucky
ope222@uky.edu
Heart Failure

Jonathan J. Perkins, MD
DeKalb Medical Center
Decatur, Georgia
jonathanjoelperkins@gmail.com
Acute Coronary Syndrome

---

*Deceased.

Saranne E. Perman, MD
Lexington Clinic
Family Medicine
Jessamine Medical and Diagnostics Center
Nicholasville, Kentucky
spearman1@gmail.com
Hearing & Vision Impairment

Marybeth Porter, MD
Clinical Instructor and Academic Generalist Fellow
Department of Family Medicine
Medical University of South Carolina
Charleston, South Carolina
portem@musc.edu
Substance Use Disorders

Nicole Powell-Dunford, MD, MPH FAAP
Deputy Commander for Clinical Services
US Army Health Clinic Schofield
Barracks
Wahiawa, Hawaii
Nicole.c.powell-dunford.mil@mail.mil
Cancer Screening in Women

Ramakrishna Prasad, MD, MPH, AAHIVS
Clinical Assistant Professor of Medicine
HIV/AIDS Program
Division of Infectious Diseases
Faculty
UPMC Shadyside Family Medicine Residency Program
Pittsburgh, Pennsylvania
prasadr@upmc.edu
HIV Primary Care

Brian A. Primack, MD, PhD, EdM, MS
Assistant Professor
Departments of Medicine and Pediatrics
School of Medicine
University of Pittsburgh
Pittsburgh, Pennsylvania
bprimack@pitt.edu
Anemia

Annelle B. Primm, MD, MPH
Deputy Medical Director
CEO and Medical Director's Office
American Psychiatric Association
aprimm@psych.org
Depression in Diverse Populations & Older Adults

Rachel M. Radin, MA, MS
Doctoral Candidate
Department of Medical and Clinical Psychology
Developmental Research Laboratory on Eating and Weight
    Behaviors
Uniformed Services University of the Health Sciences
Bethesda, Maryland
Rachel.Radin@usuhs.edu
Eating Disorders

Kelly L. Evans-Rankin, MD, CAQSM
Assistant Professor
University of Kentucky College of Medicine
Department of Family and Community Medicine
knev222@uky.edu
Common Upper & Lower Extremity Fractures

Wade M. Rankin, DO, CAQSM
Assistant Professor
University of Kentucky College of Medicine
Department of Family and Community Medicine
wademrankin@uky.edu
Common Upper & Lower Extremity Fractures

Lisa M. Ranzenhofer, PhD
Postdoctoral Research Fellow
Weight Control and Diabetes Research Center
The Miriam Hospital / Brown University Warren Alpert
    Medical School
Providence, Rhode Island
lisa_ranzenhofer@brown.edu
Eating Disorders

Brian V. Reamy, MD
Senior Associate Dean for Academic Affairs & Professor of
    Family Medicine
F. Edward Hébert School of Medicine
Uniformed Services University
brian.reamy@usuhs.edu
Dyslipidemias

Eva B. Reitschuler-Cross, MD
Assistant Professor of Medicine
University of Pittsburgh School of Medicine
University of Pittsburgh Medical Center
Division of General Medicine
Section of Palliative Care and Medical Ethics
Pittsburgh, Pennsylvania
reitschulercrosseb@upmc.edu
Hospice & Palliative Medicine

J. Scott Roth, MD, FACS
Professor of Surgery
Chief, Gastrointestinal Surgery
University of Kentucky
College of Medicine
Lexington, Kentucky
sroth@uky.edu
Hepatobiliary Disorders

Lauren M. Sacha, PharmD, BCPS
Staff Pharmacist
UPMC St. Margaret
Pittsburgh, Pennsylvania
sachalm@upmc.edu
Pharmacotherapy Principles for the Family Physician

Ruth S. Shim, MD, MPH
Vice Chair
Education and Faculty Development
Department of Psychiatry
Lenox Hill Hospital
New York, New York
rshim@nshs.edu
Depression in Diverse Populations

Gregory N. Smith, MD
Vice Chair for Operations Department of Family Medicine
University of Pittsburgh School of Medicine
Pittsburgh, Pennsylvania
Prenatal Care

Jeannette E. South-Paul, MD
Andrew W. Mathieson UPMC Professor and Chair
Department of Family Medicine
University of Pittsburgh School of Medicine
Pittsburgh, Pennsylvania
soutjx@upmc.edu
Osteoporosis
Elder Abuse
Health & Healthcare Disparities

Sukanya Srinivasan, MD, MPH
Private Practice
Penn Plum Family Medicine
Pittsburgh, Pennsylvania
srinivasans@upmc.edu
Well-Child Care

M. Sharm Steadman, PharmD, BCPS, FASHP, CDE
Professor
Department of Family & Preventive Medicine
University of South Carolina
Columbia, South Carolina
Sharm.steadman@uscmed.sc.edu
Anxiety Disorders

Mark B. Stephens, MD, MS, FAAFP, CDR, MC, USN
Associate Professor, Chair
Department of Family Medicine
Uniformed Services University of the Health Sciences
Bethesda, Maryland
mstephens@usuhs.mil
Physical Activity in Adolescents

Marian Swope, MD
Associate Professor of Psychiatry
Program Director
Child and Adolescent Psychiatry
University of Kentucky College of Medicine
Lexington, Kentucky
maswop1@uky.edu
Behavioral Disorders in Children

Andrew B. Symons, MD, MS
Vice Chair for Medical Student Education
Clinical Assistant Professor of Family Medicine
Department of Family Medicine
State University of New York (SUNY)
at Buffalo School of Medicine and Biomedical Sciences
Buffalo, New York
symons@buffalo.edu
Neonatal Hyperbilirubinemia

Marian Tanofsky-Kraff, PhD
Associate Professor
Department of Medical and Clinical Psychology
Director
Developmental Research Laboratory on Eating and Weight
  Behaviors
Uniformed Services University of the Health Sciences
Bethesda, Maryland
marian.tanofsky-kraff@usuhs.edu
Eating Disorders

Elizabeth G. Tovar, PhD, RN, FNP-C
Assistant Professor
University of Kentucky College of Nursing
Family Nurse Practitioner
Department of Family and Community Medicine
University of Kentucky
Lexington, Kentucky
elizabeth.gressle@uky.edu
The Patient-Centered Medical Home

Belinda Vail, MD, MS, FAAFP
Professor
Vice Chair and Residency Director
Department of Family Medicine
University of Kansas School of Medicine
Kansas City, Kansas
bvail@kumc.edu
Diabetes Mellitus

Jacqueline S. Weaver-Agostoni, DO, MPH
Director
Predoctoral Education
University of Pittsburgh Department of Family Medicine
UPMC Shadyside
Pittsburgh, Pennsylvania
agostonijs@upmc.edu
Acute Coronary Syndrome

Charles W. Webb, DO, FAAFP, CAQ Sports Medicine
Director
Primary Care Sports Medicine Fellowship
Assistant Professor
Department of Family Medicine and Orthopedics
Oregon Health & Science University
Portland, Oregon
webbch@ohsu.edu or webbo18@aol.com
Low Back Pain in Primary Care

Richard Welsh, MSW, LCSW
Professor
Department of Psychiatry
University of Kentucky College of Medicine;
Professor
College of Social Work
University of Kentucky
Lexington, Kentucky
rjwels0@email.uky.edu
Behavioral Disorders in Children

Stephen A. Wilson, MD, MPH, FAAFP
Assistant Professor
Family Medicine
University of Pittsburgh School of Medicine
Director
Medical Decision Making
UPMC St Margaret Family Medicine Residency
Director
Faculty Development Fellowship
University of Pittsburgh Department of Family Medicine
Pittsburgh, Pennyslvania
wilsons2@upmc.edu
Acute Coronary Syndrome
Health Maintenance for Adults

Steven R. Wolfe, DO, MPH
Dean
LECOM/Allegheny Health Network Clinical Campus
Osteopathic Program Director, Forbes Family Medicine
Assistant Clinical Professor
LECOM and Temple University
Swolfe1@wpahs.org
Caring for Gay, Lesbian, Bisexual, & Transgend Patients

Yaqin Xia, MD, MHPE
Department of Family Medicine
University of Pittsburgh School of Medicine
Pittsburgh, Pennsylvania
xiay@upmc.edu
Movement Disorders

David Yuan, MD, MS
Clinical Faculty
UPMC St. Margaret's
Pittsburgh, Pennsylvania
yuand@upmc.edu
Health Maintenance for Adults
Elder Abuse

Richard Kent Zimmerman, MD, MPH, MA
Professor
Department of Family Medicine and Clinical Epidemiology,
    School of Medicine, and Department of Behavioral and
    Community Health Sciences
Graduate School of Public Health
University of Pittsburgh
Pittsburgh, Pennsylvania
zimmrk@upmc.edu
Routine Childhood Vaccines

Preface

Current Diagnosis & Treatment: Family Medicine is the fourth edition of this single-source reference for house staff and practicing family physicians who provide comprehensive and continuous care of individuals of both sexes throughout the lifespan. The text is organized according to the developmental lifespan, beginning with childhood and adolescence, encompassing a focus on the reproductive years, and progressing through adulthood and the mature, senior years.

OUTSTANDING FEATURES

- Evidence-based recommendations
- Culturally related aspects of each condition
- Conservative and pharmacologic therapies
- Complementary and alternative therapies when relevant
- Suggestions for collaborations with other healthcare providers
- Attention to the mental and behavioral health of patients as solitary as well as comorbid conditions
- Recognition of impact of illness on the family
- Patient education information
- End-of-life issues

INTENDED AUDIENCE

Primary care trainees and practicing physicians will find this text a useful resource for common conditions seen in ambulatory practice. Detailed information in tabular and text format provides a ready reference for selecting diagnostic procedures and recommending treatments. Advanced practice nurses and physician's assistants will also find the approach provided here a practical and complete first resource for both diagnosed and undifferentiated conditions, and an aid in continuing management.

Unlike smaller medical manuals that focus on urgent, one-time approaches to a particular presenting complaint or condition, this text was envisioned as a resource for clinicians who practice continuity of care and have established a longitudinal, therapeutic relationship with their patients. Consequently, recommendations are made for immediate as well as subsequent clinical encounters.

ACKNOWLEDGMENTS

We wish to thank our many contributing authors for their diligence in creating complete, practical, and readable discussions of the many conditions seen on a daily basis in the average family medicine and primary care practice. Furthermore, the vision and support of our editors at McGraw-Hill for creating this resource for primary care have been outstanding and critical to its completion.

Jeannette E. South-Paul, MD, FAAFP
Samuel C. Matheny, MD, MPH, FAAFP
Evelyn L. Lewis, MD, MA, FAAFP

Well-Child Care

Sukanya Srinivasan, MD, MPH
Donald B. Middleton, MD

ESSENTIALS OF WELL-CHILD CARE

Providing a comprehensive patient-centered medical home for children and assisting in the progressive transition to adulthood are integral components of family medicine. The provision of well-child care through a series of periodic examinations forms the foundation for the family physician to build lasting relationships with the entire family, a critical distinction between the family physician and other medical specialists.

Enhanced nutrition, mandated safety standards, and expanded schedules for immunizations have significantly improved the health of US children, but serious childhood health problems persist. Inadequate prenatal care leading to poor birth outcomes, poor management of developmental delay, childhood obesity, lack of proper oral health, and learning disabilities are some examples of ongoing issues.

A key reference guide for childhood health promotion is the third edition (currently in revision) of *Bright Futures: Guidelines for Health Supervision of Infants, Children, and Adolescents*, funded by the US Department of Health and Human Services. The guidelines give providers a comprehensive system of care that addresses basic concerns of child rearing such as nutrition, parenting, safety, and infectious disease prevention with focused attention on evidence-based health components and interventions.

One widely accepted schedule for routine well-child visits (**Table 1-1**) is available in *Bright Futures* (http://brightfutures.aap.org/clinical_practice.html) (currently in revision). Seven visits are suggested during the first year, followed by an additional four visits by 2 years of age, and yearly visits until adulthood, coinciding with critical junctures during growth and development. Table 1-1 provides a structured framework for anticipatory guidance, exam features, and developmental screening recommendations at appropriate intervals.

The most important components of a preventive well-child visit include the following: (1) developmental/behavioral assessment; (2) physical examination, including measurement of growth; (3) screening tests and procedures; and (4) anticipatory guidance. The specific goal of each visit is to assess each component, identify concerns about a child's development and intervene with early treatment, if available, or monitor closely for changes. Another essential, recognized component is adherence to the most recent schedule of recommended immunizations from the Advisory Committee on Immunization Practices (of the US Public Health Service) and the Centers for Disease Control and Prevention (ACIP/CDC) (see Chapter 7).

The overall purpose of well visits is to engage the caregivers to partner with the physician to optimize the physical, emotional, and developmental health of the child. Family physicians need to comfortably identify common normal variants as well as abnormal findings that may require referral. Parents should be encouraged to use these dedicated well visits to raise questions, share observations, and advocate for their child, as they know their child best. Parents should be advised to bring in a list of questions during each visit and maintain their own records, especially for immunizations and growth, for each child.

Supplemental preventive health visits may be required if the child is adopted or living with surrogate parents; is at high risk for medical disorders as suggested by the conditions observed during pregnancy, delivery, neonatal history, growth pattern, or physical examination; or exhibits psychological disorders, or if the family is socially or economically disadvantaged or if the parents request or require additional education or guidance.

▶ General Considerations

Well-child care ideally begins in the preconception period. Family physicians have the opportunity to provide preconception counseling to any woman, especially one who presents for gynecological examination before pregnancy.

Table 1–1. Proposed schedule of routine well-care visits.

American Academy of Pediatrics
DEDICATED TO THE HEALTH OF ALL CHILDREN™

Recommendations for Preventive Pediatric Health Care

Bright Futures/American Academy of Pediatrics

Bright Futures.
prevention and health promotion for infants, children, adolescents, and their families™

Each child and family is unique; therefore, these Recommendations for Preventive Pediatric Health Care are designed for the care of children who are receiving competent parenting, have no manifestations of any important health problems, and are growing and developing in satisfactory fashion. Additional visits may become necessary if circumstances suggest variations from normal.

Developmental, psychosocial, and chronic disease issues for children and adolescents may require frequent counseling and treatment visits separate from preventive care visits.

These guidelines represent a consensus by the American Academy of Pediatrics (AAP) and Bright Futures. The AAP continues to emphasize the great importance of continuity of care in comprehensive health supervision and the need to avoid fragmentation of care.

Refer to the specific guidance by age as listed in Bright Futures guidelines (Hagan JF, Shaw JS, Duncan PM, eds. Bright Futures Guidelines for Health Supervision of Infants, Children and Adolescents. 3rd ed. Elk Grove Village, IL: American Academy of Pediatrics; 2008).

The recommendations in this statement do not indicate an exclusive course of treatment or standard of medical care. Variations, taking into account individual circumstances, may be appropriate.

Copyright © 2014 by the American Academy of Pediatrics.

No part of this statement may be reproduced in any form or by any means without prior written permission from the American Academy of Pediatrics except for one copy for personal use.

Table 1–1. Recommendations for Preventive Pediatric Health Care (Bright Futures/AAP periodicity schedule).

KEY: ● = to be performed   ★ = risk assessment to be performed with appropriate action to follow, if positive   ←→ = range during which a service may be provided

Reproduced with permission from Bright Futures. American Academy of Pediatrics, copyright 2008 (http://brightfutures.aap.org/pdfs/aap%20bright%20futures%20periodicity%20sched%20101107.pdf).

Prospective parents should be counseled about appropriate nutrition, including 0.4 mg of folic acid supplementation daily for all women of childbearing age. Prior to conception, referral for genetic screening and counseling should be offered on the basis of age, ethnic background, or family history. Prescription drug and supplement use should be reviewed. Exposure to cigarette smoke, alcohol, illicit drugs, or chemicals such as pesticides should be strongly discouraged. Clinicians should verify and complete immunization against hepatitis B, pertussis, tetanus, rubella, and varicella, and discuss prevention of infection from toxoplasmosis (often transmitted by contact with kittens), cytomegalovirus, and parvovirus B19.

Medical problems such as diabetes, epilepsy, depression, or hypertension warrant special management prior to conception, especially since medications may need to be changed before pregnancy. The "prenatal" visit provides an opportunity to discuss cultural, occupational, and financial issues related to pregnancy; to gather information about preparations for the child's arrival; to discuss plans for feeding and child care; and to screen for domestic violence. The prenatal visit is a good opportunity to promote breastfeeding, emphasizing the health benefits for both mother and infant. A social history should include the family structure (caregivers, siblings, etc) and socioeconomic status. Familiarity with the family's background enables the physician to dedicate visits with the newborn infant to providing parents with specific guidance about child care.

Once the child is born, the prenatal and neonatal records should be reviewed for gestational age at birth; any abnormal maternal obstetric laboratory tests; maternal illnesses such as diabetes, preeclampsia, depression, or infections that occurred during pregnancy; maternal use of drugs or exposure to teratogens; date of birth; mode of delivery; Apgar scores at 1 and 5 minutes; and birth weight, length, and head circumference. Repeated screening of parents during well-child visits for depression and tobacco use with an offer of counseling and treatment can have profound benefits for the child.

COMPONENTS OF PREVENTIVE WELL-CHILD CARE

▶ Developmental/Behavioral Assessment

Young children who experience toxic stress such as maltreatment, neglect, poverty, or a depressed parent are at increased risk for later life health problems such as asthma, heart disease, cancer, and depression. During the prenatal and early childhood years, the neuroendocrine-immune network creates end-organ setpoints that lead to these disorders. Because well-timed adjustments to the child's environment can reduce the risk for later disease, the clinician should attempt to uncover toxic stressors at each preventive health visit.

Table 1–2. Developmental "red flags."[a]

Age (months)	Clinical Observation
2	Not turning toward sights or sounds
4–5	No social smiling or cooing
6–7	Not reaching for objects
8–9	No reciprocating emotions or expressions
9–12	No imitative sound exchange with caregivers
18	No signs of complex problem-solving interactions (following 2-step directions)
18–24	Not using words to get needs met
36–48	No signs of using logic with caregivers No pretend play with toys

[a]Serious emotional difficulties in parents or family members at any time warrant full evaluation.
Reproduced with permission from Brazelton TB, Sparrow J. *Touchpoints: Birth to Three.* 2nd ed. Boston, MA: Da Capo Press; 2006.

Watching a newborn develop from a dependent being into a communicative child with a unique personality is an amazing process that caregivers and clinicians can actively promote. Early identification of developmental disorders is critical for the well-being of children and their families. Unfortunately, primary care physicians fail to identify and appropriately refer many developmental problems, even though screening tools are available. Because the period of most active development occurs during the first 3 years, clinicians must assess and document developmental surveillance for every preventive care visit and preferably at every other office visit as well regardless of purpose. **Table 1-2** lists some developmental "red flags."

Surveillance includes asking parents if they have any concerns about their child's development, taking a developmental history, observing the child, identifying any risk factors for developmental delay, and accurately tracking the findings and progress. If the family shows concerns, reassurance and reexamination is appropriate if the child is at low risk.

As a result of concerns identified during surveillance and specifically at the 9-, 18-, and 30-month visits, a formal developmental screening tool should be administered to uncover problems such as those listed in **Table 1-3**. These visits occur when parents and clinicians can readily observe strides in the different developmental domains: fine and gross motor skills, language and communication, problem solving/adaptive behavior, and personal-social skills. Developmental tests screen children who are apparently normal, confirm or refute any concerns, and serve to monitor children at high risk for developmental delay. Each test approaches the task of identifying children in a different

Table 1–3. Prevalence of developmental disorders.

Disorder	Cases per 1000
Attention deficit/hyperactivity disorder	75–150
Learning disabilities	75
Behavioral disorders	60–130
Mental retardation	25
Autism spectrum disorders	2–11
Cerebral palsy	2–3
Hearing impairment	0.8–2
Visual impairment	0.3–0.6

Data from Levy SE, Hyman SL. Pediatric assessment of the child with developmental delay. *Pediatr Clin North Am.* 1993;40:465 and CDC. Prevalence of autism spectrum disorders—autism and developmental disabilities monitoring network, 14 sites, United States, 2002. *MMWR* (*Morbidity and Mortality Weekly Report*). 2007; 6:1–40.

way; no screening tool is universally deemed appropriate for all populations and all ages. A report in the United States during 2006–2008 found that about one in six children had a developmental disability.

Table 1-4 lists several useful developmental screening tests. The historical gold standard Denver Developmental Screening Test–revised requires trained personnel about 20–30 minutes of office time to administer. Proper use is not widespread in practice. The Parents' Evaluation of Developmental Status, the Ages and Stages Questionnaire, and the Child Development Review-Parent Questionnaire are all parent-completed tools that take less than 15 minutes to complete and are easily used in a busy clinical practice but are unfortunately proprietary. Shortened, customized lists of developmental milestones should not replace the use of validated developmental assessment tools, a list of which is available from the National Early Childhood Technical Assistance Center (NECTAC).

If the screening tool results are concerning, the physician should inform the parents and schedule the child for further developmental or medical evaluation or referral to subspecialists such as neurodevelopmental pediatricians, pediatric psychiatrists, speech-language pathologists, and physical and occupational therapists. In approximately one-fourth of all cases, an etiology is identified through medical testing, such as genetic evaluation, serum metabolite studies, and brain imaging.

If screening results are within normal limits, the physician has an opportunity to focus on optimizing the child's potential. Parents can be encouraged to read to their children

Table 1–4. Developmental screening tools.

Test	Age	Time (minutes)	Source
Office Administered			
Denver II	0–6 years	30	www.denverii.com
Battelle Developmental Inventory Screening Tool (BDI-ST)	0–8 years	15	www.riverpub.com
Brigance Screens-II	0–90 months	15	www.curriculumassociates.com
Bayley Infant Neuro-developmental Screen (BINS)	3–24 months	10	www.harcourtassessment.com
Parent Administered			
Ages & Stages Questionnaires (ASQ)	4–60 months (every 4 months)	15	www.brookespublishing.com
Parents' Evaluation of Development Status (PEDS)	0–8 years	< 5	www.pedstest.com
Child Development Inventory (CDI)	1.5–6 years	45	www.childdevrev.com
Language and Cognitive Screening			
Early Language Milestone (ELM)	0–3 years	5–10	www.proedinc.com
Capute Scales (Cognitive Adaptive Test/Clinical Linguistic Auditory Milestone Scale [CAT/CLAMS])	3–36 months	15–20	www.brookespublishing.com
Modified Checklist for Autism in Toddlers	16–48 months	5–10	www.firstsigns.com

Data from Mackrides PS, Ryherd SJ. Screening for developmental delay. *Am Fam Physician* 2011; 84(5):544–549.

on a regular basis, sing and play music, limit television and other media device use altogether in toddlers and to no more than 2 hours daily for older children, and directly engage in age-appropriate stimulating activities such as exercise or game playing. Clinicians should encourage the parents and patients to report on positive behaviors and activities at every visit.

At both the 18- and 24-month visits, clinicians should formally screen for autism spectrum disorders (ASDs). Increasing public awareness and concern about ASD has made this recommendation key. The Modified Checklist for Autism in Toddlers (M-ChAT) is a widely used, validated autism-specific screening tool. Autistic disorder is a pervasive developmental disorder resulting in various social, language, and/or sensorimotor deficits with an incidence as high as 1 in 88 children. Early diagnosis and intervention may help many autistic persons achieve some degree of independent living. The differential diagnosis includes other psychiatric and developmental disorders; profound hearing loss; metabolic disorders, such as lead poisoning; and genetic disorders, such as fragile X syndrome and tuberous sclerosis. MMR (measles-mumps-rubella) vaccine does not cause autism, but failure to take folic acid during pregnancy is linked to an increased risk.

The school years offer an excellent opportunity to evaluate the child's development through grades, standardized test results, and athletic or extracurricular activities. Participation in activities outside the home and school also help gauge the child's development. For example, a critical event during adolescence is learning to drive a motor vehicle.

▶ Physical Examination

A general principle for well-child examinations (newborn to 4 years old) is to perform maneuvers from least to most invasive. Clinicians should first make observations about the child-parent(s) interaction, obtain an interval history, and then perform a direct examination of the child. Some parts of the examination are best accomplished when the infant is quiet so they may be performed "out of order." Although most communication about the child's health is between the physician and the parent(s), clinicians should attempt to communicate directly with the patient to gauge whether he or she is developmentally appropriate and to develop familiarity directly with that patient.

A physical examination of the newborn should include the following:

- **General observation**: evidence of birth trauma, dysmorphic features, respiratory rate, skin discolorations, or rashes
- **Head, ears, eyes, nose, and throat (HEENT) examination**: mobile sutures, open fontanelles, head shape, ears, bilateral retinal red reflexes, clarity of lens, nasal patency, absence of cleft palate or lip, and palpation of clavicles to rule out fracture

- **Cardiovascular examination**: cardiac murmurs, peripheral pulses, capillary refill, and cyanosis
- **Pulmonary examination**: use of accessory muscles and auscultation of breath sounds
- **Abdominal examination**: masses, distention, and the presence of bowel sounds
- **Extremity examination**: number and abnormalities of digits, and screening for congenital dislocation of the hips using Ortolani and Barlow maneuvers
- **Genitourinary examination**: genitalia and anus
- **Neurologic examination**: presence of newborn reflexes (eg, rooting, grasping, sucking, stepping, and Moro reflex), resting muscle tone

To track the child's physical and developmental progress, a comprehensive interval history and physical examination is important at each encounter, even if the parents do not report concerns. The child's weight (without clothes or shoes), height, and head circumference (until 3 years of age) are measured and plotted on standard CDC growth charts at each visit. A child's rate of growth will usually follow one percentile (25th, 50th, etc) from birth through school age. A child can appropriately cross percentiles upward (eg, a premature infant who then "catches up") or inappropriately (eg, a child who becomes obese). Any child who drops more than two percentiles over any period of time should be evaluated for failure to thrive (see Chapter 2).

By 15 months of age, children experience stranger anxiety and are much less likely to be cooperative. Clinicians can minimize the child's adverse reactions by approaching the child slowly and performing the examination while the child is in the parent's arms, progressing from least to most invasive tasks. Touching the child's shoe or accompanying stuffed animal first and then gradually moving up to the chest while distracting the child with a toy or otoscope light is often helpful. After the first year of life, the pace of the infant's growth begins to plateau. At the 15- to 18-month visit, the infant most likely will be mobile and may want to stand during the examination. To engage the child, the clinician can ask where to do the examination or which body part to examine first.

Beginning at 2 years of age, the body mass index (BMI) is plotted; at age 3 years the child's blood pressure is measured. Eye examination for strabismus (also known as "cross-eye"; measured by the cover/uncover test) allows early treatment to prevent amblyopia. By age 3 or 4 years, documentation of visual acuity should be attempted. Hearing, now tested at birth, is informally evaluated until the age of 4 years, when audiometry should be attempted. At least 75% of speech in 3-year-olds should be intelligible. Speech delay should trigger referral. Physicians need to assess gait, spinal alignment, and injuries, looking particularly for signs of child abuse or neglect. **Table 1-5** highlights the important components of

Table 1–5. Highlights of physical examination by age.

Age of Child	Essential Components of Examination
2 weeks	Presence of bilateral red reflex Auscultation of heart for murmurs Palpation of abdomen for masses Ortolani/Barlow maneuvers for hip dislocation Assessment of overall muscle tone Reattainment of birth weight
2 months	Observation of anatomic abnormalities or congenital malformations (effects of birth trauma resolved by this point) Auscultation of heart for murmurs
4–6 months	Complete musculoskeletal examination (neck control, evidence of torticollis) Extremity evaluation (eg, metatarsus adductus) Vision assessment (conjugate gaze, symmetric light reflex, visual tracking of an object to 180°) Bilateral descent of testes Assessment for labial adhesions
9 months	Pattern and degree of tooth eruption Assessment of muscle tone Presence of bilateral pincer grasp Observation of crawling behavior
12 months	Range of motion of the hips, rotation, and leg alignment Bilateral descent of testes
15–18 months	Cover test for strabismus Signs of dental caries Gait assessment Any evidence of injuries

Table 1–6. Commonly screened components of newborn screening panels.[a]

Diseases Screened	Incidence of Disease in Live Births
Congenital hypothyroidism	1:4000
Duchenne muscular dystrophy	1:4500
Congenital adrenal hyperplasia	1:10,000–1:18,000
Phenylketonuria	1:14,000
Galactosemia	1:30,000
Cystic fibrosis	1:44,000–1:80,000 (depending on population)
Biotinidase deficiency	1:60,000

[a]Screening panel requirements vary in each state.
Data from Kaye CI and Committee on Genetics. *Newborn Screening Fact Sheets.* (technical report; available at www.pediatrics.org/cgi/content/full/118/3/1304). See also *Baby's First Test* (http://babysfirst-test.org/) for complete listing of disease tests by state.

the physical examination at each age. The examiner should comment on the child's psychological and intellectual development, particularly during adolescence, when mood and affect evaluations should be recorded.

► **Screening Laboratory Tests**

Every state requires newborns to undergo serologic screening for inborn errors of metabolism (**Table 1-6**), preferably at age 2–3 days. Funded by the Department of Health and Human Services (DHSS), Baby's First Test (www.babysfirst-test.org) is an unbiased website that provides information for providers about the mandated screening requirements in each state. Examples of commonly screened conditions are hypothyroidism, phenylketonuria, maple syrup urine disease, congenital adrenal hyperplasia, and cystic fibrosis. Most institutions routinely screen newborns for hearing loss [US Preventive Services Task Force (USPSTF) recommendation for universal screening level B]. The USPSTF assigned

a level I (insufficient evidence) to universal screening of newborns for risk of chronic bilirubin encephalopathy with a transcutaneous bilirubin.

The American Academy of Pediatrics (AAP) recommends screening for anemia with fingerstick hemoglobin or hematocrit at age 12 months. Although the USPSTF assigned a level I to screening for iron deficiency, it did recommend iron dietary supplementation for age 6–12 months. Because of the high prevalence of iron deficiency anemia in toddlers (about 9%), repeat screenings may be necessary in high-risk situations. Measurement of hemoglobin or hematocrit alone detects only those patients with iron levels low enough to become anemic, so dietary intake of iron should be assessed. Pregnant adolescents should be screened for anemia. A positive screening test at any age is an indication for a therapeutic trial of iron. Thalassemia minor is the major differential consideration. A sickle cell screen is indicated in all African American children.

The AAP recommends universal lead screening at ages 12 and 24 months. If the child is considered to be at high risk, annual lead screening begins at age 6 months. Risk factors include exposure to chipping or peeling paint in buildings built before 1950, frequent contact with an adult with significant lead exposure, having a sibling under treatment for a high lead level, and location of the home near an industrial setting likely to release lead fumes. Although many agencies require a one-time universal lead screening at 1 year of age because high-risk factors are often absent in children with lead poisoning, the USPSTF recommends against screening children at average risk and assigns a level I to screening for high-risk children.

Tuberculosis (TB) screening using a purified protein derivative (PPD) is offered on recognition of high-risk factors at any age. Routine testing of children without risk factors is not indicated. Children require testing if they have had contact with persons with confirmed or suspected cases of infectious TB, have emigrated from endemic countries (Asia or the Middle East), or have any clinical or radiographic findings suggestive of TB. Human immunodeficiency virus (HIV)-infected children require annual PPD tests. Children at risk for HIV due to exposure to high-risk adults (HIV-positive, homeless, institutionalized, etc) are retested every 2–3 years. Children without specific risk factors for TB but who live in high-prevalence communities may be tested at ages 1 year, 4–6 years, and 11–12 years.

The AAP recommends universal dyslipidemia screening at ages 10 and 20 years. A cholesterol level may be obtained after age 2 years if the child has a notable family history. The National Cholesterol Education Program (NCEP) recommends screening in a child with a parent who has a total cholesterol of ≥240 mg/dL or a parent or grandparent with the onset of cardiovascular disease before age 55 years. Clinical evaluation and management of the child are to be initiated if the low-density lipoprotein (LDL) cholesterol level is ≥130 mg/dL. The USPSTF assigns a level I to cholesterol screening during childhood.

The AAP recommends an HIV test for all 20-year-olds.

▶ Anticipatory Guidance

A. Nutrition

All mothers should be strongly encouraged to breastfeed their infants. A widely accepted goal is exclusive breastfeeding for at least the first 6 months of life. Vitamin D supplement (400 U/d) is indicated for breastfed children. Parents who choose to bottle-feed their newborn have several choices in formulas, but should avoid cow's milk, because of risks like anemia. Commercial formulas are typically fortified with iron and vitamin D, and some contain fatty acids such as docosahexaenoic acid (DHA) and arachidonic acid (ARA) which are not as yet proven to promote nervous system development. Soy-based or lactose-free formulas can be used for infants intolerant of cow's milk formulas.

An appropriate weight gain is 1 oz/d during the first 6 months of life and 0.5 oz/d during the next 6 months. This weight gain requires a daily caloric intake of ~120 kcal/kg during the first 6 months and 100 kcal/kg thereafter. Breast milk and most formulas contain 20 cal/oz. Initially, newborns should be fed on demand or in some cases as for twins on a partial schedule. Caregivers need to be questioned about the amount and duration of the child's feedings and vitamin D and fluoride intake at every visit.

Healthy snacks and regular family mealtimes may help reduce the risk of obesity. Fruit juice is best avoided altogether; water is preferred for hydration. Ideal calorie intake is somewhat independent of weight but does change according to activity level. Children age 1 year should take in about 900 kcal/d; age 2–3 years, 1000; age 4–8 years, 1200 for girls and 1400 for boys; age 9–13 years, 1600 for girls and 1800 for boys; and age 14–18, 1800 for girls and 2200 for boys.

Solid foods such as cereals or pureed baby foods are introduced at 4–6 months of age when the infant can support her or his head and the tongue extrusion reflex has extinguished. Delaying introduction of solid foods until this time appears to limit the incidence of food sensitivities. The child can also continue breast- or bottle-feeding, limited to 30 oz/d, because the solids now provide additional calories. Around 1 year of age, when the infant can drink from a cup, bottle-feeding should be discontinued to protect teeth from caries. No specified optimum age exists for weaning a child from breastfeeding. After weaning, ingestion of whole or 2% cow's milk may promote nervous system development.

Older infants can tolerate soft adult foods such as yogurt and mashed potatoes. A well-developed pincer grasp allows children to self-feed finger foods. With the eruption of primary teeth at 8–12 months of age, children may try foods such as soft rice or pastas.

With toddlers, mealtimes can be a source of both pleasure and anxiety as children become "finicky." The normal child may exhibit specific food preferences or be disinterested in eating. An appropriate growth rate and normal developmental milestones should reassure frustrated parents. Coping strategies include offering small portions of preferred items first and offering limited food choices. Eating as a family gives toddlers a role model for healthy eating and appropriate social behaviors during mealtimes.

B. Elimination

Regular patterns for voiding and defecation provide reassurance that the child is developing normally. Newborn infants should void within 24 hours of birth. An infant urinates approximately 6–8 times a day. Parents may count diapers in the first few weeks to confirm adequate feeding. The older child usually voids 4–6 times daily. Changes in voiding frequency reflect the child's hydration status, especially when the child is ill.

Routine circumcision of male infants is not currently recommended, so parents who are considering circumcision require additional guidance. Although a circumcised boy has a decreased incidence of urinary tract infections [odds ratio (OR) 3–5] and a decreased risk of phimosis and squamous cell carcinoma of the penis, some clinicians raise concerns about bleeding, infection, pain of the procedure, or damage to the genitalia (incidence of 0.2–0.6%). Therefore, the decision about circumcision is based on the parents' personal preferences and cultural influences. When done, the procedure is usually performed after the second day of life, on a physiologically stable infant. Contraindications include ambiguous genitalia, hypospadias, HIV, and any overriding medical conditions. The denuded mucosa of the phallus appears raw for the first week postprocedure, exuding a small amount of serosanguineous drainage on the diaper. Infection occurs in <1% of cases. Mild soap and water washes are the best method of cleansing the area. By the 2-week checkup, the phallus should be completely healed with a scar below the corona radiata. The parents should note whether the infant's urinary stream is straight and forceful.

Newborns are expected to pass black, tarry meconium stools within the first 24 hours of life. Failure to pass stool in that period necessitates a workup for Hirschsprung disease (aganglionic colon) or imperforate anus. Later the consistency of the stool is usually semisolid and soft, with a yellow-green seedy appearance. Breastfed infants typically defecate after each feeding or at least 2 times a day. Bottle-fed infants generally have a lower frequency of stooling. Occasionally, some infants may have only one stool every 2 or 3 days without discomfort. If the child seems to be grunting forcefully with defecation or is passing extremely hard stools, treatment with lubricants such as, glycerin is recommended. Any appearance of blood in the stools is abnormal and warrants investigation. Anal fissure is common.

With the introduction of solid foods and maturation of intestinal function, stool becomes more solid and malodorous. Treatment of mild to moderate constipation may include the use of Karo syrup mixed in with feedings (1–2 tsp in 2 oz of milk) or psyllium seed or mineral oil (15–30 mL) for older children. Older children and adolescents should ingest high-fiber foods such as fruits and vegetables and drink water to reduce the risk of constipation. Children who are severely constipated may require referral.

C. Sleep Patterns

An important issue for new parents is the development of proper sleeping habits for their child. Newborns and children experience different stages of sleep/wakefulness cycles, including deep, light, or rapid-eye-movement (REM) sleep; indeterminate state; wide-awake, alert state; fussy; and crying. On average, a baby experiences a cycle every 3–4 hours, and the new parents' first job is to learn their baby's unique style. Newborns sleep an average of 18–20 hours in each 24-hour period.

At first, feeding the baby whenever he or she wakes up is the most appropriate response. Because babies often have their days and nights "reversed," tiring nighttime awakenings are commonplace because of frequent feedings. When the baby is 3 or 4 weeks old, feedings can be delayed for a bit of play and interaction. The goal is to space out the baby's awake time to 3 or more hours between feedings and a long sleep at night.

By 2–3 months, the baby's pattern of sleeping and feeding should be more predictable and parents can institute some routines that allow the child to self-comfort. After feeding, rocking, and soothing, parents should be encouraged to lay the baby down in the crib when she or he is quiet but not asleep. A soothing, consistent bedtime ritual allows babies to learn to settle down by themselves and lays the foundation for other independent behaviors in the future.

All newborn infants should be placed on their backs to sleep to reduce the risk of sudden infant death syndrome (SIDS). Risk factors include prone and side positions for infant sleep, smoke exposure, soft bedding and sleep surfaces, and overheating. Cosleeping (bed sharing) slightly increases the overall risk of SIDS, especially for infants less than 11 weeks old. The issue of cosleeping is often difficult to address as it is viewed as a common and necessary practice in some cultures. Evidence also suggests that pacifier use and room sharing (without bed sharing) are associated with decreased risk of SIDS. Although the cause of SIDS is unknown, immature cardiorespiratory autonomic control and failure of arousal responsiveness from sleep are important factors. With the "back to sleep" campaign, prone sleeping among all US infants has decreased to less than 20%, and the incidence of SIDS has decreased to 40%.

An unintended consequence of the supine sleep position has been increased incidence of positional head deformity or plagiocephaly. Providers need to recognize physical examination distinctions between this cosmetic deformity and the more significant concern of craniosynostosis. Parents should be counseled early about strategies to minimize plagiocephaly, including use of supervised prone positioning ("tummy time") and avoidance of prolonged car seat or rocker use. Early referral and treatment in severe cases typically results in satisfactory outcomes.

Sleep disorders are extremely common in young children and adolescents. Good sleep hygiene offers the best solution to these difficulties.

D. Oral Health

The poor state of oral health in many children is a continued major concern. Tooth decay remains one of the most common chronic diseases of childhood, even more common than asthma. Medically and developmentally compromised children and children from low-income families are at highest risk. Affected children remain at higher risk for cavities throughout their childhood and adulthood. To minimize early-childhood caries, children should not be put to sleep with a bottle or by breastfeeding. Parents should also be discouraged from inappropriately using the bottle or "sippy cup" as a pacifier. Dietary sugars along with cariogenic bacteria, most often acquired from the mother, who should never clean off a pacifier by inserting it into her own mouth, lead to accelerated decay in the toddler's primary teeth. Ingestion of water after feeding may help reduce cavities.

Current recommendations encourage establishing regular dental care around 6–9 months of age in high-risk children and at 1 year of age for all others. Children should continue with regular biannual dental appointments thereafter. Primary prevention includes provision of a diet high in calcium and fluoride supplementation for those with an unfluoridated water supply (<0.6 ppm) from age 6 months through age 16 years. Once primary teeth erupt, parents should use a soft-bristled brush or washcloth with water to clean the teeth twice daily. A pea-sized amount of fluoride containing toothpaste is adequate. Infants should drink from a cup and be weaned from the bottle at around 12–14 months of age. Pacifiers and thumb sucking are best limited after teeth have erupted. All children need limits on the intake of high-sugar drinks and juices, especially between meals. Fluoride applications 2–6 times per year on erupted teeth markedly reduce the incidence of caries (http://www .ada.org/goto/fluoride).

E. Safety

Accidental injury and death are the major risks to a healthy child. Safety should be stressed at every well-child visit. Poison avoidance; choking hazards; and water, pet, gun, and automobile safety are critical areas to review. The Injury Prevention Program (TIPP) from the American Academy of Pediatrics provides an excellent framework for accident prevention.

▶ Issues in Normal Development

Anticipatory guidance can be helpful to caregivers in preparation for normal growth and development and when their child exhibits variations from ideal behavior. *Bright Futures* provides extensive information about anticipatory guidance throughout childhood and adolescence. Important anticipatory guidance topics include safety, school readiness, school refusal, bullying, physical activity, media (TV, smartphones, etc) use, drug addiction, sexuality, and intellectual pursuits. Selected behavioral issues that are commonly encountered in young children include infantile colic, temper tantrums, and reluctant toilet training.

A. Infantile Colic

Colic is a term often used to describe an infant who is difficult to manage or fussy despite being otherwise healthy. Colic may be defined as 3 or more hours of uncontrollable crying or fussing at least 3 times a week for at least 3 weeks. Many parents complain of incessant crying well before 3 weeks have passed. Other symptoms include facial expressions of pain or discomfort, pulling up of the legs, passing flatus, fussiness with eating, and difficulty falling or staying asleep. Symptoms classically worsen during the evening hours. Because the diagnosis depends on parental report, the incidence of colic varies from 5% to 20%. It occurs equally in both sexes and peaks around 3–4 weeks of age.

The cause of colic is unknown, but organic pathology is present in <5% of cases. Possible etiologies include an immature digestive system sensitive to certain food proteins, an immature nervous system sensitive to external stimuli, or a mismatch of the infant's temperament and those of caregivers. Feeding method is probably unrelated. Clinicians can provide reassurance to caregivers by informing them that colicky children continue to eat and gain weight appropriately, despite the prolonged periods of crying, and that the syndrome is self-limited and usually dissipates by 3–4 months of age. Colic has no definite long-term consequences; therefore, the main problem for caregivers is to cope with anxiety over the crying child. A stressed caregiver who is unable to handle the situation is at risk for abusing a child.

No definitive treatment can be offered for colic. Little evidence supports the use of simethicone or acetaminophen drops. Switching to a hypoallergenic (soy) formula is effective when the child has other symptoms suggestive of cow's milk protein allergy. Breastfeeding mothers can attempt to make changes in their diets (eg, avoidance of cruciferous vegetables such as broccoli and cabbage) to see if the infant improves. Both clinicians and caregivers have proposed many "home remedies." Both reducing stimulation and movement such as a car ride or walk outdoors are recommended. Frequent burping, swaddling, massage, a crib vibrator, and background noise from household appliances or a white-noise generator are moderately effective. Rigorous study of these techniques is difficult, but clinicians can suggest any or all because the potential harm is minimal.

B. Temper Tantrums

A normal part of child development, temper tantrums encompass excessive crying, screaming, kicking, thrashing, head banging, breath-holding, breaking or throwing objects, and aggression. Between the ages of 1 and 3 years, a child's growing sense of independence is in conflict with physical limitations and parental controls and hampered because of limited vocabulary and inability to express feelings or experiences. This power struggle sets the stage for the expression of anger and frustration through a temper tantrum. Tantrums can follow minor frustrations or occur for no obvious reason, but are mostly self-limited. A child's tendency toward impulsivity or impatience or a delay in the development of motor skills or cognitive deficits and parental inconsistency—excessive restrictiveness, overindulgence, or overreaction—may increase the incidence of tantrums. Tantrums that produce a desired effect have an increased likelihood of recurrence.

As much as possible, parents should provide a predictable home environment. Consistency in routines and rules will help the child know what to expect. Parents should prepare the child for transitions from one activity to another, offer some simple choices to satisfy the child's growing need for control, acknowledge the child's wants during a tantrum, and act calmly when handling negative behaviors to avoid reinforcement. Physical (corporeal) punishment is not advised.

Most importantly, ignoring attention-seeking tantrums and not giving in to the demands of the tantrum will, in time, decrease the recurrence. Children who are disruptive enough to hurt themselves or others must be removed to a safe place and given time to calm down in a nonpunitive manner. Most children learn to work out their frustrations with their own set of problem-solving and coping skills, thus terminating tantrums. Persistence of tantrums beyond age 4 or 5 years requires further investigation and usually includes referral or group education and counseling.

C. Toilet Training

Some indicators of readiness for toilet use include an awareness of impending urination or defecation, prolonged involuntary dryness, and the ability to walk easily, to pull

Table 1–7. Medical problems commonly diagnosed in childhood.

Problem	Definition	Prevalence	Risk Factors	Assessment	Treatment
Developmental dysplasia of hips	Spectrum of abnormalities that cause hip instability, ranging from dislocation to inadequate development of acetabulum	8–25 cases per 1000 births	Female gender; Breech delivery; Family history; Possibly birth weight >4 kg	Screening clinical examination at birth and well-child visits of marginal use. Diagnosis: ultrasound in infants <6 months; radiographs >6 months	Abduction splints in infants <6 months; open or closed reduction more effective in those >6 months; optimal treatment remains controversial; consider orthopedic referral
Congenital heart disease	Major—large VSDs, severe valvular stenosis, cyanotic disease, large ASDs. Minor—small VSDs, mild valvular stenosis, small ASDs	5–8 cases per 1000 newborns, 50% with major disease and 50% with minor disease	Maternal diabetes or connective tissue disease; congenital infections (CMV, HSV, rubella, etc); drugs taken during pregnancy; family history; Down syndrome	Major disease presents shortly after birth. Minor disease can present with murmur, tachycardia, tachypnea, pallor, peripheral pulses; EKG, CXR, echocardiogram	Cardiology evaluation; medication; surgical treatment options
Cryptorchidism	Testicles are absent (agenesis, vascular compromise) or undescended	2–5% of full-term and 30% of premature male infants; prevalence varies geographically	Disorders of testosterone secretion; abdominal wall defects; trisomies	Increased risk of inguinal hernia, testicular torsion, infertility, and testicular cancer	Hormonal or surgical treatment, or both; can start at age 6 months; complete before age 2 years
Pyloric stenosis	Hypertrophic (elongated, thickened) pylorus, progresses to obstruction of gastric outlet	3 cases per 1000 live births	Male infants; first-born infants; unconjugated hyperbilirubinemia	Diagnosis by clinical examination, ultrasound, or upper GI series; electrolyte abnormalities (metabolic alkalosis)	Surgical repair; fluid, electrolyte resuscitation
Hypospadias	Ventral location of urethral meatus (anywhere from proximal glans to perineum)	~1 case per 250 male births	Advanced maternal age; maternal diabetes mellitus; Caucasian ethnicity; delivery before 37 weeks' gestation	Check for other abnormalities (cryptorchidism) and intersex conditions (congenital adrenal hyperplasia)	Circumcision contraindicated; urology referral, usually within 3–6 months
Strabismus	Anomaly of ocular alignment (one or both eyes, any direction)	~2–4% of population	Family history; low birth weight; retinopathy of prematurity; cataract	Clinical tests: corneal light reflex, red reflex, cover test, and cover/uncover test	Child should be referred to pediatric ophthalmologist for early treatment to reduce visual loss (amblyopia)

ASD, atrial septal defect; CMV, cytomegalovirus; CXR, chest x-ray; EKG, electrocardiogram; GI, gastrointestinal; HSV, herpes simplex virus; VSD, ventricular septal defect.

clothes on and off easily, to follow instructions, to identify body parts, and to initiate simple tasks. These indicators are not likely to be present until 18–30 months of age. Once the child becomes interested in bathroom activities or watching his or her parents use the toilet, parents should provide a potty chair. Parents can then initiate toilet training by taking the diaper off and seating the child on the potty at a time when she or he is likely to urinate or defecate. Routine sittings on the potty at specified times, such as after meals when the gastrocolic reflex is functional, may be helpful. The child who is straining or bending at the waist may be escorted to the bathroom for a toileting trial. If the child eliminates in the potty or toilet, praise or a small reward may reinforce that behavior. Stickers, storybooks, or added time with the parents can be used for motivation.

With repeated successes, transitional diapers or training pants may be used until full continence is achieved. The training process may take days to months, and caregivers can expect accidents. Accidents need to be dealt with plainly; the child should not be punished or made to feel guilty or forced to sit on the toilet for prolonged periods. Significant constipation can be treated medically, because it may present a barrier to training. About 80% of children achieve success at daytime continence by age 30 months.

As with many child-rearing issues, consistency and a nurturing environment give the child a sense of security. Training should not start too early or during times of family stress. Parents can be asked to describe specific scenarios, so concrete anticipatory guidance may be given to deal with any barriers. Toilet training, as with most behavior modification, has a higher chance of success if positive achievements are rewarded and failures are not emphasized.

Medical Concerns Outside Normal Development

Beyond the normal variations in child development, the family physician may need to identify and treat significant medical problems. Early diagnosis and referral lead to prevention of potentially serious sequelae and improved quality of life. Some of the major abnormalities detected in the young child (**Table 1-7**) underscore the importance of regular and thorough well-child-care visits with the family physician.

Media Use

Children should limit TV and computer use to no more than 2 hours per day. Parents must be aware of the content of viewed programs, videogames, and websites to reduce childhood exposure to violence and socially inappropriate content such as drug use. Safe use of handheld phones and computer devices should be routinely discussed with all parents and older children and adolescents.

Cohen GJ. Committee on psychosocial aspects of child and family health: the prenatal visit. *Pediacrics.* 2009;124(4):1227–1232.

Hagan JF, Shaw JS, Duncan PM, eds. *Bright Futures: Guidelines for Health Supervision of Infants, Children, and Adolescents.* 3rd ed. Elk Grove Village, IL: American Academy of Pediatrics; 2008.

Johnson SB, Riley AW, Granger DA, Riis J. The science of early toxic stress for pediatric practice and advocacy. *Pediatrics.* 2013;131:319–327.

Letourneau NL, Dennis CL, Benzies K, et al. Postpartum depression is a family affair: addressing the impact on mothers, fathers, and children. *Issues Ment Health Nurs.* 2012;33(7):445–457.

Olson LM, Tanner JL, Stein MT, Radecki L. Well-child care: looking back, looking forward. *Pediatr Ann.* 2008;37:143–151.

Patterson BL, Gregg WM, Biggers C, Barkin S. Improving delivery of EPSDT well-child care at acute visits in an academic pediatric practice. *Pediatrics.* 2012;130(4):e988–e995.

Tanner JL, Stein MT, Olson LM, Frintner MP, Radecki L. Reflections on well-child care practice: a national study of pediatric clinicians. *Pediatrics.* 2009;124(3):849–857.

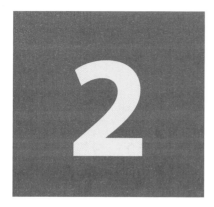

Failure to Thrive

James C. Dewar, MD

Stephanie B. Dewar, MD

ESSENTIALS OF DIAGNOSIS

- ▶ Persistent weight loss over time.
- ▶ Growth failure associated with disordered behavior and development.
- ▶ Weight less than third percentile for age.
- ▶ Weight crosses two major percentiles downward over any period of time and continues to fall.
- ▶ Median weight for age of 76–90% (mild undernutrition), 61–75% (moderate undernutrition), or <61% (severe undernutrition).

▶ General Considerations

Failure to thrive (FTT) is an old problem that continues to be an important entity for all practitioners who provide care to children. Growth is one of the essential tasks of childhood and is an indication of the child's general health. Growth failure may be the first symptom of serious organ dysfunction. Most frequently, however, growth failure represents inadequate caloric intake. Malnutrition during the critical period of brain growth in early childhood has been linked to delayed motor, cognitive, and social development. Developmental deficits may persist even after nutritional therapy has been instituted.

There is no unanimously established definition of FTT. Practitioners must also recognize the limitations of the different definitions of FTT. In a European study, 27% of well children met one criterion for FTT in the first year of life. This illustrates the poor predictive value of using a single measurement in diagnosis. Competing definitions of FTT include the following:

- **Persistent weight loss over time.** Children should steadily gain weight. Weight loss beyond the setting of an acute illness is pathological. However, the assessment and treatment for FTT need to be addressed *before* the child has had persistent weight loss.

- **Growth failure associated with disordered behavior and development.** This old definition is useful because it reminds the practitioner of the serious sequelae and important alarm features in children with undernutrition. Currently, FTT is more commonly defined by anthropometric guidelines alone.

- **Weight less than the third to fifth percentile for age.** This is a classic definition. However, this definition includes children with genetic short stature and whose weight transiently dips beneath the third percentile with an intercurrent illness.

- **Weight crosses two major percentiles downward over any period of time.** Thirty percent of normal children will drop two major percentiles within the first 2 years of life as their growth curve shifts to their genetic potential. These healthy children will continue to grow on the adjusted growth curve. Children with FTT do not attain a new curve, but continue to fall. The most accurate assessment for FTT is a calculation of the child's median weight for age. This quick calculation enables the clinician to assess the degree of undernutrition and plan an appropriate course of evaluation and intervention. The median weight for age should be determined using the most accurate growth chart for the area in which the child lives. The median should not be adjusted for race, ethnicity, or country of origin. Differences in growth are more likely due to inadequate nutrition in specific geographic or economically deprived populations. Determinations of nutritional status are as follows:

- **Mild undernutrition:** 76–90% median weight for age. These children are in no immediate danger and may be safely observed over time (**Table 2-1**).

Table 2-1. Degree of undernutrition.

Percentage of Median Weight for Age (%)	Degree of Undernutrition	Recommendation
76–90	Mild	Observe as outpatient
61–75	Moderate	Urgent outpatient evaluation Close weight follow-up
>61	Severe	Hospitalization Nutrition support In-hospital evaluation

- **Moderate undernutrition:** 75% median weight for age. These children warrant immediate evaluation and intervention with close follow-up in an outpatient setting.
- **Severe malnutrition:** <61% median weight for age. These children may require hospitalization for evaluation and nutritional support.

Failure to thrive is one of the most common diagnoses of early childhood in the United States. It affects all socio-economic groups, but children in poverty are more likely to be affected and more likely to suffer long-term sequelae. Ten percent of children in poverty meet criteria for FTT. As many as 30% of children presenting to emergency departments for unrelated complaints can be diagnosed with FTT. This group of children is of most concern. They are least likely to have good continuity of care and most likely to suffer additional developmental insults such as social isolation, tenuous housing situations, and neglect. Because FTT is most prevalent in at-risk populations that are least likely to have good continuity of care it is crucial to address growth parameters at every visit, both sick and well. Many children with FTT may not present for well-child visits. If that is the only visit at which the clinician considers growth, then many opportunities for meaningful intervention may be lost.

▶ **Pathogenesis**

All FTT is caused by undernutrition. The mechanism varies. The child may have increased caloric requirements because of organic disease. The child may have inadequate intake because not enough food is made available, or there may be mechanical difficulty in eating. Also, adequate calories may be provided, but the child may be unable to utilize them either because the nutrients cannot be absorbed across the bowel wall or because of inborn errors of metabolism.

When diagnosing FTT it is essential to consider the etiology. Over the past decades FTT has been better understood as a mixed entity in which both organic disease and psychosocial factors influence each other. With this understanding, the old belief that a child who gains weight in the hospital has nonorganic FTT has been debunked.

A. Organic FTT

Organic causes are identified in 10% of children with FTT. In-hospital evaluations reveal an underlying organic etiology in about 30% of children. The data are misleading. More than two-thirds of these children are diagnosed with gastroesophageal reflux disease (GERD). The practitioner risks one of two errors in diagnosing GERD as the source of failure to thrive. Physiological reflux is found in at least 70% of infants. It may be a normal finding in an infant who is failing to thrive for other reasons. Further, undernutrition causes decreased lower esophageal segment (LES) tone, which may lead to reflux as an effect rather than a cause of FTT.

B. Nonorganic FTT

Nonorganic FTT, weight loss in which no physiological disease is identified, constitutes 80% of cases. Historically, the responsibility for this diagnosis fell on the caregiver. The caregiver was either unable to provide enough nutrition or emotionally unavailable to the infant. In either circumstance the result was unsuccessful feeding. Psychosocial stressors were thought to create a neuroendocrine milieu preventing growth even when calories were available. Increased cortisol and decreased insulin levels in undernourished children inhibit weight gain.

C. Mixed FTT

Most FTT is *mixed*. There is a transaction between both physiological and psychosocial factors that creates a vicious cycle of undernutrition. For example, a child with organic disease may initially have difficulty eating for purely physiological reasons. However, over time, the feedings become fraught with anxiety for both parents and child and are even less successful. The child senses the parents' anxiety and eats less and more fretfully than before. The parents, afraid to overtax the "fragile" child, may not give the child the time needed to eat. They may become frustrated that they are not easily able to accomplish this most basic and essential care for the child. Parents of an ill child may perceive that other aspects of care are more important than feeding, such as strict adherence to a medication or therapy regimen.

Children with organic disease underlying FTT often gain weight in the hospital when fed by emotionally uninvolved parties such as nurses, volunteers, or physicians. Weight gain in the hospital should not be mistaken for parental neglect in the home. The primary care provider should pay close attention to the psychosocial stressors on the feeding dyad.

Conversely, the child who seems to be failing to thrive for purely psychosocial reasons often has complicating organic issues. The undernourished child is lethargic and irritable, especially at feeding times. Undernutrition decreases LES tone and may worsen reflux. The undernourished child is more difficult to feed and retains fewer calories. Poor nutrition adversely affects immunity. Children with FTT often have recurrent infections that increase their caloric requirements and decrease their ability to meet them.

The mixed model reminds the clinician that FTT is an interactive process involving physiologic and psychosocial elements and, more importantly, both caregiver and child. A fussy child may be more difficult for a particular parent to feed. A "good" or passive baby may not elicit enough feeding. Physical characteristics also affect parent-child relationships; organic disease may not only make feeding difficult but may engender a sense of failure or disappointment in the parent. It is crucial to remember that caregivers have unique relationships with each of their children. Therefore, a parent whose first child is diagnosed with FTT is not doomed to repeat the cycle with the second child. Conversely, an experienced caregiver who has fed previous children successfully may care for a child with FTT.

► Prevention

Failure to thrive may be prevented by good communication between the primary care provider and the family. The practitioner should regularly assess feeding practices and growth and educate parents about appropriate age-specific diets. As a general rule, infants who are feeding successfully gain about:

- 30 g/d at 0–3 months
- 20 g/d at 3–6 months
- 15 g/d at 6–9 months
- 12 g/d at 9–12 months
- 8 g/d at 1–3 years

In addition, growth parameters need to be recorded at every visit, sick or well. Weight should be documented for all children. Recumbent length is measured for children younger than 2 years old. Height is measured for children older than 3 years old. Between the ages of 2 and 3 years either height or length may be recorded. Length measurements exceed heights by an average of 1 cm. With a good growth chart in hand, the primary care provider can monitor growth and intervene early if problems arise.

Clinicians should investigate the economic stresses on families to ensure adequate access to nutrition for the family.

► Clinical Findings

A. Symptoms and Signs

The importance of a complete, long-term growth curve in making the diagnosis of FTT cannot be overemphasized. In acute undernutrition, the velocity of weight gain decreases while height velocity continues to be preserved. The result is a thin child of normal height. Chronic undernutrition manifests as "stunting"; both height and weight are affected. The child may appear proportionately small. Review of a growth curve may reveal that weight was initially affected and increase the suspicion for FTT. In interpreting growth charts, it is important to remember that healthy children may cross up to two major percentile lines up to 39% of the time between birth and 6 months of age and up to 15% of the time between 6 and 24 months of age. Children with length above the 50th percentile seldom have endocrine disease.

Children should be plotted on an appropriate growth curve. Growth curves are gender-specific and are available at the CDC website. Growth curves should not be used for specific countries of origin. Specific growth curves are available for children with genetic disorders such as trisomy 21 (Down syndrome) or Turner syndrome. However, these curves are not well validated. These curves draw from a small group of children, and the nutritional status of the participants was not assessed. These curves may be useful for the clinician in discussing an affected child's growth potential with the child's family.

B. History

1. General history—The clinician's most valuable tool in the diagnosis of FTT is the history. While taking the history, health care providers have the opportunity to establish themselves as the child's advocate and the parents' support. Care must be exercised to avoid establishing an adversarial relationship with the parents. It is useful to begin by asking the parents their perception of their child's health. Many parents do not recognize FTT until the clinician brings it to their attention.

The history and physical examination can uncover significant organ dysfunction contributing to growth failure. For example, the child who feeds poorly may have a physical impediment to caloric intake such as cleft palate or painful dental caries. Poor suck (ie, inadequate ability to suck) may also raise concerns for neurological disease. Recurrent upper or lower respiratory tract infections may suggest cystic fibrosis (CF), human immunodeficiency virus (HIV), or immunodeficiency. Sweating during feeding should prompt consideration of an underlying cardiac problem even in the absence of cyanosis. Chronic diarrhea can indicate malabsorption. Symptoms of chronic infection, eosinophilic disease, celiac disease, and pancreatic insufficiency should be elicited.

The health care provider must elicit more subtle aspects of past medical history as well, focusing particularly on developmental history and intercurrent illnesses. Delay in achievement of milestones should prompt a close neurologic examination. Inborn errors of metabolism and cerebral palsy can present with growth failure. A history of recurrent serious illness and FTT may be the only indicators of inborn errors of metabolism. Recurrent febrile illness without a clear source may also indicate occult urinary tract infection. A history of snoring or sleep disturbances should prompt an evaluation for tonsillar and adenoidal hypertrophy, which has been identified as a cause of FTT.

Past medical history must include a complete perinatal history (**Table 2-2**). Children with lower birth weights and those with specific prenatal exposures are at higher risk for growth problems. Of all children with diagnosed FTT, 40% have birth weights below 2500 g; only 7% of all births are below 2500 g.

Table 2-2. History taking.

Questions	Differential
Perinatal Infection Movement	Congenital infection Genetic disorders
Feeding behavior Diaphoresis Poor suck, swallow Length of feedings	Cardiac problem Neurologic, mechanical (submucosal cleft)
Diet history Infant Breastfeeding: time of nursing, sensation of letdown, fullness of breasts Formula fed: assess how parents are mixing formula, feeding techniques Older children 24-hour diet history Prospective 72-hour diet diary Dysphagia	Inadequate milk production Inappropriate diet Inappropriate interaction to stimulate feeding Inappropriate caloric intake Eosinophilic or allergic disorder reflux
Growth history Onset in infancy Onset of FTT after addition of solids Onset after infancy, recent drop	Genetic disorder: CF, syndromic, metabolic, urinary tract anomalies Celiac, eosinophilic Inflammatory bowel disease, celiac
Stooling history Diarrhea Constipation	Malabsorption: celiac, inflammatory bowel disease, eosinophilic enteritis Maldigestion: pancreatic insufficiency Cystic fibrosis, undernutrition, celiac
Voiding history	Poor stream in boys: posterior urethral valves

Low birth weight may be caused by infection, drug exposure, or other maternal and placental factors. The child with symmetric growth retardation is of particular concern. Infants exposed *in utero* to rubella, cytomegalovirus (CMV), syphilis, toxoplasmosis, or malaria are at high risk for low birth weight, length, and head circumference. These measurements portend poor catchup growth potential. Short stature is often accompanied by developmental delay and mental retardation in these children.

Children with asymmetric intrauterine growth retardation (preserved head circumference) have better potential for catchup growth and appropriate development. Fetal growth is affected by both maternal factors and exposure to toxins. Drugs of abuse such as tobacco, cocaine, and heroin have been correlated with low birth weight. Placental insufficiency caused by hypertension, preeclampsia, collagen vascular disease, or diabetes may result in an undernourished baby with decreased birth weight. Finally, intrauterine physical factors may reduce fetal growth; uterine malformation, multiple gestation, and fibroids may all contribute to smaller babies.

Maternal HIV infection is also a significant risk factor for FTT. Most children born to HIV-positive mothers have normal birth weights and lengths. However, children who are infected frequently develop FTT within the first year of life.

Family history is essential. A family history of atopy, eczema, or asthma raises the suspicion of eosinophilic enteritides. A family history of autoimmune disease should heighten the concern for celiac disease. Metabolic diseases are generally recessive, and an absence of family history should not be regarded as reassuring.

An examination of the family's relationships with the child and one another can uncover valuable information. Children described as "difficult" or "unpredictable" by their mothers have been noted to be slow or poor feeders by independent observers. Maternal depression and history of abuse are strong risk factors for FTT; addressing these issues is integral to establishing a functional feeding relationship between parent and child. Finally, a thorough assessment of economic supports may reveal that nutritious foods are unobtainable or difficult to access. Social financial supports are often inadequate to meet children's needs. Tenuous housing or homelessness may make it impossible to keep appropriate foods readily available.

2. Feeding history—A careful feeding history is part of the history of present illness. It often sheds more light on the problem than a battery of laboratory tests. When assessing an infant, it is essential to know what formula the infant is taking, in what volume, and how frequently. Caregivers should describe the preparation of formula. Caregivers may be inadvertently mixing dilute formula. In calculating caloric intake, the practitioner should remember that breast milk and formula have 20 cal/oz. Baby foods range from 40 to

120 calories per jar. An 80-cal/4-oz jar is a good average to use when making calculations.

The examiner should ask how long it takes the baby to eat; slow eating may be associated with poor suck or decreased stamina secondary to organic dysfunction. Parental estimation of the infant's suck may also be helpful. Parents should be asked about regurgitation after eating. The clinician should also inquire about feeding techniques. Bottle propping may indicate a poor parent-child relationship or an overtaxed parent.

The breastfed baby merits special mention. The sequelae of unsuccessful breastfeeding are profound. Infants may present with severe dehydration. Parents rarely recognize that the infant is failing to thrive. Mothers are often discharged from the hospital before milk is in and may be unsure about what to expect when initially learning how to breastfeed. The neonatal period is the most critical period in the establishment of breastfeeding. The primary care provider should educate the breastfeeding mother prior to hospital discharge. Milk should be in by day 3 or 4. The neonate should feed at least 8 times in a 24-hour period and should not be sleeping through the night. A "good" baby (an infant who sleeps through the night) should raise concerns of possible dehydration. Breastfed babies should have at least six wet diapers a day. Whereas formula-fed infants may have many stool patterns, the successful breastfed neonate should have at least four yellow seedy stools a day. After 4 weeks of life, the stool pattern may change to once a day or less.

Breastfed babies should be seen within the first week of life to evaluate infant weight and feeding success. Weight loss is expected until day 5 of life. Infants should regain their birth weight by the end of the second week of life. Any weight loss greater than 8% should elicit close follow-up. Weight loss greater than 10–12% should prompt an evaluation for dehydration. Primary care providers should ask about the infant's suck and whether the mother feels that her breasts are emptied at the feeding. The successful infant should empty the mother's breast and be content at the end of the nursing session. When breastfed infants are not gaining weight, it may be useful to observe the breastfeeding or obtain consultation with a lactation specialist.

The evaluation of older children also requires a thorough diet history. An accurate diet history begins with a 24-hour diet recall. Parents should be asked to quantify the amount of each food that their child has eaten. The 24-hour recall acts as a template for a 72-hour diet diary, the most accurate assessment of intake; the first 48 hours of a diet diary are the most reliable. All intakes must be recorded including juices, water, and snacks. The child who consumes an excessive amount of milk or juice may not have the appetite to eat more nutrient-rich foods. A child needs no more than 16–24 oz of milk and should be limited to <12 oz of juice per day.

It is as important to assess mealtime habits as the meals themselves. Activity in the household during mealtime may be distracting to young children. Television viewing may preempt eating. Excessive attention to how much the child eats can increase the tension and ultimately decrease the child's intake. Most toddlers cannot sit for longer than 15 minutes; prolonging the table time in the hopes of increasing the amount eaten may only exacerbate the already fragile parent-child relationship. Many toddlers snack throughout the day, but some are unable to take in appropriate calories with this strategy.

The primary care provider should also discuss the family's beliefs about a healthy diet. Some families have dietary restrictions, either by choice or culturally, that affect growth. Many have read the dietary recommendations for a healthy adult diet, but a low-fat, low-cholesterol diet is not an appropriate diet for a toddler. Until the age of 2 years children should drink whole milk, and their fat intake should not be limited.

C. Physical Examination

In addition to reviewing the growth curve, the clinician must complete a physical examination. A weight, length, or height as appropriate for the child's age, and head circumference are indicated for all children. Growth parameters may be roughly interpreted using the following guidelines:

- **Acute undernutrition**: low weight, normal height, normal head circumference
- **Chronic undernutrition**: short height, normal weight for height, normal head circumference
- **Acute or chronic undernutrition**: short height, proportionately low weight for height, normal head circumference
- **Congenital infection or genetic disorder impairing growth**: short height, normal to low weight for height, small head circumference

The general examination provides a wealth of information. Vital signs should be documented. Bradycardia and hypotension are worrisome findings in the malnourished child and should prompt consideration of immediate hospitalization. It is important to document observations of the parent-child interaction. It is also useful to note both the caregiver's and the child's affects. Parental depression has been associated with higher risk of FTT. Occasionally the examiner may find subtle indications of neglect such as a flat occiput, indicating that the child is left alone for long periods. However, a flat occiput may be a normal finding when caregiver's follow current infant sleeping recommendations.

Children with undernutrition often have objective findings of their nutritional state. Unlike the genetically small child, children with FTT have decreased subcutaneous fat. If undernutrition has been prolonged, they will also have muscle wasting; in infants it is easier to assess muscle wasting in the calves and thighs rather than in the interosseous muscles. It is also important to remember that infants suck rather than chew; therefore they will not have the characteristic facies of temporal wasting. Nailbeds and hair should be carefully noted as nutritional deficiencies may cause pitting or lines in the nails. Hair may be thin or brittle. Skin should be examined for scaling and cracking, which may be seen with both zinc and fatty acid deficiencies. Presence of eczema may indicate allergic diathesis and eosinophilic enteritis.

The physical examination should be completed with special attention directed to the organ systems of concern uncovered in the history. However, examination of some organ systems may reveal abnormalities not elicited through history. A thorough abdominal examination is of particular importance. Organomegaly in the child with FTT suggests possible inborn errors of metabolism and requires laboratory evaluation. The examiner should note the genitourinary (GU) examination. Undescended testicles may indicate panhypopituitarism, and ambiguous genitalia may indicate congenital adrenogenital hyperplasia (CAH). A careful neurologic examination may reveal subtly increased or decreased muscle tone consistent with cerebral palsy and, therefore, increased caloric requirements or inability to coordinate suck and swallow, respectively.

Children with undernutrition have been repeatedly shown to have behavioral and cognitive delays. Unfortunately, the Denver Development Screen II is an inadequate tool to assess the subtle but real delays in these children. It has been suggested that the Bayley test may be a more sensitive tool when assessing these children. Even with nutritional and social support, behavioral and cognitive lags may not resolve. Children who have suffered FTT remain sensitive to undernutrition throughout childhood; one study found a significant decrease in fluency in children with a remote history of undernutrition when they did not eat breakfast. Children with a normal nutritional history were not found to be similarly affected.

The immune system is affected by nutritional status. Children with FTT may present with recurrent mucosal infections: otitis media, sinusitis, pneumonia, and gastroenteritis. Immunoglobulin A (IgA) production is extremely sensitive to undernutrition. Children with more severe malnutrition may be lymphopenic (lymphocyte count <1500) or anergic.

Undernourished children are frequently iron-deficient, even in the absence of anemia. Iron and calcium deficiencies enhance the absorption of lead. In areas in which there is any concern for lead exposure, lead levels should be assessed as part of the workup for FTT.

D. Laboratory Findings

No single battery of laboratory tests or imaging studies can be advocated in the workup of FTT. Testing should be guided by the history and physical examination. Fewer than 1% of "routine laboratory tests" ordered in the evaluation of FTT provide useful information for treatment or diagnosis.

Tests that had been advocated as markers of nutritional status have limitations. Albumin has an extremely long half-life (21 days) and is a poor indicator of recent undernutrition. Prealbumin, which has been touted as a marker for recent protein nutrition, is decreased in both acute inflammation and undernutrition.

Children with more severe malnutrition may be lymphopenic (lymphocyte count <1500) or anergic.

Undernourished children are frequently iron deficient, even in the absence of anemia. Iron and calcium deficiencies enhance the absorption of lead. In areas in which there is any concern for lead exposure, lead levels should be assessed as part of the workup for FTT.

Laboratory evaluation is indicated when the history and physical examination suggest underlying organic disease. Children with developmental delay and organomegaly or severe episodic illness should have a metabolic workup, including urine organic and serum amino acids; there is a 5% yield in this subset of patients. Children with a history of recurrent respiratory tract infections or diarrhea should have a sweat chloride testing. A history of poorly defined febrile illnesses or recurrent "viral illness" may be followed up with a urinalysis, culture, and renal function to evaluate for occult urinary tract disease. In children with diarrhea, it may be useful to send stool for *Giardia* antigen, qualitative fat, white blood cell (WBC) count, occult blood, ova and parasites (O&P), rotavirus, and α_1-antitrypsin. Rotavirus has been associated with a prolonged gastroenteritis and FTT. Elevated α_1-antitrypsin in the stool is a marker for protein enteropathy.

For children who develop FTT after the addition of solid foods, an evaluation for celiac disease is warranted regardless of whether diarrhea is present. Fifteen percent of celiac patients present with constipation. Tissue transglutaminase along with a total IgA level may be useful for diagnosis (**Table 2-3**).

Infectious diseases need to be specifically addressed. Worldwide, tuberculosis (TB) is one of the most common causes of FTT. A Mantoux test and anergy panel must be placed on any child with risk factors for TB exposure. The possibility of HIV must also be entertained. FTT is frequently a presenting symptom of HIV in the infant.

▶ Differential Diagnosis

It is essential to differentiate a small child from the child with FTT. No criterion is specific enough to exclude those who are small for other reasons. Included in the differential diagnosis of FTT are familial short stature, Turner syndrome, normal growth variant, prematurity, endocrine dysfunction, and genetic syndromes limiting growth.

The child with FTT has a deceleration in weight first. Height velocity continues unaffected for a time. Children with familial short stature manifest a simultaneous change in their height and weight curves. Height velocity slows first

Table 2-3. Laboratory evaluation.

CBC with differential	Anemia: possible inflammatory bowel disease or celiac Eosinophilia: possible eosinophilic enteritis
CMP	Low albumin: chronic inflammation Elevated transaminases: chronic undernutrition, metabolic disorder Bicarbonate: renal disease
Antigliadin Ab	Children <3 years to evaluate for celiac
Tissue transglutaminase with total IgA	Older children to evaluate for celiac
Urinalysis	Chronic urinary tract infection
Sweat chloride	Cystic Fibrosis

(it can even plateau) in endocrine disorders such as hypothyroidism. The preterm infant's growth parameters need to be adjusted for gestational age; head circumference is adjusted until 18 months, weight until 24 months, and height through 40 months.

The family history is helpful in differentiating the child with FTT from the child with constitutional growth delay or familial short stature. Midparental height, which can be calculated from the family history, is a useful calculation of probable genetic potential:

- **For girls**: (father's height in in − 5 + mother's height)/2 ± 2 in
- **For boys**: (mother's height in in + 5 + father's height)/2 ± 2 in

If the child's current growth curve translates into an adult height that falls within the range of midparental height, reassurance may be offered.

It is most difficult to differentiate the older child with constitutional growth delay from the child with FTT. These children typically have reduced weight for height, as do children with FTT. However, unlike children with FTT, they ultimately gain both weight and height on a steady curve. Family history is often revealing in constitutional growth delay. Querying parents about the onset of their own pubertal signs may seem intrusive, but often gives the clinician the information needed to reassure parents about their child's growth.

Breastfeeding infants may be growing normally and not follow the CDC growth curves. After 4–6 months their weight may decrease relative to their peers. After 12 months their weight may catch up to that of age-matched formula-fed infants. However, a decrease in weight in early infancy is a symptom of unsuccessful breastfeeding and FTT should be considered.

Complications

Developmental delay may persist in children with FTT well past the period of undernutrition. Studies have repeatedly shown that these children, as a group, have more behavioral and cognitive problems in school than their peers, even into adolescence. One caveat about these studies is that many investigators defined FTT by that classic definition: growth failure associated with disordered behavior and development. These studies do not doom every child with FTT to scholastic and social failure, but the clinician must be vigilant and act as the child's advocate. Formal developmental screening is especially important in the child with a history of FTT. Intervention should be offered early rather than waiting "to see if the child catches up." Children with FTT are generally successful but may need specific supports on the road to achieving that success.

Treatment

A. Nutrition

The cornerstone of therapy is nutrition. The goal of treatment is catchup growth. Children with FTT may need 1.5–2 times the usual daily calories to achieve catch-up growth. For an infant this is roughly 150-200 cal/kg per day. There are many formulas for calculating caloric requirements. One simple estimate is:

$$\text{kcal/kg} = 120 \text{ kcal/kg} \times \text{median weight for current height/current weight (kg)}$$

It is important that this nutrition include adequate protein calories. Children with undernutrition require 3 grams of protein per kilogram of body weight per day to initiate catchup growth and may need as much as 5 g/kg. In severe malnutrition the protein needs can double this amount. High-calorie diets should continue until the child achieves an age-appropriate weight for height. Infant formula can often be mixed in a more concentrated way to facilitate caloric intake at a lower volume.

It is almost impossible for any child to take in twice the usual volume of food. Some solutions are to offer higher-calorie formulas (24–30 cal/oz) to infants. For older children it is possible to replace or add higher-calorie foods. Heavy cream may be substituted for milk on cereal or in cooking. Cheese may be added to vegetables. Instant breakfast drinks may be offered as snacks. It is advisable to enlist a dietician in designing a high-calorie diet for the child with FTT. Achieving an effective nutritional plan may require structured trials of meal timing and rewards as well food types, colors, temperatures, and textures.

Tube feedings are sometimes indicated in the child with FTT. Some children may benefit from nighttime feedings through a nasogastric or a percutaneous endoscopic gastrostomy tube. This solution is particularly useful in children with underlying increased caloric requirements, for example, children with cystic fibrosis and cerebral palsy. Children with mechanical feeding difficulties may also require tube feeding for some period of time. Early intervention with an occupational or speech therapist is recommended for a child who is primarily tube-fed. Without therapy the child may develop oral aversions or fail to develop appropriate oral-motor coordination. Parents need to be educated at the onset of nutritional therapy. Catchup growth is expected within the first month. However, some children may not show accelerated weight gain until after the first 2 weeks of increased nutrition. Children usually gain 1.5 times their daily expected weight gains during the catchup phase. Children's weight improves well before their height increases. This change in body habitus does not indicate overfeeding; rather it indicates successful therapy. It does not matter how quickly the child gains; the composition of weight gain will be 45–65% lean body mass.

B. Medications

Few medications are indicated in the treatment of FTT. Those few are nutritional supports. Children with FTT should be supplemented with iron. Zinc has also been shown to improve linear growth. It is sufficient to supplement children with a multivitamin containing zinc and iron. Vitamin D supplementation should also be considered. Vitamin D replacement is especially important in dark-skinned children and in children who are not regularly exposed to sunlight.

C. Social Support

Social support is essential. The services offered must be tailored to the family and the child. Certainly frequent visits with the primary care provider are useful; weight gain can be measured and concerns addressed. Home visits by social services have been shown to decrease hospitalizations and improve weight gain. Children with developmental delay need early assessment and intervention by the appropriate therapists.

These interventions, if performed early in childhood, have longlasting ramifications throughout the lifespan.

D. Indications for Referral or Hospital Admission

Most FTT can and should be managed by the primary care provider. A trusting relationship between the clinician and the family is an invaluable asset in the treatment of FTT. Parents struggling with the diagnosis often believe that the health care system views them as neglectful. This anxiety creates barriers to open and honest communication about the child's feeding and developmental status. However, suspicions may be allayed when primary care providers enlist themselves as allies in the treatment.

The primary indication for referral is the treatment of an underlying organ dysfunction that requires specialized care. Referral is also warranted when the primary care provider feels that specialized testing is needed, for example, endoscopic biopsies for the further evaluation of celiac disease or eosinophilic enteritis. The clinician may also wish to reevaluate the child who fails to begin catchup growth after 1–2 months of nutritional intervention.

Most children with FTT can be managed in the outpatient setting. A few may need hospitalization at some point during their evaluation. Indications for admission at initial evaluation are bradycardia or hypotension, which often indicate severe malnutrition. Children who are <61% of the median weight for their age should be admitted for nutritional support. Children with FTT who are admitted electively during the usual workweek have a shorter length of stay and less unhelpful lab and imaging studies. Children with hypoglycemia should be admitted. A low serum glucose is worrisome for severe malnutrition and metabolic disease.

If the clinician suspects abuse or neglect, the child should be admitted. About 10% of children with FTT are abused. These children ultimately experience poorer developmental outcomes than other children with FTT if unrecognized. When abuse is documented social services must be involved.

Another group of children who may be considered for hospital admission are those who have failed to initiate catchup growth with outpatient management. A hospital stay of several days will allow the clinician to observe feeding practices and enable the family to internalize the plan of care. Further testing for organ dysfunction may be indicated during this hospitalization. It can also be a time to enlist other health professionals in the treatment plan; occupational therapists and social workers are often helpful allies in the treatment of FTT.

Bonuck K, Parikh S, Bassila M. Growth failure and sleep disordered breathing: a review of the literature. *Int J Pediatr Otorhinolaryngol.* 2006; 70:769–778.

Cole SZ, Lanham JS. Failure to thrive: an update. *Am Fam Physician.* 2011; 83(7):829–834.

Ficicioglu C, Haack K. Failure to thrive: when to suspect inborn errors of metabolism. *Pediatrics* 2009; 124:972–979.

Frank DA: Failure to thrive. *Pediatr Clin North Am* 1988; 35(6): 1187-1206.

Jaffee AC. Failure to thrive: current clinical concepts. *Pediatr Rev.* 2011; 32(3):100–107. [PMID: 23509161]

Maggioni A. Nutritional management of failure to thrive. *Pediatr Clin North Am.* 1995; 42(4):791–810.

Olsen EM, Petersen J, Skovgaard AM, et al. Failure to thrive: the prevalence and concurrence of anthropometric criteria in a general infant population. *Arch Dis Child.* 2007; 92(2):109–114.

Prasse K, Kikano G. An overview of pediatric dysphagia. *Clin Pediatr.* 2009;48(3):247–251.

Rudolph MC. What is the long term outcome for children who fail to thrive? A systematic review. *Arch Dis Child,* 2005; 90(9):925–931.

Thompson RT. Increased length of stay and costs associated with weekend admissions for failure to thrive. *Pediatrics.* 2013; 131;e805.

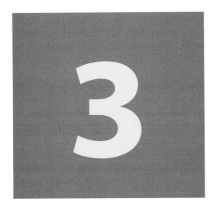

Neonatal Hyperbilirubinemia

Andrew B. Symons, MD, MS

Martin C. Mahoney, MD, PhD, FAAFP

ESSENTIALS OF DIAGNOSIS

► Visible yellowing of the skin, ocular sclera, or both are present in neonatal jaundice; however, because visual estimates of total bilirubin are prone to error, quantitative testing (serum or transcutaneous) should be completed in infants noted to be jaundiced within the first 24 hours of life.

► Risk of subsequent hyperbilirubinemia can be assessed by plotting serum bilirubin levels onto a nomogram; all bilirubin levels should be interpreted according to the infant's age (in hours).

General Considerations

Nearly every infant is born with a serum bilirubin level higher than that of the normal adult. Approximately 60% of newborns are visibly jaundiced during the first week of life. The diagnostic and therapeutic challenge for the physician is to differentiate normal physiologic jaundice from pathologic jaundice, and to institute appropriate evaluation and therapy when necessary.

Several factors are considered as major predictors for the development of severe hyperbilirubinemia among infants of ≥35 weeks' gestation. Among the most significant clinical characteristics associated with severe hyperbilirubinemia are predischarge levels in the high-risk zone on the serum bilirubin nomogram (**Figure 3-1**) and jaundice noted within 24 hours of birth. Other risk factors include various forms of hemolytic disease [eg, ABO incompatibility, glucose-6-phosphate dehydrogenase (G6PD) deficiency], elevated end-tidal carbon monoxide, gestation age of 35–36 weeks, a sibling who required phototherapy, cephalohematoma or significant bruising, exclusive breastfeeding, East Asian race, maternal age ≥25 years, and male gender.

While the American Academy of Pediatrics currently recommends universal predischarge bilirubin screening using total serum bilirubin (TSB) or total cutaneous bilirubin (TcB) measurements, the United States Preventive Services Task Force (USPSTF) determined that the evidence is insufficient to recommend screening infants for hyperbilirubinemia to prevent chronic bilirubin encephalopathy; the American Academy of Family Physicians concurs with the USPSTF position. In clinical practice, however, testing is completed for the vast majority of infants.

American Academy of Pediatrics Subcommittee on Hyperbilirubinemia. Management of hyperbilirubinemia in the newborn infant 35 or more weeks of gestation. *Pediatrics.* 2004;114:297. [PMID: 15231951]

US Preventive Services Task Force. Screening of infants for hyperbilirubinemia to prevent chronic bilirubin encephalopathy: US preventive services task force recommendation statement. *Pediatrics.* 2009; 124. [PMID: 20704172]

Pathogenesis

A. Physiologic Jaundice

The three classifications of neonatal hyperbilirubinemia are based on the following mechanisms of accumulation: increased bilirubin load, decreased bilirubin conjugation, and impaired bilirubin excretion. In the newborn, unconjugated bilirubin is produced faster and removed more slowly than in the normal adult because of the immaturity of the glucuronyl transferase enzyme system. The main source of unconjugated bilirubin is the breakdown of hemoglobin in senescent red blood cells. Newborns have an increased erythrocyte mass at birth (average hematocrit of 50% vs 33% in the adult) and a shorter lifespan for erythrocytes (90 days vs 120 days in the adult). The newborn cannot readily excrete unconjugated bilirubin, and much of it is reabsorbed by the intestine and returned to the enterohepatic circulation.

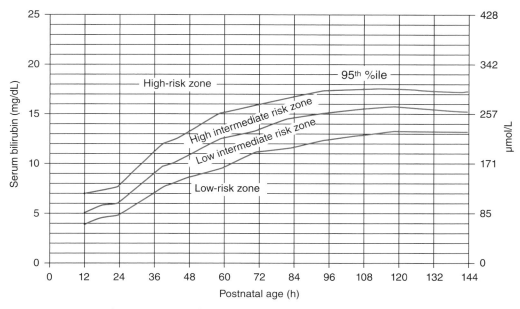

▲ **Figure 3-1.** Nomogram for designation of risk in 2840 well newborns of ≥36 weeks' gestational age with birth weight of ≥2000 g or ≥35 weeks' gestational age and birth weight of ≥2500 g based on the hour-specific serum bilirubin value. (*Reproduced with permission from American Academy of Pediatrics Subcommittee on Hyperbilirubinemia. Management of hyperbilirubinemia in the newborn infant 35 or more weeks of gestation. Pediatrics. 2004;114:297.*)

Increased production and decreased elimination of bilirubin lead to a *physiologic jaundice* in most normal newborns. Bilirubin is a very effective and potent antioxidant, and physiologic jaundice may provide a mechanism for protecting the newborn from oxygen free-radical injury. The average full-term white newborn experiences a peak serum bilirubin concentration of 5–6 mg/dL (86–103 μmol/L), which begins to rise after the first day of life, peaks on the third day of life, and falls to normal adult levels by days 10–12. African American infants tend to have slightly lower peaks in serum bilirubin. In Asian infants, serum bilirubin levels rise more quickly than in white infants and tend to reach higher peaks on average (8–12 mg/dL; 135–205 μmol/L). This leads to a longer period of physiologic jaundice among Asian and Native American newborns. Preterm infants (<37 weeks' gestation) of all races may take 4–5 days to reach peak serum bilirubin levels, and these peaks may be twice those observed among full-term infants.

B. Breastfeeding and Breast Milk Jaundice

Infants who are breastfed may experience exaggerated bilirubin levels as a result of two separate phenomena associated with breastfeeding and breast milk.

Breastfed infants may experience relative starvation in the first few days of life, due to delayed release of milk by the mother and/or difficulties with breastfeeding. This nutritional inadequacy can result in increased enterohepatic circulation of bilirubin, leading to elevated serum bilirubin levels in the first few days of life. Termed *breastfeeding jaundice*, this finding is considered abnormal and can be overcome by offering frequent feedings (10–12 times per day) and by avoiding water supplementation in breastfed infants.

Breast milk is believed to increase the enterohepatic circulation of bilirubin; however, the specific factor(s) in breast milk that is (are) responsible for this action is (are) unknown. For the first 5 days of life, the serum bilirubin level in breastfed infants parallels that in nonbreastfed infants. Beginning at approximately day 6, *breast milk jaundice* occurs in breastfed infants as serum bilirubin either rises a little for a few days or declines more slowly. Approximately two-thirds of breastfed infants may be expected to have hyperbilirubinemia from 3 weeks to 3 months of age, with as many as one-third exhibiting clinical jaundice. Breast milk jaundice (unlike breastfeeding jaundice) is considered a form of normal physiologic jaundice in healthy, thriving breastfed infants.

C. Pathologic Jaundice

Exaggerated physiologic jaundice occurs at serum bilirubin levels between 7 and 17 mg/dL (between 104 and

291 μmol/L). Bilirubin levels above 17 mg/dL in full-term infants are no longer considered physiologic, and further investigation is warranted.

The onset of jaundice within the first 24 hours of life or a rate of increase in serum bilirubin exceeding 0.5 mg/dL (8 μmol/L) per hour is potentially pathologic and suggestive of hemolytic disease. Conjugated serum bilirubin concentrations exceeding 10% of total bilirubin or 2 mg/dL (35 μmol/L) are also not physiologic and suggest hepatobiliary disease or a general metabolic disorder.

Differentiating between pathologic and physiologic jaundice requires consideration of historical as well as clinical factors. Important historical features increasing the likelihood that jaundice is pathologic include family history of hemolytic disease, ethnicity suggestive of inherited disease (eg, G6PD deficiency), onset of jaundice in the first 24 hours of life, and jaundice lasting >3 weeks. Clinical assessment requires careful attention to general appearance, vital signs, weight loss, feeding patterns, stool and urine appearance, activity levels, and hepatosplenomegaly, which may be indicative of inborn errors in metabolism, sepsis, or other conditions. A rapid rise in serum bilirubin levels and lack of response to phototherapy are also indicative of pathologic jaundice. Cholestatic jaundice, manifesting as pale-colored stool and dark urine, indicates the need to explore for the presence of biliary atresia or other pathology.

The primary concern with severe hyperbilirubinemia is the potential for neurotoxic effects as well as general cellular injury, which can occur at TSB levels exceeding 20–25 mg/dL. The term *kernicterus* refers to the yellow staining of the basal ganglia observed postmortem among infants who died with severe jaundice. (Bilirubin deposition in the basal ganglia can also be imaged using magnetic resonance techniques.) The American Academy of Pediatrics (AAP) has recommended that the term *acute bilirubin encephalopathy* be used to describe the acute manifestations of bilirubin toxicity seen in the first weeks after birth and that the term *kernicterus* be reserved for the chronic and permanent clinical sequelae of bilirubin toxicity.

Although kernicterus was a common complication of hyperbilirubinemia in the 1940s and 1950s due to Rh erythroblastosis fetalis and ABO hemolytic disease, it is rare today, with the use of Rh immunoglobulin and with the intervention of phototherapy and exchange transfusion. With early discharge to home, however, a small resurgence of kernicterus has been observed in countries in which this complication had essentially disappeared. The reported incidence of chronic kernicterus in the United States is ~1 case/27,000 live births and 1 case/44,000 live births in Canada.

Bilirubin can interfere with various metabolic pathways and may also impair cerebral glucose metabolism. The concentration of bilirubin in the brain and the duration of exposure are important determinants of the neurotoxic effects of bilirubin. Bilirubin can enter the brain when not bound to albumin, so infants with low albumin are at increased risk of developing kernicterus. Conditions that alter the blood-brain barrier such as infection, acidosis, hypoxia, sepsis, prematurity, and hyperosmolarity may affect the entry of bilirubin into the brain.

In infants without hemolysis, serum bilirubin levels and encephalopathy do not correlate well. In infants with hemolysis, TSB levels of >20 mg/dL are associated with worse neurologic outcomes, although some infants with concentrations of 25 mg/dL are normal. Kernicterus has been detected in 8% of infants with associated hemolysis who had TSB levels of 19–25 mg/dL, 33% of infants with levels of 25–29 mg/dL, and 73% of infants with levels of 30–40 mg/dL. It should be noted that the majority of cases of kernicterus described in recent years have been among neonates who had TSB levels of >30 mg/dL at the time of diagnosis, which is well above the recommended treatment thresholds of 15 or 20 mg/dL.

In its acute form, kernicterus (eg, acute bilirubin encephalopathy) may present in the first 1–2 days with poor sucking, stupor, hypotonia, and seizures, although 15% of affected infants may be asymptomatic. During the middle of the first week, hypertonia of extensor muscles, opisthotonus (backward arching of the trunk), retrocollis (backward arching of the neck), and fever may be observed. After the first week, the infant may exhibit generalized hypertonia. Some of these changes disappear spontaneously or can be reversed with exchange transfusion. In most infants with moderate (10–20 mg/dL) to severe (>20 mg/dL) hyperbilirubinemia, evoked neurologic responses return to normal within 6 months. A minority of infants (ranging between 6% and 23%) exhibit persistent neurologic deficits.

In its chronic form, kernicterus may present in the first year with hypotonia, active deep-tendon reflexes, obligatory tonic neck reflexes, dental dysplasia, and delayed motor skills. After the first year, movement disorders, upward gaze, and sensorineural hearing loss may develop. It has been suggested that long-term effects of severe hyperbilirubinemia on intelligence quotient (IQ) are more likely in boys than in girls. Seidman and colleagues studied 1948 subjects from Hadaasah Hebrew University Medical Center in Jerusalem born in 1970–1971 and drafted into the Israeli army 17 years later and found a higher risk of lowered IQ (< 85) among males with a history of TSB exceeding 20 mg/dL [odds ratio (OR) 2.96; 95% confidence interval (CI) 1.29–6.79] (Seidman et al. 1991).

Carceller-Blanchard A, Cousineau J, Delvin EE. Point of care testing: transcutaneous bilirubinometry in neonates. *Clin Biochem.* 2009;42(3). [PMID:18929553]

Kaplan M, Shchors I, Algur N, et al. Visual screening versus transcutaneous bilirubinometry for predischarge. jaundice assessment. *Acta Paediatr.* 2008;97:759–763.

Kuzniewicz M, Newman TB. Interaction of hemolysis and hyperbilirubinemia on neurodevelopmental outcomes in the collaborative perinatal project. *Pediatrics*. 2009;123:3. [PMID: 19255038]

Seidman DS et al. Neonatal hyperbilirubinemia and physical and cognitive performance at 17 years of age. *Pediatrics*. 1991;88:828. [PMID: 1896294]

Sgro M, Campbell DM, Kandasamy S, Shah V. Incidence of chronic bilirubin encephalopathy in Canada, 2007–2008. *Pediatrics*. 2012;130:4. [PMID: 22966025]

▶ **Clinical Findings**

In 2004, the AAP issued an updated practice parameter for the management of hyperbilirubinemia among newborns of ≥35 weeks' gestation. Elements of these recommendations are summarized below and can be accessed in full at http://www.aap.org.

A. Symptoms and Signs

Clinically, jaundice usually progresses from head to toe. Visual estimates of total bilirubin are prone to error, especially in infants with pigmented skin. TSB or total cutaneous bilirubin (TcB) levels should be measured in infants who develop jaundice within the first 24 hours, and all bilirubin levels should be interpreted according to the infant's age (in hours). TcB measurement devices may provide an alternative to frequent blood draws for the accurate assessment of serum bilirubin, although current guidelines indicate variability in the accuracy of TcB instruments from different manufacturers.

Evaluation of infants who develop abnormal signs such as feeding difficulty, behavior changes, apnea, and temperature changes is recommended regardless of whether jaundice has been detected in order to rule out underlying disease. Clinical protocols for evaluating jaundice, with assessments to be performed no less than every 8–12 hours in the newborn nursery, should be in place.

B. Laboratory Findings

When a pathologic cause for jaundice is suspected, laboratory studies should be promptly completed:

- When jaundice is noticed within the first 24 hours, clinicians should consider a sepsis workup, evaluation for rubella and toxoplasmosis infection, assessment of fractionated serum bilirubin levels, and blood typing to rule out erythroblastosis fetalis. Results of thyroid and galactosemia testing, obtained during the newborn metabolic screening, also should be reviewed.

- If the level of conjugated bilirubin is >2 mg/dL, a reason for impaired bilirubin excretion should be sought. If conjugated bilirubin is <2 mg/dL, hemoglobin levels and reticulocyte counts should be evaluated. A high hemoglobin concentration indicates polycythemia, whereas a low hemoglobin concentration with an abnormal reticulocyte count suggests hemolysis. If the reticulocyte count is normal, the infant must be evaluated for a nonhemolytic cause of jaundice.

- Infants with a poor response to phototherapy and those whose family history is consistent with the possibility of glucose-6-phosphate dehydrogenase (G6PD) deficiency require further testing.

- Maternal prenatal testing should include ABO and Rh (D) typing and a serum screen for unusual isoimmune antibodies. If the mother has not had prenatal blood grouping, or is Rh-negative, a direct Coombs test, blood type, and Rh (D) typing of the infant's cord blood should be performed. Institutions are encouraged to save cord blood for future testing, particularly when the mother's blood type is group O.

C. Neonatal Jaundice after Hospital Discharge

Follow-up should be provided to all neonates discharged less than 48 hours after birth. This evaluation by a health care professional should occur within 2–3 days of discharge.

Approximately one-third of healthy breastfed infants have persistent jaundice beyond 2 weeks of age. A report of dark urine or light-colored stools should prompt a measurement of direct serum bilirubin. If the history and physical examination are normal, continued observation is appropriate. If jaundice persists beyond 3 weeks, a urine sample should be tested for bilirubin, and a measurement of total and direct serum bilirubin should be obtained.

American Academy of Pediatrics Subcommittee on Hyperbilirubinemia. Management of hyperbilirubinemia in the newborn 35 or more weeks of gestation. *Pediatrics*. 2004;114:297. [PMID: 15231951]

Maisels MJ, Bhutani VK, et al. Hyperbilirubinemia in the newborn infant ≥35 weeks' gestation: an update with clarification. *Pediatrics*. 2009;124:1193–1198. [PMID: 19786452]

▶ **Prediction & Prevention**

Shorter hospital stays after delivery limit the time for hospital-based assessment of infant feeding, instruction about breastfeeding, and the detection of jaundice. Hyperbilirubinemia and problems related to feeding are the main reasons for hospital readmission during the first week of life. Among 25,439 infants discharged between 2008 and 2009 from a large medical center in Israel, 143 (0.56%) were readmitted for phototherapy.

Because bilirubin levels usually peak on day 3 or 4 of life, and as most newborns are discharged within 48 hours, most cases of jaundice occur at home. It is therefore important that infants be seen by a health care professional within a few days of discharge to assess for jaundice and overall well-being. This is important in near-term infants (35–36 weeks' gestation) who are at particular risk for hyperbilirubinemia because of both relative hepatic immaturity and inadequate nutritional intake.

Measuring TSB before discharge and then plotting this value on a nomogram (see **Figure 3-1**) can be useful for predicting the risk of subsequent moderately severe hyperbilirubinemia (>17 mg/dL) and identify neonates for whom close follow-up is warranted. A study of 17,854 live births reported that neonates in the high-risk group (95th percentile for TSB) at 18–72 hours of life had a 40% chance of developing moderately severe hyperbilirubinemia on discharge, whereas for those in the low-risk group (40th percentile for TSB), the probability for subsequently developing moderately severe hyperbilirubinemia was zero.

Bromiker R, Bin-Nun A, Schimmel MS, Hammerman C, Kaplan M. Neonatal hyperbilirubinemia in the low-intermediate-risk category on the bilirubin nomogram. *Pediatrics.* 2012;130(3): e470–e475. [PMID: 22926183]

Kuzniewicz MW, Escobar GJ, Wi S, et al. Risk factors for severe hyperbilirubinemia among infants with borderline bilirubin levels: a nested case-control study. *J Pediatr.* 2008;153:2. [PMID: 18534217]

▶ **Treatment**

A. Suspected Pathologic Jaundice

Treatment decisions for both phototherapy (**Figure 3-2**) and exchange transfusion (**Figure 3-3**) are based on TSB levels; management options should be discussed with the parents or guardians of the infant. Intensive phototherapy should produce a decline in TSB of 1–2 mg/dL within 4–6 hours, and the decline should continue thereafter. If the TSB does not respond appropriately to intensive phototherapy, exchange transfusion is recommended. If levels are in a range that suggests the need for exchange transfusion (see **Figure 3-3**), intensive phototherapy should be attempted while preparations for exchange transfusion are made. Exchange transfusion is also recommended in infants whose TSB levels rise to exchange transfusion levels despite intensive phototherapy. In any of the preceding situations, failure of intensive phototherapy to lower the TSB level strongly suggests the presence of hemolytic disease or other pathologic processes and strongly warrants further investigation or consultation.

In infants with isoimmune hemolytic disease, administration of intravenous gamma globulin (0.5–1 g/kg over 2 hours) is recommended if the TSB is rising despite intensive phototherapy or the TSB is within 2–3 mg/dL of the exchange level. If necessary, this dose can be repeated in 12 hours.

Figure 3-2 summarizes the management strategy for hyperbilirubinemia in infants of ≥35 weeks' gestation. Management decisions regarding phototherapy and exchange transfusion (see **Figure 3-3**) are based on the infant's age, risk factors, and TSB levels.

B. Phototherapy and Exchange Transfusion

1. Phototherapy—This procedure involves exposing the infant to high-intensity light in the blue-green wavelengths. Light interacts with unconjugated bilirubin in the skin,

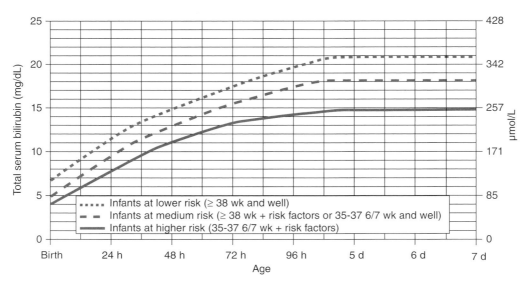

▲ **Figure 3-2.** Guidelines for phototherapy in hospitalized infants of ≥35 weeks' gestation. (*Reproduced with permission from American Academy of Pediatrics Subcommittee on Hyperbilirubinemia. Management of hyperbilirubinemia in the newborn infant 35 or more weeks of gestation. Pediatrics. 2004;114:297.*)

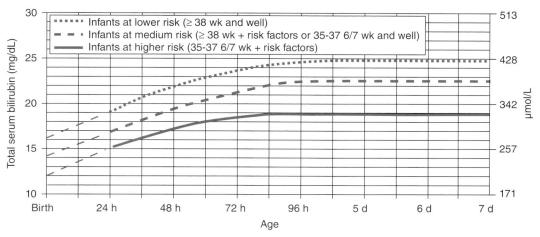

▲ **Figure 3-3.** Guidelines for exchange transfusion in infants of ≥35 weeks' gestation. (*Reproduced with permission from American Academy of Pediatrics Subcommittee on Hyperbilirubinemia. Management of hyperbilirubinemia in the newborn infant 35 or more weeks of gestation. Pediatrics. 2004;114:297.*)

converting it to less toxic photoisomers that are excreted in the bile and urine without conjugation. The efficacy of phototherapy is strongly influenced by the energy output in the blue spectrum, the spectrum of the light, and the surface area of the infant exposed to phototherapy. Commonly used light sources for providing phototherapy are special blue fluorescent tubes, compact fluorescent tubes, and halogen spotlights; however, light-emitting diodes (LEDs) have been shown to be as efficacious as conventional sources, with less heat emission.

Eye protection is placed on the infant, and the bank of lights is placed 15–20 cm from the naked infant. Exposure is increased by placing a fiberoptic blanket under the infant, lightening units all around the infant, or a white sheet around the bassinet to serve as a reflecting surface. If slight warming of the infant is noted, the tubes can be moved away a bit. Phototherapy may be interrupted briefly for parental visits or breastfeeding.

In infants with TSB levels of >25 mg/dL, phototherapy should be administered continuously until a response is documented, or until exchange therapy is initiated. If the TSB is not responding to conventional phototherapy (a *response* is defined as a sustained reduction in TSB of 1–2 mg/dL in 4–6 hours), the intensity should be increased by adding more lights; the intensity of the lights should also be increased while exchange transfusion is prepared. With commonly used light sources, overdose is impossible, although the infant may experience loose stools. Phototherapy is continued until the TSB level is lower than 14–15 mg/dL. The infant may be discharged after the completion of phototherapy. Rebound of TSB following cessation of phototherapy is usually <1 mg/dL.

2. Exchange transfusion—This procedure rapidly removes bilirubin from the circulation. Circulating antibodies against erythrocytes are also removed. Exchange transfusion is particularly beneficial in neonates with hemolysis. One or two central catheters are placed. Small aliquots of blood (8–10 mL per pass) are removed from the infant's circulation and replaced with equal amounts of donor red cells mixed with plasma. The procedure is repeated until twice the infant's blood volume is replaced (~160–200 mL/kg). Serum electrolytes and bilirubin are measured periodically during the procedure. In some cases the procedure must be repeated to lower serum bilirubin levels sufficiently. Infusing salt-poor albumin at a dose of 1 g/kg 1–4 hours before exchange transfusion has been shown to increase the amount of bilirubin removed during the procedure.

Complications of exchange transfusion include thrombocytopenia, portal vein thrombosis, necrotizing enterocolitis, electrolyte imbalance, graft-versus-host disease, and infection. Mortality from exchange transfusion approaches 2%, and an additional 12% of infants may suffer serious complications. Therefore, exchange transfusion should be reserved for neonates who have failed intensive phototherapy and should be performed by clinicians and facilities with proper experience.

If exchange transfusion is being considered, the bilirubin/albumin ratio is used in conjunction with the TSB level and other factors in determining the need for exchange transfusion (see **Figure 3-3**).

C. Suspected Nonpathologic Jaundice

For the management of breastfeeding jaundice, interruption of breastfeeding in healthy full-term newborns is generally discouraged. Frequent breastfeeding sessions (at least 8–10 times in 24 hours) are advised. However, if the mother and physician wish, they may consider using supplemental formula feedings or temporarily interrupting breastfeeding and replacing it with formula feedings. Phototherapy may be initiated, depending on TSB levels.

As discussed previously, breast milk jaundice is seen initially after day 6 of life in the majority of healthy breastfed infants between 3 weeks and 3 months of age. This is a form of normal physiologic jaundice.

Bhutani VK, Johns L. Kernicterus in the 21st century: frequently asked questions. *J Perinatol.* 2009; 29:S1. [PMID: 19177056]

Dijk PH, Hulzebos CV. An evidence-based view on hyperbilirubinaemia. *Acta Paediatrica.* 2012; 101:s464 [PMID: 22404885]

Maisels MJ, McDonagh AF. Phototherapy for neonatal jaundice. *N Engl J Med.* 2008;358:920–928. [PMID: 18305267]

Murki S et al. Light emitting diodes versus compact fluorescent tubes for phototherapy in neonatal jaundice: a multi-center randomized controlled trial. *Indian Pediatr.* 2010;47:2. [PMID: 19578227]

▷ Conclusions

Because up to 60% of all newborns are noted to be clinically jaundiced, all family physicians who care for neonates will encounter this common clinical entity. In the overwhelming majority of cases, this jaundice is entirely benign. However, it is important that the family physician recognize cases in which jaundice could represent a pathologic process or the risk for development of severe hyperbilirubinemia.

Infants who are discharged prior to 48 hours of age, particularly those who are born at <35 weeks' gestation, should be seen in the office within 2 days of discharge to evaluate jaundice and overall clinical status.

Parental education should emphasize the need to monitor the infant for jaundice, the generally benign course of most cases of jaundice, and associated symptoms such as poor feeding, lethargy, dark urine, and light-colored stools. Family physicians should encourage parents to contact the office with specific questions and concerns. An example of a parent information sheet in English and Spanish is available at http://www.aap.org/family/jaundicefaq.htm

Maisels MJ, Bhutani VK, et al. Hyperbilirubinemia in the newborn infant ≥35 weeks' gestation: an update with clarification. *Pediatrics.* 2009;124. [PMID: 19786452]

Moerschel SK, Cianciaruso LB, Tracy LR. A practical approach to neonatal jaundice. *Am Fam Physician.* 2008;77:9. [PMID: 18540490]

Moyer VA, et al. Accuracy of clinical judgment in neonatal jaundice. *Arch Pediatric Adolesc Med.* 2000;154:391. [PMID: 1076879]

Breastfeeding & Infant Nutrition

Tracey D. Conti, MD

Mamta Patel, MD

Samidha Bhat, MD

▶ General Considerations

Nutrition is a critical capstone for the proper growth and development of infants. Breastfeeding of term infants by healthy mothers is the optimal mechanism for providing the caloric and nutrient needs of infants. Preterm infants can also benefit from breast milk and breastfeeding, although supplementation and fortification of preterm breast milk may be required. Barring some unique circumstances, human breast milk can provide nutritional, social, and motor developmental benefits for most infants.

Despite increased emphasis on breastfeeding education, according to the 2012 Breastfeeding Report Card published by the Centers for Disease Control, breastfeeding initiation 6- and 12-month continuance rates rose by only approximately two percentage points. Most women presently of childbearing age were not breastfed and report having no maternal relatives who breastfed their children. Because evidence clearly suggests familial influences in the development of infant feeding practices, practitioners may find it difficult to encourage breastfeeding behaviors among women with no direct familial breastfeeding experience. Efforts to alter knowledge, attitudes, and behaviors regarding breastfeeding must effectively address the numerous psychosocial barriers. Health care providers are critical conduits for maternal and familial education. All members of the health care team, including physicians, midwives, and nurses, are valuable sources of important evidence-based information as well as psychological support for mothers in search of guidance regarding infant feeding practices. Numerous studies have shown the superiority of breast milk and the health advantages that breastfed children have. Literature has shown a lower incidence of diarrheal illness, ear infections, and allergies among breastfed infants Exclusive breastfeeding for at least 4 months in infants at risk for developing atopic disease decreases the cumulative incidence of atopic dermatitis. Lower rates of childhood obesity, type 2 diabetes, sudden infant death syndrome (SIDS), and leukemia have also been associated with breastfeeding. There are likewise financial advantages to breastfeeding. Other, somewhat controversial, investigations suggest higher intelligence among breastfed infants.

There are also maternal benefits to breastfeeding. Mothers who breastfeed are less likely to develop premenopausal breast cancer. An association with decreased rates of type 2 diabetes and ovarian cancer also exists. Studies are also focusing on the relationship between breastfeeding and the rates of postpartum depression and cardiovascular disease. Most importantly, however, is the bonding relationship that breastfeeding promotes between mother and infant.

All major maternal-child health professional organizations recommend exclusive breastfeeding for the first 6 months of life prior to the introduction of age-appropriate solid foods, followed by continued breastfeeding for the next 6 months.

The American Academy of Pediatrics (AAP) Committee on Nutrition recommends breastfeeding for the first year of life with supplemental vitamin D at birth and the addition of supplemental iron at age 4 months and possible addition of fluoride at age 6 months for infants living in regions of fluoride-poor water. Vitamin D supplementation is particularly applicable in regions with limited sunlight and for infants of mothers with decreased daily intake of cow's milk. Further recommendations include delaying introduction of cow's milk until after 1 year and delaying addition of reduced-fat milk until 2 years of age. To this end, new mothers should be encouraged to continue prenatal vitamins containing supplemental iron, calcium, and vitamin D. Supplemental solid foods should be considered at or around 6 months of age once the infant demonstrates appropriate readiness.

Centers for Disease Control and Prevention. *Breastfeeding Report Card-United States, 2012* (http://www.cdc.gov/breastfeeding/data/reprtcard.htm; accessed Jan. 22, 2013).

US Department of Health and Human Services, Healthy People 2010 Objectives for Breastfeeding. *Healthy People 2010 Midcourse Review.* Washington, DC: US Department of Health and Human Services.

Crampton R, Zain-Ul-Abideen M, Whalen B. Optimizing successful breastfeeding in the newborn. *Curr Opin Pediatr.* 2009;21:386–396.

Anatomy of the Human Breast & Breastfeeding

Women are able to produce milk when they reach childbearing age. There is no evidence that breast function, breast milk production, or composition differs among younger women. The principal external structures of the mature human female breast are the nipple, areola, and Montgomery tubercles. The areola is the darker part of the breast, and the nipple is the central most structure through which milk ducts open and milk is expressed. The areola contains the Montgomery tubercles, through which sebaceous and sweat glands (Montgomery glands) open, producing lubricating substances for the nipple.

Underlying structures include adipose tissue, mammary gland cells, and contractile myoepithelial cells surrounding the gland cells (allowing for milk ejection). Milk produced within the alveoli is ejected into the milk ducts, which open out directly to the nipple. It was previously assumed that milk was stored in lactiferous sinuses; however, more recent research has revealed that these sinuses do not exist.

Infant breastfeeding draws the nipple and areola into the mouth, causing elongation of the nipple. The elongated nipple is compressed between the palate and the tongue, and milk is expressed less than 0.05 seconds after the nipple has elongated. Stimulation of the areola is essential for the oxytocin-mediated hormonal cascade that controls milk ejection.

Physiology of Breastfeeding

Two principal hormones are required for breast milk production—oxytocin and prolactin—controlled by the hypothalamic-pituitary axis. Oxytocin production and secretion are regulated by the posterior pituitary and are stimulated by suckling. Oxytocin production in response to suckling is intermittent and stimulates ejection ("letdown") of breast milk. Oxytocin does not appear to affect breast milk production, although numerous stressors can negatively impact breast milk letdown. Evidence suggests that lactogenesis may be delayed and letdown reduced following stressful vaginal delivery or cesarean section.

Milk production is controlled primarily by the release of prolactin. Prolactin is secreted through a feedback loop under dopaminergic control with the primary action on prolactin receptors on mammary epithelium. Suckling likewise stimulates prolactin release. Furthermore, prolactin acts as an inhibitor of ovulation through hormonal feedback control, although breastfeeding is considered a relatively unreliable contraceptive mechanism.

Several additional hormones are required for milk production: cortisol, human growth hormone, insulin, thyroid and parathyroid hormones, and feedback inhibitor of lactation (FIL). Not entirely understood, FIL appears to act at the level of breast tissue to inhibit continued breast milk production when the breast is not completely emptied.

Milk production begins during the postpartum period with prolactin production and concomitant decreased estrogen and progesterone production following placental delivery. Milk production will persist under this hormonal control for the first several days; however, continued milk production beyond the initial 48 hours postpartum requires suckling. Although mothers continue to produce milk between feedings once suckling has initiated the feedback loop, milk production significantly increases during breastfeeding.

Neville MC. Anatomy and physiology of lactation. *Pediatr Clin North Am.* 2001;48:13. [PMID: 11236721]

Breast Milk

A. Stages of Production

Production of human breast milk among healthy mothers who deliver full-term infants occurs in three phases—colostrum, transitional milk, and mature milk. Colostrum is a thick, yellow substance produced during the first several days postpartum. Healthy mothers produce approximately 80–100 mL daily. Colostrum is rich in calcium, antibodies, minerals, proteins, potassium, and fat-soluble vitamins. This milk has immunologic qualities that are vital to the infant, and it possesses gastrointestinal properties to facilitate secretion of meconium. Production of colostrum is followed for the next 5–6 days with transitional milk, which provides essential components more closely resembling mature breast milk. Most women will notice a significant change evidenced by the fullness of their breasts and the change in the consistency of the milk. True milk is white and sometimes has a bluish tint. The consistency is similar to that of cow's milk with a sweet taste. Mature breast milk, produced beginning at or near postpartum day 10, produces key components, discussed in the next section.

Numerous factors may affect the supply of breast milk, including anxiety, medications, maternal nutritional status, amount of sleep, exercise, breastfeeding frequency, tactile stimulation, and fluid intake. Breastfeeding mothers should be encouraged to consume generous amounts of fluids and express breast milk every 2–3 hours. The hormonal feedback loop that controls the production and release of prolactin and oxytocin is initiated by suckling or other tactile stimulation of the breast. The greater the amount of suckling or other tactile breast stimulation, the greater the milk supply.

B. Components

Mature human breast milk contains protein, carbohydrate, and fat components and provides approximately 20 kcal/oz and 1 g of protein. The principal protein elements of both mature and premature breast milk are casein (40%) and whey (60%). Breast milk contains approximately 2.5 g/L of casein. Also called "curds," this protein forms calcium complexes. Higher concentrations of this protein are found in cow's milk. Whey (approximately 6.4 g/L) is a protein component composed of α-lactalbumin, lactoferrin, lysozyme, immunoglobulins, and albumin.

Free nitrogen, which is vital for amino acid synthesis, is also a significant component of mature breast milk and is integral for multiple biochemical pathways, including production of uric acid, urea, ammonia, and creatinine. It is also a key component of insulin and epidermal growth factor.

Mature breast milk contains ~70 g/L of lactose, the primary carbohydrate. Lactose is composed of galactose and glucose, and its concentration continues to increase throughout breastfeeding. Human milk fat likewise increases with continued breastfeeding. Mature breast milk provides approximately 40 g/L of lactose and includes triacylglycerides, phospholipids, and essential fatty acids.

The principal electrolytes in breast milk are sodium, potassium, magnesium, and calcium. Calcium appears to be mediated through the parathyroid hormone–related protein, which allows for mobilization of calcium stores from bone in otherwise healthy women. Bone calcium levels return to normal after termination of breastfeeding. Sodium and potassium concentrations in breast milk are regulated through corticosteroids.

Iron absorption is particularly high in newborns and infants, although the relative concentration of iron in mature breast milk is low. For infants younger than 6 months of age, the concentration of iron in breast milk is sufficient and supplementation is not necessary; however, recommendations for infants older than 6 months include supplemental iron from green vegetables, meats, and iron-rich cereals. The recommended daily amount of supplemental elemental iron is 1 mg/kg. Iron is an essential component in the synthesis of hemoglobin.

Vitamin K, a lipid-soluble vitamin and an important component in the clotting cascade, is routinely provided in the immediate postpartum period as a 1-mg intramuscular injection. There is evidence that oral vitamin K may produce similar benefit as well as maternal supplementation of 5 mg/d of oral vitamin K for 12 weeks following delivery.

Another lipid-soluble component, vitamin D, is essential for bone formation. Women who have limited exposure to sunlight or suboptimal vitamin D intake will produce little or no vitamin D in breast milk. The recommended daily intake of vitamin D is 400 IU (international units). Practitioners must be cognizant of mothers with special diets (ie, vegetarian diets) whose low vitamin D intake might indicate a need for supplemental vitamin D.

Other elemental minerals in breast milk (eg, zinc, copper, selenium, manganese, nickel, molybdenum, and chromium) are found in trace amounts but nonetheless are essential for a multitude of biochemical processes.

C. Composition of Preterm Breast Milk

The composition of breast milk in mothers of preterm infants is different from that in mothers of term infants. This difference persists for approximately 4 weeks before the composition approaches that of term infant breast milk. The difference in preterm milk composition reflects the increased nutrient demands of preterm infants. Preterm breast milk contains higher concentrations of total and bound nitrogen, immunoglobulins, sodium, iron, chloride, and medium-chain fatty acids. However, it may not contain sufficient amounts of phosphorus, calcium, copper, and zinc. Preterm infants are more likely to require fortification with human milk fortifiers (HMFs) to correct these deficiencies.

Lovelady CA, et al. Effect of exercise on immunologic factors in breast milk. *Pediatrics*. 2003;111:E148. [PMID: 12563088]

▶ Breastfeeding Technique

Preparation for breastfeeding should begin in the preconception period or at the first contact with the patient. Most women choose their method of feeding prior to conception. Psychosocial support and education may encourage breastfeeding among women who might not otherwise have considered it. Evidence for this strategy, however, is anecdotal and requires further investigation.

There are numerous potential supports available to women who are considering feeding behaviors. Practitioners are encouraged to identify members of the patient's support network and provide similar education to minimize the potential barriers posed by uninformed support individuals.

One commonly perceived physical barrier is nipple inversion. Women who have inverted nipples will have difficulty with the latch-on process (discussed later in this section). Nipple shields are relatively inexpensive devices that can draw the nipple out. Manual or electric breast pumps may also be used to draw out inverted nipples, typically beginning after delivery.

Breastfeeding should begin immediately in the postpartum period, ideally in the first 30–40 minutes after delivery. This is easier to accomplish if the infant is left in the room with the mother before being bathed and before the newborn examination is performed. It is also safe to allow breastfeeding before administration of vitamin K and erythromycin ophthalmic ointment.

Certain clinical situations preclude initiation of breastfeeding in the immediate postpartum period (eg, cesarean delivery, maternal perineal repair, maternal or fetal distress). In such cases breastfeeding should be initiated as early as possible. Only when medically necessary should a supplemental feeding be initiated. If a mother has expressed a desire to breastfeed, the practitioner should coordinate an interim feeding plan, emphasizing that bottle feeding not be started. Acceptable alternatives include spoon, cup, or syringe feeding.

Breastfed children commonly feed at least every 2–3 hours during the first several weeks postpartum. Infants should not be allowed to sleep through feedings; however, if necessary, feeding intervals may be increased to every 3–4 hours overnight. The production of breast milk is on a supply-demand cycle. Breast stimulation through suckling and the mechanism of breastfeeding signals the body to produce more milk. When feedings are missed or breasts are not emptied effectively, the feedback loop decreases the milk supply. As the infant grows, feedings every 3–4 hours are acceptable. During growth spurts, the amount of milk needed for the rate of growth often exceeds milk production. Feeding intervals often must be adjusted to growth periods until the milk supply "catches up."

Although feeding intervals may be increased during nighttime periods, a common question becomes when to stop waking the infant for night feedings. Anecdotal evidence suggests that after the first 2 weeks postpartum, in the absence of specific nutritional concerns, the infant can determine its own overnight feeding schedule. Typically, most infants will begin to sleep through the night once they have reached approximately 10 lb.

Positioning of the infant is critical for effective feeding in the neonatal period, allowing for optimal latch-on. In general, infant and mother should face each other in one of the following three positions: the cradle (the most common), the football, or lying side by side. The cradle hold allows the mother to hold the infant horizontally across the front of her chest. The infant's head can be on the left or right side of the mother depending on which side it is feeding. The infant's head should be supported with the crook of the mother's arm. The football hold is performed with the mother sitting on a bed or chair, the infant's bottom against the bed or chair and its body lying next to the mother's side, and the infant's head cradled in her hand. The side position allows the mother to lie on her left or right side with the infant lying parallel to her. Again, the infant's head is cradled in the crook of the mother's elbow. This position is ideally suited for women postcesarean delivery as it reduces the pain associated with pressure from the infant on their incisions. It must be stressed that choice of position is based on mother and infant comfort. It is not unusual to experiment with any or all positions before determining the most desirable. It is likewise not uncommon to find previously undesirable positions more effective and comfortable as the infant grows and the breastfeeding experience progresses. All breastfeeding positions should allow for cradling of the infant's head with the mother's hand or elbow allowing for better head control in the latch-on stage. The infant should be placed at a height (often achieved with a pillow) appropriate for preventing awkward positioning, maximizing comfort, and encouraging latch-on.

Many of the difficulties with breastfeeding result from improper latch-on. Latch-on problems are often the source of multiple breastfeeding complaints among mothers, ranging from breast engorgement to sore, cracked nipples. Many women discontinue breastfeeding secondary to these issues. The latch-on process is governed by primitive reflexes. Stroking the infant's cheek will cause it to turn toward the side on which the cheek was stroked. This reflex is useful if the infant is not looking toward the breast. Tickling the infant's bottom lip will cause its mouth to open wide in order to latch on to the breast. The mother should hold her breast to help position the areola to ease latch-on. It is important that the mother's fingers be behind the areola to prevent a physical barrier to latch-on. Once the infant's mouth is opened wide, the head should be pulled quickly to the breast. The infant's mouth should encompass the entire areola to compress the milk ducts. If this is done improperly, the infant will compress the nipple, leading to pain and eventually cracking, with minimal or no milk expression. The mother should not experience pain with breastfeeding but if it does occur, she should break the suction by inserting a finger into the side of the infant's mouth and then latch the infant on again. This process should be repeated as many times as necessary until proper latch-on is achieved.

One issue that continually concerns parents is whether the infant is receiving adequate amounts of breast milk. Several clinical measures can be used to determine whether infants are receiving enough milk. Weight is an excellent method of assessment. Pre- and postfeed measurement of an infant with a scale that is of high quality and measures to the ounce is a very accurate means of determining weight. The problem is that this type of scale is not available to most families. Weight can also be evaluated on a longer-term basis. Infants should not lose more than ~8% of their birth weight after delivery and should gain this weight back in 2 weeks. Most infants with difficulties, however, will decompensate before this 2-week period. Breastfed infants should be evaluated 2–3 days after discharge, especially if discharged prior to 48 hours postdelivery. A more convenient way to determine the adequacy of the infant's milk intake is through clinical signs such as infant satisfaction postfeeding and bowel and bladder volumes. In most cases infants who are satisfied after feeding will fall asleep. Infants who do not receive enough milk will usually be fussy or irritable or continuously want to suck at the breast, their finger, and so on. Breastfed infants usually will stool after most feeds but at a minimum 5–6 times a day. After the first couple of days, the stool should turn from meconiumlike to a mustard-colored seedy type. If breastfed infants are still passing meconium or do not have an adequate amount of stool, parents and the health care team should evaluate whether they are taking in enough milk. Infants should also urinate approximately 3 or 4 times a day. This may be difficult to assess with the era's superabsorbent diapers; therefore, the diaper should be carefully examined.

Problems Associated with Breastfeeding

An inadequate milk supply can lead to disastrous outcomes if not identified and treated. There are two types of milk inadequacies: inability to produce milk and maintain an adequate supply of it. Inadequacy type 1 is quite rare, but examples include surgeries in which the milk ducts are severed or the Sheehan syndrome. There is no specific treatment to initiate milk production in affected women. The inability to maintain an adequate milk supply has numerous etiologies, ranging from dietary deficiencies to engorgement. The key in preventing adverse events is early recognition and effective treatment. One of the mainstays of treatment is to work with the body's own feedback loop of supply and demand to increase the supply. As more milk is needed, more milk will be produced. This is effectively done by using a breast pump. Pumping should be performed after the infant has fed.

Engorgement is caused by inadequate or ineffective emptying of the breasts. As milk builds up in the breasts, they become swollen. If the condition is not relieved, the breasts can become tender and warm. Mastitis can also develop. The mainstay of treatment is to empty the breasts of milk, either by the infant or, if that is not possible, by mechanical means. Usually when the breast is engorged, the areola and nipple are affected and proper latch-on becomes difficult if not impossible. A warm compress may be used to facilitate letdown, and the breast can be manually expressed enough to allow the infant to latch on. If this is not possible or is too painful, the milk can be removed with an electric breast pump. Between feedings a cold pack can be used to decrease the amount of swelling. There have been reports of reduced pain and swelling due to chilled cabbage leaves placed inside the bra to provide a cold pack that conforms to the shape of the breast. However, there is no evidence of any medicinal properties in the cabbage that affect engorgement. Mastitis, if occurring, is treated with antibiotics. Mothers can continue to breastfeed with the affected breast, so care should be taken to choose an antibiotic that is safe for the infant.

Sore nipples are a common problem for breastfeeding mothers. In the first few weeks there may be some soreness associated with breastfeeding as the skin becomes accustomed to the constant moisture. No pain should be associated with breastfeeding; if there is pain, it is usually secondary to improper latch-on, which can be corrected. With severe cracking there will occasionally be bleeding. Breastfeeding can be continued with mild bleeding, but if severe bleeding occurs, the breast should be pumped and the milk discarded to prevent gastrointestinal upset in the infant. Certain remedies can be used in the event of cracking.

Keeping the nipples clean and dry between feedings can help prevent and heal cracking. The mother's own milk or a pure lanolin ointment can also be used as a salve. Mothers should be warned not to use herbal rubs or vitamin E because of the risk of absorption by the infant. Another cause of sore nipples is candidal infection. This usually occurs when an infant has thrush. Sometimes treating the infant will resolve the problem, but occasionally the mother will need to be treated as well. Taking the same nystatin liquid dose that the infant is using twice a day will resolve the infection. Again, keeping the nipples clean and dry can help.

Blebs, small pimple or blisterlike lesions on the nipple, can also be a cause of sore nipples. They may occur secondary to the formation of new epithelial cells covering the opening of the milk duct. Treatment includes moisturizing the nipples with lanolin and gentle exfoliation. This condition can be exacerbated by a candidal infection as well and would require the same treatment stated previously. If these lesions do not heal, they may require surgical débridement.

Another controversial issue in breastfeeding is silicone implantation. According to the American Society of Plastic surgeons, approximately 2 million women had breast implants during 2000–2007. Although minimal research has been done on the effects of silicone implants on lactation, there are a few areas of concern including implants leaking material in breast milk, the baby absorbing the silicone from the milk if it is spilled, and additional risk of infant exposure to the silicone. Because of its presence in the environment, it is difficult to distinguish between normal and abnormal maternal levels. It has been found that silicon is present in higher concentrations in cow milk and formula than in milk of humans with implants. An additional study directly assayed the silicone polymer and found that levels in the milk of women with implants were not significantly different from those in other human milk samples. The American Academy of Pediatrics, in its policy statement on silicone breast implants and breastfeeding, concluded that the "Committee on Drugs does not feel that the evidence currently justifies classifying silicone implants as a contraindication to breastfeeding." Safety of breastfeeding by women with silicone breast implants has not been adequately studied, and women who receive implants should be forewarned of this fact. However, the potential health risks of artificial feeding have been shown, and until there is better evidence, women with implants should be encouraged to breastfeed.

Other breastfeeding issues include medications, nutrient supplementation, and mothers returning to work. These issues are broad in scope; in fact, whole books have been dedicated to these subjects. The most important issue to understand when considering medication use during pregnancy is that limited research has been done in this area and that there is insufficient information on most medicines to advocate their use. Health care providers should try to use the safest medications possible that will allow mothers to continue breastfeeding. If this is not possible, mothers should be encouraged to pump the milk and discard it to maintain the milk supply.

Nutrient supplementation is another controversial issue. Vitamin D is recommended for supplementation in either dark-skinned women or women who do not receive much sunlight. The iron found in breast milk, although in low concentrations, is highly absorbable. Infants who are breastfed do not need additional sources of iron until they are 4–6 months old. This is the time when most children are started on cereal. Choosing an iron-fortified cereal will satisfy the additional iron requirement.

Return to work is the major reason why women discontinue breastfeeding. Planning this return from birth and pumping milk for storage help women to continue breastfeeding. Employers who provide time and a comfortable place for mothers to pump milk at work will also improve breastfeeding rates. Although the goal is to increase the number of women who begin breastfeeding and continue it throughout the first year of the infant's life, many women cannot or do not choose to breastfeed. Their decision must be supported, and they must be educated on alternative methods of providing nutrition for their infants.

Johnston ML, Esposito N. Barriers and facilitators for breastfeeding among working women in the United States. *J Obstet Gynecol Neonatal Nurs.* 2007;36:9–20.

Maternal Nutrition & Breastfeeding

Many studies focus on maternal nutrition and breastfeeding. It is well known that adequate fluid intake is necessary for milk production. Studies seem to suggest that the benefits of infant nutrition outweigh the risk of any maternal effects of breastfeeding.

Often some maternal foods that are strong in flavor, such as garlic, broccoli, and onions, can provide a flavor to breast milk that is displeasing to the infant or can create increased flatulence. These food types should be avoided if they interfere with feeding. Also, some women are concerned about creating allergies in their infants from the food that they consume while breastfeeding. Currently there is lack of evidence that maternal dietary restrictions (eg, avoiding peanuts) during pregnancy or lactation plays a significant role in prevention of atopic disease in infants. Antigen avoidance during lactation does not prevent atopic disease, with the possible exception of eczema, although more data are needed to substantiate conclusion.

Vegetarian Diet & Breastfeeding

The number of Americans choosing a vegetarian diet has increased dramatically in the past decade. With these increasing numbers, more research has been conducted in an effort to evaluate the feasibility of a vegetarian diet in infancy. A *vegetarian diet* is defined as a diet consisting of no meat. This definition does not encompass the variety of vegetarian diets that are consumed. A pure vegetarian or "vegan" consumes only plant food. In general, most pure vegetarians also do not use products that result from animal cruelty such as wool, silk, and leather. Lactoovovegetarians consume dairy products and eggs in addition to plants, and lactovegetarians consume only dairy products with their plant diet.

There is wide variety in each of these diets and therefore wide variety in the type and amount of food necessary for adequate nutrition. Milk from breastfeeding mothers who are vegetarians is adequate in all nutrients necessary for proper growth and development. Although all required nutrients can be found in any vegetarian diet, in infancy the amount necessary may be difficult to provide without supplementation. The American Dietetic Association stated that a lactoovovegetarian diet is recommended in infancy. If this diet is not desired by parents or is not tolerated by children, then supplementation may be necessary. Vitamin B_{12}, iron, and vitamin D are nutrients that may need to be supplemented, depending on environmental factors.

Contraindications to Breastfeeding

Although considered the optimal method of providing infant nutrition during the first year of life, breastfeeding may be contraindicated in some mothers. Scenarios that may preclude breastfeeding include mothers who actively use illicit drugs such as heroin, cocaine, alcohol, and phencyclidine (PCP); mothers with human immunodeficiency virus (HIV) infection or acquired immune deficiency syndrome (AIDS); and mothers receiving pharmacotherapy with agents transmitted in breast milk and contraindicated in children, particularly potent cancer agents. Some immunizations for foreign travelers and military personnel may also be contraindicated in breastfeeding mothers. Infants with galactosemia should also not breastfeed.

Infant Formulas

The historical record reveals that methods of replacing, fortifying, and delivering milk and milk substitutes date back to the Stone Age. Evidence suggests that the original infant "formulas" of the early and middle twentieth century consisted of 1:1 concentrations of evaporated milk and water with supplemental cod liver oil, orange juice, and honey. As the number of working mothers steadily increased during this time, the use of infant formulas became more popular.

Since the mid-1980s, more sophisticated neonatal medical practices have led to the development of countless infant formula preparations to meet a wide variety of clinical situations. Formulas exist as concentrates and powders that require dilution with water and as ready-to-feed preparations. Commonly, formula preparations provide 20 cal/oz with standard dilutions of 1 oz concentrate to 1 oz water and 1 scoop powder formula to 2 oz water for liquid concentrates and powders, respectively. Formulas exist as cow's milk–based, soy-based, and casein-based preparations.

A. Cow's Milk–Based Formula Preparations

This is the preferred, standard non–breast milk preparation for otherwise healthy term infants who do not breastfeed or for whom breastfeeding has been terminated prior to 1 year of age. Cow's milk–based formula closely resembles human breast milk and is composed of 20% whey and 80% casein with 50% more protein per deciliter (dL) than breast milk as well as iron, linoleic acid, carnitine, taurine, and nucleotides. Formulas containing docosahexaenoic acid and arachidonic acid have recently been marketed to promote eye and brain development. So far no randomized trials have shown any benefit, although no harm has been established.

Approximately 32 oz will meet 100% of the recommended daily allowance (RDA) for calories, vitamins, and minerals. These formula preparations are diluted to a standard 20 cal/oz and are typically whey-dominant protein preparations with vegetable oils and lactose. There are also multiple lactose-free preparations. Few standard formula preparations satisfy the RDA for fluoride, and exclusively formula-fed infants may require 0.25 mg/d of supplemental fluoride.

B. Soy-Based Formula Preparations

Indicated primarily for vegetarian mothers and lactose-intolerant, galactosemic, and cow's milk–allergic infants, soy-based formulas provide a protein-rich formula that contains more protein per deciliter than either breast milk or cow's milk formula preparation. Because the proteins are plant-based, vitamin and mineral composition is increased to compensate for plant-based mineral antagonists while supplementing protein composition with the addition of methionine. Soy-based formulas tend to have a sweeter taste owing to a carbohydrate composition that includes sucrose and corn syrup. There is no proven benefit of soy-based formulas for milk protein allergy. Soy-based formulas should not be used for preterm infants because they cause less weight gain and increase the risk of osteopenia of prematurity. ProSobee, Isomil, and I-Soyalac are common soy-based preparations.

C. Casein Hydrolysate–Based Formula Preparations

This poor-tasting, expensive formula preparation is indicated principally for infants with either milk and soy protein allergies or intolerance. Other indications include complex gastrointestinal pathologies. This formula, which contains casein-based protein and glucose, is not recommended for prolonged use in preterm infants owing to inadequate vitamin and mineral composition and proteins that may be difficult to metabolize. Standard preparations provide 20–24 cal/oz.

D. Premature Infant Formula Preparations

Indicated for use in preterm infants of <1800 g birth weight, and with 3 times the vitamin and mineral content of standard formula preparations, these formulations provide 20–24 cal/oz. Premature infant preparations are approximately 60% casein and 40% whey, with 1:1 concentrations of lactose and glucose as well as 1:1 concentrations of long- and medium-chain fatty acids. Commercially available preparations include Enfamil Premature with Iron, Similac Natural Care Breast Milk Fortifier, and Similac Special Care with Iron. Similac Neo-Care, designed for preterm infants weighing >1800 g at birth, provides 22 cal/oz in standard dilution.

▶ Human Milk Fortifiers for Preterm Infants

Human milk fortifiers (HMFs) are indicated for preterm infants of <34 weeks' gestation or <1500 g birth weight once feeding has reached 75% full volume. HMFs are designed to supplement calories, protein, phosphorus, calcium, and other vitamins and minerals.

Enfamil-HMF is mixed to 24 cal/oz by adding one 3.8-g packet to 25 mL of breast milk, increasing the osmolality to >350 mOsm/L. Increased osmolality may enhance gastrointestinal irritability and affect tolerance. Practitioners may recommend a lower osmolality for the first 48 hours, beginning with one packet of Enfamil-HMF in 50 mL of breast milk, producing 22 cal/oz. The maximum caloric density from this HMF is 24 cal/oz. Practitioners may add emulsified fat blends to increase caloric needs.

Similac Natural Care is a liquid milk fortifier that is typically mixed in a 1:1 ratio with breast milk. Other alternatives may include feedings with breast milk and fortifier. The osmolality of Similac Natural Care is lower than that of Enfamil—280 mOsm/L. This liquid fortifier may be preferable, particularly for infants whose mothers have low milk production.

Other specially formulated formulas are available, including antireflux and hypoallergenic formulas. Reflux seldom requires treatment unless there is poor weight gain. Antireflux formulas decrease emesis and regurgitation, but long-term benefit in terms of growth and development has not been established. Hypoallergenic formulas have been shown to promote slightly greater weight gain in the first year of life. They have also shown improvement in atopic symptoms.

Websites

Information on breastfeeding is available at the following websites:

American Academy of Pediatrics. *A Woman's Guide to Breast-feeding*: http://www.aap.org/family/brstguid.htm
La Leche League: http://www.lalecheleague.org
Resources for breastfeeding products and information: http://www.breastfeedingbasics.org, http://www.breastfeeding.hypermart.net, and http://www.medela.com

Common Acute Infections in Children

James C. Dewar, MD

Stephanie B. Dewar, MD

Infectious diseases are a major cause of illness in children. The widespread use of antibiotics and immunizations has greatly reduced morbidity and mortality from serious bacterial infections, but infections remain one of the most common types of problems encountered by physicians who care for children.

▼ GENERAL

FEVER WITHOUT A SOURCE

▶ General Considerations

Fever is the primary indication of an infectious process in children of all ages. Other than fever, however, few young children display signs or symptoms indicative of an underlying disease. Even after a careful history and a complete physical examination, a portion of children will have no clear source of infection. Most of these children will have a viral infection; however, the physician must identify those children at risk for serious bacterial infection while minimizing the risks of laboratory evaluation, treatment with antibiotics, and hospitalization. A *serious bacterial infection* (SBI) is defined as bacteremia, meningitis, urinary tract infection (UTI), pneumonia, bacterial enterocolitis, abscess, or cellulitis.

Children are generally divided into three groups for evaluation purposes: neonates (aged ≤1 month), young infants (aged <2–3 months), and young children (aged 3 months to 3 years). There is no consensus statement or guideline available for physicians in the workup and management of febrile illnesses in children. Hamilton (2013) published a useful set of guidelines that are summarized in **Table 5-1**.

Neonates younger than 1 month of age can be the most challenging to diagnose as they are unable to localize infections. The rate of serious bacterial infection in nontoxic

febrile neonates is still assumed to be between 5% and 15%. However, existing screening protocols lack the sensitivity and negative predictive value to identify infants at low risk for these infections. For this reason, it is generally accepted that all febrile infants younger than 1 month of age be admitted to the hospital, undergo a complete sepsis workup, and be treated with parenteral antibiotics pending the results of the workup. Most of these infants will be found to have a viral infection; however, some will have a serious bacterial infection such as UTI, in which *Escherichia coli* is the most common pathogen; bacteremia, with group B *Streptococcus, Enterobacter, Listeria, Streptococcus pneumoniae, E. coli, Enterococcus,* or *Klebsiella* pathogens; or meningitis. The remainder may have nonbacterial gastroenteritis, aseptic meningitis, or bronchiolitis.

In evaluating infants aged >1 month, those who are at low risk for a serious bacterial infection should be identified first. The criteria for low risk are being previously healthy, having no focal source of infection found on physical examination, and having a negative laboratory evaluation, defined as a white blood cell (WBC) count of 5000–15,000/mm³, <1500 bands/mm³, normal urinalysis, and, if diarrhea is present, <5 WBCs per high-power field in the stool. Chest radiography is included in some sets of criteria. Lumbar puncture should be performed if the patient is ill-appearing, if neurologic signs are present, or if empiric antibiotics are to be used. Additional low-risk criteria are the appearance of being nontoxic and socially well adjusted with reliable follow-up. (see **Table 5-1**) Low-risk, nontoxic-appearing infants may be treated as outpatients, with close follow-up. Empiric antibiotics are generally recommended, but may be withheld if the infant can be followed closely. All toxic-appearing or non-low-risk infants should be hospitalized and treated with parenteral antibiotics.

Similar criteria may be used to evaluate children aged 3 months to 3 years. The most common serious bacterial

Table 5-1. Evaluation and treatment of febrile children.

Infant aged ≤1 month
Admit for evaluation (blood, urine, CSF, ± stool, ± CXR and treatment with empiric antibiotics (ampicillin and gentamicin, or ampicillin and cefotxime

Infant aged 2–3 months
Consider rapid influenza testing in flu season
Toxic or non–low risk: admit and evaluate as above and treat with ceftriaxone
Nontoxic, low risk:
CBC and blood culture
Urinalysis and urine culture
Lumbar puncture if WBC >15,000 or <5000
Consider empiric antibiotics
Return for reevaluation within 24 hours
Low-risk criteria:
Clinical
Previously healthy, term infant with uncomplicated nursery stay
Nontoxic appearance
No focal bacterial infection on examination (except otitis media)
Laboratory
WBC count 5000–15,000/mm^3, ≤1500 bands/mm^3
Negative gram stain of unspun urine (preferred), or negative urine leukocyte esterase and nitrite, or ≤5 WBCs/HPF
CSF ≤8 WBCs/mm^3 and negative gram stain

Child aged 3 months to 3 years
Consider rapid influenza testing in flu season
Toxic: admit and evaluate as above and treat with ceftriaxone
Nontoxic:
CBC and blood culture rarely recommended
Urinalysis and urine culture obtain via cathetherization or clean catch
Lumbar puncture rarely recommended
CXR if T >39°C, respiratory distress, tachypnea, rales, WBC count >>20,000/mm^3
Symptomatic treatment for fever
Consider empiric antibiotics
Return if fever persists ≥48 hours or if condition deteriorates
Admit for inpatient monitoring if good outpatient follow-up not available

CSF, cerebrospinal fluid; CXR, chest x-ray; HPF, high-power field; IM, intramuscular; SaO$_2$, oxygen saturation; WBC, white blood cell.
Data from Hamilton J. Evaluation of fever in infants and young children. *Am Fam Physician.* 2013;87:254

infections in this group are bacteremia and UTIs. UTIs are present in nearly 5% of febrile infants younger than 12 months of age, with an incidence slightly higher in girls and uncircumcised boys and in those with higher temperatures. After 12 months of age, the prevalence of UTI is lower but should continue to be tested for in girls aged ≤24 months. The rate of bacteremia is still significant and more likely if the temperature is ≥39°C (≥102.2°F). The most common organisms isolated are *S. pneumoniae, Haemophilus influenzae* type b (Hib), and *Neisseria meningitidis*. The rate of infection with *H. influenzae and S. pneumonia* has fallen

dramatically since the introduction of the Hib and Prevnar vaccines. Occult pneumonia is rare in febrile children who have a normal WBC count and no signs of lower respiratory infection, such as cough, tachypnea, rales, or rhonchi. As in younger infants, toxic-appearing or non-low-risk infants should be hospitalized and treated with parenteral antibiotics as the rate of serious bacterial infections in toxic-appearing children in this age group has been reported to be as high as 10–90%. Low-risk, non-toxic-appearing children in this age group may be treated as outpatients. The use of empiric antibiotics pending culture results is left to the physician's discretion. There is general consensus that bacteremia is a risk factor for development of infectious complications, such as meningitis. However, pneumococcal bacteremia responds well to oral antibiotics, so these drugs can be used in children who appear well despite having positive blood cultures.

▶ Clinical Findings

A. Symptoms and Signs

Fever is defined as temperature of ≥38°C (≥100.4°F). Rectal measurement is the most accurate way to measure temperature. Teething is not a cause for elevated temperature. A history of any recent immunizations should be obtained. A careful, complete physical examination is necessary to exclude focal signs of infection. The skin should be examined for exanthems, cellulitis, abscesses, or petechiae. A petechial rash may herald a serious bacterial infection, most often caused by *N. meningitidis*. Common childhood infections such as pharyngitis and otitis media should be sought, and a careful lung examination should be done to rule out pneumonia. The abdomen should be examined for signs of peritonitis or tenderness. A musculoskeletal examination should be done to rule out osteomyelitis or septic arthritis. The neurologic examination should be directed toward the level of consciousness and should look for focal neurologic deficits. Nuchal rigidity may be absent even in the presence of meningitis, especially in young infants. However, infants may demonstrate "paradoxical irritability," where they prefer to be left alone rather than held, as a subtle sign of meningeal irritation.

The most important clinical decision is which infants appear toxic and therefore need more aggressive evaluation and treatment. *Toxic* in the present context is defined as a picture consistent with the sepsis syndrome—lethargy, signs of poor perfusion, marked hypoventilation or hyperventilation, or cyanosis. *Lethargy* is defined as an impaired level of consciousness as manifested by poor or absent eye contact or by failure of the child to recognize parents or to interact with people or objects in the environment.

B. Laboratory Findings

The laboratory investigation includes WBC count and differential, urinalysis and urine culture, blood culture, lumbar puncture with routine analysis and culture, and chest x-ray if there are respiratory symptoms or an elevation of the WBC. If the child has diarrhea, stool cultures should be obtained.

Treatment

All infants younger than 1 month of age should undergo complete sepsis evaluation and be treated in the hospital with intravenous (IV) antibiotics, either: (1) ampicillin plus gentamicin, or (2) ampicillin plus ceftoxime.

Ceftriaxone is an appropriate antibiotic for hospitalized older infants and children and for infants and children treated as outpatients. In infants 2–3 months of age, a single intramuscular (IM) dose of ceftriaxone may be given. The child should be reevaluated in 24 hours and a second dose of ceftriaxone given. If blood cultures are found to be positive, the child should be admitted for further treatment. If the urine culture is positive and there is a persistent fever, the child should be admitted for treatment. If the child is afebrile and well, outpatient antibiotics may be used.

Table 5-1 presents guidelines that may be useful for investigating and treating febrile children.

Hamilton J. Evaluation of fever in infants and young children. *Am Fam Physician.* 2013;87:254–260.

Huppler A. Performance of low-risk criteria in the evaluation of young infants with fever: review of the literature. *Pediatrics.* 2010; 125(2):228–233.

INFLUENZA

ESSENTIALS OF DIAGNOSIS

▶ Nonspecific respiratory infection in infants and young children.

▶ In older children, respiratory symptoms: coryza, conjunctivitis, pharyngitis, dry cough.

▶ In older children, pronounced high fever, myalgia, headache, malaise.

General Considerations

Influenza virus causes a respiratory infection of variable severity in children. Although influenza itself is a benign, self-limited disease, its sequelae, primarily pneumonia, can cause serious illness and occasionally death, especially in those children aged <2 years and with other medical conditions, including asthma.

Pathogenesis

Influenza is caused by various influenza viruses. Types A and B cause epidemic illness, whereas type C produces sporadic cases of respiratory infections. Infection with influenza virus confers limited immunity that lasts several years, until the natural antigenic drift of the virus produces a pathogen that is genetically distinct enough to escape this protection. Because every virus is new for infants, the attack rate is highest in infants and young children, with 30–50% showing serologic evidence of infection in a normal year.

Prevention

Annual influenza vaccination is the most effective way to prevent influenza and its complications. All people aged >6 months should receive annual influenza vaccination. Children aged 6 months to 8 years require two doses of flu vaccine the first season of vaccination, 1 month apart. Children aged ≥9 years and those previously immunized need only receive one dose each year. The unit dose for children aged 6–35 months is 0.25 mL. The unit dose for children aged ≥36 months is 0.5 mL. The vaccine must be repeated annually. The vaccine should be given prior to the onset of influenza activity in the community and throughout the season. Physicians should begin offering the vaccine as soon as it is available.

Chemoprophylaxis with an antiviral medication can reduce the risk of complications from influenza and should be initiated as early as possible for any patient with confirmed or suspected influenza who is hospitalized; has severe, complicated, or progressive illness; or is at high risk for complications, such as children aged <2 years or those with chronic conditions, including asthma.

Clinical Findings

A. Symptoms and Signs

Influenza in infants and young children causes a nonspecific respiratory infection often characterized by fever and cough. Occasionally the fever is high enough and the child toxic enough in appearance to prompt hospitalization and workup for sepsis. In older children and adolescents, the disease presents with the abrupt onset of respiratory symptoms, such as upper respiratory infection (URI) symptoms, conjunctivitis, pharyngitis, and dry cough. The features that distinguish influenza from the usual URI are high fever and pronounced myalgia, headache, and malaise. The acute symptoms typically last for 2–4 days, but the cough and malaise may persist for several days longer. Physical findings are nonspecific and include pharyngitis, conjunctivitis, cervical lymphadenopathy, and occasionally rales, wheezes, or rhonchi in the lungs.

B. Special Tests

Diagnosis of influenza is generally based on clinical criteria. The virus can be identified by nasopharyngeal swabs sent for rapid influenza diagnostic tests (RIDTs). These tests have high specificity (>90%) but low sensitivity (20–70%). Therefore, positive tests are generally reliable in a community when influenza activity is high and might be useful in deciding whether to institute antiviral therapy. Reverse transcription–polymerase chain reaction (RT-PCR) is the most accurate and sensitive test for detecting influenza viruses, but the time required for testing and the limited availability may limit its usefulness for medical management of individual patients.

Complications

Otitis media and pneumonia are the most common complications from influenza in children. Up to 25% of children develop otitis media after a documented influenza infection. Influenza may cause a primary viral pneumonia, but the more serious pneumonic complications are caused by bacterial superinfection. Encephalopathy, transverse myelitis, myositis, myocarditis, pericarditis, and Reye's syndrome, while rare, may also occur.

Treatment

Antiviral treatment with a neuraminidase inhibitor (zanamivir or oseltamivir) is recommended for all persons with suspected or confirmed influenza who are at higher risk for complications because of age or underlying medical conditions. This would include children aged <5 years, especially those <2 years and those with underlying medical conditions, such as asthma, sickle cell disease, diabetes mellitus, cerebral palsy (CP), epilepsy, or intellectual disability. The benefits of treatment are greater if initiated within 2 days of the onset of symptoms; however, anyone requiring hospitalization should be treated regardless of the length of symptoms. Oseltamivir can be used in children beginning at age 2 weeks at a dose of 3 mg/kg given twice daily. Zanamivir can be used for children aged ≥7 years. Zanamivir is administered via an inhaler device twice daily. Both are given as a 5-day course. Because of resistance in recent viral strains, amantadine and rimantadine are no longer recommended.

Prognosis

Influenza is ordinarily a benign self-limited disease. Morbidity and mortality are related either to postinfluenza pneumonia or to exacerbation of underlying chronic illness caused by the virus.

Fiore AE, et al. Antiviral agents for the treatment and chemoprophylaxis of influenza: recommendations of the Advisory Committee on Immunization Practices (ACIP), 2011. *MMWR* (Centers for Disease Control and Prevention *Morbidity and Mortality Weekly Report*). 2011;60:1–25.

EAR, NOSE, & THROAT INFECTIONS

OTITIS MEDIA

 ESSENTIALS OF DIAGNOSIS

► Preexisting upper respiratory infection (URI; 93%).
► Fever (25%).
► Ear pain (depending on age).
► Bulging, immobile tympanic membrane that is dull gray, yellow, or red in color.
► Perforated tympanic membrane with purulent drainage (most diagnostic).

General Considerations

Acute otitis media (AOM) is the most common reason why children are prescribed antibiotics. Almost all children have had at least one episode of AOM by age 3 years. Although common, the number of visits for AOM has been decreasing in the United States. Much of this decrease is attributed to improved clinician understanding of AOM and the routine vaccination of children. Most of the advice on managing AOM presented below is applicable to children aged >6 months who are otherwise healthy. Children with immune deficiencies, anatomic abnormalities, and ear-nose-throat (ENT) surgeries may require more aggressive treatment.

Pathogenesis

The middle ear is more prone to bacterial infection in children mainly because of the position and length of the eustachian tube. *S. pneumoniae*, nontypeable *Haemophilus influenzae*, and *Moraxella catarrhalis* are the most frequent bacterial pathogens along with respiratory viruses. *S. pneumoniae* is a frequent cause of recurrent or persistent otitis media.

Prevention

Routine use of pneumococcal conjugate and influenza vaccines has decreased the incidence of AOM and the need for surgical treatment of AOM. Breastfeeding for at least 6 months also decreases the incidence of AOM in infants. Other modifiable risk factors include daycare attendance, tobacco exposure, air pollution exposure, pacifier use, and poverty.

Clinical Findings

A. Symptoms and Signs

Signs and symptoms must be used together to make an accurate diagnosis of AOM. Most patients have nonspecific antecedent upper respiratory symptoms. Onset of ear pain for <2 days is the most frequent specific symptom. Nonverbal children may hold, tug, or rub their affected ears. Caregivers may also note a purulent discharge from the ear. Frequent but less specific symptoms include fever, crying, and changes in behavior or sleep. When symptoms are present, mild bulging of the tympanic membrane (TM) or intense erythema of the TM confirms the diagnosis of AOM. Children with severe TM bulging or new otorrhea without otitis externa can be diagnosed with AOM on the basis of examination alone. Other signs that can indicate abnormal mobility or position of the TM include opacity, nonvisualization of the bony landmarks, and air/fluid levels. Clinicians should confirm the presence of a middle ear effusion through pneumatic otoscopy or tympanometry to finalize the diagnosis of AOM whenever possible.

▶ Differential Diagnosis

The primary illness that may be confused with AOM is acute URI. Otitis externa can be distinguished from AOM by tenderness, redness, swelling, and exudates in the external auditory canal. More benign middle ear effusions that can occur after a previous AOM or from eustachian tube dysfunction from a URI or allergies should be distinguished from an episode of AOM by the lack of acute symptoms. These patients do not benefit from treatment with antibiotics.

▶ Complications

Complications of otitis media fall into two main categories: suppurative and nonsuppurative.

Suppurative complications may arise from direct extension of the infection into the surrounding bones or into the adjacent brain, such as mastoiditis, venous sinus thrombosis, and brain abscess. They may also arise from hematogenous spread of the bacteria from the middle ear, primarily sepsis and meningitis. The most frequent suppurative complications are TM perforation or chronic suppurative AOM. In most children, TM perforation will resolve spontaneously in 3 months. *Nonsuppurative* complications are primarily those that arise from middle ear effusion and inflammation and scarring of the structures of the middle ear. This includes hearing loss, balance problems, and cholesteatoma formation.

▶ Treatment

All children with AOM should be assessed for pain. The most frequently used medications are oral acetaminophen and ibuprofen. They have the advantage of being readily available, effective, and easy to administer. Topical anesthetics can work as well in children aged >5 years. Caregivers should be instructed on the appropriate dosing of analgesics to maximize effectiveness and minimize side effects.

Antibiotic treatment for AOM is effective for reducing pain and hastening recovery. Overprescription of antibiotic therapy can have negative consequences for the patient and the population. It is important that antibiotic treatment be targeted for those patients that will benefit the most. Children aged >6 months with severe signs of AOM or severe symptoms for at least 48 hours or temperature >39°C (102°F) should be prescribed antibiotics. Children younger than 24 months with bilateral AOM and less severe signs and symptoms should receive antibiotics. Unilateral AOM in children aged 6–24 months without severe signs and symptoms can initially be treated with antibiotics or be observed. When children are older than 24 months and have nonsevere AOM, they also can be prescribed antibiotics or be observed. Children who are observed should be ensured ready follow-up and administration of antibiotics if they do not improve or worsen in 48–72 hours. The decision surrounding AOM treatment should be made with the child's caregiver.

The choice of initial antibiotic therapy for most patients is amoxicillin dosed at 80–90 mg/kg daily. For penicillin-allergic children, most second- and third-generation cephalosporins have little cross reactivity. Cefdinir, cefuroxime, and cefpodoxime are preferred unless there is a documented severe reaction. Macrolides or clindamycin can be used when amoxicillin and cephalosporins are not preferred, but they provide inferior antimicrobial coverage. The duration of therapy should be 10 days for children aged <2 years or those with severe AOM. A 7-day course is sufficient for other patients.

Topical antibiotic treatment can be used in AOM with perforation. Quinolones have been shown to be effective. IM or IV ceftriaxone once daily can be used, but the optimal dosing is not known. One to three doses is likely to be effective. Children who have AOM and purulent conjunctivitis, have previously received amoxicillin in the last 30 days, or have failed treatment with amoxicillin before have a greater chance of failure with amoxicillin. They should receive amoxicillin-clavulanate if possible. Caregivers of children with AOM who receive antibiotics should be instructed to report if the patient fails to improve in 48–72 hours. These children should be reassessed and considered for a change in treatment.

Prophylactic antibiotics are no longer recommended for reducing recurrent episodes of AOM. Tympanostomy can be useful for children with recurrent AOM. *Recurrent* AOM is defined as three episodes in 3 months or four episodes in 6 months with the most recent episode in the latest 6 months. Surgery has been shown to be effective in reducing episodes of AOM and improving quality of life.

▶ Prognosis

In general, children with otitis media recover uneventfully. Middle ear effusions may persist for ≤3 months.

Halter R, Kelsberg M. Is antibiotic prophylaxis effective for recurrent acute otitis media? *J Fam Pract.* 2004;53:999–1000.

Lieberthal A, et al. The diagnosis and management of acute otitis media. *Pediatrics.* 2013;131(3):2012–3488.

Paradise JL, Dollaghan CA, Campbell TF, et al. Tubes for otitis media do not improve developmental outcomes. *J Fam Practice.* 2003; 52:939–940.

BACTERIAL PHARYNGITIS

Sore throat is a common problem in pediatrics, leading to millions of physician office visits each year. However, obtaining a clear diagnosis as to the cause of this problem is far from simple. The most important diagnosis to make is infection with group A β-hemolytic streptococci (GABHS or GAS), which is responsible for approximately 25% of cases of pharyngitis. Antibiotic treatment has only a modest effect on the course of the disease, but adequate treatment with antibiotics effectively prevents the important complication of rheumatic fever.

Viruses of many sorts cause the vast majority of cases, including some cases of exudative pharyngitis. Adenoviruses can cause pharyngoconjunctival fever, with exudative pharyngitis and conjunctivitis. Herpesviruses and coxsackie viruses can cause ulcerative stomatitis and pharyngitis. Most viruses, however, cause signs and symptoms that overlap with those of GAS.

Infectious mononucleosis can cause pharyngitis and is described in detail later. Rarely, *Neisseria gonorrhea* can cause acute pharyngitis in children and should be considered in sexually active teenagers and abused children. Group C and G streptococcus can also cause pharyngitis. This can often be epidemic and foodborne.

Group A Streptococcal Infection

ESSENTIALS OF DIAGNOSIS

▶ Moderate to severe tonsillar swelling often with exudates.

▶ Moderate to severe tender anterior cervical lymphadenopathy.

▶ Scarlatiniform rash (depending on the strain of bacteria).

▶ Absence of moderate to severe viral symptoms (cough, nasal congestion).

▶ General Considerations

Approximately 20–30% of all cases of sore throat in children are due to GAS infection. The infection is uncommon in children aged <3 years unless there is close contact with a contagious person. It occurs most often from November to May in temperate climates.

▶ Clinical Findings

A. Symptoms and Signs

Clinical symptoms and signs overlap those of viral pharyngitides and URIs. The Centor criteria have been validated for adults but not for children. Attia et al. (1999) proposed a predictive model for GAS after examining a large number of signs and symptoms. The findings most highly correlated with GABHS are: (1) moderate to severe tonsillar swelling, (2) moderate to severe tender anterior cervical lymphadenopathy, (3) scarlatiniform rash, and (4) the absence of moderate to severe coryza. If conditions 1 through 4 are present, the likelihood of GAS is 95%. In the absence of conditions 1 through 3 but in the presence of moderate to severe coryza, the likelihood of GABHS is <15%. When conditions 1 through 3 are present, the probability of GAS is ~65%

B. Laboratory Findings

A positive throat culture is the standard test to confirm GAS pharyngitis, but it takes about 24 hours to report a positive test. Rapid antigen detection tests (RADTs) and throat culture should be used in the ambulatory setting to complement clinical evaluation. Positive RADTs confirm the presence of GAS. Negative RADTs should be confirmed by throat culture because of the higher false-negative rates with this test. Another complicating factor is the inability of either rapid antigen testing or culture to distinguish between a true streptococcal infection and a viral infection in a child who is an otherwise asymptomatic GAS carrier. Carrier rates among asymptomatic children may be as high as 20%, depending on the age of the child and the season of the year.

▶ Complications

Complications of GAS fall into two main categories: nonsuppurative and suppurative. The nonsuppurative complications are rheumatic fever and poststreptococcal glomerulonephritis.

Acute rheumatic fever follows about 3% of cases of untreated GABHS. The cause is immunologic and still not fully understood.. There is great geographic variability in the incidence of this disease. Rheumatic fever can be prevented by treatment of GAS, even if treatment is delayed for ≤9 days, but a full 10 days of treatment is necessary for complete prevention.

Poststreptococcal glomerulonephritis likewise seems to be caused by a poorly understood antigen-antibody reaction. Unlike rheumatic fever, glomerulonephritis is not prevented by treatment of GAS. Hematuria following URIs should prompt further investigation.

The major suppurative complications are peritonsillar abscess (see later), cervical lymphadenitis, and mastoiditis.

Treatment

Treatment of acute GAS pharyngitis with antibiotics may expedite resolution of symptoms and prevent complications as well as prevent transmission. Only confirmed cases of GAS pharyngitis should be treated with antibiotics to avoid drug side effects and prevent the development of antibiotic-resistant strains of bacteria. Penicillin or amoxicillin are the strongly preferred treatments. Narrow-spectrum cephalosporins, clindamycin, and macrolides can be used as alternative medications when indicated by drug intolerance or allergy. All antibiotics should be dosed for 10 days except azithromycin, which has a 5-day course of treatment.

The painful throat symptoms of pharyngitis can be lessened by local treatment with topical anesthetics or warm saline rinses in older children. Treatment with acetaminophen or ibuprofen can work better for systemic symptoms such as fever and for symptoms in younger children.

A test for cure is not recommended for patients who respond to treatment. Some studies show lower than expected rates of GAS eradication even after clinical response and high asymptomatic carrier rates. At present these conditions are not considered to present enough risk to warrant the expense and risk of GAS eradication except in rare epidemic outbreaks of nonsuppurative complications. Asymptomatic household or school contacts of infected children should not be tested or empirically treated. Children should not return to school or daycare until they have been treated with antibiotics for at least 24 hours and their symptoms are controlled.

Prognosis

Streptococcal pharyngitis is ordinarily a benign, self-limited disease. Morbidity and mortality are related primarily to the previously mentioned complications. Antibiotic treatment can eliminate many but not all of these.

Attia M, et al. Multivariate predictive models for group A beta-hemolytic streptococcal pharyngitis in children. *Acad Emerg Med.* 1999;6:8. [PMID: 9928970]

Centers for Disease Control and Prevention. *CDC Academic Detailing Sheet,* March 2006.

Pichichero ME. Pathogen shifts and changing cure rates for otitis media and tonsillopharyngitis. *Clin Pediatr.* 2006;45:493–502.

Shulman S, et al. *Clinical Practice Guideline for the Diagnosis and Management of Group A Streptococcal Pharyngitis: 2012 Update.* Infectious Disease Society of America, CID 2012:55 (Nov. 15)

INFECTIOUS MONONUCLEOSIS

ESSENTIALS OF DIAGNOSIS

► Fever.

► Pharyngitis.

► Generalized lymphadenopathy.

General Considerations

Infectious mononucleosis is a clinical syndrome often caused by Epstein-Barr virus (EBV). Although ordinarily a benign illness, it has several important, if unusual complications.

Pathogenesis

Although EBV is by far the most common cause of mononucleosis, 5–10% of mononucleosislike illnesses are caused by cytomegalovirus (CMV), *Toxoplasma gondii,* or various other viruses, including HIV. EBV infects 95% of the world's population. It is transmitted in oral secretions. The incubation period is around 30–50 days. Viral shedding is highest for 1 year after the acute infection, but infection is lifelong. Most infants and young children have unapparent infections, or infections that are indistinguishable from other childhood respiratory infections. In developed countries, about one-third of infections occur in adolescence or early adulthood, and of those infected, about one-half develop clinically apparent disease. Infection occurs earlier in other countries but is rare before the age of 1 year.

The infection begins in the cells of the oral cavity, and then spreads to adjacent salivary glands and lymphoid tissue. Eventually the virus infects the entire reticuloendothelial system, including the liver and spleen.

Prevention

Because the virus is ubiquitous and is shed intermittently by nearly every adult, there is no effective prevention for this illness. No vaccine is presently available.

Clinical Findings

A. Symptoms and Signs

After the incubation period, there is often a 1–2-week prodromal period of nonspecific respiratory symptoms, including fever and sore throat. Typical symptoms include fever, sore throat, myalgia, headache, nausea, and abdominal pain.

Physical findings include pharyngitis, often with exudative tonsillitis and palatal petechiae similar to those of streptococcal pharyngitis. Lymphadenopathy is seen in 90% of cases, most often in the anterior and posterior cervical chains and less often in the axillary and inguinal chains. Epitrochlear adenopathy is a highly suggestive finding. Splenomegaly is found in ~50% of cases and hepatomegaly in 10–25%. Symptomatic hepatitis, with or without jaundice, may occur but is unusual. Various rashes, most often maculopapular, are seen in less than half of patients, but nearly all patients develop a rash if they are given ampicillin or amoxicillin.

B. Laboratory Findings

At the onset of the illness, the WBC count is usually elevated to 12,000–25,000/mm^3; 50–70% of these cells are lymphocytes, and 20–40% are atypical lymphocytes. Although 50–80% of patients have elevated hepatic transaminases, jaundice occurs in only ~5%.

The most commonly performed diagnostic test is a rapid heterophile antibody test. The diagnosis may be ambiguous because this test is 25% negative during the first week of symptoms and ≤10% negative in the second week of symptoms. In children aged <12 years, heterophile antibody testing is positive in only 25–50% of infected patients. The test may remain positive for 1 year or more after acute infection. A positive test in the presence of typical clinical symptoms is highly sensitive and specific. Heterophile tests are usually negative when viruses other than EBV are causing symptoms. In the early days of the infection, looking for atypical lymphocytes in a complete blood count (CBC) may be a reasonable approach. Definitive diagnosis of EBV infection can require serial immunoglobulin M and G (IgM and IgG) antibody testing. Testing for other causes of infectious mononucleosis is usually performed only when there is identified specific risk of exposure or transmission to vulnerable populations such as pregnant women.

C. Imaging Studies

No imaging studies are routinely useful in this illness. Ultrasound shows splenomegaly more accurately than physical examination but is usually performed only to assess the risk of splenic rupture in patients who are active in sports.

▶ **Differential Diagnosis**

Streptococcal pharyngitis is the chief illness in the differential diagnosis. Strep testing can identify asymptomatic carriers that complicate the diagnosis. Children with mononucleosis generally have more widespread lymphadenopathy than those with GAS pharyngitis. More rarely, symptoms consistent with infectious mononucleosis can also occur with HIV, cytomegalovirus (CMV), human herpesvirus 6 (HHV6), and toxoplasmosis.

▶ **Complications**

Mononucleosis is normally a benign illness. The most serious complication is spontaneous splenic rupture. This occurs in 0.5–1% of patients, almost always during the first 3 weeks of the illness. The risk of splenic rupture is elevated with trauma, and all patients with this illness should avoid contact sports for at least 3 weeks. Clinical symptoms should be resolved, and the athlete should feel well enough to participate before returning to play. Those with documented splenomegaly should not resume athletic activity until resolution has been confirmed by ultrasound.

Other complications are unusual and include rare cases of airway obstruction (1%), symptomatic hepatitis (rare), and a variety of neurologic complications (1–5%), including meningitis, encephalitis, and cranial, autonomic, or peripheral neuritis. Hemolytic anemia may occur in ~3% of cases.

Aplastic anemia is rare. Mild neutropenia and thrombocytopenia are common early in the disease, but severe cytopenias are rare.

▶ **Treatment**

Treatment is generally symptomatic and supportive with fluids and analgesics. Systemic corticosteroids can be used to lessen symptom severity and hasten recovery in more serious cases. Upper airway obstruction and severe hematologic complications generally warrant the use of steroids. A commonly recommended daily dose of prednisone is 1–2 mg/kg (≤60 mg) for 1 week. Antiviral medications have not shown a consistent benefit.

▶ **Prognosis**

Symptoms typically last about 2–4 weeks. Fatigue may be the last symptom to leave. Most patients resume normal activities after 2 months.

Bell AT, Fortune B. What test is the best for diagnosing infectious mononucleosis? *J Fam Practice*. 2006;55:799–800.
Luzuriaga K, Sullivan JL. Infectious mononucleosis. *N Engl J Med*, 2010;362:1993–2000.
Putakian M, et al. Mononucleosis and athletic participation: an evidence-based review. *Clin J Sports Med*. 2008;18:309–315.

PERITONSILLAR ABSCESS

 ESSENTIALS OF DIAGNOSIS

▶ Severe sore throat.

▶ Odynophagia.

▶ High fever.

▶ Unilateral pharyngeal swelling with deviation of the uvula.

▶ **General Considerations**

Peritonsillar abscess is the most common deep-space head and neck infection in children, accounting for almost half of these infections. It is most commonly caused by infection with GAS. The exact cause is unknown, but it is assumed that the infection usually spreads from the tonsil itself into the deep spaces behind the tonsil, where it produces a collection of pus. It can occur in children of all ages, as well as in adults, but it affects older children and adolescents more than younger children. It is almost always unilateral.

▶ **Clinical Findings**

A. Symptoms and Signs

Most children with peritonsillar abscess have had symptoms of pharyngitis for 1–7 days before presenting with symptoms related to the abscess. Many of these children have been treated with antibiotics for pharyngitis before developing the abscess. The most common symptoms are severe throat or neck pain, painful swallowing, high fever, and poor oral intake. The most common physical signs are cervical adenopathy, uvular deviation, and muffled voice with trismus. There is usually unilateral tense swelling of the anterior tonsillar pillar on the affected side. Symptoms are less clear and the examination more difficult in younger children, and young children who cannot cooperate may have to be examined under sedation.

B. Laboratory Findings

The WBC count is usually elevated, with a left shift. Throat cultures for streptococci are positive in only ~16% of specimens.

C. Imaging Studies

Computed tomography and ultrasound studies of the neck often show the abscess, but the diagnosis is generally made by history and physical examination.

▶ Differential Diagnosis

The chief disease in the differential diagnosis is epiglottitis. This infection is uncommon in an era of widespread immunization against *H. influenzae* type B, but the clinical picture may be identical in young children. Examination in the operating room under sedation may be necessary to establish the diagnosis, especially if the patient manifests tripoding, drooling, and stridor.

▶ Complications

Prompt treatment is necessary, because untreated abscesses may spread into other deep spaces in the head and neck. The airway may be compromised by swelling, especially in younger children. If the abscess ruptures into the throat, aspiration of pus may cause pneumonia.

▶ Treatment

The treatment is drainage of the abscess, either by incision or by needle aspiration. This is generally done by an otolaryngologist or a surgeon familiar with the anatomy of the neck. Tonsillectomy is often done at the discretion of the surgeon, either at the time of the acute infection or shortly thereafter. Antibiotics effective against streptococci and staphylococci, such as ampicillin/sulbactam or clindamycin, are indicated, initially intravenously. Once cultures of the pus indicate the causative organism, treatment may be focused according to its antibiotic sensitivities. Systemic corticosteroids may speed recovery, but the evidence is limited to children aged >12 years.

▶ Prognosis

Children generally recover uneventfully once appropriate treatment has begun, but they may be at increased risk for a second infection.

Galioto N. Peritonsillar abscess. *Am Fam Physician.* 2008; 77(2): 199–202,209.

Ozbek C, Aygenc E, Tuna EU, et al. Use of steroids in the treatment of peritonsillar abscess. *J Laryngol Otol.* 2004;118:439.

Schraff S, et al. Peritonsillar abscess in children: a 10-year review of diagnosis and management. *Int J Pediatr Otorhinolaryngol.* 2001; 57:213. [PMID: 11223453]

▼ INFECTIONS OF THE LOWER RESPIRATORY TRACT

CROUP (ACUTE LARYNGOTRACHEITIS)

 ESSENTIALS OF DIAGNOSIS

▶ URI prodrome.

▶ Barking cough.

▶ Symptoms worst on the first or second day, with gradual resolution.

▶ Lungs clear.

▶ Inspiratory stridor, respiratory distress, cyanosis in severe cases.

▶ General Considerations

Croup (laryngotracheitis and spasmodic croup) is an illness of infants and children aged <6 years. It is most common between 7 and 36 months, and slightly more common in boys than in girls. About 5% of children will have croup during their second year of life

▶ Pathogenesis

Croup is caused by an infection of the upper airways—the larynx, trachea, and the upper levels of the bronchial tree—and obstruction of these airways caused by edema produces most of the classic symptoms of the disease. Nearly all cases of croup are caused by viruses; parainfluenza viruses are the most common agents, along with adenovirus, respiratory syncytial virus (RSV), and (rarely) *Mycoplasma pneumoniae.*

▶ Clinical Findings

A. Symptoms and Signs

Most children with croup present after several days of prodromal URI symptoms, which are followed by the rapid onset of a barking, "seal-like" cough, and inspiratory stridor. This is somewhat frightening to both patients and parents; however, respiratory distress is generally only mild to moderate. The symptoms are generally worst on the first or second day, peak at night, and gradually resolve over the next several days. If the symptoms progress beyond this point, the child may develop worsening respiratory distress, more pronounced and more constant stridor, and cyanosis.

The lungs are usually clear. The degree of subcostal and intercostal retractions, the degree of stridor, and the presence of cyanosis are important clues to the severity of the illness. If the child is cyanotic and in respiratory distress, manipulation of the pharynx (eg, attempts to examine the pharynx using a tongue depressor) may trigger respiratory arrest. This maneuver should therefore be avoided until the clinician is in a position to manage the child's airway by endotracheal intubation only with an experienced team.

B. Laboratory Findings

Laboratory studies are rarely useful in the evaluation of routine croup. The WBC count is usually normal or slightly elevated; however, counts of >15,000/mm^3 may be seen. The blood oxygen saturation may be normal or decreased, depending on the severity of the disease.

C. Imaging Studies

The chest x-ray is usually normal, but anteroposterior soft-tissue x-rays of the neck may show subglottic narrowing, causing the classic "steeple" sign.

▶ Differential Diagnosis

Croup must be differentiated from other respiratory illnesses that cause obstruction in the region of the larynx. Epiglottitis generally lacks the URI prodrome and the croupy cough. The child prefers to sit forward, may be drooling and reluctant to lie down, and may have a high fever. Lateral neck film will demonstrate a swollen epiglottis. Children who have both foreign-body and angioneurotic edema have onset of symptoms suddenly and lack fever or other signs of infection. Children with bacterial tracheitis have persistent worsening of symptoms and signs of upper airway obstruction despite treatment. There may be evidence of soft densities on lateral neck radiograph consistent with purulent exudate within the trachea.

▶ Complications

Approximately 15% of children with croup experience complications of varying severity. These are usually related to extension of the infection to other parts of the respiratory tract, such as otitis media or viral pneumonia. Bacterial pneumonia is unusual, but bacterial tracheitis may occur. Children with severe croup may develop complications of

hypoxemia, if this is not adequately treated. Death is unusual and is generally due to laryngeal obstruction.

▶ Treatment

The published croup scoring systems may be useful for research purposes, but they do not present validated criteria for determining the best course of treatment for an individual child. High fever, toxic appearance, worsening stridor, respiratory distress, cyanosis or pallor, hypoxia, and restlessness or lethargy are all symptoms of more severe disease and should prompt the physician to admit the child for inpatient treatment.

Most children with croup may be treated at home. The mainstay of treatment has long been held to be cool, moist air, although research has not confirmed the effectiveness of this treatment. Corticosteroids have been shown to decrease the croup score and the time spent in emergency rooms and hospitals. A single IM dose of dexamethasone, at 0.6 mg/kg, may be effective in reducing the severity of moderate to severe croup in patients treated at home. Because the onset of action for dexamethasone is ~6 hours, a single dose of racemic epinephrine may be given before the child is sent home. An oral course for home treatment may be considered but has not been shown to be as effective as the IM route.

Patients who require hospitalization often receive supplemental oxygen in order to correct hypoxemia. Racemic epinephrine has long been the mainstay of treatment for patients with significant respiratory distress. Numerous studies have confirmed its effectiveness. The drug is administered via nebulizer and face mask. It action duration is 1–2 hours. Although racemic epinephrine is the drug most commonly used, L-epinephrine is equally effective, less expensive, and more widely available. Numerous studies have shown systemic dexamethasone to be effective in reducing both the severity and duration of the disease and the need for intubation. Because of its long action, the drug can be given as a single dose, which remains effective for the remainder of the course of the disease. The dose is 0.6 mg/kg, IM, and it should be given as early as possible in the course of hospitalization. Nebulized steroids and oral dexamethasone are more effective than placebo but less effective than IM dexamethasone. Children hospitalized for treatment of croup should be observed carefully for any signs of respiratory distress. Intubation and mechanical ventilation are necessary in a small percentage of children with this disease.

▶ Prognosis

The natural history of croup is that recurrences are common. However, as children grow, the airways grow larger and are less affected by edema, and symptoms tend to become less severe over time.

Cherry J. Croup. *N Engl J Med*. 2008 358;4:384–391.

BRONCHIOLITIS

ESSENTIALS OF DIAGNOSIS

▶ URI symptoms.
▶ Wheezing.
▶ Cough.
▶ Dyspnea.
▶ Tachypnea.

General Considerations

Bronchiolitis is a disorder of the lower respiratory tract that occurs most often in infants and young children. It is seen most commonly in the first 2 years of life, with more than one-third of children affected. The peak age is ~6 months. It is the leading cause of infant hospitalization and is most commonly caused by respiratory syncytial virus (RSV). Older children and adults may contract the same infection, but because they have larger airways, they do not experience the same degree of airway obstruction. In fact, an older sibling or a parent is often the source of the infant's infection.

Pathogenesis

Bronchiolitis is almost always viral in etiology. RSV causes more than half of cases; others are caused by parainfluenza virus, influenza, and human metapneumonovirus (HMPV). Pathologically, edema and accumulated cellular debris cause obstruction of small airways. This obstruction causes a ventilation-perfusion mismatch with wasted perfusion, a right-to-left shunt, and hypoxemia early in the course of the disease.

Prevention

Palivizumab is available in the United States for prevention of RSV disease in high-risk infants. The drug has been shown to decrease hospitalization rates among high-risk infants with and without chronic lung disease. The decision to use this drug is based on the age of the child at the onset of RSV season and the child's medical history. The American Academy of Pediatrics (AAP) recommends prophylaxis with palivizumab for children aged <2 years with chronic lung disease who have required medical treatment in the preceding 6 months, or who have cyanotic or complicated congenital heart disease; for infants who were born at or before 28 weeks' gestation during their first RSV season; for infants aged <6 months of age who were born at 29–32 weeks' or for <6-month-old infants born at 32–35 weeks' gestation who have two or more of these risk factors: daycare attendance, school-age siblings, exposure to environmental air pollutants, congenital abnormalities of the airways, or severe neuromuscular disease. Palivizumab is given in a dose of 15 mg/kg IM once every 30 days during the local RSV season, in five doses or less. Infants born between 32 and 35 weeks' gestation need only receive prophylaxis up to 90 days of age or a maximum of three doses, whichever comes first.

Clinical Findings

A. Symptoms and Signs

Bronchiolitis is an acute infectious illness that begins with URI symptoms. It may progress to respiratory distress wheezing, cough, and dyspnea. The infant may be irritable and feed poorly, but there are rarely any other systemic symptoms. The temperature may be elevated or below normal.

Physical examination shows the child to be tachypneic, with a respiratory rate as high as 60–80 breaths per minute, and often in severe respiratory distress. Alar flaring, retractions, and the use of accessory muscles of respiration may be evident. Examination of the lungs often shows a prolonged expiratory phase with diffuse wheezes. Diffuse fine rales may be present. The lungs are often hyperinflated with shallow respirations, and breath sounds may be nearly inaudible if the obstruction is severe.

B. Laboratory Findings

Pulse oximetry may reveal hypoxemia and aid in the decision concerning need for hospitalization. A nasopharyngeal swab may be done for RSV rapid viral antigen testing; however, results may have little impact on management.

C. Imaging Studies

The use of chest radiography is not routinely recommended but may show signs of hyperinflation with scattered areas of consolidation. These may represent postobstructive atelectasis or inflammation of alveoli. It may not be possible to exclude early bacterial pneumonia solely on the basis of radiographic findings.

Differential Diagnosis

The differential diagnosis for the wheezing infant includes viral bronchiolitis along with other pulmonary infections (eg, pneumonia, chlamydia, TB), laryngotracheomalacia, foreign body, gastroesophageal reflux, congestive heart failure, vascular ring, allergic reaction, cystic fibrosis, mediastinal mass, bronchogenic cyst, and tracheoesophageal fistula.

Complications

Complications such as bacterial pneumonia and respiratory failure are more common and more severe in children with underlying cardiac or pulmonary disease. Fewer than 400 deaths occur annually, but are highest in infants aged <6 months, and in those who are premature or have underlying cardiopulmonary disease or immunodeficiency.

Treatment

The treatment of bronchiolitis is primarily supportive with the focus on providing adequate hydration and oxygenation while the patient recovers from the illness. This may require hospitalization. Some patients may benefit from routine suctioning of the nasopharynx, especially prior to attempting to take oral feeds. Bronchodilators such as albuterol or racemic epinephrine may transiently improve the clinical status of patients with bronchiolitis but have not been shown to decrease the need for hospitalization, shorten the length of hospitalization, or decrease the time to illness resolution. Their use is not routinely recommended, but they may be used only after proven benefit in a trial of therapy in each patient. Corticosteroids and leukotriene receptor antagonists have not been shown to decrease the length of illness or need for hospitalization and thus are not routinely recommended. Nebulized hypertonic saline may reduce the length of hospitalization but is not currently routinely recommended. Patients with evidence of lobar pneumonia on chest radiograph may benefit from a course of antibiotics. Ribavirin is no longer recommended for children with bronchiolitis.

Prognosis

There appears to be a relationship between bronchiolitis and reactive airway disease, although the exact connection is unclear. Some studies have shown an increased incidence of airway hyperreactivity that may persist for years in children who have had bronchiolitis.

American Academy of Pediatrics, Committee on Infectious Diseases: American Academy of Pediatrics, Bronchiolitis Guidelines Committee. Updated guidance for palivizumab prophylaxis among infants and young children at increased risk of hospitalization for respiratory syncytial virus infection. *Pediatrics.* 2014 Aug;134(2):e620-638. doi:10.1542/peds.2014–1666. [PMID: 25070304]
Seehusen DA. Effectiveness of bronchodilators for bronchiolitis treatment. *Am Fam Physician.* 2011:83(9):1045–1047.
Zorc JJ, Hall CB. Bronchiolitis: recent evidence on diagnosis and management. *Pediatrics.* 2010;125(2):342–349.

PERTUSSIS

ESSENTIALS OF DIAGNOSIS

▶ URI symptoms.

▶ Paroxysms of coughing, often with "whoops" on inspiration.

▶ Posttussive emesis

▶ Dyspnea.

▶ Seizures.

General Considerations

Pertussis is a bacterial infection that affects airways lined with ciliated epithelium. The disease is most common in unimmunized infants and in adults, because immunity wanes 5–10 years after the last immunization. Pertussis causes serious disease in children and mild or asymptomatic disease in adults. Infants aged <6 months have greater morbidity than older children, and those aged <2 months have the highest rates of pertussis-related hospitalization, pneumonia, seizures, encephalopathy, and death. Pertussis is highly contagious, with attack rates as high as 100% in susceptible individuals exposed at close range.

Pathogenesis

The most common cause of pertussis is *Bordetella pertussis,* but adenoviruses, *Bordetella parapertussis, Mycoplasm pneumonieae, Chlamydia trachomatis,* and RSV can cause a similar disease. The organisms attack ciliated epithelium, producing toxins and resulting in inflammation and necrosis of the walls of small airways. This leads to plugging of airways, bronchopneumonia, and hypoxemia.

Prevention

The key to prevention of pertussis is immunization. Unfortunately, immunization does not confer complete protection. A total of 27,550 cases of pertussis were still reported in 2010. Up to 80% of immunized household contacts of symptomatic cases acquire infection as a result of waning immunity. All infants and toddlers should be routinely immunized as previously recommended by the CDC. In addition, since 2006, a vaccine combining acellular pertussis vaccine with tetanus and diphtheria toxoids (Tdap) has been available for use in children aged >7 years for all subsequent doses of vaccine, including the recommended adolescent booster dose given at age ≥11 years. Tdap is also recommended for all adults to replace the next booster dose of Td vaccine and for adults (including those who are 65 years or older) who have close contact with infants less than 12 months of age.

Clinical Findings

A. Symptoms and Signs

Children aged <2 years show the most typical symptoms of the disease, paroxysms of coughing, inspiratory "whoops" (which give the disease its colloquial name "whooping cough"), vomiting induced by coughing, and dyspnea lasting more than 1 month. Some will have seizures. Children aged >2 years have lower incidences of all these symptoms and a shorter duration of disease, whereas adults often have atypical symptoms. High fever is unusual in all ages.

Pertussis has an incubation period lasting 7–10 days with a range of 5–21 days. The disease progresses through the following three stages:

1. The *catarrhal stage,* which is characterized by symptoms typical of a common cold.

2. The *paroxysmal stage*, which lasts 2–4 weeks, occasionally longer. During this stage, episodes of coughing increase in severity and number. The typical paroxysm is 5–10 hard coughs in a single expiration, followed by the classic whoop as the patient inspires. Young infants seldom manifest the whoop. Coughing to the point of vomiting is common. Fever is absent or minimal.

3. During the *convalescent stage,* the paroxysms gradually decrease in frequency and number. The patient may experience a cough for several months after the disease has otherwise resolved.

Pertussis can usually be diagnosed in the paroxysmal stage, but it requires a certain level of suspicion. A cough lasting more than 2 weeks and associated with posttussive vomiting should prompt the physician to consider the diagnosis.

B. Laboratory Findings

A high WBC count ($20,000$–$50,000/mm^3$) with an absolute lymphocytosis is suggestive of pertussis in infants and young children, but is often absent in adolescents and adults.

Culture is considered the gold standard for diagnosis of pertussis. The organism can be obtained for culture by a nasopharyngeal swab but may be difficult to grow secondary to its fastidious nature. False negatives may occur in a previously immunized person, if antimicrobial therapy has been started, if >3 weeks has elapsed since the onset of the cough, or if the specimen is not handled appropriately.

Polymerase chain reaction (PCR) assays on nasopharyngeal samples are increasingly available for detection of pertussis. These have improved sensitivity and quicker turnaround time than cultures.

Convalescent serology may be helpful to confirm the diagnosis, especially later in the illness. An elevated IgG antibody to pertussis toxin after 2 weeks of the onset of cough is suggestive of recent B pertussis infection.

Direct fluorescent antibody (DFA) staining is no longer recommended.

▶ Differential Diagnosis

Any illness that causes cough should be considered in the differential diagnosis. Older children and children who have been immunized against the disease may have milder, atypical symptoms, and the only clue to the disease may be the long duration of symptoms.

▶ Complications

Complications of pertussis among infants include pneumonia, seizures, encephalopathy, hernia, subdural bleeding, conjunctival bleeding, and death. Mortality rates of approximately 1% are seen in infants aged <2 months and 0.5% in those aged 2–11 months. Complications among adolescents and adults include syncope, sleep disturbances, incontinence,

rib fractures, and pneumonia. Adults have increased complications with increasing age.

▶ Treatment

Treatment is primarily supportive, involving hydration, pulmonary toilet, and oxygen. Young infants and children may require hospitalization, especially those aged <6 months. Hospitalized patients should be placed in droplet isolation until antibiotics have been given for at least 5 days or until 3 weeks after the onset of the cough if antibiotics are not administered.

Antibiotics given during the catarrhal phase may shorten the course of the illness. Once the cough is established, antibiotics are recommended to limit the spread of the organism to others but will not shorten the course of illness. Azithromycin or erythromycin are recommended for treatment and can be used to eliminate the bacteria from the respiratory tract. Clarithromycin may also be used in patients aged >1 month, and trimethoprim-sulfamethoxazole may be used in infants aged >2 months as alternatives. Any infant aged <1 month who is treated with a macrolide should be monitored for development of infantile hypertrophic pyloric stenosis (IHPS). All household contacts of patients with pertussis should receive chemoprophylaxis and be monitored for development of the illness.

During a pertussis epidemic, newborns should receive their first immunization at 4 weeks of age, with repeat doses given at 6, 10, and 14 weeks of age. Partially immunized children aged <7 years should complete the immunization series at the minimum intervals, and completely immunized children aged <7 years should receive one booster dose, unless they have received one in the preceding 3 years. Unimmunized or boosted older children and adults should receive Tdap.

▶ Prognosis

The prognosis of pertussis depends primarily on the age of the patient. Mortality is rare in adults and children. The mortality rate for children aged <6 months is highest, but with proper care may be minimized. Most mortality is due to pneumonia and cerebral anoxia.

Pickering LK, ed. *Red Book: 2012 Report of the Committee on the Infectious Diseases,* 29th ed. Elk Grove Village, IL: American Academy of Pediatrics; 2012: 553–566.

PNEUMONIA

 ESSENTIALS OF DIAGNOSIS

▶ Fever.

▶ Acute respiratory symptoms.

▶ Tachypnea.

General Considerations

Pneumonia, infection of the lung parenchyma, occurs more often in young children than in any other age group. The diagnosis can generally be made clinically, and the majority of patients can be treated successfully with oral antibiotics and recover at home. Occasionally, the child may require hospitalization, and a small percentage will experience a complicated course.

Pathogenesis

Viruses are a leading cause of pneumonia in children of all ages. Bacterial infections are more common in developing countries and in children with complicated infections.

Age is an important consideration in determining the potential etiology of pneumonia. Neonates aged <20 days are most likely to have infections with pathogens that cause other neonatal infection syndromes, including group B streptococci, gram-negative enteric bacteria, CMV, and *Listeria monocytogenes.*

Children between the ages of 3 weeks and 3 months may have infections caused by *C. trachomatis,* normally acquired from exposure at the time of birth, to infection in the mother's genital tract. In addition, RSV, parainfluenza, and *B. pertussis* and *S. pneumonia* also cause pneumonia at this age.

Respiratory viruses such as RSV, parainfluenza, human metapneumonovirus, influenza, and rhinovirus are the most common cause of pneumonia in children between the ages of 4 months and 4 years. *S. pneumoniae* and nontypeable *H. influenzae* are common bacterial causes. *M. pneumoniae* mainly affects older children in this age group. Tuberculosis should be considered in children who live in areas of high tuberculosis prevalence.

Mycoplasma pneumoniae is the most common cause of pneumonia in children aged 5–15 years. *Chlamydia pneumoniae* is also an important cause in this age group. *Pneumococcus* is the most likely cause of lobar pneumonia. As in younger children, tuberculosis should be considered in areas of high prevalence.

Prevention

The only significantly effective form of prevention is immunization. Children should be immunized with vaccines for *H. influenzae* type b, *S. pneumonia*, and pertussis. Children aged >6 months should be immunized against influenza annually. Parents and caretakers of infants aged <6 months should be immunized against influenza and pertussis. High-risk infants should receive immune prophylaxis against RSV.

Clinical Findings

A. Symptoms and Signs

The hallmark symptoms of pneumonia are fever and cough; however, few children with these symptoms have pneumonia.

Young infants are particularly likely to have nonspecific signs and symptoms. Tachypnea is an important finding. This is defined by a respiratory rate of >60 breaths per minute in infants aged <2 months, >50 in infants aged 2–12 months, and >40 in children aged >12 months. Evidence of increased work of breathing, such as subcostal or intercostal retractions, nasal flaring, and grunting, may indicate more severe disease. Auscultatory findings are variable and include decreased breath sounds, wheezes, rhonchi, and crackles. The absence of these various pulmonary findings is helpful in predicting that a child will not have pneumonia, but their presence is only moderately predictive of the presence of pneumonia.

B. Laboratory Findings

Laboratory findings are seldom helpful in the diagnosis of pneumonia. A WBC count of >17,000/mm^3 indicates a higher likelihood of bacteremia, although blood cultures are rarely positive except in complicated infections, and oxygen desaturation indicates more severe disease. Sputum culture is the most accurate way to ascertain the cause of the infection, although obtaining a sputum sample from a child is not always possible.

C. Imaging Studies

While a chest radiograph is not necessary for the pediatric patient who is well enough to be treated in the outpatient setting, it is generally recommended for those children with hypoxia or significant respiratory distress or who have failed initial antibiotic therapy. These patients are at increased risk of complications of pneumonia, including parapneumonic effusions, necrotizing pneumonia, and pneumothorax. Routine follow-up chest radiographs are not necessary for children who recover uneventfully.

Differential Diagnosis

The differential diagnosis of pneumonia includes asthma, foreign-body aspiration, bronchiolitis, cystic fibrosis, and congenital heart disease.

Treatment

The appropriate treatment of childhood pneumonia depends on the age of the child and severity of the illness. Neonates should all be treated as inpatients. Infants aged 3 weeks to 3 months may be treated as outpatients if they are not febrile or hypoxemic, do not appear toxic, or have an alveolar infiltrate or a large pleural effusion. Older infants and children may be treated as outpatients if they do not appear seriously ill.

The choice of antibiotics depends on the age of the child and the most likely cause of infection. Neonates should be treated with ampicillin and gentamicin, with or without cefotaxime, as appropriate for a neonatal sepsis syndrome.

High-dose amoxicillin should be used in children between 2 months and 5 years of age if a bacterial etiology is suspected. Otherwise, treatment may be withheld if a viral infection is considered to be the most likely cause. For children sick enough to require hospitalization, intravenous ampicillin is appropriate. For children who appear septic or who manifest alveolar infiltrates or large pleural effusions, cefotaxime or ceftriaxone should be used. If *S. aureus* is suspected, either vancomycin or clindamycin should also be provided.

Macrolides are also appropriate first-line choices for school-aged children and adolescents who are evaluated and treated as outpatients and with findings compatible with atypical pathogens. Doxycycline may be used in children aged >8 years. Children who are ill enough to require inpatient treatment should be treated with a macrolide, plus either cefotaxime or ceftriaxone. The recommended duration of treatment is 10 days, depending on the clinical response.

Influenza antiviral therapy should be given to those children who have moderate to severe pneumonia consistent with influenza, particularly during community outbreaks.

Prognosis

Worldwide, pneumonia is an important cause of death in children. In developed countries, however, the death rate for childhood pneumonia has dropped dramatically with the development of antibiotics.

Bradley J, et al. Executive summary: the management of community-acquired pneumonia in infants and children older than 3 months of age: clinical practice guidelines by the Pediatric Infectious Disease Society and the Infectious Disease Society of America. *Clin Infect Dis.* 2011;53(7):617–630.

GASTROINTESTINAL & GENITOURINARY INFECTIONS

GASTROENTERITIS

ESSENTIALS OF DIAGNOSIS

▶ Diarrhea.
▶ Vomiting may be present or absent.

General Considerations

Diarrheal diseases are among the most common illnesses and perhaps the leading cause of death among children worldwide. It is estimated that there are 1 billion illnesses and 3–5 million deaths from these illnesses each year. In the United States, there are an estimated 20–35 million cases of diarrhea annually, with 1.5 million outpatient visits to physicians and over 200,000 hospitalizations but only 300 deaths per year. Gastroenteritis may be caused by any of a large number of viruses, bacteria, or parasites. Most infections are caused by ingestion of contaminated food or water.

Pathogenesis

Four families of viruses can cause gastroenteritis. All are spread easily through fecal-oral contact, and many are associated with localized outbreaks in hospitals, daycare centers, and schools. Rotavirus is a common cause of gastroenteritis during winter months. It primarily affects children between 3 months and 2 years of age, and by age 4 or 5 years, nearly all children have serologic evidence of infection. Norwalk virus is the most common cause of gastroenteritis among older children and, along with astroviruses and enteric adenoviruses, causes year-round, often localized outbreaks of disease.

Bacteria may cause either inflammatory or noninflammatory diarrhea. Common causes of inflammatory diarrhea are *Campylobacter jejuni,* enteroinvasive or enterohemorrhagic *E. coli, Salmonella* species, *Shigella* species, and *Yersinia enterocolitica.* Noninflammatory diarrhea may be caused by enteropathogenic or enterotoxigenic *E. coli* or by *Vibrio cholerae.*

The most common parasitic cause of diarrhea in the United States is *Giardia lamblia.* Numerous other parasites, including *Cryptosporidium* and *Entamoeba histolytica,* along with helminthes such as *Strongyloides stercoralis,* may cause diarrhea. Most parasitic infections cause chronic diarrhea and are beyond the scope of this chapter.

Prevention

The most effective prevention measure is for children to have access to uncontaminated food and water. Careful hand washing and good sanitation practices also help prevent the spread of infection among children. An increased rate of breastfeeding has been shown to decrease the incidence of gastroenteritis among all children in small communities.

In 2006, the Advisory Committee on Immunization Practices (ACIP) recommended that the new oral rotavirus vaccine (RotaTeq®) be given to all children at 2, 4, and 6 months of age. This immunization schedule has been shown to be effective for two seasons after administration, but no studies have been done to establish whether it is effective for longer. It should be noted that, unlike the initial rotavirus vaccine, which was withdrawn from the market, the new vaccine has not been shown to be associated with an increased rate of intussusception. In 2008, a second oral vaccine (Rotarix®) was licensed as a two-dose series, given at 2 and 4 months of age. The ACIP does not express a preference for one vaccine over the other.

Clinical Findings

A. Symptoms and Signs

The cardinal sign of gastroenteritis is diarrhea, with or without vomiting. Systemic symptoms and signs may include fever and malaise. Fever and severe abdominal pain are more common with inflammatory diarrhea. The estimated degree of dehydration should be established before beginning treatment.

In most children with viral gastroenteritis, fever and vomiting last <2–3 days, although diarrhea may persist for ≤5–7 days. Most cases of diarrhea caused by foodborne toxins last 1–2 days. Many, but not all, bacterial infections persist for longer periods of time.

B. Laboratory Findings

Stool cultures for bacteria and examination for parasites should be analyzed if the stool is positive for blood or leukocytes, if diarrhea persists for >1 week, or if the patient is immunocompromised. The presence of fecal leukocytes indicates an inflammatory infection, although not all such infections produce a positive test. Blood indicates a hemorrhagic or inflammatory infection. In a child who appears significantly dehydrated, serum electrolytes should be tested, especially if the child is hospitalized for fluid therapy.

Complications

Diarrheal diseases are for the most part benign, self-limited infections. Mortality is caused primarily by dehydration, shock, and circulatory collapse. Bacterial pathogens may spread to remote sites and cause meningitis, pneumonia, and other infections. *E. coli* O157:H7 may cause hemolytic-uremic syndrome.

Treatment

The keys to treatment of gastroenteritis are rehydration, or avoidance of dehydration, and early refeeding. Children who are severely (>9%) dehydrated or who appear toxic or seriously ill should be hospitalized for rehydration and treatment. Otherwise, children may be managed at home. Vomiting is the chief obstacle to rehydration or maintenance of hydration. Children who are vomiting should be given frequent (every 1–2 minutes) very small amounts (≤5 mL) of rehydration solution to avoid provoking further attacks of emesis (**Table 5-2**).

Children who have diarrhea but are not dehydrated should continue on whatever age-appropriate foods they were taking before the illness. In those who are dehydrated but not severely so, oral rehydration has been shown to be the preferred method of rehydration. Juices, water flavored with drink mix, and sports drinks do not have the recommended concentrations of carbohydrates and electrolytes

Table 5-2. Evaluation of dehydration in children.

While the degree of dehydration is often misjudged by clinicians, the following scale is one of several that can be helpful in estimating the severity in infants and young children:

<3%—usually subclinical

Mild to moderate dehydration (3–9%):
  Thirsty, eager to drink
  Decreased tears
  Slightly dry mucous membranes
  Sunken eyes
  Cool extremities
  Decreased urine output

Severe dehydration (>9%):
  Thready/absent pulses
  Prolonged capillary refill
  Prolonged or absent capillary refill
  Cold extremities
  Apathetic, lethargic, unconscious
  Minimal urine output

Data from Franado-Villar D. *Pediatr Rev.* 2012; 33; 487

and should be avoided. The World Health Organization's or UNICEF's reduced-osmolarity rehydration solution is the preferred therapy. Children who are mildly (<3%) dehydrated should be given 50 mL/kg of solution, plus replacement of ongoing losses from stool or emesis, over each 4-hour period. Children who are moderately (3–9%) dehydrated should be given 100 mL/kg, plus losses, over each 4-hour period. Refeeding with age-appropriate foods should begin as soon as the child is interested in eating. Therapy with antidiarrheal and antiemetic medications has been shown to have minimal effect on the volume of diarrhea. Additionally, these drugs have an unacceptably high rate of side effects, and their use is not recommended.

Even when diagnosed, many bacterial infections do not require treatment. *Campylobacter* (erythromycin) and *Shigella* (trimethoprim sulfamethoxazole or cephalosporin) infections may require treatment. Infections with *Salmonella* should not be treated with antibiotics unless the child is aged <3 months or manifests bacteremia or disseminated infection. Treatment of *E. coli* O157:H7 infection does not reduce the severity of the illness and may increase the likelihood of hemolytic-uremic syndrome. Other *E. coli* infections should be treated only if they are severe or prolonged. *Giardia* infections should be treated.

Probiotics such as *Lactobacillus* may reduce the duration of the diarrhea, especially if caused by rotavirus, and are most effective when started early in the illness.

Prognosis

With proper rehydration and refeeding, morbidity and mortality from viral gastroenteritis is minimal. Morbidity and mortality from bacterial infections is dependent on the virulence of the organism and complications from distant spread or remote effects, such as hemolytic-uremic syndrome.

Committee on Infectious Diseases American Academy of Pediatrics. Prevention of rotavirus diseases: updated guidelines for use of rotavirus vaccine. *Pediatrics.* 2009;123(5):1412–1420.

URINARY TRACT INFECTIONS

 ESSENTIALS OF DIAGNOSIS

▶ Common bacterial cause of febrile illness in young children.

▶ Symptoms are often nonspecific in young children.

▶ Urinalysis is not always reliable; appropriate culture is needed for final diagnosis.

▶ General Considerations

Urinary tract infections (UTIs) are the most common serious bacterial infection in children aged <2 years. Among febrile young children, between 3% and 5% have a UTI, and among infants UTIs account for approximately 5% of unfocused febrile illnesses. UTI is the most frequent site of SBIs in young children. UTI may also be a marker for urinary tract anomalies in young children. UTIs may lead to renal scarring, which may cause hypertension and renal insufficiency later in life.

▶ Pathogenesis

In the first 8–12 weeks of life, some UTIs may be caused by hematogenous spread of bacteria from a remote source. Otherwise, the infections are caused by bacteria ascending the urethra into the bladder. From the bladder, bacteria may ascend the ureters to cause pyelonephritis.

The most common pathogens responsible for UTIs are enteric bacteria. *E. coli* is found in 70–90% of infections. *Pseudomonas aeruginosa* is the most common nonenteric gram-negative pathogen, and *Enterococcus* species are the most common gram-positive organisms seen. Group B *Streptococcus* is occasionally found in neonates. *S. aureus* is rarely seen in children who do not have indwelling catheters and suggests seeding from a distant focus, such as renal abscess, osteomyelitis, or endocarditis.

▶ Clinical Findings

A. Symptoms and Signs

The most important factors in prevalence of UTI are the patient's age and gender. In newborns, preterm infants are several times more likely to have a UTI than full-term infants. In febrile infant girls, the most important factors are white race, age <12 months, fever ≥39°C, fever for ≥2 days, and no other source of infection. More than two of these risk factors should prompt serious consideration of UTI. In infant boys, circumcision is the most important risk factor. Nonblack race, fever ≥39°C, fever for >24 hours, and no other source of infection are other important risk factors. Uncircumcised febrile infant boys always have a >1% risk of UTI. Circumcised febrile infant boys have a significant risk of UTI with more than two of the other risk factors. The usual age at which children experience a first symptomatic infection is 1–5 years. In this age group girls are 10–20 times more likely to have a UTI than boys. Two-thirds of young children with a febrile UTI have acute pyelonephritis.

Among children aged <2 years, symptoms are often lacking or nonspecific. Parents may become suspicious if the child appears to be in pain while urinating, but otherwise fever may be the only presenting complaint. Among children who have developed language skills, typical UTI symptoms, such as dysuria, urgency, and urinary frequency, may be seen.

B. Laboratory Findings

To be most reliable, urine must be collected by a clean catch, catheterization, or suprapubic aspiration. Urine collected in an adhesive collection bag is often contaminated. Bag urinalysis is mostly helpful when negative. Bag urine culture is helpful retrospectively only if negative. The final diagnosis of UTI depends on an appropriately collected culture result of ≥50,000 colony-forming units (CFUs) per milliliter of a uropathogen combined with a urinalysis suggestive of pyuria.

Urine should be analyzed for pyuria and bactiuria. Dipstick urinalyisis is a component of urine evaluation. A positive urine nitrite test is very specific, but a negative test is not helpful for bactiuria. Leukocyte esterase testing is very sensitive but not as specific for UTI. Fever from other conditions, vigorous activity, or contamination can produce a positive leukocyte esterase test. Microscopic urinalysis for pyuria is positive if there are ≥5 WBCs per high-powered field in a spun urine. Unspun unrinalysis using a counting chamber is more sensitive. Significant bactiuria correlating to a UTI is confirmed by the presence of bacteria on examination of least 10 oil immersion fields of gram-stained unspun fresh urine.

Urine collected for analysis should be sent for culture. A culture is considered positive if there is growth of a single uropathogen of at least 50,000 CFUs/mL. Lactobacillus, coagulase-negative staphylococcus, and corynebacterium are seldom considered pathogens. The diagnosis of asymptomatic bactiuria should be considered for positive cultures without evidence of pyuria. The sensitivity and specificity of laboratory urine testing for UTI increases significantly as more components of the evaluation are concordant. Relying on a single test to diagnose UTI is not preferred.

C. Imaging Studies

The goal of imaging is to diagnose the presence of urinary tract anomalies that require further evaluation.

Children of any age with a UTI who have a family history of renal or urologic disease, poor growth, or hypertension should undergo a renal and bladder ultrasound. Renal and bladder ultrasound should be performed on febrile infants aged ≤24 months with their first UTI. Older children with recurrent febrile UTIs should also be studied. This evaluation should include assessment of the renal parenchyma and renal size. If a child is not seriously ill or responds quickly to treatment, it may be preferable to delay the ultrasound until UTI treatment is completed to ensure the most accurate assessment of ureter and kidney size. More seriously ill children should be imaged in the first 2 days of treatment to assess for serious complications such as abscess formation.

The optimal treatment of vesicoureteral reflux (VUR) is not presently known. Recent evidence contraindicates a voiding cystourethrogram (VCUG) on all children with a first febrile UTI. VCUG should be performed on children with recurrent febrile UTIs or if ultrasound findings are suggestive of ongoing VUR (renal scarring or poor renal growth or hyrdronephrosis). VCUG should be performed after the patient's symptoms have resolved.

▶ Differential Diagnosis

Urinary tract infection should be considered in any child who presents with a febrile illness in whom the cause of the fever cannot be readily ascertained by physical examination. In premenarcheal girls, chemical urethritis may cause dysuria. Prolonged exposure to bubble baths is a frequent source. Trauma can also cause dysuria, including sexual abuse. Systemic symptoms of infection are absent in these children. In older children, sexually transmitted diseases (STDs) can cause acute urinary symptoms.

▶ Complications

Acute complications of UTI include sepsis, renal abscess, and disseminated infection, including meningitis. Recurrent pyelonephritis can cause renal scarring, which can lead to hypertension or renal insufficiency later in life.

▶ Treatment

A. Acute Infection

Infants aged <2 months with UTI should be hospitalized and treated with intravenous antibiotics as indicated for sepsis until cultures identify the causative organism and the best antibiotic for treatment. Infants aged 2 months to 2 years may be treated as outpatients with oral antibiotics unless they appear toxic, are dehydrated, or are unable to retain oral intake. Older children can usually be treated as outpatients unless they appear seriously ill. The initial choice of antibiotic

may be a sulfonamide, trimethoprim-sulfamethoxazole, a cephalosporin, or amoxicillin-clavulanate. Nitrofurantoin, which is excreted in the urine but does not reach therapeutic blood levels, should not be used to treat febrile children with a UTI. Ideally, the choice of antimicrobial agent should be driven by local patterns of infection and susceptibility. The duration of treatment should be 7–14 days. Treatment courses of ≤3 days have been shown to be inferior in children.

If the child responds clinically to treatment within 2 days, no further immediate follow-up is needed. A child who is not improving after 2 days of treatment should be reevaluated. Retesting and hospital treatment should be considered. Antibiotic treatment should be guided by the patient's urine culture results as they become available.

B. Prevention of Recurrent Infection

Prevention of long-term sequelae focuses on prevention of recurrent infection. Caregivers should be made aware to have patients promptly evaluated for future unexplained febrile illnesses. Infants and children with abnormal ultrasounds or grade III–V VUR should be considered for consultation with a pediatric urologist. In children with structurally normal urinary tracts, treatment of chronic constipation has been shown to decrease the recurrence of UTI, as has behavioral correction of voiding dysfunction associated with incomplete emptying of the bladder. Improving hygiene, especially in girls, has not been shown to decrease UTI rates. Based on retrospective studies, circumcision of boys has been claimed to be associated with decreased UTI rates.

For some children with recurrent UTIs, long-term prophylactic antibiotic treatment may be effective in reducing the frequency of infections. However, there are no clear guidelines as to when this treatment should be considered.

DeMuri GP, Wald ER. Imaging and antimicrobial prophylaxis following the diagnosis of urinary tract infection in children. *Pediatr Infect Dis J.* 2008;27:553–554.

Farhat W, McLorie G. Urethral syndromes in children. *Pediatr Rev.* 2001; 22:17.

Hoberman A, Charron M, Hickey RW, et al. Imaging studies after a first febrile urinary tract infection in young children. *N Engl J Med.* 2003; 348:195.

Keren R. Imaging and treatment strategies for children after first urinary tract infection. *Curr Opin Pediatr.* 2007;19:705–710.

La Scola C, De Mutiis C, Hewitt IK, et al. Different guidelines for imaging after first UTI in febrile infants: yield, cost, and radiation. *Pediatrics.* 2013; 131:e665.

Shah G, Upadhyay J. Controversies in the diagnosis and management of urinary tract infections in children. *Pediatr Drugs.* 2005;7:339–346.

Shaikh N, et al. Prevalence of urinary tract infection in childhood: a meta-analysis. *Pediatr Infect Dis J.* 2008;27:302–308.

Subcommittee on Urinary Tract Infection, Steering Committee on Quality Improvement and Management, Roberts KB. Urinary tract infection: clinical practice guideline for the diagnosis and management of the initial UTI in febrile infants and children 2 to 24 months. *Pediatrics.* 2011;128:595.

6

Skin Diseases in Infants & Children

Mark A. Knox, MD
Barry Coutinho, MD

▼ INFECTIONS OF THE SKIN

IMPETIGO

ESSENTIALS OF DIAGNOSIS

▶ Nonbullous: yellowish crusted plaques.
▶ Bullous: bullae, with minimal surrounding erythema, rupture to leave a shallow ulcer.

▶ General Considerations

Impetigo is a bacterial infection of the skin. More than 70% of cases are of the nonbullous variety.

▶ Pathogenesis

Most cases of nonbullous impetigo are caused by *Staphylococcus aureus,* although group A β-hemolytic streptococci are found in some cases. Coagulase-positive *S. aureus* is the cause of bullous impetigo; methicillin-resistant *S. aureus* (MRSA) has been isolated from patients. Impetigo can develop in traumatized skin, or the bacteria can spread to intact skin from its reservoir in the nose.

▶ Clinical Findings

Nonbullous impetigo usually starts as a small vesicle or pustule, followed by the classic small (<2-cm) honey-colored crusted plaque. The infection may be spread to other parts of the body by fingers or clothing. There is usually little surrounding erythema, itching occurs occasionally, and pain is usually absent. Regional lymphadenopathy is seen in most patients. Without treatment, the lesions resolve without scarring in 2 weeks.

Bullous impetigo is usually seen in infants and young children. Lesions begin on intact skin on almost any part of the body. Flaccid, thin-roofed vesicles develop, which rupture to form shallow ulcers.

▶ Differential Diagnosis

Nonbullous impetigo is unique in appearance. Bullous impetigo is similar in appearance to pemphigus and bullous pemphigoid. Growth of staphylococci from fluid in a bulla confirms the diagnosis.

▶ Complications

Cellulitis follows ~10% of cases of nonbullous impetigo but rarely follows bullous impetigo. Either type may rarely lead to septicemia, septic arthritis, or osteomyelitis. Scarlet fever and poststreptococcal glomerulonephritis, but not rheumatic fever, may follow streptococcal impetigo.

▶ Treatment

Localized disease is effectively treated with mupirocin ointment. Topical 1% retapamulin ointment is a newer, second-line option. Patients with widespread lesions or evidence of cellulitis should be treated with systemic antibiotics effective against staphylococci and streptococci. If infection with MRSA is a possibility, trimethoprim-sulfamethoxazole should be considered where community-acquired MRSA is a likely cause, while intravenous vancomycin is the preferred drug for hospitalized patients.

▶ Patient Education

Further information is available at the following link:
http://www.uptodate.com/contents/impetigo-the-basics?source=see_link

FUNGAL INFECTIONS

▶ General Considerations

Fungal infections of the skin and skin structures may be generally grouped into three categories: dermatophyte infections, other tinea infections, and candidal infections.

▶ Pathogenesis

Dermatophytoses are caused by a group of related fungal species—primarily *Microsporum*, *Trichophyton*, and *Epidermophyton*—that require keratin for growth and can invade hair, nails, and the stratum corneum of the skin. Some of these organisms are spread from person to person; some are zoonotic, spreading from animals to people; and some infect people from the soil. Other fungi can also cause skin disease, such as *Malassezia furfur* in tinea versicolor. Finally, *Candida albicans*, a common resident of the gastrointestinal tract, can cause diaper dermatitis and thrush.

▶ Clinical Findings

A. Symptoms and Signs

1. Dermatophytoses

A. TINEA CORPORIS—Infection of the skin produces one or more characteristic gradually spreading lesions with an erythematous raised border and central areas that are generally scaly but relatively clearer and less indurated than the margins of the lesions. The central clearing helps differentiate these lesions from those of psoriasis. Small lesions may resemble those of nummular eczema. The lesions may have a somewhat serpiginous border, but they are usually more or less round in shape, hence the common name of "ringworm." They can range in size from one to several centimeters.

B. TINEA CAPITIS—Fungal infection of the scalp and hair is the most common dermatophytosis in children. This presents as areas of alopecia with generally regular borders. Typically, the hair shafts break off a few millimeters from the skin surface, distinguishing this from alopecia areata. The infection may also produce a sterile inflammatory mass in the scalp, called a *kerion*, which may be confused with a bacterial infection.

2. Nondermatophyte infections

A. TINEA VERSICOLOR—Tinea versicolor is normally seen in adolescents and adults. The causative organism, *Malassezia furfur,* is part of the normal skin flora. The infection most often becomes evident during warm weather, when new lesions develop. A warm, humid environment, excessive sweating, and genetic susceptibility are important factors for developing this infection. Because treatment does not eradicate the fungus from the skin, it often recurs annually, during the summer months, in susceptible individuals. In chronically warm climates, it is a perennial problem, with new crops of lesions developing unpredictably throughout the year. The lesions are characteristically scaly macules, usually reddish brown in light-skinned people but often hyper- or hypopigmented in people of color. They can be found almost anywhere on the body but are seen most commonly on the torso. The lesions are rarely pruritic. The individual lesions may enlarge and coalesce to form larger lesions with irregular borders.

3. Candidal infections

A. THRUSH—Thrush is a common oral infection in infants. Isolated incidents of this disease are common in immunocompetent infants, but recurrent infections in infants or infections in children and adolescents may indicate an underlying immune deficiency. The infection presents as thick white plaques on the tongue and buccal mucosa. These can be scraped off only with difficulty, revealing an erythematous base.

A. CANDIDAL DIAPER DERMATITIS—This infection is most common in infants aged 2–4 months. *Candida* is a common colonist of the gastrointestinal tract, and infants with diaper dermatitis should be examined for signs of thrush. The fungus does not ordinarily invade the skin, but the warm, humid environment of the diaper area provides an ideal medium for growth. The infection is characterized by an intensely erythematous plaque with a sharply demarcated border. Advancing from the border are numerous satellite papules, which enlarge and coalesce to enlarge the affected area.

B. Special Tests

Dermatophyte and other tinea infections are usually diagnosed clinically. Examination of potassium hydroxide preparations of scrapings from the affected area, which show hyphae, confirms the diagnosis. Fungal cultures may be helpful when the diagnosis is suspected but cannot otherwise be confirmed. Diagnosis of candidal infections is generally made by clinical findings.

▶ Treatment

Tinea corporis is treated with topical antifungal medications. Nystatin, miconazole, clotrimazole, ketoconazole, and terbinafine creams are all effective. Rarely, widespread infection requires systemic therapy.

Topical therapy is ineffective in tinea capitis, although shampoos containing 2% ketoconazole or 1% selenium sulfide have been shown to reduce fungal colony counts and are sometimes recommended for use 2–3 times per week as adjunct therapy (Ali, et al. 2007). The gold standard for treatment has long been griseofulvin, but because of the 6-week duration of therapy required, other treatments of shorter duration are becoming more popular. Although not approved by the FDA for this use, fluconazole, itraconazole, and terbinafine have been shown to be at least as effective, if not more so, and require shorter courses of therapy, generally 2–4 weeks (Ali, et al. 2007). Ketoconazole is not recommended because of rare incidents of hepatotoxicity.

Ali S, Graham TAD, Forgie SED. The assesment and management of tinea capitis in children. *Pediatr Emerg Care.* 2007; 23: 662–665.

Tinea versicolor can be treated with topical selenium sulfide lotion or any of the previously listed topical creams. In older children, systemic treatment can also be given, with either ketoconazole or fluconazole as single doses. Ketoconazole may be given monthly as prophylaxis if recurrences are frequent (Crespo-Erchiga and Florencia 2006).

Crespo-Erchiga V, Florencia VD. Malassizia yeasts and pityriasis versicolor. *Curr Opin Infect Dis*, 2006;19:139–147.

Candidal infections are most often treated with nystatin. Diaper dermatitis responds well to topical nystatin cream. If intense inflammation is present, topical steroids for a few days may be helpful. Thrush is usually treated with nystatin suspension. Up to 2 weeks may be needed for complete resolution of the infection. In resistant cases, the mouth may be painted with gentian violet. Clotrimazole lozenges are an effective alternative, but most children who develop thrush are too young to use the lozenges appropriately.

Prognosis

All these infections in immunocompetent children respond well to treatment. However, left untreated, they can cause widespread and significant skin disease.

Patient Education

Further information is available at the following links:

http://familydoctor.org/familydoctor/en/diseases-conditions/tinea-infections.html

http://www.mayoclinic.com/health/tinea-versicolor/DS00635

http://familydoctor.org/familydoctor/en/diseases-conditions/diaper-rash.html

▼ PARASITIC INFESTATIONS

SCABIES

ESSENTIALS OF DIAGNOSIS

- ► Intense pruritus.
- ► Small erythematous papules.
- ► Burrows are pathognomonic but may not be seen.

Pathogenesis

Scabies is a common infestation caused by the mite *Sarcoptes scabiei*. The disease is acquired by physical contact with an infected person. Transmission of the disease by contact with infested linens or clothing is less common, because the mites can live off the body for only 2–3 days. The female mite burrows between the superficial and deeper layers of the epidermis, laying eggs and depositing feces as she goes along. After 4–5 weeks, her egg laying is complete, and she dies in the burrow. The eggs hatch, releasing larvae that move to the skin surface, molt into nymphs, mature to adults, mate, and begin the cycle again. Pruritus is caused by an allergic reaction to mite antigens.

Clinical Findings

A. Symptoms and Signs

Diagnosis is based primarily on clinical suspicion, as physical findings are highly variable and the disease can mimic a wide variety of skin conditions. The classic early symptom is intense pruritus. The usual finding is 1- to 2-mm erythematous papules, often in a linear pattern. The finding of burrows connecting the papules is diagnostic but is not always seen. In infants, the disease may involve the entire body—including the face, scalp, palms, and soles—and pustules and vesicles are common. In older children and adolescents, the lesions are most often seen in the interdigital spaces, wrist flexors, umbilicus, groin, and genitalia. Severe infestation may produce widespread crusted lesions.

B. Special Tests

Superficial scrapings under mineral oil may show entire mites, eggs, or fecal pellets. However, success in finding these is limited and a negative examination does not rule out the disease.

Treatment

Permethrin 5% cream, applied to the entire body (excluding the face in older children), is the preferred treatment in subjects aged ≥2 months. Treatment will kill mites and eliminate the risk of contagion within 24 hours. However, pruritus may continue for several days to 2 weeks after treatment. The entire family should be treated at the same time, and all clothing and bedding should ideally be machine-washed in hot water (>60°C). A single 200-µg/kg oral dose of ivermectin, repeated in 2 weeks, is now an effective treatment option in patients aged >5 years who weigh >15 kg, with no serious adverse reactions.

Currie BJ, McCarthy JS. Permethrin and ivermectin for scabies. *N Engl J Med.* 2010;362:717–725.

Patient Education

Further information is available at the following link:
http://kidshealth.org/PageManager.jsp?lic=44&article_set=22947

LICE (PEDICULOSIS)

ESSENTIALS OF DIAGNOSIS

▶ Pruritus.
▶ Visualization of lice on the body or nits in hair.

Pathogenesis

Three varieties of lice cause human disease. *Pediculus humanus corporis* causes infestations on the body, and *P. humanus capitis* causes infestation on the head. *Phthirus pubis*, or crab lice, infests the pubic area. All are spread by physical contact, either with an infested person or with clothing, towels, or hairbrushes that have been in recent contact with an infested person. Symptoms are caused by an allergic reaction to louse antigens that develop after a period of sensitization. Body lice can be a vector for other disease, such as typhus, trench fever, and relapsing fever. Infestation with pubic lice is highly correlated with infection by other sexually transmitted diseases. Nits are the eggs of the louse. They are cemented to hairs, are usually <1 mm in length, and are translucent. Body lice lay their nits in the seams of clothing. The nits can remain viable for ≤1 month and will hatch when exposed to body heat when the clothing is worn again.

Prevention

Body lice are associated primarily with poor hygiene and can be prevented by regular bathing and washing of clothing and bedding. Patients with hair lice must not share clothing, hair accessories, combs, brushes, or towels.

Clinical Findings

The cardinal symptom of louse infestation is pruritus, which develops as the person becomes sensitized. Excoriations in the infested area are common. The lice themselves can usually be seen easily. Head and pubic lice are easily seen, but body lice are present on the body only when feeding.

Treatment

Permethrin 5% cream, applied for 8–12 hours, is the treatment of choice for body lice. Clothing and bedding should be heat-washed, because exposure to hot water will kill the nits. Permethrin 1% cream rinse is used to treat head and pubic lice.

Newer treatments for head lice include a single application of spinosad 0.9% topical suspension in children aged ≥4 years, or topical ivermectin 0.5% in patients aged ≥6 months. Malathion 0.5% lotion may be considered when permethrin resistance is suspected. Use of nit removal combs have not been proven as effective alternatives or adjuncts to topical pediculicides.

Gunning K, Pippitt K, et al. Pediculosis and scabies: treatment update. *Am Fam Physician*. 2012; 86(6):535

Patient Education

Further information is available at the following link:
http://familydoctor.org/familydoctor/en/diseases-conditions/head-lice.html

▼ INFECTIOUS DISEASES WITH SKIN MANIFESTATIONS

BACTERIAL INFECTIONS

Scarlet Fever (Scarlatina)

ESSENTIALS OF DIAGNOSIS

▶ Symptoms of streptococcal pharyngitis.
▶ "Sandpaper" rash.
▶ Circumoral pallor.
▶ "Strawberry" tongue (red or white).

General Considerations

Scarlet fever is an infection caused by certain strains of group A streptococci. The infection most commonly begins as a typical streptococcal pharyngitis, but it can also follow streptococcal cellulitis or infection of wounds or burns.

Clinical Findings

The classic feature of scarlet fever is the rash. It develops 12–48 hours after the onset of pharyngitis symptoms, usually beginning in the neck, axillae, and groin and becoming generalized within 24 hours. The rash is a fine, faintly erythematous exanthem that is often more easily felt than seen, giving it the name of "sandpaper" rash. The rash itself is seldom present on the face, but there is often flushing of the face except for the area around the mouth (circumoral pallor). The tongue is often erythematous and swollen. In the early stages of the disease, the tongue may have swollen papillae protruding through a white coating (white "strawberry" tongue). Later in the illness, the coating desquamates, leaving the tongue red and the papillae swollen (red "strawberry" tongue). After about 1 week, desquamation begins on the face and progresses downward over the body, finally involving the hands and feet.

Differential Diagnosis

Kawasaki disease and any of the viral exanthems may be confused with scarlet fever.

Complications

Scarlet fever is generally a benign disease. In severe cases, bacteremia and sepsis may occur, and rheumatic fever may follow an untreated infection. Glomerulonephritis may also be a sequel.

Treatment

Treatment of scarlet fever is no different from treatment of the primary streptococcal infection (see Chapter 5).

Patient Education

Further information is available at the following link:
http://www.mayoclinic.com/health/scarlet-fever/DS00917

VIRAL INFECTIONS

Roseola (Exanthem Subitum)

ESSENTIALS OF DIAGNOSIS

▶ Sudden onset of high fever.
▶ No diagnostic signs.
▶ Development of rash as fever breaks after 3–4 days.

Pathogenesis

Human herpesvirus 6 (HHV6) causes the vast majority of cases of clinical roseola, although other viruses cause some cases as well. It is rare in infants aged <3 months and in children aged >2 years; most cases occur in infants between the ages of 6 and 12 months. Infections occur year round.

Clinical Findings

A. Symptoms and Signs

The hallmark of roseola is the abrupt onset of high fever, often 39.4°–41.1°C (103°–106°F). Febrile seizures occur in up to one-third of patients. Despite the high fever, children usually look relatively well. Mild signs of the upper respiratory infection may be seen, but there are no diagnostic signs. After 3–4 days, the fever breaks suddenly, followed by the appearance of a rash. This is usually a macular or maculopapular rash that starts on the trunk and spreads to the arms and neck and then often to the face and legs. The rash resolves within 3 days, but it may be more transient.

B. Laboratory Findings

Laboratory findings are usually normal.

Differential Diagnosis

In the early stages of the disease, many children with high fever and seizures are admitted to the hospital for workup of suspected meningitis or sepsis. After the rash appears, the diagnosis is obvious in retrospect.

Complications

Rare cases of encephalitis or fulminant hepatitis have been reported.

Treatment & Prognosis

Treatment is entirely symptomatic. Unless the patient develops one of the rare complications listed earlier, roseola is a benign, self-limited infection.

Patient Education

Further information is available at the following link:
http://www.mayoclinic.com/health/roseola/DS00452

Varicella (Chickenpox)

ESSENTIALS OF DIAGNOSIS

▶ Prodrome of upper respiratory–like symptoms.
▶ Rash consists of small vesicles on erythematous base.
▶ Vesicles rupture with crusting.

General Considerationss

Prior to widespread immunization of children, approximately 90% of adults in the United States manifested serologic evidence of varicella infection, regardless of whether they had clinically apparent disease.

Pathogenesis

The varicella-zoster virus is a herpesvirus. After resolution of the initial infection, the virus produces a latent infection in the dorsal root ganglia. Reactivation produces herpes zoster ("shingles").

Prevention

Childhood immunization should prevent most disease. The vaccine is given in two doses—the first between 12 and 18 months of age, and the second between 4 and 6 years of age. Varicella-zoster immune globulin can help prevent infection in immunocompromised children, nonimmune pregnant women who are exposed to the virus, and newborns exposed to maternal varicella.

Centers for Disease Control. *MMWR*. 57 (51,52):Q1–Q4. Jan. 2, 2009.

Clinical Findings

The usual incubation period of varicella is about 14 days. Most children experience a prodromal phase of upper respiratory–like symptoms for 1–2 days before the onset of the rash. Fever is usually moderate. Almost all infected children will develop a rash. The extent of the rash is highly variable. Lesions usually begin on the trunk or head but eventually can involve the entire body. The classic lesion is a pruritic erythematous macule that develops a clear central vesicle. After 1–2 days, the vesicle ruptures, forming a crust. New lesions develop daily for 3–7 days, and typically lesions are scattered over the body in various states of evolution at the same time. Ulcerative lesions on the buccal mucosa are common. The infection is contagious from the onset of the prodrome until the last of the lesions has crusted over.

Differential Diagnosis

Varicella usually presents as an unmistakable clinical picture, but the rash may be missed in children with mild disease.

Complications

In immunocompetent children, the most common complication is bacterial superinfection of the lesions, causing cellulitis or impetigo. Other, more serious complications are most common in children aged <5 years or adults aged >20 years. Meningoencephalitis and cerebellar ataxia can occur. These normally resolve within 1–3 days without sequelae. Viral hepatitis is common but normally subclinical. Varicella pneumonia is uncommon in healthy children; it usually resolves after 1–3 days but may progress to respiratory failure in rare cases.

Treatment

Treatment is ordinarily symptomatic, including antipruritic medications if needed. Aspirin should be avoided, to prevent development of Reye syndrome. Patients with signs of disseminated varicella, such as encephalitis and pneumonia, should be treated with intravenous acyclovir.

Prognosis

Varicella is normally a benign, self-limited disease. Complications in immunocompetent children are rare.

Patient Education

Further information is available at the following link:
  http://familydoctor.org/familydoctor/en/diseases-conditions/chickenpox.html

Erythema Infectiosum (Fifth Disease)

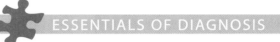

ESSENTIALS OF DIAGNOSIS

▶ Prodrome of mild upper respiratory–like symptoms.
▶ Rash begins as erythema of cheeks, then becomes more generalized—macular at first, then reticular.
▶ Rash lasts 1–3 weeks.

General Considerations

Erythema infectiosum (fifth disease) is a common childhood infection that rarely causes clinically significant disease.

Pathogenesis

The disease is caused by parvovirus B19. It appears sporadically but often in epidemics in communities. Children are infectious during the prodromal stage, which is inapparent or mild and usually indistinguishable from an upper respiratory infection. The rash is an immune-mediated phenomenon that occurs after the infection, so children with the rash are not infectious and should not be restricted from school or other activities.

Clinical Findings

Erythema infectiosum begins with a prodromal stage of upper respiratory symptoms, headache, and low-grade fever. This stage may be clinically inapparent.

The rash occurs in three phases, often transient enough to go unnoticed. The first stage is facial flushing, described as a "slapped cheek" appearance. Shortly afterward, the rash becomes generalized over the body, initially as a faint erythematous, often confluent, macular rash. In the third stage, the central regions of the macules clear, leaving a distinctive faint reticular rash. The rash comes and goes evanescently over the body and can last from 1 to 3 weeks. There are rarely any other associated findings.

Differential Diagnosis

Erythema infectiosum is usually clinically recognizable, but it may be confused with other viral exanthems.

Complications

Arthritis is rare in children but may occur in adolescents. Thrombocytopenic purpura and aseptic meningitis are rare complications.

Fetal hydrops and fetal demise may be seen in fetuses whose mothers contract the infection. It is estimated that ≤5% of infected fetuses will be affected by the virus.

Treatment & Prognosis

There is no known treatment for this disease. Except for rare complications in children, this is a benign infection. Fetal complications are unusual.

Patient Education

Further information is available at the following link:
http://familydoctor.org/familydoctor/en/diseases-conditions/fifth-disease.html

INFLAMMATORY DISORDERS OF THE SKIN

ATOPIC DERMATITIS

 ESSENTIALS OF DIAGNOSIS

▶ Pruritus is the cardinal symptom.
▶ Lesions are excoriated, are scaly, and may become lichenified.

General Considerations

Atopic dermatitis is a common skin disorder in children, affecting 10–15% of the population. It appears during the first year of life in 60% of cases and during the first 5 years in 85%.

Pathogenesis

The cause of atopic dermatitis is unclear. It has a strong association, both in the individual and in families, with allergic rhinitis and asthma, and is classified as an atopic disorder. Food allergies, primarily to cow's milk, wheat, eggs, soy, fish, and peanuts, have been implicated in 20–30% of cases. In recent years, however, there has been a shift in thinking about cause and effect. Rather than being a primary allergic disorder that leads to changes in skin architecture, many authorities now consider atopic dermatitis to be primarily an epidermal barrier defect, which allows allergens, including food

allergens, to penetrate the skin and stimulate an immune response (Bieber 2008).

Bieber T. Atopic dermatitis. *N Engl J Med.* 2008;358:1483–1494.

Clinical Findings

The diagnosis is based on the presence of three of the following major criteria: (1) pruritus, (2) lesions with typical morphology and distribution, (3) facial and extensor involvement in infants and children, (4) chronic or chronically relapsing dermatitis, and (5) personal or family history of atopic disease.

Pruritus is the hallmark of the disease, usually preceding the skin lesions, which usually develop as a reaction to scratching. The skin becomes excoriated, develops weeping and crusting, and later may become scaly or lichenified. Secondary bacterial infection is common. In infants, the lesions usually involve the face but may appear in a generalized pattern over much of the body. In young children, the extensor surfaces of the extremities are often involved. In older children and adults, the disease often moves to involve the flexion areas of the extremities instead. The disease typically is chronic, although remissions and relapses are common.

Differential Diagnosis

Atopic dermatitis may be confused with seborrheic dermatitis, especially in infants, in whom facial lesions are common. Atopic dermatitis seldom follows the distribution of oil glands, as is typical with seborrheic dermatitis. It may also be confused with psoriasis, contact dermatitis, scabies, and cutaneous fungal infections.

Complications

The most common complication is secondary bacterial infection. Low-grade bacterial infection should be considered as a factor in lesions that do not respond well to usual therapies.

Treatment

Nonpharmacologic measures are important in the treatment of this disease. Long baths and bathing in hot water exacerbate dryness of the skin and should be avoided. Use of soaps that do not contain fragrances may be helpful, or it may be necessary to use nonsoap cleansers instead. Moisturizers that contain fragrances and other irritants will aggravate the problem. If secondary infection is suspected, systemic antibiotics effective against streptococci and staphylococci should be given.

Topical corticosteroids are the mainstay of treatment. The lowest potency preparation that is effective should be used, especially on the face and the diaper area, which are more sensitive to the skin atrophy associated with the prolonged use of higher-potency steroids. The use of high-potency steroids over large areas of the body has the potential for significant systemic absorbtion and suppression of the hypothalamic-pituitary-adrenal axis (Pariser 2009). Systemic steroids are useful for severe acute flares. Antipruritic medications may be useful, but these all have significant sedative side effects. Doxepin, a tricyclic antidepressant with strong antihistaminic effects, is often useful in patients with severe manifestations. Cyclosporine and mycophenolate are useful for the most refractory cases (Denby and Beck 2012).

Tacrolimus and pimecrolimus, topical immune modulators, are less effective than high-potency topical steroids. Whether they are as effective or less effective than medium-potency steroids is unclear. In most patients, there is little or no systemic absorption of either of these drugs, although pimecrolimus appears to produce lower blood concentrations than tacrolimus (Pariser 2009). Because these drugs do not cause skin atrophy, they may be useful for prolonged treatment of facial lesions. In February 2005, the Food and Drug Administration issued a "black box" warning for these drugs, prompted by concerns of cancer related to lymphoproliferative changes seen in some posttransplantation patients. A joint taskforce of the American Academy of Allergy, Asthma, and Immunology and the American College of Allergy, Asthma, and Immunology reviewed the data the same year and concluded that the evidence did not support a causal link between these drugs and lymphoma.

Denby KS, Beck LA. Update on systemic therapies for atopic dermatitis. *Curr Opin Allergy Clin Immunol.* 2012; 12:421–426.
Fonacier L, Spergel JM, Leung DYM. The black box warning for topical calcineurin inhibitors: looking outside the box. *Ann Allerg Asthma Immunol.* 2006; 97:117–120.
Pariser D. Topical corticosteroids and topical calcineurin inhibitors in the treatment of atopic dermatitis: focus on percutaneous absorption. *Am J Therap.* 2009; 16:264–273.

Prognosis

Although it is usually fairly easily controlled, atopic dermatitis is a chronic skin disorder. It often becomes less severe as children grow into school age, but relapses and persistence of some disease into adulthood is common.

Patient Education

Further information is available at the following link:
http://familydoctor.org/familydoctor/en/diseases-conditions/eczema-and-atopic-dermatitis.html

SEBORRHEIC DERMATITIS

ESSENTIALS OF DIAGNOSIS

▶ Inflamed lesions with yellowish or brownish crusting.
▶ Lesions may be localized or generalized.

General Considerations

Seborrheic dermatitis is a common inflammatory disorder of the skin. It is most common in infancy and adolescence, when the sebaceous glands are more active. It generally resolves or becomes less severe after infancy, but localized lesions or mild, generalized scalp disease may be seen throughout adulthood.

Pathogenesis

The exact cause of seborrheic dermatitis is unknown. Infection with *Malassezia* yeasts has been implicated, and the disease may be caused by an abnormal inflammatory or immune response to the fungus.

Clinical Findings

The typical lesions of seborrheic dermatitis are inflammatory macular lesions, usually with brownish or yellowish scaling. Inflammation may begin during the first month of life, and it usually becomes evident within the first year. In infants, the lesions may be generalized, but in older children, lesions are most common in areas where sebaceous glands are concentrated, such as the scalp, face, and axillae. Marginal blepharitis may be seen. Cradle cap is a common variant seen in infants, either by itself or in association with other lesions. This is seen as scaling and crusting of the scalp, often with extremely heavy buildup of scale in untreated infants.

Differential Diagnosis

Atopic dermatitis is the main element in the differential diagnosis. The disease may also be confused with psoriasis and other cutaneous fungal infections.

Complications

Secondary infection, either bacterial or fungal, is a common complication.

Treatment

Topical treatment with antifungal creams or shampoo is the mainstay of treatment. Topical steroids may be used for intense inflammation. Short courses of treatment with oral antifungal drugs, such as fluconazole, may be useful for control of severe or widespread disease. Scalp lesions usually respond to antiseborrheic shampoos, such as selenium sulfide. Cradle cap is treated by soaking the scales with mineral oil and then gently débriding them with a toothbrush or washcloth. Following débridment, cleansing with baby shampoo is normally adequate for control; antiseborrheic or antifungal shampoos are rarely necessary.

Gupta AK, Nicol K, Batra R. Role of antifungal agents in the treatment of seborrheic dermatitis. *Am J Clin Dermatol.* 2004;5:417–422.

Prognosis

Seborrheic dermatitis generally resolves or lessens in severity after infancy, but localized lesions or mild, generalized scalp disease may be seen throughout adulthood.

Patient Education

Further information is available at the following link:

http://familydoctor.org/familydoctor/en/diseases-conditions/seborrheic-dermatitis.html

ACNE VULGARIS

 ESSENTIALS OF DIAGNOSIS

► Comedones, open or closed.
► Papules, pustules, or nodules.

General Considerations

Acne vulgaris is an extremely common skin disease in older children and adolescents. The prevalence of this disorder increases with age: 30–60% of 10–12-year-olds and 80–95% of 16–18-year-olds are affected.

Pathogenesis

Acne is caused by the interaction of several factors in the pilosebaceous unit of the skin. The basic abnormality is excessive sebum production caused by sebaceous gland hyperplasia and generally related to androgenic influences. Hyperkeratinization of the hair follicle results in obstruction of the follicle and the formation of a microcomedone. Sebum and cellular debris accumulate, forming an environment that can become colonized by *Propionibacterium acnes*. The presence of the bacteria provokes an immune response that includes the production of inflammatory mediators. Lesions are most commonly seen in areas of the body that have the highest concentration of sebaceous glands. The face is the most common site for lesions to develop, but the chest, back, neck, and upper arms may be affected as well.

Although the androgenic influences that cause the increase in sebum production are generally related to puberty, numerous factors can cause or aggravate acne. Mechanical obstruction or irritation (eg, by shirt collars) can be a factor. Cosmetics can occlude follicles and trigger eruptions. Medications, most commonly anabolic steroids, corticosteroids, lithium, and phenytoin, can cause or aggravate acne. Hyperandrogenic states, such as polycystic ovary syndrome, are often associated with acne. Emotional stress has been shown to exacerbate the problem. Finally, the role of diet has long been controversial. No specific foods have been found to aggravate acne, despite common assumptions. However, acne is almost uniformly a disease of Western cultures, and some authorities are studying the role of the high-glycemic-index Western diet in its development. This diet leads to higher levels of insulinlike growth factor, which has androgenic effects.

Clinical Findings

Several types of lesions characterize this disease, and they can occur in varying combinations and degrees of severity. Microcomedones can evolve into visible comedones, either open ("blackheads") or closed ("whiteheads"). Inflammatory papules and pustules may develop. Nodules are pustules with diameters of >5 mm. Hyperpigmentation and scarring may develop at the sites of more severe lesions.

Multiple classification systems have been devised to characterize this disorder. The disease may be classed as comedonal, papulopustular (inflammatory), and nodulocystic (also inflammatory, but more severe). The American Academy of Dermatology defines three levels of severity. In mild acne, there are a few to several papules and pustules, but no nodules. In moderate acne, there are several to many papules and pustules and a few to several nodules. In severe disease, there are extensive papules and pustules, along with many nodules.

Differential Diagnosis

The diagnosis is usually straightforward. The physician should consider drug-induced acne if the patient is taking any medications. Severe acne in athletes raises the possibility of anabolic steroid use. In women, severe acne, hirsutism, and other signs of virilization suggest an underlying hyperandrogenic condition.

Complications

The primary morbidity of acne is psychological. This can be a serious problem for the adolescent patient. Hyperpigmentation and scarring may result from more severe disease, especially from nodulocystic acne.

Treatment

The various treatments for acne are aimed at reducing infection and inflammation, normalizing the rate of desquamation of follicular epithelium, or correcting hormone excesses or other systemic factors. Treatments work better in combination than singly.

A. Topical Antibiotics

Antibiotics are directed at the infectious component of acne. By reducing infection, they also have a beneficial effect on the inflammatory component of the disease. *P. acnes* has been developing antibiotic resistance worldwide, and this may be responsible for some treatment failures

Available topical antibiotic preparations include erythromycin, clindamycin, benzoyl peroxide, topical dapsone, and azelaic acid. Available evidence shows that erythromycin and clindamycin work better in combination with benzoyl peroxide than either agent alone, and this also limits the development of resistance. The different strengths of benzoyl peroxide appear to be about equally effective.

B. Oral Antibiotics

It is generally believed that oral antibiotics are more effective than topical agents and therefore more useful in severe disease. However, because few, if any, good-quality comparisons of the two modalities exist, it is impossible to be certain of this. Tetracycline is the mainstay of oral antibiotic treatment. Side effects are minimal—primarily gastrointestinal upset. Doxycycline may be taken with food to minimize gastric upset, but this agent is more photosensitizing than tetracycline. Minocycline is a more effective agent against *P. acnes* than the other tetracyclines, but it is more expensive and has a higher incidence of serious side effects, such as vertigo and lupuslike syndrome. It is generally best reserved for disease that does not respond to first-line agents. All tetracyclines bond to calcium in bone and teeth and can cause staining of dental enamel. They should not be given to children younger than 10 years of age. Erythromycin is an alternative when tetracyclines cannot be used.

C. Topical Retinoids

Retinoids are derivatives of vitamin A. They prevent the formation of comedones by normalizing the desquamation of the follicular epithelium. Tretinoin has been in use much longer than the other agents, adapalene and tazarotene. All agents have the main adverse effect of excessive drying, burning, and inflammation of the skin. This can be ameliorated by changing to a lower concentration of the agent or by periodically skipping a day of application. Although tretinoin has been rated pregnancy category C, and there are no clear indications of teratogenicity, the role of topical retinoids in pregnancy is a matter of debate. Tazarotene has been designated pregnancy category X.

All agents are available in various strengths and vehicles. The choice of vehicle is determined by the patient's skin type.

D. Isotretinoin

Isotretinoin is a metabolite of vitamin A that reduces sebaceous gland size, decreases sebum production, and normalizes desquamation of follicular epithelium. It is effective for severe nodular acne and for acne unresponsive to other treatments. Adverse effects are common, including dry eyes, dry skin, headache, and mild elevation in liver enzymes and serum lipids. Benign intracranial hypertension is less common but must be considered if the patient develops headaches. Despite commonly held beliefs, evidence does not support the idea that depression is a side effect of this drug. Isotretinoin is extremely teratogenic, with major malformations occurring in 40% of infants exposed during the first trimester, so it must be used only after a negative pregnancy test—preferably after two negative tests—and with strict attention to contraception. Enrollment in the iPLEDGE program is a prerequisite to prescription of isotretinoin in the United States.

E. Hormonal Therapy

Because of the antiandrogenic effect of the progestin component, combined oral contraceptives are effective in reducing the severity of acne in women. Although some newer brands have been explicitly marketed for this indication, they have not been proved superior to older, less expensive brands.

F. Combination Therapy

Agents for the treatment of acne work best in combination. The choice of agents can be tailored to the severity of the disease. Because of the time required for complete turnover of the epithelium, at least 6–8 weeks of treatment should be given before assessing the effectiveness of the regimen. If the disease is not adequately controlled, the regimen may be intensified (eg, by increasing the concentration of a retinoid, changing from a topical to an oral antibiotic, or adding another agent). Patients should be advised that total suppression of lesions may not be possible; otherwise, the patient's assessment can be used as a guide to decide whether more intensive treatment is necessary.

There are several guidelines for combination therapy:

For patients with comedones only, retinoids are the first line of therapy. These are applied once a day to the entire area involved.

For most patients with mild to moderate acne, combination treatment with topical antibiotics plus topical retinoids is the first-line treatment.

For moderate to severe inflammatory acne, oral antibiotics can be substituted for topical agents.

For severe nodulocystic acne or for disease unresponsive to other regimens, isotretinoin is the treatment of choice.

G. Other Treatments

Intralesional steroids may be used as an adjunct for treating acne nodules. Laser and photodynamic therapy are newer options for acne treatment, although studies are of variable quality.

▶ Prognosis

Although in general, acne diminishes at the end of adolescence, it may persist into adult life.

Haider A, Shaw J. Treatment of acne vulgaris. *JAMA*. 2004;292:726. [PMID: 15304471] (Comprehensive review of available treatments.)

Liao D. Management of acne. *J Fam Practice*. 2003; 52:43. [PMID: 12540312] (Evidence-based review of treatment.)

Thiboutot D, Gollnick H, et al. New insights into the management of acne: an update from the Global Alliance to Improve Outcomes in Acne group. *J Am Acad Dermatol*. 2009; 60 (5 suppl):S1–S50.

Routine Childhood Vaccines

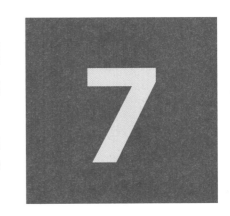

Richard Kent Zimmerman, MD, MPH
Donald B. Middleton, MD

Routine vaccination during childhood is among the most significant of all medical advances. Although many vaccine preventable diseases such as *Haemophilus influenza b* infection are now rarely encountered, others such as pertussis persist despite widespread vaccination. Concerns about vaccine efficacy, safety, and duration of protection continue to interfere with universal acceptance of some vaccines such as mumps-measles-rubella (MMR) vaccine despite demonstrated effectiveness. Important concerns about vaccination include the child's age and underlying medical conditions, disease burden, vaccine efficacy and adverse reactions, and official recommendations.

General Rules for Vaccination

To achieve optimal protection, the clinician should vaccinate all patients in accordance with the timeline of the Centers for Disease Control and Prevention (CDC) universal vaccine schedule (**Figure 7-1**). With few exceptions all vaccine doses count for all time. Prolonged delay between vaccine doses does not necessitate restarting a vaccine series. Doses should not be given early, with the exception that a 4-day grace period be allowed. Storage and management issues are covered in CDC publications.

HEPATITIS B VACCINE

In the United States the estimated number of persons chronically infected with hepatitis B virus (HBV) is 1.25 million, 36% of whom acquired HBV during childhood. HBV infection becomes chronic in 90% of infected infants, with 30–60% of those infected before the age of 4 years, and 5–10% of those infected as adults. Each year in the United States, HBV kills about 6000 people. Up to 25% of infants infected with HBV will eventually die of HBV-related cirrhosis or liver cancer. Under universal hepatitis B vaccination, reported new cases of HBV fell to 3374 in 2010.

Hepatitis B virus transmission occurs primarily by blood exposure or by sexual contact with infected persons. The source of infection is not identified in 30–40% of cases. Some cases may result from in apparent contamination of skin lesions or mucosal surfaces; hepatitis B surface antigen (HBsAg) has been found in impetigo, in saliva, on toothbrush holders of persons chronically infected with HBV, and on used blood sugar testing stylets. Infants and children can transmit HBV.

Rationale for Routine Hepatitis B Vaccination

Although anti-HBV antibody levels diminish over time, most persons maintain protection through immunologic memory in lymphocytes. Immunologic memory and the long incubation period of HBV infection allow most immunized persons to mount a protective anamnestic immune response. Therefore low or absent serum antibody levels do not accurately predict susceptibility to HBV.

The number of vaccine doses administered, intervals between doses, genetics, prematurity, and underlying medical conditions affect immunogenicity. After the third dose of hepatitis B (HepB) vaccine, more than 95% of children seroconvert. Efficacy for HepB vaccine is high. Immunosuppression and prematurity with low birth weight are associated with lower rates of seroconversion. HepB vaccination should be delayed in preterm infants weighing <2 kg until 1 month of age or hospital discharge, whichever is first, unless the mother is HBsAg-positive or has unknown HBsAg status, in which case HepB vaccine should be given within 12 hours of birth.

Adverse Reactions

Of all children infected with HBV, 3–9% have pain at the injection site; 8–18% have mild, transient systemic adverse

For those who fall behind or start late, provide catch-up vaccination at the earliest opportunity as indicated by the orange bars in the figure. School entry and adolescent vaccine age groups are in bold.

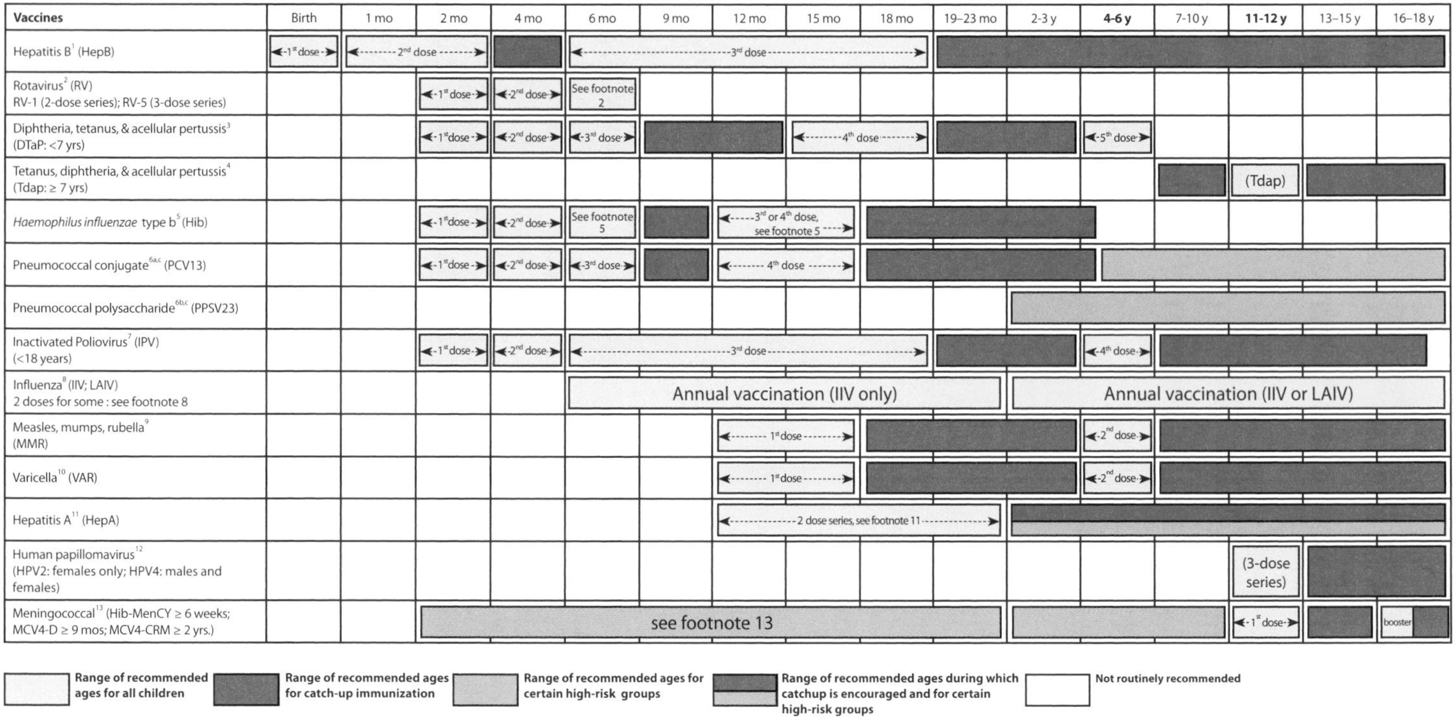

This schedule includes recommendations in effect as of January 1, 2013. Any dose not administered at the recommended age should be administered at a subsequent visit, when indicated and feasible. The use of a combination vaccine generally is preferred over separate injections of its equivalent component vaccines. Vaccination providers should consult the relevant Advisory Committee on Immunization Practices (ACIP) statement for detailed recommendations, available online at http://www.cdc.gov/vaccines/pubs/acip-list.htm. Clinically significant adverse events that follow vaccination should be reported to the Vaccine Adverse Event Reporting System (VAERS) online (http://www.vaers.hhs.gov) or by telephone (800-822-7967).Suspected cases of vaccine-preventable diseases should be reported to the state or local health department. Additional information, including precautions and contraindications for vaccination, is available from CDC online (http://www.cdc.gov/vaccines) or by telephone (800-CDC-INFO [800-232-4636]).

This schedule is approved by the Advisory Committee on Immunization Practices (http://www.cdc.gov/vaccines/acip/index.html), the American Academy of Pediatrics (http://www.aap.org), the American Academy of Family Physicians (http://www.aafp.org), and the American College of Obstetricians and Gynecologists (http://www.acog.org).

NOTE: The above recommendations must be read along with the footnotes of this schedule.

▲ **Figure 7-1.** Recommended immunization schedule for persons aged 0–18 years, 2013, United States.

events such as fatigue and headache; and 1–6% have temperature higher than 37.7°C (99.8°F).

Recommendations

The comprehensive US hepatitis B vaccination policy includes: (1) prevention of perinatal HBV infection, (2) routine vaccination of infants, (3) catch-up immunization of adolescents not previously vaccinated, and (4) unvaccinated adults aged 19–59 years with diabetes mellitus (type 1 and type 2) as soon as possible after a diagnosis of diabetes is confirmed. Routine postvaccination testing is not indicated except for anti-HBs and HBsAg testing at age 9–18 months for infants born to HBsAg-positive mothers. An adequate antibody response is a titer of ≥10 mIU/mL.

HEPATITIS A VACCINE

All infants should receive two doses of hepatitis A vaccine. The first dose is given at age 12–15 months and the second dose, 6 months later. Side effects include localized swelling and redness.

PERTUSSIS VACCINE

More than 41,000 cases of pertussis were reported in the United States in 2012, representing hundreds of thousands of infections. Waning immunity after childhood pertussis vaccination, partial protection, and alterations in pertussis surface proteins are apparent reasons for disease perpetuation. Most pertussis-related hospitalizations and deaths occur in infants too young to be fully vaccinated. Infants aged <12 months suffer a case/fatality rate of 0.6%.

Pertussis is highly contagious; 70–100% of susceptible household contacts and 50–80% of susceptible school contacts become infected following exposure. Contagion lasts from 1 week after exposure to 3 weeks after the onset of symptoms. Transmission is by respiratory droplets or occasionally by contact with freshly contaminated objects. Adults and adolescents are the primary source of pertussis infection for young infants. The reported incidence rate among adults and adolescents has risen.

Paroxysmal cough can last for months, with significant disruption of daily activities. Complications of pertussis include pneumonia, the leading cause of death, and seizures. Encephalopathy, due to hypoxia or minute cerebral hemorrhages, occurs in ~1% of cases, is fatal in about one-third of those afflicted, and causes permanent brain damage in another one-third.

Rationale for Vaccination

Before routine pertussis vaccination, peaks in whooping cough incidence occurred approximately every 3–4 years, infecting virtually all children. In the United States between 1925 and 1930, 36,013 persons died as a result of pertussis-related

complications. With widespread pertussis vaccination, the incidence of pertussis dropped by >95%, although it has been increasing in recent years, partly as a result of improved diagnostic technics. Diphtheria, tetanus, acellular pertussis (DTaP) vaccines have efficacy rates ranging from 80% to 89%. All available pertussis containing vaccines also vaccinate against tetanus and diphtheria.

Adverse Reactions

Minor adverse reactions associated with DTaP/Tdap vaccination include injection site edema, fever, and fussiness. Uncommon adverse reactions with DTaP are persistent crying for ≥3 hours, an unusual high-pitched cry, seizures (usually febrile seizures without any permanent sequelae), and hypotonic-hyporesponsive episodes. The extremely rare anaphylactic reaction to DTaP is a contraindication to further doses of DTaP. Rarely, temporary swelling of the entire limb has occurred after the fourth or fifth DTaP dose, or a sterile abscess can follow DTaP vaccination.

Recommendations

Five doses of DTaP vaccine are recommended for all children prior to school entry. Only four doses are needed if the fourth dose is given after the child's fourth birthday. To reduce the incidence of adolescent pertussis and secondarily infection of infant siblings, the Advisory Committee on Immunization Practices (ACIP) recommends a single dose of tetanus toxoid, reduced diphtheria toxoid, and reduced acellular pertussis (Tdap) vaccine for persons aged 11 years and older. In addition, ACIP recommends a Tdap dose during each pregnancy, preferably at week 27–36 of gestation, regardless of prior Tdap administration.

PNEUMOCOCCAL CONJUGATE VACCINE

Prior to the introduction of pneumococcal conjugate vaccine (PCV), *Streptococcus pneumoniae,* a gram-positive diplococcus with >90 different polysaccharide capsules, caused ~17,000 cases of invasive disease (bacteremia, meningitis, or infection in a normally sterile site), in the United States, including 200 deaths annually among children aged <5 years. Respiratory tract droplets spread infection. *S. pneumoniae* is a common cause of community-acquired pneumonia, sinusitis, otitis media, and bacterial meningitis.

Rationale for Vaccination

Two vaccines protect against pneumococcus: the 23-valent polysaccharide vaccine (PPSV23) and the 13-valent conjugate vaccine (PCV13). PPSV23 does not produce an anamnestic response and thus may not induce longlasting immunity and is not effective in children aged <2 years. PCV13 elicits a T cell reaction leading to an anamnestic response so is effective in infants and induces longlasting immunity. This vaccine reduces nasopharyngeal carriage rates and transmission of *S. pneumoniae,* leading to herd immunity, including older adults. PCV13 vaccine efficacy against invasive disease is estimated at 94% for vaccine serotypes. Efficacy against clinical pneumonia is 11%; against clinical pneumonia with radiographic infiltrate, 33%; and against pneumonia with radiographic consolidation of ≥2.5 cm (most typical of *S. pneumoniae*), 73%.

Adverse Reactions

No serious adverse reactions are associated with PCV13: 10–14% develop redness and 15–23% develop tenderness at the injection site. Fever of ≤38°C (≤100.4°F) occurs in 15–24% of vaccinees. PPSV23 causes injection site redness, pain, and swelling in ≤60%.

Recommendations

The ACIP recommends four doses of PCV13 for routine infant immunization. All children aged 2–5 years who have not received PCV13 and all children aged 6–17 years with chronic renal failure or nephrotic syndrome, functional or anatomic asplenia (eg, sickle cell disease or splenectomy), or immunosuppressive conditions (eg, congenital immunodeficiency or HIV), or who are receiving chemotherapy with alkylating agents, antimetabolites, or long-term systemic corticosteroids should receive one dose of PCV13. Children aged ≥2 years with the conditions listed previously should receive a dose of PPSV23 in addition to PCV13 (see ACIP recommendations for details). One-time PPSV23 revaccination after 5 years is recommended for immunocompromised and asplenic children. The ACIP recommends that adults aged ≥19 years with immunocompromising conditions, functional or anatomic asplenia, cerebrospinal fluid (CSF) leaks, or cochlear implants receive a dose of PCV13.

HAEMOPHILUS INFLUENZA b (Hib) VACCINE

All infants should receive either three doses {if PRP-OMP [poly (ribosylribitol phosphate) – outer membrane protein] is given} or four doses (other types) of Hib vaccine. Combination vaccines that contain Hib serve to reduce the overall number of injections. Side effects are generally mild, including localized redness, pain, and swelling and low-grade fever.

POLIOVIRUS VACCINE

Poliovirus spreads to 73–96% of susceptible household contacts, primarily via the fecal-oral route (oral-oral possible). The incubation period ranges from 3 to 35 days.

Up to 90% of cases of poliovirus infection are subclinical; approximately 5% are nonspecific viral illness with complete recovery, 1–2% are nonparalytic aseptic meningitis, and <2%

are paralytic poliomyelitis. The case/fatality rate is 2–5% in children and 15–30% in adults.

Rationale for Vaccination

In 1994, the Americas were declared free of indigenous poliomyelitis, but poliovirus was isolated from a few Amish children in the United States in 2005, indicating a need for continued vigilance. Poliovirus vaccination is recommended because of outbreaks in other countries, importation of wild poliovirus, and its highly contagious nature.

Recommendations

Prior to school entry, four doses of all-inactivated poliovirus vaccine (IPV) (oral poliovirus vaccine doses count) are recommended for all children. A fourth dose is not necessary if the third dose is administered at age ≥4 years.

INFLUENZA VACCINE

During the influenza season, hospitalizations increase because of pneumonia and other complications. Preschoolers, especially infants younger aged <1 year, are at high risk. Complications include bacterial pneumonia, primary viral pneumonia (uncommon), worsening of chronic respiratory and cardiac diseases, sinusitis, otitis media, and rarely Reye syndrome associated with concomitant salicylate use. Children have an increased risk of encephalopathy and death. Influenza is extremely contagious, transmitted from person to person usually via the airborne route. Persons such as students in crowded environments are at high risk. The incubation period is 2 days (range, 1–5 days). Young children can shed virus for ≤6 days before onset of symptoms, have the highest attack rate (14–40% yearly, especially high in preschoolers), and frequently infect other family members.

Vaccine Types

Two types of influenza vaccines are currently licensed for children: inactivated influenza vaccine (IIV) intramuscular and live attenuated influenza vaccine (LAIV) intranasal. The LAIV contains cold-adapted virus that replicates somewhat in the nasopharynx, where the temperatures are cooler, but inefficiently in lower airways where temperatures are warmer. Licensed vaccines include both trivalent and newer quadrivalent vaccines that contain two type A viruses and two type B viruses that should reduce illness due to both lineages of B strains.

Vaccine Efficacy

The effectiveness of influenza vaccine depends primarily on the match between the vaccine virus strains and wild circulating viruses during the influenza season and on the immunocompetence of the vaccine recipient. IIV has moderate efficacy (44–57%) in children aged 1–5 years and good efficacy (≥77%) in older children and adolescents. Immunity from IIV is time-limited. Hence, annual vaccination just prior to the influenza season is recommended. Protection develops within 2 weeks after vaccination. In healthy children, LAIV was 94% efficacious against culture-confirmed influenza for two doses and 89% for one dose.

▶ Safety of & Adverse Reactions to Influenza Vaccines

A. Inactivated Influenza Vaccine

Local reactions to IIV are injection site soreness for <2 days. In persons previously exposed to influenza disease or vaccination, IIV and placebo have similar rates of systemic reactions such as fever. In young children not previously exposed to influenza vaccine, fever, malaise, and myalgia can occur after IIV. A study from the Vaccine Safety Datalink found no serious reactions from IIV among 251,600 children aged <18 years.

B. Live Attenuated Influenza Vaccine

Persons vaccinated with LAIV shed vaccine virus. In one daycare study, 80% of vaccinees aged 8–36 months shed vaccine virus for a mean of 7.6 days. One unvaccinated contact contracted the vaccine virus, which retained its temperature-sensitive, attenuated properties; the transmission rate was estimated at 0.6–2.4%. Adverse events to LAIV included nasal congestion and rhinorrhea (20–75%), headache (2–46%), fever (0–26%), vomiting (3–13%), abdominal pain (2%), and myalgia (0–21%); these were reported more commonly by vaccines than by placebo recipients, were self-limited, and were more common after the first dose.

▶ Recommendations

All children aged ≥6 months should receive routine annual influenza vaccination. IIV is licensed by the US Food and Drug Administration (FDA) for children aged ≥6 months. Currently, the FDA licenses LAIV for healthy children aged ≥2 years. LAIV is not intended for children with chronic cardiopulmonary conditions such as asthma, chronic metabolic disease, renal failure, hemoglobinopathies, or immunosuppression, including HIV or on long-term aspirin therapy. The FDA recommends IIV for all these individuals.

Children aged <9 years who have not had any previous influenza vaccine should receive two doses, at least 4 weeks apart in the first year of vaccination or in the second year, if two doses were not administered in the first year. Children previously vaccinated with two doses subsequently require only one dose each year. The IIV dosage varies by age: 0.25 mL intramuscularly for children aged 6–35 months and 0.5 mL intramuscularly for those aged ≥3 years. In 2014, CDC stated a preference for LAIV in children ages 2-8 years when LAIV was readily available.

MEASLES, MUMPS, & RUBELLA (MMR) VACCINE

Measles can cause severe morbidity, be acutely fatal, or cause a delayed fatal encephalopathy (subacute sclerosing panencephalitis) in adolescence. Outbreaks start with an imported measles case that spreads among persons unvaccinated because of philosophic or religious exemptions; the attack rate among unvaccinated household contacts is ≥90%. Infected persons can transmit measles from 4 days prior to 4 days after rash onset. Worldwide measles kills about 160,000 people per year. Mumps produces excruciating, bilateral parotitis and sometimes pancreatitis, orchitis, cerebellar ataxia, or death. Rubella causes posterior cervical adenopathy, arthralgia, and minimal rash, but it can also result in devastating *congenital rubella syndrome.*

▶ Rationale for Vaccination

The first dose of MMR protects 95% of children, necessitating a second vaccine dose for all. After two doses, >99% of persons are immune. To avoid interference from transplacentally conferred maternal antibodies, MMR vaccine is ideally given at age 12 months. Immunity is probably lifelong in almost all persons who initially seroconvert; the rate of waning immunity is <0.2% per year.

▶ Adverse Reactions

Pain, irritation, and redness at the injection site are common but mild. Reactions to measles vaccine include fever [usually <38.8°C (102°F)] between days 7 and 12, transient rash between days 5 and 20, or transient thrombocytopenia (1 in 25,000 to 2 million doses). Adverse reactions to rubella vaccine include generalized lymphadenopathy in children and transient arthralgia in young women; and to mumps vaccine, adverse reactions include transient orchitis in young men. MMR does not cause autism.

▶ Recommendations

The MMR vaccine is given routinely subcutaneously to all healthy children at age 12–15 months with a second dose at age 4–6 years. A second dose is especially important for students planning to attend college.

VARICELLA VACCINE

Varicella-zoster virus (VZV) causes chickenpox, a generally benign illness. However, the hospitalization rate is 5 cases per 1000 population. Because transmission rates are as high as 90% and communicability via aerosol droplets begins 1–2 days prior to rash onset, prevention of spread requires universal vaccination. Complications include secondary skin infection (impetigo and invasive group A streptococcal disease), pneumonia, and other severe disorders. The lifetime risk for herpes zoster (shingles) is 10–50%.

Rationale for Vaccination

Before universal VZV vaccination was available, the majority of individuals hospitalized each year for VZV-related complications were 1–4 years old. Because VZV vaccination reduces hospitalization, routine vaccination is cost-effective; each $1 spent on universal immunization avoids approximately $5 in costs. Varicella vaccine contains live attenuated virus and is 97% effective against moderate to severe disease. Postvaccination breakthrough disease is usually mild, producing fewer than 30 pox lesions. A two-dose vaccination strategy was adopted to reduce breakthrough cases.

Adverse Reactions

Following subcutaneous injection, local pain and erythema occur in 2–20% after the first dose and ≤47% after the second dose. Later, 5–41 days after administration, 4–10% develop a median of five varicellalike, short-lived (2–8 days) lesions. A brief, low-grade fever develops in 12–30% of vaccinees. Vaccine virus can rarely be transmitted to healthy immunocompetent persons. Persons with previously unrecognized prior immunization or VZV infection are not at increased risk from a dose of vaccine. Shingles is less common among vaccinees.

Recommendations

The ACIP recommends the first dose for age 12–15 months and the second dose for age 4–6 years with catch-up vaccination through 18 years of age for previously uninfected or unvaccinated children. Serologic tests are not required. Immunocompromised persons require no special precautions to avoid vaccinees except avoidance of direct contact with a vaccine-induced rash.

Postexposure Prophylaxis

Varicella-zoster virus vaccine is effective in modifying varicella if given within 3–5 days of exposure to wild varicella. Artificial varicella-zoster immune globulin (VariZIG) is recommended for exposed immunosuppressed patients, pregnant women, and infants of mothers who develop varicella 5 days before to 2 days after delivery and may be effective if given within 10 days of exposure.

MENINGOCOCCAL CONJUGATE VACCINE

In the pre–conjugate vaccine era, *Neisseria meningitidis,* the most common cause of bacterial meningitis in children and young adults in the United States, caused approximately 2200–3000 cases of invasive disease annually, at an incidence of 0.8–1.5 cases per 100,000 persons. Death occurs in about 10% of cases, and sequelae such as limb loss, neurologic disabilities, and hearing loss occurs in 11–19%.

Often colonizing the throat, *N. meningitidis* is transmitted via respiratory tract droplets and occurs sporadically most often in children aged <5 years. Serogroup B accounts for >30% of meningococcal disease, mostly in children aged <2 years. Serogroup Y accounts for approximately 30% of sporadic cases, while serogroups A and C cause most outbreaks. In the prevaccine era, the incidence of meningococcal disease for college freshmen living in dormitories was 5.1 per 100,000, compared with 0.7 per 100,000 for other undergraduates and 1.4 per 100,000 in 18–23-year-olds in the general population. College freshman living in dormitories or wishing protection against meningococcus should be vaccinated with meningococcal conjugate vaccine for groups A, C, Y, and W-135 (MCV4).

Vaccine Types

The meningococcal (groups A, C, Y, and W-135) conjugate vaccine (MCV4) is recommended for all adolescents at age 11–12 years, with a booster dose at age 16 years and catch-up vaccination for ages 13–18 years; for all persons aged 2–55 years with high-risk medical indications, including asplenia or terminal complement deficiencies; and for travelers to hyperendemic areas such as sub-Saharan Africa. It provides long-term immunity and induces higher antibody levels than does polysaccharide vaccine (MPSV4). Two MCV4 brands exist for somewhat different age ranges; see package inserts, the computer program *Shots by STFM* (www.immunizationed.org), or CDC information for details. A combination vaccine with serogroups Y and C and Hib is FDA-approved for infants aged ≥6 weeks. Serogroup B vaccine was licensed in the US in 2014 and recommendations for its use are pending. MCV4 is available for infants at high risk; see CDC or Shots for details.

Following intramuscular injection, the most common adverse events are mild local pain, headache, and fatigue. Mild to moderate systemic reactions such as fever, fussiness, and drowsiness are infrequent.

ROTAVIRUS VACCINE

Prior to the introduction of rotavirus vaccine, rotavirus caused 2–3 million cases of gastroenteritis, 60,000 hospitalizations, and a reported 20–60 deaths annually in the United States.

Two live oral rotavirus vaccines are licensed in the United States: pentavalent (RV5) and monovalent (RV1). RV5 contains five reassortant viruses from bovine and human strains, whereas RV1 contains human strain type G1P1A. The vaccines reduce hospitalization for rotavirus gastroenteritis by 85–100% and reduce rotavirus of any severity by 74–87%. The duration of immunity is not clear but appears to wane in the second season after administration.

All infants should receive either three doses of RV5 or two doses of RV1 by age 32 weeks. Doses are given 2 months apart. Side effects include vomiting, diarrhea, irritability, and fever. Intussusception after either RV1 or RV5 is rare.

HUMAN PAPILLOMA VIRUS (HPV) VACCINE

To prevent anogenital cancers, all adolescents aged ≥11 years should receive three doses of HPV vaccine. Two vaccines, HPV2 and HPV4, are available. Both contain HPV 16 and 18. Also containing cancer-preventing sero types 6 and 11, HPV4 prevents genital warts. Side effects include local pain and swelling and syncope, necessitating 15–20 minutes of postvaccination observation. A nine valent HPV vaccine is currently under consideration for FDA approval.

Centers for Disease Control and Prevention. General recommendations on immunization. Recommendations of the Advisory Committee on Immunization Practices (ACIP). *MMWR* 2011; 60(RR02): 1-60.

Centers for Disease Control and Prevention. Epidemiology and prevention of vaccine-preventable diseases, 12th ed., 2nd printing. In: Atkinson W, Wolfe S, Hamborsky J, eds. Washington, DC: Public Health Foundation; 2012.

Centers for Disease Control and Prevention: Recommended immunization schedule for persons age 0 through 18 years –2013, United States (available at http://www.cdc.gov/vaccines/schedules/hcp/imz/child-adolescent.html).

Pickering LD, ed. *Red Book: 2012 Report of the Committee on Infectious Diseases*, 29th ed. American Academy of Pediatrics, 2012.

Behavioral Disorders in Children

Richard Welsh, LCSW

Marian Swope, MD

ATTENTION DEFICIT–HYPERACTIVITY DISORDER

 ESSENTIALS OF DIAGNOSIS

▸ Neurodevelopmental abnormalities with an early age of onset.

▸ Deficits on measures of attention and cognitive function.

▸ Hyperactivity.

▸ Impulsivity.

General Considerations

Up to 20% of school-aged children in the United States have behavioral problems, at least half of which involve attention and/or hyperactivity difficulties. Attention Deficit Hyperactivity Disorder (ADHD) is the most common and well-studied of the childhood behavioral disorders.

Clinical Findings

Individuals diagnosed with ADHD are likely to experience significant difficulties with executive functioning, which impairs academic performance, social relationships, self-control, and memory. Brown (2005) outlines six executive function deficits that are observed in individuals diagnosed with ADHD: (1) organizing and prioritizing (difficulty getting started on tasks); (2) focusing and sustaining attention (easily distracted); (3) regulating alertness, sustaining effort (drowsiness); (4) managing frustration (low frustration tolerance or disproportionate emotional reactions); (5) working memory (difficulty retrieving information); and (6) self-regulation (difficulty inhibiting verbal and behavior responses).

Brown TE. *Attention Deficit Disorder: The Unfocused Mind in Children and Adults.* New Haven, CT: Yale University Press; 2005.

There is no single diagnostic test or tool for ADHD. The diagnostic criteria included in the *Diagnostic and Statistical Manual of Mental Disorders,* fifth edition (*DSM-5*) are the current basis for the identification of individuals with ADHD. There is rarely a need for extensive laboratory analysis, but screening for iron deficiency and thyroid dysfunction is reasonable.

The American Academy of Child and Adolescent Psychiatry and the American Academy of Pediatrics (AAP), with input from members of the American Academy of Family Physicians, have formulated evidence-based practice guidelines to aid in the improvement of current diagnostic and treatment practices.

American Academy of Child and Adolescent Psychiatry. http://aappolicy.aappublications
American Academy of Pediatrics website. org/cgi/content/full/pediatrics;105/5/1158).

Differential Diagnosis

The diagnosis is made by parent interview, direct observation, and the use of standardized and scored behavioral checklists such as the Connors Parent and Teacher Rating Scales, Child Behavior Checklist (CBCL), Vanderbilt ADHD Diagnostic Parent and Teacher Scales, Achenbach, along with computerized tests (Gordon Diagnostic Testing, Connors Continuous Performance Task, and Test of Variables of Attention) measuring impulsivity and inattention that are specific for ADHD and should include input from both parents and teachers.

Complications

Attention deficit–hyperactivity disorder is often associated with other Axis I diagnoses. From 35% to 60% of referred

ADHD children have oppositional defiant disorder (ODD), and 25-50% will develop conduct disorder (CD). Of these, 15–25% progress to antisocial personality disorder in adulthood. Of all referred ADHD children, 25–40% have a concurrent anxiety disorder. As many as 50% of referred children with ADHD eventually develop a mood disorder—most commonly depression, diagnosed in adolescence. The diagnosis of bipolar disease in childhood increases the risk of concurrent label of ADHD because of the overlap of behaviors. About half the children with Tourette syndrome have ADHD.

There is a definite association among ADHD, academic problems, and learning disabilities. Between 20% and 50% of children with ADHD have at least one type of learning disorder.

▶ Treatment

A. Pharmacotherapy

1. Stimulants—Stimulant medications are the most frequently researched and the safest and most effective treatments for the symptoms of ADHD, but they are not a "cure." The fact that stimulants are controlled substances (schedule II) with an abuse potential justifies the close scrutiny of their use. About 65% of children with ADHD show improvement in the core symptoms of hyperactivity, inattention, and impulsivity with their first trial of a stimulant, and ≤95% will respond when given appropriate trials of various stimulants. The management of these medications can be complex, and treatment failures may more often be the result of improper treatment strategies than effective medication.

Perhaps the most important step is the choice of medications. Stimulants most commonly used include methylphenidate (Ritalin, Concerta, Metadate CD, Ritalin LA, Methylphenidate ER, Daytrana), dexmethylphenidate (Focalin), dextroamphetamine (Dexedrine, Vyvanse), and mixed amphetamine salts (Adderall). In more recent years, novel drug delivery systems have been developed for stimulants and these formulations have become routine in clinical practice.

Absolute contraindications to the use of stimulants include concomitant use of monoamine oxidase (MAO) inhibitors, psychosis, glaucoma, underlying cardiac conditions, existing liver disorders, and a history of stimulant drug dependence. Adverse cardiovascular effects of stimulants have consistently documented mild increases in pulse and blood pressure of unclear clinical significance. Caution should be used in treating patients who have a family history of early cardiac death of arrhythmias or a personal history of structural abnormalities, palpitations, chest pain, and shortness of breath or syncope of unclear origin either before or during treatment with stimulants.

Because stimulants are Schedule II controlled substances, prescriptions with no refills are usually written monthly; however, several states allow 3-month prescriptions. Growth and vital signs should be checked and documented, and it is vital to monitor the medication effects and the child's progress. Issues to address include: (1) adequacy and timing of the dosage, (2) compliance with the regimen, (3) changes in school or non-school-related activities that may affect medical therapy, and (4) maintenance of appropriate growth. An initial dropoff in weight gain may occur during titration phase, but over 2 years this reverses, resulting in no long-term sustained growth suppression from stimulant use. Drug holidays are no longer standard procedure, but parents may opt for their children to have periods off the medications to minimize potential unknown drug effects or to assess the continuing need for the medication.

2. Nonstimulants—Many nonstimulant medications are being used for ADHD, alone and in combination with neurostimulants. Nonstimulant agents are less widely studied and are summarized here to inform the physician about their use. They vary from the tricyclic antidepressants to α-agonists (Tenex, Intuniv and Clonidine, Kapvay) to the highly selective catecholamine reuptake inhibitor atomoxetine (Strattera). Nonstimulants are often used to treat both ADHD and comorbid states, and their effectiveness alone is generally less than that of the neurostimulants. Fear and misunderstanding about the effects of neurostimulants make these nonstimulant agents attractive to parents.

B. Psychotherapeutic Interventions

1. Behavioral modification—Behavioral modifications are designed to improve specific behaviors, social skills, and performance in specific settings. Behavioral approaches require detailed assessment of the child's responses and the conditions that elicited them. Strategies are then developed to change the environment and the behaviors while maintaining and generalizing the behavioral changes. The most prudent approach to the treatment of ADHD is multimodal. The combination of psychosocial interventions and medications produces the best results.

2. Educational interventions—The education of children with ADHD is covered by three federal statutes: the Individuals with Disabilities Education Act (IDEA), Section 504 of the Rehabilitation Act of 1973, and the Americans with Disabilities Act (ADA) of 1990. The diagnosis of ADHD alone does not suffice to qualify for special education services. The ADHD must impair the child's ability to learn. A 1991 Department of Education Policy Clarification Memorandum specifies three categories by which ADHD children may be eligible for special education: (1) health impaired (other documented condition such as Tourette syndrome), (2) specific learning disability (could be ADHD alone if there is a significant discrepancy between a child's cognitive ability or intelligence and his or her academic performance), and (3) seriously emotionally disturbed. It is therefore vital to document all comorbid conditions in these children.

3. Parent education and training—Parental understanding of ADHD is vital to successful treatment. Parents must know the difference between nonadherence and inability to perform. They need to understand that ADHD is not a choice but a result of nature. Many parents respond well to referral to local and national support groups such as Children and Adults with Attention Deficit/Hyperactivity Disorder (CHADD) or the Attention Deficit Disorder Association (ADDA).

Parent training programs such as developed by Russell Barkley and others provide confused and overwhelmed parents with specific management strategies shown to be effective in reducing noncompliance. In these group training sessions, parents are taught skills in how to more effectively communicate with their children, learn how to consequate noncompliance, and enhance school performance.

Prognosis

Follow-up studies of children with ADHD show that adult outcomes vary greatly. There are three general outcome groups. The largest group is the 50–60% of affected children who continue to have concentration, impulsivity, and social problems in adulthood. About 30% of affected children function well in adulthood and have no more difficulty than controlled normal children. The final group represents about 10–15% who, in adulthood, have significant psychiatric or antisocial problems. Predictors for bad outcomes include comorbid CD, low IQ, and concurrent parental pathology.

OPPOSITIONAL DEFIANT DISORDER

 ESSENTIALS OF DIAGNOSIS

▶ Age-inappropriate display of angry, irritable, and oppositional behaviors that has occurred for at least 6 months.

▶ Behaviors are *not* part of a psychotic or mood disorder, nor is the diagnosis made if the criteria for CD are met.

▶ Physical aggression is *not* typical, nor are significant problems with the law.

▶ Progression to CD is rare.

▶ Not associated with any known physical or biochemical abnormality.

General Considerations

The cause is generally related to social, parental, and child factors. A correlation exists between ODD and living in crowded conditions such as high-rise buildings with inadequate play space. There are strong correlations between the way parents act and oppositional behavior. Mothers, especially, demonstrate high levels of anxiety and depression. Family relationships, especially the marital relationship, tend to be strained. This sets up a vicious cycle as the child becomes increasingly insecure and more difficult to handle, conditions that prompt the parents to react with more rejection and anger.

Prevalence

The reported prevalence of ODD varies from 2% to 16% of children and adolescents. Studies show an increasing rate of diagnosis from late preschool or early school-aged children to grade school to middle school to high school and then a decrease in college-aged individuals. Unlike gender differences in CD and ADHD, they are minimal in ODD, and boys are only slightly more likely to receive a diagnosis of ODD than girls. Conclusive data on racial or cultural differences do not exist, but worldwide ODD and CD are more prevalent among families of low socioeconomic status who tend to live in close quarters.

Clinical Findings

Common manifestations of ODD include persistent stubbornness, résistance to directions, and unwillingness to negotiate and compromise with others. Defiant behaviors include persistent testing of limits, arguing, ignoring orders, and denying blame for most misdeeds. Hostility usually takes the form of verbal abuse and aggression. The most common setting is the home, and behavioral problems may not be evident to teachers or others in the community. Because the symptoms of the disorder are most likely to be manifested toward individuals that the patient knows well, they are rarely apparent during clinical examination. Children and adolescents with ODD do not see themselves as the problem but instead view their behavior as a reasonable response to unreasonable demands.

Differential Diagnosis

Diagnosis is made by parents, patient, or teacher history and direct observation.

Behavioral checklists are available that can identify the pattern of ODD. They include the Child Behavioral Checklist. It is rare that any medical testing or neuropsychiatric testing is necessary, unless comorbid states are present. The *DSM-5* presents specific diagnostic criteria for ODD.

Complications

Oppositional defiant disorder is common among children and adolescents with ADHD. The combination of ADHD, ODD, family adversity, and low verbal IQ are predictors of progression to more serious CD and antisocial behaviors as adults. However, although ≤50% of ADHD children have

ODD behaviors, only ~15% of those diagnosed with ODD have ADHD.

Approximately 15% of ODD children have anxiety disorders, and approximately 10% have depression of mood disorders. Addressing these problems can often help with the oppositional behaviors.

▶ Treatment

A. Behavioral Therapy

The vast majority of these patients and their families can be managed with behavioral therapies, especially parental training and family therapy.

B. Medications for Oppositional Defiant Disorder

Medication for youth with ODD should not be the sole intervention and are primarily adjunctive, palliative, and noncurative. Medications may be beneficial in the context of other diagnoses and as such may be helpful adjuncts to a treatment package for symptomatic treatment and to treat comorbid conditions. For example, stimulants and atomoxetine may be useful in treating ODD in the context of another principal diagnosis such as ADHD. ODD behaviors in the context of an anxiety disorder or a depressive disorder may be successfully treated with a selective serotonin reuptake inhibitor (SSRI). Aggressive and oppositional behaviors complicate a wide range of other diagnoses in this age range. Therefore medications should target specific syndromes as much as possible.

Loeber R et al. Oppositional defiant and conduct disorder: a review of the past 10 years, part 1. *J Am Acad Child Adolesc Psychiatr.* 2000;39:1468. [PMID: 11128323]
Steiner H, Remsing L. Work Group on Quality Issues. Practice parameter for the assessment and treatment of children and adolescents with oppositional defiant disorder. *J Am Acad Child Adolesc Psychiatr.* 2007; 46(1):126–141. [PMID: 17195736]

C. Pharmacotherapy for Comorbid Conditions

There is no accepted pharmacologic treatment for oppositional behaviors, but comorbid conditions such as ADHD or depression must be properly addressed and appropriately treated. For children who do not respond to nonmedical interventions or are extremely impaired, it is best to consult a pediatric psychiatrist. Medications used for ODD, comorbid with other conditions, include clonidine, lithium, carbamazepine, valproic acid, and risperidone; all have significant risks, and their use should be monitored carefully.

▶ Prognosis

The most serious consequence of ODD is the development of more dangerous conduct problems. Although the majority of children with ODD will not develop CD, in some cases

ODD appears to represent a developmental precursors of CD. This seems to hold true for boys more than for girls. For children in whom such symptoms subsequently decrease with maturity, the prognosis is good. If oppositional behaviors progress and begin to involve the violation of others' rights, then the child will probably progress to CD.

American Academy of Child and Adolescent Psychiatry. *ODD: A Guide for Families.* eAACAP on AACAP.org; 2009.
Lavigne JV et al. Oppositional defiant disorder with onset in pre-school years: longitudinal stability and pathways to other disorders. *J Am Acad Child Adolesc Psychiatr.* 2001;40:1393. [PMID: 11765284]

CONDUCT DISORDER

 ESSENTIALS OF DIAGNOSIS

▶ A repetitive and persistent pattern of behavior in which the basic rights of others and major age-appropriate societal norms are violated.

▶ Behaviors may be characterized by aggression toward people and animals, destruction of property, deceitfulness or theft, and serious violation of rules.

▶ General Considerations

Conduct disorder also constitutes a public health concern by contributing to school and gang violence, weapon use, substance abuse, and high dropout rates. It is therefore important to identify these behaviors and intervene as early as possible.

The risk of CD is higher in children whose biological or adoptive parents have antisocial personality disorder, and siblings of children with CD have a higher risk for developing the condition as well. CD is also more common in children whose biological parents have ADHD, CD, alcohol dependence, mood disorders, and schizophrenia.

There is no doubt that the caregiver-child interaction contributes to disruptive behavior. Factors in these relationships include: (1) low levels of parental involvement in the child's activities, (2) poor supervisions, and (3) harsh and inconsistent disciplinary practices. The child views behavioral problems as strategies to secure attention and becomes closer to the caregiver or parent. Neighborhood and peer factors also contribute to the incidence of CD. Poverty, living in crowded conditions in a high-crime neighborhood, and having a "deviant" peer group all increase the risk of CD.

▶ Prevalence

The prevalence of CD varies from 1% to 10% overall, depending on the studied population, with ranges of 6–16%

in boys and 2–9% in girls younger than 18 years. CD tends to increase from middle childhood to adolescence. Although certain behaviors (eg, physical fighting) decrease with age, the most serious aggressive behaviors (eg, robbery, rape, and murder) increase during adolescence. The differing incidence of CD in boys and girls does not occur until after age 6 years, and boys and girls with CD manifest differing behaviors. Boys exhibit more fighting, stealing, vandalism, and school discipline problems, whereas girls are more likely to lie, be truant, run away, and abuse substances.

Clinical Findings

There are four main groupings of behaviors in CD: (1) aggression toward people or animals, (2) destruction of property, (3) deceitfulness or theft, and (4) serious violation of rules. Behavioral disorders must be differentiated from normal reactions to abnormal circumstances. The *DSM-5* states that the diagnosis of CD should not be made when behaviors are in response to the social context. Screening questions might include asking about troubles with police, involvement in physical fights, suspensions from school, running away from home, sexual activity, and the use of tobacco, alcohol, and drugs.

Differential Diagnosis

A clear majority (75%) of children with CD have at least one other psychiatric diagnosis. Of all children with CD, 30–50% also have ADHD. A significant proportion of children present with symptoms of both ADHD and CD, and both conditions should be diagnosed when this occurs. Comorbid ADHD and CD are consistently reported to be more disabling than either disorder alone. Finally, children with comorbid ADHD and CD appear to have a much worse long-term outcome than those with either disorder alone.

Other psychiatric diagnoses commonly seen in association with CD include anxiety disorders, mood disorders, substance abuse, schizophrenia, somatoform disorder, and obsessive-compulsive disorder. This is not surprising, considering that these diagnoses are more common in the parents of children with CD.

Intermittent explosive disorder features sudden aggressive outbursts that are usually unprovoked. These individuals do not intend to hurt anyone but say that they "snapped" and, without realizing it, attacked another person. Intermittent explosive disorder is distinguished from CD in that these episodes are the only signs of behavioral problems and these individuals do not engage in other rule violations. The treatise by Green (2010) is an excellent reference for diagnosis and treatment recommendations.

Green R. *The Explosive Child*. New York, NY: Harper Collins, 2010.

Treatment

A key element in the initial treatment of these children is to obtain parental involvement. Although many parents of children with CD have problems themselves, they do not want their children to follow their path. All parties need to be aware of the possibility of a poor prognosis without the interventions of the caregiver.

A. Behavioral Interventions

Behavioral interventions are similar to those for ODD. Collaborative resources such as school counselors, residential care, juvenile court designated workers, and the Department of Social Services can provide wraparound services for children and adolescents who are generally unmotivated and resistive to any type of intervention that may be necessary.

B. Psychopharmacology

Psychopharmacological interventions alone are insufficient to treat youth with CD. Medications are best seen as adjunctive treatments. Very often, youths with CD have other diagnoses. Because aggression, mood lability, and impulsivity may be seen in a wide range of comorbid diagnoses, these symptoms may be targets for pharmacological interventions. Antidepressants, anticonvulsants, lithium carbonate, α-agonists, and antipsychotics have been used clinically. The potential side effects of various classes of medications may potentially outweigh their benefits.

Steiner H. Practice parameters for the assessment and treatment of children and adolescents with conduct disorder. *J Am Acad Child Adolesc Psychiatr*. 1997; 36(10):122S–139S. [PMID: 9334568]

Prognosis

The social burden and public health concerns associated with CD make diagnosis and treatment of this condition very important. About 40% of children with early-onset CD are diagnosed in adulthood with antisocial personality disorder or psychopathology. Overall, approximately 30% of children with CD continue to demonstrate a repetitive display of illegal behaviors. Antisocial behavior rarely begins in adulthood, and the family cycle of such behaviors is difficult to break.

American Academy of Child and Adolescent Psychiatry. *Your Child*. 2000.
American Academy of Child and Adolescent Psychiatry. *Your Adolescent*. 2009.

Seizures

Donald B. Middleton, MD

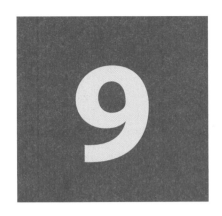

ESSENTIALS OF DIAGNOSIS

- ▶ Occurrence of an aura.
- ▶ Alteration in or impaired consciousness or behavior.
- ▶ Abnormal movement.
- ▶ Interictal trauma or incontinence.
- ▶ Eyewitness account.
- ▶ Presence of fever.
- ▶ Postictal confusion, lethargy, sleepiness, or paralysis.
- ▶ Diagnostic electroencephalogram.
- ▶ Abnormality on neuroimaging.

General Considerations

Despite an alarming appearance, a single seizure rarely causes injury or permanent sequelae or signals the onset of epilepsy. The lifetime risk for seizure is about 10%, but only 2% of the population develops unprovoked, recurrent seizures (epilepsy). *Epilepsy* is usually defined as repetitive, often stereotypic seizures, but even a single seizure coupled with a significant abnormality on neuroimaging or a diagnostic electroencephalogram (EEG) can signify epilepsy. Seizure incidence is high in childhood, decreases in midlife, and then peaks in the elderly. The annual number of new seizures during childhood is 50,000–150,000, only 10,000–30,000 of which constitute epileptic seizures. In 2010, active epilepsy afflicted 1% of all adults in the United States and 1.9% of those with family incomes below $35,000. During childhood the incidence of partial seizures is 20 per 100,000; generalized tonic-clonic seizures, 15 per 100,000; and absence seizures, 11 per 100,000.

Only ~30% of children get a medical evaluation after a single seizure. In contradistinction, >80% of children with a second seizure obtain medical assistance. Approximately 50% of adults with epilepsy have seen a neurologist. A recognizable, treatable seizure etiology; a negative family history; a normal physical examination; a lack of head trauma; a normal EEG; and normal neuroimaging indicate a low risk for seizure recurrence. Each year approximately 3% of 6-month-old to 6-year-old children have a febrile seizure, the most common childhood seizure entity. The likelihood of these children developing epilepsy is extremely low even if the febrile seizure recurs.

Pathogenesis

A seizure results from an abnormal, transient outburst of involuntary neuronal activity. Anoxic degeneration, focal neuron loss, hippocampal sclerosis (common in temporal lobe epilepsy), and neoplasia are examples of pathologic central nervous system (CNS) changes that can produce seizures. Why a seizure spontaneously erupts is unclear, but abnormal ion flow in damaged neurons initiates the event.

Seizures are either generalized (a simultaneous discharge from the entire cortex) or partial (focal, a discharge from a focal point within the brain). Generalized seizures impair consciousness and, except for some petite mal (absence) spells, cause visible abnormal movement, usually intense muscle contractions termed *convulsions*. Because generalized convulsions occur most commonly in the absence of a focal defect, the initiating mechanism of a generalized seizure is less well understood than that of a partial seizure initiating from a focal CNS lesion. Partial seizures may either impair consciousness (complex) or not (simple) and can start with almost any neurologic complaint, termed the *aura*, including abnormal smells, visions, movements, feelings, or behaviors such as nonresponsiveness. Partial seizures can progress to and thus mimic generalized seizures, a fact that sometimes obscures the true nature of the problem because the commotion of the convulsion dominates recall of events.

The etiology of epilepsy in childhood is 68% idiopathic, 20% congenital, 5% traumatic, and 4% postinfectious, but only 1% each vascular, neoplastic, and degenerative. The latter three are much more common in adulthood: 16% vascular, 11% neoplastic, and 3% degenerative. Complex partial seizures, the most difficult type to control, afflict 21% of children; generalized tonic-clonic seizures, the easiest to control, 19%; myoclonic seizures, often difficult to recognize because of limited motor activity, 14%; absence seizures, rare in adults, 12%; simple partial seizures, 11%; other generalized seizures, 11%; simultaneous multiple types, often syndrome-associated, 7%; and other types 5%. In adults, 39% of epilepsy cases are complex partial seizures, 25% generalized, 21% simple partial, and 15% other types.

The majority of convulsions are due to an inciting event such as head trauma; CNS infection; epileptogenic drug ingestion such as some antihistamines; or metabolic abnormalities such as hypoglycemia, hyponatremia, or alcohol withdrawal, but the cause of many reactive seizures remains unknown. Nonspecific etiologies such as stress or sleep deprivation are often assumed to lower the seizure threshold. Impact seizures are common after head trauma, but the 5-year risk for epilepsy is only 2%. On the other hand, 15–30% of children with depressed skull fractures develop epilepsy. Syncopal episodes with diminished CNS perfusion often result in minor twitching or even major tonic-clonic seizures that do not portend epilepsy.

Unprovoked seizures are more likely to be epilepsy. The majority of epileptic seizures has no known cause and thus are termed *cryptogenic*. Those with identifiable causes such as prior head trauma are called *symptomatic*. If genetic inheritance is at fault, the epilepsy is *idiopathic*. Genetic predisposition to epilepsy has been determined for many entities, including tuberous sclerosis and juvenile myoclonic epilepsy, which affects 1–3 per 1000 persons and is linked to 15 different chromosomal loci. A genetic predisposition to seize is probably distributed throughout the population.

Table 9-1 presents a scheme of seizure description to guide treatment and predict outcome. Some forms of epilepsy are specially categorized as epilepsy syndromes {eg, infantile spasms (West syndrome) or benign childhood epilepsy with centrotemporal spikes [rolandic epilepsy or benign epilepsy with centrotemporal spikes (BECTS)]}. **Table 9-2** lists a general classification of epilepsy syndromes.

▶ Prevention

Primary prevention begins in pregnancy. Pregnant women must avoid addictive drug use (alcohol, cocaine, benzodiazepines), trauma (automobile safety), and infection (young kittens with toxoplasmosis). Modern obstetric techniques minimize birth trauma and cerebral anoxia, the leading cause of cerebral palsy, which is an unfortunately persistent disorder despite efforts to reduce its incidence. Family history may reveal significant errors of metabolism (Gaucher

Table 9-1. Classification of seizures.

I. Generalized
   A. Convulsive: tonic, clonic, tonic-clonic
   B. Nonconvulsive: absence (petit mal), atypical absence, myoclonic, atonic

II. Partial (focal or localization related)
   A. Simple (consciousness preserved): motor, somatosensory, special sensory, autonomic, psychic
   B. Complex (consciousness impaired): at onset, progressing to loss of consciousness
   C. Evolving to secondary generalized

III. Unclassified
   A. Syndrome-related: West syndrome (infantile spasms), Lennox-Gastaut syndrome, neonatal seizures, others
   B. Other etiology

disease) or genetic disorders, some of which are amenable to treatment. Strict attention to childhood immunization to prevent CNS infection, especially pertussis and pneumococcal, or *Haemophilus influenzae* type b infection; and to safety throughout life beginning in infancy (using car seats, wearing bicycle helmets, supervision when swimming or in the bathtub, wearing seatbelts); and to avoidance of addictive drugs (alcohol, cocaine, phencyclidine) are examples of appropriate primary seizure prevention strategies. Annual influenza vaccination decreases the potential for febrile illness and secondary seizures, especially in persons with epilepsy. A full night's sleep, regular exercise, and a well-rounded diet are extremely important in the primary prevention of seizures.

Secondary prevention requires attention to the triggers, such as drugs that lower seizure threshold or cause seizures *de novo* (**Table 9-3**). Some children seize after prolonged fasting, possibly from hypoglycemia; for example, the unfed infant who seizes on Sunday morning when the parents oversleep, the "Saturday night seizure." Stimulation from light or noise, startle responses, faints, metabolic derangements, or certain videogames, television shows, or computer programs can cause seizures. Avoidance of any known precipitant reduces the future likelihood of another event. Although a convulsion can cause significant injury on its own, accident prevention is paramount. Individuals with epilepsy should not drive until seizure-free for 6 months, swim or take baths alone, or engage in potentially dangerous activities such as climbing on a roof. Patient education and referral to sources such as the Epilepsy Foundation (http://www.epilepsyfoundation.org/) play important roles in keeping patients and families healthy and active.

▶ Clinical Findings

A. Symptoms and Signs

The clinician must decide whether a neurologic event could be a seizure, and if so, what evaluations are necessary

Table 9-2. Abbreviated classification of epilepsies and epileptic syndromes.

I. Localization-related (focal, local, partial) epilepsies and syndromes
   A. Idiopathic (genetic) with age-related onset
      1. Benign childhood epilepsy with centrotemporal spikes (rolandic or BECTS)
      2. Childhood epilepsy with occipital paroxysms
      3. Primary reading epilepsy
   B. Symptomatic (remote or preexisting cause)
   C. Cryptogenic (unknown etiology)
II. Generalized epilepsies and syndromes
   A. Idiopathic with age-related onset, in order of age at onset
      1. Benign neonatal familial convulsions
      2. Benign neonatal convulsions
      3. Benign myoclonic epilepsy in infancy
      4. Childhood absence epilepsy (pyknolepsy)
      5. Epilepsy with grand mal seizures on awakening
      6. Other
   B. Cryptogenic and/or symptomatic epilepsies in order of age at onset
      1. Infantile spasms (West syndrome)
      2. Lennox-Gastaut syndrome
      3. Other
   C. Symptomatic
      1. Nonspecific etiology
      2. Specific syndromes
         a. Diseases presenting with or predominantly evidenced by seizures
III. Epilepsies and syndromes undetermined as to whether they are focal or generalized
   A. With both types
      1. Neonatal seizures
      2. Severe myoclonic epilepsy in infancy
      3. Acquired epileptic aphasia (Landau-Kleffner syndrome)
   B. Without unequivocal generalized or focal features
      1. Sleep-induced grand mal
IV. Special syndromes
   A. Situation-related seizures
      1. Febrile convulsions
      2. Related to other identifiable situations: stress, hormonal changes, drugs, alcohol, sleep deprivation
   B. Isolated, apparently unprovoked epileptic events
   C. Epilepsies characterized by specific modes of seizure precipitation
   D. Chronic progressive epilepsia partialis continua of childhood

Data from Berg AT, Berkovic SF, Brodie MJ, et al. Revised terminology and concepts for organization of seizures and epilepsies: report of the ILAE commission on classification and terminology, 2005–2009. *Epilepsia.* 2010; 51:676–685. [PMID: 20196795]

Table 9-3. Drugs linked to seizures.

A. Over-the-counter drugs
   1. Antihistamines: cold remedies
   2. Ephedra: common in diet supplements
   3. Insect repellents and insecticides: benzene hexachloride
   4. "Health" and "diet" drugs: ginkgo
B. Prescription drugs
   1. Antibiotics: penicillins, imipenem, fluoroquinolones; acyclovir, ganciclovir; metronidazole; mefloquine; isoniazid
   2. Asthma treatments: aminophylline, theophylline, high-dose steroids
   3. Chemotherapeutic agents: methotrexate, tacrolimus, cyclosporine
   4. Mental illness agents: tricyclics, selective serotonin reuptake inhibitors, methylphenidate, lithium, antipsychotics, bupropion
   5. Anesthetics and pain relievers: meperidine, propoxyphene, tramadol; local (lidocaine) or general anesthesia
   6. Antidiabetic medications: insulin and oral agents
   7. Antiepilepsy drugs: carbamazepine
   8. Miscellaneous: some β-blockers, immunizations, radiocontrast
C. Drugs of abuse
   1. Alcohol
   2. Cocaine
   3. Phencyclidine
   4. Amphetamine
   5. LSD (lysergic acid diethylamide)
   6. Marijuana overdose
D. Drug withdrawal
   1. Benzodiazepines: diazepam, alprazolam, chlordiazepoxide; flumazenil in benzodiazepine-dependent patients
   2. Barbiturates
   3. Meprobamate
   4. Pentazocine may precipitate withdrawal from other agents
   5. Alcohol
   6. Narcotics
   7. Antiepileptic drugs: rapid drop in levels

Data from Fisher RS. *Medications that Cause Seizures.* Epilepsy Foundation; 2009 (available at http://www.epilepsy.com/epilepsy/newsletter/jul09_AEDs; accessed May 1, 2013)

(**Table 9-4**), and whether treatment is required to prevent recurrence. The consequences of diagnosing a seizure include consideration of the effects on the family, school, driving, activities, work, and plans such as pregnancy. The primary tool for seizure assessment is the history, including: (1) age at onset; (2) family history; (3) developmental status; (4) behavior profile; (5) intercurrent distress including fever, vomiting, diarrhea, or illness exposure; (6) precipitating events, including exposure to flashing lights, toxins, or trauma; (7) sleep pattern; (8) diet; and (9) licit and illicit drug use. A critical feature pointing to a partial seizure is the occurrence of an aura, although a brief aura can also accompany a generalized seizure. Any symptom can constitute an aura, which usually requires more extensive evaluation for a focal CNS lesion. Because 20% of childhood seizures occur only at night, a description of early-morning behavior, including transient neurologic dysfunction or disorientation, is important. Reports of preictal, ictal, and postictal events from both the patient and witnesses help clarify the seizure type and therapy.

Mental retardation and cerebral palsy are among the most common conditions associated with epilepsy. Other cognitive

Table 9-4. Historical evaluation of possible seizure.

I. Behavior: mood or behavior changes before and after the seizure
II. Preictal symptoms or aura
  A. Vocal: cry or gasp, slurred or garbled speech
  B. Motor: head or eye turning, chewing, posturing, jerking, stiffening, automatisms (eg, purposeless picking at clothes or lip smacking), jacksonian march, hemiballism
  C. Respiration: change in or cessation of breathing, cyanosis
  D. Autonomic: drooling, dilated pupils, pallor, nausea, vomiting, urinary or fecal incontinence, laughter, sweating, swallowing, apnea, piloerection
  E. Sensory changes
  F. Consciousness alteration: stare, unresponsiveness, dystonic positioning
  G. Psychic phenomena: delusion, déjà vu, daydreams, fear, anger
III. Postictal symptoms
  A. Amnesia
  B. Paralysis: ≤24 hours, may be focal without focal CNS lesion
  C. Confusion, lethargy, or sleepiness
  D. Nausea or vomiting
  E. Headache
  F. Muscle ache
  G. Trauma: tongue, broken tooth, head, bruising, fracture, laceration
  H. Transient aphasia

Data from the National Institute for Health and Clinical Excellence (NICE). *The Epilepsies: The Diagnosis and Management of the Epilepsies in Adults and Children in Primary and Secondary Care.* London, UK: National Institute for Health and Clinical Excellence (NICE); 2012 (Clinical Guideline 137).

Table 9-5. Some causes of seizures.

Cause	Examples
Reflex Visual	Photic stimulation, colors, television, videogames
Auditory	Music, loud noise, specific voice or sound
Olfactory	Smells
Somatosensory	Tap, touch, immersion in water, tooth brushing
Cognitive	Math, card games, drawing, reading
Motor	Movement, swallowing, exercise, eye convergence, eyelid fluttering
Other	Startle, eating, sudden position change, sleep deprivation
Genetic	Neurofibromatosis, Klinefelter syndrome, Sturge-Weber syndrome, tuberous sclerosis
Structural	Hippocampal sclerosis, neoplasia, cerebral atrophy (dementia)
Congenital	Hamartoma, porencephalic cyst
Cerebrovascular	Arteriovenous malformation, stroke
Infectious	Syphilis, tuberculosis, toxoplasmosis, HIV infection, meningitis, encephalitis
Metabolic	Porphyria, phenylketonuria, electrolyte disorder (eg, hypoglycemia, hypocalcemia, hypomagnesemia), hyperosmolality, hyperventilation, drugs
Trauma	Depressed skull fracture, concussion
Other	Collagen vascular disease (systemic lupus erythematosus), eclampsia, demyelinating disease (multiple sclerosis), blood dyscrasias (sickle cell disease, idiopathic thrombocytopenia), mental disease (autism)

disorders linked to epilepsy include attention deficit hyperactivity disorder, learning disorders, and dementia. Associated psychological difficulties such as depression; psychoses; anxiety disorders, including panic attacks; eating disorders, such as anorexia nervosa; or personality disorders are common in epilepsy and often make recognition or control of seizures difficult. In adults sleep apnea can cause recurrent seizures. The myriad causes of seizures (**Table 9-5**) require diligence to elucidate.

1. Generalized seizures—Tonic-clonic (grand mal) seizures are both the most common and the most readily recognized. A short cry just before the seizure, apnea, and cyanosis are usual. The majority of these seizures are reactive, do not recur, last <3 minutes (usual maximum 15 minutes), and have no major sequelae. Following a convulsion, Todd postictal paralysis can persist for ≤24 hours even without an underlying structural lesion. When myoclonic or tonic-clonic epilepsy begins between ages 8 and 18 years, prospects for permanent remission are poor: about 90% relapse when antiepileptic drug (AED) treatment is stopped.

More difficult to identify, typical absence spells (petit mal) are brief (10–30-second) losses of consciousness and unresponsive stare with occasional blinking, chewing, or lip smacking without collapse. Common from ages 3 to 20 years, these spells are often precipitated by photic stimulation or hyperventilation and interrupt normal activity only briefly. Up to 50% of petit mal seizures evolve into tonic-clonic seizures, especially if the onset is during adolescence. Approximately 10% of epileptic children have atypical absence spells with some motor activity of the extremities, of duration >30 seconds, and postictal confusion. Many of these children are mentally handicapped. Both types of absence spells can occur up to hundreds of times per day, creating havoc with school performance and recreational activities.

2. Partial seizures—Benign epilepsy with centrotemporal spikes (BECTS) accounts for 15% of all epilepsy, has an onset between ages 2 and 14 years, and presents with guttural noises and tonic or clonic face or arm contractions, often in the early morning. An aura of numbness or tingling in the mouth often precedes motor arrest of speech and excessive salivation in a conscious child. Although not dangerous, nocturnal BECTS may generalize into grand mal convulsions. Approximately 20% of these children have only one episode; 25% develop repetitive seizures unless treated. By age 16 years almost all are seizure-free.

The classic, albeit rare, simple partial seizure is the jacksonian march, an orderly progression of clonic motor activity, distal to proximal, indicating a focal motor cortex defect. The arm on the side to which the head turns may be extended while the opposite arm flexes, creating the classic fencer's posture. Many of these seizures generalize into clonic-tonic convulsions.

Myoclonic jerks consist of single or repetitive contractions of a muscle or muscle group and account for 7% of seizures in the first 3 years of life. Benign occipital epilepsy has an onset between ages 1 and 14 years, with a peak incidence between ages 4 and 8 years and consists of migraine like headaches with vomiting, loss of vision, visual hallucinations, or illusions. Episodes usually stop during adolescence.

Complex partial seizures usually begin after age 10 years and last 1–2 minutes each. Consciousness may be lost at onset or gradually; postictal confusion occurs in 50–75%. Behavior alteration, including hissing, random wandering, sleepwalking, and irrelevant speech; affective changes such as fearfulness or anger; and autonomic dysfunction such as vomiting, pallor, flushing, enuresis, falling, and drooling demonstrate the variety of manifestations. Especially common are changes in body or limb position, ictal confusion, and a dazed expression. The child always exhibits amnesia for these events.

Syndromes usually present with several different types of seizures closely linked in time. Myoclonic jerks, grand mal seizures, and absence spells in a mentally deficient individual suggest Lennox-Gastaut syndrome.

B. Physical Findings

Because 3% of children have simple febrile convulsions, fever is the most important physical finding. A stiff neck coupled with a fever mandates a lumbar puncture. Focal infection such as pneumonia or otitis media can cause febrile seizures. Keeping current with immunizations is the best preventive measure. Many febrile seizures are linked to viral infections like herpesvirus 6, the cause of roseola.

Abnormal neurologic findings such as focal paralysis or facial asymmetry point to the need for imaging studies. Seizures often complicate cerebral palsy or stroke. Failure to return to baseline alertness in short order should trigger more intensive evaluation. Café-au-lait spots (neurofibromatosis), adenoma sebaceum and hypopigmented spots (tuberous sclerosis), port-wine stain (Sturge-Weber), or cutaneous telangiectasia (Louis-Bar) on the skin or cherry red spots in the eyes (Tay-Sachs) clue the diagnosis. Primary or metastatic cancer is a particularly important consideration in smokers or with unexplained weight loss, HIV infection, or lymphadenopathy.

Trauma such as a fractured tooth or broken bone provides definitive evidence of seizure activity. Trauma is generally absent if syncope is at fault. Other significant complications of seizures include lacerations, dislocations, concussion, aspiration pneumonia, arrhythmias, pulmonary edema, myocardial infarction, drowning, and death. Well-intentioned but misdirected bystanders who attempt to stop the seizure or stop the tongue from "being swallowed" can lead to trauma. Lacerations or fractures can suggest child abuse; shaken baby syndrome with CNS hemorrhage can present with a seizure.

C. Laboratory Findings

The decision to perform tests is based on: (1) the patient's age (patients <6 months require action); (2) history of preceding illness, especially diabetes mellitus, gastroenteritis, and dehydration; (3) history of substance abuse or drug exposure; (4) type of seizure (eg, complex partial seizures); (5) failure to return to normality following a seizure; and (6) interictal abnormal neurologic examination. **Table 9-6** lists the usual evaluations. The majority of evidence fails to support routine testing, especially for first-time, tonic-clonic seizures.

Routine blood tests are more often abnormal in patients with isolated seizures than in those with epilepsy. Persons taking carbamazepine, diuretics, or other medications can develop hyponatremia. Glucose, magnesium, and calcium levels and complete blood counts (CBCs) usually are normal. A high creatine phosphokinase or prolactin level (performed within 10–30 minutes of the seizure) may indicate prior generalized seizure activity with the exception of absence and myoclonic types. Other helpful evaluations include toxicology screens, pregnancy tests, and psychometric studies. Lumbar puncture is required for suspected meningitis, unusual in a fully immunized person. Meningococcal meningitis is most likely to affect young infants, first-year college students residing in a dormitory room, or travelers returning from the Middle East.

An EEG is diagnostic in 30–50% of first-time seizures; accuracy improves to 90% with repetitive testing. A focally abnormal EEG suggests the need for neuroimaging. A routine EEG is not necessary for a single febrile seizure. Up to a one-third of seizure victims with normal EEGs eventually are proven to have epilepsy. Awake, asleep, hyperventilation, and light-stimulated EEG tracings are best at uncovering an abnormality. Because tracings within 48 hours of a seizure may be falsely abnormal (generalized slowing common), the optimal timing for an EEG is in debate. EEG patterns are particularly diagnostic in absence spells, BECTS, and juvenile

Table 9-6. Recommendations for evaluation of a first seizure.

Study	Recommendation	Strength of Recommendation[a]
Electroencephalogram	All patients (somewhat in debate)	A
Blood tests [electrolytes, glucose, blood urea nitrogen (BUN), creatinine, calcium, magnesium]	Individual basis: especially indicated for age ≤6 months; continued illness; history of vomiting, diarrhea, dehydration, or diuretic use	A
Toxicology screening	Possible drug or substance of abuse exposure	C
Lumbar puncture	Possible meningitis or central nervous system (CNS) infection; continued CNS dysfunction	B

CNS imaging
  Computed tomography (CT)
  Magnetic resonance imaging (MRI)
	Value limited largely to head trauma
	Best performed for:
	Prolonged postictal paralysis or failure to return to baseline
	Persistent significant cognitive, motor, or other unexplained neurologic abnormality
	Age <12 months
	Perhaps with partial seizures
	An EEG indicative of nonbenign seizure disorder
		A
		A

Prolactin level	Variable benefit; 10–30 minutes after a seizure	B
Creatine kinase level	Variable benefit	C

[a]A, supported by clinical studies and expert opinion; B, expert opinion; limited evidence for support; C, limited to specific situations; insufficient evidence for or against this evaluation.

myoclonic epilepsy. Video-EEG recording can verify a seizure diagnosis or detect psychogenic seizures. Also, 24-hour EEG monitoring often reveals an unexpectedly high seizure frequency.

Many experts advise that an EEG is indicated for all patients with first nonfebrile seizures or repetitive febrile seizures, ~5% of whom develop epilepsy. However, obtaining an EEG after the first seizure may not be worthwhile, especially as obtaining an EEG is some children is difficult and ~2% of normal children have abnormal EEGs. If the EEG is abnormal, treatment with an AED often causes new dilemmas. Seizure reoccurrence is 50% with an abnormal EEG and 25% with a normal EEG. Neuroimaging deserves similar consideration. In the absence of other abnormalities, an underlying brain tumor in children and adolescents is extremely rare, but seizures are not. In an international review of 3291 children with brain tumors, only 35 otherwise normal children (1%) had a seizure as the initial difficulty. The key is to perform a complete physical examination and provide follow-up. Parental or patient acquiescence with a decision to delay evaluation until a second seizure occurs may be advisable.

Magnetic resonance imaging (MRI) is preferred over computed tomography (CT) scanning. Although abnormalities are detected in up to one-third of MRIs, only 1–2% of these findings influence either treatment or prognosis, especially in otherwise normal children. **Table 9-7** lists recommended evaluations for neuroimaging for each seizure type.

Neuroimaging is most useful for focal neurologic abnormalities; a history of infection, deteriorating behavior or school function, or trauma; the young infant; those with persistent focal seizures (except BECTS); focal EEG abnormalities; persons aged >18 years; or SE (27% have abnormal MRI findings). Prior to CNS surgery to treat epilepsy, MRI or cerebral angiography and positron emission tomography (PET) scans are needed to assess the feasibility and extent of the procedure.

▶ **Differential Diagnosis**

Seizure mimics in infants include gastroesophageal reflux, brief shuddering, benign nonepileptic myoclonus, or the Moro reflex; in toddlers, breath-holding spells, night terrors, and benign paroxysmal vertigo; and in older persons, tics, behavior problems, hysteria, panic attacks, transient global amnesia, and hyperventilation. Persons with psychogenic seizures (pseudoseizures) must be evaluated for psychiatric disturbances, especially depression or suicidal ideation. Psychogenic seizures account for 20% of referrals to epilepsy centers and often coexist with true seizures. Malingering to avoid stressful situations such as school (bullying is a

Table 9-7. Imaging recommendations for childhood seizures.

Seizure Type	Imaging Study
Neonatal	Cranial ultrasound preferred CT acceptable
Partial	MRI preferred CT acceptable
Generalized 　Neurologically normal 　Neurologically abnormal	 MRI or CT but low yield MRI preferred CT acceptable
Intractable or refractory	MRI preferred SPECT[a] acceptable PET acceptable
Febrile	No study
Post-traumatic (seizures within 　1 wk of trauma)	CT preferred MRI acceptable

[a]SPECT, single-photon emission computed tomography.

risk factor) or true conversion reactions are included in the differential. Malingering patients may use soap to simulate frothing at the mouth, bite their tongues, or urinate or defecate voluntarily to simulate seizures. The differential diagnosis includes drugs of abuse, narcolepsy, migraine, Tourette syndrome, shuddering attacks, hereditary tremors, and cough-induced or vasovagal syncopal convulsions. Syncopal seizures, uncovered through tilt table testing, are best treated with control of syncope, not seizures. Cardiac entities such as prolonged QT interval (electrocardiogram) or aortic stenosis or hypertrophic cardiomyopathy (echocardiogram) should be considered in those with a family history of fainting or suggestive physical findings. Specialist consultation, video-EEG recording, 24-hour EEG recording, and watchful waiting almost always provide the correct diagnosis eventually.

▶ **Treatment**

Four components constitute the cornerstones of epilepsy treatment: (1) avoidance of participating factors; (2) lifestyle modifications, including daily sleep regimens and exercise; (3) AEDs; and (4) surgery for localized seizure foci.

A. First Aid and Initial Care

Acute assistance for a seizure requires placing the patient prone, removing eyeglasses, loosening clothing and jewelry, and clearing the area of harmful objects, but *not* putting any object into the patient's mouth or attempting to apply any restraint. If a patient is diabetic, sublingual glucose (tablets or solution) or sucrose may help. After the seizure, the patient should be placed on one side and observed until awake. Families should call for medical assistance if a seizure lasts longer than 3 minutes, the patient requests assistance or is injured, or a second seizure occurs. After a tonic-clonic seizure, vigorous stimulation may reduce postictal apnea and perhaps sudden death. To reduce the risk of sudden death, patients with epilepsy should be encouraged to sleep in the *supine* position. Hospitalization is necessary only if the patient is at high risk, lives alone without appropriate supervision, or remains ill. Postictal confusion, sleepiness, headache, muscle soreness, and lethargy are common. Patients and families appreciate an explanation of what transpired, information as to how to avoid further difficulties, and definite follow-up arrangements. Avoidance of seizure-provoking activities and provocative drugs or behaviors is appropriate treatment for reactive seizures.

B. Pharmacotherapy

Reactive seizures with correctable causes or unprovoked seizures that are benign or infrequent do not require AEDs. Many experts do not use AEDs for a single seizure; medication side effects include worsening seizure severity or frequency, organ damage, or even death. AEDs do not positively affect long-term prognosis or always provide seizure control: 20–30% of those on AEDs still have significant seizure activity.

All primary care physicians should have a command of basic AED use and side effect profiles. In addition to carbamazepine, phenytoin, and valproic acid, three other AEDs approved for generalized tonic-clonic and partial epilepsy are worth attention: (1) lamotrigine approved for those aged >2 years, (2) levetiracetam for those aged >1 month and for myoclonic epilepsy in those aged >12 years, and (3) topiramate approved for persons aged >2 years. **Table 9-8** provides information on selected AEDs. Some drugs [acetazolamide, adrenocorticotropic hormone (ACTH), clobazam, ezogabine, felbamate, lacosamide, nitrazepam, oxcarbazepine, perampanel, pyridoxine (vitamin B_6), rufinamide, tiagabine, vigabatrin, and zonisamide] usually require specialist guidance, whereas others, including gabapentin, pregabalin, clonazepam, ethosuximide, and primidone, are often well known to primary care physicians.

The selection of AED is based on the seizure type, which is unfortunately inaccurately identified ~25% of the time. The least toxic AED, usually carbamazepine, lamotrigine, valproic acid, or levetiracetam, is initiated. Primary generalized seizures respond best to monotherapy with valproic acid, which controls seizures in 80%. Divalproex has fewer side effects, especially gastrointestinal. Lamotrigine and carbamazepine or levetiracetam are also good choices to control tonic-clonic or partial convulsions. Ethosuximide is ideal for absence spells, with lamotrigine and valproic acid as alternatives. Sometimes difficult to control, juvenile myoclonic epilepsy responds best to valproic acid. Gabapentin or pregabalin can be added

Table 9-8. Drugs for the treatment of seizures.

Drug	Seizure Type	Pediatric Dosage (mg/kg)		Adult Starting Daily Dose [Maximal Dose (mg)]	Number of Daily Doses	Therapeutic Level (μg/mL)	Dosage Forms		
		Starting Dose	Usual Daily Dose				Pill (mg)	Liquid	Notes
Lamotrigine	GM, CPS, SPS	0.15–0.6	1–15	100 (700)	2	Variable	CT: 2, 5, 25 T: 25, 100, 150, 200	—	Gen/Tr (some forms)
Topiramate	GM, CPS, SPS	1–3	5–9	25 (400)	2	Variable	C: 15, 25 T: 25, 50, 100, 200	—	Tr only
Phenytoin	GM, CPS, SPS	5 orally, 10–20 intravenously	5–15	100 TID (700)(1500 loading dose)	1–3	10–20	C:100 EC: 30, 100 CT: 50	S:125 mg/5 mL (use not recommended)	Gen/Tr (some forms)
Carbamazepine	GM, CPS, SPS	5–10	15–30	200 TID (2000)	2–4	4–12	T: 200 CT:100 ET: 100, 200, 300,400	S:100 mg/5 mL	Gen/Tr (some forms)
Valproic acid	GM, PM, CPS, SPS, M	10–15	15–60	250 BID (3000)	2–4	50–120	C: 250 CS:125 ET: 500 DI: 125, 250, 500	SY: 250 mg/5 mL	Gen/Tr (some forms)
Ethosuximide	PM	10–20	10–40	250 BID (2000)	1–2	40–100	C: 250	SY: 250 mg/5 mL	Gen/Tr (some forms)
Clonazepam	M	0.01–0.03	0.025–0.2	0.5 TID (20)	2–3	18–80	T: 0.5, 1, 2	—	Gen/Tr
Gabapentin	Additive only; GM, CPS, SPS	10–15	25–50	100 TID (4800)	3	>2	C: 100, 300, 400, 800 T: 100, 300, 400, 600, 800	Sol: 250 mg/5 mL	Tr
Primidone Levetiracetam	GM, CPS, SPS GM, CPS, SPS, M	10 10	10–30 20–60	100 QHS (1500) 500 BID (3000)	2–4 1–2	5–15 Not established	T: 50, 250 T: 250, 500, 750, 1000 ET: 500, 750	— Sol: 300 mg/5 ml	Gen/Tr (some forms) Gen/Tr

C, capsule; CPS, complex partial seizure; CS, capsule sprinkles; CT, chewable tablet; DT, delayed-release tablet; EC, extended-release capsule; ET, extended-release tablet; Gen, generic; GM, grand mal; M, myoclonic; PM, petit mal; S, suspension; Sol, solution; SPS, simple partial seizure; SY, syrup; T, tablet; Tr, trade.

Table 9-9. Side effects of selected antiepileptic drugs.

Drug	Common Side Effects
Phenytoin	Hirsutism, coarse facial appearance, gum hyperplasia, nystagmus
Carbamazepine	Hyponatremia (in ≤10% of patients)
Valproic acid	Hair loss, weight gain, edema, pancreatitis, thrombocytopenia
Lamotrigine	Life-threatening rash (as high as ~1 out of 50 children; first 2 months of treatment)
Phenobarbital	Personality change
Topiramate	Renal stones, weight loss
Zonisamide	Renal stones
Ethosuximide	Abdominal pain, abnormal behavior
Levetiracetam	Dizziness, behavioral changes, severe rash
Gabapentin	Nausea, lethargy, behavioral changes

Reprinted with special permission from Treatment Guidelines from The Medical Letter. *Drugs for Epilepsy.* 2013; 11:9–18. [PMID 23348233]

Table 9-10. Recommended monitoring parameters for antiepileptic drugs.

Lrug	Monitoring
Carbamazepine	Complete blood count (CBC) with platelets at baseline, then twice monthly for first 2 months, and annually or as clinically indicated Blood chemistries with emphasis on hepatic and renal function and electrolytes at baseline, then at 1 months, and annually or as clinically indicated Electrocardiogram (ECG) at baseline for patients >40 years and as clinically indicated
Phenytoin	CBC at baseline and as clinically indicated Blood chemistries with emphasis on hepatic and renal functions at baseline, annually, and as clinically indicated ECG at baseline for patients >40 years and as clinically indicated Phenytoin level in 1 weeks, then in 1 month, and annually or as clinically indicated in older patients
Valproic acid	CBC with platelets at baseline, then twice monthly for first 2 months, and annually or as clinically indicated Blood chemistries with emphasis on hepatic function at baseline, then at 1 month, and annually or as clinically indicated Protime, international normalized ratio (INR), partial prothrombin time (PPT) at baseline and annually Valproic acid level weekly for 2 weeks, then annually or as clinically indicated in older patients

Data from the National Institute for Health and Clinical Excellence (NICE). *The Epilepsies: The Diagnosis and Management of the Epilepsies in Adults and Children in Primary and Secondary Care.* London, UK: National Institute for Health and Clinical Excellence (NICE); 2012 (Clinical Guideline 137).

when control of seizures is inadequate. Any new symptom or sign in a patient on an AED must trigger a search in a standard reference for AED side effects (**Table 9-9**). These are sometimes serious and often unfamiliar to primary care physicians. Many of the newer agents are also expensive. Generic carbamazepine and levetiracetam are inexpensive. Because of its side effects, phenytoin has fallen from favor but is still frequently prescribed because it is among the cheaper effective AEDs. For a patient on phenytoin, whenever any drug is added to or withdrawn from the medical regimen, a serum phenytoin level should be obtained, usually 5–7 days later. Phenobarbital should not be used. For home treatment of acute repetitive seizures, rectal diazepam gel (0.2–0.5 mg/kg) or buccal or intranasal midazolam liquid (0.25–1 mg/kg) are safe and effective.

Use of one drug to control seizures—increased to its maximum dose or to just below toxicity if necessary—is best. If one drug proves to be ineffective, another AED is started while the current AED is withdrawn slowly over ≥1 week. Polytherapy is fraught with drug side effects and often loss of seizure control, but to achieve satisfactory control, it is necessary to administer two drugs in 25% of patients. Neurologic consultation is often a superior choice to random new drug use.

Serum AED levels to guide dosage should be obtained: (1) as a check on compliance; (2) to detect toxicity, especially with multiagent regimens or in the young or mentally handicapped; (3) when the drug regimen is changed; (4) for poor seizure control; and (5) when a problem develops that can affect drug levels. **Table 9-10** provides a scheme for monitoring the effects of three common AEDs: valproic acid, phenytoin, and carbamazepine. Valproic acid levels often fail to predict either toxicity or seizure control. Whether seizure-free patients require periodic drug level monitoring is unclear. Growing children may need levels more often, but after informing patients and parents about the plan, allowing a seizure-free child to "grow out" of the AED like a slow taper-off medication seems reasonable. In some circumstances such as pregnancy or salicylate use, free-AED (nonprotein-bound) serum levels may be a better guide to dosing, especially for phenytoin and valproic acid.

Whether routine checks of hematologic or liver functions can prevent organ damage is also unclear. All patients and parents should be warned to be alert for fever, jaundice, itching, bruising, and bleeding, as signs of toxicity. Many physicians follow CBCs, liver and renal tests, and serum AED levels periodically, once or twice a year.

Some AEDs, especially carbamazepine, phenytoin, primidone, and topiramate, may interfere with oral contraceptives. Midcycle bleeding indicates possible oral contraceptive failure. Management includes alternative contraceptive methods, a higher estrogen content product, or a noninteracting AED such as gabapentin, levetiracetam, or valproic acid. Some AEDs may increase the risk of suicide, but the overall risk is low. In one large study, suicidal ideation was 0.43% on AEDs compared to 0.22% on placebo, but another study found no direct link. Some AEDs may adversely affect bone density.

No specific seizure-free time interval predicts resolution of epilepsy. A single seizure type, normal neurologic examination, normal IQ, and normal EEG all predict good outcomes if the AED is stopped. In one study of 1013 patients free of seizures for 2 years, 40% had a recurrence following drug withdrawal compared with 12% of those who maintained AED treatments. Freedom from drug side effects and daily medication must be weighed against this 28% difference with potential loss of job or driving ability or possible injury. A recent abnormal EEG would make a decision to stop therapy more difficult. Most AEDs should be slowly withdrawn over at least 6–12 weeks. During withdrawal, recurrence of the aura signals that the risk of seizure recurrence is high. Once children grow into young adulthood, assuming a 2–5-year period without seizures, attempts to stop AED treatment ought to be strongly considered.

During pregnancy, since all AEDs can cause fetal malformations, the AED that controls seizures the best, except possibly valproic acid, should be continued. A fetal sonogram can identify malformations. Folic acid, 4 mg daily, and vitamins D and K during the last 4 weeks minimize fetal problems. Serum AED levels during pregnancy are helpful. Women who take AEDs can safely breastfeed.

C. Referral or Hospitalization

Poorly controlled or complicated seizures or progressive developmental delay should prompt neurologic consultation. Hospitalization is necessary for prolonged or complicated seizures, SE, inadequate family resources, or parental or physician concern. In general, seizures are not dangerous and do not cause CNS damage, but persons with repetitive seizures must be guarded from injury and other complications.

D. Surgery and Other Treatments

Treatments that require referral and extensive evaluation prior to institution include vagal nerve stimulation, ketogenic diet, and surgery. Vagal nerve stimulation is less invasive than surgery and controls or reduces seizures in ~40% of patients with previously refractory epilepsy. The ketogenic diet reduces episodes by ~50%, but compliance is difficult.

Many experts believe that surgical correction for epilepsy is underutilized. At least 20% of patients with epilepsy are inadequately controlled with AEDs alone, and some who are controlled on AEDs will benefit from surgery because of reduced seizure frequency or AED side effects. Surgery for specific epilepsy types, including temporal lobe lesion resection, results in 80% seizure-free outcomes. Indications for surgery include recurrent uncontrolled seizures, focal EEGs, consistent focal abnormalities on neuroimaging, or major AED side effects. Unfortunately, PET or single-photon emission computed tomography (SPECT) imaging often reveals unsuspected abnormalities that may preclude surgical correction.

E. Family Counseling

Family members, caregivers, teachers, and coworkers need instruction in proper seizure first aid. Helpful information and group support are available from the American Epilepsy Society (http://www.aesnet.org), the Epilepsy Foundation of America (http://www.epilepsyfoundation.org/), or local epilepsy foundations. Vocational help and assistance to defray medical costs, such as drug manufacturer patient assistance programs, are often needed. A close physician-patient relationship, adequate sleep and exercise, stress reduction, and avoidance of alcohol or sedative drugs serve the interests of patients and their families.

A seizure per se does not lower IQ or cause brain damage. Although the negative consequences of epilepsy to daily life should not be underestimated, most otherwise normal patients lead full, productive lives. Scheduling activities for each day may help. Some children respond better to home schooling until seizures are controlled. Untreated epilepsy is often but not always debilitating. Children with epilepsy are significantly more likely to suffer from depression, attention deficit–hyperactivity disorder, developmental delay, autism, and headaches. For those who develop psychological dysfunction, especially depression, psychiatric consultation or medication is usually helpful.

F. Alternative Therapies

Few alternative therapies have evidence-based support. Pyridoxine (vitamin B_6) and magnesium have scientific grounding for specific seizure disorders. Beneficial claims for acupuncture, chiropractic, or naturopathic manipulation are unfounded. Food allergies do not cause convulsions unless they cause anaphylaxis or epilepsy. Most alternative therapy sources advise avoidance of alcohol, caffeine, and aspartame, the first two of which are logical. Proof that taurine, folic acid, vitamin B_{12}, manganese, zinc, dimethylglycine, megavitamins, or various diets reduce seizure frequency or medication requirements is absent or marginal.

Herbal remedies such as passionflower, skullcap, valerian, belladonna, causticum, cicuta, or cuprum metallicum have not been adequately studied. On the other hand, any nontoxic technique to reduce stress and bring order to a patient's life may help. Some patients have learned to control seizures with self-relaxation or special techniques such as looking at a particular piece of jewelry as an aura comes on. Those who wish to augment medical treatment with noninvasive treatments may be permitted to do so after physician review for safety and follow-up to see if the treatments appear to help over time.

▶ Febrile Convulsions

The most common seizure disorder, febrile convulsions, affects 3% of children between ages 6 months and 6 years. After age 14 years febrile seizures are rare. Despite a recurrence rate of 30%, only 3% of these individuals develop epilepsy. Those with a family history of epilepsy, abnormal neurologic or developmental status prior to the seizure, or a prolonged (>15-minute) focal seizure have at least a 15% chance of epilepsy. Commonly, a toddler with an upper respiratory infection, enterovirus, or roseola suddenly seizes during an afternoon nap. Usually short tonic-clonic convulsions, such seizures are multiple in one-third of cases. Postictal sleepiness can last several hours. Laboratory tests are unnecessary unless the child is aged <6 months or meningitis is suggested by failure to arouse, continued focal seizures, or physical findings (stiff neck, bulging fontanel, rash). Seizures that occur in the office or emergency department are suggestive of more serious infection.

Treatment consists of reassurance to worried parents that the worst has passed and that these seizures leave no permanent brain damage. Controlling fever with warm baths to reduce shivering, acetaminophen (10–15 mg/kg every 4 hours), or ibuprofen (5–10 mg/kg every 6 hours) may reduce immediate risk of recurrence. If begun at the onset of fever, buccal or intranasal midazolam, 0.25–1 mg/kg; oral or rectal valproic acid, 20 mg/kg every 8 hours for 1–3 days; or diazepam, 0.5 mg/kg every 8 hours for 1–3 days can reduce recurrence. Intravenous lorazepam is the drug of choice for prolonged febrile seizures. Hospitalization is best if seizures are prolonged beyond 30 minutes or are recurrent or complicated, if follow-up is inadequate, or if parents or the physician want observation. Chronic treatment is advised only for the child with multiple recurrences, persistent neurologic abnormality, or worrisome EEG findings.

▶ Status Epilepticus

Any recurrent or prolonged seizure uninterrupted by consciousness for more than 5 minutes is termed *status epilepticus* (SE), which is classified as either convulsive or nonconvulsive. SE carries a low risk of permanent residual brain damage that can be minimized through rapid treatment. Approximately 5% of children with febrile convulsions and 20% of all persons with epilepsy have SE at least once. Newly diagnosed epileptic patients often develop SE. Although any seizure type—including myoclonic or simple partial seizures—can cause SE, most commonly consciousness is severely impaired. A persistent grand mal seizure is readily identified as SE, but diagnosing SE in a comatose patient with no abnormal motor movement can be difficult without an EEG. Confused but ambulatory persons may be in a state absence or complex partial epilepsy SE. Diagnosis is based on EEG findings. Death is usually related to a serious underlying etiology rather than SE itself.

Management requires stabilization of vital signs. Adolescents and adults should be given 100 mg of thiamine with 50 mL of 50% glucose (children: 2–4 mL/kg of 25% glucose) and naloxone (0.1–2 mg/kg; children 0.01 mg/kg) repeated as necessary. Lorazepam, 0.1 mg/kg (maximum of

Table 9-11. Evaluation of neonatal seizures.

I. History
  A. Pregnancy related
    1. Infection: toxoplasmosis, rubella, cytomegalovirus, herpes, syphilis (TORCHS) titers; IgM level
    2. Maternal addiction: smoking, alcohol, cocaine, heroin, barbiturates
    3. Maternal behavior: inadequate prenatal care, lack of folic acid
  B. Delivery related
    1. Anoxia
    2. Trauma
  C. Family history: chromosomal disorders, errors of metabolism

II. Physical findings
  A. Recognizable patterns of malformation: eyes, ears, hands, facies, head shape
  B. Neurologic evaluation: motor, sensory, cranial nerves
  C. Odor: phenylketonuria
  D. Dermatologic signs: crusted vesicles, abnormal creases, hypopigmentation, nevi
  E. Ocular: chorioretinitis, cataracts, coloboma, cherry red spot

III. Laboratory evaluation
  A. Neuroimaging: cranial ultrasound, magnetic resonance imaging (MRI), computed tomography (CT) scan
  B. Chest radiograph
  C. Cerebral spinal fluid: culture, cell count, Gram stain, India ink, VDRL,[a] glycine, glucose, protein, xanthochromia
  D. Blood test: cultures, complete blood count, electrolytes, renal function, glucose, magnesium, calcium, karyotype, glycine, lactate, ammonia, long-chain fatty acid levels
  E. Urine: culture, glucose, protein, cells

[a]VDRL, Venereal Disease Research Laboratory.
Data from the National Institute for Health and Clinical Excellence (NICE). *The Epilepsies: The Diagnosis and Management of the Epilepsies in Adults and Children in Primary and Secondary Care.* London, UK: National Institute for Health and Clinical Excellence (NICE); 2012 (Clinical Guideline 137).

4 mg) intravenous push at 2 mg/min, is successful in stopping 80% of SE episodes in 2–3 minutes. A second dose in 10 minutes is frequently successful in the remaining 20%. Midazolam is the drug of choice for intramuscular SE control. Although the intranasal and buccal routes are particularly useful if neither the IV nor IM routes are feasible, rectal diazepam is currently the drug of choice. Poorly controlled SE responds to phenytoin, 20 mg/kg intravenous push at 50 mg/min, while monitoring the electrocardiogram and blood pressure, or its safer prodrug, fosphenytoin, given at 30 mg/kg intravenous push at 150 mg/min. Other alternatives are midazolam, levetiracetam, and propofol. Some SE in children younger than 18 months of age responds to pyridoxine, 50 mg intravenously. For other information, the clinician is referred to the Cochrane Database. Once the SE is controlled, a search for the underlying cause should be conducted.

Table 9-12. Clinical practice guidelines for management of patients with seizure disorders.

Clinical Scenario	Guideline
Febrile seizure	Children with febrile seizures, even if recurrent, should rarely be treated with antiepileptic drugs (AEDs)
Provoked seizure	Long-term prophylactic AED treatment for children with head injuries or correctable causes of seizure is not indicated
Unprovoked, tonic-clonic epileptic seizure	AED treatment should generally not be commenced routinely after a first, unprovoked tonic-clonic seizure if the history and physical examination are otherwise normal
Generalized epilepsy	The choice of first AED should be determined, where possible, by the seizure type and potential adverse effects
Focal seizure	When appropriate monotherapy fails to reduce seizure frequency, combination therapy should be considered; use of >2 drugs usually requires consultation
Monitoring for adverse effects of AEDs	Routine AED level monitoring is generally not required
Withdrawal of AEDs	Withdrawal of AED treatment should be considered for individuals who have been seizure-free for ≥2 years, especially if a recent EEG is normal
Prolonged or serial seizure	Prolonged or serial seizures can be treated with intravenous lorazepam or intranasal or buccal midazolam or rectal diazepam

Neonatal Seizures

Neonatal seizures are difficult to recognize. In the first month of life, clonic-tonic seizure activity is uncommon. Focal rhythmic twitches, recurrent vomiting, poor feeding and responsiveness, high-pitched crying, posturing, chewing, apnea, cyanosis, and excessive salivation should raise alarm. Diligent inquiry into family history, prenatal history, and maternal habits is warranted. Neurologic consultation is advisable. Often difficult to control, these seizures may have a dismal outcome. Treatment for maternal drug addiction with resultant neonatal drug withdrawal seizures, which usually leave no residual defects, includes paregoric, methadone, phenobarbital, and various benzodiazepines. **Table 9-11** lists suggested evaluations.

Prognosis

Clinical practice guidelines for management of patients with seizure disorders are presented in **Table 9-12**. Overall, roughly one-third of patients have a second seizure, and about 75% of these experience a third seizure. No adverse outcomes are likely even with ≤10 untreated seizures. A study of 220 children indicated that 92% of those treated for idiopathic seizures remained seizure-free for as long as 5 years. Eventually 70% of epileptic children and 60% of adults become seizure-free posttreatment.

Sudden unexpected death in epilepsy occurs in 1–2 persons per 1000 per year, peaking at age 50–59 years. Tonic-clonic seizures, treatment with three or more AEDs, and an intelligence quotient (IQ) of <70 are risk factors for sudden death; choice of AED and AED serum levels are not.

Appleton R, Macleod S, Martland T. Drug management for acute tonic-clonic convulsions including convulsive status epilepticus in children. Cochrane Epilepsy Group, published online; 2010 (DOI: 10.1002/14651858.CD001905.pub2). [PMID: 18646081]

Berg AT, Berkovic SF, Brodie MJ, et al. Revised terminology and concepts for organization of seizures and epilepsies: report of the ILAE commission on classification and terminology, 2005–2009. *Epilepsia.* 2010; 51:676–685. [PMID: 20196795]

Brophy GM, Bell R, Claassen J, et al. Neurocritical Care Society Status Epilepticus Guideline Writing Committee. Guidelines for the evaluation and management of status epilepticus. *Neurocrit Care.* 2012; 17(1):3–23. [PMID: 22528274]

Centers for Disease Control and Prevention. Epilepsy in adults and access to care–United States, 2010. *MMWR.* 2012; 61: 909–913. [PMID: 23151949]

Devinsky O. Sudden, unexpected death in epilepsy. *N Engl J Med.* 2011; 365:1801–1811. [PMID: 22070477]

National Institute for Health and Clinical Excellence (NICE). *The Epilepsies: The Diagnosis and Management of the Epilepsies in Adults and Children in Primary and Secondary Care.* London, UK: National Institute for Health and Clinical Excellence (NICE); 2012 (Clinical Guideline 137).

Patel H, Dunn DW, Austin JK, et al. Psychogenic nonepileptic seizures (pseudoseizures). *Pediatr Rev.* 2011; 32:e66–e72. [PMID: 21632872]

Russ SA, Larson K, Halfon N. A national profile of childhood epilepsy and seizure disorder. *Pediatrics*. 2012; 129:256–264. [PMID: 22271699]

Subcommittee on Febrile Seizures, American Academy of Pediatrics. Neurodiagnostic evaluation of the child with a simple febrile seizure. *Pediatrics*. 2011; 127(2):389–394. [PMID: 21285335]

The Medical Letter. *Drugs for Epilepsy*. 2013; 11:9–20. [PMID: 23348233]

Wilden JA, Cohen-Gadol AA. Evaluation of first nonfebrile seizures. *Am Fam Physician*. 2012; 86:334–340. [PMID: 22963022]

Wolf P. Acute drug administration in epilepsy: a review. *CNS Neurosci Ther*. 2011; 17:442–448. [PMID: 21951369]

Physical Activity in Adolescents

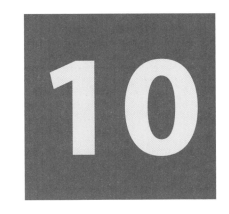

Christopher W. Bunt, MD, FAAFP

Mark B. Stephens, MD, MS, FAAFP

"Do it, move it, make it happen. No one ever sat their way to success."

—*Unknown*

The United States continues to struggle with the medical and economic consequences of physical inactivity and obesity. Despite evidence that trends in rising rates of obesity are slowing, declines in physical activity over the past several decades have largely mirrored the rise in obesity among children and adolescents. Longitudinal data from the National Health and Examination Surveys (NHES) show that the percentage of overweight and obese adolescents in the United States has increased from 5% to 18% since the mid-1980s. Obese youth are less likely to engage in physical activity and are much more likely to report chronic health problems compared with peers of normal weight. Obese adolescents are also more likely to struggle with orthopedic problems and behavioral health issues and to be obese as adults.[1]

During adolescence, levels of spontaneous physical activity drop significantly from high points in childhood. The number of US adolescents meeting recommended activity levels is low, and this figure has not changed significantly over the past 10+ years (**Table 10-1**). Adolescents spend much of their time engaged in sedentary activities. Most adolescents engage in ≥1 hour of technology-related behavior (TV, Internet, videogaming, etc) per day. In contrast, adolescents currently average a mere 12 minutes per day of vigorous physical activity. One-third of the US high-school students are not regularly active; one-half of high school seniors are not enrolled in physical education classes, and 70% of all high school students watch ≥1 hour of TV every day of the week. For students who are enrolled in physical education, the actual amount of class time devoted to physical

activity is often insignificant. Students often spend most of their time in physical education class standing around, waiting for instructions, or socializing. Teens active in school sporting activities are also more likely to be active as adults. Health-related behaviors, such as dietary habits and physical activity patterns, solidify during adolescence and persist into adulthood. Recognition of individuals who are insufficiently active, overweight, or obese during adolescence is key to promoting lifelong healthy behaviors.

Gordon-Larsen P, et al. Longitudinal physical activity and sedentary behavior trends: adolescence to adulthood. *Am J Prevent Med.* 2004; 27:277. [PMID: 15488356]

Lowry R, et al. Recent trends in participation in physical education among US high school students. *J School Health.* 2001; 71:145. [PMID: 11357870]

National Center for Health Statistics. *Prevalence of Obesity among Children and Adolescents: United States, Trends 1963–1965 through 2009–2010.* CDC, Health E-Stat. (http://www.cdc.gov/nchs/data/hestat/obesity_child_09_10/obesity_child_09_10.htm; accessed April 8, 2013).

Singh A, et al. Tracking of childhood overweight into adulthood: a systematic review of the literature. *Obes Rev.* 2008;9(5): 474–488. [PMID: 18331423]

Telama R, et al. Physical activity from childhood to adulthood: a 21-year tracking study. *Am J Prevent Med.* 2005;28(3):267–273. [PMID: 15766614]

DEFINITIONS

The following definitions apply to the discussion of physical activity and obesity (**Table 10-2**). *Physical fitness* refers to a general state of well-being that allows an individual to perform activities of daily living in a vigorous manner. Physical fitness includes health-related characteristics and skill-related characteristics. Health-related components of physical fitness include cardiorespiratory endurance, muscular strength, muscular endurance, flexibility, and body composition. Skill-related components of physical fitness include

---

[1]The opinions herein are those of the authors. They do not represent official policy of the Department of Defense, the Department of the Navy or the Air Force, or the Uniformed Services University.

Table 10-1. Trends in moderate-to-vigorous physical activity and sedentary behavior among US High School Students, 2011 national overview.

General Behaviors

13.8% of students had not participated in ≥60 minutes of any kind of physical activity that increased their heart rate and made them breathe hard some of the time on at least 1 day during the 7 days before the survey (ie, did not participate in ≥60 minutes of physical activity on any given day)

28.7% of students had been physically active doing any kind of physical activity that increased their heart rate and made them breathe hard some of the time for a total of ≥60 minutes per day on each of the 7 days before the survey (ie, were physically active for ≥60 minutes on all 7 days)

51.8% of students went to physical education (PE) classes on ≥1 day in an average week when they were in school (ie, attended PE classes)

31.5% of students attended PE classes 5 days in an average week when they were in school (ie, attended PE classes daily)

Sedentary Behaviors

31.1% of students played videogames or computer games or used a computer for nonschool work activity for ≥3 days on an average school day (ie, used computers ≥3 hours per day)

32.4% of students watched television ≥3 hours per day on an average school day

Data from the National Youth Risk Behavior Surveys, Centers for Disease Control and Prevention.

Table 10-2. Definitions of physical activity, physical fitness, and exercise.

Physical activity	Any body movement that results in the expenditure of energy
Physical fitness	A general state of overall well-being that allows individuals to conduct the majority of their activities of daily living in a vigorous manner
Health-related physical fitness	Aerobic capacity (cardiorespiratory endurance) Body composition Muscular strength Muscular endurance Flexibility
Skill-related physical fitness	Power Agility Speed Balance Coordination Reaction time
Exercise	A structured routine of physical activity specifically designed to improve or maintain one of the components of health-related physical fitness

power, speed, agility, and balance. Historically, physical education programs have emphasized skill-related activities and athletic ability. From a public health perspective, however, the health-related components of physical fitness are more important in terms of overall morbidity and mortality from chronic diseases related to physical inactivity.

Physical activity refers to any body movement resulting in the expenditure of energy. Physical activity occurs in a broad range of settings. Leisure-time activities, occupational activities, routine activities of daily living, and dedicated exercise programs all represent valid forms of physical activity. Physical activity varies along a continuum of intensity from light (eg, housework) to moderate (eg, jogging) to more vigorous (eg, strenuous bicycling). *Exercise* refers to a structured routine of physical activity that is specifically designed to improve or maintain one of the components of health-related physical fitness. Historically, society has placed more emphasis on formal exercise programs as the primary means of achieving physical fitness rather than promoting physical activity in a more general sense.

Body mass index (BMI) is the anthropometric measurement of choice for assessing body composition in children, adolescents, and adults. BMI is calculated by dividing an individual's weight (in kilograms) by the square of the individual's height (in meters). Charts and digital tools for the office (http://www.nhlbi.nih.gov/guidelines/obesity/BMI/bmicalc.htm) and for mobile devices are available for rapid calculation of BMI. Normative values for underweight, normal weight, overweight, and obesity for adolescents have been established, and are presented in **Table 10-3**. BMI-for-age charts have replaced standard weight-for-height charts as the preferred mechanism for tracking weight in children and adolescents (**Figures 10-1** and **10-2**). *Overweight* adolescents are those who fall between the 85th and 95th percentiles of BMI-for-age. *Obese* adolescents are above the 95th percentile of BMI-for-age.

Table 10-3. Definitions of overweight and obesity for adolescents and adults.

Definition	Clinical Parameter
Obesity (adults)	BMI >30
Overweight (adults)	BMI 25.1–29.9
Obesity (adolescents)	BMI >95th percentile for age
Overweight (adolescents)	95th < BMI >85th percentile for age
Underweight (adolescents)	BMI <5th percentile for age

Data from Centers for Disease Control and Prevention (http://www.cdc.gov/nccdphp/dnpa/bmi/bmi-for-age.htm).

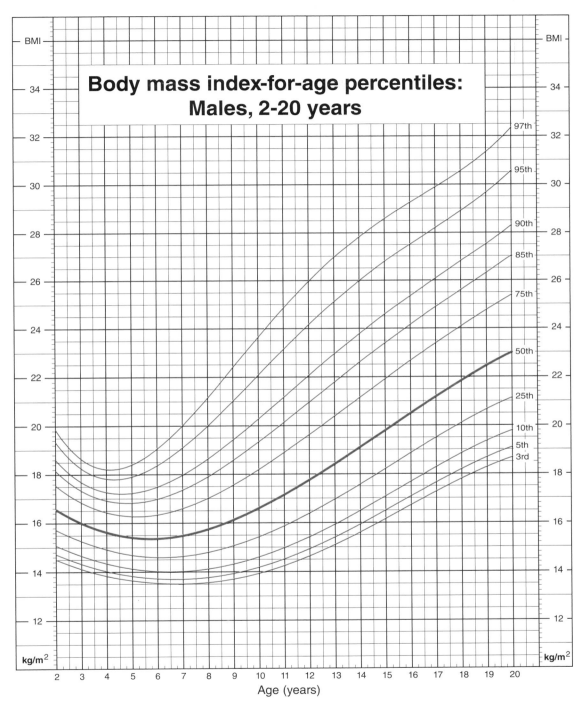

▲ **Figure 10-1.** Body mass index for age: males. [From Centers for Disease Control and Prevention, Atlanta, GA (available at http://www.cdc.gov/growthcharts/data/set1clinical/cj41l023.pdf).]

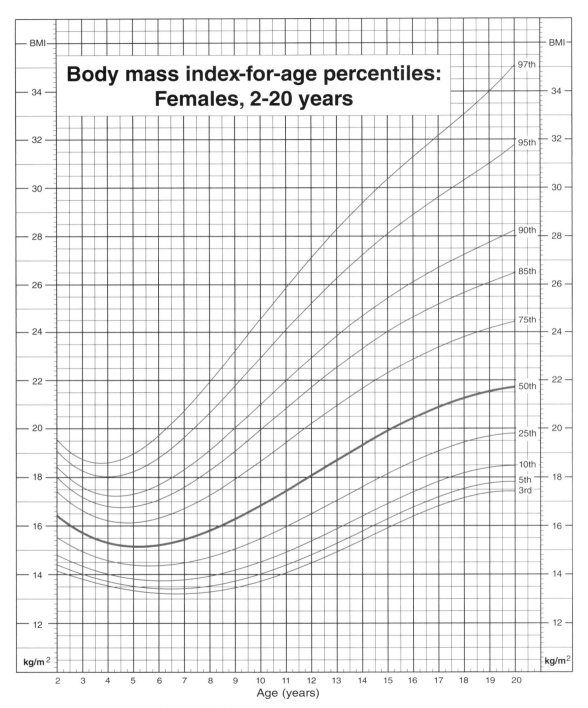

▲ **Figure 10-2.** Body mass index for age: females. [From Centers for Disease Control and Prevention, Atlanta, GA; (available at http://www.cdc.gov/growthcharts/data/set1clinical/cj41l024.pdf).]

Bouchard C, et al. Why study physical activity and health? In: Bouchard C et al. eds. *Physical Activity and Health.* Champaign, IL: Human Kinetics; 2007: 3–19.

Brener ND, et al. *School Health Profiles: Characteristics of Health Programs among Secondary Schools in Selected US sites.* (School Health Profiles 2010.) Atlanta, GA: Centers for Disease Control and Prevention; 2011 (available at http://www.cdc.gov/healthyyouth/profiles/2010/profiles_report.pdf; last accessed on April 18, 2013).

Ogden CL, Carroll MD, Kit BK, Flegal KM. *Prevalence of Obesity in the United States 2009–2010.* (NCHS Data Brief 82.) Hyattsville, MD: National Center for Health Statistics; 2012.

RISKS ASSOCIATED WITH PHYSICAL INACTIVITY

Physical inactivity is a primary risk factor for cardiovascular disease and all-cause mortality. A sedentary lifestyle also contributes to increased rates of diabetes, hypertension, hyperlipidemia, osteoporosis, cerebrovascular disease, and colon cancer. Adolescents who are less physically active are more likely to smoke cigarettes, less likely to consume appropriate amounts of fruits and vegetables, less likely to routinely wear a seatbelt, and more likely to spend increased time engaged in sedentary technology-related behaviors.

Physical activity serves numerous preventive functions. In addition to preventing chronic diseases such as hypertension, diabetes, and cardiovascular disease, sufficient levels of physical activity on a regular basis are associated with lower rates of mental illness. Teens that spend more time engaged in sedentary technology-related behaviors have higher rates of depression. Physically active adolescents have lower levels of stress and anxiety and have higher self-esteem than sedentary peers. Active adolescents also have fewer somatic complaints, and are more confident about their own future health. They have improved relationships with parents and authority figures, and also have a better body image.

Gopinath B, Hardy LL, Baur LA, Burlutsky G, Mitchell P. Physical activity and sedentary behaviors and health-related quality of life in adolescents. *Pediatrics.* 2012; 130(1):e167–e174.

Lotan M, et al. Physical activity in adolescence. a review with clinical suggestions. *Int J Adolesc Med Health.* 2004;16:13. [PMID: 15900808]

Primack B, et al. Association between media use in adolescence and depression in young adulthood: a longitudinal study. *Arch Gen Psychiatr.* 2009; 66(2):181–188. [PMID: 19188540]

Suris JC, Parera N. Don't stop, don't stop: physical activity and adolescence. *Int J Adolesc Med Health.* 2005; 17:67. [PMID: 15900813]

FACTORS INFLUENCING PHYSICAL ACTIVITY

Despite the overwhelming evidence supporting the health-related benefits of physical activity, young Americans are becoming increasingly sedentary. A complex interaction of social, cultural, gender-related, environmental, and familial factors associated with "modern living" has contributed to decreased rates of physical activity.

▶ Social Factors

Socioeconomic status is one of the strongest predictors of physical activity in both adolescents and adults. Lower socioeconomic status is associated with lower levels of spontaneous physical activity. Youth of higher socioeconomic status engage in more spontaneous physical activity, are more frequently enrolled in physical education classes, and are more likely to be active during physical education classes when compared with peers of lower socioeconomic status. This relationship persists when controlling for age, gender, and ethnicity. The Task Force on Community Preventive Services (http://www.thecommunityguide.org/pa/index.html) found strong evidence of the effectiveness of implementing programs designed to increase the length or activity levels of school-based physical education classes. Such school-based programs improve both physical activity levels and physical fitness in children and adolescents.

Social mobility also plays an important role in shaping levels of physical activity. Specifically, achieved levels of social positioning are more strongly associated with positive health behaviors and increased levels of physical activity than the social class of origin. Youth with active friends are more likely to be active. Youth with sedentary friends are more likely to be sedentary. There are also significant differences in patterns of spontaneous physical activity when youth attending public schools are compared with youth attending private secondary schools. In the public school system, individuals are more likely to enroll in physical education classes. In private schools, adolescents are more likely to participate in organized team sports. Participation in organized sports is associated with higher levels of physical activity in adulthood.

As a consequence of modern life, most Americans have become increasingly reliant on automated transportation. This has had a negative impact on the simplest form of physical activity: walking. Historically, youth walked to school. This no longer holds true. Despite the fact that one-third of American schoolchildren live less than 1 mile from their school, fewer than 25% of these children walk or bike to school. The number of children walking to school in the United States has decreased by 66% since 1977.

▶ Cultural & Ethnic Factors

Cohort studies consistently suggest that there are inherent cultural differences in levels of spontaneous physical activity. Data from the Youth Risk Behavior Survey (http://www.cdc.gov/HealthyYouth/yrbs/index.htm) and the National Longitudinal Study of Adolescent Health (http://www.cpc.unc.edu/projects/addhealth) show that minority adolescents engage in the lowest levels of physical activity. These findings are consistent for both leisure-time physical activity and activity during physical education class.

Currently, 25% of adolescents consider themselves to be "too fat." Hispanic youth are more likely to view themselves as overweight when compared with African Americans and non-Hispanic whites. Adolescents viewing themselves as overweight are significantly less physically active than normal-weight peers and are less likely to engage in healthy behaviors. Compared with non-Hispanic whites, African American and Hispanic youth are at significantly higher risk for being overweight and obese. The NHES data through 2010 reveal an obesity prevalence of 18% for non-Hispanic whites, compared to 23% for non-Hispanic blacks and 29% for Mexican Americans.

There are important cultural differences in perceptions about the inherent value of exercise. Not all cultures encourage using leisure time for fitness activities. In fact, dedicating time for exercise as an isolated activity can be viewed as either selfish or as a poor use of time. Cultural and ethnic differences also exist in television viewing habits. Hispanic and African American adolescents spend significantly more time watching television than do non-Hispanic whites.

Gender-Related Factors

There are significant differences in levels of spontaneous physical activity between male and female adolescents. Boys are generally more active than girls from childhood through adolescence. Levels of physical activity decline for both boys and girls during adolescence, but there is a disproportionate decline for girls. The reasons for this are unclear. Factors that are positively associated with an increased likelihood of physical activity among female adolescents include perceived competence at a particular activity, perceived value of the activity, favorable physical appearance during and after the activity, and positive social support for the activity.

Environmental Factors

Many of the barriers to physical activity are environmental. Of these, television, Internet surfing, and videogaming ("screen-time" activities) may be the most important for adolescents. It is estimated that between the ages of 8 and 18, youth spend an average of 4.5 hours daily engaged in technology-related sedentary behaviors. This translates to >25% of waking hours spent in front of a videomonitor. By contrast, adolescents spend <1% of their time (an estimated 12–14 minutes per day) engaged in vigorous physical activity. The impact of television, video, personal computers, and handheld gaming devices on the activity levels of youth is so significant that the American Academy of Pediatrics has released a position statement recommending that youth engage in no more than 2 hours per day of screen time.

Television is not the only environmental issue contributing to adolescent inactivity and obesity. Adolescents are more reliant than ever on labor-saving devices like elevators and escalators. Other technology-related sedentary behaviors (videogaming, smartphone activities, Internet surfing) further reduce the incentive to be physically active. Acquiring a driver's license is an important milestone during adolescence. Unfortunately, driving motorized vehicles is an additional excuse that enables sedentary behaviors. Poor community planning has resulted in a paucity of safe gymnasiums or playing fields for adolescents to access and use during their leisure time. Erosions in public infrastructure such as poorly maintained sidewalks and poorly controlled crossings (eg, lack of traffic lights and/or crossing guards) also contribute to decreased physical activity in children and adolescents. Thoughtful community planning and healthy urban design are meaningful ways to embed physical activity in the fabric of community life. An additional factor contributing to increased obesity in particular is lack of access to healthy foodstuffs. Within the urban environment in particular, there is an abundance of readily available, inexpensive and calorically dense foods.

Familial Factors

Finally, there are factors inherent within individual families that shape how active young individuals will be. Children and adolescents with overweight parents are more likely to be overweight. Interestingly, parental levels of physical activity do not accurately predict their children's levels of physical activity. Children and youth from larger families are more active than children from small families. Children whose parents watch a great deal of television are more likely to spend time watching television themselves. Children whose parents are available to provide transportation to organized sporting activities are more likely to be physically active. Interestingly, individuals *forced* to exercise as children are less likely to be physically active as adults.

Davison K, et al. Do attributes in the physical environment influence children's physical activity? A review of the literature. *Int J Behav Nutr Phys Act.* 2006; 3:19–28. [PMID: 16872543].

Forshee RA, et al. The role of beverage consumption, physical activity, sedentary behavior and demographics on body mass index of adolescents. *Int J Food Sci Nutr.* 2004;55:463. [PMID: 15762311]

Gordon-Larsen P, et al. Determinants of adolescent physical activity and inactivity patterns. *Pediatrics.* 2000; 105:E83. [PMID: 10835096]

Guide to Community Preventive Services. Behavioral and social approaches to increase physical activity: enhanced school-based physical education. (available at http://www.thecommunityguide.org/pa/behavioral-social/index.html. Last updated December 21, 2011. Accessed April 8, 2013).

Guide to Community Preventive Services. Promoting physical activity: environmental and policy approaches. (available at http://www.thecommunityguide.org/pa/environmental-policy/index.html; last updated March 30, 2010. Accessed April 8, 2013).

Katzmarzyk PT, et al. International conference on physical activity and obesity in children: summary statement and recommendations. *Appl Physiol Nutr Metab.* 2008; 33(2):371–388 [PMID: 18347694]

Mantjes JA, Jones AP, Corder K, et al. School related factors and 1 yr change in physical activity amongst 9–11 year old English school children. *Int J Behav Nutr Phys Act.* 2012;9:153.

Martin S, et al. National prevalence and correlates of walking and bicycling to school. *Am J Prevent Med.* 2007; 33(2):98–105. [PMID: 17673096]

National Center for Health Statistics. Prevalence of obesity among children and adolescents: United States, trends 1963–1965 through 2009–2010. CDC, Health E-Stat. (http://www.cdc.gov/nchs/data/hestat/obesity_child_09_10/obesity_child_09_10.htm). *J Commun Health.* 2008; 33(4):206–216.

Singh GK, Kogan MD, Siahpush M, van Dyck PC. Independent and joint effects of socioeconomic, behavioral, and neighborhood characteristics on physical inactivity and activity levels among US children and adolescents. *J Commun Health.* 2008; 33(4):206–216.

Singh GK, Yu SM, Siahpush M, Kogan MD. High levels of physical inactivity and sedentary behaviors among US immigrant children and adolescents. *Arch Pediatr Adolesc Med.* 2008; 162(8):756–763.

Sturm R. Childhood obesity: what can we learn from existing data on societal trends, Part 1. *Prevent Chron Dis.* 2005; 1–9. [PMID: 15888231]

Tammelin T, et al. Physical activity and social status in adolescence as predictors of physical inactivity in adulthood. *Prevent Med.* 2003; 37:375. [PMID: 14507496]

Veselska Z, Madarasova Geckova A, Reijneveld SA, van Dijk JP. Aspects of self differ among physically active and inactive youths. *Int J Public Health.* 2011; 56(3):311–318.

Whitt-Glover MC, Taylor WC, Floyd MF, et al. Disparities in physical activity and sedentary behaviors among US children and adolescents: prevalence, correlates, and intervention implications. *J Public Health Policy.* 2009; 30(suppl 1):S309–S334.

Yang X, et al. Risk of obesity in relation to physical activity tracking from youth to adulthood. *Med Sci Sports Exercise.* 2006; 38: 919. [PMID: 16672846]

ASSESSMENT

There are three primary ways to assess physical activity levels in adolescents: (1) direct observation, (2) activity or heart rate monitors, and (3) self-report questionnaires. Of these methods, direct observation and electronic assessment (accelerometry, actigraphy) provide the most accurate and objective measurements. However, direct observation is labor-intensive and higher-technology solutions are often prohibitively expensive. Several cost-effective alternatives are available.

The Patient-Centered Assessment and Counseling for Exercise Plus (PACE+) Nutrition program has been developed to help clinicians assess physical activity levels as well as to provide patients with proper advice regarding physical activity and proper nutrition. As part of this program, a two-question self-report screening tool has been developed as a valid self-assessment of adolescent physical activity. The combination of BMI and the PACE+ activity measure allows for a rapid clinical assessment of physical activity status, weight status, and health risks. Two other simple screening tools, the World Health Organization Health

Behavior in Schoolchildren (WHO HBSC; www.hbsc.org) and International Physical Activity Questionnaire (IPAQ short version; http://www.ipaq.ki.se/ipaq.htm) have also been validated for use when assessing adolescent physical activity levels. Additionally, electronic monitoring devices, including heart rate monitors, accelerometers, and pedometers, can provide objective assessments of physical activity levels in adolescents. While heart rate monitors and accelerometers are likely too expensive for routine clinical use, pedometers are often an affordable, cost-effective, and valid assessment method for assessing adolescents' levels of physical activity.

Prochaska JJ, Sallis JF, Long B. A physical activity screening measure for use with adolescents in primary care. *Arch Pediatr Adolesc Med.* 2001;155:554. [PMID: 11343497]

Rangul V, et al. Reliability and validity of two frequently used self-administered physical activity questionnaires in adolescents. *BMC Med Res Methodol.* 2008;8:47–57. [PMID: 18627632]

Sirard JR, Pate RR. Physical activity assessment in children and adolescents. *Sports Med.* 2001;31:439. [PMID: 11394563]

GUIDELINES & CLINICAL INTERVENTIONS

It is known that risk factors for chronic disease track from childhood through adolescence into adulthood. Overweight adolescents are more likely to become overweight adults. Because obesity levels are rising sharply among adolescents and physical activity levels are declining, there is an acute need for interventions to promote physical activity in children and adolescents. Through the years, multiple guidelines have been proposed to assist clinicians in providing activity counseling for their adolescent patients (**Table 10-4**).

▶ American College of Sports Medicine/ American Heart Association Guidelines

The most recent American College of Sports Medicine (ACSM)/American Heart Association (AHA) guidelines for physical activity in individuals aged >18 years recommend a minimum of 30 minutes of moderate-intensity activity 5 days a week or 20 minutes of vigorous activity 3 days a week. Moderate-intensity aerobic activity is equivalent to a brisk walk, while vigorous-intensity activity is exemplified by jogging. Individuals can further improve their health in a dose-response relationship by exceeding these minimum recommendations for physical activity.

Garber, CE, Blissmer B, Deschenes MR, et al. Quantity and quality of exercise for developing and maintaining cardiorespiratory, musculoskeletal, and neuromotor fitness in apparently healthy adults: guidance for prescribing exercise. *Med Sci Sports Exerc.* 2011;43(7):1334–1359.

Table 10-4. Guidelines for physical activity in adolescence.

Guideline Source	Recommendation
International Consensus Conference on Physical Activity Guidelines for Adolescents/American Academy of Pediatrics Statement (2012)	1. Physical activity 3–5 days/week 2. Activity sessions of ≥20 minutes requiring moderate to vigorous physical exertion 3. Emphasis on consideration of familial, social, and community factors when promoting activity
ACSM/AHA Consensus Statement	1. All Americans should strive to be physically active on most, preferably all days of the week according to individual abilities 2. Goal of accumulating 30 minutes of moderate to vigorous physical activity each day 3. Sedentary individuals benefit from even modest levels of physical activity 4. Sufficient levels of activity can be accumulated through independent bouts of activity throughout the day
National Strength and Conditioning Association (2009)	1. A properly designed and supervised resistance training program is relatively safe for youth 2. A properly designed and supervised resistance training program can enhance the muscular strength and power of youth 3. A properly designed and supervised resistance training program can improve the cardiovascular risk profile of youth 4. A properly designed and supervised resistance training program can improve motor skill performance and may contribute to enhanced sports performance of youth 5. A properly designed and supervised resistance training program can increase a young athlete's resistance to sports related injuries 6. A properly designed and supervised resistance training program can help improve the psychosocial well-being of youth 7. A properly designed and supervised resistance training program can help promote and develop exercise habits during childhood and adolescence
Healthy People 2020 (2012)	1. Increase the proportion of adolescents who meet current federal physical activity guidelines for aerobic physical activity and for muscle-strengthening activity 2. Increase the proportion of the nation's public and private schools that require daily physical education for all students 3. Increase the proportion of adolescents who participate in daily school physical education 4. Increase the proportion of children and adolescents who do not exceed recommended limits for screen time 5. Increase the proportion of the nation's public and private schools that provide access to their physical activity spaces and facilities for all persons outside of normal school hours (ie, before and after the school day, on weekends, and during summer and other vacations) 6. Increase the proportion of physician office visits that include counseling or education related to physical activity 7. Increase the proportion of trips made by walking 8. Increase the proportion of trips made by bicycling
Physical Activity Guidelines for Americans (2008)	1. Accumulate 60 minutes of moderate to vigorous activity every day 2. Children and adolescents should perform cardiovascular activities on 3 days of the week and muscle-strengthening or bone-strengthening activities on 3 days of the week 3. All activities should be age- and developmentally appropriate to avoid the risk for overtraining

► International Consensus Conference on Physical Activity Guidelines for Adolescents

Convened in 1993, this expert panel recommends that adolescents be physically active on most, if not all, days of the week. Adolescents should strive for activity 3–5 days per week for ≥20 minutes at levels requiring moderate to vigorous exertion. Activity should routinely occur as part of play, games, sporting activities, work, recreation, physical education, or planned exercise sessions. These guidelines also emphasize the importance of considering family, school, and community factors when counseling adolescents about physical activity. The American Academy of Pediatrics further recommends that adolescents accumulate 60 minutes of physical activity during the course of a day. Activity should be moderate in intensity and should be varied in type to include recreation, sports, or home-based, community-based, and school-based activities. Activities that are unstructured and enjoyable have the best rates of compliance.

American Academy of Pediatrics. Promoting physical activity as a way of life (available at http://www.healthychildren.org/English/ages-stages/gradeschool/fitness/Pages/Promoting-Physical-Activity-as-a-Way-of-Life.aspx. Accessed April 8, 2013).

Twisk JW. Physical activity guidelines for children and adolescents: a critical review. *Sports Med.* 2001;31:617. [PMID: 1147523]

Healthy People 2020

Healthy People 2020 contains national health objectives for promotion of adolescent general health as well as adolescent physical activity. Of the 15 objectives outlined in *Healthy People 2020*, 8 are specifically targeted to promote physical activity in adolescents. (**Table 10-4**).

US Department of Health and Human Services: *Healthy People 2020.* DHHS, Government Printing Office, 2010 (available at http://www.healthypeople.gov/2020/topicsobjectives2020/overview.aspx?topicId=2 and http://www.healthypeople.gov/2020/topicsobjectives2020/objectiveslist.aspx?topicId=33. Last updated Dec. 12, 2012. Accessed April 8, 2013).

Dietary Guidelines for Americans

Now in its seventh edition, these guidelines are the cornerstone for providing clinical nutritional advice. Emphasizing the inherent relationship between physical activity, dietary choices, and resultant weight issues, the current edition of the *Guidelines* is the second to specifically recommend physical activity as a part of routine dietary practice. Adolescents should aim to accumulate ≥60 minutes of moderate physical activity on a daily basis.

US Department of Health and Human Services; US Department of Agriculture. *Dietary Guidelines for Americans 2010.* 7th ed. Washington, DC: Government Printing Office; 2011 (available at http://www.cnpp.usda.gov/dgas2010-policydocument.htm. Last updated March 14, 2012. Accessed April 8, 2013).

Physical Activity Guidelines for Americans

In 2008, the US Department of Health and Human Services released the *Physical Activity Guidelines for Americans.* Recognizing that children and adolescents who are more active have improved health and a lower burden of disease, there are several key recommendations: (1) all adolescents should perform ≥60 minutes of moderate to vigorous physical activity every day; (2) as part of the daily physical activity, children and adolescents should perform cardiovascular activities on 3 days of the week and muscle-strengthening or bone-strengthening activities on 3 days of the week; and (3) all activities should be age- and developmentally appropriate to avoid overtraining. In December 2012, the midcourse report was released, reinforcing these recommendations for strategies to increase physical activity in youth.

US Department of Health and Human Services. *2008 Physical Activity Guidelines for Americans* (available at www.health.gov/paguidelines. Accessed Aug. 3, 2009).

US Department of Health and Human Services. *Physical Activity Guidelines for Americans Midcourse Report. Strategies to Increase Physical Activity among Youth* (available at http://www.health.gov/paguidelines/midcourse/pag-mid-course-report-final.pdf. Accessed April 8, 2013).

National Strength & Conditioning Association

While regular aerobic physical activity is a mainstay of all recommendations, family physicians should also feel safe in recommending a structured resistance training program. While commonly thought of as weight training, resistance training is a broad phrase that encompasses many activities designed to improve overall fitness. Initially written in 1985, with revisions in 1996 and 2009, the National Strength and Conditioning Association (NSCA) position statement on youth resistance training documents the benefits to the cardiovascular risk profile, psychosocial well-being, resistance to injury, and overall exercise habits for all children and adolescents completing regular resistance training.

Faigenbaum AD, Kraemer WJ, Blimkie CJ, et al. Youth resistance training: updated position statement paper from the national strength and conditioning association. *J Strength Cond Res.* 2009;23(5 suppl):S60–S79.

PROMOTING PHYSICAL ACTIVITY: HOW CAN FAMILY PHYSICIANS HELP?

Health care professionals play a central role in promoting physical activity among adolescents. Adolescents have the lowest utilization of health care services of any segment of the population. They do, however, rely on their physician as a reliable source of health care information. Clinicians should therefore consider the opportunity to provide preventive advice at each adolescent visit. Using a modification of the 5A approach to tobacco cessation, physicians should *ask* adolescents about their current levels of physical activity and *advise* adolescents about appropriate levels of physical activity. Adolescents should strive for 60 minutes of moderate to vigorous physical activity or 10,000–12,000 steps per day if using a pedometer.

When reviewing guidelines or recommending lifestyle changes with adolescent patients, it is important to promote the concept of physical activity as opposed to physical fitness. Adolescents should be aware that cumulative bouts of physical activity are just as effective as sustained periods of exercise in attaining health-related benefits. For changes to be effective in adolescence and likely to persist, physical activity should be enjoyable and social support for the activity from family, peers, and/or the local community is the key. Using established guidelines within the context of social, cultural, familial, and environmental factors, clinicians must improve preventive counseling services to adolescents.

Adams MA, Caparosa S, Thompson S, Norman GJ. Translating physical activity recommendations for overweight adolescents to steps per day. *Am J Prevent Med.* 2009; 37(2):137–140. [PMID: 19524391]

Huang J, et al. The role of primary care in promoting children's physical activity. *Br J Sports Med.* 2009; 43:19–21. [PMID: 19001016]

Joy EA. Practical approaches to office-based physical activity promotion for children and adolescents. *Curr Sports Med Rep.* 2008; 7(6):367–372.

Ma J, et al. U.S. adolescents receive suboptimal preventive counseling during ambulatory care. *J Adolesc Health.* 2005; 36:441e1. [PMID: 15841517]

US Preventive Services Task Force. *Guide to Clinical Preventive Services, Recommendations of the U.S. Preventive Services Task Force.* Washington, DC: DHHS, Agency for Healthcare Research and Quality; 2005.

Van Sluijs E, et al. Effectiveness of interventions to promote physical activity in children and adolescents: systematic review of controlled trials. *Br Med J.* 2007; 335(7622):703–712. [PMID: 17884863]

SPECIAL CONSIDERATIONS

▶ Performance-Enhancing Supplements

Since 2003 or so, the use of performance-enhancing supplements has become commonplace in adolescent populations. One-half of the US population consumes some form of nutritional supplement on a regular basis, resulting in over $44 billion in annual sales. Reasons cited for the use of dietary nutritional supplements include ensuring good nutrition, preventing illness, improving performance, warding off fatigue, and enhancing personal appearance.

Estimates suggest that roughly 5% of all adolescents have used some form of performance-enhancing nutritional supplements. Adolescents, in particular, are vulnerable to the allure of performance-enhancing products.

Creatine remains the most popular performance-enhancing supplement. It is reported to increase energy during short-term intense exercise, increase muscle mass, strength, lean body mass, and decrease lactate accumulation during intense exercise. Although it is clear that supplementation with exogenous creatine can raise intramuscular creatine stores, it is not clear how effective creatine is as a performance aid. In general, creatine supplementation may be useful for activities requiring short, repetitive bouts of high-intensity exercise. There is conflicting evidence, however, as to whether it is effective in increasing muscle strength or muscle mass. There are no scientific data regarding the safety or effectiveness of long-term use of creatine in adolescents.

Anabolic-androgenic steroids (AASs) are another important category of performance-enhancing substances used by adolescents. Testosterone is the prototypical androgenic steroid hormone. Many synthetic modifications have been made to the basic molecular structure of testosterone in an attempt to promote the anabolic, muscle-building effects of testosterone while minimizing androgenic side effects. Androstenedione is one of several oral performance-enhancing supplements that are precursors to testosterone. The effectiveness of androstenedione as a performance-enhancing supplement is debatable. To date, the largest controlled trial examining its effectiveness showed no significant gains in muscular strength compared with a standard program of resistance training. The Anabolic Steroid Control Act of 2004 expanded the definition of anabolic steroids to include androstenedione and tetrahydrogestrinone (THG)—a designer steroid whose use was implicated in accusations of steroid use by several famous US athletes—as controlled substances, making their use as performance-enhancing drugs illegal.

Despite this ban, it is estimated that 3–10% of adolescents have used anabolic steroids. Importantly, adolescents who use anabolic steroids have been shown to be more likely to engage in high-risk personal health behaviors such as tobacco use and excessive alcohol consumption. Users of other nutritional performance-enhancing supplements have also been shown to engage in similarly predictable high-risk behaviors. The American Academy of Pediatrics in 2006 published a position statement strongly discouraging the use of performance-enhancing substances.

Clinicians should be aware of the prevalence of performance-enhancing supplement use in the adolescent population. They should also be aware of health-related behaviors that often accompany the use of these products and provide preventive counseling accordingly. The preparticipation physical examination represents an excellent opportunity for clinicians to provide information about performance-enhancing products to young athletes. When counseling adolescents about the use of performance-enhancing products, it is helpful to ask the following questions:

1. Is the product *safe* to use?
2. *Why* does the adolescent want to use a particular product?
3. Is the product *effective* in helping to meet the desired goal?
4. Is the product *legal*?

Many adolescents will either experiment with or regularly use performance-enhancing products regardless of the information or advice they receive from medical professionals. Adolescents are more likely to trust peers, coaches, mainstream media sources, and family regarding the safety and effectiveness of supplements. Nevertheless, physicians must ensure that adolescents are aware of potential health risks and bans from competition that can accompany use of performance-enhancing products. As a rule, the use of performance-enhancing supplements in adolescents should be discouraged.

Gomez J. American Academy of Pediatrics Committee on Sports Medicine and Fitness. Use of performance-enhancing substances. *Pediatrics* 2005; 115:1103. [PMID: 15805399]

Evans MW, Ndetan H, Perko M, et al. Dietary supplement use by children and adolescents in the United States to enhance sport performance: results of the National Health Interview Surevey. *J Prim Prevent.* 2012; 33(1):3–12. [PMID 22297456]

Stephens MB, Olsen C. Ergogenic supplements and health-risk behaviors. *J Fam Pract.* 2001; 50:696. [PMID: 11509164]

▶ Female Athlete Triad

Although many adolescents engage in insufficient physical activity, there is a segment of the population for whom too much exercise leads to specific physiologic side effects. The term *female athlete triad* refers to the combination of disordered eating, amenorrhea, and osteoporosis that can accompany excessive physical training in young female athletes. Athletes particularly at risk include those who participate in gymnastics, ballet, figure skating, distance running, or any other sport that emphasizes a particularly lean physique.

The preparticipation physical examination represents an excellent opportunity for clinicians to screen for and prevent the female athlete triad. During this examination, screening questions for female athletes should include careful menstrual, dietary (including a history of disordered eating practices), and exercise histories. When elicited, a history of amenorrhea (particularly in a previously menstruating woman) should be taken seriously. The American College of Sports Medicine recommends that these women be considered at risk for the athlete triad and that a formal medical evaluation be undertaken within 3 months.

Hobart JA, Smucker DR. The female athlete triad. *Am Fam Physician.* 2000; 61:3357. [PMID: 10865930]

▶ Exercise & Sudden Death

Another small segment of the adolescent population is at risk during exercise. These individuals are predisposed to sudden cardiac death during physical activity. Highly publicized events among well-known athletes have focused significant media attention on this issue. Although the incidence of sudden cardiac death in young athletes is quite low, proper screening is still important. The preparticipation physical examination represents an excellent clinical opportunity to identify adolescents at risk for sudden cardiac death during physical activity.

When screening for sudden death in young athletes, the medical history should include questions about exercise-related syncope or near-syncope, shortness of breath, chest pain, and palpitations. Family history of premature death or premature cardiovascular disease is also important to obtain. A prior history of a cardiac murmur or specific knowledge of an underlying cardiac abnormality (either structural, valvular, or arrhythmic) in the athlete should be elicited as well. On physical examination, blood pressure should be recorded. The precordial fields should be auscultated in the supine, squatting, and standing positions. Murmurs that increase from squatting to standing or that increase with the Valsalva maneuver are of potential concern and merit further evaluation. The equality of the femoral pulses should be noted. While routine use of modalities such as ECGs, stress testing, and/or echocardiograms as screening efforts are not routinely recommended, if there is any suspicion that the athlete might have a symptomatic arrhythmia or be at risk for sudden cardiac death, that individual should be withheld from physical activity pending formal cardiology consultation and evaluation.

American Academy of Pediatrics. *Preparticipation Physical Evaluation.* 4th ed. 2010.

Giese EA, et al. The athletic preparticipation evaluation: cardiovascular assessment. *Am Fam Physician.* 2007:75:983. [PMID: 17427614]

O'Connor FG, et al. Sudden death in young athletes: screening for the needle in a haystack. *Am Fam Physician.* 1998; 57:2763. [PMID: 9636339]

Eating Disorders

Rachel M. Radin, MA, MS

Lisa M. Ranzenhofer, MS

Marian Tanofsky-Kraff, PhD

Evelyn L. Lewis, MD, MA, FAAFP

General Considerations

More than 8 million Americans suffer from eating disorders. Approximately 90% of them are young women; however, middle-aged women, children, and men are also affected. The prevalence of eating disorders appears to vary by the population being studied. Recently, binge eating disorder (BED), previously considered a putative diagnosis subsumed under the category "eating disorder not otherwise specified," was included as its own category of eating disorder in the *Diagnostic and Statistical Manual of Mental Disorders*, fifth edition (*DSM-5*). Its inclusion has changed the face of eating disorders. While anorexia (AN) and bulimia nervosa (BN) appear to primarily affect women, the ratio of women to men with BED is approximately 3:2. There are also significant cross-cultural differences in the prevalence and presentation of AN, BN, and BED.

Eating disorders are more prevalent in industrialized societies (where food is abundant and thinness is valued as attractive) than in developing countries. Women in Western countries traditionally have exhibited greater concern for body habitus than those in developing countries, who appear to be more accepting of and comfortable with a fuller body shape. In many of the latter societies, a fuller figure has been considered the cultural stereotype of attractiveness, although this ideal appears to change when individuals from these societies integrate into Western culture.

Westernization has affected many countries, and individuals from other cultures should not be excluded from consideration of an eating disorder diagnosis. Immigration from non-Western to Western cultures appears to place individuals at greater risk for eating disorders. Indeed, degree of acculturation into American society is associated with eating disorder risk, likely due to the adoption of Western body image ideals. As individuals (particularly girls and women) from cultures in which AN is unknown or extremely rare immigrate to Westernized societies with higher rates of AN, they tend to develop disorders as they attempt to acculturate.

Two core features are common across all eating disorders: (1) severe disturbance in eating habits, and (2) excessive concern and/or dissatisfaction with body shape and weight. However, on the surface, individuals with AN and BED present quite differently. Further, AN, BN, and BED differ in terms of prevalence, demographic correlates, and medical ramifications. Classification of both overeating and undereating disorders into a single category poses difficulties for the conceptualization and treatment of these conditions.

Dalle Grave R. Eating disorders: progress and challenges. *Eur J Intern Med*. 2011;22:2:153. [PMID: 21402245]

Hudson JI, et al. The prevalence and correlates of eating disorders in the National Comorbidity Survey Replication. *Biol Psychiatry*. 2007;61:348. [PMID: 1892232]

Normative versus Abnormal Eating

Before detailing the clinical characteristics of various eating disorders, it is necessary to identify what is meant by "normative eating." In so doing, it becomes apparent that a great deal of dieting occurs in Western culture as part of normal eating. In fact, estimates suggest that anywhere from 15% to 80% of the population may be dieting at a given time. Despite these statistics, over 65% of the adult population, and ~16% of children and adolescents aged 2–19 years, are considered overweight or obese. High prevalence of obesity appears to disproportionately affect those of racial and ethnic minorities. Approximately 75% of African American and Mexican American adults, compared to ~68% of non-Hispanic white adults, are considered overweight or obese. Similarly, ~22% of African American and Hispanic children, compared with 14% of non-Hispanic white children, are overweight.

The term "dieting" in lay culture has been used to describe a wide variety of behaviors ranging from healthful (eg, eating more vegetables, increasing exercise) to extreme (eg, prolonged fasting, self-induced vomiting). Appropriateness of dieting should be considered in light of the specific behaviors that constitute dieting. Further, consideration of dieting in the context of an individual's weight status is an important factor in evaluating whether dieting is pathological (in underweight or nonoverweight individuals) versus appropriate (in overweight individuals). It has been suggested that dieting typically precedes eating disorder onset in cases of BN, while for BED, binge eating has been reported as preceding the onset of dieting in approximately half of cases.

Women are most likely to restrict their food intake to control their weight or lose weight, but increasingly men are also engaging in dieting behavior. Perhaps most worrisome is the prevalence of dieting among adolescents and even children. Data suggest that 40% of 9-year-old girls have dieted, and even 5-year-olds voice concern about their diet that appear to be linked to cultural standards for body image. Although few individuals who diet develop an eating disorder, dieting, in combination with other factors, may be an important precipitant to the development of eating disorders. The acceptance of dieting as "normative" may prohibit recognition of problem eating.

Flegal KM, et al. Prevalence of obesity and trends in the distribution of body mass index among US adults, 1999–2010. *JAMA.* 2012;307(5):491. [PMID: 22253363]

Flegal KM, et al. Prevalence and trends in obesity among US adults, 1998–2008. *JAMA.* 2010;303(3):235. [PMID: 20071471]

Ogden CL, et al. Prevalence of obesity and trends in body mass index among US children and adolescents, 1999–2010. *JAMA.* 2012;307(5):483. [PMID: 22253364]

▶ Prevalence of Eating Disorders

The prevalence and incidence rates for eating disorders vary significantly, depending on the disorder and the population. Data suggest that the lifetime prevalence estimates of AN and BN are 0.6% and 1% respectively, whereas the lifetime prevalence of BED is 2.8%. Generally speaking, of patients with classic signs and symptoms of AN or BN, 90% are female, 95% are white, and 75% are adolescent when they develop the disorder. These data are substantiated by several cross-cultural studies that have reported few, if any, cases in rural areas of Africa, the Middle East, or Asia with the exception of Japan, the only non-Western country that has seen a substantial and persistent increase in eating disorders. AN has been implicated as a "culture-bound syndrome" because certain cultural mores are reflected in the signs and symptoms of the disorder. In adults, recent studies of racial and ethnic differences in eating disorder prevalence within a nationally representative sample suggest that the incidences of AN and BED are similar across racial and ethnic groups. However, certain other data suggest that BN is more prevalent among Hispanics and African Americans than among non-Hispanic whites. Hispanics are more likely to develop binge eating and BED than AN and BN. Several studies have shown that other abnormal eating behaviors may be as common or even more so among African Americans (eg, purging by laxatives vs vomiting, binge eating). African American women are also more likely to develop BN or BED than AN, and a recent study (Marques L et al) found a strong association between BED and obesity in this population. Given the high rates of obesity in ethnic minority populations, experts have postulated that BED is a significant problem among these groups. The predominance of non-Hispanic whites among cases of AN may contribute to cultural bias in diagnosis, with less recognition of eating disorders among ethnic minorities.

Compared to adults, the prevalence of eating disorders among adolescents is characterized by a differential racial and ethnic pattern. Among adolescents, a recent study (Swanson SA et al) of racial and ethnic differences in eating disorder prevalence within a nationally representative sample suggest that non-Hispanic white adolescents report a greater prevalence of AN compared to other racial and ethnic groups. However, Hispanic adolescents report the highest prevalence of BN in comparison to non-Hispanic white and black adolescents. Further, there is a trend for greater prevalence of BED among ethnic minorities, relative to AN and BN. BN and BED are also more prevalent among adolescent girls compared to boys. Among high school students, Hispanic and non-Hispanic white girls tend to report similar levels of eating disordered attitudes and cognitions, such as excessive shape and weight concern and extreme dieting, which may be risk factors for full-syndrome disorders. African American girls, however, report lower body weight concerns and behaviors than girls of other ethnicities. Among adolescent boys, nearly all ethnic minorities report more eating disorder symptoms and weight concerns compared to Caucasian boys. How subthreshold disturbances and risk factors manifest into differential prevalence of full-syndrome disorders across cultures is not well understood.

It is traditionally believed that AN and BN tend to affect adolescent girls of middle to upper socioeconomic status. However, some recent data suggest a lack of association between socioeconomic status the presentation of any eating disorder. Age- and sex-specific estimates suggest that about 0.5–1% of adolescent girls develop AN, whereas 5% of older adolescent and young adult women develop BN. This population also exhibits a high frequency of coexistence between AN and BN. It has been reported that as many as 50% of AN patients may exhibit bulimic behaviors while 30–80% of patients with BN have a history of AN.

Data suggest that approximately 3–5% of people surveyed in a general population have BED. Although being overweight is not a criterion for the diagnosis of BED, it has been estimated that slightly over 11% of individuals who join Weight Watchers and 30% of individuals who present to hospital-based weight control programs meet the diagnosis of BED. BED appears to afflict adults of all socioeconomic strata and education level equally. Furthermore, BED is often diagnosed in middle-aged adults.

Finally, it should be noted BED is the most prevalent eating disorder in the United States, affecting 6–10% of young women. Recent research suggests that individuals diagnosed with an eating disorder not otherwise specified (EDNOS) did not differ significantly from AN and BED in terms of eating or general pathology. However, individuals with BN exhibited greater eating and general psychopathology compared to EDNOS. Girls meeting all criteria for AN except amenorrhea did not differ from full-syndrome AN. Further, nearly 40% of individuals diagnosed with EDNOS went on to develop either AN or BN within 1–2 years. Thus, EDNOS seems to represent a heterogenous category whose symptoms overlap substantially with traditional eating disorders. Clinicians should monitor possible progression of EDNOS to full-syndrome AN, BN, or BED, especially given the paucity of treatment recommendations for EDNOS.

Alegria M, et al. Prevalence and correlates of eating disorders in Latinos in the US. *Int J Eat Dis.* 2007:40:S15. [PMID: 17584870]

Franko D. Race, ethnicity, and eating disorders: considerations for DSM-V. *Int J Eat Dis.* 2007; 40(suppl):S31–S34. [PMID: 17879288]

Hudson JI, et al. The prevalence and correlates of eating disorders in the National Comorbidity Survey Replication. *Biol Psychiatry.* 2007; 61:348. [PMID: 1892232]

Marques L, et al. Comparative prevalence, correlates of impairment, and service utilization for eating disorders across US ethnic groups: implications for reducing ethnic disparities in health care access for eating disorders. *Int J Eat Dis.* 2011; 44(5):412. [PMID: 20665700]

Swanson SA, et al. Prevalence and correlates of eating disorders in adolescents: results from the National Comorbidity Survey Replication, adolescent supplement. *JAMA.* 2011; 68:714. [PMID: 21383252]

Thomas JJ, et al. The relationship between eating disorder not otherwise specified (EDNOS) and officially recognized eating disorders: meta-analysis and implications for DSM. *Psychol Bull.* 2009;135(3); 407. [PMID: 19379023]

Wonderlich SA, et al. The validity and clinical utility of binge eating disorder. *Int J Eat Dis.* 2009; 42(8):687. [PMID: 19621466]

▶ Pathogenesis

The origins of eating disorders are extremely complex and poorly understood. However, biological, psychological, cultural, and societal factors are likely contributors to the predisposition, precipitation, and perpetuation of these disorders. Typically, individuals with eating disorders are assumed to have a biological or genetic predisposition that is activated by environmental (ie, sociocultural, psychosocial) factors.

Risk factors for developing an eating disorder include participation in activities that promote thinness (eg, ballet dancing, modeling, and athletics) and certain personality traits, such as low self-esteem, difficulty expressing negative emotions, difficulty resolving conflict, being perfectionistic, and neuroticism and/or anxiety. Mounting data also support substantial biological predispositions to AN and BN. Mothers and sisters of probands who had AN were found to have 8 times the risk of developing an eating disorder compared with the general population. Genetic studies also lend strong support to the underlying biological supposition regarding eating disorders. Twin studies have shown heritability estimates in the 50–90% range for AN and 35–50% for BN, with monozygotic twins having higher concordance than dizygotic twins. A strong association between AN and BN in families has also been found in the Virginia Twin Registry.

Eating disorders may also be precipitated by psychosocial factors in vulnerable individuals. These precipitating factors often relate to developmental tasks of adolescence and include maturation fears, particularly those related to sexual development, peer group involvement, independence and autonomy struggles, family conflicts, sexual abuse, and identity conflicts. Two other psychological factors that figure permanently in the pathogenesis of BN or BED are sexual trauma and depression. Patients with either of these disorders are predisposed to have a family and personal history of depression. Therefore, it is important to note the presence of depression or history of sexual trauma during the initial patient assessment.

Since the mid-1990s, the number of men who openly report dissatisfaction with their physical appearance has tripled. Today nearly as many men as women claim to be unhappy about their appearance, and 50% more men reportedly seek evaluation and treatment for eating disorders than they did in the 1990s. This trend may by rooted in an obsession with "six-pack abs" and bulging biceps that seems especially common among athletes and fitness enthusiasts. Pursuit of muscularity to the exclusion of healthful habits may be a precursor to eating disorder development in males. Additionally, exercise status and sexual orientation are two risk factors for eating disorders in men. Often men who develop eating disorders have a history of being overweight when they were younger. Men considered to be at increased risk of developing eating disorders include:

- Athletes, especially those participating in sports that work against gravity, such as gymnastics.

- Men with gender issues.

- Men with personality traits such as perfectionism and impulsive behaviors, and those who have anxiety.

- Obese boys who face teasing and have low self-esteem.

Increasingly, research on the risk-factors for eating disorders has indicated that eating disorder (ED) symptoms may emerge as early as middle childhood. Dieting, concerns about shape and weight, and body dissatisfaction are present in children as young as 5 years of age, and common among children aged 8 to12 years. Early factors shown to be associated with later development of AN include feeding and gastrointestinal difficulties during infancy and early childhood, maternal body dissatisfaction, and dieting and shape concerns during early and middle childhood. Similarly, early concerns with eating and weight are potential red-flags for future development of BN. Overweight status during childhood has been shown to be related to future development of both BN and BED.

Loss-of-control (LoC) *eating*, defined as the feeling of being unable to control what or how much one is eating regardless of the amount of food consumed, has been reported in young children. Loss-of control eating is fairly common among children, especially among those who are overweight (prevalence estimates among overweight youth range from 4% to 45%). LoC eating in youth is analogous to binge eating in adults, and may be a precursor for future development of BED. Children afflicted with LoC eating are at risk for gaining excess weight as they grow, and they have more disturbed eating patterns, symptoms of depression and anxiety, and behavior problems compared to children without such behaviors. Children who are at risk for becoming overweight adults, including those who are overweight and who have overweight parents, should be queried about loss of control eating to monitor potential progression to BN or BED.

Bulik CM. Prevalence, heritability, and prospective risk factors for anorexia nervosa. *Arch Gen Psychiatry.* 2006:63. [PMID: 16520436]

Keel PK, Forney, KJ. Psychosocial risk factors for eating disorders. *Int J Eat Dis.* 2013; 46(5):433. [PMID: 23658086]

Mazzeo SE, et al. A twin study of specific bulimia nervosa symptoms. *Psychol Med.* 2010; 40(7):1203. [PMID: 2882507]

Mazzeo SE, et al. Assessing heritability of anorexia nervosa symptoms using a marginal maximal likelihood approach. *Psychol Med.* 2009; 39(3):463. [PMID: 2640444]

McFarland MB, Petrie, TA. Male body satisfaction: factorial and construct validity of the body parts satisfaction scale for men. *J Couns Psychol.* 2012; 59(2):329. [PMID: 22268574]

Misra M, et al. Effects of anorexia nervosa on clinical, hematologic, biochemical, and bone density parameters in community-dwelling adolescent girls. *Pediatrics.* 2004; 114:1574. [PMID: 15574617]

Rome ES, et al. Children and adolescents with eating disorders: the state of the art. *Pediatrics.* 2003; 111:e98. [PMID: 12509603]

Tanofsky-Kraff M, et al. A prospective study of pediatric loss of control eating and psychological outcomes. *J Abnorm Psychol.* 2011;120(1):108. [PMID: 21114355]

▶ Prevention & Screening

Eating disorders are serious and complex problems, and the earlier an eating disorder is identified, the better the patient's chance of recovery. This makes a compelling argument for targeted screening of at-risk groups, including gymnasts, runners, body builders, wrestlers, dancers, rowers, and swimmers. These groups warrant close monitoring because their sports or livelihood dictate weight restriction. The populations at highest risk for AN and BN are female adolescents and young adults, and screening should occur throughout adolescence, especially at ages 14 and 18 years. This correlates with the transition to high school and college and the associated stressors.

In contrast to AN and BN, which typically emerge during adolescence, BED is most frequently detected during middle adulthood, even though many individuals report an onset of the disorder in their mid-twenties and initial binge eating behaviors can begin even earlier. Because of the relatively high prevalence of BED in community samples (3–5%), routine screening for binge eating among overweight adults may be warranted. Almost all individuals seeking treatment for weight control should be screened for BED because of the high incidence of this disorder in this group (~30–50%). Although these individuals may fall short of meeting the full criteria for BED, the problematic attitudes associated with the disorder will likely be uncovered. The tools used for screening can be very sophisticated and vary with the population being assessed. However, some are easily incorporated into the routine primary care office visit (**Table 11-1**). These questions are very helpful for the early detection of BN and BED; some individuals with these disorders can be uncovered using self-report alone. Those with AN, on the other hand, are more often resistant to self-reporting and usually require reporting by others (eg, parents or friends). Therefore, it is imperative that parents, friends, teachers, family, dentists, and physicians become educated about the possible signs and symptoms associated with these difficult-to-manage disorders to facilitate prevention or early management of these individuals. Some cases of BN may be similarly difficult to detect, because many patients with BN are of a healthy weight status, and maintain secrecy surrounding bulimic behaviors.

Table 11-1. Screening questionnaire.

1. Has there been any change in your weight?
2. What did you eat yesterday?
3. Do you ever binge? Do you feel a sense of loss of control while eating? Do you ever feel that you cannot control what or how much you are eating?
4. Have you ever used self-induced vomiting, laxatives, diuretics, or enemas to lose weight or compensate for overeating?
5. How much do you exercise in a typical week?
6. How do you feel about how you look?
7. Are your menstrual periods regular?

Data from Powers PS. Initial assessment and early treatment options for anorexia nervosa and bulimia nervosa. *Psychiatr Clin North Am.* 1996;19(4):639. [PMID: 8933600]

Clinical Findings

A. Symptoms and Signs

The multiple symptoms experienced by the patient and signs noted by the physician are related to the numerous methods used to manipulate weight. When initially screening a patient, a symptom checklist can facilitate the history-taking procedure (**Table 11-2**). Although treatment-seeking individuals will often answer questions honestly, patients with AN are usually reticent to be seen or report any problem with weight.

If the review of systems contains primarily positive results, this may be indicative of a significant problem for the patient. Most commonly, female patients with AN complain of amenorrhea, depression, fatigue, weakness, hair loss, and bone pain (which may be indicative of pathologic fracture secondary to osteopenia). Constipation or abdominal pain, or both, occur frequently but may be commonly mistaken as symptoms of endometriosis or pelvic inflammatory disease, which are disorders common to both anorexia and bulimia. Unlike AN, BN may be missed initially by the inexperienced clinician because these patients may present with normal or near-normal body weight or be slightly underweight. In addition to constipation and gastrointestinal pain, patients with BN may present with menstrual irregularity, food and fluid restrictions, abuse of diuretics and laxatives (causing dizziness and bloody diarrhea), misuse of diet pills (leading to palpitations and anxiety), frequent vomiting (resulting in throat irritation and pharyngeal trauma), sexually transmitted diseases (which appear to be related to impulsive, risk-taking behaviors associated with this disorder), and

bone pain. Mouth sores, weaknesses, dental caries, heartburn, muscle cramps, dizziness and fainting, hair loss, easy bruising, and cold intolerance are some of the more obvious presenting complaints.

B. Diagnostic Criteria

The hallmark of AN is the refusal to eat anything except minimal amounts of food, resulting in low body weight (given the contexts of age, sex, developmental trajectory, and physical health). The hallmark of BN is the attempt to restrict food intake that eventually leads to out-of-control eating episodes followed by inappropriate compensatory behaviors (eg, vomiting). The commonalities among the eating disorders include disturbance in body image (both body shape and body weight overconcern) and an excessive drive for thinness.

Perhaps the most substantial change to the *DSM-5* is the recognition of BED as its own category of eating disorder. In its previous iteration, the *DSM-IV-TR*, BED was described under Appendix B: Criteria Sets and Axes Provided for Further Study, and diagnosable under "eating disorder not otherwise specified."

1. Anorexia nervosa—The diagnostic criteria for AN are defined and listed in the *DSM-5*. The hallmark of AN is the restriction of energy intake, leading to *significantly low body weight*, which is defined as a weight that is less than minimally normal or, for children and adolescents, less than minimally expected. A significant change from the *DSM-IV-TR* to the *DSM-5* is the removal of the word "refusal" regarding the maintenance of one's body weight at or above a minimally normal level (criterion A). "Refusal" implies an intentional effort by the patient, which can be difficult to assess. Rather, criterion A has been reworded to focus on more observable behaviors. Patients with AN exhibit an intense fear of weight gain or persistent behavior that interferes with weight gain (criterion B) and body image disturbance or a persistent lack of recognition of the seriousness of low body weight (criterion C), which may include any or all of its three components: emotional (eg, self-disgust), perceptual (eg, "my thighs are too fat"), and cognitive (eg, "people will hate me if I'm fat"). The onset of AN is typically between ages 14 and 18 years, although middle-childhood cases have been reported. A major change in the diagnostic criteria for AN is the removal of amenorrhea, or the absence of at least three menstrual cycles (under criterion D). This criterion was removed, as it does not apply to males, or to females who are premenarchal, postmenopausal, or taking oral contraceptives. Additionally, some individuals may develop all other symptoms of AN but still report some menstrual activity.

Two subtypes of AN are identified: a binge eating–purging type and a restricting type (specified to occur during the previous 3 months). The former subtype includes patients who engage in diuretic laxative abuse, vomiting, and overuse of enemas to eliminate calories. Patients who do not engage

---

Table 11-2. Evaluation of eating disorders: the history.

History should include questions on the following:

Weight (minimum/maximum, as well as ideal)

Menstrual history and pattern (if applicable: age of menarche, date of last period)

Body image (thin, normal, heavy; satisfaction/dissatisfaction with current weight)

Exercise regimen (amount, intensity, response to inability to exercise)

Eating habits

Sexual history [if applicable, a history of current sexual activity, number of partners, and review of health habits and sexual practices that might place the patient at risk for sexually transmitted diseases (STDs)]

Current and past medication

Laxative/diuretic/diet pill use, ipecac, cigarettes, alcohol, drugs

Substance abuse (eg, cigarettes, alcohol, drugs)

Binge eating and purging behavior (identify a binge: feeling of "loss of control," how much, what kinds of food; presence of triggers–foods, time of day, feelings; frequency of binge eating; identify vomiting methods–finger, toothbrush)

Psychiatric history (substance abuse, mood/anxiety/personality disorders)

Suicidal ideation

in either binge eating or purging behaviors are categorized as having the restrictive subtype. AN binge eating–purging subtype differs from BN in weight criteria, size of the binge (usually smaller), and consistency of purging (less frequent).

2. Bulimia nervosa—BN is slightly more common than AN and largely seen in collegiate women, although the disorder usually starts in the late teenage years. Dieting often precedes and is associated with BN. This results in out-of-control eating and is followed by inappropriate compensatory behaviors. Patients with BN may be slightly more difficult to initially identify than those with AN, because most are within normal weight range for age and height. However, some may be overweight or slightly underweight.

The *DSM-5*-defined criteria for BN include recurrent episodes of binge eating in which more food than normal is consumed in a discrete period of time. The patient must also engage in recurrent inappropriate compensatory behaviors. Both criteria occur on average once a week for 3 months (marking a reduction in frequency criteria from the *DSM-IV-TR*, previously diagnosed as twice weekly for 3 months). Frequency criteria for binge eating and purging episodes were reduced to once a week, as individuals who report episodes once a week were found to be similar to those reporting episodes twice a week or more. Subtypes of BN (purging and nonpurging) were deleted from the current iteration of the DSM, as the available data suggest that individuals with the nonpurging subtype (eg, fasting and excessive exercise) more closely resembled individuals with BED. Further, defining nonpurging inappropriate behaviors was difficult to assess.

3. Binge eating disorder—The most recent of the eating disorder diagnostic categories is BED. Previously described within the *DSM-IV-TR* under Appendix B: Criteria Sets and Axes Provided for Further Study, and diagnosable under "eating disorder not otherwise specified," the *DSM-5* now recognizes BED as its own category of eating disorder. Extensive research supports the clinical utility and validity of the diagnosis.

Evidence suggests that BED affects women and men (3:2) more evenly, impacts a broader age range of individuals (aged 20–50 years), and likely affects African Americans and Hispanics as often as non-Hispanic whites. Most people with BED are obese and have a history of "yoyo" dieting. The *DSM-5*-defined criteria for BED include the hallmark symptom of binge eating in the absence of compensatory behaviors. Patients report feeling a sense of "loss of control" while consuming larger amounts of food than is typical for most people in a discrete period of time. The episodes are associated with rapid eating, eating until uncomfortable, eating large amounts of food when they are not hungry, and eating alone. The patient typically experiences intense feelings of guilt and shame surrounding these eating episodes. Episodes occur at least once per week for a duration of 3 months, marking

a reduction in the frequency criterion listed from the *DSM-IV-TR* (from twice per week for a duration of 6 months). BED is characterized by a comparable elevated level of disordered eating attitudes (eg, overvaluation of shape and weight) as the classic eating disorders of AN and BN.

4. Other specified feeding or eating disorder—A considerable change to the *DSM-5* is the removal of the category "eating disorders not otherwise specified" (EDNOS) and replacement with the following two categories: "other specified feeding or eating disorder" or "unspecified feeding or eating disorder." As the previous catchall category of EDNOS specified fairly vague criteria, changes to the *DSM-5* are intended to minimize the use of these catchall diagnoses, and to specify diagnose that more accurately describe an individual's symptoms and behaviors in an effort to more appropriately tailor treatment recommendations. The *DSM-5*-defined criteria for an "other specified feeding or eating disorder" include atypical AN, marked by all criteria for AN except that an individual's current weight is within or above the normal range; BN of low frequency and/or limited duration (< once a week, and/or <3 months); BED of low frequency and/or limited duration (< once a week, and/or <3 months); purging disorder (marked by purging behavior in the absence of binge eating characteristic of BN); and night eating syndrome (recurrent episodes of eating after awakening from sleep or excessive consumption following an evening meal).

5. Unspecified feeding or eating disorder—This category applies to presentations in which symptoms characteristic of a feeding and eating disorder that cause clinically significant distress or impairment in all areas of functioning predominate, but do not meet the full criteria for any of the *DSM-5* feeding or eating disorders. This category is used in situations in which the clinician chooses *not* to specify the reason why the criteria are not met for a specific feeding and eating disorder, and includes presentations in which there is insufficient information to make a more specific diagnosis (eg, in emergency room settings).

C. Physical Examination

Whenever suspicion of an eating disorder is raised, a detailed physical and dental examination should be conducted (**Table 11-3**). Complications of AN and BN can affect most organ systems; however, early in the diagnosis the "good-looking" or "normal-weight" patient may elude diagnosis by even the most astute physician. Multilayered, baggy clothing worn by adolescents may be representative of the latest fads in fashion or a significant eating disturbance. Just as baggy clothing may be used to conceal cachexia, patients may use increased fluid consumption and the addition of undergarment weights to normalize their weight prior to weigh-ins.

A thorough physical examination addresses several issues. It may indicate the presence of another condition

Table 11-3. Key components of the physical examination in patients with eating disorders.

Assessment of vital signs
Body temperature [hypothermia: <35.5°C (96°F)]
Heart rate (bradycardia: <50 bpm)
Blood pressure (hypotension: 90/50 mmHg)
Weight (taken with the patient dressed in a hospital gown) and height assessment should factor in previous height and weight percentiles, anticipated growth, and average weights of healthy adolescents of the same sex, height, and sexual maturation [prepared from National Center for Health Statistics (NCHS) data]
Evaluation of body mass index (BMI)
    Quetelet BMI (weight-to-height relationship: defined as weight in kilograms divided by height in meters squared; this BMI is then compared with reference data; percentile tables for BMI for age and sex based on NCHS data have been developed for children and adolescents)
Gynecologic examination (if applicable)
    Pelvic evaluation (atrophic vaginitis)
    Breast evaluation (atrophy)
    Pregnancy testing (where appropriate)
    Sexually transmitted disease testing (where appropriate)

Data from Fisher M, et al. Eating disorders in adolescents: a background paper. *J Adolesc Health*. 1995; 16:420. [PMID: 7669792]

[eg, Crohn disease or central nervous system lesion (papilledema)] or emphasize to the patient that the body is adapting to an unhealthy state. This objective evidence can be particularly effective, because the use of "scare tactics" to motivate healthy behaviors is usually futile.

One of the most significant disturbances associated with patients undergoing evaluation for eating disorders will be detected by assessing pulse, resting, and other static measurements. These should be assessed at the initial evaluation and at each follow-up. Patients with AN often have significant bradycardia [<60 beats per minute (bpm) in ≤91% of patients in various series]. Of those with AN, 85% may have hypotension with pressures lower than 90/60–90/50 mmHg, secondary to a chronic volume-depleted state. Symptomatic orthostatic hypotension has been suggested as a reason for hospitalization. Cardiac arrhythmias are also common. Abuse of laxatives and diuretics causes the most serious damage for bulimic patients. The misuse of syrup of ipecac to induce vomiting is extremely dangerous in this population and often results in irreversible cardiomyopathy. Assessment of vital signs is critical and often leads to the detection of cardiac arrhythmias (resulting from hypokalemia), metabolic acidosis, hypotension, and faint pulse.

Height, weight, and BMI should also be recorded regularly and at each visit. This is helpful in establishing the patient's weight trends, because few individuals with AN are overweight prior to the onset of their disease. These weight trends also help identify the patient's failure to gain weight during normal adolescent growth spurts. It is vitally important to obtain accurate readings. Therefore, patients should be weighed in a hospital gown, not in personal clothing, because of the various strategies they employ to disguise their weight loss.

Careful examination of the patient's body should also be performed. Signs of AN such as brittle hair and nails, dry scaly skin, loss of subcutaneous fat, fine facial and body hair (lanugo hair), carotene pigmentation, breast atrophy, and atrophic vaginitis may be readily observable. Physical examination findings more representative of bulimic patients include the callused finger (Russell sign) used to induce vomiting, dry skin, and dull hair. Periodontal diseases are well-recognized sequelae of BN and may present as erosion of tooth enamel, mouth sores, dental caries, gum inflammation, chipped teeth, and sialadenosis (swelling of the parotid glands). BED patients are typically (but not always) overweight or obese and may present with common obesity-related health comorbidities.

American Academy of Pediatrics, Committee on Adolescence. Identification and management of eating disorders in children and adolescents. *Pediatrics*. 2010; 126(6):1240. [PMID: 21115584]

D. Laboratory Findings

There are no confirmatory laboratory tests specific to the diagnosis of eating disorders, and reported findings may be normal. Nonetheless, screening or baseline evaluations are recommended and should include a complete blood count with differential, urinalysis, blood chemistries (electrolytes, calcium, magnesium, and phosphorus), thyroid function tests, an amenorrhea evaluation, and baseline electrocardiogram, as indicated. Generally speaking, laboratory abnormalities are due to the weight control habits or methods used by the patient, or the resulting complications.

In the early stages of AN, laboratory findings may show elevated BUN, which may be secondary to dehydration; leukopenia due to increased margination of neutrophils; and pancytopenia. In addition, low circulatory levels of luteinizing hormone (LH) and follicle-stiulating hormone (FSH), osteopenia and osteoporosis, deficiency of gonadotropin-releasing hormone, low estradiol, elevated cortisol, low triiodothyronine (T_3) and free thyroxine (T_4), an increase in reverse T_3, and hypoglycemia with diminished circulating insulin levels may be observed.

Laboratory testing in BN patients is also usually normal. However, when an abnormality is present (ie, metabolic alkalosis), it is usually due to the effects of binge eating and purging. Significant hypokalemia due to purging places the patient at high risk for cardiac arrhythmias, the most common cause of death in BN. Hypophosphatemia, metabolic acidosis (secondary to laxative abuse), and osteopenia and osteoporosis (in BN patients with a past history of AN) are also possible findings.

Laboratory findings in male patients with AN are characterized by low testosterone, diminished LH and FSH, and decreased testicular volume. Likewise, libido and sexual functioning are diminished in these patients during the starved state. Also of note is the presence of osteopenia in male adolescents and young men with eating disorders. Although relatively common, this is usually an unrecognized clinical problem in these patients.

American Academy of Pediatrics, Committee on Adolescence. Identification and management of eating disorders in children and adolescents. *Pediatrics*. 2010;126(6):1240. [PMID: 21115584]
Gowers S, Bryant-Waugh R. Management of child and adolescent eating disorders: the current evidence base and future directions. *J Child Psychol Psychiatry*. 2004; 45:63. [PMID: 14959803]

▶ Differential Diagnosis

In patients presenting with weight loss, other differential diagnoses, both medical and psychiatric, must be considered. Eating disorder symptoms may be caused by numerous medical disorders, including brain tumors, malignancy, connective tissue disease, malabsorption syndrome, hyperthyroidism and infection, gastrointestinal disease (IBD, Crohn disease, ulcerative colitis), menstrual irregularities, cystic fibrosis, and substance abuse (eg, cocaine, amphetamines).

The psychiatric differential diagnosis includes affective and major depressive disorders, schizophrenia, obsessive-compulsive disorder, and somatization disorder. However, the diagnosis of an eating disorder is made by confirming, by history and mental state examination, the core psychopathology of a morbid fear of fatness, and not by ruling out all conceivable medical causes of weight loss or binge-purge behavior. Because eating disorders and affective disorders have both been shown to have an increased incidence in first-degree relatives of anorexics, a thorough family history should also be performed.

American Academy of Pediatrics, Committee on Adolescence. Identification and management of eating disorders in children and adolescents. *Pediatrics*. 2010;126(6):1240. [PMID: 21115584]
Berg KC, et al. Assessment and diagnosis of eating disorders: a guide for professional counselors. *J Couns Dev*. 2012; 90 (3):262.
Carney CP, Andersen AE. Eating disorders. Guide to medical evaluation and complications. *Psychiatry Clin North Am*. 1996;19:657. [PMID: 8933601]
Davis AJ, Grace E. *Dying to Be Thin: Patients with Anorexia and Bulimia*. Continuing Education Monograph of the North American Society for Pediatric and Adolescent Gynecology; 1999.

▶ Complications

Complications of eating disorders are listed in **Table 11-4**.

Table 11-4. Complications of eating disorders.

Cardiovascular: bradycardia, congestive heart failure, dysrythmias, electrocardiographic abnormalities, ipecac-induced cardiomyopathy, mitral valve prolapse, pericardial effusion, orthostatic hypotension
Dermatologic: acrocyanosis, brittle hair and nails, carotene pigmentation, edema, hair loss, lanugo hair, Russell sign
Endocrine: amenorrhea, diabetes insipidus, growth retardation, hypercortisolism, hypothermia, low T_3 syndrome, pubertal delay
Gastrointestinal: acute pancreatitis, Barrett esophagus, bloody diarrhea, constipation, delayed gastric emptying, esophageal or gastric rupture, esophagitis, fatty infiltration and focal necrosis of liver, gallstones, intestinal atony, Mallory-Weiss tears, parotid hyptertrophy, perforation/rupture of the stomach, perimolysis and increased incidence of dental caries, superior mesenteric artery syndrome
Hematologic: bone marrow suppression, impaired cell-mediated immunity, low sedimentation rate
Neurologic: corical atrophy, myopathy, peripheral neuropathy, seizures
Skeletal: osteopenia, osteoperosis, osteoporotic fracture

▶ Treatment

Overall, eating disorders present an unusual challenge for clinicians. Much of the denial, resistance, and anger of the patient and occasionally the family may now be directed at the physician. However, awareness that patients with these disorders are frequently ambivalent, desiring but often afraid of recovery and making the physician the target of their emotions and of the inner conflict, serves to facilitate the building of a trusting relationship, the foundation of effective therapy.

A. Early-Stage Eating Disorders

A developmental perspective cannot be overemphasized for the early detection, and possible prevention, of eating disorders. The only factor consistently associated with more promising treatment outcomes for AN and other eating disorders is early detection and shorter duration of illness. Although many cases of early eating disturbance do not progress to full-syndrome eating disorders, the number of girls and boys in elementary, middle, and high schools engaging in extreme dieting (eg, fasting, excessive exercise) and disordered eating behaviors (eg, binge eating, purging behaviors) is alarmingly high. In fact, many of these individuals fall into the *DSM-5* categories of other specified feeding or eating disorders, or unspecified feeding or eating disorders. Such behaviors should be monitored. Many cases of eating disorders are characterized by a prodromal period of dieting and excessive weight and eating concern that place vulnerable individuals at risk for full-syndrome eating disorders.

Management of the early or mild stages of an eating disorder diagnosis begins with the assessment of weight loss or weight control and establishment of a working relationship and rapport with the patient and family. Next, the physician focuses on the patient's methods of weight loss or weight control. This opens the door to educating the patient on the importance of maintaining good health—including a discussion of normal eating, nutrition, and exercise—and assisting the patient in establishing a goal weight that will serve as a boundary for excessive weight loss.

In addition to the institution of an appropriate diet and weight goal, patients may also be instructed on beginning and maintaining a food diary. This assists the physician in identifying patterns and triggers for dysfunctional habits and gives patients a way to exert some control over their eating behavior.

Another important component of treatment is to acknowledge the possibility of relapse and have a plan in place. Discussing some of the potential triggers of relapse—relationship problems, family issues (eg, divorce, separation), academic and peer pressure—and the strategies to cope with them can help patients avoid feelings of hopelessness when they are experienced. The patient who relapses should be reevaluated within 3–6 weeks. Information obtained on the follow-up visit is helpful in determining whether weight is changing precipitously, if there are changes in physical examination findings, or, most importantly, if the dysfunctional eating habits are more entrenched. These markers help determine whether the patient will require referral.

B. Established Eating Disorders

Patients who clearly meet the criteria for an established eating disorder typically require management by a multidisciplinary team that includes a physician (family physician, pediatrician, or internist), nutritionist or dietician, nurse, mental health professional, and other support staff.

The role of any family physician who is not an integral part of an established eating disorder treatment team is to coordinate and facilitate transfer. This role is critical because the trust in the primary care physician may not be readily transferred to the team of specialists. It is essential that the family physician remain involved in the patient's treatment by providing regular medical assessments, supporting the patient and family, clarifying the tasks performed by each of the team members, reinforcing the importance of the referral, and preventing premature discontinuation of treatment.

Among the various approaches to the management of eating disorders are family therapy, short-term psychotherapies such as cognitive behavioral therapy (CBT), and interpersonal psychotherapy (IPT), behavior modification, and psychoactive medications. According to the condition of the patient (**Table 11-3**), they may be applied in the inpatient or outpatient setting.

1. Anorexia nervosa—Few empirically validated treatments have shown substantial efficacy for AN. Some patients, through medical management and nutritional change, along with psychotherapy, are able to maintain a requisite weight for medical stability; however, many patients retain subthreshold eating pathology and underweight status.

The primary treatment goals for AN are medical stability and weight stabilization. In the female patient, this means a weight at which ovulation and menses can occur; in the male patient, it entails return to normal hormone levels and sex drive; and in adolescents and children, return to normal physical and sexual maturation. Other goals include treating medical and physical complications; motivating patients to cooperate and participate in treatment education regarding healthy nutrition and eating patterns; treating underlying eating disordered psychopathology and fear of weight gain that accompanies AN, as well as comorbid psychiatric conditions; encouraging and supporting family participation; and, ultimately, preventing relapse. Because of the variation and severity of symptoms presented, a comprehensive approach to available services and their clinical dimensions must be considered by the multidisciplinary team. Treatment approach will also vary with the age of the patient. Younger patients are often more successfully treated by utilizing family therapy that involves the parent in refeeding and using the family for balancing food intake, exercise, bedrest, and privileges.

The cornerstone of the multidisciplinary approach to treatment is inpatient or outpatient psychiatric management. While physicians manage the medical comorbidities and nutritionists help reestablish normal eating patterns, mental health professionals target treatment of the underlying psychological causes and symptoms of eating disorders, including distorted cognitions, body image issues, self-image and ego strength problems, and comorbid conditions (ie, mood and anxiety disorders). They use various behavioral or psychological therapies. The chronic and complex characteristics of AN are also inherent problems in the use of psychosocial modalities for treatment. Although behavior modification and family therapy are often effective during the acute refeeding program, psychodynamic therapies and short-term therapies are not. However, psychotherapy is deemed very helpful once malnutrition is corrected. Clinicians use the CBT approach to restructure or modify distorted beliefs and attitudes regarding strict food rituals and dichotomous thinking (viewing the world as "black or "white" or "all or none"). Individual psychodynamic and group therapy are also used by many therapists to address underlying personality disturbances after the acute phase of weight restoration has occurred.

The treatment services available range from intensive inpatient settings, through partial hospital and residential programs, to varying levels of outpatient care. The pretreatment patient evaluation (weight, cardiac, and metabolic status) is essential in determining where treatment will occur. For example, patients who are significantly malnourished, weighing <75% of their individually estimated ideal body weight, are likely to require a 24-hour hospital program. For these patients, hospitalization should occur before the onset of medical instability (ie, marked orthostatic hypotension,

Table 11-5. Criteria[a] for hospitalization.

Severe malnutrition (weight, 75% ideal body weight)
Dehydration
Electrolyte disturbance
Cardiac dysrhythmia
Physiologic instability (eg, severe bradycardia, hypotension, hypothermia,
   orthostatic changes)
Arrested growth and development
Failure of outpatient treatment
Acute food refusal
Uncontrollable binge eating and purging
Acute medical complications of malnutrition, such as syncope, seizures,
   cardiac failure
Acute psychiatric emergencies, such as suicidal ideation or acute psychosis,
   and any comorbid diagnosis that interferes with treatment, such as
   severe depression, obsessive-compulsive disorder, or severe family
   dysfunction

---

[a]Any one or more of the criteria listed above would justify hospitalization.
Reproduced with permission from Fisher M, et al. Eating disorders in adolescents: a background paper. *J Adolesc Health.* 1995; 16:420.

bradycardia of <40 bpm, tachycardia >110 bpm, hyperthermia, seizures, cardiac dysrhythmia, or failure), which could otherwise result in greater risks when refeeding and a more problematic prognosis overall. In such patients, hospitalization is based on psychiatric and behavioral grounds such as acute food refusal, uncontrollable binge eating and purging, failure of outpatient management, and comorbid psychiatric diagnosis (**Table 11-5**).

For milder cases of AN, successful alternatives to intensive inpatient programs have been partial hospitalization and day treatment programs. These programs typically involve a high level of parental participation and are indicative of the patient's motivation to participate in treatment. Initially, these programs require the patient's presence and participation for 14 hours a day. However, as patients approach their target weights, they can be seen in outpatient sessions 3 times per week. Once the target weight is reached, follow-up is less frequent.

Patients selected for outpatient treatment are highly motivated and have brief symptom duration; cooperative, supportive families; no serious medical complications; and BMI > 17.5. Their management should also be orchestrated by a multidisciplinary team that includes a primary care physician (family practitioner, pediatrician), nutritionist, psychotherapist, family therapist, and support staff, because success is highly dependent on careful monitoring of weight obtained in a hospital gown and after voiding, orthostatic vital signs, temperature, urine-specific gravity, and the patients' eating disorder symptoms and behaviors. As an initial step, a clearly and concisely written behavioral contract with the patient and family (if appropriate) can be established. The contract

serves as an agreement to maintain an acceptable minimum weight and vital signs or be hospitalized. Criteria for treatment failure and hospitalization are also included. However, it should be noted that although behavioral contracts are encouraged, they may not be as effective in the outpatient setting because they are more difficult to monitor. Nonetheless, they are helpful in achieving the goal of outpatient management, which is to prompt the patient to self-monitor and assume responsibility for appropriate eating.

For the patient with AN, daily structure is key and should include three meals and several snacks each day. Parents should ensure that healthy foods are readily available and that mealtimes are planned. Although this results in a gradual increase in caloric intake, it may still be necessary to limit physical activity to facilitate weight gain of ≤1 lb per week. This incremental weight increase prevents the gastric dilation, edema, and congestive heart failure experienced by patients who have restricted their eating for a prolonged period of time.

Psychotropic medications are not useful in treatment of AN when patients are in a malnourished state. However, they are frequently used after sufficient weight restoration has occurred for maintenance and the treatment of other associated psychiatric symptoms. Psychotropic medications other than selective serotonin reuptake inhibitors (SSRIs) are most often used. They include neuroleptics for obsessive-compulsive symptoms and anxiety disorders, and acute anxiety agents to reduce anticipatory anxiety associated with eating.

2. Bulimia nervosa—Few patients with uncomplicated BN require hospitalization. Indications for the few patients (<5%) who require inpatient care include severe disabling symptoms that have not responded to outpatient management, binge-purge behavior causing severe physiologic or cardiac disturbances (eg, dysrhythmias, dehydration, metabolic abnormalities), and psychiatric disturbances (eg, suicidal ideation or attempts, substance abuse, major depression). If hospitalization is warranted, the treatment focus is on metabolic restoration, nutritional rehabilitation, and mood stabilization. These patients may also require assistance with laxative, diuretic, and illicit drug withdrawal. Hospitalization is usually brief, and management then transfers to partial hospitalization programs or outpatient treatment facilities. Partial hospitalization programs usually require the patient to be present 10 hours per day, 5 days a week. Support is usually provided in a group format and family participation is often required. Many of the treatment modalities for BN resemble those for AN. However, the primary focus differs significantly. Although some bulimia patients may be slightly underweight, most are of normal weight; hence nutritional rehabilitation targets the patient's pattern of binging and purging in weight restoration. Therefore, nutritional counseling serves as an adjuvant to other treatment modalities and has been noted to enhance the effectiveness of the overall treatment program.

Interventions targeting the psychosocial aspects surrounding BN address the issues of binging and purging, food restriction, attitudes related to eating patterns, body image and developmental concerns, self-esteem and sexual difficulties, family dysfunction, and comorbid conditions (eg, depression). The most efficacious psychosocial approach is CBT, a relatively short-term approach specifically focused on the eating disorder symptoms and underlying cognitions (eg, low self-esteem, body image concerns) of BN. Patients managed with CBT demonstrate profound decrements in three very characteristic behaviors: binge eating, vomiting, and laxative abuse. However, the percentage of patients who can achieve total abstinence from binge-purge behavior is invariably small. IPT, also a short-term treatment, is considered a second line of treatment.

Other types of individual psychotherapy that are used in clinical practice include psychodynamic approaches that may be helpful in treating some of the underlying causes of BN. Group psychotherapy is moderately successful. The efficacy of this approach is increased when it is combined with nutritional counseling and frequent clinic visits. Family or marital therapy should also be considered in conjunction with other treatment modalities for adolescents living at home, older patients from dysfunctional homes, and patients experiencing marital discord.

Another important aspect of eating disorder management is pharmacotherapy with antidepressants (eg, SSRIs). These agents were first used in the acute phase of treatment for BN because of its well-established comorbid association with clinical depression. It was later reported that nondepressed patients also responded to these medications. Multiple clinical studies have shown the SSRIs to have an antibulimic (reduction in binge eating and vomiting rates) effect independent of their antidepressant effect. Therapists have also noted improvement in mood and anxiety symptoms. Other antidepressant medications used in the treatment of BN include the tricyclic antidepressants (imipramine/desipramine), the monoamine oxidase inhibitors (MAOIs; phenelzine and isocarboxazid). The MAOIs should be used with great caution and only in patients with severe BN. At this time, fluoxetine is the only SSRI approved by the Food and Drug Administration for the treatment of BN. A 20-mg per day dose is used to initiate treatment, with doses of 40–60 mg/d required for maintenance.

3. Binge eating disorder—Although most individuals with BED are obese, normal-weight people are also affected. Therefore, treatment usually focuses on the distress experienced by individuals rather than on their weight problem. CBT, IPT, and group approaches are effective. CBT, which teaches techniques to monitor eating habits and alternative responses to difficult situations, appears to be the most efficacious. For patients with greater eating-related and psychosocial distress, IPT appears to be a particularly potent treatment. The great majority of those affected can be treated as outpatients and hospitalization is rarely needed.

Similar to BN, pharmacotherapy has demonstrated effectiveness for the treatment of BED. SSRIs appear to foster reductions in binge eating, psychiatric symptoms, and the severity of the illness. Medications aiming to reduce weight among overweight and obese BED patients, including topiramate, have also shown promising results for weight reduction. There is mixed support for whether combining psychotherapy (CBT) with pharmacologic interventions enhances remission rates. However, specific medications (orlistat, topiramate) have been shown to enhance weight loss achieved with CBT and behavioral weight loss.

American Psychiatric Association. *Clinical Guidelines for Eating Disorders* (available at http://psychiatryonline.org/content.aspx?bookid=28&sectionid=39113853).

Berkman ND. Management of eating disorders. *Evid Rep Technol Assess.* (full report) 2006;135:1. [PMID: 17628126]

Fisher M. Treatment of eating disorders in children, adolescents, and young adults. *Pediatr Rev.* 2006; 27:5. [PMID: 16387924]

Reas DL, Grilo CM. Review and meta-analysis of pharmacotherapy for binge-eating disorder. *Obesity.* 2008; 19(9):2024. [PMID: 19186327]

▶ Prognosis

The prognosis for full recovery of patients with AN is modest. Many individuals demonstrate symptomatic improvement over time, but a substantial number have persistent problems with body image, disordered eating, and psychological challenges. A review of multiple carefully conducted follow-up studies of hospitalized populations (at ≥4 years after the onset of illness) showed that the outcomes for 44% could be rated as good (weight restored to within 15% of recommended weight for height; regular menses established), 24% were poor (weight never reached 15% of recommended weight for height; menses absent or sporadic), approximately 28% fell between the good and poor groups, and approximately 5% had died (early mortality). Approximately two-thirds of patients continued to have morbid food and weight preoccupation and psychiatric symptoms, and ~ 40% continued to have bulimic symptoms. Longer duration of illness, lower initial weight, previous treatment failure, vomiting, family dysfunction, and being married have all been associated with a worse prognosis. Adolescents have better outcomes than adults, and younger adolescents have better outcomes than older adolescents.

The outcomes for patients with BN are more promising. Generally speaking, the short-term success rate for patients treated with psychosocial modalities and medication is reported to be 50–70%, with relapse rates between 30% and 50% after 6 months to 6 years of follow-up. Data also suggest that slow, steady progress continues when the follow-up period is extended to 10–15 years. BN is associated with lower mortality and higher rates of recovery compared to AN.

Characteristically, patients with BN who have onset at an early age, milder symptoms at start of treatment, and a good support system, and those more likely to be treated as outpatients often have a better prognosis. Typically, individuals with BN have one or more relapses during recovery, whereas those with AN generally have a more protracted and arduous course, requiring long-term, intensive therapy. Outcomes for BED are less certain. Without treatment, BED is often characterized by a chronic, fluctuating course, but many patients are able to decrease the frequency of binge eating with proper treatment.

Arcelus J, et al. Mortality rates in patients with anorexia nervosa and other eating disorders. A meta-analysis of 36 studies. *Arch Gen Psychiatry*. 2011;68(7):724. [PMID: 21727255]

Becker AE, et al. Genes and/or jeans? Genetic and socio-cultural contributions to risk for eating disorders. *J Addict Dis*. 2004; 23:81. [PMID: 15256346]

Keel PK, Brown, TA. Update on course and outcome in eating disorders. *Int J Eat Dis*. 2010; 43(3):195. [PMID: 20186717]

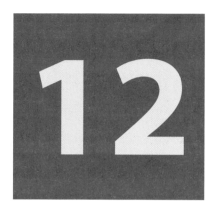

Adolescent Sexuality

Amy Crawford-Faucher, MD, FAAFP

Adolescence, generally between 12 and 19 years, is a time of complex physical, cognitive, psychosocial, and sexual changes, and physical development occurs in advance of cognitive maturity. Not until maturity is reached in all of these realms does the adolescent acquire mature decision-making skills and the ability to make healthy decisions regarding sexual activity. Sexuality involves more than just anatomic gender or physical sexual behavior, but incorporates how individuals view themselves as male or female, how they relate to others, and the ability to enter into and maintain an intimate relationship on a giving and trusting basis. Adolescent sexual development forms the basis for further adult sexuality and future intimate relationships. Adolescents who are sexually active before having achieved the capacity for intimacy are at risk for unwanted or unhealthy consequences of sexual activity.

DEVELOPMENT

▶ Physical Changes

Rapid changes in their bodies often make adolescents feel uncomfortable and self-conscious. Puberty usually starts between 9 and 12 years for girls and between 11 and 14 years for boys. In girls, these hormonal changes result in the development of breasts, growth of pubic and axillary hair, body odor, and menstruation (often irregular or unpredictable for the first 18–24 months). Boys develop increased penis and testicular size; facial, pubic, and axillary hair; body odor; and a deepened voice, and experience nocturnal ejaculations ("wet dreams"). As adolescents are learning to adjust and grow comfortable with their changing bodies, questions concerning body image are common (eg, penis size, breast size and development, distribution of pubic hair, and changing physique in general).

▶ Cognitive Changes

The shift from concrete thinking to abstract thinking (the cognitive development of formal operations) begins in early adolescence (11–12 years) and usually reaches full development by 15–16 years—so 10–14-year-olds should not be expected to function with full capacity for abstract thinking. In contrast to younger children, adolescents:

- Show an increased ability to generate and hold in mind more than one complex mental representation.
- Show an appreciation of the relativity and uncertainty of knowledge.
- Tend to think in terms of abstract rather than only concrete representations; they think of consequences and the future (abstract) versus a sense of being omnipotent, invincible, infallible, and immune to mishaps (concrete).
- Show a far greater use of strategies for obtaining knowledge, such as active planning and evaluation of alternatives.
- Are self-aware in their thinking and able to reflect on their own thought processes and evaluate the credibility of the knowledge source.
- Understand that fantasies are not acted out.
- Have the capacity to develop intimate, meaningful relationships.

▶ Psychosocial Changes

Core psychosocial developmental tasks of adolescence include the following:

- Becoming emotionally and behaviorally independent rather than dependent, especially in developing independence from the family.
- Acquiring educational and other experiences needed for adult work roles and developing a realistic vocational goal.
- Learning to deal with emerging sexuality and to achieve a mature level of sexuality.

- Resolving issues of identity and achieving a realistic and positive self-image.
- Developing interpersonal skills, including the capacity for intimacy, and preparing for intimate partnerships with others.

Psychosocial development includes both internal (introspective) and external forces. Peers, parents or guardians, teachers, and coaches all influence adolescent expectations, evaluations, values, feedback, and social comparison. Failure to accomplish the developmental tasks necessary for adulthood results in identity or role diffusion: an uncertain self-concept, indecisiveness, and clinging to the more secure dependencies of childhood.

As part of this maturation process, it is natural for adolescents to explore sexual relationships and sexual roles in their social interactions. The adolescent's task is to successfully manage the conflict between sexual drives and the recognition of the emotional, interpersonal, and biological results of sexual behavior.

▶ Sexual Changes

Gender identity forms a foundation for sexual identity. Gender identity, the sense of maleness or femaleness, is established by age 2 years and solidifies as adolescents experience and integrate sexuality into their identity. Sexual identity is the erotic expression of self as male or female and the awareness of self as a sexual being who can be involved in a sexual relationship with others. The task of adolescence is to integrate sexual orientation into sexual identity. Heterosexual orientation is taken for granted by society. For lesbian and gay individuals, this creates a clash between outside cultural expectations and their inner sense of self. Same-sex orientation emerges during adolescence but is far more subtle and complex; it includes behavior, sexual attraction, erotic fantasy, emotional preference, social preference, and self-identification—felt to be a continuum from completely heterosexual to completely homosexual (see Chapter 62).

Currently in US society, the primary developmental task of the gay adolescent is to adapt to a socially stigmatized sexual role. Societal antihomosexual attitudes are associated with significant psychological distress for gay, lesbian, and bisexual (GLB) persons and have a negative impact on mental health, including a greater incidence of depression and suicide (as many as one-third have attempted suicide at least once), lower self-acceptance, and a greater likelihood of hiding sexual orientation. When GLB adolescents disclose their orientation to their families, they may experience overt rejection at home as well as social isolation among their peers. GLB adolescents often lack role models and access to support systems. They are more likely to run away and become homeless, which puts them at higher risk for unsafe sex, drug and alcohol use, and exchanging sex for money or drugs. Although the research is limited,

transgendered persons are reported to experience similar problems. Negative attitudes within society toward gay, lesbian, bisexual, and transgendered (GLBT) individuals lead to antigay violence (see Chapter 58).

Adolescents with questions or concerns about sexual orientation need the opportunity to discuss their feelings, their experiences, and their fears of exposure to family and friends. GLBT adolescents need reassurance about their value as a person, support regarding parental and societal reactions, and access to role models. Parents, Families, and Friends of Lesbians and Gays (PFLAG) is a nationwide organization whose purpose is to assist parents with information and support (see Chapter 62).

Problems with sexual identity may manifest in extremes—sexually acting out or repression of sexuality. Frequent sexual activity and various sexual partners are negative risk factors for physical or psychological health, and can suggest poor integration of sexual identity in adolescents.

American Academy of Child & Adolescent Psychiatry. *Normal Adolescent Development, Part I. Facts for Families*, no. 57; (available at http://www.aacap.org/AACAP/Families_and_ Youth/Facts_for_Families/Facts_for_Families_Pages/Normal_ Adolescent_Development_Part_I_57.aspx) Dec. 2011 (accessed April 19, 2013).

Christie D, Viner R. Adolescent development. *Br Med J.* 2005; 330(7486):301–304.

Leibowitz SF, Tellingator C. Assessing gender identity concerns in children and adolescents: evaluation, treatments and outcomes. *Curr Psychiatry Rep.* 2012; 14(2):111–120.

SEXUAL BEHAVIOR & INITIATION OF SEXUAL ACTIVITY

Early- to middle-stage adolescents begin to experience sexual urges that may be satisfied by masturbation. Masturbation is the exploration of the sexual self and provides a sense of control over one's body and sexual needs. Masturbation starts in infancy, providing children with enjoyment of their bodies. Parents are typically uncomfortable observing this behavior. In early adolescence, masturbation is an important developmental task, allowing the adolescent to learn what forms of self-stimulation are pleasurable and integrating this with fantasies of interacting with another. Sexual curiosity intensifies. With older adolescents, the autoeroticism of masturbation develops into experimentation with others, including intercourse.

Typical reasons for sexual activity in early to midadolescence are curiosity, peer pressure, seeking approval, physical urges, and rebellion. Sexual activity can be misinterpreted by the adolescent as evidence of independence from the family or individuation. Adolescent girls may misinterpret sexual activity as a measure of a meaningful relationship. When sexual activity is used to satisfy needs such as self-esteem, popularity, and dependence, it delays or prevents development of a capacity for intimacy and is associated with casual and less responsible sexual activity. Appropriate education, parental support, and a positive sexual self-concept are associated with a later age of first intercourse, a higher consistent use of contraceptives, and a lower pregnancy rate. Parental supervision and establishing limits, living with both parents in a stable environment, high self-esteem, higher family income, and orientation toward achievement are associated with delayed initiation of sexual activity.

Commitment to a religion or affiliation with certain religious denominations appears to affect on sexual behavior. For example, an adolescent's frequent attendance at religious services is associated with a greater likelihood of abstinence. On the other hand, for adolescents who are sexually active, frequency of attendance is associated with decreased contraceptive use by girls and increased use by boys.

Evidence suggests that school attendance reduces adolescent sexual risk-taking behavior. Worldwide, as the percentage of girls completing elementary school has increased, adolescent birth rates have decreased. In the United States, adolescents who have dropped out of school are more likely to initiate sexual activity earlier, fail to use contraception, become pregnant, and give birth. Among those who remain in school, greater involvement with school, including athletics for girls, is related to less sexual risk taking, including later age of initiation of sex and lower frequency of sex, pregnancy, and childbearing.

Schools structure students' time, creating an environment that discourages unhealthy risk taking, particularly by increasing interactions between children and adults. They also affect selection of friends and larger peer groups. Schools can increase belief in the future and help adolescents plan for higher education and careers, and they can increase students' sense of competence, as well as their communication and refusal skills. Schools often have access to training and communications technology and also provide an opportunity for the kind of positive peer learning that can influence social norms.

Evaluation of school-based sex education programs that typically emphasize abstinence, but also discuss condoms and other methods of contraception, indicates that the programs either have no effect on—or, in some cases, result in—a delay in the initiation of sexual activity. There is strong evidence that providing information about contraception does not increase adolescent sexual activity by hastening the onset of sexual intercourse, increasing the frequency of sexual intercourse, or increasing the number of sexual partners. More importantly, providing this information results in increased use of condoms or contraceptives among adolescents who were already sexually active.

Factors associated with early age of first intercourse and lack of contraceptive use are early pubertal development, a history of sexual abuse, lower socioeconomic status, poverty, lack of attentive and nurturing parents, single-parent homes, cultural and familial patterns of early sexual experience, lack of school or career goals, and dropping out of school. Additional factors include low self-esteem, concern for physical appearance, peer group pressure, and pressure to please partners.

Compared with those not sexually active, sexually active male adolescents used more alcohol, engaged in more fights, and were more likely to know about HIV and AIDS. Similarly, sexually active female adolescents used more alcohol and cigarettes. Both sexually active male and female adolescents had higher levels of stress. Alcohol and drug use is associated with greater risk taking, including unprotected sexual activity.

Kirby DB, et al. The "safer choices" intervention: its impact on the sexual behaviors of different subgroups of high school students. *J Adolesc Health.* 2004; 35:442. [PMID: 15581523]

SCOPE OF THE PROBLEM

▶ Prevalence & Consequences of Sexual Activity

Approximately 47% of all US adolescents have ever had sex. Most teens become sexually active in their later teen years; 70% have had sexual intercourse by the time they turn 19. Approximately 33% of all 15–19-year-olds have had sexual intercourse in the past 3 months. For adolescents who want to have intercourse, the primary reasons given are sexual curiosity (50% of boys; 24% of girls) and affection for their partner (25% of boys; 48% of girls). For adolescents who agree to have intercourse but do not really want to, the primary reasons given are peer pressure (~30%), curiosity (50% of boys; 25% of girls), and affection for their partner (>33%). With little sex education, adolescents are poorly prepared to openly discuss their need for contraception, negotiate safe sex, and negotiate the types of behavior in which they are willing to participate. Sexual behavior that contradicts personal values is associated with emotional distress and lower self-esteem. As adolescents are learning to develop appropriate interpersonal skills, damage to self-esteem can be significant when sexual activity is exchanged for attention, affection, peer approval, or reassurance about their physical appearance. Furthermore, early unsatisfactory sexual experiences can set up patterns for repeated unsatisfactory sexual experiences into adulthood.

▶ Unintended Pregnancy

Close to 80% of teen pregnancies in the United States are not planned. Although teen pregnancy rates have fallen dramatically since 1990 (from 117 per thousand in 1990 to 34.3 per thousand in 2010), nearly 34% of teen girls will have at least one pregnancy by the time they turn 22. Despite similar rates of adolescent sexual activity, the United States has the highest rate of adolescent pregnancy among developed nations. Compared to American teens, European teens are more likely to use contraception, and to use the most reliable contraception.

Unintended pregnancy is socially and economically costly. Medical costs include lost opportunity for preconception care and counseling, increased likelihood of late or no prenatal care, increased risk for a low-birth-weight infant, and increased risk for infant mortality. The social costs include reduced educational attainment and employment opportunity, increased welfare dependence, and increased risk of child abuse and neglect. In addition to the adolescent being confronted with adult problems prematurely, the parents' ability to lead productive and healthy lives and to achieve academic and economic success is compromised.

Although women in their 20s account for more than half of all induced abortions, in 2008, 26% of adolescent pregnancies ended in abortion. Adolescents who terminate pregnancies are less likely to become pregnant over the next 2 years; more likely to graduate from high school; and more likely to show lower anxiety, higher self-esteem, and more internal control than adolescents who do not terminate pregnancies. For an adolescent, postponement of childbearing improves social, psychological, academic, and economic outcomes of life (see Chapter 16).

Sexually Transmitted Infections

Adolescents (10–19 years old) and young adults (20–24 years old) have the highest rates of sexually transmitted diseases, including gonorrhea and chlamydia. Additionally, 26% of new HIV cases are diagnosed in young people aged 13–24 years; 4 of 5 of these are in young males. Education about transmission and increased access and use of condoms can help prevent sexually transmitted diseases.

Sexual Abuse

More than 100,000 children are victims of sexual abuse each year. Sexual abuse contributes to sexual and mental health dysfunction as well as public health problems such as substance abuse. Victims of sexual abuse may have difficulty establishing and maintaining healthy relationships with others. Additionally, they may engage in premature sexual behavior, frequently seeking immediate release of sexual tension, and have poor sexual decision-making skills.

Although only a relatively small proportion of rapes are reported, a major national study found that 22% of women and approximately 2% of men had been victims of a forced sexual act.

Delinquency and homelessness are associated with a history of physical, emotional, and sexual abuse, as well as negative parental reactions to sexual orientation. Homelessness is associated with exchanging sex for money, food, or drugs. Additionally, homeless adolescents are at high risk for repeated episodes of sexual assault.

Centers for Disease Control and Prevention. *Sexually Transmitted Diseases Surveillance. STDs in Adolescents and Young Adults.* Atlanta, GA: CDC; 2011.

Facts on American Teens' Sexual and Reproductive Health (available at http://www.gutmacher.org/pubs/FB-ATSRH.html. Accessed April 19, 2013).

Hamilton BE, Ventura SJ. *Birth Rates for U.S. Teenagers Reach Historic Lows for All Ages and Ethnic Groups.* NCHS Data Brief 89. Hyattsville, MD: National Center for Health Statistics. 2012.

US Department of Health and Human Services. *Adolescent Health in the United States, 2007.* US Government Bookstore, 2008. DHHS Publication PHS 2008-1034.

US Department of Health and Human Services: *Child Maltreatment 2007: Reports from the States to the National Child Abuse and Neglect Data System.* Washington, DC: Government Printing Office; 2009.

SOURCES OF INFORMATION

The Family

While parents are not the primary source of information about sexuality, they do influence their adolescent's sexual attitudes; parent-adolescent communication can mitigate the strength of peer influence on sexual activity. Warm parent-child relationships with parental supervision and monitoring can lead to decreased sexual activity. However, parental control can be associated with negative effects if it is excessive or coercive. Adolescent sexuality can be very threatening to adults, who may not have resolved their own issues concerning sexuality. With escalating stresses, the self-esteem of parents may decline, making them either highly impulsive or overly controlling or rigid. Heightened levels of anxiety contribute to blocked communication.

The Family Physician

Because many parents are uncomfortable discussing sexuality with their children, family physicians must be proactive in initiating and facilitating conversations about the topic.

Providing a handout (**Table 12-1**) for parents might help facilitate home discussions about sexuality. If information is not available at home, the family physician is uniquely positioned to serve as a resource and should take a proactive approach by creating the proper environment for discussion, initiating the topic of sexuality, and providing anticipatory guidance for both adolescents and their families (**Table 12-2**).

A. Creating the Environment

- Ensure confidentiality for the preadolescent or adolescent for discussions about sexuality.

- Interview adolescents without the parent or guardian in the room to help create a trusting environment.

- Provide an office letter to the parent to outline policies regarding confidentiality and accessibility for adolescents.

Many states have laws regarding the ability of adolescents to seek health care for specific issues—such as contraception,

Table 12-1. How to talk to your child about sex.

1. **Be available.** Watch for clues that show they want to talk. If your child doesn't ask, look for ways to bring up the subject. For example, you may know a pregnant woman, watch the birth of a pet, or see a baby getting a bath. Use a TV program or film to start a discussion. Libraries and schools have good books on sex that are geared to different ages.
2. **Answer their questions.** Answer honestly and without showing embarrassment, even if the time and place do not seem appropriate. A short answer may be best for the moment. Then return to the subject later. Not knowing enough about the subject to answer a question can be an opportunity to learn with your child. Tell your child that you'll get the information and continue the discussion later, or do the research together. Answer the question that is asked, but don't overload the child with too much information at once.
3. **Identify components accurately.** Use correct names for body parts and their functions to show that they are normal and okay to talk about.
4. **Practice talking about sex.** Discuss sex with your partner, another family member, or a friend. This will help you feel more comfortable when you do talk with your child.
5. **Talk about sex more than once.** Children need to hear things repeatedly over the years, because their level of understanding changes as they grow older. Make certain that you talk about feelings and not just actions. It is important not to think of sex only in terms of intercourse, pregnancy, and birth. Talk about feeling oneself as man or woman, relating to others' feelings, thoughts, and attitudes, and feelings of self-esteem.
6. **Respect their privacy.** Privacy is important, for both you and your child. If your child doesn't want to talk, say, "OK, let's talk about it later," and do. Don't forget about it. Avoid searching a child's room, drawers, or purse for "evidence," or listening in on a telephone or other private conversation.
7. **Listen to your children.** They want to know that their questions and concerns are important. Laughing at or ignoring children's questions may stop them from asking again. They will get information, accurate or inaccurate, from other sources. Listen, watch their body language to know when they are ready for you to talk, and repeat back to them what you think you heard.
8. **Share your values.** If your jokes, behaviors, or attitudes don't show respect for sexuality, then you cannot expect your child to be sexually healthy. Children learn attitudes about love, caring, and responsibility from you, whether you talk about it or not. Tell your child what your values are about sex and about life. Parents need to know what their children value in their lives, and children need to know that their parents are concerned about their health and future well-being.
9. **Help teach your child how to make decisions.** It is important for you to: (a) have your child identify the problem, (b) analyze the situation, (c) search for options or solutions, (d) think about possible consequences to these options, (e) choose the best option, (f) take action, and then (g) watch for the results.

Data from http://www.plannedparenthood.org/parents/ and http://www.familydoctor.org/familydoctor/en/teens/puberty-sexuality/ questions-and-answers-about-sex.html.

Table 12-2. Office approach to adolescent health care.

1. Establish comfortable, friendly relationships that permit discussion in an atmosphere of mutual trust well before sensitive issues arise. Ensure confidentiality before the need arises. Establish separate discussions with parents and adolescents as a matter of routine.
2. Take a firm, proactive role to initiate developmentally appropriate discussions of sexuality. Recognize and use teachable moments regarding sexuality.
3. Provide anticipatory guidance and resources to facilitate family discussions about sexuality and cue families and preteens about upcoming physical and psychosocial developmental changes.
4. Enhance communication skills. Use reflective listening. With a nonjudgmental manner, accept what adolescents have to say without agreeing or disagreeing.
5. Use a positive approach when discussing developmental changes and needed interventions, complimenting pubertal changes.
6. Increase knowledge of family systems and the potential impact of physicians on the family.
7. Discuss topics about sexuality incrementally over time to improve assimilation and decrease embarrassment. Avoid scientific terms. Keep answers to questions thorough yet simple. Be cautious about questions that might erode trust.
8. Know your limitations. Use other professional staff and referrals when necessary.

Data from Croft CA, Asmussen L. A developmental approach to sexuality education: implications for medical practice. *J Adolesc Health.* 1993;14:109.

mental health, substance abuse, and pregnancy—without parental presence or approval. Family physicians need to be familiar with the nuances of these laws in their practicing state.

B. Proactive Approach

- Provide anticipatory guidance to parents of adolescents when they present for their own health needs.
- Cue preteens about the upcoming physical changes of puberty.
- Discuss sexuality topics incrementally, in developmentally appropriate forms (**Table 12-3**).

C. Asking the Question

Family physicians can initiate the topic of sexuality with adolescents during health maintenance or perhaps even acute care visits. For instance, physicians might ask their adolescent patients whom they are dating and to whom they are attracted. Because abstract thinking is still undergoing development, adolescents need explicit examples to understand ideas. History taking must be specific and directive. Instructions should be concrete. Answers to questions should be simple and thorough.

Concerns in early adolescence typically relate to body image and what is "normal," both physically and socially.

Information and reassurance about pubertal changes are critical parts of physical examinations. Conversations may include addressing concerns about obesity, acne, and body image that affect self-perception of acceptability and attractiveness. Discussions about how to handle peer pressure are always helpful. The adolescent's understanding of safer sexual practices as well as the ability to negotiate the behavior in which they are willing or unwilling to participate should be explored.

Although it is important to avoid making assumptions about sexual orientation, an adolescent who presents with depression and suicidal ideation should be questioned about this. Hiding one's orientation increases stress. It is important to be aware of community resources for GLBT adolescents such as psychologists and counselors, GLBT community support groups, and organizations such as PFLAG.

Caring for adolescents can be exciting and challenging. Physicians should recognize that their own projections of unfinished sexual issues from their adolescence may surface

Table 12-3. Adolescent sexual development.

	8–12 Years	≥13 Years
Sexual knowledge	Knows correct terms for sexual parts, commonly uses slang; understands sexual aspects of pregnancy; increasing knowledge of sexual behavior (eg, masturbation, intercourse); knowledge of physical aspects of puberty by age 10	Understands sexual intercourse, contraception, and sexually transmitted diseases (STDs)
Body parts and function	Should have complete understanding of sexual, reproductive, and elimination functions of body parts; all need anticipatory guidance on upcoming pubertal changes for both sexes, including menstruation and nocturnal emissions	Important to discuss health and hygiene, as well as provide more information about contraceptives, STDs/HIV, and responsible sexual behaviors' access to health care is important
Gender identity	Gender identity is fixed; encouragement to pursue individual interests and talents regardless of gender stereotypes is important	Discuss men and women's social perception; males tend to perceive social situations more sexually than females and may interpret neutral cues (eg, clothing, friendliness) as sexual invitations
Sexual abuse prevention	Assess their understanding of an abuser and correct misconceptions; explain how abusers, including friends, relatives, and strangers, may manipulate children; help them identify abusive situations, including sexual harassment; practice assertiveness and problem-solving skills; teach them to trust their body's internal cues and to act assertively in problematic situations	Teach them to avoid risky situations (eg, walking alone at night, unsafe parts of town); discuss dating relationships, particularly date/acquaintance rape and its association with alcohol and drug use, including date rape drugs; encourage parents to provide transportation home immediately if their teenagers are ever in difficult or potentially dangerous situations and also to consider enrolling their children in a self-defense class (eg, karate)
Sexual behavior	Sex games with peers and siblings: role play and sex fantasy, kissing, mutual masturbation, and simulated intercourse; masturbation in private; shows modesty, embarrassment–hides sex games and masturbation from adults; may fantasize or dream about sex; interested in media sex; uses sexual language with peers; considers making decisions in the context of relationships; should be provided with information about contraceptives, STDs/HIV, and responsible sexual behaviors	Pubertal changes continue—most girls menstruate by 16, boys are capable of ejaculation by 15; dating begins; sexual contacts are common—mutual masturbation, kissing, petting; sexual fantasy and dreams; sexual intercourse may occur in ≤70% by age 19; encourage parents to share attitudes and values; provide access to contraceptives; respect need and desire for privacy; set clear rules about dating and curfews
Developmental issues;[a] most sexual concerns are related to the developmental tasks	Early adolescence (Tanner I, II): physical changes, including menstruation and nocturnal emissions; often ambivalent over issues of independence and protection and family relationships; egocentric; beginning struggles of separation and emerging individual identity; seemingly trivial concerns to adults can reach crisis proportions in young adolescents; common concerns include fears of too slow or too rapid physical development, especially breasts and genitalia; concern and curiosity about their bodies; sexual feelings and sexual behavior of their peer group as well as adults around them; although masturbation is very healthy and normal, reassurance may be needed given persistence of myths and mixed messages	Middle adolescence (Tanner III, IV): peer approval; experimentation and risk-taking behavior arise from developmental task of defining oneself socially; sexual intercourse may be viewed as requisite for peer acceptance; curiosity, need for peer approval, self-esteem, and struggle for independence from parents can lead to intercourse at this stage; feelings of invincibility lead to sexual activity that is impulsive and lacking discussion about sexual decision making, such as contraception, preferences for behavior, relationship commitment, or safe sex; increasing insistence on control over decisions; increasing conflict with parents

(Continued)

Table 12-3. Adolescent sexual development. (Continued)

8–12 Years	≥13 Years
Developmental tasks: 1. Independence and separation from the family 2. Development of individual identity 3. Beginning to shift from concrete to abstract thinking	Developmental tasks: 1. Development of adult social relationships with both sexes 2. Continued struggle for independence 3. Continued development of individual identity 4. Continued shifting from cognitive to abstract thinking Late adolescence (Tanner V): With cognitive maturation, issues regarding peer acceptance and conflicts with parents regarding independence lessen; intimacy, commitment, and life planning, including thoughts of future parenthood; self-identity continues to solidify, moral and ethical values, exploration of sexual identity; crises over sexual orientation may surface at this stage; increasing ability to recognize consequences of own behavior Developmental tasks: 1. Abstract (futuristic) thinking 2. Vocational plans 3. Development of moral and ethical values 4. Maturation toward autonomous decision making

ᵃThese are general categories; adolescents vary in their physical, psychosocial, and cognitive development.
Data from Gordon BN, Schroeder CS. Sexuality: *A Developmental Approach to Problems*. New York, NY: Plenum Press; 1995; and Alexander B, et al. Adolescent sexuality issues in office practice. *Am Fam Physician*. 1991;44:1273.

in caring for adolescent patients. This can make discussions, particularly about sensitive subjects such as drugs, alcohol, nicotine, and sex, difficult. Recognizing and addressing these issues or referring adolescents to colleagues with greater experience and comfort with these matters would be appropriate.

The role of family physicians is to provide a supportive, sensitive, and instructive environment in which they neither ignore nor judge adolescent sexual activity but reassure, listen to, clarify, and provide correct information about this important aspect of adolescent development. Ideally the goal should be to delay sexual activity until adolescents have the knowledge and tools needed to make healthy decisions about sex. However, identifying adolescents at risk, educating them about safer sex, establishing sexual limits, and providing information about support and educational resources for adolescents who are currently sexually active are critical activities for the family physician.

Martino SC, Elliott MN, Corona R, et al. Beyond the big talk: the roles and breadth and repetition in parent-adolescent communication about sexual topics. *Pediatrics*. 2008; 121; e612–e618.

Websites

For Patient Information

American Academy of Family Physicians. *Information from Your Family Doctor: Sex: Making the Right Decision*; 2010 (available at http://www.familydoctor.org/handouts/276.html).
American Academy of Family Physicians. *Sexual Health for Teens* (available at http://kidshealth.org/PageManager.jsp?dn=familydoctor&lic=44&ps=203&cat_id=20014).
Parents, Families and Friends of Lesbians and Gays (PFLAG). http://www.pflag.org

For Provider Information

Gay and Lesbian Medical Association (GLMA). http://www.glma.org

Menstrual Disorders

LTC Mary V. Krueger, DO, MPH

Menstrual disorders are a heterogeneous group of conditions that are both physically and psychologically debilitating. Although they were once considered nuisance problems, it is now recognized that menstrual disorders take a significant toll on society, in days lost from work, as well as the pain and suffering experienced by individual women. These disorders may arise from physiologic (eg, pregnancy), pathologic (eg, stress, excessive exercise, weight loss, endocrine or structural abnormalities), or iatrogenic (eg, secondary to contraceptive use) conditions.

Irregularities in menstruation may manifest as complete absence of menses, dysfunctional uterine bleeding, dysmenorrhea, or premenstrual syndrome. Vaginal bleeding is addressed in Chapter 34. Since it is essential to know what is normal in order to define that which is abnormal, normal menstrual parameters are listed in **Table 13-1**.

AMENORRHEA

ESSENTIALS OF DIAGNOSIS

▶ Primary amenorrhea: the absence of menses by 15 years of age in patient with secondary sex characteristics, or absence of menses by 13 years of age in a patient without secondary sex characteristics.

▶ Secondary amenorrhea: absence of menses for at least 6 months in a woman with previously normal menses, or at least 12 months or six cycles without a period in a woman with previously irregular menses.

▶ General Considerations

Amenorrhea is a symptom, not a diagnosis, and may occur secondary to a number of endocrine, physiologic, and anatomic abnormalities. Classifying amenorrhea into primary and secondary amenorrhea can aid in evaluation and simplify diagnosis.

▶ Primary Amenorrhea

The clinician must be sensitive to the fact that the adolescent patient may be uncomfortable discussing her sexuality, especially in the presence of a parent. The most common causes of primary amenorrhea are gonadal dysgenesis, hypothalamic hypogonadism, pituitary disease, and anatomic abnormality.

▶ Prevention

Primary amenorrhea may be prevented by maintaining an appropriate body weight and treating the underlying conditions.

▶ Clinical Findings

A. Signs and Symptoms

The history and physical exam (H&PE) are the most important steps in diagnosing primary amenorrhea. Key elements of the history are listed in **Table 13-2**. This targeted history will help narrow the differential and eliminate unnecessary testing. Physical examination should focus on appearance of secondary sexual characteristics and pelvic examination findings—specifically the presence or absence of a uterus. BMI should also be calculated and compared with prior visits to assess both for rapid weight loss or weight gain. Presence or absence of breast development and presence or absence of the uterus and cervix are decision points for further testing and diagnostic categories.

B. Laboratory Findings

Choice of laboratory examination should be guided by history and physical findings and are listed here on the basis

Table 13-1. Normal menstrual parameters.

Age of menarche	<16 years old
Age of menopause	>40 years old; mean age 52
Length of menstrual cycle	22–45 days
Length of menstrual flow	3–7 days
Amount of menstrual flow	<80 cc

of etiology. A pregnancy test should be performed on all individuals presenting for primary amenorrhea that have secondary sexual characteristics and functional anatomy. Although the initial cycles after menarche are often anovulatory, pregnancy can occur before the first recognized menstrual cycle. Patients with a normal pelvic examination but absent breast development should receive serum FSH (follicle-stimulating hormone) measured to distinguish peripheral (gonadal) from central (pituitary or hypothalamic) causes of amenorrhea. A high FSH suggests gonadal dysgenesis. A karyotype should be performed to differentiate patients with Turner's syndrome (45 X) that is most common from other variations. It is important to identify patients with a 46 XY karyotype, since these individuals have a high peripubertal risk for gonadoblastoma and dysgerminoma. If the uterus is absent, serum testosterone and karyotype should be performed. Elevated testosterone

Table 13-2. Key historical elements in the evaluation of primary amenorrhea.

• Recent medical history
• History of head trauma (damage to the hypothalamic-pituitary axis)
• History of weight loss and amount of regular physical activity (female athlete triad)
• Timeline of development of secondary sexual characteristics (if present)
• Past medical history
  • Diabetes
  • Juvenile rheumatoid arthritis
  • Inflammatory bowel disease
  • Malignancy
  • Chronic infection
	• Family history
	  • Time of menarche in the patient's mother and sister(s)
	  • Family history of gonadal dysgenesis
	• Medications
	  • Medication or supplement use (particularly hormonal)
	• Social history
	  • Sexual activity
	  • History of psychosocial deprivation/abuse
	• Symptoms
	  • Anosmia (Kallmann syndrome)
	  • Monthly abdominal pain (imperforate hymen, transverse vaginal septum)
	  Headache
	  Visual changes
	  Lactation (in the absence of pregnancy)

Table 13-3. Etiologies of primary amenorrhea.

Physiologic
Constitutional delay
Pregnancy
Pathologic
Absent breast development, normal pelvic examination findings
Hypothalamic failure
Anorexia nervosa, excessive weight loss, excessive exercise, stress
Chronic illness (juvenile rheumatoid arthritis, diabetes, irritable bowel syndrome)

Gonadotropin deficiency
Kallmann syndrome (associated with anosmia)
Pituitary dysfunction after head trauma or shock
Infiltrative or inflammatory processes
Pituitary adenoma
Craniopharyngioma

Gonadal failure
Gonadal dysgenesis (ie, Turner syndrome)

Normal breast development, normal pelvic examination findings
Hypothyroidism
Hyperprolactinemia

Normal breast development, abnormal pelvic examination findings
Testicular feminization
Anatomic abnormalities (uterovaginal septum, imperforate hymen)

in the presence of a Y chromosome indicates presence of functional testicular tissue that should be excised to prevent later neoplastic transformation. In patients with both normal breast development and a pelvic examination, serum prolactin and TSH should be measured to rule out hyperprolactinemia and hypothyroidism. If these values are in the normal range, investigation should proceed according to the secondary amenorrhea algorithm. The etiologies for primary amenorrhea are listed in **Table 13-3**.

C. Imaging Studies

Radiographic studies are targeted toward the diagnosis suggested by history, physical, and laboratory studies. Magnetic resonance imaging (MRI) is indicated in patients with suspected pituitary pathology. Computerized visual field testing may be added if examination or MRI indicates optic chiasm compression. Pelvic imaging should be performed in patients with suspected pelvic anomalies. Transverse vaginal septum, imperforate hymen, or vaginal agenesis can be detected or confirmed through imaging.

▶ Treatment

A. Medical Therapy

Successful treatment of primary amenorrhea is based on correct diagnosis of the underlying etiology. The patient should be counseled as to the cause of her amenorrhea, implications for future fertility, risks of malignancy (if applicable), and treatment options. Patients with functional hypothalamic amenorrhea due to physical or psychological stress can reverse this by weight gain, resolution of emotional issues, or decrease in intensity of exercise. For patients with hypothyroidism, thyroid replacement should be started at a low dose and titrated up, with caution to avoid overreplacement. Patients with pituitary adenomas should be treated with the dopamine agonists bromocriptine or cabergoline, the former having the best established safety record and approved for use in pregnancy. Metformin can be used in patients with polycystic ovarian syndrome (PCOS) who are insulin-resistant. Cyclical estrogen-progesterone and combined estrogen-progesterone oral contraceptive pills, patches, or vaginal ring can be used in patients with gonadal dysgenesis or hypoestrogenic state. Only providers experienced in this field should perform induction of puberty in patients with constitutional delay. Estrogen is responsible for epiphyseal closure as well as the adolescent growth spurt; mistimed administration could have significant effects on the final achieved height in these patients. For patients who desire fertility, ovulation induction with clomiphene citrate, exogenous gonadotropins, or pulsatile GnRH (gonadotropin-releasing hormone) may be required.

B. Surgical Intervention

Structural anomalies should be addressed surgically. In those patients with congenital absence of a uterus, investigation should be undertaken for associated renal anomalies. Gonadectomy should be performed after puberty in patients with Y chromosome material to prevent the development of subsequent gonadal neoplasia.

C. Behavioral Modification

Patients with hypothalamic failure due to rapid weight loss, excessive exercise, or stress should receive counseling to address the underlying cause of these problems.

▶ Secondary Amenorrhea

The most common type of amenorrhea, secondary amenorrhea, is diagnosed when a woman with previously normal menses goes at least 6 months without a period, or when a woman with previously irregular menses goes at least 12 months or at least six cycles without a period.

▶ Clinical Findings

A. Signs and Symptoms

Pertinent history in the evaluation of secondary amenorrhea includes: (1) previous menstrual history (timing and quality of menses), (2) pregnancies (to include terminations and complicated deliveries), (3) symptoms of endocrine disease, (4) medication history, (5) weight loss or gain, (6) exercise level, (7) history of instrumentation or surgery to genital tract, and (8) masculinizing characteristics noticed by patient or family. Physical examination should assess pubertal development and secondary sexual characteristics while looking for evidence of hyperandrogenism. These latter findings may include oily skin, acne, striae, clitoromegaly, and hirsutism.

B. Laboratory Findings

After the exclusion of pregnancy, initial labs should include fasting glucose, thyroid-stimulating hormone (TSH), and prolactin levels. In the absence of significant abnormalities in these values, a progestin challenge test should be performed to assess the patient's estrogen status. FSH should be measured on women who do not experience withdrawal bleeding within 2 weeks. A high FSH value (>30 IU/L) is indicative of ovarian failure, whereas normal or low values indicate either an acquired uterine anomaly (Asherman syndrome) or hypothalamic-pituitary failure. Ovarian failure is confirmed with a low serum estradiol level (<30 pg/mL). A serum luteinizing hormone (LH) and FSH should be drawn on women who do not experience withdrawal bleeding after the progesterone challenge and have a normal estrogen level. An elevated LH value is highly suggestive of PCOS (polycystic ovary syndrome), especially in a woman with clinical features of virilization. If the LH level is normal, an LH/FSH ratio should be determined. This ratio is elevated (>2.5) in women with PCOS even when FSH and LH values are within normal limits. This diagnosis can be confirmed by measurement of serum testosterone and dehydroepiandrosterone sulfate (DHEA-S), which should be normal or just mildly elevated in PCOS. An increased testosterone/DHEA-S ratio is suggestive of an adrenal source. This finding warrants further study with determination of 17-hydroxyprogesterone. This level is elevated in late-onset congenital adrenal hyperplasia and Cushing syndrome. Cushing syndrome may be excluded with a 24-hour urinary free cortisol and dexamethasone suppression testing.

C. Imaging Studies

Hysterosalpingogram is indicated with history of uterine instrumentation and/or suggestion of anatomic anomaly as source of amenorrhea. Computed tomographic (CT) scanning of the adrenal glands and ultrasound of the ovaries should be performed in women with clinical features of virilization and increased testosterone (>200 ng/dL) or DHEAS-S (>7 μg/mL). A CT or MRI of the pituitary should be performed if pituitary pathology is suspected.

▶ Differential Diagnosis

The differential diagnosis of secondary amenorrhea can be broken down into those etiologies with and those without evidence of hyperandrogenism.

A. With Evidence of Hyperandrogenism

1. Polycystic ovary syndrome (PCOS)—Responsible for 20% of secondary amenorrhea, PCOS is the most common reproductive female endocrine disorder, occurring in 5–7% of women. PCOS is associated with an increased risk of type 2 diabetes, abdominal obesity, hypertension, hypertriglyceridemia, and cardiovascular events.

2. Autonomous hyperandrogenism—Tumors of adrenal or ovarian origin may secrete androgens. Virilization is more pronounced than in PCOS and may manifest as frontal balding, increased muscle bulk, deep voice, clitoromegaly, and severe hirsutism.

3. Late-onset or mild congenital adrenal hyperplasia—This rare condition may be diagnosed with the finding of an increased 17-hydroxyprogesterone level in the setting of secondary amenorrhea and hyperandrogenism.

B. Without Evidence of Hyperandrogenism on Examination

1. Medication use—History should be reviewed for use of contraceptives, particularly progesterone-only preparations. These may take the form of oral contraceptives (OCPs), implants, injectables, or intrauterine devices. It is important to inform women on progestin-only pills that 20% of patients will become amenorrheic within the first year of use. Rates are even higher for those using injectable progesterone, with 55% of women at 1 year and 68% of women at 2 years reporting amenorrhea.

2. Functional hypothalamic amenorrhea—Amenorrhea in this setting, seen in patients who have experienced rapid weight loss, severely restricted calorie intake, stress or rigorous exercise, may be part of the female athlete triad of amenorrhea, disordered eating, and osteoporosis.

3. Hypergonadotropic hypogonadism—Premature ovarian failure (cessation of ovarian function before 40 years of age) may be autoimmune or idiopathic, or may occur secondarily to radiotherapy or chemotherapy (cyclophosphamide is associated with destruction of oocytes).

4. Hyperprolactinemia—Pituitary adenomas may present with amenorrhea and galactorrhea, and are responsible for 20% of cases of secondary amenorrhea. Prolactin secreted by these tumors acts directly on the hypothalamus to suppress GnRH secretion. Dopamine receptor–blocking agents, hypothalamic masses, and hypothyroidism are less common causes of hyperprolactinemia.

5. Thyroid disease—Profound hypothyroidism or hyperthyroidism affects the feedback control of LH, FSH, and estradiol on the hypothalamus, causing menstrual irregularities.

6. Hypogonadotropic hypogonadism—Head trauma, severe hypotension (shock), infiltrative or inflammatory processes, pituitary adenoma, or craniopharyngioma may damage the pituitary, resulting in decreased or absent gonadotropin (LH and FSH) release. These patients will often display symptoms relating to deficiency of other pituitary hormones as well.

Treatment

Treatment depends on correct diagnosis of the underlying etiology. As in primary amenorrhea, the goals of treatment are to establish a firm diagnosis, to restore ovulatory cycles and treat infertility (when possible), to treat hypoestrogenemia and hyperandrogensim, and to assess and address risks associate with a persistent hypoestrogenemic state.

A. Treating the Underlying Causes of Amenorrhea

Patients with identified hypothyroidism should be treated with thyroxine replacement. Patients with hyperprolactinemia secondary to prolactinoma may be treated with either surgical resection or dopamine agonist therapy. Bromocriptine is often used in women who desire to conceive, since there is no increased incidence of congenital malformations, and it has been used successfully for over 20 years. Patients found to have empty sella or Sheehan syndrome should be treated with replacement of pituitary hormones.

Women whose amenorrhea is secondary to absent ovarian function before 40 years of age have premature ovarian failure. Those who experience ovarian failure before 30 years of age should undergo karyotype testing to screen for Y chromosome elements, which are associated with malignancies. These patients are at a high risk of osteoporosis and cardiovascular disease because of their hypoestrogenemic state. Estrogen replacement should be considered, with progesterone for those patients with an intact uterus, to prevent these sequelae.

Women with adrenal or ovarian androgen-secreting tumors should undergo appropriate surgical intervention. Likewise, women found to have Asherman syndrome as a cause for their amenorrhea should undergo lysis of adhesions followed by endometrial stimulation with estrogen. These patients are at increased risk of placenta accreta in subsequent pregnancies.

Patients with PCOS may achieve resumption of menses with weight loss. The assistance of a registered dietician should be sought to improve success rates in this daunting task. Metformin, a biguanide insulin sensitizer, has been used to treat PCOS, with reports of success in both inducing ovulation and improving laboratory markers for cardiovascular risk.

DYSMENORRHEA

 ESSENTIALS OF DIAGNOSIS

► Affects 50% of all women, and between 20% and 90% of all adolescent women.

► Primary defined as painful menses in absence of pelvic disease; secondary defined as painful menses caused by pelvic disease.

General Considerations

Dysmenorrhea is the most common gynecologic complaint and is a leading cause of morbidity in women of reproductive age, resulting in absence from work and school, as well as nonparticipation in sports.

Pathogenesis

Primary dysmenorrhea is caused by the release of prostaglandin $F_2\alpha$ from the endometrium at the time of menstruation, and rarely occurs until ovulatory menstrual cycles are established. Prostaglandins induce smooth-muscle contraction in the uterus, causing pressure within the uterus to exceed that of the systemic circulation. Ischemia ensues, causing an anginal equivalent in the uterus. The cause of secondary dysmenorrhea varies with the underlying disease.

Clinical Findings

A. Symptoms and Signs

Symptoms of primary dysmenorrhea include pain beginning with the onset of menstruation and lasting 12–72 hours, characterized as crampy and intermittent in nature, with radiation to the low back or upper thighs. Headache, nausea, vomiting, diarrhea, and fatigue may accompany the pain. Symptoms are usually worst on the first day of menses and then gradually resolve. The patient may report that her dysmenorrhea began gradually, with the first several years of menses, and then intensified as her periods became regular and consistently ovulatory. Conversely, patients with *secondary amenorrhea* report symptoms beginning after age 20, lasting 5–7 days, and progressive worsening of pain with time. These patients may also report pelvic pain that is not associated with menstruation.

B. Physical Findings

A pelvic examination with cervical smear and cultures should be performed in all patients presenting with a chief complaint of dysmenorrhea. Findings of cul-de-sac induration and uterosacral ligament nodularity on pelvic examination are indicative of endometriosis. Adenexal masses could indicate endometriosis, neoplasm, hydrosalpinx, or scarring from chronic pelvic inflammatory disease (PID). Likewise, uterine abnormalities or tenderness should raise the examiner's index of suspicion for the underlying pathology as the cause for dysmenorrhea.

C. Laboratory Findings

Any woman with acute onset of pelvic pain should have a pregnancy test. Women with a history consistent with primary dysmenorrhea do not require additional initial labs. In those who fail to respond to therapy for primary dysmenorrhea or in those whom a diagnosis of secondary dysmenorrhea is suspected, a complete blood count (CBC) and an erythrocyte sedimentation rate (ESR) may help in detection of the underlying infection or inflammation.

D. Imaging Studies

Patients with abnormal findings on pelvic examination who do not respond to therapy for primary dysmenorrhea or who have a history suggestive of pelvic pathology should undergo pelvic ultrasound.

E. Special Examinations

In patients whom endometriosis is suggested, diagnostic laparoscopy may be indicated. Because of the high rates of treatment and diagnostic failure with laparoscopy, some authors recommend empirically treating patients with a presumptive diagnosis of endometriosis with GnRH analogs for 3 months. Proponents argue that this provides both diagnostic and therapeutic functions, while forgoing surgical complications.

Treatment

A. Medical Therapies

Treatment for primary dysmenorrhea focuses on reducing endometrial prostaglandin production. This can be accomplished with NSAIDs (nonsteroidal anti-inflammatory drugs), which inhibit prostaglandin synthesis, or with contraceptives that suppress ovulation. It is recommended to allow at least three full cycles to assess efficacy of either of these approaches. In patients who do not experience success with these means, an alternate diagnosis, such as endometriosis, should be considered. Medical therapies are listed in **Table 13-4** with respect to their degree of efficacy.

B. Physical Modalities

Physical modalities utilizing heat, acupuncture/acupressure, and spinal manipulation have been proposed for inclusion in the treatment of dysmenorrhea. A heated abdominal patch was demonstrated to have efficacy similar to ibuprofen (400 mg) for the treatment of dysmenorrhea, with quicker, but not greater, relief observed with the combination of ibuprofen and heat. Acupuncture relieved pain in 91% of patients with dysmenorrhea, compared to 36% relief for control patients in a study with sham acupuncture. A systematic review of spinal manipulation in the treatment of dysmenorrhea failed to find evidence for the effectiveness of this approach.

Table 13-4. Medications for the treatment of primary dysmenorrhea.

	Medication	Mechanism of Action	Primary Side Effects/ Complications	Strength of Recommendation [a]	Comments
Effective	NSAIDs: diclofenac, ibuprofen, mefenamic acid, naproxen, ASA	Inhibits prostaglandin synthesis (Fenemates also block prostaglandin action)	GI upset, GI bleed	A	Most effective when started before onset of pain; fenemates show enhanced action in some studies due to dual mechanism of action
	Danazol	Suppression of menses	Amenorrhea, vaginal dryness, jaundice, eosinophilia	B	Significant side effects; primarily for severe endometriosis
	Hormonal contraceptives: oral, injectable, implantable, intravaginal administration	Reduced prostaglandin release during menstruation	Irregular menses, mood swings, acne, DVT	B	Use with caution in patients >35 years old and smokers; not for patients desiring fertility
	COX-2 inhibitors	Inhibits prostaglandin synthesis	Cardiovascular risk, acute renal failure	B	Contains sulfa moiety; consider safer, less expensive NSAIDs first
	Levonorgestrel intrauterine device (Mirena)	Thins uterine lining through inhibition	Hypertension, acne, weight gain	B	Effective for 5 y
Probably effective	Leuprolide acetate (Lupron)	Suppression of menses	Weight gain, hirsuitism, elevation of BP	B	Very expensive with significant side-effects. Not 1st line.
	Depo-medroxyprogesterone acetate (Depo-Provera)	Suppression of menses	Amenorrhea, hypermenorrhea	B	Weight gain may be significant
	Glyceryl trinitrate patches	Tocolytic	Headache	B	Less effective than NSAID; more side effects, low tolerability
Uncertain efficacy	Nifedipine (Procardia)	Induction of uterine relaxation	Hypotension, peripheral edema	C	Moderate to good pain reduction but high rate side effects
	Transdermal contraceptive patch	Reduced prostaglandin release during menstruation	Local irritation, irregular menses	B	Less effective than OCPs, efficacy varies with pt weight

[a]A, consistent, good-quality, patient-oriented evidence; B, inconsistent or limited-quality patient-oriented evidence; C, consensus, disease-oriented evidence, usual practice, opinion, or case series.

C. Supplements and Herbals

A number of supplements and herbal formulations have been touted as relieving the symptoms of dysmenorrhea. While some small trials have showed promising results, the data are not strong enough at this time to recommend widespread use. A systematic review of Chinese herbal therapy for treatment of dysmenorrhea showed promising results with self-designed formulas in small studies, but not with commonly used herbal health products. Results were limited by poor methodological quality and small sample size.

D. Behavior Modification

Strenuous exercise and caffeine intake are both lifestyle factors that can modulate prostaglandin-induced uterine contractions. Strenuous exercise can increase uterine tone, resulting in increased periods of uterine "angina" with accompanying increases in prostaglandins. Decreasing strenuous exercise in the first few days of a woman's menses may reduce her dysmenorrhea. Conversely, caffeine decreases uterine tone by increasing uterine cyclic adenosine monophosphate levels.

E. Surgical Therapy

If a patient continues to have significant dysmenorrhea with this treatment, further testing for causes of secondary dysmenorrhea should be considered, and surgical options, such as interruption of pelvic nerve pathways, should be explored when applicable.

PREMENSTRUAL SYNDROME

ESSENTIALS OF DIAGNOSIS

▶ A cluster of affective, cognitive and physical symptoms that occurs before the onset of menses, during the luteal phase of the menstrual cycle.

▶ Absence of a symptom-free week in the time period immediately following menses suggests that a chronic psychiatric disorder may be present.

General Considerations

While 40% of women experience PMS symptoms significant enough to interfere with daily life, 5% of women experience severe impairment. Evaluation, diagnosis, and treatment of PMS should be undertaken prudently, as it is often mistaken for other disorders, and sometimes treated with counterproductive and even harmful approaches. The clinician must be sensitive in addressing issues of reduced self-worth, frustration, and depression that may be present in women suffering from this condition.

Pathogenesis

Premenstrual syndrome is assumed to be secondary to interactions between the ovarian hormones, estrogen and progesterone, and central neurotransmitters. Serotonin is the central neurotransmitter most often implicated in the manifestations of PMS. This would explain the cyclical mood changes that are synchronized with the changes in ovarian hormone levels. Systemic symptoms, such as bloating, may be produced through the peripheral effects of these hormones. Trace elements and nutrients are also speculated to have a role in the pathogenesis of PMS symptoms, but their role is less clear.

Clinical Findings

A. Symptoms and Signs

Symptoms may include irritability, bloating, depression, food cravings, aggressiveness, and mood swings. Abraham's classification of premenstrual syndrome (**Table 13-5**) helps the clinician to organize history taking for patients with PMS.

Factors associated with an increased risk of PMS include stress, alcohol use, exercise, smoking, and the use of certain medications. It is not clear whether some of these factors are causative or are forms of self-medication used by sufferers. A prospective symptom diary kept for at least 2 months is helpful in assessing the relation of symptoms to the luteal phase of menses. The absence of a symptom-free week early

Table 13-5. Abraham's classification of symptoms of premenstrual syndrome.

A: Anxiety
Nervous tension
Mood swings
Irritability
Anxiety
C: Cravings
Headache
Craving for sweets
Increased appetite
Heart pounding
Fatigue
Dizziness or faintness
D: Depression
Depression
Forgetfulness
Crying
Confusion
Insomnia
H: Water-related symptoms
Weight gain
Swelling of extremities
Breast tenderness
Abnormal bloating

in the follicular phase, the time period just after menses, suggests that a chronic psychiatric disorder may be present. A record of symptoms that are temporally clustered before menses and that decline or diminish 2–3 days after the start of menses is highly suggestive of PMS. Patients with PMS experience fluid retention and fluctuating weight gain in relation to their menses. Mild edema may or may not be evident on physical examination.

B. Laboratory Findings

There are no laboratory evaluations recommended in the diagnosis of PMS. Nutrient deficiency tests are not recommended, as they do not adequately assess the patient's physiologic state.

C. Radiologic Studies

There are no radiologic studies recommended in the assessment of PMS.

Treatment

The treatment goals for PMS are to minimize symptoms and functional impairment while optimizing the patient's overall health and sense of well-being. Therapy should take an integrative approach, including education, psychological

Table 13-6. Selected pharmacological and supplemental therapies for PMS.

Medication	Mechanism of Action	Indication(s) for Use in PMS	Dosing	Primary Side Effects/ Complications	Evidence Supporting Use
Mefenamic acid	Inhibits prostaglandin synthesis; competes for prostaglandin binding sites	Pain relief	500 mg loading dose, then 250 g PO QID for ≤7 days	Diarrhea, nausea, vomiting, drowsiness with pro- longed use: decreased renal blood flow and renal papillary necrosis	RCCT
GnRH agonists (nafre- lin, leuprolide)	LH and FSH transient stimulation then prolonged suppression	Severe PMS; relief of all symptoms in 50% of patients	Nafrelin—200 mg intrana- sal BID; leuprolide— 3.75 mg depot IM every 4 weeks or 0.5 mg SQ daily	Vaginal dryness, accelerated bone loss (drugs can be given with additional back therapy to avoid these symptoms), hot flashes	Controlled clinical trial
Danazol	Suppresses LH and FSH	Severe PMS	200 mg PO daily in luteal phase	Acne, weight gain, hirsut- ism, virilization	RCCTs
Alprazolam (second- line since it appears to treat only depressive symp- toms and has high addictive potential)	Depressant effect on central nervous system	Depression caused by PMS	0.25 mg PO TID during late luteal phase of cycle	Drowsiness, increased appetite, withdrawal (discontinue if patient exhibits withdrawal symptoms)	RCCT
SSRIs: fluoxetine, sertraline, parox- etine, venlafaxine, citalopram	Serotonin reuptake inhibitor	Depression, anger, and anxiety caused by PMS	Varies with drug: all month or just during luteal phase (start day 14, end at start of menses)	Nervousness, insomnia, drowsiness, nausea, anorexia	EBM review
Diuretics (metolazone, spironolactone)	Reduction in retained fluid	Bloating, edema, breast tenderness (espe- cially in women with >1.5 kg premen- strual weight gain)	Metolazone—2.4 mg/d PO; spironolactone— 25 mg PO QID	Electrolyte imbalance	EBM review
Bromocriptine	Dopamine agonist	Breast tenderness and fullness	2.5 mg PO BID-TID	Postural hypotension, nausea	Use not supported by RCCTs
Hormonal contracep- tives	Suppression of estrogen and progesterone	General symptoms	Varies by formulation	Varies by formulation	Use not supported by RCCTs for treatment of PMS
Vitamin B₆	Precursor in coenzyme for the biosynthesis of dopamine and serotonin	Depression and general symptoms	50 mg po qd or bid	Ataxia, sensory neuropathy	EBM review
γ-Linoleic acid	Prostaglandin E1 pre- cursor that inhibits prostaglandin production and metabolism	Breast tenderness, bloating, weight gain, edema	3 g/d in late luteal phase of menstrual cycle	Headache, nausea	Efficacy not supported
Calcium	Restoration of calcium homeostatsis	Depression, anxiety, and dysphoric states	800-1600 mg QD in divided doses	Bloating, nausea	RCCT

EBM, evidence-based medicine; RCCT, randomized controlled clinical trials.

support, exercise, diet, and pharmacological intervention, if necessary. By providing education about the prevalence and treatability of PMS, the clinician can destigmatize the disease and encourage the patient to take ownership of the treatment plan.

Many first-line treatments for PMS, although not based on well-designed prospective trials, also have general health benefits, are inexpensive, and have few side effects. These include dietary modifications, as recommended by the American Heart Association and moderate exercise at least 3 times a week. Patients should begin to see the results of these lifestyle changes 2–3 months after initiation. Patients should be counseled to expect improvement in their symptoms, rather than cure. Multiple approaches may be required before finding the optimal treatment.

For those patients with continued symptoms, secondary treatment strategies may be employed. Dietary supplements, specifically vitamin B_6, calcium, and magnesium, have been suggested to correct possible deficiencies. Current therapies are listed in **Table 13-6**, with their levels of supporting evidence, primary benefits, and potential side effects.

Alternative therapies include herbal medicine, dietary supplements, relaxation, message, reflexology, manipulative therapy, and biofeedback. Although some small trials have shown promising results, there is no compelling evidence from well-designed studies supporting the use of these therapies in the treatment of PMS.

Cho, SH, Hwang EW. Acupuncture for primary dysmenorrhoea: a systematic review. *Br J Obstet Gynecol.* 2010; 117:509.

Proctor M, Hing W, Johson T, Murphy P. Spinal manipulation for primary and secondary dysmenorrhea. *Cochrane Database Syst Rev.* 2009;(1).

Zhu X, et al. Chinese herbal medicine for primary dysmenorrhoea. *Cochrane Database Syst Rev.* 2008;(2):CD005288 (review). [PMID: 18425916]

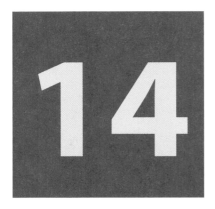

Sexually Transmitted Diseases

Robin Maier, MD, MA

Peter J. Katsufrakis, MD, MBA

ESSENTIALS OF DIAGNOSIS

► Privacy, confidentiality, and legal disease reporting concerns affect detection and treatment.

► Suspicion or diagnosis of one sexually transmitted disease (STD) should prompt screening tests for others.

► Diagnosis of an STD should always include identification and treatment of partners, and education to reduce risk of future infection.

General Considerations

Sexually transmitted diseases (STDs) include sexually transmitted infections and the clinical syndromes they cause. There are an estimated 20 million new STDs in the United States annually, almost half of them among persons aged 15–24 years.

Although all sexually active individuals are susceptible to infection, adolescents and young adults are most commonly affected. Reasons for this include: (1) an attitude of invincibility, (2) lack of knowledge about the risks and consequences of STDs, and (3) barriers to health care access.

This chapter emphasizes the clinical presentation, diagnostic evaluation, and treatment of STDs commonly found in the United States. Readers of this chapter should be able to:

• Differentiate common STDs on the basis of clinical information and laboratory testing.

• Treat STDs according to current guidelines.

• Intervene in patients' lives to reduce risk of future STD acquisition.

The discussion draws greatly from the most recent Centers for Disease Control and Prevention (CDC) guidelines for treatment of STDs. The authors are indebted to the individuals who worked to develop these recommendations.

Federal and state laws create disease-reporting requirements for many STDs. Gonorrhea; *Chlamydia*; chanchroid; syphilis; Hepatitis A, B, C; and HIV (including AIDS) are all nationally notifiable. Clinicians should contact their local health department for pertinent reporting information.

Privacy and confidentiality concerns are different for STDs than for general medical information. Patients generally experience greater anxiety about information pertaining to a possible diagnosis of an STD, and this may limit their willingness to disclose clinically pertinent information. Conversely, legal requirements for disease reporting and health department partner notification programs can inadvertently compromise patient confidentiality if not handled with the utmost professionalism. Furthermore, although minors generally require parental consent for nonemergent medical care in all states, minors can be diagnosed and treated for STDs without parental consent. Additionally, many US states' legislations may permit physicians to prescribe treatment for the heterosexual partners of men or women with *Chlamydia* or gonorrhea without examining the partner. Thus, laws in different jurisdictions create additional options and complexities in treating STDs. Practitioners need to be familiar with local requirements.

Centers for Disease Control and Prevention; Workowski KA, Berman SM. Sexually transmitted disease treatment guidelines, 2010. *MMWR Recomm Rep.* 2010;59(RR-12):1–110.

Centers for Disease Control and Prevention. *Sexually Transmitted Disease Surveillance, 2011.* Atlanta, GA: US Department of Health and Human Services; 2012.

Forhan SE, Gottlieb SL, Sternberg MR, et al. Prevalence of sexually transmitted infections among female adolescents aged 14 to 19 in the United States. *Pediatrics.* 2009; 124(6):1505. [PMID: 19933728]

Prevention

Intervening in patients' lives to reduce their risk of disease due to STDs is no less important than reducing risk due to smoking, inadequate exercise, poor nutrition, and other health risks. STD risk assessment should prompt providers to undertake discussion of risk reduction, and thus disease prevention. Physicians' effectiveness depends on their ability to obtain an accurate sexual history employing effective counseling skills. Specific techniques include creating a trusting, confidential environment; obtaining permission to ask questions about STDs; demonstrating a nonjudgmental, optimistic attitude; and combining information collection with patient education, using clear, mutually understandable language (see Chapter 17). Prevention is facilitated by an environment of open, honest communication about sexuality.

A. Counseling

The US Preventive Services Task Force (USPSTF) recommends high-intensity behavioral counseling to prevent sexually transmitted infections (STIs) for all sexually active adolescents and for adults at increased risk for STIs, for example, adults with current STIs or infections within the past year who have multiple current sexual partners, or who are members of a population with a high rate of STIs. Recommendations for changes in behavior should be tailored to the patient's specific risks and needs; simple suggestions such as keeping condoms available have been shown to be effective. Brief counseling using personalized risk reduction plans and culturally appropriate videos can significantly increase condom use and prevent new STDs, and can be conducted even in busy public clinics with minimal disruption to clinic operations. Effective interventions to reduce STDs in adolescents can extend beyond the examination room and include school-based and community-based education programs. Characteristics of successful interventions include multiple sessions, most often in groups, with total duration from 3 to 9 hours, or two 20-minute counseling sessions before and after HIV testing. Individuals with chronic infections [eg, herpes simplex virus (HSV) and HPV] will need counseling tailored to help them accurately understand their infection and effectively manage symptoms and transmission risk.

Lin JS, Whitlock E, O'Connor E, Bauer V. Behavioral counseling to prevent sexually transmitted infections: a systematic review for the U.S. Preventive Services Task Force. *Ann Intern Med.* 2008; 149(7):497–508, W96-9. (Summary for patients in *Ann Intern Med.*)

USPSTF. *The Guide to Clinical Preventive Services 2012: Recommendations of the US Preventive Services Task Force* (available at www.ahrq.gov2008 Oct 7;149(7):I36. [PMID: 18838722]

B. Condoms

For sexually active patients, male condoms are effective in reducing the sexual transmission of HIV infection. When used correctly and consistently, male latex condoms can reduce the risk of other STIs, including *Chlamydia,* gonorrhea, and *Trichomonas.* Condoms may afford some protection against transmission of HSV, and may mitigate some adverse consequences of infection with HPV, as their use has been associated with higher rates of regression of cervical intraepithelial neoplasia and clearance of HPV in women.

Effectiveness depends on correct, consistent use. Patients should be instructed to use only water-based lubricants. Providers may need to demonstrate how to place a condom on the penis via a suitable model, especially for persons who may be inexperienced with condom use.

Spermicide is not recommended for STI/HIV prevention. Some may confuse contraception with disease prevention; nonbarrier methods of contraception such as hormonal contraceptives or surgical sterilization do not protect against STDs. Women employing these methods should be counseled about the role of condoms in prevention of STDs.

Crosby R, Bounse S. Condom effectiveness: where are we now? *Sex Health.* 2012;9(1):10-177. [PMID: 22348628]

C. Vaccination

Vaccination for hepatitis B virus (HBV) is indicated for all unvaccinated adolescents, all unvaccinated adults at risk for HBV infection, and all adults seeking protection from HBV infection. Other settings where all unvaccinated persons should receive vaccination include correctional facilities, drug abuse treatment and prevention services centers, health care settings serving men who have sex with men, and HIV testing and treatment facilities. Additionally, individuals with chronic liver disease (including chronic HBV or hepatitis C infection), end-stage renal disease, diabetes mellitus, and potential occupational or travel exposure should be vaccinated. The prevalence of past exposure to HBV in homosexual men and injection drug users may render prevaccination testing cost effective, although it may lower compliance. For this reason, if prevaccination testing is employed, patients should receive their first vaccination dose when tested. If employed, HBV core antibody testing is an effective screen for immunity.

Vaccination for hepatitis A virus (HAV) is indicated for homosexual or bisexual men, persons with chronic liver disease (including hepatitis B and C), and IV drug users; additionally, some individuals with occupational or travel exposure should be vaccinated. In cases of sexual or household contact with someone with HAV, hepatitis A vaccine or immune globulin should be administered as soon as possible after exposure. (For additional information on hepatitis A and B, see Chapter 31.)

Two HPV vaccines are available and licensed for females aged 9-26 years to prevent cervical precancers and cancers, the quadrivalent HPV (Gardasil) and the bivalent HPV vaccine (Cervarix). Universal vaccination of females aged 11–12 years is recommended with either vaccine, as is catchup vaccination for females aged 13–26 years. In order to prevent genital warts and anal cancers, all males may receive the quadrivalent HPV vaccine at ages 9–26. The quadrivalent HPV vaccine (Gardasil) is universally recommended for males aged 11–12 years, as is catchup vaccination for males aged 13–21 years. Gardasil is also recommended for high risk males (men who have sex with men and those who are immunocompromised) ages 22–26. Experimental vaccines are also being explored for other STDs.

Society of Teachers of Family Medicine. Shots by STFM 2013 (available at http://www.immunizationed.org/shotsonline.aspx; accessed April 6, 2013).

D. Partner Treatment

Following treatment of an individual patient, treatment of asymptomatic partners of a diagnosed patient is commonly employed in STD treatment. For patients with multiple partners, it may be difficult to identify the source of infection. Partner treatment should be recommended for sexual contacts occurring prior to diagnosis within the time intervals indicated for each disease:

- Chancroid, 10 days
- Granuloma inguinale, 60 days
- Lymphogranuloma venereum, 60 days
- Syphilis, 3 months plus the duration of symptoms for patients diagnosed with primary syphilis (even if the contact tests seronegative); 6 months plus the duration of symptoms for patients diagnosed with secondary syphilis, and 1 year for patients with early latent syphilis
- Chlamydial infection, 60 days
- Gonorrhea, 60 days
- Epididymitis, 60 days
- Pelvic inflammatory disease (PID), 60 days
- Pediculosis pubis, 30 days
- Scabies, 30 days

Although in general physicians must examine a patient directly before prescribing treatment, when prior medical evaluation and counseling is not feasible, or resource limitations constrain evaluation and diagnosis, other partner management options may be considered. One of these is partner-delivered therapy, in which patients diagnosed with *Chlamydia* or gonorrhea deliver the prescribed treatment to their partners; this option is affected by state laws and regulations.

Repeat testing at 3 months following treatment is indicated for persons with *Chlamydia* or gonorrhea, due to the increased incidence of reinfection. Patients should also be instructed to avoid sexual contact for the duration of therapy

to prevent further transmission. Patients taking single-dose azithromycin for *Chlamydia* infection should be instructed to avoid sexual contact for 7 days. Patients must also be instructed to avoid contact with their previous partner(s) until both patient and partner complete treatment.

E. Screening

Some form of STD screening, such as questions asked during the history interview or included in routine history forms, should be a universal practice for *all* patients, with periodic and regular updating. Content, frequency, and additional screening should be determined by individual patient circumstances, local disease prevalence, and research documenting effectiveness and cost-benefit. **Table 14-1** summarizes current recommendations for STD screening from the USPSTF.

Table 14-1. US Preventive Services Task Force (USPSTF) recommendations for STD screening.[a]

Infection	Recommendation
Chlamydia	Screen *all* pregnant women and sexually active women aged ≤24 years; screen all sexually active or pregnant women aged ≥25 years who are at increased risk for sexually transmitted infection (eg, having a prior history of STD, having new or multiple sex partners, inconsistent condom use, or who exchange sex for money or drugs)
Gonorrhea	Screen all sexually active women, including those who are pregnant, for gonorrhea infection if they are at increased risk for infection (eg, aged <25 years), previous gonorrhea, or other STD, new or multiple sex partners, inconsistent condom use, sex work, and drug use
Hepatitis B	Screen all pregnant women at their first prenatal visit
HIV	Screen all pregnant women
Screen all adolescents and adults aged 15-65 years for HIV
Screen younger adolescents and older adults believed to be at increased risk for HIV infection
Syphilis	Screen all pregnant women
Screen persons at increased risk for syphilis infection (eg, men who have sex with men and engage in high-risk sexual behavior, commercial sex workers, persons who exchange sex for drugs, and those in adult correctional facilities)

[a]The USPSTF does not presently recommend routine screening for hepatitis C, human papillomavirus, or herpes simplex.
Data from US Preventive Services Task Force (available at http://www.uspreventiveservicestaskforce.org/adultrec.htm; accessed March 27, 2013).

1. Chlamydia and gonorrhea—Annual screening of all sexually active women aged <25 years is recommended, as is screening of older women with risk factors (eg, those who have a new sex partner or multiple sex partners).

The benefits of *Chlamydia trachomatis* screening in women have been demonstrated in areas where screening programs have reduced both the prevalence of infection and rates of PID. Evidence is insufficient to recommend routine screening for *C. trachomatis* in sexually active young men, based on feasibility, efficacy, and cost-effectiveness. However, screening of sexually active young men should be considered in clinical settings with a high prevalence of *Chlamydia* (eg, adolescent clinics, correctional facilities, and STD clinics).

2. Pregnancy—Recommendations for screening pregnant women vary somewhat depending on the source. According to the CDC, pregnant women should receive a serologic test for syphilis, Hepatitis B surface antigen, and HIV at the onset of prenatal care. High-risk women should repeat HIV and syphilis testing early in the third trimester, and should repeat hepatitis B surface antigen and syphilis testing again at delivery. Furthermore, pregnant women at risk for HBV infection should be vaccinated for hepatitis B.

Providers of obstetric care should test for *Neisseria gonorrhoeae* at the onset of care if local prevalence of gonorrhea is high or if the woman is at increased risk, and testing should be repeated in the third trimester if the woman is at continued risk. Providers should test for *Chlamydia* at the first prenatal visit. Women aged <25 years and those at increased risk for chlamydial infection (ie, those who have multiple partners or who have a partner with multiple partners) should also be tested again in the third trimester. Evidence does not support routine testing for bacterial vaginosis. For asymptomatic pregnant women at high risk for preterm delivery, the current evidence is insufficient to assess the balance of benefits and harms of screening for bacterial vaginosis. Symptomatic women should be evaluated and treated.

3. HIV—HIV screening is recommended for patients aged 15–65 years in all health care settings after the patient is notified that testing will be performed unless the patient declines. CDC recommends that younger adolescents and older adults at increased risk also be screened. Repeat annual testing for HIV is indicated for any high-risk patient, including patients with a diagnosed STD or with a history of behaviors that could expose them to HIV. Testing is also indicated for patients who present with a history and findings consistent with the acute retroviral syndrome (ARS), symptoms of which are listed in **Table 14-2**. Appropriate testing regimens include an HIV1 screening antibody test such as enzyme immunoassay, with a confirmatory test such as the Western immunoblot. HIV2 prevalence in the United States is very low, so routine testing is not indicated, although several commercial antibody tests screen for both

Table 14-2. Acute retroviral syndrome: associated signs and symptoms.

| **More common** |
| Fever |
| Myalgia |
| Arthralgia |
| Headache |
| Photophobia |
| Diarrhea |
| Sore throat |
| Lymphadenopathy |
| Maculopapular rash |
| **Less common** |
| Acute meningoencephalitis |
| Peripheral neuropathy |
| Fatigue |
| Night sweats |
| Weight loss |
| Decreased libido |
| Muscle wasting |

Data from Primary HIV Infection. In *DynaMed* [database online]. EBSCO Publishing (available at http://web.ebscohost.com/dynamed/detail?vid=14&sid=61579187; updated Feb. 13, 2013; accessed April 7, 2013).

HIV1 and HIV2; HIV2 should be considered for persons coming from areas of high HIV2 prevalence (eg, parts of West Africa, particularly Cape Verde, Ivory Coast, Gambia, Guinea-Bissau, Mali, Mauritania, Nigeria, and Sierra Leone).

Early diagnosis of ARS may present a very narrow window of opportunity to alter the course of HIV infection in the recently infected patient, and to block the source of most presumed new HIV transmission. Symptoms are common and nonspecific, rendering diagnosis difficult without a high index of suspicion; they include fever, malaise, lymphadenopathy, pharyngitis, and skin rash. Appropriate testing should include a nucleic acid test for HIV such as HIV-RNA polymerase chain reaction (PCR); routine HIV antibody tests are not sufficient, because they seldom will have become positive during ARS. Individuals with positive HIV tests should be referred immediately to an expert in HIV care.

All HIV-infected individuals pose particular challenges for STD risk reduction. Reducing high-risk behaviors of known HIV-infected patients is a top priority, both to decrease the further spread of HIV and to limit the exposure of HIV patients to additional STDs. Persons with HIV also have substantial medical, psychological, and legal needs that are beyond the scope of this chapter.

4. Other STDs—Accepted national guidelines directing screening for other STDs do not exist. If undertaken, additional screening should be guided by local disease prevalence and an individual patient's risk behaviors.

Centers for Disease Control and Prevention; Workowski KA, Berman SM. Sexually transmitted disease treatment guidelines, 2010. *MMWR Recomm Rep.* 2010;59(RR-12):1–110.

US Preventive Services Task Force. The Guide to Clinical Preventive Services 2013. AHRQ. 2013. (available at http://www.uspreventiveservicestaskforce.org/adultrec.htm; accessed March 27, 2013).

SEXUALLY TRANSMITTED INFECTIONS & SYNDROMES

ESSENTIALS OF DIAGNOSIS

▶ Presenting clinical syndromes often guide diagnosis and treatment.

▶ History and findings can justify presumptive treatment while awaiting laboratory confirmation of a diagnosis.

Patients who are infected with STDs rarely present with accurate knowledge of their microbiological diagnosis. More commonly, patients present with clinical syndromes consistent with one or more diagnoses, so that providers frequently employ syndromic evaluation and treatment. This approach is useful for several reasons, including the fact that more than one disease may be present, and has been employed commonly in resource-poor settings with limited access to advanced diagnostic technology. The following recommendations for testing strategies and use of empiric treatment pending laboratory results should be adapted to take into consideration local availability of specific tests, the probability of the diagnosis based on the history and examination, disease-associated morbidity, the risk of further transmission while awaiting diagnosis, and the likelihood that an untreated patient will return for laboratory test results and treatment. Treatment information is summarized in **Table 14-3,** and additional treatment information appears within the text description of specific diseases where applicable.

GENITAL ULCER DISEASES

ESSENTIALS OF DIAGNOSIS

▶ Herpes is the most common cause of genital ulcers in the United States.

▶ Most persons infected with herpes simplex virus type 2 (HSV2) have *not* been diagnosed with genital herpes.

▶ All persons with genital ulcers need laboratory evaluation for syphilis and HSV [rapid plasma reagin (RPR) or Venereal Disease Research Laboratories (VDRL) dark-field microscopy; and culture or PCR tests for HSV]

▶ **General Considerations**

In the United States, herpes simplex is the most common cause of genital ulcer disease (GUD); syphilis is less common, and other causes such as chancroid, lymphogranuloma venereum, and granuloma inguinale are very uncommon. Because this is not true throughout the world, physicians treating international travelers or recent arrivals to the United States may need to consider a broad spectrum of potential etiologies. The approach to diagnosis needs to include consideration of the likelihood of the different etiologies based on the patient's history, physical examination, and local epidemiology. Furthermore, all types of GUD are associated with increased risk of HIV transmission, making HIV testing a necessary part of GUD evaluation.

Herpes Simplex

At least 50 million persons in the United States have genital HSV2 infection.

The majority of persons infected with HSV2 have not been diagnosed with genital herpes. Many such persons have mild or unrecognized infections but shed virus intermittently in the genital tract. The majority of genital herpes infections are transmitted by persons unaware that they have the infection or who are asymptomatic when transmission occurs. Herpes simplex virus type 1 is causing an increasing proportion of anogenital herpes and in some populations, such as young women and men who have sex with men (MSM), may now account for the majority of first episode anogenital infections.

▶ **Clinical Findings**

A. Symptoms and Signs

A first episode of genital herpes classically presents with blisters and sores, with local tingling and discomfort. Visible lesions may be preceded by a prodrome of tingling or burning. Some patients also report dysesthesia or neuralgic pain in the buttocks or legs and malaise with fever. The clinical spectrum of disease can include atypical rashes, fissuring, excoriation, and discomfort of the anogenital area, cervical lesions, urinary symptoms, and extragenital lesions. Recent data suggest that a minority of patients who acquire HSV2 have symptoms associated with initial infection, although overt disease may follow. In immunocompromised persons, HSV can manifest as large, chronic, hyperkeratotic ulcers. If lesions persist despite antiviral therapy, acyclovir-resistant HSV should be suspected.

Both HSV1 and HSV2 cause genital disease, although HSV1 produces fewer clinical recurrences and may be less severe. Symptoms during recurrences are generally less intense and shorter in duration. Infectious virus is shed intermittently and unpredictably in some asymptomatic patients. Latex condoms, when used correctly and consistently, may reduce the risk of genital HSV transmission.

B. Laboratory Findings

Diagnosis of HSV is based on either culture of the vesicle base or ulcer, or PCR test for HSV DNA. PCR assays for HSV DNA are more sensitive and have been increasingly used. Cytologic detection of cellular changes of herpes virus infection is insensitive and nonspecific, both in genital lesions (Tzanck smear) and cervical Papanicolaou (Pap) smears, and so should not be relied on. Type-specific serologic assays may be useful in patients with recurrent symptoms and negative HSV cultures, those with a clinical diagnosis of genital herpes without laboratory confirmation, or in patients who have a partner with genital herpes.

▶ Treatment

Treatment of HSV can be episodic (ie, in response to an episode of disease) or suppressive, with daily medication continuing for months or years. Treatment for an initial outbreak consists of 7–10 days of oral medication (see Table 14-3). Episodic treatment is effective when medication is started during the prodrome or on the first symptomatic day. No benefit will be seen if treatment of recurrences is delayed; thus, patients should be given a prescription to have available for use when needed.

Suppressive therapy is traditionally indicated for patients with frequent recurrences, although this may be individualized

Table 14-3. STD treatment guidelines for adults and adolescents.

Disease	Recommended Regimens	Dose, Route
Chlamydia (nonpregnant)	Azithromycin **or** doxycycline	1 g orally, single dose 100 mg PO BID × 7 days
Chlamydia (in pregnancy)	Azithromycin **or** amoxicillin	1 g orally, single dose 500 mg PO TID × 7 days
Gonorrhea	Ceftriaxone **plus** chlamydia treatment listed above, as appropriate for pregnancy status	250 mg IM, single dose
Pelvic inflammatory disease (nonpregnant, outpatient)	Ceftriaxone **plus** doxycycline ± metronidazole	250 mg IM, single dose 100 mg PO BID × 14 days 500 mg PO BID × 14 days
Pelvic inflammatory disease (nonpregnant, inpatient)	Doxycycline **plus** cefoxitin **or** cefotetan	100 mg PO Q12hours 2 g IV Q6hours 2 g IV Q12hours
Pelvic inflammatory disease (in pregnancy)	Hospitalize and treat parenterally	
Cervicitis	Treat for chlamydia and consider concurrent gonorrhea treatment if prevalence is high	
Nongonococcal urethritis	Treat for chlamydia	
Epididymitis (initial therapy)	Ceftriaxone **plus** doxycycline	250 mg IM, single dose 100 mg PO BID × 10 days
Epididymitis (if gonorrhea negative, or likely caused by enteric organism)	Levofloxacin **or** ofloxacin	500 mg PO daily × 10 days 300 mg PO BID × 10 days

(Continued)

Table 14-3. STD treatment guidelines for adults and adolescents. (Continued)

Disease	Recommended Regimens	Dose, Route
Trichomoniasis	Metronidazole	2 g PO, single dose
	or	
	tinidazole (avoid during pregnancy)	2 g PO, single dose
Vulvovaginal candidiasis (choice between OTC intravaginal, prescription intravaginal, or oral treatment) (*Note:* During pregnancy, only 7-day topical azole treatments are recommended.)	**Over-the-counter (OTC) intravaginal** butoconazole	2% cream 5 g intravaginally × 3 days
	or	
	clotrimazole	1% cream 5 g intravaginally × 7–14 days
	or	**or**
	miconazole	2% cream 5 g intravaginally × 3 days
	or	
	tioconazole	2% cream 5 g intravaginally × 7 days
	Prescription intravaginal	**or**
	butoconazole	4% cream 5 g intravaginally × 3 days
	or	**or**
		100 mg vaginal suppository, one daily × 7 days
		or
		200 mg vaginal suppository, one daily × 3 days
		or
		1200 mg vaginal suppository, once 6.5% ointment 5 g intravaginally, once 2% cream (single-dose bioadhesive product), 5 g intravaginally, once
	nystatin	100,000-unit vaginal tablet, daily × 14 days (less effective)
	or	
	terconazole	0.4% cream 5 g intravaginally × 7 days
	Oral treatment	**or**
	fluconazole (contraindicated in pregnancy)	0.8% cream 5 g intravaginally × 3 days
		or
		80 mg vaginal suppository, daily × 3 days 150 mg oral tablet once
Bacterial vaginosis (nonpregnant)	Metronidazole	500 mg PO BID × 7 days (no alcohol for 9 days)
	or	
	metronidazole gel 0.75%	One applicator vaginally daily × 5 days
	or	
	clindamycin cream 2%	One applicator vaginally at bedtime × 7 days (oil-based, can weaken latex condoms)
Bacterial vaginosis (in pregnancy)	Metronidazole	500 mg PO BID × 7 days
	or	**or**
	clindamycin	250 mg PO 3× daily for 7 days 300 mg PO BID × 7 days
Chanchroid	Azithromycin	1 g PO single dose
	or	
	ceftriaxone	250 mg IM single dose
	or	
	ciprofloxacin (contraindicated in pregnancy)	500 mg PO BID × 3 days
	or	
	erythromycin base	500 mg PO 3 × daily for 7 days
Lymphogranuloma venereum (nonpregnant)	Doxycycline	100 mg PO BID × 21 days
Lymphogranuloma venereum (in pregnancy)	Erythromycin base	500 mg PO 4 × daily for 21 days

(Continued)

Table 14-3. STD treatment guidelines for adults and adolescents. (Continued)

Disease	Recommended Regimens	Dose, Route
HPV external genital/perianal warts (may choose either patient-applied or provider-administered treatments) (*Note:* Podofilox, imiquimod, sinecatechins, and podophyllin are all contraindicated in pregnancy.)	**Patient-applied** podofilox 0.5% soln or gel **or** imiquimod 5% cream **or** sinecatechins 15% ointment **Provider-administered** cryotherapy (liquid nitrogen or cryoprobe) **or** podophyllin resin 10–25% in a compound tincture of benzoin **or** TCA or BCA 80–90% **or** surgical removal	
HPV cervical warts	Biopsy and consultation	
HPV vaginal warts	Cryotherapy with liquid nitrogen (not cryoprobe) **or** TCA or BCA 80–90%	
HPV urethral meatus warts (*Note:* Podophyllin is contraindicated in pregnancy.	Cryotherapy with liquid nitrogen **or** podophyllin 10–25% in compound tincture of benzoin	
HPV anal warts	Cryotherapy with liquid nitrogen **or** TCA or BCA 80–90% **or** surgical removal	
HSV first episode (*Note:* Acyclovir is preferred in pregnancy.)	Acyclovir **or** famciclovir **or** valacyclovir	400 mg PO 3 × daily for 7–10 days **or** 200 mg PO 5 × daily for 7–10 days 250 mg PO 3 × daily for 7–10 days 1 g PO BID for 7–10 days
HSV episodic therapy for recurrent episodes (*Note:* Acyclovir is preferred in pregnancy.)	Acyclovir **or** famciclovir **or** valacyclovir	400 mg PO 3 × daily for 5 days **or** 800 mg PO BID × 5 days **or** 800 mg PO 3 × daily for 2 days 125 mg PO BID × 5 days **or** 1000 mg PO BID × 1 day **or** 500 mg PO once, followed by 250 mg PO BID for 2 days 500 mg PO BID × 3 days **or** 1 g PO daily × 5 days

(Continued)

Table 14-3. STD treatment guidelines for adults and adolescents. (Continued)

Disease	Recommended Regimens	Dose, Route
HSV suppressive therapy (*Note:* Acyclovir is preferred in pregnancy.)	Acyclovir **or** famcyclovir **or** valacyclovir	400 mg PO BID 250 mg PO BID 500 mg PO daily **or** 1 g PO daily
Syphilis: primary, secondary, and early latent	Benzathine penicillin G (*Note:* Nonpregnant patients without HIV coinfection can consider doxycycline or tetracycline as an alternative.)	2.4 million units IM
Syphilis: late latent and unknown duration	Benzathine penicillin G (*Note:* Nonpregnant patients without HIV coinfection can consider doxycycline or tetracycline as an alternative.)	7.2 million units, administered as 3 doses of 2.4 million units IM, at 1- week intervals
Neurosyphilis	Aqueous crystalline penicillin G	18–24 million units daily, administered as 3–4 million units IV Q4h × 10–14 days (*Note:* Penicillin allergy requires desensitization.)
Pediculosis pubis: "crab lice" (*Note:* Wash clothes and bedding.)	Permethrin 1% cream rinse **or** Pyrethrins with piperonyl butoxide	Apply to affected areas and wash off after 10 minutes Apply to affected areas and wash off after 10 minutes
Scabies (*Note:* Wash clothes and bedding.)	Permethrin 5% cream **or** ivermectin (contraindicated in pregnancy)	Apply to entire body from neck down; wash off after 8–14 hours 0.2 mg/kg PO once and repeated after 2 weeks

BCA, bichloroacetic acid; HPV, human papillomavirus; HSV, human simplex virus; soln, solution; TCA, trichloroacetic acid.
Data from the Centers for Disease Control and Prevention; Workowski KA, Berman SM. Sexually transmitted disease treatment guidelines, 2010. *MMWR Recomm Rep.* 2010;59(RR-12):1–110.

with respect to the stress and disability caused by recurrences. Available experience suggests that long-term suppression is safe and is not associated with development of antiviral resistance. Suppressive therapy seems to reduce but not eliminate asymptomatic shedding. Daily treatment with valacyclovir (500 mg) has been shown to decrease the rate of HSV2 transmission in discordant heterosexual couples in which the source partner has a history of genital HSV2 infection. Suppression does not change the natural history of a patient's infection; however, because the frequency of recurrences diminishes with time, suppression may be particularly useful during the time period immediately following initial infection. Available therapies appear to be safe in pregnant women, although data for valacyclovir and famciclovir are limited.

Syphilis

General Considerations

Syphilis cases reported to the CDC had declined since the early 1950s until a resurgence was noted in the 1990s. In 1999, the CDC launched "The National Plan to Eliminate Syphilis from the United States." In 2011, 13,970 cases of primary and secondary syphilis were reported. National numbers increased every year from 2000 to 2009, and have largely held steady since then. Men who have sex with men now account for more than two-thirds of new cases of primary and secondary syphilis. More recent resurgences of syphilis in some populations and geographic areas indicate the need for continued vigilance.

Clinical Findings

A. Symptoms and Signs

Syphilis infection is characterized by stages, and accurate staging is vital to determine appropriate therapy. *Primary syphilis* is characterized by the appearance of a painless, indurated ulcer—the chancre—occurring 10 days to 3 months after infection with *Treponema pallidum*. The chancre usually heals by 4–6 weeks, although associated painless bilateral lymphadenopathy may persist for months.

Secondary syphilis has variable manifestations, but usually includes symmetric mucocutaneous macular, papular, papulosquamous, or pustular lesions with generalized nontender lymphadenopathy. In moist skin areas such as the perianal or vulvar regions, papules may become superficially eroded to form pink or whitish condylomata lata. Constitutional symptoms such as fever, malaise, and weight loss occur commonly. Less common complications include meningitis, hepatitis, arthritis, nephropathy, and iridocyclitis.

Latent syphilis is diagnosed in persons with serologic evidence of syphilis infection *without* other current evidence of disease. "Early" latent syphilis is defined as infection for less than 1 year. A diagnosis of early latent syphilis is demonstrated by seroconversion, a definitive history of primary or secondary syphilis findings within the past year, or documented exposure to primary or secondary syphilis in the past year. Asymptomatic patients with known infection of >1 year or in whom infection of <1 year cannot be conclusively demonstrated are classified as having late latent syphilis or latent syphilis of unknown duration, respectively. These two categories of syphilis are treated equivalently. The magnitude of serologic test titers cannot reliably differentiate early from late latent syphilis.

Neurosyphilis can occur at any stage of infection and is difficult to diagnose, as no single test can be used in all instances. The cerebrospinal fluid (CSF) VDRL test is highly specific but insensitive. The diagnosis depends on a combination of serologic tests, elevated CSF cell count or protein, or a reactive VDRL. CSF fluorescent treponemal antibody absorption (FTA-abs) is less specific, but highly sensitive. CSF pleocytosis [>5 white blood cells (WBCs)/mm^3] is usually evident, although HIV infection and other conditions may also cause increased WBCs in the CSF.

Tertiary syphilis is characterized by a self-destructive immune response to a persistent low level of pathogens. It can manifest as neurosyphilis, cardiovascular syphilis including aortitis, or in the form of gummas, granulomas, or psoriasiform plaques.

Patients are infectious during primary, secondary, and early latent stages of syphilis.

B. Laboratory Findings

Positive darkfield examination or direct fluorescent antibody tests of lesion exudates definitively diagnose primary syphilis. More typically, syphilis is diagnosed by positive serologic results of both a nontreponemal test (VDRL or RPR) and a treponemal test [*Treponema pallidum* particle agglutination (TPPA) or FTA-abs].

Nontreponemal tests may be falsely positive because of other medical conditions (eg, some collagen vascular diseases). When positive because of syphilis, their titers generally rise and fall in response to *T. pallidum* infection and treatment, respectively, and usually return to normal (negative) following treatment, although some individuals remain "serofast" and have persistent low positive titers. Treponemal tests usually yield persistent positive results throughout the patient's life following infection with *T. pallidum*. Treponemal test titers do not correlate with disease activity or treatment.

Lumbar puncture is indicated for: (1) neurologic or ophthalmologic signs or symptoms, (2) active aortitis or gumma, or (3) treatment failure (a fourfold increase in titer or a failure to decline fourfold or more within 12–24 months).

▶ Treatment

Treatment for syphilis as described in Table 14-3 is based on current CDC guidelines. Follow-up testing of patients diagnosed with syphilis is a vital part of care, as it determines the effectiveness of therapy and provides useful information to differentiate potential future serofast patients from those with recurrent infection.

The nontreponemal test titer should have fallen fourfold or more (eg, from 1:32 to ≤1:8) for persons with primary or secondary syphilis in 6–12 months post therapy. If it does not, consider this a treatment failure or an indication of reinfection. In evaluating such a potential treatment failure, the patient should, at minimum, receive continued serologic follow-up and repeat HIV serology if previously negative. Lumbar puncture should also be considered, and if the results are normal, the patient should be treated with 2.4 million units of benzathine penicillin weekly for 3 weeks and followed as described previously.

Chancroid

Chancroid has declined in the United States and worldwide. In 2011, a total of eight cases of chancroid were reported in only six states in the United States. These data should be interpreted with caution, however, because *Haemophilus ducreyi* is difficult to culture, and thus this condition may be substantially underdiagnosed.

Definitive diagnosis is difficult, requiring identification of *H. ducreyi* on special culture medium that is seldom readily available. Presumptive diagnosis rests on the presence of painful genital ulcer(s) with a negative HSV test and negative syphilis serology, with or without regional lymphadenopathy.

Treatment consists of oral antibiotics as listed in Table 14-3. Healing of large ulcers may require >2 weeks. If patients do not show clinical improvement after 7 days, consider the accuracy of the diagnosis, medication nonadherence, antibacterial resistance, or a combination of these. Fluctuant lymphadenopathy may require drainage via aspiration or incision.

Although definitive diagnosis generally rests on laboratory testing, history and examination (H&PE) often lead to a presumptive diagnosis. **Table 14-4** summarizes findings for different causes of GUD.

Other Causes of GUD

Granuloma inguinale or donovanosis is caused by *Calymmatobacterium granulomatis,* which is endemic in some tropical nonindustrialized parts of the world and is rarely reported in the United States. The bacterium does not grow on standard culture media; diagnosis rests on demonstration of so-called Donovan bodies in a tissue specimen. Infection causes painless, progressive, beefy red, highly vascular lesions without lymphadenopathy. Treatment is

Table 14-4. Differentiation of common causes of genital ulcers.[a]

Parameter	Herpes	Syphilis	Chancroid	Lymphogranuloma Venereum	Granuloma Inguinale
Ulcer(s) appearance	Often purulent	"Clean"	Purulent	May be purulent	"Beefy," hemorrhagic
Number	Usually multiple	Single[b]	Often multiple	Single or multiple	Multiple
Pain	Yes	No	Yes	Ulcer: no Nodes: yes	No
Preceded by	Papule, then vesicle	Papule	Papule	Papule; ulcer often unnoticed	Nodule(s)
Adenopathy	Painful with primary outbreak	Painless	Painful; may suppurate	Painful; may suppurate	No, unless secondary bacterial infection
Systemic symptoms	Often with primary outbreak	Rarely	Occasionally	Usually not	No

[a]A diagnosis based solely on medical history and physical examination is often inaccurate.
[b]Up to 40% of patients with primary syphilis have more than one chancre.

often prolonged, and relapse can occur months after initial treatment and apparent cure.

Lymphogranuloma venereum is caused by serovars L1, L2, and L3 of *C. trachomatis*. The small ulcer arising at the site of infection is often unnoticed or unreported. The most common clinical presentation is painful unilateral lymphadenopathy. Rectal exposure in women and in MSMs may result in proctocolitis (mucus or hemorrhagic rectal discharge, anal pain, constipation, fever, or tenesmus). Diagnosis rests on clinical suspicion, epidemiologic information, exclusion of other etiologies, and *C. trachomatis* tests. In addition to antibiotics, treatment may require aspiration or incision and drainage of buboes; nevertheless, patients may still experience scarring.

Domantay-Apostol GP, Handog EB, Gabriel MT. Syphilis: the international challenge of the great imitator. *Dermatol Clin.* 2008; 26(2):191–202. [PMID: 18346551]

Kapoor S. Re-emergence of lymphogranuloma venereum. *J Euro Acad Dermatol Venereol.* 2008; 22(4):409–416. [PMID 18363909]

Mattei P, Beachkofsky TM, Gilson RT, Wisco OJ. Syphilis: a reemerging infection. *Am Fam Physician.* 2012; 86(5):433–440. [PMID 22963062]

URETHRITIS

ESSENTIALS OF DIAGNOSIS

▶ Coinfection with *Chlamydia trachomatis* is common in those with *Neisseria gonorrhoeae*, justifying treatment for both.

▶ Nucleic acid amplification tests have largely supplanted cell culture tests for diagnosis.

In 2011, population studies showed a rate of *Chlamydia* infection of 457.6 cases per 100,000 and a rate of gonorrhea infection of 104.2 cases per 100,000 in the United States. Rates for both of these pathogens are higher in females than males, and are highest in the adolescent and young adult age groups.

Sexually transmitted diseases causing urethritis are typically diagnosed in men, although women may also experience urethritis as a consequence of an STD. For clinical management, urethritis can be divided into nongonococcal urethritis (NGU) and urethritis due to *N. gonorrhoeae* infection.

Nongonococcal Urethritis

One frequent cause of NGU is *C. trachomatis*. In 2011, 1,412,791 *Chlamydia* cases were reported, and although significant, these numbers likely dramatically underestimate actual cases of *C. trachomatis* infection. The spectrum of *C. trachomatis*–caused disease includes extragenital manifestations, among them ophthalmic infection and a reactive arthritis.

Causes of nonchlamydial NGU may include *Mycoplasma genitalium*, *Ureaplasma urealyticum*, *Trichomonas vaginalis*, herpes simplex, and adenovirus. Diagnosis of NGU can be based on: (1) purulent urethral discharge; (2) Gram stain of urethral secretions with ≥5 WBCs per high-power field (HPF) and no gram-negative intracellular diplococci (which, if present, would indicate gonorrhea); (3) first-void urine with positive leukocyte esterase, or >10 WBCs/HPF. Nucleic acid amplification tests (*Chlamydia* or gonorrhea) offer greater convenience and better sensitivity than culture and represent the best tests currently available.

In patients presenting with recurrent urethritis, diagnostic evaluation may be necessary to identify the etiology. In evaluating recurrent urethritis, the physician should assess medication compliance and potential reexposure; perform wet mount, culture, or both, for *T. vaginalis*; and treat as indicated by findings, or empirically as per Table 14-3.

Treatment of NGU generally employs azithromycin or doxycycline, with alternatives as listed in Table 14-3. If findings of urethritis are present, treatment is generally indicated pending results of diagnostic tests. Because diagnostic testing typically does not look for all potential causes of urethritis, patients with negative tests for gonorrhea and *C. trachomatis* may also benefit from treatment. Empiric treatment of symptoms without documentation of urethritis findings is recommended only for patients at high risk for infection who are unlikely to return for a follow-up evaluation. Such patients should be treated for gonorrhea and *Chlamydia*. Partners of patients treated empirically should be evaluated and treated. If treatment is not offered at the initial visit, diagnostic testing should employ the most sensitive test available, with follow-up treatment as indicated by test results and symptom persistence.

Gonorrhea

▶ General Considerations

In 2011, 321,849 cases of gonorrhea were reported in the United States. Rates have been moderately stable since 2004, more common in the South (135.5 cases per 100,000 population vs 104.2 cases per 100,000 for the country), and somewhat more common in women than in men (108.9 vs 98.7 cases per 100,000, respectively).

▶ Clinical Findings

A. Symptoms and Signs

If symptomatic, gonorrhea typically causes dysuria and a purulent urethral discharge; however, it may also cause asymptomatic infection or disseminated systemic disease, including pharyngitis, skin lesions, septic arthritis, tenosynovitis, arthralgias, proctitis, perihepatitis, endocarditis, and meningitis. In these cases, there is usually minimal genital inflammation.

Clinical differentiation between gonorrhea and *Chlamydia* may be difficult. Characteristically, urethral exudate in gonorrhea is thicker, more profuse, and more purulent in appearance than the exudate caused by *C. trachomatis*, which is often watery with mucus strands. However, differentiation of etiology based on clinical appearance is notoriously unreliable.

B. Laboratory Findings

Nucleic acid amplification technology (NAAT, including PCR) has largely supplanted culture for diagnosis because of enhanced sensitivity and excellent specificity. NAAT tests can be performed on endocervical swabs, vaginal swabs, urethral swabs, and urine samples. In addition, some laboratories have established performance specifications for the use of NAAT testing for gonorrhea on rectal and pharyngeal swabs. However, the use of NAAT testing in nongenital sites is rendered more challenging by the potential for cross-reactivity with nongonorrheal *Neisseria* species. In addition, gonorrhea PCR test sensitivity is quite poor in women's urine specimens—as low as 55%, and therefore endocervical swab NAAT testing is to be preferred in this population.

Diagnostic evaluation identifies disease etiology and may facilitate the public health missions of contact tracing and disease eradication. For an individual patient, however, the physician may treat empirically if follow-up cannot be ensured and test methodology is insensitive. Decisions about diagnostic testing should consider both public health goals and how information obtained will influence patient (and partner) treatment.

▶ Treatment

When treating for gonorrhea, practitioners should treat also for *C. trachomatis*, as coinfection is common. Quinolone-resistant *N. gonorrhoeae* strains are now widely disseminated throughout United States and the world. Since April 2007, quinolones have no longer been recommended in the United States for treatment of gonorrhea and associated conditions such as PID. As of October 2012, oral cephalosporins are no longer a recommended treatment for gonorrheal infection. Decreased susceptibility of *N gonorrhoeae* to cephalosporins and other antimicrobials is expected to continue to spread; therefore, state and local surveillance for antimicrobial resistance is crucial for guiding local therapy recommendations. Ceftriaxone 250 mg IM is currently effective for the treatment of uncomplicated gonorrhea at all anatomic sites.

Treatment failures should be followed by (repeat) culture and sensitivity testing, and any resistance should be reported to the public health department.

Centers for Disease Control and Prevention; Workowski KA, Berman SM. Sexually transmitted disease treatment guidelines, 2010. *MMWR Recomm Rep.* 2010;59(RR-12):1–110.

Centers for Disease Control and Prevention. *Sexually Transmitted Disease Surveillance, 2011.* Atlanta, GA: US Department of Health and Human Services; 2012.

EPIDIDYMITIS

The cause of epididymitis varies with age. In men aged ≤35 years, it is most commonly due to gonorrhea or *C. trachomatis*, or to gram-negative enteric organisms in men who engage in unprotected insertive anal intercourse. In men aged >35 years, epididymitis is seldom sexually transmitted, and is more likely caused by gram-negative enteric organisms; increased risk in this case is found in patients who have undergone recent urologic surgery, or who have anatomic abnormalities. Patients usually present with unilateral testicular pain and inflammation with onset over several days. The clinician must differentiate epididymitis from testicular torsion, since the latter is a surgical emergency requiring immediate correction. The laboratory evaluation of suspected epididymitis includes Gram stain, nucleic acid amplification test, and serologic testing for HIV and syphilis.

PROCTITIS, PROCTOCOLITIS, & ENTERITIS

Proctitis, proctocolitis, and enteritis may arise from anal intercourse or oral-anal contact. Depending on organism and anatomic location of infection and inflammation, symptoms can include pain, tenesmus, rectal discharge, and diarrhea. Etiologic agents of proctitis include *C. trachomatis* (lymphogranuloma venereum), *N. gonorrhea, T. pallidum*, and HSV. Other agents may cause proctitis or enteritis including *Giardia lamblia, Campylobacter, Shigella*, and *Entamoeba histolytica*. In HIV-infected patients, additional etiologic agents include cytomegalovirus, *Mycobacterium avium* intracellulare, *Salmonella, Cryptosporidium, Microsporidium*, and *Isospora*. Symptoms may also arise as a primary effect of HIV infection.

Diagnosis involves examination of stool for ova, parasites, occult blood, and WBCs; stool culture; and anoscopy or sigmoidoscopy.

Treatment should generally be based on results of diagnostic studies. However, if the onset of symptoms occurs within 1–2 weeks of receptive anal intercourse, and there is evidence of purulent exudates or polymorphonuclear neutrophils on Gram stain of anorectal smear, the patient can be treated presumptively for gonorrhea and chlamydial infection. If painful perianal ulcers are present or mucosal ulcers are detected on anoscopy, presumptive therapy should include a regimen for genital herpes and lymphogranuloma venereum.

VAGINITIS

ESSENTIALS OF DIAGNOSIS

▶ A careful history, examination, and laboratory testing should be performed to determine the etiology of vaginal complaints. Information on sexual behaviors and practices, gender of sex partners, menses, vaginal hygiene practices (eg, douching or use of douche products), and other medications should be elicited.

▶ Examination of vaginal discharge by wet mount, potassium hydroxide (KOH) preparation, pH, and odor.

▶ Disease-specific point-of-care test or vaginal fluid culture if indicated.

Patients with vaginitis may present with vaginal discharge, vulvar itching, irritation, or all of these, and sometimes with complaints of abnormal vaginal odor. Common etiologies include *Candida albicans, T. vaginalis*, and bacterial vaginosis. Diagnostic evaluation typically includes physical examination and evaluation of a saline wet mount and potassium hydroxide (KOH) preparation. Differences between common causes of vaginitis are summarized in **Table 14-5** and described next.

Vulvovaginal Candidiasis

Vulvovaginal candidiasis (VVC) is typically caused by *C. albicans*, although occasionally other species are identified. More than 75% of all women will have at least one episode of VVC during their lifetime. The diagnosis is presumed if the patient has vulvovaginal pruritus and erythema with or without a white discharge, and is confirmed by wet mount or KOH preparation showing yeast or pseudohyphae, or culture showing a yeast species.

Vulvovaginal candidiasis can be classified as uncomplicated, complicated, or recurrent. Uncomplicated VVC encompasses sporadic, nonrecurrent, mild to moderate symptoms due to *C. albicans* that, in an otherwise healthy patient, are responsive to routine therapy. Complicated VVC implies recurrent or severe local disease in a patient with impaired immune function (eg, diabetes or HIV), or infection with resistant yeast species. Recurrent VVC is defined as four or more symptomatic episodes annually.

Treatment is summarized in Table 14-3. Uncomplicated candidiasis should respond to short-term or single-dose therapies as listed. Complicated VVC may require prolonged treatment. Treatment of women with recurrent vulvovaginal candidiasis should begin with an intensive regimen (7–14 days of topical therapy or a multidose fluconazole regimen) followed by 6 months of maintenance therapy to reduce the likelihood of subsequent recurrence. Symptomatic candidal vaginitis is more frequent in HIV-infected women and correlates with severity of immunodeficiency.

Vulvovaginal candidiasis is seldom acquired through sexual intercourse. There are no data to support treatment of sex partners. Some male sex partners have balanitis and may benefit from topical antifungal agents.

Trichomoniasis

Vaginitis due to *T. vaginalis* presents with a thin, yellow, or yellow-green frothy malodorous discharge and vulvar irritation that may worsen following menstruation. However, many women have minimal or no symptoms at all. Diagnosis can often be made via prompt examination of a freshly obtained wet mount, which reveals the motile trichomonads. Although culture is more sensitive, it may not be as readily available, and results are delayed. Point-of-care tests (eg, Osom *Trichomonas* Rapid Test and Affirm VPIII) are also available and tend to be more sensitive than vaginal wet prep. Partners of women with *Trichomonas* infection require treatment.

Table 14-5. Common causes of vaginitis.

Diagnostic Test	Findings Characteristics of		
	Candida albicans	*Trichomonas vaginalis*	Bacterial Vaginosis
pH	<4.5	>4.5	>4.5
KOH to slide	Yeast or pseudohyphae		Amine or "fishy" odor
Saline to slide	Yeast or pseudohyphae	Motile *T. vaginalis* organisms	"Clue" cells
Culture	Yeast species	*T. vaginalis*	Nonspecific (not recommended)

Bacterial Vaginosis

Bacterial vaginosis arises when normal vaginal bacteria are replaced with an overgrowth of anaerobic bacteria. Although not thought to be an STD, it is associated with having multiple sex partners or a new sex partner.

Diagnosis can be based on the presence of three of four clinical criteria: (1) a thin, homogeneous vaginal discharge; (2) a vaginal pH value of >4.5; (3) a positive "whiff" test (fishy odor when KOH is added to vaginal discharge); and (4) the presence of clue cells in a wet mount preparation.

Treatment is recommended for women with symtoms. Potential benefits of therapy include reducing the risk for infectious complications associated with bacterial vaginosis during pregnancy and reducing the risk for other infections. Routine treatment of sex partners is not recommended.

Cervicitis

Cervicitis is characterized by purulent discharge from the endocervix, which may or may not be associated with vaginal discharge or cervical bleeding. The diagnostic evaluation should include testing for *Chlamydia*, gonorrhea, bacterial vaginosis, and *Trichomonas*. Absence of symptoms should not preclude additional evaluation and treatment, as approximately 70% of chlamydial infections and 50% of gonococcal infections in women are asymptomatic.

Nucleic acid amplification tests are the preferred diagnostic test for gonorrhea and *Chlamydia* and can be performed on vaginal, cervical, or urine specimens (although, urine testing for gonorrhea has only 55% sensitivity and so cervical specimens are preferred). Empiric treatment should be considered in areas with high prevalence of *C. trachomatis* or gonorrhea, or if follow-up is unlikely.

Centers for Disease Control and Prevention; Workowski KA, Berman SM. Sexually transmitted disease treatment guidelines, 2010. *MMWR Recomm Rep.* 2010;59(RR-12):1–110.

Cook RL, et al. Systematic review: noninvasive testing for Chlamydia trachomatis and Neisseria gonorrhoeae. *Ann Intern Med.* 2005; 142:914. [PMID: 15941699]

PELVIC INFLAMMATORY DISEASE

 ESSENTIALS OF DIAGNOSIS

▶ Diagnosis is challenging, requiring the clinician to balance underdiagnosis with overtreatment.

▶ Consequences of untreated PID can include chronic pain, infertility, and death.

Pelvic inflammatory disease (PID) is defined as inflammation of the upper genital tract, including pelvic peritonitis, endometritis, salpingitis, and tuboovarian abscess due to infection with gonorrhea, *C. trachomatis*, or vaginal or bowel flora; etiology is often polymicrobial. Diagnosis is challenging because of often vague symptoms, lack of a single diagnostic test, and the invasive nature of technologies needed to make a definitive diagnosis. Lower abdominal tenderness and uterine, adnexal, or cervical motion tenderness with signs of lower genital tract inflammation increase the specificity of a PID diagnosis. Other criteria enhance the specificity of the diagnosis (but reduce diagnostic sensitivity):

• Fever >38.3°C (>101°F)

• Abnormal cervical or vaginal discharge

• Abundant WBCs in saline microscopy of vaginal secretions

• Elevated sedimentation rate

• Elevated C-reactive protein

• Cervical infection with gonorrhea or *C trachomatis*

Definitive diagnosis rests on techniques that are not always readily available and that are rarely used to make the diagnosis. These include laparoscopic findings consistent with PID, evidence of endometritis on endometrial biopsy, and ultrasonographic findings showing thickened fluid-filled tubes with or without free pelvic fluid or tuboovarian complex.

Determination of appropriate therapy should consider pregnancy status, severity of illness, and patient compliance. Less severe disease can generally be treated with oral antibiotics in an ambulatory setting, whereas pregnant patients and those with severe disease may need hospitalization. Options are listed in Table 14-3.

Centers for Disease Control and Prevention; Workowski KA, Berman SM. Sexually transmitted disease treatment guidelines, 2010. *MMWR Recomm Rep.* 2010; 59(RR-12):1–110.

Trigg BG, Kerndt PR, Aynalem G. Sexually transmitted infections and pelvic inflammatory disease in women. *Med Clin N Am.* 2008; 92(5):1083–1113.

HPV INFECTION & EXTERNAL GENITAL WARTS

 ESSENTIALS OF DIAGNOSIS

▶ Diagnosis of genital warts is usually made by visual inspection. Biopsy may be indicated if diagnosis is uncertain.

▶ Treatment is directed toward genital warts or to precancerous lesions caused by HPV. In the absence of lesions, treatment is not recommended for subclinical genital HPV infection, which often clears spontaneously.

▶ General Considerations

It is estimated that >79 million Americans are infected with HPV, with 15 million new infections and 453,000 initial visits to physicians for genital warts occurring annually. Even this estimate may be low; overall HPV prevalence among US females aged 14–59 years was estimated to be 42.5%, based on 2003–2006 National Health and Nutrition Examination Survey (NHANES) data. Over 100 types of HPV have been identified, and over 40 types cause genital lesions. Types 6, 11, and others typically produce benign exophytic warts, whereas types 16, 18, 31, 33, 35, and others are associated with dysplasia and neoplasia. Thus, cervical and anogenital squamous cancer can be considered STDs; other cancers may also be sexually transmitted.

▶ Clinical Findings

Diagnosis is almost always based on physical examination with bright light and magnification, and rarely requires biopsy. If the diagnosis is uncertain, consider referral to a physician with extensive experience in external genital warts. Biopsy should be considered for >1-cm warts; indurated, ulcerated, or fixed to underlying structures; atypical in appearance; pigmented; or resistant to therapy. Application of 3–5% acetic acid as an aid to visualization is seldom useful, and the resulting nonspecific acetowhite reaction may lead to overdiagnosis of genital warts.

Human papillomavirus is the primary cause of cervical cancer, and screening guidelines for cervical cancer screening including the use of HPV testing, are reviewed in Chapter 26. Genital warts are not an indication for screening more frequently.

Because of the increased incidence of anal cancer in HIV-infected homosexual and bisexual men and high-risk women, screening for anal cytologic abnormalities may be considered. However, there are limited data on the natural history of anal intraepithelial neoplasias, the reliability of screening methods, the safety of and response to treatments, and the programmatic considerations that would support this screening approach.

▶ Treatment

The therapeutic goal in treatment of external genital warts is elimination of warts. Treatment strives to eliminate symptoms, and a potential theoretical benefit is reduced likelihood of transmission. Clinicians should be certain of the diagnosis prior to instituting therapy, and should not apply treatments to skin tags, pearly penile papules, sebaceous glands, or other benign findings that do not require (and will not respond to) genital wart treatment.

No evidence suggests any treatment is superior to others. The possibility of spontaneous resolution may justify no treatment, if that is the patient's wish.

Treatments can be categorized as provider-applied or patient-applied. Physicians should familiarize themselves with at least one or two treatments in each category, as described in Table 14-3. Most treatments work via tissue destruction. Imiquimod uses a different mechanism; by inducing production of interferon, it may be more effective than other therapies in treating some genital warts or other skin conditions, including molluscum contagiosum. Patients unresponsive to an initial course of treatment may require another round of treatment, more aggressive treatment, or referral to a specialist.

Although most HPV infections will clear spontaneously within 2 years and cause no harm, patients with HPV need to understand the possibility of chronic infection, including its natural history and treatment options, and should receive adequate education and counseling to achieve optimal treatment outcomes. The chronic nature of HPV infection combined with the serious, albeit relatively infrequent, complication of cancer creates significant challenges to patient coping and provider counseling.

Centers for Disease Control and Prevention. *Fact Sheet: Incidence, Prevalence and Cost of Sexually Transmitted Infections in the United States* (available at http://www.cdc.gov/std/stats/STI-Estimates-Fact-Sheet-Feb-2013.pdf; accessed April 9, 2013).

Saslow D, Solomon D, Lawson HW, et al. ACS-ASCCP-ASCP Cervical Cancer Guideline Committee (2012), American Cancer Society, American Society for Colposcopy and Cervical Pathology, and American Society for Clinical Pathology screening guidelines for the prevention and early detection of cervical cancer. *CA J.* 2012; 62:147–172. [PMID: 22431528]

MOLLUSCUM CONTAGIOSUM

Molluscum contagiosum appears in individuals of all ages and from all races, but has been reported more commonly in the white population and in males. Lesions are due to infection with poxvirus, which is transmitted through direct skin contact, as occurs among children in a nursery school and among adults during sexual activity. Diagnosis is typically based on inspection, which reveals dimpled or umbilicated flesh-colored or pearly papules several millimeters in diameter; if needed, a smear of the core stained with Giemsa reveals cytoplasmic inclusion bodies. Lesions usually number fewer than 10–30, but may exceed 100, especially in HIV-infected patients who may have verrucous, warty papules, as well as mollusca of >1 cm diameter. Lesions usually resolve spontaneously within months of appearance, but can be treated with cryotherapy, cautery, curettage, or removal of the lesion's core, with or without local anesthesia.

Villa L, Varela JA, Otero L, et al. Molluscum contagiosum: a 20-year study in a sexually transmitted infections unit. *Sex Transm Dis.* 2010; 37(7):423–424. [PMID: 20414149]

HEPATITIS

Vaccines for prevention of viral hepatitis and indications were described previously. Diagnostic and treatment considerations of viral hepatitis are reviewed in Chapter 32.

ECTOPARASITES

Pediculosis pubis results from infestation with "crab lice" or *Phthirus pubis*. Affected patients usually present with pubic or anogenital pruritus, and may have identified lice or nits. The physician should be able to identify lice or nits with careful examination, and their absence calls into question the diagnosis despite compatible history.

Scabies, resulting from infestation with *Sarcoptes scabiei*, usually presents with pruritus not necessarily limited to the genital region. The intensity of pruritus may be increased at bedtime, and may be out of proportion to modest physical findings of erythematous papules, burrows, or excoriation from scratching. A classic finding on physical examination is the serpiginous burrow present in the web space between fingers, although this finding is frequently absent in individuals with scabies.

Scabies can be sexually transmitted in adults; sexual contact is not the usual route of transmission in children. Pruritus may persist for weeks after treatment. Retreatment should be deferred if intensity of symptoms is diminishing and no new findings appear. In HIV-infected patients with uncomplicated scabies, treatment is the same as for HIV-uninfected patients. However, HIV-infected patients are at risk for a more severe infestation with Norwegian scabies, which should be managed with expert consultation.

Centers for Disease Control and Prevention; Workowski KA, Berman SM. Sexually transmitted disease treatment guidelines, 2010. *MMWR Recomm Rep.* 2010;59(RR-12):1–110.

GENERAL PRINCIPLES OF THERAPY

 ESSENTIAL FEATURES

▶ Presumptive treatment while awaiting laboratory test results is common practice.

▶ Coexisting HIV infection may modify STD treatment regimens.

▶ Patient education and partner treatment are essential to reduce disease spread.

Treatments may be empirically targeted to agents most likely causing the presenting clinical syndrome, or targeted to a specific infection diagnosed definitively. Regardless, there are overarching concerns affecting STD treatment that pertain to adherence and treatment success, HIV status, partner treatment, test of cure, and pregnancy.

Adherence considerations may favor shorter or single-dose regimens. For example, although single-dose azithromycin is more expensive than 7-day doxycycline therapy, reduced medication compliance and attendant costs of follow-up evaluation for patients treated with doxycycline may favor the use of azithromycin.

With HIV coinfection, treatments are generally the same as for uninfected patients unless stated otherwise. One potential difference is that HSV often causes more significant and prolonged symptoms in HIV-infected than in uninfected patients, so that HIV-infected patients may require longer treatment or higher medication dosages, or both. Syphilis treatment is the same as for HIV-uninfected patients regardless of stage. However, careful follow-up is important, as treatment failure or progression to neurosyphilis may be more common in the presence of HIV.

Ulcerative and nonulcerative STDs can increase the risk of HIV transmission approximately three- to fivefold.

Pregnancy imposes constraints and special considerations for therapy. Where applicable, these are noted in the treatment recommendations in Table 14-3.

As described previously, patients often present with a clinical syndrome potentially attributable to more than one infectious agent, and optimally focused therapy depends on microbiological identification. However, delaying therapy may allow symptoms to continue, resulting in untreated infection or continued spread (if the patient fails to return for follow-up or heed advice to avoid sexual contact until cured), and contribute to increased long-term morbidity. Consequently, it may be desirable to treat at the initial presentation for the infectious agents considered most likely.

Websites

American Social Health Association (ASHA): http://www.ashastd .org/
CDC STD Treatment Guidelines: http://www.cdc.gov/std/

SEXUAL ASSAULT

Management of victims of sexual assault encompasses much more than treatment or prevention of STDs. Providers must heed legal requirements and effectively manage the psychological trauma, while not compromising the best course of medical care.

Proper medical management of sexual assault victims includes collection of evidence, diagnostic evaluation, counseling, and medical therapies to treat infection and unintended pregnancy. The diagnostic evaluation should include the following:

- Nucleic acid amplification tests for *Neiserria gonorrhoeae* and *C. trachomatis* from specimens collected from any sites of penetration or attempted penetration.

- Vaginal wet mount and culture for *T. vaginalis*; wet mount can also detect sperm which are motile for ~6 hours.

- Serum tests for syphilis, hepatitis B, and HIV.

- Pregnancy testing.

Evaluation for STDs may be repeated in 1–2 weeks after the initial evaluation to detect organisms that may have been undetected, unless the patient was treated prophylactically. Repeat testing for syphilis and HIV should be performed at 6 weeks, 3 months, and 6 months. Providers should also consider testing for hepatitis C virus, transmission of which has been documented following sexual assault.

Prophylactic treatment for STDs may be offered or recommended as compliance with follow-up visits is poor. Hepatitis B vaccine should be administered according to the routine schedule; hepatitis B immune globulin is not necessary unless the perpetrator is known to be infected with HBV. Azithromycin, 1 g orally, plus ceftriaxone 250 mg intramuscularly, plus metronidazole 2 g orally, may be offered to treat *C. trachomatis, N. gonorrhea*, and *Trichomonas*. Gastrointestinal side effects, especially when combined with postcoital oral contraceptive pills, may make this regimen intolerable, and alternative therapies or watchful waiting may be preferable.

Need for and benefit from HIV postexposure prophylaxis is difficult to predict. If instituted, the greatest benefit results from initiation of therapy as soon after exposure as possible. For guidance in deciding whether to begin postexposure HIV prophylaxis and in selecting appropriate treatment and monitoring, providers may contact the National Clinician's Post-Exposure Prophylaxis Hotline (PEPline) at 888-HIV-4911 (888-448 4911).

After the neonatal period, STDs in children most commonly result from sexual abuse. In addition to vaginal gonococcal infection, pharyngeal and anorectal infection may occur and are often asymptomatic. Specific diagnostic techniques should rely only on existing guidelines as data on nucleic acid amplification tests for *Chlamydia* and gonorrhea are limited and performance may be test-dependent. Specimen preservation is essential for future testing when needed.

Alter MJ, Bell BP, et al. A comprehensive immunization strategy to eliminate transmission of hepatitis B virus infection in the United States: recommendations of the Advisory Committee on Immunization Practices (ACIP) Part II: immunization of adults. MMWR Recomm Rep. 2006;55(RR-16):1.

Black CM, et al. Multicenter study of nucleic acid amplification tests for detection of *Chlamydia trachomatis* and *Neisseria gonorrhoeae* in children being evaluated for sexual abuse. *Pediatr Infect Dis J.* 2009; 28:608–613. [PMID: 19451856]

Luce H, Schrager S, Gilchrist V. Sexual assault of women. *Am Fam Physician.* 2010;81(4):489–495. [PMID: 20148503]

Health Maintenance for Adults

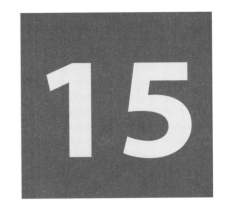

Stephen A. Wilson, MD, MPH, FAAFP

Lora Cox-Vance, MD

Paul R. Larson, MD, MS

Rachel Simon, PharmD, BCPS

David Yuan, MD, MS

On average, each day longer you live, the longer you are likely to live, yet the closer to dying you become. The goal of health maintenance (HM) is to help people live longer and healthier lives.

General Considerations

In this chapter, the findings and positions of the United States Preventative Service Task Force (USPSTF) are emphasized because it generates the most comprehensive and evidence-based recommendations of any organization. Hence, knowing the USPSTF grading system for its recommendations is important (**Table 15-1**). The USPSTF is sponsored by the Agency for Healthcare Research and Quality (AHRQ) and is the leading independent panel of private-sector experts in prevention and primary care.

This chapter describes prevention then presents HM by the age groups 18-39, 40-49, 50-59, 60-74, and ≥75 years of age. USPSTF Grade A and B recommendations are emphasized with highlights to some areas of special interest or controversy, including sections on immunizations and aspirin.

Health maintenance involves three types of prevention: primary, secondary, and tertiary (**Figure 15-1**).

Prevention

A. Primary Prevention

Targets individuals who may be *at risk* to develop a medical condition and intervenes to prevent the onset of that condition (eg, childhood vaccination programs, water fluoridation, smoking prevention programs, clean water, and sanitation). The disease does *not* exist. The *goal is to prevent development* of disease.

B. Secondary Prevention

Targets individuals who have developed an *asymptomatic* disease and institutes treatment to prevent complications (eg, routine Papanicolaou smears; screening for hypertension, diabetes, or hyperlipidemia). The disease does exist, but the person is unaware (*asymptomatic*). The *goal is to identify and treat* people with disease.

C. Tertiary Prevention

Treatment targets individuals with a *known* disease, with the goal of limiting or preventing future complications (eg, rigorous treatment of diabetes mellitus, post–myocardial infarction treatment with β-blockers and aspirin). The disease exists and there are symptoms. The *goal is to prevent complications.*

Secondary and tertiary prevention require some type of screening. This raises important issues: (1) who should be screened, (2) for which disease(s), and (3) with what test(s) (**Table 15-2**).

1. The disease—The disease must have a period of being detectable before the symptoms start so that it can be found and treated; for instance, colon cancer has no early symptoms but can be detected with screening. The disease cannot appear too quickly, such as a cold and certain lung cancers. The disease must be common in the target population; for instance, stomach cancer is not screened for in the United States (uncommon), but it is screened for in Japan, where is it is more common.

2. The test—*Ideally* the screening test will identify all people with disease and only people with disease will test positive. In *reality*, screening tests are acceptable if they do the job well enough—sensitive enough to have few false negatives and specific enough to have few false positives. Screening tests should also be cost-efficient, easy, reliable, and as painless as possible.

3. Treatment—When screening for disease, treatment must be available, be acceptable, and have benefits that outweigh the risk. Mortality is the most often used endpoint. If a group

Table 15-1. USPSTF grade definitions.

Grade	Definition	Suggestions for Practice
A	USPSTF recommends the service. There is high certainty that the net benefit is substantial.	Offer or provide this service.
B	USPSTF recommends the service. There is high certainty that the net benefit is moderate or moderate certainty that the net benefit is moderate to substantial.	Offer or provide this service.
C	USPSTF recommends against routinely providing the service. There may be considerations that support providing the service in an individual patient. There is at least moderate certainty that the net benefit is small.	Offer or provide this service only if other considerations support the offering or providing the service in an individual patient.
D	USPSTF recommends against the service. There is moderate or high certainty that the service has no net benefit or that the harms outweigh the benefits.	Discourage the use of this service.
I statement	USPSTF concludes that the current evidence is insufficient to assess the balance of benefits and harms (risks) of the service. Evidence is lacking, of poor quality, or conflicting, and the balance of benefits and risks cannot be determined.	Read the clinical considerations section of USPSTF recommendation statement. If the service is offered, patients should understand the uncertainty about the balance of benefits and harms.

of people who are screened and then treated live longer or better than a group of people who are not screened, then the screening test may be good for that population. If the two groups of people die at the same rate, there is usually no point in screening for the disease.

SCREENING

A. Health Maintenance: Across the Ages What *Not* to *Do*

Conditions for which the USPSTF recommends *against routine screening* in asymptomatic adults:

- Aspirin to prevent myocardial infarction in men aged <45 years
- Asymptomatic bacteriuria in men and nonpregnant women
- Bacterial vaginosis in asymptomatic pregnant women at low risk for preterm delivery
- BRCA-related cancers in women not at increased risk
- Cancers: cervix (if hysterectomy), ovary, pancreas, prostate, testicular
- Carotid artery stenosis
- Chronic obstructive pulmonary disease
- Electrocardiography (ECG)
- Genital herpes
- Gonorrhea in low-risk men and women
- Heart disease in low-risk patients using ECG, electron-beam computed tomography (EBCT)
- Hemochromatosis
- Hepatitis B

Person's health	Disease natural progression	
Well ↓ ↓ ↓ ↓ ↓ ↓ ↓ ↓ Sick	Absent → → → → → → → → → Present	
	Primary Prevention	*Secondary Prevention*
		Tertiary Prevention

▲ **Figure 15-1.** The three types of disease prevention.

Table 15-2. Wilson-Jungner criteria for appraising the validity of a screening program.

1. The condition being screened for is an important health problem
2. The natural history of the condition is well understood
3. There is a detectable early stage
4. The earlier the stage, the more beneficial is the treatment
5. A suitable test is available for the early stage
6. The test is acceptable
7. Intervals for repeating the test are determined
8. Adequate health service provision is made for the extra clinical workload resulting from screening
9. The risks, both physical and psychological, are less than the benefits
10. The costs are balanced against the benefits

- Routine aspirin or nonsteroidal anti-inflammatory drugs (NSAIDs) for primary prevention of colorectal cancer for average risk
- Scoliosis
- Stress echocardiogram
- Syphilis

Vitamin supplements with β-carotene to prevent cancer and cardiovascular disease (CVD)

B. Health Maintenance: Across the Ages—Insufficient Evidence

Conditions for which the USPSTF found *insufficient* evidence to promote routine screening in asymptomatic adults at low risk:

- Abuse of elderly and vulnerable adults
- Cancers: bladder, oral, skin
- *Chlamydia* in men
- Clinical breast examination beyond screening mammography, women aged ≥40 years
- Dementia
- Diabetes mellitus if blood pressure (BP) <135/80 mmHg
- Drug abuse
- Family violence
- Gestational diabetes mellitus
- Glaucoma
- Lung cancer
- Peripheral artery disease with the ankle-brachial index
- Suicide risk
- Thyroid disease
- Vitamin supplementation with A, C, E, multivitamins to prevent cancer and heart disease
- Vitamin D and calcium supplementation to prevent fractures: men, premenopausal women

C. Health Maintenance: Across the Ages—Aspirin

The role of aspirin in health maintenance and promotion varies according to whether it is used for primary or secondary/tertiary prevention. For the latter, it is generally beneficial (**Table 15-3**). For primary prevention it is not that simple (**Tables 15-4, 15-5, and 15-6**). The USPSTF recommends against the routine use of aspirin and nonsteroidal anti-inflammatory drugs (NSAIDs) to prevent colorectal cancer in persons at average risk for colorectal cancer (grade D recommendation).

D. Health Maintenance: Ages 18–39

Table 15-7 summarizes USPSTF grade A and grade B screening and counseling recommendations for average-risk 18–39-year-olds. Below the screening tests in focus are as follows: hypertension, cervical cancer, *Chlamydia*, lipid disorders, depression, tobacco, and specific screening for those at increased risk.

1. Hypertension—Hypertension is the most common condition seen in family medicine. It contributes to many adverse health outcomes, including premature deaths, heart attacks, renal insufficiency, and stroke. Blood pressure measurement identifies individuals at increased risk for cardiovascular disease. Treatment of hypertension decreases the incidence of cardiovascular disease events.

Hypertension is defined as elevated blood pressure, either systolic blood pressure (SBP) or diastolic blood pressure (DBP), on at least two separate occasions separated by one to several weeks. In persons

- *18–60 years of age*—elevation is either a SBP of ≥140 mmHg or a DBP of ≥90 mmHg.
- *≥60 years of age*—elevation is either a SBP of ≥150 mmHg or a DBP of ≥90 mmHg.
- *≥18 years of age with chronic kidney disease*—defined as an estimated or measured glomerular filtration rate of <60 mL/min per 1.73 m² in individuals aged <70 years–elevation is either a SBP of ≥140 mmHg or a DBP of ≥90 mmHg.
- Of *any age with albuminuria* (>30 mg of albumin/g of creatinine)—elevation is either a SBP of ≥140 mmHg or a DBP of ≥90 mmHg.

The Eighth Report of the Joint National Committee on Prevention, Detection, Evaluation, and Treatment of High Blood Pressure (JNC8) recommends screening every 2 years in persons with blood pressure of <120/80 mmHg and every year with systolic blood pressure of 120–139 mmHg or diastolic blood pressure of 80–90 mmHg. The American Heart Association (AHA) has issued similar recommendations beginning at age 20.

Hypertension should be treated. Treatment is addressed in Chapter 35.

2. Cervical cancer—Cervical cancer screening is discussed in detail in Chapter 27.

3. *Chlamydia* screening—The USPSTF recommends screening for *Chlamydia* infection in all sexually active women aged ≤24 years, or women aged ≥25 years at increased risk. The optimal screening interval for nonpregnant women is unknown. The CDC recommends at least annual screening for women at increased risk. *Chlamydia trachomatis* infection is the most common sexually transmitted bacterial infection in the United States. In women, genital infection

Table 15-3. Indications for aspirin (ASA) therapy summary of available guidelines & recent evidence in selected disease states and Concomitant Therapies

Topic	Available Guidelines and Recent Evidence

Diabetes secondary prevention	ADA Diabetes Guidelines 2010
	  Men > 50 (women > 60) years of age *and* one of the following: family history of CVD, smoking, hypertension, dyslipidemia, albuminuria
	Br Med J. 2009 meta-analysis
	  No difference in risk of major CV events, CV mortality, or all-cause mortality between ASA and placebo → role of ASA in this population questioned
	  Decreased risk of MI in men, but not in women (significant study heterogeneity)

Heart failure secondary prevention	ACC/AHA Update to Heart Failure Guidelines 2009 No recommendation at this time, due to controversial evidence Aspirin may negate the positive effect of angiotensin-converting enzyme (ACE) inhibitor therapy

Dual therapy (ASA + warfarin) secondary prevention	ACCP Antithrombotic and Thrombolytic Therapy Guidelines 2008
	  Patients with mechanical heart valves
	  1. And a history of coronary artery disease, peripheral arterial disease, or other risk factors for atherosclerotic disease (1B)
	  2. Who have additional risk factors for thromboembolism: atrial fibrillation, hypercoagulable state, or low ejection fraction (1B)
	    a. Consider if bioprosthetic heart valves and additional risk factors for thromboembolism (2C)
	    b. Particularly in patients with a history of atherosclerotic disease.
	    c. Following clopidogrel discontinuation in patients on triple therapy.
	    d. No dual therapy if at high risk for bleeding history of GI bleed or age > 80 (2C)

Dual antiplatelet therapy (ASA + clopidogrel) secondary and tertiary prevention	ACCP Antithrombotic and Thrombolytic Therapy Guidelines 2008: primary prevention
	  Recommend against routine use of aspirin and clopidogrel (1A)
	ACCP Antithrombotic and Thrombolytic Therapy Guidelines 2008: secondary prevention
	  NSTE ACS: clopidogrel × 12 months (1A)
	  Symptomatic coronary artery disease (2B)
	  PCI with bare-metal stent: clopidogrel × 12 months (1A)
	  PCI with drug-eluting stent: clopidogrel × 12 months (1B)
	  Indefinitely if low risk of bleeding and combination tolerable (2C)

Triple therapy (ASA + clopidogrel + warfarin) tertiary prevention	ACCP Antithrombotic and Thrombolytic Therapy Guidelines 2008
	  PCI with bare-metal stent and strong indication for warfarin: clopidogrel × 4 weeks (2C)
	  PCI with drug-eluting stent and strong indication for warfarin: clopidogrel × 12 months (2C)
	  Consider warfarin INR goal of 2.0–2.5

ACC, American College of Cardiology; ACCP, American College of Chest Physicians; ADA, American Diabetes Association; AHA, American Heart Association; CVD, cardiovascular disease; CV, cardiovascular; GI, gastrointestinal; MI, myocardial infarction; NSTE ACS, non–ST-elevated acute coronary syndrome; PCI, percutaneous coronary intervention.

ACCP 2008 Grades of Recommendation	1A	1B	1C	2A	2B	2C
Definition	Strong recommendation, high-quality evidence	Strong recommendation, moderate-quality evidence	Strong recommendation, low- or very-low-quality evidence	Weak recommendation, high-quality evidence	Weak recommendation, moderate-quality evidence	Weak recommendation, Low- or very-low-quality evidence

Table 15-4. Evidence for use of aspirin for primary prevention of cardiovascular events and associated increased risk of adverse events in men versus women.

Prevention Outcome & Increased Risk	Men	Women
Cardiovascular events	✓	✓
Myocardial infarctions	✓	
Ischemic stroke		✓
Cardiovascular mortality or all-cause mortality		
Hemorrhagic stroke	✓	
Gastrointestinal bleeding	✓	✓

Data from US Preventive Services Task Force. Aspirin for the prevention of cardiovascular disease: US Preventive Services Task Force recommendation statement. *Ann Intern Med.* 2009;150:396–404.

may result in urethritis, cervicitis, pelvic inflammatory disease (PID), infertility, ectopic pregnancy, and chronic pelvic pain. Infection during pregnancy is related to adverse pregnancy outcomes, including miscarriage, premature rupture of membranes, preterm labor, low birth weight, and infant mortality. The benefits of screening and subsequent treatment in high-risk pregnant and nonpregnant individuals are substantial.

The USPSTF identified no evidence of the benefits of screening women who are not at increased risk for *Chlamydia* infection. In this low-risk population it is moderately certain that the benefits outweigh the risks of screening to only a small degree. Nucleic acid amplification tests

(NAATs) for *Chlamydia* have high specificity and sensitivity as screening tests and may be used with either urine or vaginal swabs.

Screening of pregnant women for *Chlamydia* infection is recommended for all women at the first prenatal visit. For those who remain at increased risk or acquire a new risk factor, such as a new sexual partner, screening should be repeated during the third trimester.

4. Lipid disorders—Men aged >35 years should be screened for lipid disorders. This age may be reduced to 20 if there is an increased risk for coronary heart disease. Screening for women does not need to start until age 45.

The optimal interval for screening is uncertain. Reasonable options include every 5 years, with shorter intervals for those with risk factors (eg, diabetes mellitus) or lipid levels close to those warranting therapy.

High levels of total cholesterol (TC) and low-density lipoprotein-cholesterol (LDL-C) and low levels of high-density lipoprotein–cholesterol (HDL-C) are independent risk factors for coronary heart disease. The risk is highest in those with a combination of risk factors. Therefore, a careful review of the complete risk factor profile is necessary to assess the benefit of screening and subsequent lowering of high cholesterol levels with medications. (Please see Chapter 37 for a full discussion of lipid disorders.)

5. Depression screening—Depression is common and a leading cause of disability in both adolescents and adults. Screening for depression improves the accurate identification of depressed patients in primary care settings. The USPSTF concluded that the net benefit of screening adults for depression is higher (moderate) when staff-assisted depression care supports are in place to ensure accurate diagnosis, effective treatment, and follow-up. In the

Table 15-5. When to use aspirin for primary prevention of MI (men) and stroke (women) per age and 10-year Framingham risk for event.

Men (years)	10-year MI risk	< 45	45–59	60–69	70–79	> 80	Risk:benefit consideration for patients with GI risk
Women (years)	10-year stroke risk	<55	55–59	60–69	70–79	> 80	
Framingham Score	4–8%		✓			Evidence lacking	GI risk > benefit
	3–7%						
	9–11%		✓	✓		Evidence lacking	GI risk = benefit
	8–10%						
	>12%		✓	✓	✓	Evidence lacking	GI risk < benefit
	>11%						

Data from US Preventive Services Task Force. Aspirin for the prevention of cardiovascular disease: US Preventive Services Task Force recommendation statement. *Ann Intern Med.* 2009; 150:396-404.

Table 15-6. When to add proton pump inhibitor therapy to ASA.

Aspirin Therapy: Proton pump inhibitor therapy recommended based on gastrointestinal risk factors	
One of the following	**Two of the following**
Concomitant other NSAID use	**Age >60 years**
History of ulcer complication	**Corticosteroid steroid use**
History of ulcer disease	**Dyspepsia**
Concomitant antiplatelets	**Gastroesophageal reflux disease symptoms**
Concomitant anticoagulants	
History of gastrointestinal bleeding	

Data from Bhatt DL, Scheiman JS, Abraham NS, et al. ACCF/ACG/AHA 2008 Expert consensus document on reducing the gastro-intestinal risks of antiplatelet therapy and NSAID use. *Circulation.* 2008;118;1894-1909.

absence of such care supports, the net benefit may be small. Numerous formal screening tools are available, but there is insufficient evidence to recommend one tool over another. All positive screens should trigger a full diagnostic interview.

6. Tobacco use counseling—Cessation of tobacco use may be the single most important lifestyle intervention for the maintenance and improvement of health. All adults should be assessed for tobacco use and tobacco cessation interventions provided for those who use tobacco products. Tobacco use, cigarette smoking in particular, is the leading cause of preventable death in the United States, resulting in >400,000 deaths annually from cardiovascular disease, respiratory disease, and cancer. Smoking during pregnancy results in the deaths of approximately 1000 infants annually and is associated with an increased risk for premature birth and intrauterine growth retardation. Environmental tobacco smoke may contribute to death in ≤38,000 people annually.

Cessation of tobacco use is associated with a corresponding reduction in the risk of heart disease, stroke, and lung disease. Tobacco cessation at any point during pregnancy yields sub-stantial health benefits for the expectant mother and fetus.

Smoking cessation interventions, including brief (<10 minutes) behavioral counseling sessions and pharma-cotherapy delivered in primary care settings, are effective in increasing the proportion of smokers who successfully quit and remain abstinent for 1 year. Even minimal counseling interventions (<3 minutes) are associated with improved smoking cessation rates. One of several screening strategies aimed at engaging patients in smoking cessation discussions is the "5A" behavioral counseling framework:

1. *Ask* about tobacco use.
2. *Advise* to quit through clear personalized messages.
3. *Assess* willingness to quit.
4. *Assist* to quit.
5. *Arrange* follow-up and support.

7. Screening and counseling specifically for persons aged 18–39 years at increased risk—

- HIV—screen once for all persons aged 15–65 years, more for those at increased risk (A).
- Syphilis—screen for men and women at increased risk (A).
- BRCA mutation testing for breast and ovarian cancer (B).
- Gonorrhea—screen women who are pregnant or at increased risk (B).
- Healthy diet—screen adults with hyperlipidemia and other risk factors for coronary heart disease (CHD) (B).
- Intimate-partner violence—screen women of childbear-ing age (B).
- Sexually transmitted infections—provide behavioral counseling for sexually active adolescents and adults at increased risk (B).
- Skin cancer—provide behavioral counseling for children, adolescents, and young adults aged 18–24 years (B).
- Type 2 diabetes mellitus—screen men and women with sustained blood pressure of ≥135/80 mmHg (B).
- Lipid disorders in adults—screen women aged 20–44 and men aged 20-34 years at increased risk for CHD (B).

▶ **E. Health Maintenance: Ages 40–49 with Emphasis on Breast Cancer and Lipid Screening**

Tables 15-8, 15-9, and 15-10 summarize USPSTF recom-mendations for average-risk 40–49-year-olds.

1. Breast cancer—Please see Tables 15-9 and 15-10 and Chapter 27 for discussion of screening for breast cancer.

2. Lipid screening—All women aged ≥45 years should be screened for lipid disorders. Women aged 20–44 years should be screened if they are at increased risk for coronary heart disease (CHD). *Increased risk*, for this recommenda-tion, is defined by the presence of any of the following risk factors: diabetes, previous personal history of CHD or non-coronary atherosclerosis (eg, abdominal aorta aneurysm, peripheral artery disease, carotid artery stenosis), a family history of cardiovascular disease before age 50 years in male relatives or age 60 years in female relatives, tobacco use, hypertension, obesity (BMI >30). (Further discussion of dyslipidemia is found in section on health maintenance for ages 18–39 years (above) and in Chapter **XX**.)

Table 15-7. Health promotion & preventive screening for adults aged 18–39.

Grade	Recommended Health Promotion or Screening
A	**Asymptomatic bacteriuria**: screen—*pregnant women*
A	**Chlamydia**: Screen—*Women* Ages 24 and *Younger* OR Women Ages 25 and *Older* at Increased Risk
A	**Folic acid**: Supplementation—all *women* planning or capable of pregnancy
A	**HIV**: Screening—age 15–65 once, more frequently for high-risk people
A	**HIV**: Screen—*pregnant women*
A	**Hepatitis B virus**: Screen—*pregnant women*
A	**High Blood Pressure**: Screen—Adults 18 and Over
A	**Lipid disorders in adults**: Screen—men aged ≥35 years
A	**Rh(D) blood typing**: Screen—*pregnant women*, first pregnancy-related visit
A	**Syphilis**: Screen—*pregnant women*
A	**Syphilis**: Screen—men and women at increased risk
A	**Tobacco use**: Counsel and interventions for adults
A	**Tobacco use**: Counsel and interventions for *pregnant women*
B	**Alcohol misuse**: Screen and behavior counseling interventions in primary care—adults
B	**BRCA-related cancer**: Risk assessment, genetic counseling, and genetic testing—*women at increased risk*
B	**Breastfeeding**: Primary care interventions to promote—all *pregnant women and new mothers*
B	**Chlamydia**: Screen—*pregnant women* aged ≤24 years *or pregnant women* aged ≥25 years who are at increased risk
B	**Depression**: Screen—adolescents, aged 12–18 years, in clinical practices with systems of care
B	**Depression**: Screen—adults aged ≥18 years—when staff-assisted depression care supports are in place
B	**Gonorrhea**: Screening—pregnant women and women at increased risk
B	**Healthy diet**: Counsel—adult with hyperlipidemia and other risk factors for CVD
B	**Hepatitis C virus infection**: Screen—adults at high risk and adults born between 1945 and 1965
B	**Intimate-partner violence**: Screen—*women of childbearing age*
B	**Iron-deficiency anemia**: Screen—asymptomatic *pregnant women*
B	**Obesity**: Screen for and management of—all adults
B	**Rh(D) blood typing**: Screen—antibody testing unsensitized Rh(D-negative *pregnant women*
B	**Sexually transmitted infections**: Behavioral counseling—sexually active adolescents and adults at increased risk
B	**Skin cancer**: Behavioral counseling—persons aged 10–24 years
B	**Type 2 diabetes mellitus**: Screen men and women with sustained blood pressure >135/80 mmHg

Table 15-8. Health promotion & preventive screening for adults aged 40–49.

Intervention	Target Group,[a] Screening Interval[b]	Grade	Recommendation
Aspirin to prevent CVD[c]		A	Aspirin daily when the potential benefit due to a reduction in myocardial infarctions outweighs the potential harm due to an increase in gastrointestinal hemorrhage
Physical exam blood pressure (BP)	Every 1–2 years depending on BP	A	Screen every 2 years in persons with BP <120/80 mmHg and every year in persons with BP 120-130/80-90 mmHg
Testing Lipid disorders	Men > 35, Q5y Women > 45 if risk for CHD, every 5 years	A	For women, the risk factors include diabetes, previous personal history of CHD or non-coronary atherosclerosis, a family history of cardiovascular disease before 50 in males and 60 in females, tobacco, hypertension, obesity (BMI >30)
Pap smear	Every 1–3 years	A	Screen for cervical cancer in women who have been sexually active and have a cervix
HIV	If high risk	A	Risks include men having sex with men, unprotected sex with multiple partners, injection drug use, sex worker, history of sex with partners who are HIV+, bisexual, or injection drug users, history of STI, transfusion between 1978 and 1985
Syphilis	If high risk	A	Risks include men who have sex with men and engage in high risk sexual behavior, commercial sex workers, persons who exchange sex for drugs, and those in adult correctional facilities
Chlamydia	If high risk	A	Risks factors include a history of *Chlamydia* or other STI, new or multiple sexual partners, inconsistent condom use, and exchanging sex for money or drugs
Counsel Tobacco use		A	Ask all adults about tobacco use and provide tobacco cessation interventions for those who use tobacco products
Testing Mammogram	Against routine screening in normal-risk women aged 40–49 years	C	Offer mammography to an individual patient if she is at higher risk of breast cancer (http://www.cancer.gov/bcrisktool/), then screen biennially
Diabetes Mellitus Type 2	All with sustained blood pressure >135/80 mmHg	B	Screen asymptomatic adults with sustained blood pressure greater than 135/80 mmHg.
Counsel Obesity: BMI>30		B	Clinicians screen all adult patients for obesity and offer intensive counseling and behavioral interventions to promote sustained weight loss for obese adults
Alcohol misuse		B	Screen for risky or hazardous drinking and provide behavioral counseling interventions to reduce alcohol misuse by adults
Depression	If there are systems in place to ensure accurate diagnosis, effective treatment, and follow-up	B	Screening adults for depression in clinical practices that have systems in place to assure accurate diagnosis, effective treatment, and follow up
STI	If high risk	B	Screen adults with STI in past year or multiple current sexual partners

[a]Target group: in none noted, includes men and women aged 40–49.
[b]Screening interval: if none noted, unknown.
BMI, body mass index; CHD, coronary heart disease; CVD, cardiovascular disease; HIV, human immunodeficiency virus; Q5y, every 5 years; STI, sexually transmitted infection.
Data from USPSTF. *Screening for Breast Cancer. Recommendations and rationale.* US Preventive Services Task Force; Feb.2002 (available at http://www.ahrq.gov/clinic/3rduspstf/breastcancer/brcanrr.pdf).

Table 15-9. Insufficient evidence for clinical breast examinations and breast self-examinations.

Intervention	Target Group	Grade	Recommendation
Clinical breast exam	Women	I	Could not determine benefits of CBE alone or the incremental benefit of adding CBE to mammography
Breast self-exam	Women	D	Against teaching breast self-examination (BSE)

Data from USPSTF. *Screening for Breast Cancer. Recommendations and rationale.* US Preventive Services Task Force; Feb. 2002 (available at http://www.ahrq.gov/clinic/3rduspstf/breastcancer/brcanrr.pdf).

F. Health Maintenance: Ages 50–59

Table 15-11 summarizes USPSTF recommendations for average-risk 50–59-year-olds, with major changes in recommendations for prostate and lung cancer screening.

1. Colorectal cancer screening—This should occur from age 50 to 75 years using a variety of tests, as follows:

Sensitivity—Hemoccult II < fecal immunochemical tests < Hemoccult SENSA ≈ flexible sigmoidoscopy < colonoscopy

Specificity—Hemoccult SENSA < fecal immunochemical tests ≈ Hemoccult II < flexible sigmoidoscopy = colonoscopy

Screening with fecal occult blood testing, sigmoidoscopy, or colonoscopy reduces mortality, assuming 100% adherence to any of these regimens: (1) annual high-sensitivity fecal occult blood testing, (2) sigmoidoscopy every 5 years combined with high-sensitivity fecal occult blood testing

Table 15-10. USPSTF (2009) breast cancer screening recommendations in women using film mammography.

Population	Ages 40–49 Years	Ages 50–74 Years	Ages ≥75 Years
Recommendation	Do not screen routinely. Individualize decision to begin biennial screening according to the patient's context, risk and values.	Screen every 2 years	No recommendation
	Grade: C	Grade: B	Grade: I (insufficient evidence)
Risk assessment	Recommendation applies to women aged ≥40 years not at increased risk by virtue of a known genetic mutation or history of chest radiation. Increasing age is the most important risk factor for most women.		
Screening tests	Standardization of film mammography has led to improved quality. Refer patients to facilities certified under the Mammography Quality Standards Act (MQSA).		
Timing of screening	Evidence indicates that biennial screening is optimal. This preserves most of the benefit of annual screening and cuts the risk nearly in half. A longer interval may reduce the benefit.		
Benefit/riskbalance	There is convincing evidence that screening with film mammography reduces breast cancer mortality, with a greater absolute reduction for women aged 50–74 years than for younger women. Harms (risks) of screening include psychological risks, additional medical visits, imaging, and biopsies in women without cancer, inconvenience due to false-positive screening results, risks of unnecessary treatment, and radiation exposure. Risks seem moderate for each age group. False-positive results are a greater concern for younger women; treatment of cancer that would not become clinically apparent during a woman's life (overdiagnosis) is an increasing problem as women age.		
Nothing specific recommended (grade I)			Among women aged ≥75 years, evidence of benefit is lacking.

Table 15-11. Health promotion & preventive screening for adults aged 50–59.

USPSTF Grade	Recommended Health Promotion or Screening
A[a]	**Aspirin to prevent CVD** in **men:** Ages 45–79 years to reduce risk of MI when potential benefit outweighs potential harm of an increase in GI hemorrhage
A[a]	**Aspirin to prevent CVD** in **women:** Ages 55–79 years to reduce risk of ischemic strokes when potential benefit outweighs potential harm of an increase in GI hemorrhage
A[a]	**Cervical cancer:** Screen sexually active women aged ≤21 years Q3y as long as normal
A[a]	**Chlamydia:** Screen women aged ≤24 years or women aged ≥25 years who at increased risk
A	**Colorectal cancer:** Screen adults aged 50–75 years
A	**HIV:** Screen adults and adolescents aged 15-65 years once, more frequently for those with high-risk behaviors
A	**High blood pressure:** Screen adults aged ≥18 years
A	**Lipid disorders in adults:** Screen men aged ≥35 years
A	**Lipid disorders in adults:** Screen women ≥45, increased risk for CHD
A	**Syphilis:** Screen men and women at increased risk
A[a]	**Tobacco use:** Counseling and interventions for adults
B	**Alcohol misuse:** Screening and behavioral counseling
B	**BRCA mutation testing for breast and ovarian cancer:** Women, increased risk
B	**Breast cancer:** Preventive medication discussion—women, increased risk
B[a]	**Breast cancer:** Screening with mammography for women 50–74 years
B[a]	**Depression:** Screen adults aged ≥18 years when staff-assisted depression care supports *are* in place
B	**Gonorrhea:** Screen pregnant women and women at increased risk
B	**Healthy diet:** Counsel adults with hyperlipidemia and other risk factors for CVD
B	**Lung cancer:** Annual screening for lung cancer with low-dose computed tomography in adults ages 55–80 years who have a 30-pack/yr smoking history and currently smoke or have quit within the past 15 years; screening should be discontinued once a person has not smoked for 15 years or develops a health problem that substantially limits life expectancy or the ability or willingness to undergo curative lung surgery
B	**Obesity:** Screening and intensive counseling for obese men and women
B	**Sexually transmitted infections:** Behavioral counseling for sexually active adolescents and adults at increased risk
B	**Type 2 diabetes mellitus:** Screen men and women if sustained BP ≥135/80 mmHg
D[a]	**Prostate cancer screening**

CVD, cardiovascular disease; Q3h, every 3 hours.
[a]See earlier discussions and tables.

every 3 years, or (3) screening colonoscopy at intervals of 10 years. Evidence is insufficient regarding screening with fecal DNA or CT colonography.

For a more complete discussion of colorectal cancer screening, see Chapter **XX**.

2. Hypertension—Screen every 2 years if blood pressure is <120/80 mmHg and every year with systolic blood pressure of 120–139 mmHg or diastolic blood pressure of 80–90 mmHg.

3. Aspirin—Benefits must outweigh risks. See earlier discussion of acetylsalicylic acid (ASA) and Tables 15-3, 15-4, 15-5, and 15-6. Aspirin should not be initiated to prevent stroke in women aged <55 years of age. Aspirin should not be used to prevent colorectal cancer in persons at average risk for colorectal cancer.

4. Prostate cancer screening (USPSTF recommendation D)—As discussed earlier, an effective screening test should detect disease early, and early treatment should improve morbidity and mortality. There is no conclusive evidence that treatment of prostate cancers detected by screening improves outcomes. Recognition of the fact that most men *with prostate cancer* do not die and the limitations of currently available prostate screening tests has led to fluidity regarding the best prostate screening practices. As new data become available, the guidelines from major organizations seem to be increasingly similar with some nuances.

The USPSTF recommends against prostate cancer screening (recommendation D), based on their conclusion of the current evidence that there is very small potential benefit and significant potential risk from screening. The American Academy of Family Physicians (AAFP) supports the USPSTF guidelines.

The American Cancer Society (ACS) recommends that men make an informed decision with their physicians as to whether they should be tested for prostate cancer. Starting at age 50 years, men should discuss the pros and cons of testing with a physician. If they are African American or have a father or brother who had prostate cancer before age 65, men should discuss testing with a physician starting at age 45. If men decide to be tested, they should opt for the prostate-specific antigen (PSA) blood test with or without a rectal exam. How often they are tested will depend on their PSA level.

The American Urologic Association (AUA) guidelines are as follows:

- PSA screening in men under age 40 years is not recommended.
- Routine screening in men aged 40–54 years at average risk is not recommended.
- For men aged 55–69 years, the decision to undergo PSA screening involves weighing the benefits of preventing prostate cancer mortality in 1 man for every 1000 men screened over a decade against the known potential risks

associated with screening and treatment. For this reason, *shared decision making is recommended for men aged 55–69 years* who are considering PSA screening, and proceeding according to patients' values and preferences.

- To reduce the harms of screening, a routine screening interval of ≥2 years may be preferred over annual screening in those men who have participated in shared decision making and decided on screening. As compared to annual screening, it is expected that 2-year screening intervals will preserve most of the benefits and reduce the risk of overdiagnosis and false positives.
- Routine PSA screening is not recommended in men over age 70 or any man with a <10–15-year life expectancy.

The reasons for these changes away from the prior recommendations to screen are based on new, large, long-running studies. Also, epidemiologic data factor in as well. Prostate cancer is the most common nondermatologic cancer in US males. If they live to be 90 years old, one out of six US males will be diagnosed with prostate cancer. Risk factors for development of prostate cancer include advanced age, family history, and race. Nearly 70% of prostate cancer diagnoses occur in men aged ≥65 years. The risk of developing prostate cancer is nearly 2.5 times greater in men with a family history of prostate cancer in a first-degree relative. Rates of prostate cancer occurrence are lower in Asian and Hispanic males than in non-Hispanic Caucasian males. African-American men are at twice the risk of white men. While US men have an approximately 16% lifetime risk of being diagnosed with prostate cancer, they have only ~3% risk of dying from it.

Digital rectal examination (DRE) and prostate-specific antigen (PSA) testing are the most commonly used prostate cancer screening tools. Physician-performed DRE is limited in that it allows only a portion of the prostate gland to be palpated and has poor interrater reliability. Sensitivity of DRE is low (53–59%), and positive predictive value (PPV) is only 18–28%. The PPV of PSA for prostate cancer screening is similarly low, at ~30%. Proposed prostate cancer screening methods include using PSA cutoff of 4 ng/mL, measuring PSA velocity, and percent free PSA. No currently available data demonstrates a mortality benefit with any of these. Whether DRE adds value to PSA screening is debatable, if not doubtful. DRE should not be used as a standalone test to screen for prostate cancer.

Both DRE and PSA screening can lead to detection of clinically insignificant prostate cancers, exposing patients to undue psychological distress and potentially harmful procedures and treatments, such as biopsy and radical prostatectomy. Unfortunately, DRE and PSA screening can also miss aggressive prostate cancers.

5. Lung cancer screening—The USPSTF assigns a B recommendation to annual screening for lung cancer with low-dose computed tomography in adults aged 55–80 years who have a 30-pack/yr smoking history and currently smoke or have

Table 15-12. Health promotion and preventive screening for adults aged 60–74.

Group	Recommendations
Women 60–74 years	**Pap smear:** At least every 3 years (A) **Mammogram:** Every 1–2 years (B) **Colorectal cancer:** Screening[a] (A) **Osteoporosis screening**: All women aged ≥65 years and high-risk women starting at age 60: screen using DEXA or bone densitometry testing (B) **Weight and BMI:** Screen for obesity using BMI (body mass index) (B) **Blood pressure:** Annually for all adults (A) **Tobacco:** Counsel about quitting (A) **Alcohol:** Counsel to reduce alcohol misuse (B) **Aspirin chemoprevention:** Postmenopausal women and all with increased coronary heart disease risk (A)
Men 60–74 years	**Cholesterol:** Test every 5 years (A) **Abdominal aortic aneurysm (AAA):** Ultrasound once in men who have ever smoked (B,C) **Colorectal cancer:** Screening[a] (A) **Weight and BMI:** Screen for obesity using BMI (body mass index) (B) **Blood pressure:** Annually for all adults(A) **Tobacco:** Counsel about quitting (A) **Alcohol:** Counsel to reduce alcohol misuse (B)

[a]See colon cancer screening discussion in section on health maintenance for adults aged 50–59 years.

quit within the past 15 years. Screening should be discontinued once a person has not smoked for 15 years or develops a health problem that substantially limits life expectancy or the ability or willingness to undergo curative lung surgery. This has been a controversial recommendation because of concerns about radiation exposure (high false positive findings on initial screen leading to more CT scanning; the 25-year recommendation is based on studies of 3 years of screening), cost-benefit concerns, and the unsure role of screening in people who continue to smoke (eg, whether a negative screen will impede the desire to quit, whether a false-positive screen will result in increased quit rates). The AAFP has not endorsed this recommendation. Like all USPSTF recommendations, it will be reevaluated as new data emerge.

▶ G. Health Maintenance: Ages 60–74

Table 15-12 summarizes USPSTF recommendations for average-risk 60–74-year-olds.

Screening tests in focus: Abdominal aortic aneurysm (AAA) and osteoporosis.

1. Screening for abdominal aortic aneurysm (AAA), men only:

- One-time screening for AAA by ultrasonography in men aged 65–75 who have ever smoked (B).
- No recommendation for or against screening for AAA in men aged 65–75 years who have never smoked (C).
- Against routine screening for AAA in women (D), due to false-positive rate and lower prevalence of AAA.

2. Screening for osteoporosis in postmenopausal women:

- All women aged ≥65 years should be screened routinely for osteoporosis (B).
- Women at increased risk[1] for osteoporotic fractures should begin screening at age 60 (B).
- No recommendation for or against routine osteoporosis screening in postmenopausal women aged <60 or in women aged 60–64 years who are not at increased risk for osteoporotic fractures (C).

Screening should occur every 3 years even if treatment is initiated.

Osteoporosis Risk Assessment Tools

- Foundation on Osteoporosis Research and Education (FORE) 10-year Risk Calculator at https://riskcalculator.fore.org/default.aspx
- FRAX® WHO Fracture Risk Assessment Tool at http://www.shef.ac.uk/FRAX/tool.jsp?country=9
- The Osteoporosis Risk Assessment Instrument (ORAI) uses age, weight, and the use of estrogen as an aid to selecting postmenopausal patients for bone density testing (Cadarette, et al. 2000).

---

[1]Risk factors: Low body weight (<70 kg) is the single best predictor of low bone mineral density; next best is no current use of estrogen therapy; others supported by less evidence include smoking, weight loss, family history, decreased physical activity, alcohol or caffeine use, or low calcium and vitamin D intake.

Cadarette SM, Jaglal SB, Kreiger N, McIsaac WJ, Darlington GA, Tu JV. *Can Med Assoc J.* 2000;162(9):1289–1294.

▶ ## H. Health Maintenance: Age ≥75

Perhaps the most important aspect of health maintenance in people aged ≥75 years is lifestyle. HM recommendations for this age group are summarized in **Table 15-13** and discussed below.

In patients aged ≥75 years, health maintenance decisions become more complex. The focus remains both primary and secondary prevention; however, there are relatively few studies evaluating the utility and impact of HM interventions in this population. Therefore, it becomes increasingly important to work with geriatric patients to make informed, individualized HM decisions. Among patients aged ≥75 years, there exist wide variations in the number and severity of comorbid conditions, functional status, life expectancy, and

Table 15-13. Health promotion & preventive screening for adults aged ≥75 years.

Condition	USPSTF Recommendations (Grade)	Alternate Recommendations from Other Organizations
Tobacco abuse	Recommended (A)	
Alcohol misuse	Recommended (A)	
Nutrition screening and counseling	Recommended (B)—for patients with risk factors for cardiovascular disease	
Hypertension	Recommended (A)	
Hyperlipidemia	Recommended (A)	
Aspirin for prevention of cardiovascular disease	Recommended (A)—in men aged ≤79 years	
Aspirin for prevention of ischemic stroke	Recommended (A)—in women aged ≤79 years	
Diabetes	Recommended (B) for BP ≥135/80 mmHg	
Obesity	Recommended (B)	
Depression	Recommended (B)—if supportive care available	
Falls	Recommended (B)—use of exercise, physical therapy, vitamin D supplementation if high risk, community-dwelling	AGS: All older adults should be screened for falls within the last year
Colon cancer	Not recommended routinely (C),—consider in select patients aged 75–85 years; recommendation against (D) ages >85	ACG: Indefinite screening after age 50
Prostate cancer	Recommendation against (D)—PSA	AUA[a], ACS: DRE and PSA annually for men aged ≥50 years with life expectancy ≥10 years
Breast cancer	Neither for nor against (I)	AGS: mammogram every 3 years for adults aged ≥75 years if life expectancy ≥4 years[a]
Cervical cancer	Recommendation Against (I)	
Hearing Impairment	Neither for nor against (I)	
Vision impairment	Neither for nor against (I)	
Dementia	Neither for nor against (I)	Dementia

ACG, American College for Gastroenterology; ACS, American Cancer Society; AGS, American Geriatrics Society; AUA, American Urologic Association; CDC, Centers for Disease Control and Prevention; USPSTF, US Preventive Services Task Force.
[a]Guideline currently under revision.

Table 15-14. Immunizations for adults aged ≥18 years: general recommendations.

Age (yrs)	Tdap/Td Q10y	HPV 0, 2, 6 mo	Varicella 0, ≥4 wk Live[a]	Zoster 1 Dose Live[a]	MMR 1-2 Doses Live[a]	Influenza 1 Dose/yr Nasal=Live[a]	Pneumococcal 1 Dose	HAV 0, 6-12 mo	HBV 0, 1, 6 mo	Meningococcal 1-2 Doses (5 yr Apart)
18–39 →	Tdap × 1, then Td	Age ≥26	Patients without immunity		Patients without immunity	Nasal or IM				
Give →	√	√	√		√	√				
40–49 →	Tdap × 1, then Td		Patients without immunity		Patients without immunity	Nasal or IM				
Give →	√		√		√	√				
50–59 →	Tdap × 1, then Td		Patients without immunity		Patients without immunity	Nasal or IM				
Give →	√		√		√	√				
→	<65 Tdap × 1 then Td Q10y ≥65 Td only		Patients without immunity	√	Born before 1957 and without immunity	≥65 priority IM only	≥65: if received dose ≥65 and 5 y passed, give 2nd dose			
Give →	√		√	√	√	√	√			
>75 →	Td	+	Patients without immunity			IM				
Give →	√		√	√		√				

[a]Separate *live* vaccines by 28 days or give on the same day.

HAV, hepatitis A virus; HBV, hepatitis B virus; HPV, human papillomavirus; IM, intramuscularly; mo, months; Q10y, every 10 years; Td, tetanus + diphtheria; Tdap, tetanus + diphtheria + pertussis; wk, weeks; yr, years.

Table 15-15. Immunizations for adults aged ≥18 years: compelling and special indications.

Condition	Tdap/Td Every 10 years	HPV 0, 2, 6 months	Varicella 0, ≥4 week Live[a]	Zoster 1 Dose Live[a]	MMR 1-2 Doses Live[a]	Influenza 1 dose/year Nasal=Live[a]	Pneumococcal 1 Dose	HAV 0, 6-12 months	HBV 0, 1, 6 months	Meningococcal 1-2 Doses (5 years Apart)
Asthma							√			
Cigarette smoking							√			
Pregnancy	Tdap postpartum 2 years from last Td		Do not give; could cause harm	Do not give; could cause harm	Only postpartum; could cause harm before	√				
Health care workers	Tdap × 1, 2 years from last Td				2 doses (if not immune)	√		If work with HAV	√	
Contact with children	Infants <12 mo Tdap × 1, 2 years from last Td					Children <5 years				
International travel to certain countries					2 doses (if not immune)			√	√	√ 2 doses if residing in endemic countries
Students in post–secondary school					2 doses (if not immune)					Students living in dormitories
Immuno-suppressed						√	2 doses (5 years apart)			
Nursing home residents						√	√			
Certain chronic disease states[b]						√	√			
Renal disorders							2 doses (5 years apart)			
Asplenia							2 doses (5 years apart)			√
Chronic liver disease								√		
MSM								√	√	
Illegal drug use								√	√	

[a]Separate *live* vaccines by 28 days or give on the same day.
[b]Including chronic pulmonary, cardiovascular, hepatic, renal, hematological, neurologic, neuromuscular, or metabolic disorders (including diabetes).
HAV, hepatitis A virus; HBV, hepatitis B virus; HPV, human papillomavirus; MSM, men who have sex with men; Q10y, every 10 years; Td, tetanus + diphtheria; Tdap, tetanus + diphtheria + pertussis.
Data from Centers for Disease Control and Prevention. Recommended adult immunization schedule–United States, 2009. *MMWR* 2009;57(53).

patients' overall goals of care and preferences. Each of these factors must be considered when discussing HM interventions in older patients. Consideration of both benefits and risks of any HM intervention is also essential.

Guidelines regarding cancer screening in patients aged ≥75 years especially require individualized, patient-specific discussions and decisions. The United States Preventive Task Force (USPSTF) suggests that the benefits of colon cancer screening in adults aged 75–85 years do not outweigh the risks, and explicitly recommends against it in patients aged >85 years. The American College for Gastroenterology (ACG) recommends colon cancer screening beginning at age 50 and does not suggest when to discontinue screening.

For breast cancer screening, USPSTF recommends neither for nor against mammography in women aged ≥75 years. The American Geriatric Society (AGS) recommends screening mammography every 3 years after age 75 with no upper age limit for women with an estimated life expectancy of ≥4 years. The American Cancer Society (ACS) and USPSTF agree that older women with previously negative Pap results do not benefit from ongoing screening for cervical cancer after the age of 75.

Prostate cancer screening remains a controversial topic, with USPSTF advising against the use of prostate-specific antigen (PSA) for prostate cancer. A detailed discussion of prostate cancer and prostate cancer screening is included elsewhere in this chapter.

The American Geriatric Society recommends screening all older adults for a history of falls within the last year, and USPSTF recommends the use of exercise, physical therapy, and vitamin D supplementation in community-dwelling older adults at increased risk for falls. USPSTF recommends neither for nor against screening for vision impairment, hearing impairment or dementia in asymptomatic patients aged ≥75 years.

▶ I. Health Maintenance: Adult Immunizations

Tables 15-14 and **15-15** summarize the vaccination recommendations for adults.

American Cancer Society. *Cancer Facts and Figures, 2014* (available at http://www.cancer.org/research/cancerfactsstatistics/cancerfactsfigures2014/index; accessed Feb. 24, 2014).

American College of Cardiology Foundation/American Heart Association Task Force on Practice Guidelines. 2009 focused update incorporated into the ACC/AHA 2005 Guidelines for the Diagnosis and Management of Heart Failure in Adults. *Circulation.* 2009;119:e391–497.

American Geriatrics Society. *AGS Position Statement: Breast Cancer Screening in Older Women* (available at http://www.americangeriatrics.org/products/positionpapers/brstcncr.shtml; accessed Feb. 24, 2014).

American Urologic Association. *Prostate Specific Antigen Best Practice Statement: 2009 Update* (available at http://www.auanet.org/content/guidelines-and-quality-care/clinical-guidelines/main-reports/psa09.pdf; accessed March 25, 2013).

Becker R, et al. The primary and secondary prevention of coronary artery disease. *Chest.* 2008;133;S776–S814.

Bhatt DL, et al. ACCF/ACG/AHA 2008 expert consensus document on reducing the gastrointestinal risks of antiplatelet therapy and NSAID use. *Circulation.* 2008;118;1894–1909.

Buse JB, et al. Primary prevention of cardiovascular diseases in people with diabetes mellitus: a scientific statement from the American Heart Association and the American Diabetes Assocation. *Circulation.* 2007;115:114–126.

Catalona WJ, et al. Comparison of digitial rectal examination and serum prostate specific antigen in the early detection of prostate cancer: results of a multicenter clinical trial of 6,630 men. *J Urol.* 1994;11:1283–1290.

De Berardis G, et al. Aspirin for primary prevention of cardiovascular events in people with diabetes: meta-analysis of randomized controlled trials. *Br Med J.* 2009;339:b4531.

Esserman L, et al. Rethinking screening for breast cancer and prostate cancer. *JAMA.* 2009;302(15):1685–1692.

FORE https://riskcalculator.fore.org/default.aspx (accessed Feb. 24, 2014).

FRAX® http://www.shef.ac.uk/FRAX/tool.jsp?country=9 (accessed Feb. 24, 2014).

Jemal A, et al. Cancer statistics, 2007. *CA Cancer J Clin.* 2007;57:43–66.

Lanza FL, Chan FK, Quigley EM, and the Practice Parameters Committee of the American College of Gastroenterology. *Am J Gastroenterol.* 2009;104:728–738.

Lefevre M. Prostate cancer screening: let patients decide. *Am Fam Physician.* 2008:78(12):1388–1389.

Lim L, et al. Screening for prostate cancer in U.S. men; ACPM position statement on preventive practice. *Am J Prevent Med.* 2008; 34(2):164–170.

Lin K, et al. Benefits and harms of prostate-specific antigen screening for prostate cancer: an evidence update for the U.S. Preventive Services Task Force. *Ann Intern Med.* 2008;149:192–199.

Miller AB, Baines CJ, To T, Wall C. Canadian National Breast Screening Study: 1. Breast cancer detection and death rates among women aged 40 to 49 years. *Can Med Assoc J.* 1992; 147:1459–1476.

Mistry K, Cable G. Meta-analysis of prostate-specific antigen and digital rectal examination as screening tests for prostate carcinoma. *J Am Board Fam Practice.* 2003;16(2):95–101.

National Cancer Institute Surveillance Epidemiology and End Results Program. *Cancer Stat Fact Sheets—Cancer of the Prostate, 2006* (accessed Nov. 3, 2009 at http://seer.cancer.gov/statfacts/html/prost.html).

Rex DK, Johnson DA, Anderson JC, et al. American College of Gastroenterology Guidelines for Colorectal Cancer Screening 2008. *Am J Gastroenterol.* 2009;104(3):739–750.

Ross A, Clark M. Cancer screening in the older adult. *Am Fam Physician.* 2008;78(12):1369–1374.

Salem D, O'Gara P, Madias C. Valvular and structural heart disease. *Chest.* 2008;133;S593–S629.

Saslow D, et al. American Cancer Society Guideline for the Early Detection of Cervical Neoplasia and Cancer. *CA Cancer J Clin.* 2002;52:342–362.

Smith DS, Catalona WJ. Interexaminer variability of digital rectal examination in detecting prostate cancer. *Urology.* 1995; 45(1):689–697.

Smith R, et al. Cancer screening in the United States, 2009: a review of current American Cancer Society guidelines and issues in cancer screening. *CA Cancer J Clin.* 2009; 59:27–41.

Spalding, M, Sebesta S. Geriatric screening and preventive care. *Am Fam Physician.* 2008; 78(2):206–215.

Takahashi P, et al. Preventive health care in the elderly population: a guide for practicing physicians. *Mayo Clin Proc.* 2004; 79:416–427.

Terret C, et al. Effects of comorbidity on screening and early diagnosis of cancer in elderly people. *Lancet Oncol.* 2009; 10:80–87.

United States Preventive Services Task Force. *Guide to Clinical Preventive Services, Recommendations for Adults* (available at http://www.uspreventiveservicestaskforce.org/adultrec.htm; accessed Feb. 24, 2014).

Walter L, Covinsky K. Cancer screening in elderly patients: a framework for individualized decision making. *JAMA.* 2001; 285(21):2750–2756.

Websites

http://epss.ahrq.gov/ePSS/search.jsp (accessed 02/24/2014)
http://generalmedicine.suite101.com/article.cfm/screening_tests
http://info.cancerresearchuk.org/cancerstats/types/breast/riskfactors
http://www.ahrq.gov/CLINIC/uspstf/uspsprca.htm
http://www.ahrq.gov/clinic/uspstfix.htm
http://www.asccp.org/pdfs/consensus/algorithms_cyto_07.pdf
http://www.gptraining.net/training/tutorials/management/audit/screen.htm
http://www.immunizationed.org/default.aspx
http://www.auanet.org/advnews/press releases/article.cfm?articleNo=290
http://www.cancer.org/healthy/findcancerearly/cancerscreening-guidelines/american-cancer-society-guidelines-for-the-early-detection-of-cancer
http://www.cdc.gov/vaccines/schedules/hcp/adult.html
http://www.cdc.gov/vaccines/schedules/hcp/imz/adult.html
http://www.immunizationed.org/default.aspx
http://www.shef.ac.uk/FRAX/tool.jsp?country=9
http://riskcalculator.fore.org/default.aspx

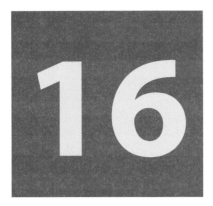

Preconception Care

Essam Demian, MD, FRCOG

Number of births in the United States (from preliminary data) in the year 2013 was 3,957,577. Although most infants are born healthy, it is of critical importance that the infant mortality rate in the United States ranks 34th among developed nations. Preconception care has been advocated as a measure to improve pregnancy outcomes. In 2006, the Centers for Disease Control and Prevention (CDC) published a report aimed at improving preconception care. This report outlined the following 10 recommendations: (1) individual responsibility across the life span, (2) consumer awareness, (3) preventive visits, (4) intervention for identified risks, (5) interconception care, (6) prepregnancy checkup, (7) health insurance coverage for women with low incomes, (8) public health programs and strategies, (9) research, and (10) monitoring improvements. Preconception care can be provided most effectively as part of ongoing primary care. It can be initiated during visits for routine health maintenance, during examinations for school or work, at premarital or family planning visits, after a negative pregnancy test, or during well child care for another family member.

Hamilton B E, et al. Births: preliminary data for 2013. *Natl Vital Stat Rep*. 2014;63(2):1.

Johnson K, et al. Recommendations to improve preconception health and health care-United States. A report of the CDC/ATSDR preconception care work group and the select panel on preconception care. *MMWR Recomm Rep*. 2006; 55(RR-6):1. [PMID: 16617292]

NUTRITION

A woman's nutritional status before pregnancy may have a profound effect on reproductive outcome. Obesity is the most common nutritional disorder in developed countries. Obese women are at increased risk for prenatal complications such as hypertensive disorders of pregnancy, gestational diabetes, and urinary tract infections. They are more likely to deliver large-for-gestational age infants and, as a result, have a higher incidence of intrapartum complications. Maternal obesity is also associated with a range of congenital malformations, including neural tube defects, cardiovascular anomalies, cleft palate, hydrocephalus, and limb reduction anomalies. Because dieting is not recommended during pregnancy, obese women should be encouraged to lose weight prior to conception.

On the other hand, underweight women are more likely than women of normal weight to give birth to low-birth-weight infants. Low birth weight may be associated with an increased risk of developing cardiovascular disease and diabetes in adult life (the "fetal origin hypothesis").

At the preconception visit, the patient's weight and height should be assessed and the history should include inquiries regarding anorexia, bulimia, pica, vegetarian eating habits, and use of megavitamin supplements.

Vitamin A is a known teratogen at high doses. Supplemental doses exceeding 5000 IU/d should be avoided by women who are or may become pregnant. The form of vitamin A that is teratogenic is retinol, not β-carotene, so large consumption of fruits and vegetables rich in β-carotene is not a concern.

***Folic acid supplementation* is recommended to avoid** *neural tube defects* (NTDs), including spina bifida, anencephaly, and encephalocele, which affect approximately 4000 pregnancies each year in the United States. Although anencephaly is almost always lethal, spina bifida is associated with serious disabilities including paraplegia, bowel and bladder incontinence, hydrocephalus, and intellectual impairment.

Since the mid-1980s, multiple studies conducted in various countries have shown a reduced risk of NTDs in infants whose mothers used folic acid supplements. The strongest evidence was provided by the Medical Research Council Vitamin Study in the United Kingdom, which showed a 72% reduction of recurrence of NTDs with a daily dose of 4 mg of folic acid started 4 weeks prior to conception and continued through the first trimester of pregnancy. Additionally, other studies showed a reduction in the incidence of first occurrence NTD with lower doses of folic acid (0.36–0.8 mg). Since 1992, the CDC has recommended that all women of childbearing age who are capable of becoming pregnant take 0.4 mg of folic acid daily to reduce the risk of NTDs in pregnancy. Also, patients who experienced a previous pregnancy affected by an NTD should be advised to take 4 mg of folic acid daily starting 1–3 months prior to planned conception and continuing through the first 3 months of pregnancy.

Prenatal folic acid may also have beneficial effects on child neurodevelopment. A study in 2013 revealed that maternal use of folic acid around the time of conception was associated with a lower risk of autistic disorder in children.

MRC Vitamin Study Research Group. Prevention of neural tube defects: results of the Medical Research Council Vitamin Study. *Lancet.* 1991; 338:131. [PMID: 1677062]

Stothard KJ, et al. Maternal overweight and obesity and the risk of congenital anomalies: a systematic review and meta-analysis. *JAMA.* 2009; 301(6):636. [PMID: 19211471]

Suren P, et al. Association between maternal use of folic acid supplements and risk of autism spectrum disorders in children. *JAMA.* 2013; 309(6):570. [PMID 23403681]

EXERCISE

An increasing number of women opt to continue with their exercise programs during pregnancy. Among a representative sample of US women, 42% reported exercising during pregnancy. Walking was the leading activity (43% of all activities reported), followed by swimming and aerobics (12% each).

Available data suggest that moderate exercise is safe for pregnant women who have no medical or obstetric complications. A meta-analysis review of the literature on the effects of exercise on pregnancy outcomes found no significant difference between active and sedentary women in terms of maternal weight gain, infant birth weight, length of gestation, length of labor, or Apgar scores.

Exercise may actually reduce pregnancy-related discomforts and improve maternal fitness and sense of self-esteem. The American College of Obstetricians and Gynecologists (ACOG) recommends that exercise in the supine position and any activity that increases the risk of falling (gymnastics, horseback riding, downhill skiing, and vigorous racquet sports) be avoided during pregnancy. Contact sports (such as hockey, soccer, and basketball) should also be avoided as they can result in trauma to both the mother and the fetus. Scuba diving is contraindicated during pregnancy because the fetus is at risk for decompression sickness. Absolute contraindications to exercise during pregnancy are significant heart or lung disease, incompetent cervix, premature labor or ruptured membranes, placenta previa or persistent second- or third-trimester bleeding, and preeclampsia or pregnancy-induced hypertension.

ACOG Committee on Obstetric Practice. ACOG Committee Opinion, no.267, Jan. 2002 (reaffirmed 2009): Exercise during pregnancy and the postpartum period. *Obstet Gynecol.* 2002; 99:171. [PMID: 11777528]

MEDICAL CONDITIONS

▶ Diabetes

Congenital anomalies occur 2–6 times more often in the offspring of women with diabetes mellitus and have been associated with poor glycemic control during early pregnancy. Preconceptional care with good diabetic control during early embryogenesis has been shown to reduce the rate of congenital anomalies to essentially that of a control population. In a meta-analysis of 18 published studies, the rate of major anomalies was lower among preconception care recipients (2.1%) than nonrecipients (6.5%).

According to the American Diabetes Association recommendations, the goal for blood glucose management in the preconception period and in the first trimester is to reach the lowest A_{1c} level possible without undue risk of hypoglycemia to the mother. A_{1c} levels that are less than 1% above the normal range are desirable. Suggested pre- and postprandial goals are as follows: before meals, capillary plasma glucose 80–110 mg/dL; 2 hours after meals, capillary plasma glucose <155 mg/dL.

Prior to conception, a baseline dilated eye examination is recommended, because diabetic retinopathy can worsen during pregnancy. Hypertension, frequently present in diabetic patients, needs to be controlled. Angiotensin-converting enzyme inhibitors, angiotensin receptor blockers, and diuretics should be avoided as they have been associated with adverse effects on the fetus. Insulin is used almost exclusively in pregnancy for patients with either type 1 or type 2 diabetes. Despite the emerging evidence about the safety of oral hypoglycemic drugs during pregnancy, the ACOG recommends limiting their use for control of type 2 diabetes during pregnancy until more data become available.

▶ Hypothyroidism

Approximately 2.5% of pregnant women in the United States have hypothyroidism. Before 12 weeks' gestation, the fetal thyroid is unable to produce hormones and the fetus is dependent on maternal thyroxine that crosses the placenta. During pregnancy, maternal thyroid hormone requirements increase as early as the fifth week of gestation, typically before the first obstetrical visit. Inadequately treated maternal hypothyroidism is associated with impaired cognitive function in the offspring, as well as pregnancy complications including increased rates of miscarriage, preeclampsia, placental abruption, preterm birth, and low birth weight. Treatment with levothyroxine should be optimized before conception in women with hypothyroidism, and these patients should be advised of the need for increased dosage should they become pregnant.

Epilepsy

Epilepsy occurs in 1% of the population and is the most common serious neurologic problem seen in pregnancy. There are approximately 1 million women of childbearing age with epilepsy in the United States, of whom, around 20,000 deliver infants every year. Much can be done to achieve a favorable outcome of pregnancy in women with epilepsy. Ideally, this should start before conception. Menstrual disorders, ovulatory dysfunction, and infertility are relatively common problems in women with epilepsy and should be addressed.

Women with epilepsy must make choices about contraceptive methods. Certain antiepileptic drugs (AEDs), such as phenytoin, carbamazepine, phenobarbital, primidone, and topiramate, induce hepatic cytochrome P450 enzymes, leading to an increase in the metabolism of the estrogen and progestin present in the oral contraceptive pills. This increases the risk of breakthrough pregnancy. The American Academy of Neurology recommends the use of oral contraceptive formulations with ≥50 μg of ethinyl estradiol or mestranol for women with epilepsy who take enzyme-inducing AEDs.

Both levonorgestrel implants (Norplant) and the progestin-only pill have reduced efficacy in women taking enzyme-inducing AEDs. Other AEDs that do not induce liver enzymes (eg, valproic acid, lamotrigine, vigabatrin, gabapentin, and felbamate) do not cause contraceptive failure.

Because many AEDs interfere with the metabolism of folic acid, all women with epilepsy who are planning a pregnancy should receive folic acid supplementation at a dose of 4–5 mg/d. Withdrawal of AEDs can be considered in any woman who has been seizure-free for at least 2 years and has a single type of seizure, normal neurologic examination and intelligence quotient, and an electroencephalogram that has normalized with treatment. Because the risk of seizure relapse is greatest in the first 6 months after discontinuing AEDs, withdrawal should be accomplished before conception. If withdrawal is not possible, monotherapy should be attempted to reduce the risk of fetal malformations. Offspring of women with epilepsy are at increased risk for intrauterine growth restriction, congenital malformations that include craniofacial and digital anomalies, and cognitive dysfunction. The term *fetal anticonvulsant syndrome* encompasses various combinations of these findings and has been associated with use of virtually all AEDs. Some recent studies have indicated a higher risk for birth defects as well as for language impairment in association with valproic acid compared with other AEDs, mainly carbamazepine and lamotrigine.

Phenylketonuria

Phenylketonuria (PKU) is one of the most common inborn errors of metabolism. It is associated with deficient activity of the liver enzyme phenylalanine hydroxylase, leading to an accumulation of phenylalanine in the blood and other tissues. If untreated, PKU can result in mental retardation, seizures, microcephaly, delayed speech, eczema, and autistic-like behaviors. All states have screening programs for PKU at birth. When diagnosed early in the newborn period and when treated with a phenylalanine-restricted diet, affected infants have normal development and can expect a normal life span.

Dietary control is recommended for life in individuals with PKU, especially in women planning conception. High maternal phenylalanine levels are associated with facial dysmorphism, microcephaly, developmental delay and learning difficulties, and congenital heart disease in the offspring.

The achievement of pre- and periconceptional dietary control with a phenylalanine-restricted diet has significantly decreased morbidity in the infants of women with hyperphenylalaninemia.

American Diabetes Association. Preconception care of women with diabetes. *Diabetes Care.* 2004; 27(suppl 1):S76. [PMID: 14693933]

Koch R, et al. The Maternal Phenylketonuria International Study: 1984–2002. *Pediatrics.* 2003; 112:1523. [PMID: 14654658]

GENETIC COUNSELING

The ideal time for genetic counseling is before a couple attempts to conceive, especially if the history reveals advanced maternal age, previously affected pregnancy, consanguinity, or family history of genetic disease.

Certain ethnic groups have a relatively high carrier incidence for certain genetic disorders. For example, Ashkenazi Jews have a 1:30 chance of being a carrier for Tay-Sachs disease, a severe degenerative neurologic disease that leads to death in early childhood. Carrier status can easily be determined by a serum assay for the level of the enzyme hexosaminidase A. Screening for Tay-Sachs disease is recommended prior to conception, because testing on serum is not reliable in pregnancy and the enzyme assay on white blood cells that is used in pregnancy is more expensive and labor-intensive. Couples of Ashkenazi Jewish ancestry should also be offered carrier screening for Canavan disease, cystic fibrosis, and familial dysautonomia before conception or during early pregnancy.

Cystic fibrosis (CF) is the most common autosomal recessive genetic disorder in the non-Hispanic white population, with a carrier rate of 1:25. It is characterized by the production of thickened secretions throughout the body, but particularly in the lungs and the gastrointestinal tract. As it is becoming increasingly difficult to assign a single ethnicity to individuals, the ACOG considers it reasonable to offer CF carrier screening to all couples regardless of race or ethnicity.

Other common genetic disorders for which there is a reliable screening test for carriers are sickle cell disease in African

Americans, β-thalassemia in individuals of Mediterranean descent, and α-thalassemia in Southeast Asians. Sickle cell carriers can be detected with solubility testing (Sickledex) for the presence of hemoglobin S. However, ACOG recommends hemoglobin electrophoresis screening in all patients considered at risk for having a child affected with a sickling disorder. Solubility testing is described as inadequate because it does not identify carriers of abnormal hemoglobins such as the β-thalassemia trait or the HbB, HbC, HbD, or HbE traits. A complete blood count with indices is a simple screening test for the thalassemias and will show a mild anemia with a low mean corpuscular volume.

Fragile X syndrome is the most common cause of mental retardation after Down syndrome and is the most common inherited cause of mental retardation. It affects approximately 1 in 3600 men and 1 in 4000–6000 women and results from a mutation in a gene on the long arm of the X chromosome. In addition to mental retardation, fragile X syndrome is characterized by physical features such as macroorchidism, large ears, a prominent jaw, and autistic behaviors. Preconception screening should be offered to women with a known family history of fragile X syndrome or a family history of unexplained mental retardation, developmental delay or autism.

American College of Obstetrics and Gynecology, Committee on Genetics. ACOG Committee Opinion, no. 486, April 2011. Update on carrier screening for cystic fibrosis. *Obstet Gynecol.* 2011; 117(4):1028. [PMID 21422883]

IMMUNIZATIONS

The preconception visit is an ideal time to screen for rubella immunity, because rubella infection in pregnancy can result in miscarriage, stillbirth, or an infant with congenital rubella syndrome (CRS). The risk of developing CRS abnormalities (hearing impairment, eye defects, congenital heart defects, and developmental delay) is greatest if the mother is infected in the first trimester of pregnancy. In 2005, the United States was the first country in the Americas to declare that it had eliminated endemic rubella virus transmission. However, because of international travel, imported cases of rubella and CRS can still occur.

Immunization should be offered to any woman with a negative rubella titer and advice given to avoid conception for 1 month due to the theoretical risk to the fetus. Inadvertent immunization of a pregnant woman with rubella vaccine should not suggest the need to terminate the pregnancy as there is no evidence that the vaccine causes any malformations or CRS.

If a pregnant woman acquires varicella before 20 weeks' gestation, the fetus has a 1–2% risk of developing fetal varicella syndrome, which is characterized by skin scarring, hypoplasia of the limbs, eye defects, and neurologic abnormalities. Infants born to mothers who manifest varicella 5 days before to 2 days after delivery may experience a severe infection and have a mortality rate as high as 30%.

At the preconception visit, patients who do not have a prior history of chickenpox and who are seronegative should be offered vaccination. In 1995, the live attenuated varicella vaccine was introduced and the recommended regimen for patients aged >13 years is two doses 4 weeks apart. Patients should avoid becoming pregnant for at least 4 weeks after the second dose.

Since 1988, the CDC has recommended universal screening of pregnant women for hepatitis B. Although hepatitis B vaccine can be given during pregnancy, women with social or occupational risks for exposure to hepatitis B virus should ideally be identified and offered immunization prior to conception.

LIFESTYLE CHANGES

▶ Caffeine

Caffeine is present in many beverages, in chocolate, and in over-the-counter (OTC) medications such as cold and headache medicines. One cup of coffee contains approximately 120 mg of caffeine, a cup of tea has 40 mg of caffeine, and soft drinks such as cola contain 45 mg of caffeine per 12-oz serving. Consumption of caffeine during pregnancy is quite common, but its metabolism is slowed. Cigarette smoking increases caffeine metabolism, leading to increased caffeine intake.

Several epidemiologic studies have suggested that caffeine intake may be associated with decreased fertility, increased spontaneous abortions, and decreased birth weight. As a result, in 1980, the FDA advised pregnant women to avoid caffeine during pregnancy. However, an extensive literature review of the effects of caffeine concluded that pregnant women who consume moderate amounts of caffeine (≤5–6 mg/kg daily) spread throughout the day and do not smoke or drink alcohol have no increase in reproductive risks.

▶ Tobacco

Between 12% and 22% of pregnant women smoke during pregnancy, subjecting themselves and their infants to numerous adverse health effects. Smoking during pregnancy has been associated with spontaneous abortion, prematurity, low birth weight, intrauterine growth restriction, placental abruption, and placenta previa, as well as an increased risk for sudden infant death syndrome (SIDS). Accumulating evidence also indicates that maternal tobacco use is associated with birth defects such as oral clefts and foot deformities. Paradoxically, smoking during pregnancy has reportedly been associated with a reduced risk of preeclampsia. However, the smoking-related adverse outcomes of pregnancy outweigh this benefit.

The use of nicotine-replacement products to facilitate smoking cessation has not been sufficiently evaluated during pregnancy to determine its safety. Nicotine gum is rated category C during pregnancy, while nicotine patches, inhaler, and nasal spray are category D. If nicotine replacement therapy is used during pregnancy, products with intermittent delivery (gum or inhaler) are preferred as they provide a smaller daily dose than continuous delivery products such as the patch. If the nicotine patch is used, it is recommended that it be removed at night to limit fetal nicotine exposure. Women who are contemplating pregnancy should be advised to quit smoking prior to conception, and nicotine replacement could then be prescribed. Smoking cessation either before pregnancy or in early pregnancy is associated with improvement in maternal airway function and an infant birth weight comparable to that observed among non-smoking pregnant women.

▶ **Alcohol**

In 1981, the surgeon general of the United States recommended that women abstain from drinking alcohol during pregnancy and when planning a pregnancy, because such drinking may harm the fetus. Nevertheless, approximately 1 in 13 pregnant women will drink alcohol during pregnancy and 1 in 71 will binge-drink.

The most severe consequence of exposure to alcohol during pregnancy is fetal alcohol syndrome (FAS), characterized by a triad of prenatal or postnatal growth retardation, central nervous system (CNS) neurodevelopmental abnormalities, and facial anomalies (short palpebral fissures, smooth philtrum, thin upper lip, and midfacial hypoplasia). FAS is the major preventable cause of birth defects and mental retardation in the Western world. In the United States, the prevalence of FAS is estimated to be between 0.5 and 2 cases per 1000 births.

Some ethnic groups are disproportionately affected by FAS. American Indians and Alaska Native populations have a prevalence of FAS 30 times higher than white populations. It also appears that binge drinking produces more severe outcomes in offspring than more chronic exposure, possibly because of *in utero* withdrawal and its concomitant effects.

At the preconception visit, physicians should counsel their patients that there is no safe level of alcohol consumption during pregnancy and that the harmful effects on the developing fetal brain can occur at any time during pregnancy. High alcohol consumption in women has also been associated with infertility, spontaneous abortion, increased menstrual symptoms, hypertension, and stroke. Mortality and breast cancer are also increased in women who report drinking more than two alcoholic beverages daily.

▶ **Illicit Drugs**

Illicit drug use during pregnancy remains a major health problem in the United States. Among pregnant women aged 15–44 years, 4.4% report using illicit drugs. At the preconception visit, all patients should be questioned about drug use and offered counseling, referral, and access to recovery programs.

Marijuana is the most frequently used illicit drug in pregnancy. It does not appear to be teratogenic in humans, and there is no significant association between marijuana usage and preterm birth or congenital malformations. Prenatal exposure to marijuana is associated with increased hyperactivity, impulsivity, and inattention symptoms in children at age 10 years.

Cocaine use during pregnancy has been associated with spontaneous abortion, premature labor, intrauterine growth restriction, placental abruption, microcephaly, limb reduction defects, and urogenital malformations. Initial reports that suggested "devastating" outcomes for prenatal exposure to cocaine have not been substantiated. A meta-analysis of 36 studies concluded that cocaine exposure *in utero* has not been demonstrated to affect physical growth and that it does not appear to independently affect developmental scores from infancy to age 6 years.

Maternal use of heroin and other opiates is associated with low birth weight due to premature delivery as well as intrauterine growth restriction, preeclampsia, placental abruption, fetal distress, and SIDS.

Infants born to heroin-dependent mothers often develop a syndrome of withdrawal known as *neonatal abstinence syndrome* within 48 hours of delivery. Neonatal withdrawal is characterized by CNS hyperirritability, respiratory distress, gastrointestinal dysfunction, poor feeding, high-pitched cry, yawning, and sneezing. Methadone has long been used to treat opioid dependence in pregnancy because of its long half-life. It has been associated with increases in birth weight. However, the use of methadone is controversial because more than 60% of neonates born to methadone-maintained mothers require treatment for withdrawal. Also, a substantial number of patients on methadone maintenance continue to use street narcotics and other illicit drugs. Buprenorphine, a partial opiate agonist, may have important advantages over methadone, including fewer withdrawal symptoms and a lower risk of overdose.

Benowitz N, Dempsey D. Pharmacotherapy for smoking cessation during pregnancy. *Nicotine Tobac Res.* 2004;6(suppl 2):S189. [PMID: 15203821]

Christian MS, Brent RL. Teratogen update: evaluation of the reproductive and developmental risks of caffeine. *Teratology.* 2001;64:51. [PMID: 11410911]

Substance Abuse and Mental Health Services Administration. *Results from the 2010 National Survey on Drug Use and Health: Summary of National Findings.* NSDUH Series H-41, HHS Publication No. (SMA) 11-4658. Rockville, MD: Substance Abuse and Mental Health Services Administration; 2011.

SEXUALLY TRANSMITTED DISEASES

The latest estimates suggest that there are up to 19 million new cases of sexually transmitted diseases (STDs) in the United States each year. The preconception visit is a good opportunity to screen for genital infections such as *Chlamydia,* gonorrhea, syphilis, and HIV.

Chlamydia and gonorrhea are two of the most prevalent STDs, and both are often asymptomatic in women. In pregnancy, both *Chlamydia* and gonorrhea have been associated with premature rupture of membranes, preterm labor, postabortion and postpartum endometritis, and congenital infection.

Infants whose mothers have untreated *Chlamydia* infection have a 30–50% chance of developing inclusion conjunctivitis and a 10–20% chance of developing pneumonia. Inclusion conjunctivitis typically develops 5–14 days after delivery and is usually mild and self-limiting. Pneumonia due to *Chlamydia* usually has a slow onset without fever and can have a protracted course if untreated. Long-term complications may be significant. Ophthalmia neonatorum is the most common manifestation of neonatal gonococcal infection. It occurs 2–5 days after birth in up to 50% of exposed infants who did not receive ocular prophylaxis. Corneal ulceration may occur, and unless treatment is initiated promptly, the cornea may perforate, leading to blindness.

Congenital syphilis occurs when the spirochete *Treponema pallidum* is transmitted from a pregnant woman with syphilis to her fetus. Untreated syphilis during pregnancy may lead to spontaneous abortion, nonimmune hydrops, stillbirth, neonatal death, and serious sequelae in liveborn infected children. In 2011, a total of 360 cases of congenital syphilis were reported in the United States, a decrease from 387 cases in 2010.

Women are increasingly affected by HIV. In untreated HIV-infected pregnant women, the risk of mother-to-child transmission varies from 16% to 40%. However, it is possible to dramatically reduce the transmission rates by using highly active antiretroviral therapy (HAART) during pregnancy, by offering elective cesarean delivery at 38 weeks if the viral load at term is higher than 1000 copies/mL, and by discouraging breastfeeding. In developed countries, transmission rates as low as 1–2% have been achieved. (For more information concerning sexually transmitted diseases, see Chapter 14.)

Centers for Disease Control and Prevention (CDC). *2011 Sexually Transmitted Diseases Surveillance* (available at http://www.cdc.gov/std/stats11/Surv2011.pdf)

Medications

Therapeutic regimens for chronic illnesses are best modified, when possible, in the preconception period to include those drugs that have been used the longest and have been determined to pose the lowest risk.

Antihypertensives

Women with chronic hypertension who are receiving angiotensin-converting enzyme inhibitors or angiotensin receptor blockers should be advised to discontinue them before becoming pregnant or as soon as they know that they are pregnant because of the possible hazards to the fetus. These drugs can result in fetal renal impairment, anuria leading to oligohydramnios, intrauterine growth restriction, hypocalvaria, persistent patent ductus arteriosus, and stillbirth. Thiazide diuretics can be continued through conception and pregnancy if they were used before pregnancy as they do not adversely affect pregnancy outcomes.

Anticoagulants

Warfarin (Coumadin) readily crosses the placenta and is a known human teratogen. The critical period for fetal warfarin syndrome is exposure during weeks 6–9 of gestation. This syndrome primarily involves nasal hypoplasia and stippling of the epiphyses. Later drug exposure may also be associated with intracerebral hemorrhage, microcephaly, and mental retardation. In patients who require prolonged anticoagulation therapy, discontinuing warfarin in early pregnancy and substituting heparin will reduce the incidence of congenital anomalies, because heparin does not cross the placenta.

Antithyroid Drugs

Both propylthiouracil and methimazole are effective in the management of hyperthyroidism in pregnancy. Propylthiouracil is generally the preferred agent because in addition to inhibition of tetraiodothyronine (T_4) synthesis, it also inhibits the peripheral conversion of T_4 to triiodothyronine (T_3). Methimazole crosses the placenta in larger amounts and has been associated with aplasia cutis, a congenital defect of the scalp. If the patient is taking methimazole, it is reasonable to switch to propylthiouracil prior to conception.

Isotretinoin

Isotretinoin is indicated for severe recalcitrant nodular acne unresponsive to conventional therapy. As many as 50% of fetuses exposed to the drug develop severe congenital anomalies of the ears, CNS, heart, and thymus. In 2005, the FDA approved a computer-based risk management program called "iPledge" to prevent fetal exposure to isotretinoin (report available at http://www.ipledgeprogram.com). Female patients of childbearing age must have two negative pregnancy tests and use two appropriate forms of contraception before starting therapy. They also have to wait at least a month before considering pregnancy after completing a course of isotretinoin.

Risk Categories

The FDA has defined five risk categories (A, B, C, D, and X) that are used by manufacturers to rate their products for use during pregnancy.

A. Category A

Controlled studies in women fail to demonstrate a risk to the fetus in the first trimester (and there is no evidence of risk in later trimesters), and the possibility of fetal harm appears remote (eg, folic acid and thyroxine).

B. Category B

Either (1) animal reproduction studies have not demonstrated fetal risk but no controlled studies in pregnant women have been conducted, or (2) animal reproduction studies have shown an adverse effect (other than a decrease in fertility) that was not confirmed in controlled studies in women in the first trimester and there is no evidence of risk in later trimesters (eg, acetaminophen, penicillins, and cephalosporins).

C. Category C

Either (1) studies in animals have revealed adverse effects on the fetus (teratogenic, embryocidal, or other) but no controlled studies in women have been reported, or (2) studies in women and animals are not available. Drugs should be given only if the potential benefit justifies the potential risk to the fetus (eg, acyclovir and zidovudine).

D. Category D

Positive evidence of human fetal risk exists, but the benefits from use in pregnant women may be acceptable despite the risk, especially if the drug is used in a life-threatening situation or for a severe disease for which safer drugs cannot be used or are ineffective (eg, tetracycline and phenytoin).

E. Category X

Either (1) studies in animals or humans have demonstrated fetal abnormalities, (2) evidence of fetal risk exists on the basis of human experience, or (3) both possibilities 1 and 2, and the risk of using the drug in pregnant women clearly outweighs any possible benefit. The drug is contraindicated in women who are or may be pregnant (eg, isotretinoin, misoprostol, warfarin, and statins).

OCCUPATIONAL EXPOSURES

An increasing number of women are entering the workforce worldwide, and most are in their reproductive years. This has raised concerns for the safety of pregnant women and their fetuses in the workplace. The preconception visit is the best time to identify and control exposures that may affect parental health or pregnancy outcome. The three most common occupational exposures reported to affect pregnancy are video display terminals, organic solvents, and lead.

▶ Videodisplay Terminals

In 1980, a cluster of four infants with severe congenital malformations was reported in Canada. The cluster was linked to the fact that the mothers had all worked with videodisplay terminals (VDTs) during their pregnancy, at a newspaper department in Toronto. Many epidemiologic studies have since investigated the effects of electromagnetic fields emitted from VDTs on pregnancy outcome. Most studies found only equivocal or no associations of VDTs with birth defects, preterm labor, and low birth weight. Thus, it is reasonable to advise women that there is no evidence that using VDTs will jeopardize pregnancy.

▶ Organic Solvents

Organic solvents constitute a large group of chemically heterogeneous compounds that are widely used in industry and common household products. Occupational exposure to organic solvents can result from many industrial applications, including dry cleaning, painting, varnishing, degreasing, printing, and production of plastics and pharmaceuticals. Smelling the odor of organic solvents is not indicative of a significant exposure, because the olfactory nerve can detect levels as low as several parts per million, which are not necessarily associated with toxicity. A meta-analysis of epidemiologic studies demonstrated a statistically significant relationship between exposure to organic solvents in the first trimester of pregnancy and fetal malformations. There was also a tendency toward an increased risk for spontaneous abortion. Women who plan to become pregnant should minimize their exposure to organic solvents by routinely using ventilation systems and protective equipment.

▶ Lead

Despite a steady decline in average blood levels of lead in the US population in recent years, approximately 0.5% of women of childbearing age may have blood levels of lead of >10 μg/dL. The vast majority of exposures to lead occur in artists using glass staining and in workers involved in paint manufacturing for the automotive and aircraft industries. Other occupational sources of exposure to lead include smeltering, printing, and battery manufacturing. The most worrisome consequence of low to moderate lead toxicity is neurotoxicity. A review of the literature suggested that low-dose exposure to lead *in utero* may cause developmental deficits in the infant. However, these effects seem to be reversible if further exposure to lead is avoided. It is crucial to detect and treat lead toxicity prior to conception because the chelating agents used (dimercaprol, ethylenediaminetetraacetate, and penicillamine) can adversely affect the fetus if used during pregnancy.

DOMESTIC VIOLENCE

Domestic violence is increasingly recognized as a major public health issue. In the United States, 1.5 million women are raped or physically assaulted by an intimate partner every year. Domestic violence crosses all socioeconomic, racial, religious, and educational boundaries. Even physicians are not immune; in a survey, 17% of female medical students and faculty had experienced abuse by a partner in their adult life, an estimate comparable to that of the general population. Victims of domestic violence should be identified preconceptionally, because the pattern of violence may escalate during pregnancy. The prevalence of domestic violence during pregnancy ranges from 0.9% to 20.1%, with most studies identifying rates between 3.9% and 8.3%. Whereas violence in nonpregnant women is directed at the head, neck, and chest, the breasts and the abdomen are frequent targets during pregnancy. Physical abuse during pregnancy is a significant risk factor for low birth weight and maternal complications of low weight gain, infections, anemia, smoking, and alcohol or drug usage. If it is identified that a patient is the victim of domestic violence, the physician should assess her immediate safety and make timely referrals to local community resources and shelters.

deLahunta EA, Tulsky AA. Personal exposure of faculty and medical students to family violence. *JAMA*. 1996;275(24):1903. [PMID 8648871]

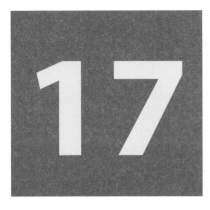

Prenatal Care

Martin Johns, MD
Gregory N. Smith, MD

Many family physicians assist pregnant women and deliver their infants as a routine part of their practice. In 2012, 15% of surveyed family physicians delivered babies and averaged 20 deliveries per year. In rural areas, 17% of family physicians delivered babies. Many more family physicians provide prenatal care without assisting in the delivery. Practicing maternity care provides an opportunity to establish relationships with an entire family, developing lifelong continuity of care. It is also a time for initiating preventive care and adopting a healthier lifestyle by making better dietary choices, quitting smoking, and abstaining from alcohol. The goal of prenatal care is to promote the birth of a healthy baby while also promoting the health of the mother and minimizing risk to her.

General Considerations

There are several key components to prenatal care including the establishment of an accurate gestational age and estimated date of delivery, the initial assessment of maternal risk factors for the development of complications, the ongoing assessment of maternal and fetal health and well-being, and patient education. Pregnant women receive 13–15 office visits for a typical low-risk pregnancy when care begins in the first trimester. After her initial visit a woman will see her provider every 4 weeks until 28 weeks' gestation, and then every 2 weeks until 36 weeks' gestation, followed by weekly visits until delivery. Women at higher risk for complications, or those who develop complications in pregnancy, may be seen more frequently. Despite a general acceptance and widespread adoption of prenatal care, there is little evidence that demonstrates proven effectiveness in reducing maternal and fetal morbidity and mortality. Observational studies comparing women who receive prenatal care and those who do not are confounded by selection bias regarding socioeconomic status, maternal education, substance abuse and other factors that affect health and risk status. A 2010 Cochrane review comparing fewer prenatal visits with the standard schedule demonstrated that

in high-income countries there was no difference in perinatal mortality in the reduced visit group; however, there was increased perinatal mortality in the reduced visit group in low-income countries. Women in all countries were less satisfied with the reduced-visits schedule. Further research to determine and define "adequate" prenatal care is ongoing.

Carroli G, Dowswell T, Duley L, et al. Alternative versus standard packages of antenatal care for low-risk pregnancy. *Cochrane Database of Systematic Reviews.* 2010, Issue 10. Art. No.: CD000934. DOI: 10.1002/14651858.CD000934.pub2

PRENATAL VISITS

Initial Visit

The initial visit should include a detailed history and physical exam establish an accurate estimated date of confinement (EDC) and identify risk factors that will require additional testing and monitoring (**Table 17-1**). History of the current pregnancy should include establishing the date of the last menstrual period (LMP). According to Nagle's rule, the average pregnancy is 280 ± 14 days from a reliable last menstrual period (LMP). Criteria for a reliable LMP include previous regular menstrual cycles of 28–35 days' length, an LMP that is normal in length, and a normal amount of menstrual flow for a patient who was off hormonal contraception for 3 months. If dates are uncertain, consider early ultrasound (US), as US-determined crown-rump length in the first trimester is accurate to within 3–5 days and helps establish estimated gestational age (EGA). However, an US done after the first trimester is no more accurate that a reliable LMP. Therefore, attention to clinical markers of EGA throughout the pregnancy is important.

Obstetrical history obtained at this visit includes date of previous pregnancies; length of gestation; method of delivery; length of labor; any complications during pregnancy, labor, and the postpartum period; and sex, size, and viability

Table 17-1. Initial prenatal visit: basic components.

1. History of current pregnancy: assessment of gestation age and symptoms
2. Prior obstetrical history
3. Gynecologic history
4. Past medical history; chronic illnesses, surgeries, medications, allergies, immunizations
5. Social history: alcohol, drugs, tobacco, occupation, home situation
6. Screen for depression and intimate-partner violence
7. Family/genetic history: ethnic background, genetic and congenital defects (include the father's children with other mothers)
8. Physical exam: general and pelvic with attention to uterine size
9. Testing: routine and other tests if indicated by history or exam (see Table 17-5)
10. Risk assessment
11. Patient education (see text)

of infant. Additionally, gynecological history describes menarche, menstrual history, prior STDs, gynecological surgeries, and treatments for infertility.

In addition to establishing LMP, the maternity practitioner should ask about the frequently seen symptoms of pregnancy: nausea, vomiting, fatigue, and breast tenderness. If they resolve prior to the end of the first trimester, suspicion for an impending miscarriage is heightened, especially when accompanied by vaginal bleeding and/or cramping. Presence of any febrile illness subsequent to the LMP should increase concern for viral illnesses that can affect the pregnancy. Women who are not immune to rubella or varicella or who have been exposed to erythema infectiosum (also known as "fifth disease") should have acute and convalescent IgM and IgG titers. A manifestation of the classic rashes associated with these diseases in conjunction with elevated titers signifies resolving infection. Infection with these viruses in nonimmune gravidas puts the fetus at risk and requires careful monitoring of fetal growth. Referral for a maternal fetal medicine evaluation should be considered.

Exploring the patient's medical history for any chronic problems is important. Preexisting medical conditions such as hypertension, thyroid disease, diabetes, and asthma, as well as psychiatric conditions such as depression and bipolar disorder can all impact the outcome of the pregnancy as well as other less common conditions. Reviewing medications taken prior to the diagnosis of pregnancy and ongoing medication usage allows timely risk assessment. Switching a patient from medications that are contraindicated in pregnancy to medications that are recognized as safe should be accomplished during the first visit. The benefits of maintaining patients on medications that control conditions such as asthma will outweigh the risks, as asthma exacerbations can be quite problematic during pregnancy. Allergies to medications should be reviewed and updated to ensure that the patient will not be inadvertently exposed to any harmful medications.

Review of the patient's immunization status is done at the first prenatal visit. During the flu season all pregnant patients without a contraindication to the flu vaccine should be immunized with the current influenza vaccine strain as the gravid patient is at increased risk for severe complications of flu. Patients not immune to rubella will need to be identified to ensure that they receive this attenuated live virus vaccine postpartum. The CDC has now recommended that all women should be vaccinated during the 3rd trimester with the Tdap vaccine to reduce risk of maternal infection by pertussis during the early postpartum period as well as maximize passive immunization of the fetus. Fathers-to-be and others who will have close contact with the infant after delivery should be encouraged to be immunized as well.

Family history should be reviewed with the patient. Securing a history of genetic or familial congenital abnormalities is critical. It is particularly important to determine the ethnic background of the patient and the father and also to ascertain whether the father has previously sired other children with any genetic or congenital defects.

Patients from certain ethnic groups are at increased risk for genetic diseases, Ashkenazi Jews, Cajuns, and others should be offered screening if not done as part of preconceptual counseling.

Asking the patient about tobacco, alcohol, and drug use should always be addressed during the initial visit. Cessation of these substances should be encouraged and patients referred to support sources in the community to help with efforts to quit. Patients with active use of opioids should be referred for conversion to methadone or suboxone and outpatient maintenance programs. The practitioner should ascertain current job status to determine whether any adaptations will be needed as the pregnancy progresses. As pregnancy increases the risk for domestic violence, the patient and her partner should be screened psychologically and, when appropriate, offered support and referral. Screening for depression with a standard "two-question screen" should be done at the initial visit and at least once each trimester to reduce the risk of postpartum depression. Patients who answer at least one question positive should then be administered an Edinburgh Postnatal Depression Test or PHQ-9 (the standardized nine-item Patient Health Questionnaire) to determine the presence or absence of depression. Patients who meet criteria for depression should be offered counseling and medication.

A thorough physical examination should be performed, including a pelvic exam to rule out any abnormalities that would preclude vaginal delivery. A speculum exam should be done to identify cervical infection or pathology and to complete Papanicolao screening. Bimanual exam facilitates comparison of uterine size with EGA as well as determination of the presence of other anatomic abnormalities. First-trimester uterine size should be consistent with EGA on the basis of LMP or other dating parameters. Uterine size approximated in centimeters is reliable. If uterine size is significantly inconsistent with the historically determined EGA, the practitioner should perform an ultrasound to determine the discrepancy. Clinical pelvimetry to determine adequacy and shape of the pelvic inlet, midpelvis, and outlet can be done during this initial bimanual exam. This exam, however, is unreliable in determining the likelihood of vaginal delivery.

After the initial history and physical examination are done, the practitioner provides trimester-appropriate patient education and determines patient risk for less-than-optimal outcomes. The healthy patient with minimal risk can receive usual counseling, routine laboratory testing, and routine follow-up. Patients with an increased risk for genetic diseases or congenital abnormalities can be referred to genetics consultants for further evaluation. Patients with obstetrical or chronic medical problems should be referred to maternal fetal medicine specialists to help with management or transfer of care.

▶ Subsequent Visits

Follow-up visits allow the maternity practitioner to determine the presence of any problems that would increase risk, address patient concerns, and cultivate the relationship with the patient (**Table 17-2**). In addition to eliciting patient questions or concerns, the practitioner should evaluate the following symptoms (possible causes in parentheses):

- Vaginal bleeding (spontaneous abortion, placenta previa, placental abruption, ectopic pregnancy, threatened abortion)
- Dysuria [urinary tract infection (UTI)]
- Cramping (threatened abortion, preterm labor)
- Headache or visual changes (preeclampsia, migraine)
- Nausea and vomiting (multiple feti or preeclampsia after first trimester)
- Vaginal discharge [sexually transmitted infections (STIs), rupture of membranes]
- Abdominal pain (ectopic, threatened abortion, biliary colic, preeclampsia)

The presence of any of these symptoms should prompt further investigation to determine the cause and appropriate

Table 17-2. Subsequent visits.

1. Patient concerns
2. Focused symptoms review
3. Ongoing alcohol, tobacco, or drug use identified at first visit
4. Depression and intimate-partner violence screens each trimester
5. Vitals: blood pressure, weight
6. Exam: fundal height, fetal heart tones, estimated fetal weight, and presentation
7. Testing (see Table 17-5)
8. Risk assessment
9. Patient education (see text)

intervention. Additionally, the practitioner should ask about fetal movement, which is normally noted between 18 and 20 weeks. Once present, any decrease in frequency should prompt further investigation immediately. Vital signs include weight and blood pressure. Practitioner-based intervention or referral to a nutritionist is indicated for patients with excessive weight gain. Blood pressures of >140/90 mmHg suggest pregnancy-induced hypertension or preeclampsia and necessitate further workup to determine cause. Physical exam should include measurement of fundal height, fetal heart tones (FHTs), and presentation and size of fetus by Leopold's maneuvers (after 32 weeks). Fundal height is a reliable predictor of gestational age. The fundus will reach the umbilicus at 20 weeks. It additionally will be 1 cm above the midline of the superior symphysis for each week of pregnancy during weeks 20–36. For a uterus that is rotated, one should measure in the midline directly across from the uterine fundus. If uterine size varies by >2 cm above or below the EGA, one should look for a cause. Consider polyhydramnios and macrosomia if above the expected fundal height, or oligohydramnios or intrauterine growth restriction (IUGR) if below the expected fundal height. By 34–36 weeks, fetal presentation can be determined. If breech is suspected or presentation is uncertain, an US should be performed to clarify presentation. For persistent breech presentation, referral for external version should be considered at 37–38 weeks to reduce risk of a cesarean section. Additional examination of other body systems should be guided by patient complaints elicited during the interview.

Social issues identified in the initial visit should be reevaluated at subsequent visits. Patients with ongoing tobacco, alcohol, or drug use should be queried at each visit and counseled to quit. Screening for depression should be done each trimester. Patients with a history of intimate-partner violence should be assessed frequently because the risk increases as pregnancy progresses.

ULTRASOUND

The use of ultrasound (US) in prenatal care has revolutionized the diagnosis and treatment of fetal conditions during gestation. Additionally, most mothers-to-be expect to have an ultrasound at 18–20 weeks EGA to determine the gender of the fetus while completing the anatomic screen (covered by most insurers regardless of clinical indication). Studies have shown that routinely performed US does not improve outcome versus clinically indicated US for suspected abnormalities in the mother or fetus (**Table 17-3**). Abnormalities identified on ultrasound will require follow-up or referral to obstetrical and/or maternal-fetal medicine (MFM) consultants for management as clinically indicated.

One particular US for the fetus is the biophysical profile (BPP), which is done to assess fetal status (**Table 17-4**). It is most commonly used to assess the fetus when the mother has gestational diabetes requiring medication, preeclampsia,

Table 17-3. Common maternal and fetal indications for ultrasound studies.

Maternal Indications	Fetal Indications
Uncertain LMP	Fetal number
Uncertain dating	Fetal presentation
Vaginal bleeding	Decreased fetal movement
Pelvic pain	Fetal viability
Threatened abortion	Aneuploidy
Ectopic pregnancy	Abnormal AFP
Uterine abnormalities	Polyhydramnios/oligohydramnios
Diabetes	IUGR
Hypertensive disorders	Macrosomia
Placenta previa	Biophysical profile
Placental abruption	Postdates (missed due dates)
Size not equal to EGA	Follow-up abnormalities on routine anatomic scan

Data from Ewigman BG, Crane JP, Frigoletto FD, et al. Effect of prenatal ultrasound screening on perinatal outcome. RADIUS study group. *N Engl J Med.* 1993; 329(12): 821-827.

Table 17-4. Scoring and management for the biophysical profile (BPP).

BPP Score	Risk of Death within 1 Week	Management
10/10 or 8/10 normal amniotic fluid volume 8/8 (no NST)	1/1,000	No fetal intervention indicated[a]
8/10 with abnormal amniotic fluid volume	89/1,00	Assess for RoM[b] and fetal renal status if normal delivery for fetal indications
6/10 normal fluid	Variable	If term delivery indicated; if remote from term, reassess 24 hours; if ≤6, deliver for fetal indication
6/10 abnormal fluid	89/1,000	Deliver for fetal indication
4/10	91/1,000	Delivery indicated
2/10	125/1,000	Delivery indicated
0/10	600/1,000	Delivery indicated

[a]Intervention for maternal or obstetrical indications (eg, postdates, hypertensive disorders).
[b]Range of motion (fetal).
Data from Manning FA. Dynamic ultrasound-based fetal assessment: the fetal biophysical profile score. *Clin Obstet Gynecol.* 1995;38(1):26-44.

or is past the due date. There are four components of the BPP ultrasound: fetal movement, fetal tone, fetal breathing, and amniotic fluid volume. These measurements are combined with the results of a nonstress test (NST). Scoring for each is either 2 for normal or 0 for abnormal result. Management based on BPP score is given in Table 17-4. Ultrasound information is best combined with clinical information based on history and examination to help guide appropriate decision making.

PRENATAL TESTING

Routine Tests in Prenatal Care

Women undergo a standard battery of diagnostic tests as part of routine prenatal care. Routine prenatal testing and the gestational ages at testing are listed in **Table 17-5**.

Urine Glucose & Protein Testing

Urine dipstick testing for glucose and protein traditionally has been performed at every prenatal visit to screen for gestational diabetes and preeclampsia. This continues to be standard care in most offices; however, there is no evidence of improved outcome or increased diagnosis of either preeclampsia or gestational diabetes through routine testing versus urine testing based on indications such as elevated blood pressure. Pregnant women whose blood pressures are elevated should undergo urine testing for protein in the form of a spot urine protein: creatinine ratio, followed by 24-hour urine protein testing if indicated. Urine testing for gestational diabetes has an unacceptably low sensitivity (7–36%) and positive predictive value (7–27%).

Alto WA. No need for glycosuria/proteinuria screen in pregnant women. *J Fam Practice.* 2005;54(11):978–983. [PMID: 16266604]
Gribble RK, Meier PR, Berg RL. The value of urine screening for glucose at each prenatal visit. *Obstet Gynecol.* 1995; 86(3): 405–410. [PMID: 7651652]
Rhode MA, Shapiro H, Jones OW 3rd. Indicated vs routine prenatal urine chemical reagent strip testing. *J Reprod Med.* 2007; 52(3):214–219. [PMID: 17465289]

Screening for Gestational Diabetes

Gestational diabetes affects 5% of pregnancies in the United States and causes significant maternal and fetal morbidity. Women with gestational diabetes have higher rates of preeclampsia, operative deliveries, shoulder dystocia, and subsequent development of type 2 diabetes. These outcomes may be improved with appropriate diagnosis and treatment of diabetes during pregnancy. All women should be screened for gestational diabetes between 24 and 28 weeks' gestation. The most common approach in the United States is a 1-hour screening glucose challenge test followed by diagnostic testing for women with abnormal test results. The glucose challenge test measures plasma glucose 1 hour after a 50-g

Table 17-5. Routine prenatal tests.

Test	Indication	When Obtained	Additional Notes
Blood type and Rh status	Prevention of alloimmunization	Initial visit	
Antibody screen	Prevention of fetal hydrops	Initial visit	RhD-negative women with a negative antibody screen should receive RhoGam at 28 weeks' gestation
Hemoglobin	Anemia	Initial visit	Women with anemia should receive iron supplementation and repeat testing after 6 weeks; consider repeat testing at 28 weeks universally
Hemoglobin electrophoresis	Hemoglobinopathy screening	Initial visit	Testing based on race alone is not reliable in areas of ethnic diversity
Cystic fibrosis screening	Testing for heterozygous carriers of common cystic fibrosis genes	Initial visit	Although not necessary to test universally, information on testing should be made available to all patients
HIV	Prevention of neonatal transmission	Initial visit	Repeat at 36 weeks for women at highest risk for infection (commercial sex workers) or in areas of high prevalence
RPR	Prevention of congenital syphilis	Initial visit	Repeated at 26–28 weeks
Rubella antibody titer	Prevention of congenital rubella syndrome in future pregnancies	Initial visit	Best obtained prior to pregnancy when vaccination is safe; vaccination should occur postpartum if patient is not immune
Hepatitis B	Prevention of neonatal hepatitis B	Initial visit	Infants born to chronic carriers of hepatitis B should receive hepatitis B immune globulin (HBIg) and vaccination against hepatitis B within 12 hours of life
Gonorrhea	Prevent neonatal transmission	Initial visit	Repeat at 36 weeks for women at high risk for reinfection or in areas of high prevalence
Chlamydia	Decrease preterm labor, prevent neonatal transmission	Initial visit	Repeat at 36 weeks for women at high risk for reinfection or in areas of high prevalence
Urine culture	Detect asymptomatic bacteriuria	11–16 weeks	Treatment of positive cultures with antibiotics should be followed by repeat testing to demonstrate eradication
1-hour glucola (50 g)	Screening for gestational diabetes	24–28 weeks	Women at increased risk for diabetes due to obesity, prior history of gestational diabetes, or strong family history of diabetes should be tested early and then retested at 28 weeks
Group B β-streptococcus culture	Screening for the presence of group B β-streptococcus	35–36 weeks	Bacteria antibiotic sensitivities should be obtained for women allergic to penicillin to guide intrapartum antibiotic therapy; clindamycin is preferred if bacteria is sensitive

oral glucose load. Women with abnormal 1-hour testing then require a diagnostic 3-hour oral glucose tolerance test (OGTT). This test uses a 100-g oral glucose load after an overnight fast with fasting, 1-, 2-, and 3-hour measurements. More than one abnormal measurement on OGTT is diagnostic of gestational diabetes.

Women at high risk for gestational diabetes due to obesity, a prior history of gestational diabetes, or a strong family history of diabetes should be screened for diabetes as early in

pregnancy as possible with a 1-hour 50-g oral glucose test and a hemoglobin A1c. Abnormal 1-hour testing should be followed by a 3-hour OGTT. High-risk women whose test results are negative before 24 weeks' gestation should be rescreened at 24–28 weeks' gestation with a 1-hour 50-g glucose test.

Women diagnosed with gestational diabetes are at a high risk for the development of type 2 diabetes over the next several years after their pregnancy. They should receive counseling on lifestyle measures to reduce the risk of type 2 diabetes. Follow-up screening for type 2 diabetes begins at the 6-week postpartum visit with a 2-hour 75-g oral glucose test (OGT). If negative, the ADA recommends that women continue to be screened for diabetes every 3 years.

Blumer I, Hader E, Hadden DR, et al. Diabetes and pregnancy: an endocrine society clinical practice guideline. *J Clin Endocrinol Metab*. 2013; 98(11):4227–4449.

Getahun D, Nath C, Ananth CV, et al. Gestational diabetes in the United States: temporal trends 1989 through 2004. *Am J Obstet Gynecol*. 2008; 198(5):525,1–e5. [PMID: 18279822]

Moyer VA. Screening for gestational diabetes mellitus. U.S. Preventive Services Task Force Recommendation Statement. *Ann Intern Med*. 2014.

Practice Bulletin no. 137: Gestational diabetes mellitus. *Obstet Gynecol*. 2013; 122(2 Pt 1):406-416.

Serlin DC, Lash RW. Diagnosis and management of gestational diabetes mellitus. *Am Fam Physician*. 2009; 80(1): 57-62 (review). [PMID: 19621846]

Screening for Birth Defects

Down syndrome is the most common chromosomal abnormality encountered in a live birth and the most common etiology of congenital intellectual disability, affecting 1 out of every 629 live births in the United States. The prevalence of Down syndrome is affected primarily by maternal age.

Second-Trimester Genetic Screening

Serum testing for Down syndrome can be performed between 16 and 20 weeks' gestation in the form of the quadruple (quad) screen. The quad screen involves measuring levels of α-fetoprotein, intact β-human chorionic gonadtropin (β-hCG), inhibin A, and unconjugated estriol. Quad screening has an 81% sensitivity rate for Down syndrome.

First-Trimester Genetic Screening

Screening for Down syndrome in the first trimester involves both ultrasound testing for nuchal translucency (NT) and serum measurement of β-hCG and pregnancy-associated plasma protein A (PAPP-A). NT is a fluid collection seen at the back of the neck. It is larger in babies with Down syndrome and is also present in several other structural anomalies such as congenital cardiac defects, diaphragmatic hernias, and abdominal wall defects. First-trimester testing has a sensitivity of 82–87% with a 5% false-positive rate.

Special training is required to perform NT screening. It is still not available in all parts of the country. Furthermore, NT measurements cannot always be made in the first trimester, depending on the position of the fetus.

Sequential First- & Second-Trimester Screening

Combining first- and second-trimester screening tests will increase sensitivity for Down syndrome. In sequential screening, women are screened for Down syndrome in the first trimester. If those results indicate a high risk for Down syndrome, genetic counseling and confirmation testing is offered. If the test indicates low risk, women can then obtain a second-trimester α-fetoprotein level, which is combined with the first-trimester results to calculate a final risk. Sequential screening increases sensitivity for detecting Down syndrome to 95% with a 5% false-positive rate. Women with positive screening tests should be referred for invasive testing via amniocentesis (second trimester) or chorionic villous sampling (first semester) if available.

ACOG Committee on Practice Bulletins. ACOG Practice Bulletin no.77: screening for fetal chromosomal abnormalities. *Obstet Gynecol*. 2007; 109(1):217–227. [PMID: 17197615]

Malone F, Canick JA, Ball RH, et al. First- and Second-Trimester Evaluation of Risk (FASTER) Research Consortium. First-trimester or second-trimester screening, or both, for Down's syndrome. *N Engl J Med*. 2005; 353(19):2001–2011. [PMID: 16282175]

Resta RG. Changing demographics of advanced maternal age (AMA) and the impact on the predicted incidence of Down syndrome in the United States: implications for prenatal screening and genetic counseling. *Am J Med Genet*. 2005;133(1):31–36. [PMID: 15637725]

PATIENT EDUCATION

Patient education is an integral part of prenatal care. Beginning with the initial prenatal visit, there are many important pregnancy-related topics to discuss with women. Many women and their partners also take an active role in learning all they can through books and the Internet. It is helpful for providers to be able to recommend good, accurate resources for patients and their families. Many offices provide written and web-based content to augment what is taught during the visit. Topics covered during visits are focused on anticipatory guidance and vary by trimester.

First Trimester

During the first trimester and specifically at the initial visit, topics often reviewed involve an overview of the practice, dietary and nutritional counseling, patient safety, and lifestyle modifications. Women should receive information regarding the setup of the practice, after-hours phone numbers, members of the care team, and patient expectations. As miscarriage is common, the warning signs and symptoms of impending pregnancy loss should be reviewed.

Dietary counseling includes recommendations on weight gain on the basis of the woman's prepregnancy body mass index (BMI). The Institute of Medicine (IOM) recommendations for weight gain in pregnancy is a helpful clinical tool, but final recommendations should be individualized to the patient. Women should eat a well-balanced diet during pregnancy that is approximately 50% carbohydrates, 20% protein, and 30% fat. There is no benefit to protein supplementation. Women have an increased caloric requirement of approximately 150 cal during the first trimester, 300 cal during the second trimester, and 500 cal in the third trimester. However, the goal should be for healthy food choices and to avoid the idea of "eating for two." All women should take a prenatal vitamin daily, primarily for folic acid to prevent neural tube defects. Folic acid supplementation should be initiated prior to pregnancy if possible, at a dose of 400 μg daily. This is the dose found in most prenatal vitamins. Women also have increased requirements for iron during pregnancy. In non-anemic patients a prenatal vitamin should supply all the iron that they require (~15–30 mg elemental iron).

Dietary counseling should also focus on foods to avoid during pregnancy. Certain fish species contain high levels of mercury and should be avoided during pregnancy. These include shark, swordfish, and king mackerel. The FDA recommends that ≤6 oz of solid white tuna be consumed weekly or ≤12 oz of canned light tuna. Other foods to avoid include unpasteurized dairy products, such as unpasteurized cheeses, undercooked meats, and uncooked delicatessen meats, due to the risk for foodborne infections and illness. Caffeine should be limited to <300 mg daily (2–3 cups of coffee), although data on caffeine and adverse pregnancy outcomes are mixed.

Along with dietary hazards, women should also avoid exposure to infections such as influenza, varicella, parvovirus B19, cytomegalovirus, toxoplasmosis, and other infections associated with animals. Environmental and work exposures to toxic substances should be reviewed with the patient, including tobacco, alcohol, and illicit drug exposure and use. Most women can continue working right up to their due date, but those with very physically demanding jobs may have to stop working, especially if they are at risk for preterm labor. Intimate partner violence affects ≤20% of pregnant women, and abuse often worsens during pregnancy. All women should be asked about the safety of their home confidentially but directly. Providers should have a working knowledge of the community resources available in their area for victims of intimate partner violence.

Lifestyle changes associated with pregnancy are a common source of questions, especially regarding sexual activity, exercise, and travel. Most couples can continue normal sexual relations throughout pregnancy but will often have to adjust positions because of the gravid uterus. Sexual intercourse is contraindicated in placenta previa, cervical insufficiency, and preterm labor.

Mild to moderate exercise is safe during pregnancy for most women. Women who are inactive prior to pregnancy can be encouraged to engage in mild exercise to promote physical health and well-being. Low-impact activities such as swimming, water aerobics, and walking are good forms of exercise in pregnancy. Women who were physically active prior to pregnancy can maintain similar levels of exercise

during pregnancy with some caveats; specifically, they should avoid activities that could increase the risk of falls and abdominal trauma such as downhill skiing and horseback riding and avoid activities that put heavy stress on the abdominal muscles such as pilates. As their center of gravity changes during pregnancy, runners should also be cautious to avoid falls. Maintaining adequate hydration and avoiding overheating are also important considerations. Exercise plans should be individualized by prepregnancy fitness.

Airline travel is safe for women with uncomplicated pregnancies up to 36 weeks' gestation. During the flight, women should wear seat belts when seated, maintain adequate hydration, and move around the cabin as much as possible to avoid venous thromboembolism. Car safety is especially important during pregnancy. Motor vehicle accidents are a leading cause of maternal morbidity and mortality and a common cause for placental abruption. Seat belts must be worn at all times. The lap belt should be worn low across the hips, under the uterus. The shoulder belt should go above the fundus and between the breasts. When taking long-distance car rides it is important to make frequent stops.

▶ **Second & Third Trimesters**

Patient education during subsequent visits involves reinforcement of previous recommendations, especially with regard to health and safety such as tobacco, alcohol, drug use, and domestic violence. Anticipatory guidance on the physiologic changes of pregnancy such as heartburn, leg swelling, and hemorrhoids should be covered. Signs and symptoms of preterm labor should be reviewed regularly along with warning signs and symptoms of preeclampsia. Fetal movement monitoring and "kick counts" should be reviewed. Up to 15% of women will call their physicians at some point during the third trimester because of perceived decreased fetal movement. Perform kick counts by having a woman eat something containing carbohydrates and then lie on her left side in a quiet room. With this technique, 10 movements over 2 hours is considered normal fetal movement.

Exclusive breastfeeding, as recommended by the WHO for the first 6 months of life, should be encouraged because of the many benefits to the mother and the baby. Women and their partners are often encouraged to sign up for childbirth classes if available. These classes allow for better understanding of the delivery hospital, the labor process, and development of a birth plan. Options for labor anesthesia and analgesia should be discussed during the third trimester.

REFERRAL & MANAGEMENT OF HIGHER-RISK PATIENTS

When pregnant women develop conditions that require higher levels of monitoring and care, it is essential for family physicians to have a close working relationship with their obstetrical consultants. The AAFP-ACOG liaison committee has published recommendations for consultations between family physicians and obstetrician-gynecologists. Guidelines for consultation in the antepartum and peripartum period for women who develop high-risk conditions should be clearly established on the basis of local referral patterns and availability of obstetrician-gynecologists and maternal-fetal medicine specialists. All family physicians and obstetricians on the medical staff should agree to these guidelines for the best care of patients. Decisions regarding consultation or transfer of care should be delineated at the time of consultation as well as explained to the patient.

AAFP-ACOG Joint Statement on Cooperative Practice and Hospital Privileges (available at http://www.aafp.org/about/policies/all/aafp-acog.html; accessed Feb. 2, 2014).

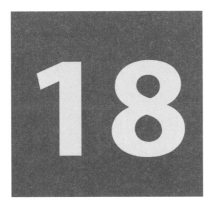

Contraception

Susan C. Brunsell, MD

General Considerations

According to the 2006–2010 National Survey of Family Growth (NSFG), approximately one-half of all pregnancies in the United States were unintended. These rates have remained relatively unchanged since 1995. However, changes in contraceptive method use among married, non-Hispanic white women have contributed to a significant decline in the proportion of unintended births among this group. Sixty-two percent of women of reproductive age are currently using contraception. Of women using a contraceptive method, the most common methods used are the oral contraceptive pills (28%) and female sterilizations (27%). Use of intrauterine devices has increased since 1995, from 0.8% to 5.6%, whereas fewer women report that their partners are using condoms as their current most effective means of contraception. Addressing family planning and contraception is an important issue for providers of care to reproductive-age women. Because of the wide range of contraceptive options available, it is important that health care providers maintain currency with the recent advances concerning counseling, efficacy, safety, and side effects.

Jones J, Mosher W, Daniels K. *Current Contraceptive Use in the Unites States, 2006-2010, and Changes in Patterns of Use Since 1995.* National Health Statistics Reports no 60. Hyattsville, MD: National Center for Health Statistics; 2012.

COMBINED ORAL CONTRACEPTIVES

According to the 2006–2010 NSFG, the combined oral contraceptive pill is the leading contraceptive method among women, with 28% of women between the ages of 15–44 choosing the pill. The availability of lower-dose combination oral contraceptives (COCs) (<50 μg ethinyl estradiol) has provided many women a highly effective, safe, and tolerable method of contraception.

Combined oral contraceptives suppress ovulation by diminishing the frequency of gonodotropin-releasing hormone pulses and halting the luteinizing hormone surge. They also alter the consistency of cervical mucus, affect the endometrial lining, and alter tubal transport. Most of the antiovulatory effects of COCs derive from the action of the progestin component. The estrogen doses are not sufficient to produce a consistent antiovulatory effect. The estrogenic component of COCs potentiates the action of the progestin and stabilizes the endometrium so that breakthrough bleeding is minimized. When administered correctly and consistently, they are >99% effective at preventing pregnancy. However, failure rates are as high as 8–10% during the first year of typical use. Noncompliance is the primary reason cited for the difference between these rates, frequently secondary to side effects such as abnormal bleeding and nausea.

Hormonal Content

The estrogenic agent most commonly used in COCs is ethinyl estradiol (EE), in doses ranging from 20 to 35 μg. Mestranol, which is used infrequently, is less potent than ethinyl estradiol such that a 50-μg dose of mestranol is equivalent to 30–35 μg of ethinyl estradiol. It appears that decreasing the dose of estrogen to 20 μg reduces the frequency of estrogen-related side effects, but increases the rate of breakthrough bleeding. In addition, there may be less margin for error with low-dose preparations such that missing pills may be more likely to result in breakthrough ovulation.

Multiple progestins are used in COC formulations. Biphasic and triphasic oral contraceptives, which vary the dose of progestin over a 28-day cycle, were developed to decrease the incidence of progestin-related side effects and breakthrough bleeding, although there is no convincing evidence that multiphasics indeed cause fewer adverse effects. As with estrogens, some progestins (norethindrone and levonorgestrel) are biologically active, while others are prodrugs that are activated by metabolism. Norethindrone acetate is converted to norethindrone, and norgestimate is metabolized into several active steroids, including levonorgestrel. Progestins that do not require hepatic transformation tend to have better bioavailability and a longer serum half-life. For example, levonorgestrel has a longer half-life than norethindrone. Norgestimate and desogestrel have lower androgenic potential than other progestins.

Drospirenone, a derivative of spironolactone, differs from other progestins because it has mild antimineralocorticoid activity. Contraceptive efficacy, metabolic profile, and cycle control are comparable to other COCs. The clinical implications of the diuretic like potential of drospirenone are not yet clear. Because of its antimineralocorticoid effects and the potential for hyperkalemia, drospirenone should not be used in women with severe renal disease or hepatic dysfunction.

Combination oral contraceptives are traditionally dosed cyclically with 21 days of hormone and 7 days of placebo during which a withdrawal bleed occurs. To address the potential of escape ovulation in the lowest estrogen formulations (20 µg), many regimens reduce the number of hormone-free days to 2–4 days. Extended cycle regimens or continuous hormonal regimens are safe and acceptable forms of contraception and may be more efficacious than cyclic regimens. Extended cycle regimens result in fewer scheduled bleeding episodes; however, they also result in more unscheduled bleeding and/or spotting episodes that decrease with time. Women who may particularly benefit from these regimens are those who have symptoms exacerbated by their menses. These include women who have seizure disorders, endometriosis, menstrual headaches, premenstrual dysphoric disorder, menorrhagia, or dysmenorrhea. There are several extended cycle regimens approved by the FDA (Sasonal, Seasonique, Lybrel); however, traditionally packaged COCs may also be prescribed as extended cycle regimens. Women are advised to use the active pills and then start a new pack, ignoring the placebo pills. This regimen gives women the option of cycling as they desire, modifying the timing of individual periods on a month-by-month basis for personal reasons.

▶ Side Effects

Side effects may be due either to the estrogen component, the progestin component, or both. Side effects attributable to progestin include androgenic effects, such as hair growth, male-pattern baldness, and nausea. Switching to an agent with lower androgenic potential may decrease or resolve these problems. Estrogenic effects include nausea, breast tenderness, and fluid retention. Weight gain is commonly assumed to be a side effect of COCs; however, multiple studies have failed to confirm a significant effect. Weight gain can be managed by switching to a different formulation; however, appropriate diet and exercise should be emphasized.

Bleeding irregularities is the side effect most frequently cited as the reason for discontinuing COCs. Patients should be counseled that irregular bleeding/spotting is common in the first 3 months of COC use and will diminish with time. Spotting is also related to missed pills. Patients should be counseled regarding the importance of taking the pill daily. If the bleeding does not appear to be related to missed pills, the patient should be evaluated for other pathology such as infection, cervical disease, or pregnancy. If this evaluation is negative, the patient may be reassured. Another approach would be to change the pill formulation to increase the estrogen or progestin component. The doses can be tailored to the time in the cycle when the bleeding occurs. If the bleeding precedes the menses, consider a triphasic pill that increases the dose of estrogen (eg, Estrostep) or progestin (eg, Ortho-Novum 7/7/7) sequentially through the cycle. If the bleeding follows the menses, consider Mircette, which has only 2 hormone-free days. Increase the estrogen and/or the progestin midcycle for midcycle bleeding (eg, Triphasil).

Combined oral contraceptives may cause a small increase in blood pressure in some patients. The risk increases with age. The blood pressure usually returns to normal within 3 months if the COC is discontinued. Both estrogens and progestins are known to affect blood pressure. Therefore, switching to a lower estrogen formulation or a progestin-only pill may not resolve the problem.

Combined oral contraceptives can be safely prescribed after a thorough medical history (including the use of tobacco products) and blood pressure documentation. While a breast examination, Pap smear, and sexually transmitted disease screening may be indicated in a particular patient, these procedures are not required before a first prescription of COCs.

▶ Major Sequelae

The use of most oral contraceptives with <50 µg of estrogen approximately triples one's risk of venous thromboembolism (VTE). COCs containing third-generation progestogens (desogestrel, gestodene, but not norgestimate) or the progestin drospirenone have a greater risk of VTE (1.5–3.0 fold) over COCs containing levonorgestrel. Bias and confounding in these studies do not explain the consistent epidemiologic findings of increased risk. Obesity, increasing age, and the factor V Leiden mutation are contributing risk factors. The best approach to identify women at higher risk of VTE before taking COCs is controversial. Universal screening for factor V Leiden is not cost-effective. Furthermore, family history of VTE has unsatisfactory sensitivity and positive predictive value for identifying carriers of other common defects. Although the absolute risk of VTE remains low, women using COCs containing desogestrel, gestodene, and drospirenone should be counseled regarding potential increased risk. An FDA Advisory Committee has concluded that the benefits of COCs likely outweigh the risks in most women.

The risk of thrombotic or ischemic stroke among users of COCs appears to be relatively low. There is no evidence that the type of progestin influences risk or mortality associated with ischemic stroke. The risk of ischemic stroke does appear to be directly proportional to estrogen dose, but even with the newer low-estrogen preparations there is still a slightly increased risk compared with nonusers. Hypertension and cigarette smoking interact with COC use to substantially increase the risk of ischemic stroke. The risk of hemorrhagic stroke in young women is low and is not increased by the use of COCs. History of migraine without focal neurologic signs is not a contraindication to hormonal contraception.

Current use of COCs is associated with an increased risk of acute myocardial infarction (AMI) among women with known cardiovascular risk factors (diabetes, cigarette smoking, hypertension) and among those who have not been effectively screened for risk factors, particularly for blood pressure. The risk for AMI does not increase with increasing duration of use or with past use of COCs.

Many epidemiologic studies have reported an increased risk of breast cancer among COC users. For current users of COCs, the relative risk of breast cancer compared with never-users is 1.24. This small risk persists for 10 years, but essentially disappears after this time period. Although COC users have a modest increase in risk of breast cancer, the disease tends to be localized. The pattern of disappearance of risk after 10 years coupled with the tendency toward localized disease suggests that the overall effect may represent detection bias or perhaps a promotional effect.

▶ Noncontraceptive Health Benefits

Most studies evaluating the relationship between COCs and ovarian cancer have shown a protective effect for oral contraceptives. There appears to be a 40–80% overall decrease in risk among users, with protection beginning 1 year after starting use, with a 10–12% decrease annually in risk for each year of use. Protection persists between 15 and 20 years after discontinuation. The mechanisms by which COCs may produce these protective effects include suppression of ovulation and the suppression of gonadotropins.

The use of COCs conveys protection against endometrial cancer as well. The reduction in risk of ≤50% begins 1 year after initiation, and persists for ≤20 years after COCs are discontinued. The mechanism of action is likely reduction in the mitotic activity of endometrial cells because of progestational effects.

Numerous epidemiologic studies demonstrate that the use of COCs will reduce the risk of salpingitis by 50–80% compared with the risk to women not using contraception or who use a barrier method. The purported mechanism for protection includes progestin-induced thickening of the cervical mucus so that ascent of bacteria is inhibited, and a decrease in menstrual flow resulting in less retrograde flow

to the fallopian tubes. There is no protective effect against the acquisition of lower genital tract sexually transmitted diseases. Other noncontraceptive benefits of COCs include decreased incidence of benign breast disease, relief from menstrual disorders (dysmenorrhea and menorrhagia), reduced risk of uterine leiomyomata, protection against ovarian cysts, reduction of acne, improvement in bone mineral density, and a reduced risk of colorectal cancer.

Maguire K. The state of hormonal contraception today: established and emerging noncontraceptive health benefits. *Am J Obstet Gynecol.* 2011;205(4 suppl):S4-S8. [PMID: 21961824]

Shulman LP. The state of hormonal contraception today: benefits and risks of hormonal contraceptives: combined estrogen and progestin contraceptives. *Am J Obstet Gynecol.* 2011;205(4 suppl):S9-S13. [PMID: 21961825]

Van Hylckma Vlieg A, Helmerhorst FM, Vanderboucke JP, Doggen CJ, Rosendaal FR. The venous thrombotic risk of oral contraceptives, effects of oestrogen dose and progestogen type: results of the MEGA case-control study. *Br Med J.* 2009;339:b2921. [PMID:19679614]

TRANSDERMAL CONTRACEPTIVE SYSTEM

A transdermal contraceptive patch containing norelgestromin, the active metabolite of norgestimate, and ethinyl estradiol is marketed by Ortho-McNeil under the trade name Ortho-Evra. The system is designed to deliver 150 μg of norelgestromin and 20 μg of ethinyl estradiol daily directly to the peripheral circulation. The treatment regimen for each cycle is three consecutive 7-day patches (21 days) followed by one patch-free week so that withdrawal bleeding can occur. The patch can be applied to one of four sites on a woman's body: abdomen, buttocks, upper outer arm, or torso (excluding the breast).

Ortho-Evra's efficacy is comparable to that of COCs. Compliance with the patch is much higher than with COC, which may result in fewer pregnancies overall. However, pregnancy is more likely to occur in women weighing >198 lb. Breakthrough bleeding, spotting, and breast tenderness are slightly higher for Ortho-Evra than COCs in the first two cycles, but there is no difference in later cycles. Amenorrhea occurs in only 0.1% of patch users. Patch-site reactions occur in 2–3% of women.

Initiation of patch use is similar to initiation of COC use. Women apply the first patch on day 1 of their menstrual cycle. Another option is to apply the first patch on the Sunday after their menses begins. This becomes their patch change day. Subsequently, they change patches on the same day of the week. After three cycles they have a patch-free week during which they can expect their menses. A backup contraceptive should be used for the first 7 days of use.

The US Food and Drug Administration (FDA) requires labeling on the Ortho-Evra patch to warn health care providers and patients that this product exposes women to higher levels of estrogen than most birth control pills.

Average concentration at steady state for ethinyl estradiol is ~60% higher in women using Ortho-Evra compared with women using an oral contraceptive containing 35 μg of ethinyl estradiol. In contrast, peak concentrations for ethinyl estradiol are ~25% lower in women using Ortho-Evra. In general, increased estrogen exposure may increase the risk of blood clots. The potential risks related to increased estrogen exposure with the patch should be balanced against the risk of pregnancy if patients have difficulty following the daily regimen associated with typical birth control pills.

Burkman RT. Transdermal hormonal contraception: benefits and risks. *Am J Obstet Gynecol.* 2007; 197(2):134.e1-6. [PMID: 17689623]

INTRAVAGINAL RING SYSTEM

The NuvaRing vaginal contraceptive ring is a flexible, transparent ring made of ethylene vinylacetate copolymers, delivering an average of 120 μg of etonorgestrel and 15 μg of ethinyl estradiol per day. A woman inserts the NuvaRing herself, wears it for 3 weeks, and then removes and discards the device. After one ring-free week, during which withdrawal bleeding occurs, a new ring is inserted. Continuous use has been studied; results are similar to those observed with COCs. Rarely, NuvaRing can slip out of the vagina if it has not been inserted properly or while removing a tampon, moving the bowels, straining, or with severe constipation. If the NuvaRing has been out of the vagina for >3 hours, breakthrough ovulation may occur. Patients may be counseled to check the position of the NuvaRing before and after intercourse.

Peak serum concentrations of etonorgestrel and ethinyl estradiol occur about 1 week after insertion and are 60–70% lower than peak concentrations produced by standard COCs. The manufacturer recommends using backup birth control for the first 7 days of use if not switching from another hormonal contraceptive. NuvaRing prevents pregnancy by the same mechanism as COCs. Pregnancy rates for users of NuvaRing are between 1 and 2 per 100 woman-years of use.

The side effects of NuvaRing are similar to that of COC pills; the main adverse effect is disrupted bleeding. Breakthrough bleeding/spotting occurs in 2.6–11.7% of cycles, and absence of withdrawal bleeding occurs in 0.6–3.8% of cycles. Fewer than 1–2% of women experience discomfort or reported discomfort from their partners with NuvaRing. NuvaRing is associated with increased vaginal secretions, which is a result of both hormonal and mechanical effects. Although 23% of ring users reported vaginal discharge, the normal vaginal flora appears to be maintained. The ring is not associated with either adverse cytologic effects or bacteriologic colonization of the vaginal canal. The contraindications to NuvaRing are similar to those of COCs. In addition, the ring may not be an appropriate choice for women with conditions that render the vagina more susceptible to irritation or that increase the likelihood of ring expulsion, such as vaginal stenosis, cervical prolapse, cystocele, or rectocele.

Bateson D, McNamee K, Briggs P. Newer non-oral hormonal contraception. *Br Med J.* 2013; 346:f341. [PMID: 23412438]
Bitzer J, Simon JA. Current issues and available options in combined hormonal contraception. *Contraception.* 2011;84 (4):341-356. [PMID: 21920188]

PROGESTIN-ONLY PILL

Progestin-only oral contraceptives (POPs), sometimes called the "minipill," are not widely used in the United States. Their use tends to be concentrated in select populations, notably breastfeeding women and those with contraindications to estrogen. Two formulations of POPs are available: one containing norgestrel, the other with norethindrone. POPs appear to prevent conception through several mechanisms, including suppression of ovulation, thickening of cervical mucus, alteration of the endometrium, and inhibition of tubal transport. Efficacy of POPs requires consistent administration. The pills should be taken at the same time every day without interruption (no hormone-free week). If a pill is taken >3 hours late, a backup method of contraception should be used for the next 48 hours. No increase in the risk for thromboembolic events has been reported for POPs. The World Health Organization has deemed this contraceptive method acceptable for use in women with a history of venous thrombosis, pulmonary embolism, diabetes, obesity, or hypertension. Vascular disease is no longer considered a contraindication to use. The most common side effects of POPs are menstrual cycle disruption and breakthrough bleeding. Other common side effects include headache, breast tenderness, nausea, and dizziness. In general, POP use protects against ectopic pregnancy by lowering the chance of conception. If POP users do get pregnant, an average of 6–10% of pregnancies are extrauterine—higher than in women not using contraception. Therefore POP users should be aware of the symptoms of ectopic pregnancy.

IMPLANTS

Implanon and Nexplanon are implantable contraceptives containing the progestin etonorgestrel, the active metabolite of desogestrel, and are approved for 3 years of use. Etonorgestrel has high progestational activity but weak androgenic activity. A single rod is inserted subdermally on the inside of the upper arm. Both implants release etonorgestrel at a rate of 60–70 μg per day initially, which decreases to 25–30 μg by the end of 3 years. Etonorgestrel levels are undetectable 1 week after removal. Nexplanon is bioequivalent to Implanon but has a preloaded applicator designed to reduce the risk of insertion errors. In addition, Nexplanon is radiopaque and can therefore be located by x-ray if necessary. Like other progestin-only contraceptives, the mechanism of action is by inhibition of ovulation and thickening of cervical mucus. The implants are effective with a pregnancy rate of <1%. Irregular bleeding is the primary reason cited for discontinuation, accounting for 13–19% of discontinuations. Other adverse effects include headache, weight gain, acne, breast and abdominal pain, mood swings, depression, and decreased libido. The implants are not associated with decreased bone mineral density or venous thromboembolic disease.

Timing of insertion depends on the patient's recent history. If she is not currently using contraception, insert during the menstrual cycle. If she is using COCs, insert during the pill-free week. If insertion occurs at other times, backup contraception is recommended for the first 7 days after insertion. Only health care providers who receive training from the manufacturer are allowed to order and insert the implant.

Mommers E. Nexplanon, a radiopaque etonorgestrel implant in combination with a next-generation applicator: 3-year results of a non-comparative multicenter trial. *Am J Obstet Gynecol.* 2012;207(5):388.e1-6. [PMID: 22939402]

INJECTABLE CONTRACEPTIVES

Injectable long-acting contraception offers users convenient, safe, and reversible birth control as effective as surgical sterilization. Depot-medroxyprogesterone acetate (DMPA) is a 3-month progestin-only formulation that can be administered by deep intramuscular injection (IM-DMPA) into the gluteus or deltoid muscle or subcutaneously (SC-DMPA). Patients using SC-DMPA can be taught to self-administer subcutaneously 4 times per year. Self-administration facilitates access to injectable contraception for many women, eliminating the need for an office visit. In addition to contraception, SC-DMPA is also indicated for the treatment of pain associated with endometriosis.

Studies have shown that DMPA acts primarily by inhibiting ovulation. With typical use, the failure rate of DMPA is 0.3 per 100 woman-years, which is comparable to that of levonorgestrel implants, copper intrauterine devices, or surgical sterilization. Neither increasing weight nor use of concurrent medications has been noted to alter efficacy, apparently because of high circulating levels of progestin.

The first injection of DMPA should be administered within 5 days of the onset of menses or within 5 days of a first-trimester abortion. If a woman is postpartum and breastfeeding, then the drug should not be administered until at least 6 weeks postdelivery. When switching from COCs, the first injection may be given any time while the active pills are being taken or within 7 days of taking the last active pill. Repeat injections of DMPA should be administered every 12 weeks. If a patient presents at 13 weeks or later, the manufacturer recommends excluding pregnancy before administering a repeat injection.

The use of DMPA has no permanent impact on fertility; however, return of fertility may be delayed after cessation of use. Fifty percent of women who discontinue DMPA to become pregnant will have conceived within 10 months of the last injection. In a small proportion of women, fertility is not reestablished until 18 months after the last injection.

Menstrual changes are the most common side effects reported by users of DMPA. After 1 year of use, approximately 75% of women receiving DMPA report amenorrhea, with the remainder reporting irregular bleeding or spotting. Some women, especially adolescents, view amenorrhea as a potential benefit of use. Women, who voice concern over this side effect, can be reassured that the amenorrhea is not harmful. Patients with persistent bleeding or spotting should be evaluated for genital tract neoplasia and infection as appropriate. If these are excluded and the symptoms are bothersome to the patient, a 1–3-month trial of low-dose estrogen can be considered. Early reinjection (eg, every 8–10 weeks) does not seem to decrease bleeding.

Other side effects attributed to DMPA include weight gain, mood swings, reduced libido, and headaches. Because of concerns regarding decreased bone mineral density (BMD) after prolonged use, the manufacturer no longer recommends use for >2 years. Reassuringly, results from several studies indicate almost complete recovery of BMD 2 years after discontinuation. Many clinicians recommend that users take supplemental calcium and vitamin D. DMPA may be used safely by smokers ≥35 years, and by other women at increased risk for arterial or venous events. Use of DMPA has not been associated with clinically significant alterations in hepatic function.

INTRAUTERINE DEVICES

Throughout the world, the most common form of reversible contraception is the intrauterine device (IUD); however, relatively few women in the United States use IUDs (~1% compared with 15–30% in Europe and Canada), although those that do express a high degree of satisfaction. Currently there are two IUDs marketed for use in the United States. The most common IUD used is the copper-T 380A (Paragard) made of polyethylene with fine-wire copper wrapped around the stem and copper in the sleeves of each horizontal arm. It is approved for 10 years of use. The levonorgestrel IUD (Mirena) has a polyethylene frame that releases 20 µg of levonorgestrel per day for as long as 5 years. Both IUDs are visible on x-ray.

The contraceptive action of IUDs is probably a result of a combination of factors. The IUD induces an inflammatory, foreign-body reaction within the uterus that causes prostaglandin release. This release results in altered uterine activity, inhibited tubal motility, and a direct toxic effect on sperm. The copper present in the copper-T enhances the contraceptive effects by inhibiting transport of ovum and sperm. IUDs containing a progestin produce a similar effect and, in addition, thicken cervical mucus and suppress ovulation. IUDs are not abortifacients; they prevent fertilization. The IUD is one of the most effective methods of reversible contraception available. Among women who use the IUD perfectly (checking strings regularly to detect expulsion), the probability of pregnancy in the first year of use is 0.6% for the copper-T, and 0.1% for the levonorgestrel IUD. The progestational activity of the levonorgestrel IUD reduces menstrual blood loss and has been used to treat excessive uterine bleeding. The IUD may be inserted on any day of the month provided that the woman is not pregnant.

The main benefits of the IUD are a high level of effectiveness, lack of associated systemic metabolic effects, and provision of long-acting, reversible contraception. The most common reason cited for discontinuing the IUD is bleeding. Bleeding can be minimized with the use of a NSAID. However, if persistent or severe, the patient should be evaluated for infection or perforation. Patients can be reassured that the amount of bleeding and cramping usually decreases with time.

Expulsion occurs in 2–10% of women in the first year of use, with most expulsions occurring in the first 3 months. Nulliparity, abnormal amount of menstrual flow, and severe dysmenorrhea are risk factors for expulsion. In addition, the expulsion rate may be higher when the IUD is inserted at the time of the menses. Pregnancy may be the first sign of expulsion. Therefore, patients should be instructed to check for the IUD strings after each menstrual cycle. If a pregnancy does occur with an IUD in place, the IUD should be removed as soon as possible. In the presence of an IUD 50–60% of pregnancies spontaneously abort. The risk drops to 20% when the IUD is removed. Septic abortion is 26 times more common in women with an IUD. The copper-T IUD protects against ectopic pregnancy, whereas the progesterone IUD increases the risk of ectopic pregnancy almost twofold.

A common myth about IUDs is that they increase the risk of pelvic inflammatory disease (PID). However, it is now known that the risk of PID is highest in the first 20 days after insertion of an IUD, and then returns to the baseline rate. The risk is eliminated if screening and treatment of sexually transmitted infections are done before insertion. Therefore, bacterial contamination associated with the insertion process is the likely cause of infection, not the IUD itself. IUD insertion should be delayed in a woman with active cervicitis. However, women with positive *Chlamydia* cultures after IUD insertion are unlikely to develop PID, even with retention of the IUD, if the infection is promptly treated. The levonorgestrel IUD may lower the risk of PID by thickening cervical mucus and thinning the endometrium. Routine antibiotic prophylaxis is not recommended before IUD insertion.

The incidental finding of actinomyces on cervical cytology is more common in IUD users than in other women. If actinomyces is detected on Pap smear and the patient has signs or symptoms of PID, the IUD should be removed immediately and the patient treated with doxycycline. If the patient is asymptomatic, antibiotic treatment is not recommended and the Pap smear is repeated in 1 year.

The following conditions are contraindications to insertion of an IUD: pregnancy; current or recent cervicitis, PID, or endometritis; uterine or cervical malignancy; undiagnosed vaginal or uterine bleeding; or an IUD already in place. Conditions commonly assumed to be contraindications but are *not* included are diabetes mellitus, valvular heart disease, history of ectopic pregnancy (except for the levonorgestrel IUD), nulliparity, treated cervical dysplasia, irregular menses, breastfeeding, corticosteroid use, age <25 years, and multiple sexual partners. Women with multiple sexual partners should be counseled to use condoms to reduce their risk of sexually transmitted disease.

Winner B, et al. Effectiveness of long-acting reversible contraception. *N Engl J Med*. 2012;366(21):1998-2007. [PMID: 22621627]

BARRIER CONTRACEPTION

The percentage of women who used a method of contraception at their first premarital intercourse increased from 43% in the 1970s to 78% in 2006–2010. Most of this increase was due to an increase in use of the male condom at first premarital intercourse, from 22% in the 1970s to 68% in 2006–2010 (NSFG 2006–2010). Condoms are inexpensive, easy to use, and available without a prescription. Most commercially available condoms are manufactured from either latex or polyurethane. While polyurethane and latex condoms offer similar protection against pregnancy, breakage and slippage rates appear to be higher with the polyurethane condom. Natural membrane condoms (made from sheep intestine) are also available; however, they do not offer the same degree of protection from STDs. Because couples vary widely in their ability to use condoms consistently and correctly, the failure rate also varies. The percentage of women experiencing an unintended pregnancy within the first year of use ranges from 3% with perfect use to 14% with typical use. Women relying on condoms for contraception and protection from STDs should be reminded that oil-based lubricants reduce the integrity of a latex condom and facilitate breakage. Because vaginal medications (eg, for yeast infections) often contain oil-based ingredients, they can damage latex condoms as well.

There are several vaginal barrier contraceptives available that are easy to use and effective. The contraceptive efficacy of all barrier methods depends on their consistent and correct use. The percentage of women experiencing an unintended pregnancy within the first year of typical use ranges from 15% to 32%.

The female condom is a soft, loose-fitting, latex sheath with two flexible rings at either end. One ring is inserted into the vagina and lies adjacent to the cervix. The other ring remains outside of the vagina, against the perineum. Sperm is captured within the condom. The sheath is coated on the inside with a silicone-based lubricant. It is available without a prescription and is intended for one-time use. Female and male condoms should not be used together because the two condoms can adhere to one another, causing slippage and displacement. With correct and consistent use, the female condom can decrease the transmission of STDs, including HIV/AIDS.

The diaphragm is a dome-shaped latex rubber cup with a flexible rim. It is inserted, with a spermicide, into the vagina before intercourse. Once it is in position, the diaphragm provides contraceptive protection for 6 hours. If a longer interval has elapsed, insertion of additional spermicide is required. After intercourse the diaphragm must be left in place for 6 hours, but no longer than 24 hours. Use of the diaphragm has been associated with an increase risk of urinary tract infections (UTI). Spermicide exposure is an important risk factor for UTI (due to alterations in vaginal flora), although mechanical factors in diaphragm use also may contribute to the risk of UTI. Use of the diaphragm requires an appointment with a health care provider for education, fitting, and a prescription. Oil-based vaginal products should not be used with the latex diaphragm.

The cervical cap is cup-shaped silicone device that fits around the cervix. The device can be placed anytime before intercourse, with spermicide, and can be left in place for ≤48 hours. The advantages of the cervical cap over the diaphragm are that it can be left in place longer, and it is more comfortable. Like the diaphragm, the cap is manufactured in different sizes, and must be fitted by a clinician. The cap needs to be placed directly over the cervix to be effective, so it should not be used if a woman finds the placement to be difficult or uncomfortable.

The contraceptive sponge is a small, pillow-shaped polyurethane sponge containing a spermicide. The sponge protects for ≥12–24 hours, regardless of how many times intercourse occurs. After intercourse, the sponge must be left in place for ≥6 hours before it is removed and discarded. The sponge comes in one universal size and does not require a prescription.

Spermicides are an integral component of several of the barrier contraceptives. Nonoxynol-9, the active chemical agent in spermicides available in the United States, is a surfactant that destroys the sperm cell membrane. It is available in a various formulations, including gel, foam, creme, film, suppository, or tablet. Spermicide use may lower the chance of infection with a bacterial STD by as much as 25%. However, women at high risk for acquiring HIV should not use products containing nonoxynol-9. Some studies have shown that it causes vaginal lesions, which could then be entry points for HIV.

EMERGENCY CONTRACEPTION

As many as half of the unintended pregnancies in the United States result from condom failure, missed birth control pills, or incorrect or inconsistent use of barrier contraception. Optimal use of emergency contraception could reduce unintended pregnancy in the United States by as much as 50%. Emergency contraception, available as combined oral contraceptives, progestin-only pills, and the copper intrauterine device, are safe and effective. When taken as directed, emergency contraceptive pills (ECPs) can reduce the risk of pregnancy by 75–89% after a single act of unprotected intercourse, while a copper IUD inserted within 5 days of intercourse can reduce the risk by 99%.

Emergency contraception (EC) is appropriate when no contraception was used or when intercourse was unprotected as a result of contraceptive accidents (eg, condom slippage). Since pill regimens involve only limited exposure to hormones, ECPs are safe. They have not been shown to increase the risk of venous thromboembolism, stroke, myocardial infarction, or other cardiovascular events. In addition, ECPs will not disrupt an implanted pregnancy and will not cause birth defects. ECPs work primarily by inhibiting ovulation, with some effects on sperm motility and thickening of cervical mucus. They will not disrupt an implanted pregnancy. Unfortunately, ECPs do not protect against sexually transmitted diseases.

Combined oral contraceptive for use as EC is frequently referred to as the *Yuzpe method*. Commercially available COCs containing ethinyl estradiol and levonorgestrel or norgestrel can be used as emergency contraception. Each of two doses separated by 12 hours must contain ≥100 µg ethinyl estradiol plus 0.5 mg levonorgestrel or 1.0 mg norgestrel (eg, four white Lo/Ovral pills per dose). When used correctly, the Yuzpe method decreases expected pregnancies by 75%. More specifically, 8 out of every 100 women who have unprotected intercourse once during the second or third week of their cycles will become pregnant; however, 2 out of 100 will become pregnant if the Yuzpe method is used. The most common adverse effects are nausea (50%) and vomiting (20%). Antiemetics taken 30–60 minutes before each dose help minimize these symptoms. Other side effects include delayed or early menstrual bleeding. Some women also experience heavier menses.

The most common progestin-only method of emergency contraception consists of 1.5 mg of levonorgestrel taken in one or two doses ("plan B one-step" or "next choice"). The progestin-only regimen is more effective than the Yuzpe method, preventing ≤85% of expected pregnancies. In addition, nausea occurs in <25% of patients, and vomiting is reduced to ~5% in women on the progestin-only regimen. Treatment is effective when initiated ≤5 days after unprotected intercourse, and a single 1.5-mg dose is as effective as two 0.75-mg doses 12 hours apart. Progestin-only emergency contraception is available without a prescription to women aged ≥17 years.

Ulipristal ("Ella"), a progesterone receptor modulator, was approved by the FDA as a one-dose emergency contraception in 2010. It is effective when taken ≤5 days after unprotected intercourse. Its action mechanism is delay or inhibition of ovulation. Ulipristal requires that a prescription be dispensed.

To prevent pregnancy, a copper-containing IUD can be inserted ≤5 days after unprotected intercourse. The IUD is highly effective and can be used for long-term contraception. An IUD is not recommended for anyone at risk for sexually transmitted diseases or ectopic pregnancy, or if long-term contraception is not desired. The IUD is the most effective method of EC, with failure rates of <1%.

Screening patients for ECP use is based on the time of unprotected intercourse and the date of the last normal menstrual period. There are no preexisting disease contraindications, and inadvertent use in pregnancy has not been linked to birth defects. Neither a pregnancy test nor a pelvic examination is required, although it may be done for other reasons (eg, screening for STDs). In contrast, IUD insertion for emergency contraception is an office-based procedure that requires appropriate counseling and screening as for any patient desiring an IUD for contraception.

Counseling regarding the availability of emergency contraception can occur anytime that contraception or family planning issues are discussed. It is especially appropriate if the patient is relying on barrier methods or does not have a regular form of contraception. The counseling can be reinforced when patients present with contraceptive mishaps. Information that should be discussed includes the definition of emergency contraception, indications for use, mechanism of action, lack of protection against STDs, instructions on use, and follow-up plans including ongoing contraception.

American Academy of Pediatrics, Committee on Adolescence. Emergency contraception. *Pediatrics.* 2012; 130(6):1174-1182. [PMID: 23184108]
Prine L. Emergency contraception, myths and facts. *Obstet Gynecol Clinics North Am.* 2007; 34:127-136.

SPECIAL POPULATIONS

▶ Adolescents

Adolescent pregnancy continues to be a serious public health problem in the United States. Almost 1 in 10 adolescent females becomes pregnant each year, with 74–95% described as unintended. Improved contraceptive practices has contributed to an almost 40% decrease in the teen pregnancy rate. The general approach to adolescent contraception should focus on keeping the clinician-patient encounter interactive. Several suggestions include: avoiding "yes/no" questions, keeping clinician speaking time short and focused, and avoiding the word "should."

Abstinence deserves emphasis, especially in young teenagers. Counseling should focus not on "just say no" but rather "know how to say no." Oral contraceptives (COCs) and condoms are the most common contraceptive methods chosen by teens. These methods should be promoted simultaneously as an approach to pregnancy and STD prevention. COC use is associated with health benefits that are especially important during adolescence including treatment for acne and menstrual cycle irregularity, decreased risk of pelvic inflammatory disease and functional ovarian cysts, and decreased dysmenorrhea. The main concern that adolescents have regarding COCs is the development of side effects, especially weight gain. They can be reassured that many studies have proven that COCs do not cause weight gain. Another issue that may contribute to the reluctance of adolescents to seek contraception is fear of a pelvic examination. Contrary to popular belief, a pelvic examination is not necessary when contraception is prescribed, especially if it will delay the sexually active teens' access to needed pregnancy prevention. Adolescents should be counseled regarding missed pills and given anticipatory guidance about breakthrough bleeding and amenorrhea. Adolescents miss on average up to three pills per month, and the risk of contraceptive failure is twice as high among teenagers as it is among women aged >30 years. These data underscore the potential benefits of offering adolescents long-acting reversible contraception (injectables, implants, and IUDs) to reduce unintended pregnancy in this high-risk group.

In some respects, DMPA ("Depo-Provera") is an ideal contraceptive for adolescents. The dosing schedule allows flexibility and minimal maintenance, and the failure rate is extremely low. However, concerns regarding bone loss in long-term users have prompted the recommendation that use not exceed 2 years. Although available data on adolescents are scant, they indicate that this group may be especially vulnerable to bone mineral density loss. It is not known whether bone loss before achieving peak bone density is recoverable, or to what extent the loss impacts the future risk of fracture. In addition, adolescents are likely to demonstrate other risk behaviors for bone loss, including early sexual activity, smoking, alcohol use, and poor diet choices. Until the results of larger studies are available, definitive recommendations in teenagers cannot be made.

The etonorgestrel implant has many advantages for the teen who desires contraception: ease of use, discreet, improvement of acne, reduction of dysmenorrhea, and outstanding efficacy. Despite common misperceptions, implants are not associated with increased risk of venous thromboembolism or decreased bone mineral density. Unfortunately, despite its ease of use, high efficacy, and safety, many young women choose to discontinue this method early because of problems with unpredictable irregular bleeding.

Contraceptive efficacy, convenience, and high continuation rate makes the IUD an excellent contraception method for appropriately selected adolescents. The CDC medical elligibility criteria for birth control classify women from menarche to age 20 and nulliparous women as category 2, where the advantages of using the method generally outweigh the theoretical or proven risks. The two major disadvantages include menstrual irregularity including heavier bleeding, and pelvic cramping. Both of these side effects tend to mitigate with time.

Vaginal barrier contraceptives are not ideal choices for several reasons. Many adolescents are not prepared to deal so intimately with their own bodies and do not wish to prepare so carefully for each episode of intercourse. However, they can be an effective method for highly motivated, educated adolescents.

A discussion of emergency contraception (EC) should be part of contraceptive counseling for all adolescents. To increase the availability of EC, teens may be provided with a replaceable supply of EC pills to keep at home. Several studies in adolescents have shown that direct access to emergency contraception increases its rate of use, but does not result in repetitive use. Although concern for improper use persists, women who are provided education on the method, use the method correctly, and incorrect use does not pose a health risk beyond unintended pregnancy.

Breastfeeding Women

The lactational amenorrhea method is a highly effective, temporary method of contraception. However, to maintain effective protection against pregnancy, another method must be used as soon as menstruation resumes, the frequency or duration of breastfeeds is reduced, bottle-feeding or regular food supplements are introduced, or the baby reaches 6 months of age. Other good contraceptive options for lactating women include barrier methods, progestin-only methods, or an IUD. Some experts recommend that breastfeeding women delay using progestin-only contraception until 6 weeks postpartum. This recommendation is based on a theoretical concern that early neonatal exposure to exogenous steroids should be avoided if possible. The combined pill is not a good option for lactating women because estrogen decreases breastmilk supply.

Perimenopausal Women

Women aged >40 years have the second highest proportion of unintended pregnancies, exceeded only by girls 13–14 years old. Although women still need effective contraception during perimenopause, issues including bone loss, menstrual irregularity, and vasomotor instability also need to be addressed. Oral contraceptives offer many

benefits for healthy, nonsmoking perimenopausal women. They have been found to decrease the risk of postmenopausal hip fracture, regularize menses in women with dysfunctional uterine bleeding, and decrease vasomotor symptoms.

For perimenopausal women with cardiovascular risk factors, progestin-only methods may be preferred, including progestin-only pills, levonorgestrel (or copper) IUDs, contraceptive implants, and DMPA. Barrier methods or sterilization may also be appropriate in select women. Control of dysfunctional uterine bleeding can be obtained with injectable progestogens or the levonorgestrel IUD. Low-dose estrogen can be added to these methods if estrogen replacement is desired and appropriate.

Physiologically, menopause is the permanent cessation of menstruation as a consequence of termination of ovarian follicular activity. Determining the exact onset of menopause in a woman using hormonal contraception can be tricky. Many clinicians measure the level of follicle-stimulating hormone (FSH) during the pill-free interval to diagnose menopause. However, because suppression of ovulation can vary from month to month, a single FSH value is unreliable. In addition, in women using COCs, FSH levels can be suppressed even on the seventh pill-free day. Given that most women do not become menopausal until after age 50, and considering the limited utility of FSH testing, one approach to managing this transition avoids FSH testing entirely. Women continue to use their COCs until age 50–52, at which time they can discontinue use or transition to hormone replacement therapy.

Cornet A. Current challenges in contraception in adolescents and young women. *Curr Opin Obstet Gynecol.* 2013; 25(suppl 1): S1-S10. [PMID 23370330]

Hartmen LB, Monasterio E, Hwang L. Adolescent contraception: review and guidance for pediatric clinicians. *Curr Probl Pediatr Adolesc Health Care.* 2012;42(9):221-263. [PMID: 22959636]

The World Health Organization (WHO) has published comprehensive tables of medical conditions and personal characteristics that may affect contraceptive choice. These tables can be found online (http://whqlibdoc.who.int/publications/2010/9789241563888_eng.pdf). In 2010, the Centers for Disease Control and Prevention (CDC) adapted the WHO tables for US clinicians and patients. The CDC tables are available at http://www.cdc.gov/reproductivehealth/UnintendedPregnancy/USMEC.htm.

Adult Sexual Dysfunction

19

Charles W. Mackett, III, MD

▶ Disturbance in one or more aspects of the sexual response cycle.

▶ Cause is often multifactorial, associated with medical conditions, therapies, and lifestyle.

▶ General Considerations

Sexual dysfunction is a disturbance in one or more of the aspects of the sexual response cycle. It is a common problem that can result from communication difficulties, misunderstandings, and side effects of medical or surgical treatment, as well as underlying health problems. Because sexual difficulties often occur as a response to stress, fatigue, or interpersonal difficulties, addressing sexual health requires an expanded view of sexuality that emphasizes the importance of understanding individuals within the context of their lives and defining sexual health across physical, intellectual, emotional, interpersonal, environmental, cultural, and spiritual aspects of their lives and their sexual orientation. Sexual dysfunction is extremely common. A survey of young to middle-aged adults found that 31% of men and 43% of women in the general population reported some type and degree of sexual dysfunction. The prevalence is even higher in clinical populations.

Recognition of sexual dysfunction is important. It may be the initial manifestation of significant underlying disease or provide a marker for disease progression and severity. It should be a consideration when managing a number of chronic medical conditions.

Sexual dysfunction is positively correlated with low relationship satisfaction and general happiness. Despite this, only 10% of affected men and 20% of affected women seek medical care for their sexual difficulties. The key to identification of sexual function disorders is to inquire about their presence. A discussion of sexual health can be initiated in various ways. Educational· material or self-administered screening forms convey the message that sexual health is an important topic that is discussed in the clinician's office. **Table 19-1** lists several questionnaires that can be incorporated into self-administered patient surveys for office practices.

Sexual history can be included as part of the social history, as part of the review of systems under genitourinary systems, or in whatever manner seems most appropriate to the clinician. There are many other opportunities to bring a discussion of sexual health into the clinical encounter, as outlined in **Table 19-2**. Clinician anxiety may be reduced by asking the patient for permission prior to taking the sexual history.

Once the history confirms the existence of sexual difficulties, obtain as clear a description as possible of the following elements: the aspect of the sexual response cycle most involved, the onset, the progression, and any associated medical problems. Asking patients what they believe to be the cause can help the clinician identify possible etiologies. Asking patients what they have tried to do to resolve the problems and clarifying the patient's expectations for resolution can help facilitate an appropriate therapeutic approach. Involving the partner in diagnosis and subsequent management can be very valuable.

Sexual dysfunction is associated with many factors, conditions, therapies, and lifestyle choices (**Table 19-3**). In some instances the underlying medical condition may be the cause of the sexual dysfunction (eg, arterial vascular disease causing erectile dysfunction). In other instances the sexual dysfunction contributes to the associated condition (eg, erectile dysfunction leads to loss of self-esteem and depression). Sexual difficulties can begin with one aspect of the sexual response cycle and subsequently affect other aspects

Table 19-1. Sexual health screening questionnaires.

Sexual Health Inventory for Men (SHIM)
International Index of Erectile Function (IIEF)
World Health Organization (WHO) Intensity Score
Androgen Deficiency in the Aging Male (ADAM)
Female Sexual Function Index (FSFI)
Sexual Energy Scale
Brief Index of Sexual Function Inventory (BISF-W)
Changes in Sexual Functioning Questionnaire (CSFQ)

(eg, arousal difficulties causing depression, which can then negatively affect sexual interest).

Nusbaum MR, Hamilton CD. The proactive sexual health inquiry. *Am Fam Physician.* 2002; 66:1705. [PMID: 12449269]

DISORDERS OF DESIRE

General Considerations

Difficulties with sexual desire are the most common sexual concern. Over 33% of women and 16% of men in the general population report an extended period of lack of sexual interest. Other investigators have reported prevalence rates as high as 87% in specific populations. Women who were younger, separated, non-white, less educated, and of lower socioeconomic status reported the highest rates. Men from the same demographics as well as increasing age reported the highest rates.

Table 19-2. Sexual health inquiry.

Review of systems or social history.
What sexual concerns do you have?
Has there been any change in your (or partner's) sexual desire or frequency of sexual activity?
Are you satisfied with your (or partner's) present sexual functioning?
Is there anything about your sexual activity (as individuals or as a couple) that you (or your partner) would like to change?
Counseling about healthy lifestyle (smoking or alcohol cessation, exercise program, weight reduction).
Discussing effectiveness and side effects of medications.
Inquire before and after medical event or procedures likely to impact sexual function (myocardial infarction, prostate surgery).
Inquire when there is an imminent or recent lifecycle change such as pregnancy, new baby, teenager, children leaving the home, retirement, menopause, "discovery" of past abuse.

Data from Nusbaum MRH. *Sexual Health.* American Academy of Family Physicians; 2001; Nusbaum MR, Hamilton C. The proactive sexual health inquiry: key to effective sexual health care. *Am Fam Physician.* 2002;66:1705; and Nusbaum M, Rosenfeld J. *Sexual Health across the Lifecycle: A Practical Guide for Clinicians.* Cambridge University Press, 2004:20.

Table 19-3. Factors associated with sexual dysfunction.

Aging
Chronic disease
   Diabetes mellitus
   Heart disease
   Hypertension
   Lipid disorders
   Renal failure
   Vascular disease
Endocrine abnormalities
   Hypogonadism
   Hyperprolactinemia
   Hypo/hyperthyroidism
Lifestyle
   Cigarette smoking
   Chronic alcohol abuse
Neurogenic causes
   Spinal cord injury
   Multiple sclerosis
   Herniated disk
Penile injury/disease
   Peyronie plaques
   Priapism
Pharmacologic agents
Psychological issues
   Depression
   Anxiety
   Social stresses
Trauma/injury
   Pelvic trauma/surgery
   Pelvic radiation

Classification

Decrease in sexual desire can be related to decrease or loss of interest in or an aversion to sexual interaction with self or others. It can be primary or secondary, generalized, or situational in occurrence. Sexual aversion is characterized by persistent or extreme aversion to, and avoidance of, sexual activity. Separating these difficulties can be difficult. For example, a patient who has experienced sexual trauma may have difficulties with subsequent partners and ultimately develop an aversion to sexual activity.

A common situation in clinical practice is when partners differ in their level of sexual desire. Although most couples negotiate a workable solution, it may cause relationship dissatisfaction. It can also be a marker for extrarelationship affairs or domestic violence.

Pathogenesis

Changes in or a loss of sexual desire can be the result of biological, psychological, social, or interpersonal factors. Numerous medical conditions directly or indirectly affect sexual desire (**Table 19-4**). Illnesses and medications that

Table 19-4. Common medical conditions that may affect sexual desire.

Pituitary/hypothalamic
Infiltrative diseases/tumors
Endocrine
   Testosterone deficiency
     Castration, adrenal disease, age-related bilateral
      salpingo oophorectomy, adrenal disease
   Thyroid deficiency
   Endocrine-secreting tumors
   Cushing syndrome
   Adrenal insufficiency
Psychiatric
   Depression and stress
   Substance abuse
Neurologic
   Degenerative diseases/trauma of the central nervous system
Urologic/gynecologic (indirect cause)
   Peyronie plaques, phimosis
   Gynecologic pain syndromes
Renal
   End-stage renal disease, renal dialysis
Conditions that cause chronic pain, fatigue, malaise
   Arthritis, cancer, chronic pulmonary or hepatic disease

Table 19-5. Drugs most commonly associated with sexual dysfunction.

Drug Class	Negative Effect on Sexual Response Cycle
Antihypertensives	Arousal difficulties

Diuretics
  Thiazides
  Spironolactone
	Arousal and desire

Sympatholytics
  Central agents (methyldopa, clonidine)
  Peripheral agents (reserpine)
	
	Arousal and desire
	Arousal and desire

α-Blockers	Arousal and orgasm
β-Blockers (particularly nonselective agents)	Arousal and desire

Psychiatric medications
  Antipsychotics
  Antidepressants
    Tricyclic antidepressants
    MAO inhibitors
    SSRIs
  Anxiolytics
    Benzodiazepines
	
	Multiple phases of sexual function
	
	Arousal and desire
	Multiple phases of sexual function
	Arousal and orgasm
	
	Arousal difficulties

Antiandrogenic agents
  Digoxin
  H$_2$ receptor blockers
	
	Arousal and desire
	Arousal and desire

Others
  Alcohol (long-term, heavy use)
  Ketoconazole
  Niacin
  Phenobarbital
  Phenytoin
	
	Arousal and desire
	Arousal and desire
	Arousal and desire
	Arousal and desire
	Arousal and desire

MAO, monoamine oxidase; SSRI, selective serotonin reuptake inhibitor.

decrease relative androgen levels, increase the level of sex hormone–binding globulin, or interfere with endocrine and neurotransmitter functioning can negatively affect desire. In both men and women, sexual desire is linked to levels of androgens, testosterone, and dehydroepiandrosterone (DHEA). In men, testosterone levels begin to decline in the fifth decade and continue to do so steadily throughout later life. For both genders, DHEA levels begin to decline in the 30s, decrease steadily thereafter, and are quite low by age 60.

Decreased sexual desire is a common manifestation of some psychiatric conditions, particularly affective disorders. Several medications can negatively affect desire and the sexual response cycle (**Table 19-5**). The agents most commonly associated with these changes are psychoactive drugs, particularly antidepressants, and medications with antiandrogen effects. Many psychosocial issues affect sexual desire. Factors as widely varied as religious beliefs, primary sexual interest in individuals outside the main relationship, specific sexual phobias or aversions, fear of pregnancy, lack of attraction to partner, and poor sexual skills in the partner can all diminish sexual desire.

▶ **Clinical Findings**

A. Symptoms and Signs

Evaluation of decreased sexual desire should include a detailed sexual problem history, which may clarify difficulties with sexual desire, identify predisposing conditions, and help establish a therapeutic plan. In addition to loss of desire, a diminished sense of well-being, depression, lethargy, osteoporosis, loss of muscle mass, and erectile dysfunction are other manifestations of androgen deficiency.

Physical examination should be directed toward the identification of unrecognized conditions such as endocrine abnormalities (eg, hypogonadism, hypothyroidism).

B. Laboratory Findings

Assessment of hormone status may be helpful. In men, assess androgen status. In women, assess both androgens and estrogen status.

Assessment of the total plasma testosterone level, obtained in the morning, is the most readily available study.

In most men, levels below 300 ng/dL are symptomatic of hypogonadism; however, 200 ng/dL might be a more appropriate cutoff for diagnosis in older men. Free testosterone more accurately reflects bioavailable androgens. Levels less than 50 pg/mL suggest hypogonadism. If low testosterone is confirmed, further endocrine assessment and imaging is indicated to determine the specific underlying etiology.

▶ Treatment

Treatment is directed at the underlying etiology and consists of both nonspecific and specific therapy. Educating couples about the impact of extraneous influences—fatigue, preoccupation with child rearing, work-related stress, and interpersonal conflict—can improve awareness of these issues. Encouraging couples to set time aside for themselves, to schedule "dates," can be very effective. Educating partners about gender generalities and encouraging communication about sexual desires can be helpful. The quality of the relationship appears to be a critical component in women's sexual response cycle.

An emotionally and physically satisfying relationship enhances sexual desire and arousal and has a positive feedback on the quality of the relationship. The importance of allowing time for sexual relations, incorporating the senses, understanding what is pleasing to one's partner, and incorporating seduction cannot be overemphasized.

The impact of potentially reversible medical conditions or medications on sexual desire should be addressed. Treating organic etiologies such as depression, hypothyroidism, hyperprolactinemia, and androgen deficiency can often restore sexual interest.

When medications affect desire, treatment approaches can include lowering the dosage, suggesting drug holidays, discontinuing potentially offensive medications, or switching to a different agent. Where continuation of therapy is indicated, adding specific agents to address the sexual manifestations can be useful. Hormone supplementation may be considered.

A. Androgen Replacement

The goal of replacement therapy is to raise the level to the lowest physiologic range that promotes satisfactory response (**Table 19-6**). Oral testosterone is not recommended due to the prominent first-pass phenomenon and the potential for significant liver toxicity. Intramuscular injections result in dramatic fluctuations in blood levels. Topical preparations offer the advantage of consistent levels in the normal range. Local skin reactions are common with patches. Topical gels tend to have fewer skin side effects.

Table 19-6. Androgen therapy: agents, routes, and dosages.

Route/Agent	Dosage for Women	Dosage for Men (mg/d)
Oral[a] Methyltestosterone Fluoxymesterone Estratest and Estratest HS Dehydroepiandrosterone	10 mg: ¼–½ tablet daily or 10 mg Monday, Wednesday, Friday 2 mg: ½ tablet daily or 1 tablet every other day Either 1.25 or 0.625 mg 25–75 mg 3 times weekly to daily[a]	10–50 5–20
Buccal Methyltestosterone[c]	5–25 mg daily USP tablet, 0.25 mg[b]	5–25
Sublingual Methyltestosterone Testosterone micronized USP tablet	0.25 mg[b]	
Transdermal Testosterone patch Topical testosterone Testosterone micronized	2.5–5.0 mg applied every day or every other day 1% vaginal cream daily to clitoris and labia 1–2% gel daily to clitoris and labia[b]	4–6 5–10 (Androderm)
Intramuscular Testosterone enanthate Testosterone propionate	200 mg/mL: 0.25–0.5 mL every 3–5 weeks 100 mg/mL: 0.25–0.5 mL every 3–4 weeks	50–400 mg every 2–4 weeks 25–50 mg 2–3 times weekly

[a]Oral methyltestosterone, aside from the combination estratest, should be used only short term due to the risk of hepatotoxicity.
[b]Must be compounded by a pharmacist.
[c]Guay A. Advances in the management of androgen deficiency in women. *Med Aspects Hum Sex*. 2001;1:32–8.
Data from Nusbaum M, Rosenfeld J. *Sexual Health Across the Lifecycle: A Practical Guide for Clinicians*. Cambridge University Press; 2004: Chapters 6 and 7.

A diagnosis of androgen insufficiency is appropriate only in women who are adequately estrogenized, whose free testosterone is at or below the lowest quartile of the normal range for the reproductive age (20–40 years), and who present with clinical symptoms.

Androgen supplementation can be helpful for desire and arousal difficulties in both men and women. Dehydroepiandrosterone sulfate (DHEAS) is available over the counter and is dosed at 25–75 mg/d on the basis of response. Transdermal testosterone can be compounded as 1–2% cream, gel, or lotion that can be applied to the labial and clitoral area. Oral methyltestosterone, available as Estratest for women, has been used safely for years. Oral administration of methyltestosterone is a less preferred route, given erratic absorption, and concerns about liver effects.

Exogenous estrogens and progestins lower physiologically available androgens and can contribute to decreased sexual interest. Addition of androgens, methyltestosterone, or DHEAS can offset this negative impact. If no benefit occurs from this change, the physician should reassess the quality of the sexual relationship and also consider discontinuing the exogenous hormones. All oral contraceptive agents lower bioavailable androgen levels as a result of high sex hormone–binding globulin levels. Changing to oral contraceptive pills with greater androgen activity, such as those containing norgestrel, levonorgestrel, and norethindrone acetate, may be an effective change (**Table 19-7**).

B. Contraindications and Risk of Testosterone Therapy

Because testosterone treatment may stimulate tumor growth in androgen-, estrogen-, or progesterone-dependent cancers, it is contraindicated in men with prostate cancer and in men and women with a history of breast cancer. Although it is known that testosterone accelerates the clinical course of prostate cancer, there is no conclusive evidence that testosterone therapy increases the incidence of prostate cancer.

Certain patient populations such as the elderly and patients who have a first-degree relative with prostate cancer may be at increased risk. Preexisting sleep apnea and hyperviscosity, including deep venous thrombosis or pulmonary embolism, are relative contraindications to testosterone use. Serious hepatic and lipid changes have been associated with the use of oral preparations. Benign prostatic hypertrophy, lipid changes, gynecomastia, sleep apnea, and increased oiliness of skin or acne are other reported side effects.

If androgen therapy is initiated for both men and women, close follow-up is recommended to assess androgen levels, lipid profile, hematocrit levels, and liver function. Periodic assessment of the prostate-specific antigen level may be considered. Until more data regarding long-term use are available, it is probably most prudent to check androgen, hematocrit, liver, and lipid levels every 3–6 months.

Frank JE, et al. Diagnosis and treatment of female sexual dysfunction. *Am Fam Physician*. 2008; 74(5):635–642. [PMID:18350761]
Snyder PJ. Hypogonadism in elderly men—what to do until the evidence comes. *N Engl J Med*. 2004; 350–440. [PMID: 14749451]

DISORDERS OF EXCITEMENT & AROUSAL

▶ General Considerations

Arousal disorders affect 18.8% of women and 5% of men in the general population. Prevalence of arousal difficulties is much higher in patient populations with coexisting illnesses such as depression, diabetes, and heart disease. Abuse also has a negative effect on arousal and sexual health.

▶ Pathogenesis

Arousal difficulties most likely result from a mix of organic and psychogenic etiologies. Organic causes include vascular, neurogenic, and hormonal etiologies. Vascular arterial or inflow problems are by far the most common. Regardless of the primary etiology, a psychological component frequently coexists. Optimal function requires an intact nervous system and responsive arterial vasculature. Sexual stimulation results in nitric oxide release, which initiates a cascade of events leading to a dramatic increase in blood flow to the penis, vagina, and clitoris. Nitric oxide causes an increase in the production of cyclic guanosine monophosphate (cGMP). As cGMP concentrations rise, vascular smooth muscle relaxes, allowing increased arterial blood flow. The cGMP buildup is countered by the enzyme phosphodiesterase type 5 (PDE5).

Inhibiting the action of PDE5 results in higher levels of cGMP, causing increased and sustained vasodilation.

Table 19-7. Relative androgenicity of progestational components of oral contraceptive agents.

Least
Norethindrone (0.4–0.5 mg)[a]
Norgestimate (0.18–0.25 mg)
Desogestrel (0.15 mg)
Ethynodiol diacetate (1.0 mg)
Medium/neutral
Norethindrone (0.5–1.0 mg)[a]
Greatest
Levonorgestrel (0.1–0.15 mg)
Norgestrel (0.075–0.5 mg)
Norethindrone acetate (1.0–1.5 mg)

[a]Norethindrone (0.35 mg) without estrogen, in progestin-only oral contraceptive pills, has medium relative androgenicity.
Data from Nusbaum MRH. *Sexual Health*. American Academy of Family Physicians; 2001; and Burham T, Short R, eds. *Drug Facts and Comparisons*. Mosby; 2001.

Arousal disorders appear to increase with age, but chronic illnesses and therapeutic intervention are more likely the root cause. Lifestyle factors such as tobacco, alcohol, exercise, and diet also contribute.

► Clinical Findings

A. Symptoms and Signs

The first step in assessment is to ensure that arousal is the primary problem. Some men may complain of erectile difficulties but on detailed questioning may lack desire or may have premature ejaculation. Detailed information about the onset, duration, progression, severity, and association with medical conditions, medications, and psychosocial factors will enable the provider to identify if the patient's problem has a primarily organic or psychogenic etiology.

Physical examination should be focused and directed by the history. The clinician should assess overall health, including lifestyle topics such as exercise, tobacco use, and alcohol use. Screening for manifestations of affective, cardiovascular, neurologic, or hormonal etiology should be performed.

B. Laboratory Findings

If not previously done, a lipid profile and fasting blood glucose may identify unrecognized systemic disease that can predispose to vascular disease. Measurement of androgen levels (including DHEA) should be performed if androgen supplementation is being considered.

► Treatment

Chronic medical conditions should be treated to reverse or slow their progression. Medications contributing to arousal problems (eg, antihypertensive agents) should be replaced with other agents, if possible, or reduced in dosage. Potentially reversible causes should be addressed.

Glucose control, moderating alcohol consumption, exercise, and smoking cessation are important lifestyle changes necessary to maintain healthy sexual response. Nitric oxide appears to be androgen sensitive, so correction of androgen levels may be necessary before PDE5 inhibitors will be successful. Sexual lubricants such as Astroglide, Replens, and K-Y jelly can add lubrication and enhance sensuality.

A. Oral Agents

Sildenafil, vardenafil, tadalafil, and avanafil are PDE5 inhibitors and provide first-line treatment for male erectile dysfunction. Inhibitors do not result in spontaneous erection and require erotic or physical stimulation to be effective. PDE5 inhibitors are contraindicated in patients who take organic nitrates of any type. Nitrates are nitric oxide donors. The concomitant use of a PDE5 inhibitor and a nitrate can result in profound hypotension. PDE5 inhibitors are also contraindicated in patients with recent cardiovascular events or who are clinically hypotensive.

The side effects of PDE5 inhibitors are related to the presence of PDE5 in other parts of the body and cross-reactivity with other PDE enzyme subtypes. A transient disturbance in color vision, characterized typically by a greenish-blue hue, is due to a slight cross-reactivity with PDE5 isoenzyme in the retina. Because of this cross-reactivity, PDE5 inhibitors should not be used in patients with retinitis pigmentosa. Side effects tend to be mild and transient, and include headache, flushing, dyspepsia, and rhinitis.

PDE5 inhibitors are not approved by the FDA for use in women, and their role in treating female arousal difficulties remains controversial. Studies of genital stimulation devices and topical warming gels have shown these adjuncts to be beneficial to sexual functioning.

B. Vacuum Constriction Devices

These devices are effective for most causes of erectile dysfunction, are noninvasive, and are a relatively inexpensive treatment option. The device consists of a cylinder, vacuum pump, and constriction band. The flaccid penis is placed in the cylinder. Pressing the cylinder against the skin of the perineum forms an airtight seal. Negative pressure from the pump draws blood into the penis, resulting in increased firmness. When sufficient blood has entered the erectile bodies, a constriction band is placed around the base of the penis, preventing the escape of blood. Following intercourse the band is removed. Side effects include penile pain, bruising, numbness, and impaired ejaculation.

C. Intracavernosal Injection

With this method, synthetic formulations of prostaglandin E_1 (alprostadil alone or in combination with other vasoactive agents) is injected directly into the corpus cavernosum. This results in spontaneous erection. Intracavernosal injection is effective in producing erection in most patients with erectile dysfunction, including some who failed to respond to oral therapy.

D. Penile Prosthesis

In patients not responding to other therapies, a permanent penile prosthesis has proven to be safe and effective in many patients. Current models have a 7–10-year life expectancy or longer. Overall patient satisfaction is excellent.

► Sexual Pain Syndromes

Sexual pain syndromes can negatively affect arousal. Sexual pain syndromes occur in 14% of women and 3% of men in the general population, and >70% of samples of female patients. Peyronie plaques or other penile deformity, priapism, and lower urinary tract symptoms (LUTSs) can be etiologic in male sexual pain syndrome. For women, vaginitis, vestibulitis, pelvic pathology, vaginismus, and inadequate vaginal lubrication may cause sexual pain. Sexual pain syndromes negatively affect desire, arousal, and thus orgasm.

Heidelbaugh JJ. Management of erectile dysfunction. *Am Fam Physician*. 2010:81(3):305–312. [PMID: 20112889]

Nusbaum MRH, et al. The high prevalence of sexual concerns among women seeking routine gynecological care. *J Fam Practice*. 2000; 49:229 [PMID: 1073548]

DISORDERS OF EJACULATION & ORGASM

Premature ejaculation affects 29% of men in the general population, and orgasm difficulties affect 8% of men and 24% of women. Over 80% of women in patient populations report difficulties with orgasm.

Premature ejaculation results from a shortened plateau phase. In addition to heightened sensitivity to erotic stimulation and, often, learned behavior from rushed sexual encounters, organic etiology is also likely. The ejaculatory reflex involves a complex interplay between central serotonergic and other neurons. Premature ejaculation is speculated to be a dysfunction of serotonergic receptors.

Although premature ejaculation tends to improve with age by the natural lengthening of the plateau phase, it persists for many men. Like erectile dysfunction, premature ejaculation is often associated with shame and depression. Orgasmic difficulties can feed back negatively on arousal and then desire. Difficulty achieving orgasm affects a greater number of women than men and typically results from a prolonged arousal phase caused by inadequate stimulation. Medications can also interfere. Selective serotonin reuptake inhibitors (SSRIs) raise the threshold for orgasm, which makes them highly effective treatment options for men with premature ejaculation, but highly problematic for both genders who have difficulty achieving orgasm. Medications that lower the threshold for orgasm can be very problematic for men with premature ejaculation but can be very effective for treating problems with orgasm. These include cyproheptadine, bupropion, and possibly PDE5 inhibitors, which can be helpful for men with delayed ejaculation. Psychotropic agents and alcohol often delay ejaculation. Medications for treating sexual side effects of psychotropic agents or for women having difficulty with orgasm are also useful for treating delayed ejaculation (**Table 19-8**).

Retrograde ejaculation is caused by abnormal function of the internal sphincter of the urethra and can result from anatomic disruption (eg, transurethral prostatectomy), sympathetic nervous system disruptions (eg, damage from surgery), lymph node invasion, or diabetes. Retrograde ejaculation can result from interference with the sphincter function from medications such as antipsychotics, antidepressants, and antihypertensive agents as well as alcohol use.

Table 19-8. Antidotes for psychotropic-induced sexual dysfunction.

Drug	Dosage
Yohimbine	5.4–16.2 mg, 2–4 hours prior to sexual activity
Bupropion	100 mg as needed or 75 mg TID
Amantadine	100–400 mg as needed or daily
Cyproheptadine	2–16 mg a few hours before sexual activity
Methylphenidate	5–25 mg as needed
Dextroamphetamine	5 mg sublingually 1 hour prior to sex
Nefazodone	150 mg 1 hour prior to sex
Sildenafil	50–100 mg as needed

Data from Nusbaum MRH: *Sexual Health*. American Academy of Family Physicians; 2001; and Maurice W. Ejaculation/orgasm disorders. In: *Sexual Medicine in Primary Care*. Mosby; 1999:192.

Dextroamphetamine, ephedrine, phenylpropanolamine, and pseudoephedrine are potentially effective in treating retrograde ejaculation.

Evaluation should include a history of sexual problems, medications, and quality of the relationship. Treatment approaches include discontinuing, decreasing the dosage of, or drug holidays from offending medications. Small studies have shown a benefit from rescue agents that can be added as standing (or as needed) medications (see Table 19-8). SSRIs are the treatment of choice for premature ejaculation. It is helpful if women become familiar with the type of stimulation they require for orgasm and communicate that to their partners. An excellent reference for patients is the book by Heiman and LoPiccolo (1988).

The resolution phase is typically not problematic for either gender, but misunderstandings of age-related changes can occur. Men, and their partners, need to understand that with increasing age the refractory period to sexual stimulation lengthens, sometimes up to 24 hours. Men may require more direct penile stimulation for sexual response as they age.

Heiman JR, LoPiccolo J. *Becoming Orgasmic: A Sexual & Personal Growth Program for Women*. Englewood Cliffs, NJ: Prentice-Hall; 1988.

McMahon CG, et al. Disorders of orgasm and ejaculation in men. *J Sex Med*. 2004:1(1)58–65. [PMID: 16422984]

SEXUAL ACTIVITY & CARDIOVASCULAR RISK

Sexual activity and intercourse are associated with physiologic changes in heart rate and blood pressure. A patient's ability to meet the physiologic demands related to sexual activity should be assessed, particularly if the patient is not accustomed to the level of activity associated with sex or may be at increased risk for a cardiovascular event. Typical sexual intercourse is associated with an oxygen expenditure of 3–4 metabolic equivalents (METS), whereas vigorous sexual intercourse can expend 5–6 METS. Patients unaccustomed to the level of exercise associated with sexual activity and who have risk factors for cardiovascular events should be considered for cardiovascular screening. Men with erectile dysfunction are at significantly increased risk for cardiovascular, cerebrovascular, and peripheral vascular disease.

Jackson G, et al. The second Princeton consensus on sexual dysfunction and cardiac risk: new guidelines for sexual medicine. *J Sex Med*. 2006; 3(1)28–36. [PMID: 11556163]

Acute Coronary Syndrome

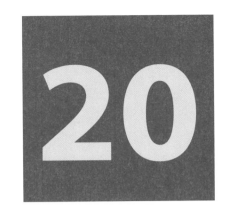

Stephen A. Wilson, MD, MPH, FAAFP
Jacqueline Weaver-Agostoni, DO, MPH
Jonathan J. Perkins, MD

General Considerations

Acute coronary syndrome (ACS) encompasses unstable angina, ST elevation myocardial infarction (STEMI), and non-ST-elevation myocardial infarction (NSTEMI). It is the symptomatic cardiac end product of cardiovascular disease (CVD) resulting in reversible or irreversible cardiac injury, and even death.

Diagnosis

The diagnosis of ACS requires two of the following: ischemic symptoms, diagnostic electrocardiogram (ECG) changes, or elevated serum marker of cardiac injury.

A. Symptoms

By themselves, signs and symptoms are not sufficient to diagnose or rule out ACS, but they start the investigatory cascade. Having known risk factors for coronary artery disease (CAD) (**Table 20-1**) or prior ACS increases the likelihood of ACS. Up to one-third of people with CAD progress to ACS with chest pain. While chest pain is the predominant symptom of ACS, it is not always present. Symptoms include the following:

- Chest pain
  - Classic: substernal pain that occurs with exertion and alleviates with rest (In a person with a history of CAD, this called "typical" or "stable" angina)
  - Dull, heavy pressure in or on the chest
  - Sensation of a heavy object on the chest
  - Initiated by stress, exercise, large meals, sex, or any activity that increases the body's demand on the heart for blood
  - Lasting >20 minutes
  - Radiating to the back, neck, jaw, left arm or shoulder

- Accompanied by feeling clammy or sweaty
- Associated with sensation of dry mouth (women)
- Not affected by inspiration
- Not reproducible with chest palpation
- Right-sided chest pain, occasionally
  - More common in African-American patients
- Pain high in the abdomen or chest, nausea, extreme fatigue after exercise, back pain, and edema can occur in anyone, but are more common in women
- Extreme fatigue or edema after exercise
- Shortness of breath
  - This can be the only sign in the elderly
  - More common in African-American than white patients
  - More common in women than men
- Levine's sign—chest discomfort described as a clenched fist over the sternum (the patient will clench his/her fist and rest it on or hover it over his/her sternum)
- Angor anami—great fear of impending doom/death
- Nausea, lightheadedness, or dizziness
- Less commonly
  - Mild, burning chest discomfort
  - Sharp chest pain
  - Pain that radiates to the right arm or back
  - A sudden urge to defecate in conjunction with chest pain

Chest pain that is present for days, is pleuritic, is positional, or radiates to the lower extremities or above the mandible is less likely to be cardiac in origin.

B. Physical Findings

Examination findings that increase the probability that symptoms are from ACS include hypotension, diaphoresis,

Table 20-1. Risk factors for coronary artery disease.

Nonmodifiable/Uncontrollable

Male sex
Age: men ≥45 years old
    women ≥55 years old or postmenopausal
Positive family history of CAD

Modifiable with Demonstrated Morbidity and Mortality Benefits

Hypertension	Overweight and obesity
Left ventricle hypertrophy	Physical inactivity
Dyslipidemia	Smoking (risk abates after 3 years' quit)
HDL <35 mg/dL	Low fruit and vegetable intake
LDL >130 mg/dL	Excessive alcohol intake[a]
Diabetes mellitus	

Potentially Modifiable but without Demonstrated Mortality and Morbidity Effects

Stress	Elevated uric acid
Depression	Lipoprotein(a)
Hypertriglyceridemia	Fibrinogen
Hyperhomocysteinemia	Elevated high-sensitivity C-reactive protein
Hyperreninemia	

[a]>2 drinks/day in men, >1 drink per day in women and lighter-weight persons; 1 drink = 0.5 oz (15 mL) of ethanol: 12 oz beer, 5 oz wine, or 1.5 oz 80-proof whiskey.

and systolic heart failure indicated by a new S_3 gallop, new or worsening mitral valve regurgitation, pulmonary edema, and jugular venous distention.

Chest pain reproducible with palpation is significantly less likely to be ACS.

C. Diagnostic Testing

Anyone suspected of having ACS should be evaluated with a 12-lead electrocardiogram (ECG) and serum cardiac biomarkers (eg, troponin, CPK-MB).

Notable ECG findings are as follows:

- ST-T segment (>1–mm elevation or depression) and T-wave (inversion) changes suggest ischemia.

- Q wave suggests accomplished infarction.

- ST elevation is absent in unstable angina and NSTEMI.

- New bundle branch block or sustained ventricular tachycardia indicates a higher risk of progression to infarction.

Accurate ECG interpretation is essential for diagnosis, risk stratification, and guiding the treatment plan. Many findings are non-specific, and the pre-existing presence of bundle branch block (BBB), interventricular conduction delay (IVCD), or Wolff-Parkinson-White syndrome reduce the diagnostic reliability of an ECG in patients with chest pain. If there is a recent ECG for comparison the presence of a new BBB or IVCD raises the suspicion of ACS.

A normal ECG does not exclude ACS. Up to 25–50% of people with angina or silent ischemia have a normal ECG; 10% of ACS is subsequently diagnosed with an MI after an initial normal ECG.

Cardiac biomarkers are blood tests that indicate myocardial damage. Troponins T and I are preferred because of their high sensitivity and specificity for myocardial injury. Troponin I is most preferred because troponin T is more likely to be elevated by renal disease, polymyositis, or dermatomyositis. Newer highly sensitive troponin I assays have a 97–99%, negative predictive value of depending on the chosen cutoff value, as early as 3 hours after the onset of symptoms. However, the specificity is lower, resulting in a tradeoff–fewer false negatives afford earlier diagnosis at the cost of more false positives. The potential impact of this will be discussed in the treatment section of this chapter. Troponin remains elevated for 7–10 days, and can therefore help identify prior recent infarctions.

When initial ECG and cardiac markers are normal, they should be repeated within 6–12 hours of symptom onset. If they are normal a second time, exercise or pharmacological cardiac stress testing should be done to evaluate for inducible ischemia. Exercise stress testing (EST) is preferred, but stress testing with chemicals (dobutamine, dipyridamole, or adenosine) can be used to simulate the cardiac effects of exercise in those unable to exercise enough to produce a test adequate for interpretation.

Exercise stress testing is the main test for evaluating those with suspected angina or heart disease (**Table 20-2**). Interpretation of the test is based on the occurrence of signs of stress-induced impairment of myocardial contraction, including ECG changes (**Table 20-3**) and/or symptoms and signs of angina. The false-positive rate is 10%.

Table 20-2. Exercise stress testing.

Indications	Contraindications
Confirm suspected angina	Cardiac failure
Evaluation of extent of myocardial ischemia and prognosis	Any febrile illness
Risk stratification after myocardial infarction	Left ventricular outflow tract obstruction or hypertrophic cardiomyopathy
Detection of exercise-induced symptoms (eg, arrhythmias or syncope)	Severe aortic or mitral stenosis
• Evaluation of outcome of interventions (eg, PCI or CABG)	Uncontrolled hypertension
• Assessment of cardiac transplant	Pulmonary hypertension
• Rehabilitation and patient motivation	Recent myocardial infarction
	Severe tachyarrhythmias
	Dissecting aortic aneurysm
	Left mainstem stenosis or equivalent
	Complete heart block

Reproduced with permission from Grech ED. Pathophysiology and investigation of coronary artery disease. *Br Med J.* 2003;326:1027–1031.

Table 20-3. Main endpoints for abnormal exercise ECG.

Target heart rate achieved (>85% of maximum predicted heart rate)
ST segment depression >1 mm (downsloping or planar depression of greater predictive value than upsloping depression)
Slow ST recovery to normal (>5 minutes)
Decrease in systolic blood pressure >20 mmHg
Increase in diastolic blood pressure >15 mmHg
Progressive ST segment elevation or depression
ST segment depression >3 mm without pain
Arrhythmias (atrial fibrillation, ventricular tachycardia)

Features Indicative of a Strongly Positive Exercise Test
Exercise limited by angina to <6 minutes of Bruce protocol
Failure of systolic blood pressure to increase >10 mmHg, or fall with evidence of ischemia
Widespread marked ST segment depression >3 mm
Prolonged recovery time of ST changes (>6 minutes)
Development of ventricular tachycardia
ST elevation in absence of prior myocardial infarction

Reproduced with permission from Grech ED. Pathophysiology and investigation of coronary artery disease. *BMJ.* 2003; 326:1027–1031.

Adding *radionuclide myocardial perfusion imaging* (**Table 20-4**) to EST can improve sensitivity, specificity, and accuracy, especially in patients with a nondiagnostic exercise test or limited exercise ability. *Acute rest myocardial perfusion imaging* is very similar, but is performed during or shortly after resolution of angina symptoms that were not induced by a stress test. Radionucleatide EST can

Table 20-4. Some indications for the use of radionuclide perfusion imaging rather than exercise electrocardiography.

Complete left bundle-branch block
Electronically paced ventricular rhythm
Preexcitation (Wolff-Parkinson-White) syndrome or other, similar electro-cardiographic conduction abnormalities
More than 1 mm of ST-segment depression at rest
Inability to exercise to a level high enough to give meaningful results on routine stress electrocardiography[a]
Angina and a history of revascularization[b]

The guidelines were developed by the American College of Cardiology, the American Heart Association, the American College of Physicians, and the American Society of Internal Medicine.
[a]Patients with tins factor should be considered for pharmacologic stress tests.
[b]In patients with angina and a history of revascularization, characterizing the ischemia, establishing the functional effect of lesions, and determining myocardial viability are important considerations.
Reproduced with permission from Lee TH, Boucher CA. *N Engl J Med.* 2001;344(24):1840–1845.

be advantageous in women because EST is less accurate in women compared to men.

Chest radiography (CXR) is used to assess for non-ACS causes of chest pain (eg, aortic dissection, pneumothorax, pulmonary embolus, pneumonia, rib fracture).

Echocardiography can be used to determine left ventricle ejection fraction, assess cardiac valve function, and detect regional wall motion abnormalities that correspond to areas of myocardial damage. Its high sensitivity and low specificity make it most useful to exclude ACS if the study is normal. It can also be used as an adjunct to stress testing. Since stress-induced impairment of myocardial contraction precedes ECG changes and angina, *stress echocardiography*, done and interpreted by experienced clinicians, can be superior to EST.

Cardiac magnetic resonance imaging does not yet have a clinical role because its sensitivity and specificity for detecting significant CAD plaque do not eclipse angiography, the gold standard.

Electron-beam computed tomography (EBCT) currently lacks utility since a positive test does not correlate well to an ACS episode. The future role of EBCT may change as more studies are done with higher resolution CT machines.

Coronary angiography is the gold standard. Main indications are in **Table 20-5.** Risks include death (1 in 1400), stroke (1 in 1000), coronary artery dissection (1 in 1000), arterial access complications (1 in 500), and minor risks such as arrhythmia; 10–30% of angiography studies are normal.

Pathogenesis & Epidemiology

Cardiovascular disease (CVD) includes all diseases of the heart and vascular (eg, stroke and hypertension).

Table 20-5. Main indications for coronary angiography.

Uncertain diagnosis of angina (coronary artery disease cannot be excluded by noninvasive testing)
Assessment of feasibility and appropriateness of various forms of treatment (percutaneous intervention, bypass surgery, medical)
Class I or U stable angina with positive stress test or class III or W angina without positive stress test
Unstable angina or non-Q-wave myocardial infarction (medium- and high-risk patients)
Angina not controlled by drug treatment
Acute myocardial infarction–especially cardiogenic shock, ineligibility for thrombolytic treatment, failed thrombolytic reperfusion, re-infarction, or positive stress test
Life threatening ventricular arrhythmia
Angina after bypass surgery or percutaneous intervention
Before valve surgery or corrective heart surgery to assess occult coronary artery disease

Reproduced with permission from Grech ED. Pathophysiology and investigation of coronary artery disease. *Br Med J.* 2003; 326:1027–1031.

CAD, synonymous with coronary heart disease (CHD), affects the coronary arteries by diminishing their ability to be a conduit for carrying oxygenated blood to the heart.

A. Atherosclerosis Progression

Atherosclerotic disease is the thickening and hardening (loss of elasticity) of the arterial wall due to the accumulations of lipids, macrophages, T lymphocytes, smooth-muscle cells, extracellular matrix, calcium, and necrotic debris. **Figures 20-1–20-3** grossly depict the multifactorial and complex depository, inflammatory, and reactive processes that collaborate to occlude coronary arteries.

B. Genetic Predisposition

Traditional risk factors for CAD include high LDL cholesterol, low HDL cholesterol, hypertension, family history of CAD, diabetes, smoking, menopause for women, and age >45 for men. Some inherited risk factors (eg, dyslipidemia and propensity for diabetes mellitus) are modifiable; others (eg, age and sex) are not. Genes affect the development and progression of disease and its response to risk factor modification and lifestyle decisions; nature (genetics) meets nurture (environment) and they responsively interrelate (**Table 20-6**). Obesity is an excellent example of the dynamics of the interplay between genetics and environment.

▶ Prevention: Primary, Secondary, & Tertiary

The cascade of events of CHD that lead to ACS can be interrupted, delayed, or treated. *Primary prevention* tries to prevent disease before it develops, namely, prevent or delay development of risk factors (eg, prevent the onset of smoking, obesity, diabetes, or hypertension). *Secondary prevention* attempts to prevent disease progression by identifying and treating risk factors or preclinical, asymptomatic disease (eg, treat hypertension or nicotine addiction *before* the occurrence of ACS). *Tertiary prevention* is treatment of established disease to restore and maintain highest function, minimize negative disease effects, and prevent complications, that is, help recover from and prevent recurrence of ACS (eg, treatment of hypertension and lowering LDL target from 100 mg/dL to 70 mg/dL after the occurrence of ACS).

Primary prevention of ACS should begin in childhood by preventing tobacco use, eating a diet rich in fruits and vegetable and low in saturated fats, exercising regularly for 20–30 minutes 5 times a week, and maintaining a BMI of 18–28 kg/m². Compared to waiting to initiate secondary and tertiary strategies, these primary prevention strategies yield a larger impact on decreasing lifetime risk of death from ACS and years of productive life lost to ACS.

Secondary and tertiary preventions involve increasingly aggressive management of those who have known risk factors for or have experienced ACS (**Figure 20-4** and **Table 20-7**). Although the association between cholesterol and ACS death is weaker in those aged >65 years, HMG-CoA reductase inhibitor drugs (statins) still positively impact morbidity and mortality in this demographic. This may be due to their effects that go beyond their lipid lowering: pleiotropic effects such as anti-inflammation and endothelial stabilizing.

Some once touted therapies have been found to be ineffective. Because of a lack of effect and potential harm, estrogen ± progestin *hormone replacement therapy* should not be used as primary, secondary, or tertiary prevention of CAD. *Antibiotics* and the *antioxidants folate, vitamin C, and vitamin E* do not improve ACS morbidity and mortality.

▶ Cardiac Rehabilitation

Cardiac rehabilitation, an example of tertiary prevention, is a multidisciplinary attempt to prevent future ACS by focusing on three areas: exercise, risk factor modification, and psychosocial intervention. Optimal medical management is part of this process. Patient adherence to the plan is integral to long-term success.

Exercise-based rehabilitation programs reduce both all-cause and cardiac mortality in patients with a history of myocardial infarction, surgical intervention [percutaneous coronary intervention (PCI), coronary artery bypass graft (CABG)], or stable CAD.

Risk factor modification addresses the content of Figure 20-4 and Table 20-7; involves dietician-guided nutritional training; and emphasizes smoking cessation via counseling, drug therapy (bupropion, varenicline), nicotine replacement, and formal cessation programs.

Psychosocial intervention emphasizes the identification and management of the psychological and social effects

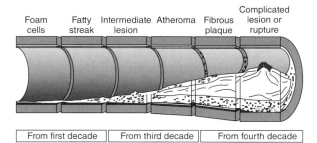

▲ Figure 20-1. Atheromatous plaque progression. (Reproduced with permission from Grech ED. Pathophysiology and investigation of coronary artery disease. *Br Med J.* 2003; 326:1027.)

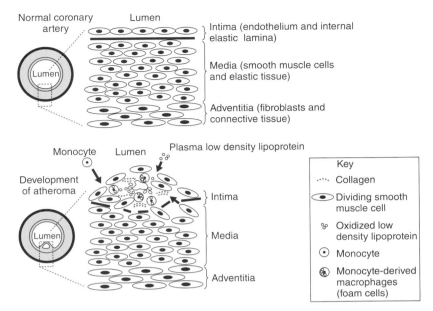

▲ **Figure 20-2.** Mechanism of plaque development. (Reproduced with permission from Grech ED. Pathophysiology and investigation of coronary artery disease. *Br Med J.* 2003; 326:1027.)

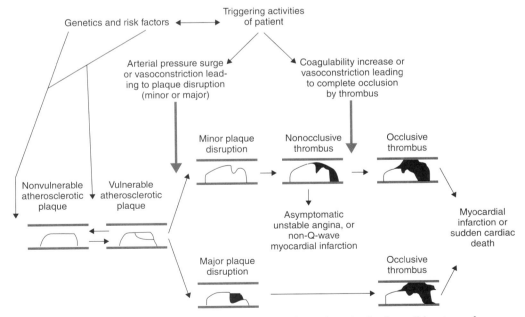

▲ **Figure 20-3.** Mechanism of coronary artery thrombosis. Hypothetical methods of possible trigger for coronary thrombosis: (1) physical or mental stress leads to hemodynamic changes leads to plaque rupture, (2) activities causing an increase in coagulability, and (3) stimuli leading to vasoconstriction. The role of coronary thrombosis in unstable angina, MI, and sudden cardiac death has been well described. (From Muller JE, et al. Triggers, acute risk factors and vulnerable plaques: the lexicon of a new frontier. *J Am Coll Cardiol.* 1994;23:809. Reproduced with permission from the American College of Cardiology. Chasen CA, Muller JE. Triggers of myocardial infarction. *Cardiol Special Ed.* 1997; 3:57.)

Table 20-6. Genetic and environmental influences on CHD predisposition.

Gene-Environment Interaction	Favorable Genes	Unfavorable Genes
Favorable environment	Low risk	Moderate risk
Unfavorable environment	Moderate risk	High risk

Reproduced with permission from Scheuner MT. Genetic predisposition to coronary artery disease. *Curr Opin Cardiol.* 2001;16:251–260.

that can follow ACS. These effects can include depression, anxiety, family issues, and job-related problems. Depression has been linked to worse mortality in patients with CHD. Psychosocial intervention alone does not affect total or cardiac mortality, but does decrease depression and anxiety, which may impact quality of life.

▶ Differential Diagnosis of ACS Signs & Symptoms

These are listed as follows:

- Anemia
- Aortic aneurysm
- Aortic dissection
- Cardiac tamponade
- Cardiac valve rupture
- Cardiomyopathy
- Cholecystitis
- Costochondritis
- Coronary artery anomaly or aneurysm
- Diaphragramatic irritation/inflammation due to
  - Hepatitis
  - Infection
  - Mass effect from nearby cancer
  - Pancreatitis
  - Pulmonary edema/effusion
- Drug use (eg, cocaine)
- Duodenal ulcer
- Esophageal spasm
- Esophagitis
- Gastritis
- Generalized anxiety disorder (GAD)
- Gastroesophageal reflux disease (GERD)
- Hiatal hernia
- High-altitude exposure
- Hyperthyroidism
- Panic attack
- Peptic ulcer disease
- Pericardial effusion
- Pericarditis
- Pleurisy/pleuritis
- Pneumothorax
- Prinzmetal's angina (coronary vasospasm)—more common in women

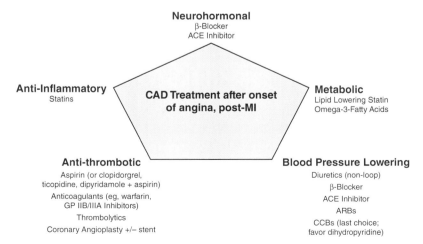

▲ **Figure 20-4.** Tertiary revention for CAD (ACE, angiotensin-converting enzyme; ARB, angiotensin receptor blocker; CCB, calcium channel blocker; GP, glycoprotein).

Table 20-7. Guide to comprehensive risk reduction for patients with coronary artery disease.

Risk Intervention	Recommendations			
Smoking: *Goal:* complete cessation	Strongly encourage patient and family to stop smoking. Provide counseling, nicotine replacement, bupropion, and formal cessation programs as appropriate.			
Lipids: *Primary goal* LDL <100 mg/dL *Secondary goals* HDL >35 mg/dL TG <200 mg/dL	Start AHA Step II Diet in all patients: (30% fat, <200 mg/d cholesterol) Assess fasting lipid profile. • In post-MI patients, lipid profile may take 4–6 weeks to stabilize. Add drug therapy according to the following table:			
	LDL <100 mg/dL	LDL 100–130 mg/dL	LDL >130 mg/dL	HDL <35 mg/dL
	No medication unless post-MI; if post-MI, use statin and target LDL <70 mg/dL	Consider adding drug therapy to diet, as follows:	Add drug therapy to diet, as follows:	Emphasize weight management and physical activity Advise smoking cessation
		Statins as 1st-line suggestion drug therapy		If needed to achieve LDL goals, consider statin, fibrate, fish oil
	TG <200 mg/dL	TG 200–400 mg/dL	TG >400 mg/dL	
	Statin Resin Omega-3-fatty acids (fish oil)	Statin Omega-3-fatty acids (fish oil)	Consider combined drug therapy (statin, resin, fish oil)	
	If LDL goal not achieved, consider combination therapy			
Physical activity: Minimum goal 30 minutes 3–4 times per week	Assess risk, preferably with exercise test, to guide prescription Encourage minimum of 30–60 minutes of moderate-intensity activity 3–4 times weekly (walking , jogging, cycling, or other aerobic activity) supplemented by an increase in daily lifestyle activities (eg, walking breaks at work, using stairs, gardening, household work) Maximum benefit 5–6 hours a week Advise medically supervised programs for moderate- to high-risk patients			
Weight management *Ideal BMI:* 18.5–25 kg/m^2	Start intensive diet and appropriate physical activity intervention, as outlined above, in patients >120% of ideal weight for height Particularly emphasize need for weight loss in patients with hypertension, elevated triglycerides, or elevated glucose levels Desirable waist-to-hip ratio for men, <0.9: for middle-aged and elderly women, <0.8			
Antiplatelet agents/ anticoagulants	Start aspirin 80– 325 mg/d, if not contraindicated Manage warfarin to international normalized ratio of 2–3.5 for post-MI patients not able to take or fails aspirin, then consider ticlopidine, clopidogrel, or dipyridamole + aspirin			
ACE inhibitors post-MI	Start post-MI in stable patients, within 24 hours in patients with anterior MI, CHF, renal insufficiency, EF <40%, (LV dysfunction) Maximize dose as tolerated indefinitely Use to manage blood pressure or symptoms in all other patients			
β-blockers	Post-MI, as tolerated			
estrogens	No role; more evidence of harm than help			
Blood pressure *Goal:* ≤140/90 mmHg **Optimal: 115/75**	Initiate lifestyle modification: weight control, physical activity, and alcohol moderation in all patients with blood pressure >140 mmHg systolic or 90 mmHg diastolic Add blood pressure medication, individualize to other patient requirements and characteristics (ie, age, race, need for drugs with specific benefits) if blood pressure is ≥140 mmHg systolic or ≥90 mmHg diastolic in 3 months if initial blood pressure is >160 mmHg systolic or 100 mmHg diastolic			

ACE, angiotensin-converting enzyme; BMI, body mass index; CHD, coronary heart disease; CHF, congestive heart failure; EF, ejection fraction; IV, left ventricular; LFTs, liver function tests; MI, myocardial infarction; TFTs, thyroid function tests; TG, triglycerides; UA, uric acid.
Data from Smith SC Jr, Blair SN, Bonow RO, et al. AHA/ACC guidelines for preventing heart attack and death in patients with atherosclerotic cardiovascular disease. *J Am Coll Cardiol.* 2001; 38:1581–1583.

- Pulmonary embolus
- Pulmonary hypertension
- Radiculopathy
- Shoulder arthropathy
- Stress reactional anxiety
- Supraventricular tachycardia
- Vasculitis

▶ ACS Complications

There are four major complications: (1) death, (2) myocardial infarction (MI), (3) hospitalization, and (4) cardiac disability—lifestyle and activity options are diminished because the heart is unable to supply the oxygenated blood that the body needs to fulfill its demand because the coronary arteries are unable to supply the heart muscle.

There is one important formula to keep in mind for management of ACS:

Treatment: time = tissue!

ACS causes myocardial infarction (MI) in three ways:

1. Atheromatous plaque buildup increases till the artery is totally occluded.

2. An atheromatous plaque ruptures or tears, leading to occlusions via inflammatory response and thrombus formation as platelets adhere to the site to seal off the plaque.

3. Superimposition of thrombus on a disrupted atherosclerotic plaque.

The *goal of treatment* is to save cardiac muscle by reducing myocardial oxygen demand and/or increasing oxygen supply.

All patients with ACS should be hospitalized, be medically stabilized, and receive further cardiac evaluation to determine STEMI versus NSTEMI versus unstable angina and then treatment appropriate to the diagnosis. Immediate PCI can be beneficial for STEMI, but can be safely delayed in low-risk NSTEMI. All ACS patients should receive medical management, which begins with the mnemonic **HOBANACS**:

Heparin (low-molecular-weight heparin→fewer MIs and deaths)

Oxygen

Beta-blocker (β-blocker; if hemodynamically stable: metoprolol, timolol, propranolol, or carvedilol if decreased ejection fraction)

Aspirin (initially 160–325 mg each day then 70–162 mg daily indefinitely)

Nitroglycerin (for pain; stop if hypotension occurs)

ACE inhibitor (angiotensin-converting enzyme inhibitor; within the first 24 hours if anterior-location infarct, heart failure, or ejection fraction of ≤40%, unless contraindicated)

Clopidogrel (up to 1 year; not within 5 days of CABG)

Statins (HMG-CoA-reductase inhibitors; goal LDL <70 mg/dL)

Morphine may be added for pain and anxiety relief. It also provides some afterload reduction.

Anticoagulation with *heparin* starts with low-molecular-weight heparin if PCI is not planned. Unfractionated heparin should be used if creatinine clearance <60 mL/minute or if early PCI or CABG is planned within 24 hours. Fondaparinux is as effective as enoxaparin with less major bleeding and lower long-term mortality.

Beta-blockers decrease the workload on the heart by slowing it down and decreasing blood pressure. The goal should be <130/85 mmHg or < 130/80 mmHg if diabetes or chronic kidney disease is present; optimal blood pressure may be 115/75 mmHg.

Aspirin (ASA) should be continued indefinitely. Once ACS is stabilized, a dose of 81 mg per day should suffice. If ASA is not tolerated, clopidogrel should be used. If there is a history of gastrointestinal bleeding and either ASA or clopidogrel is used, drugs to decrease the risk of recurrent gastrointestinal bleeding (eg, proton-pump inhibitors) should be given.

Clopidogrel requires a loading dose (300–600 mg) followed by the daily maintenance dose (75 mg). If there is no plan for PCI, it should be added to aspirin and anticoagulant therapy as soon as possible after admission. If PCI is likely, it can be added before the procedure. Duration of treatment should be for at least 3 months and ideally up to 1 year. Ticagrelor (180 mg load then 90 mg twice daily) compared to clopidogrel resulted in lower all-cause mortality, vascular mortality, and MI rate without increase in major bleeding or stroke. Prasugrel (5–10 mg daily) compared to clopidogrel has not shown lower risk of death from cardiovascular causes, myocardial infarction, or stroke, and bleeding risks are similar.

Platelet glycoprotein IIB/IIIA (GP IIB/IIIA) receptor inhibitors should be used judiciously if there is no plan for revascularization: 100 STEMIs need to be treated to prevent one MI or death, but for every one prevention there is one major bleeding complication. Specifically, abciximab should be used only if PCI is planned.

Reperfusion–PCI, CABG, medications can also be used. If cardiac tissue is to survive, blood flow must be restored. STEMI (active infarctions) require medical thrombolysis or emergent angioplasty to achieve this. Primary PCI is the recommended method of reperfusion. If PCI or CABG cannot be initiated within 120 minutes, then thrombolytic, fibrinolytic agents should be started within 30–60 minutes. When medical therapy is used because PCI/CABG cannot be initiated within 120 minutes, if blood flow is still not restored, then proceed to PCI/CABG as soon as possible without a "cooling off" period A cooling-off period (ie, delaying PCI or CABG because of failed medical thrombolysis, increases mortality without decreasing bleeding complications).

While there is a modest decrease in recurrent ischemia, *early PCI* within 24 hours of symptom onset for lower-risk NSTEMI patients does not decrease mortality compared to *late PCI* within 36 hours. Higher-risk patients (ST >1-mm depression, T wave inversion, impaired renal function, hemodynamically unstable, TIMI[1] score > 4, GRACE[2] >140, presence of heart failure) with NSTEMI benefit from early PCI within 24 hours. There is no difference in NSTEMI mortality between PCI in 70 minutes compared to 21 hours in higher-risk patients (TIMI score is >4).

The 2-year risk of death or recurrent MI is the same for PCI and CABG, but approximately 5% with a CABG get less angina.

Post-MI care should center around tertiary care (see cardiac rehabilitation, illustrated in Figure 20-4, and Table 20-7). Optimal blood pressure is closer to 115/75 mmHg, since in 40–70-year-olds each increment of 20 mmHg in systolic BP or 10 mmHg in diastolic BP doubles the risk of CVD across the entire BP range from 115/75 mmHg to 185/115 mmHg.

Cyclooxygenase-2 (COX2) nonsteroidal anti-inflammatory drugs and naproxen should be avoided because they increase risk for ACS.

For some individuals, using warfarin (goal INR 2.0–3.0) together with aspirin or warfarin alone (goal INR 3.0–4.0) results in a better all-cause mortality than taking aspirin alone. It reduces the risk of myocardial infarction and stroke but increases the risk of major bleeding.

CULTURAL CONSIDERATIONS

Cultural issues can affect the diagnosis, treatment, and outcome of ACS. Some clinical symptoms are more common in certain patient populations (see prior symptoms list). Overall, atypical symptoms are more prevalent in women and elderly patients. Symptoms may include jaw and neck pain, dyspnea, fatigue, dry mouth, palpitations, indigestion, cough, and nausea and emesis. Maybe because atypical symptoms occur more frequently in women and older adults, they tend to experience delaying diagnosis, less aggressive treatment, and increased rates of in-hospital mortality.

Other notable differences exist between patient populations that relate to diagnosis and treatment of cardiac disease. Both men and women with ACS respond to early invasive treatment. Women tend to have a more severe first ACS, are less likely to receive thrombolysis, and are at greater risk for death and hospital readmission at 6 months. Patients with symptoms of acute MI are less often hospitalized if they are nonwhite or have a normal or nondiagnostic ECG. Patients experiencing ACS who are women <55 years of age, are nonwhite, have shortness of breath as their chief complaint, or have a normal or indeterminate ECG and are less often hospitalized, thus increasing their morality. After ACS, women are more likely than men to experience depression and hence its ramifications.

Patients are more likely to adhere to treatment plans that they can afford. This should be taken into account when deciding which medication to prescribe and which diets and exercise plans to recommend. Emphasize free and low-cost exercise options; remember that some diet approaches are less expensive than others.

PROGNOSIS

An estimated 60% of myocardial infarction deaths occur within the first hour of symptom onset. Prognosis following a survived MI without subsequent intervention carries a mortality rate of 10% the first year and 5% each additional year. Sudden death, more common in patients with a lower ejection fraction, following ACS occurs in 1.4% of patients during the first month, and decreases to 0.14% per month after 2 years.

When either troponin T or I level is normal at 2, 4, and 6 hours after the onset of chest pain in patients with a normal ECG, the 30-day risk of cardiac death and nonfatal acute MI is nearly zero.

Normal troponin T levels at 10–12 hours after symptom onset in patients with chest pain and a normal ECG indicate a low risk of adverse events for the next 12 months. Even slight elevations in cardiac troponin levels in patients with unstable angina and NSTEMI help identify high-risk patients who may benefit the most from early invasive treatment.

Website-accessible scoring systems can help risk-stratify patients with chest pain and help determine prognosis given a range of different circumstances by analyzing individual patient characteristics and test results. Prognostic tools are valuable when educating patients about possible outcomes, and when discussing and deciding on treatment options.

Balady GJ et al. Core components of cardiac rehabilitation/secondary prevention programs: 2007 update: a scientific statement from the American Heart Association Exercise, Cardiac Rehabilitation, and Prevention Committee, the Council on Clinical Cardiology; the Councils on Cardiovascular Nursing, Epidemiology and Prevention, and Nutrition, Physical Activity, and Metabolism; and the American Association of Cardiovascular and Pulmonary Rehabilitation. *Circulation.* 2007;115:2675–2682.

---

[1]TIMI: *Thrombolysis In Myocardial Infarction* calculators (http://www.mdcalc.com/timi-risk-score-for-uanstemi https://www.essentialevidenceplus.com/content/rules/153).
[2]GRACE: Global Registry of Acute Coronary Events calculator (http://www.outcomes-umassmed.org/grace/).

Fihn SD et al. 2012 ACCF/AHA/ACP/AATS/PCNA/SCAI/STS guideline for the diagnosis and management of patients with stable ischemic heart disease: Executive Summary—a report of the American College of Cardiology Foundation/American Heart Association Task Force on Practice Guidelines, and the American College of Physicians, American Association for Thoracic Surgery, Preventive Cardiovascular Nurses Association, Society for Cardiovascular Angiography and Interventions, and Society of Thoracic Surgeons. *J Am Coll Cardiol.* 2012; 60:e44–e164 (available at http://dx.doi.org/10.1016/j.jacc.2012.07.013).

Montalescot G et al. Immediate vs delayed intervention for acute coronary syndromes: a randomized clinical trial. *JAMA* 2009; 302:947;302(9):947–954. doi:10.1001/jama.2009.1267.

Seventh Report of the Joint National Committee on Prevention, Detection, Evaluation and Treatment of High Blood Pressure (JNC7).

Smith SC Jr et al. AHA/ACC guidelines for secondary prevention for patients with coronary and other atherosclerotic vascular disease: 2006 update: endorsed by the National Heart, Lung, and Blood Institute. *Circulation.* 2006; 113(19):2363–2372.

Websites
For Information on ACS & CVD

American Academy of Family Physicians: http://www.aafp.org and http://familydoctor.org

American College of Cardiology: http://www.acc.org

American Heart Association: http://www.americanheart.org

Centers for Disease Control: http://www.cdc.gov

Family Practice Notebook: http://fpnotebook.com/CV/index.htm

National Heart, Lung, and Blood Institute: http://www.nhlbi.nih/health/public/heart/other/chdfacts.htm

Mayo Clinic.com: http://www.mayoclinic.com

MEDLINE Plus: http://www.medlineplus.gov

Medtronic: http://www.medtronic.corn/cad

Merck Manual: http://www.merck.com/mrkshared/mmanual/home.jsp

National Institutes of Health–health topics: http://health.nih.gov/

Risk Assessment Tool for Estimating 10-year Risk of Developing Hard CHD (myocardial infarction and coronary death): http://hp2010.nhlbihin.net/atpIII/calculator.asp?usertype=prof

UPMC patient information: http://patienteducation.upmc.com/

For Informaion on Other Cardiac Disorders

https://www.essentialevidenceplus.com/content/poem/110991 Early angiography not crucial in low risk NSTEMI patients (TIMACS).

https://www.essentialevidenceplus.com/content/poem/111003 Highly sensitive troponin I more accurate for AMI diagnosis (APACE).

http://www.mdcalc.com/timi-risk-score-for-uanstemi

http://www.nhlbi.nih.gov/health/public/heart/other/chdfacts.htm

Heart Failure

Michael King, MD, MPH

Oscar Perez, Jr., DO

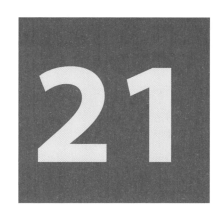

▶ Left ventricular dysfunction by echocardiography

▶ Dyspnea on exertion and fatigue are common, but paroxysmal nocturnal dyspnea, orthopnea, and peripheral edema are more diagnostic.

▶ Third heart sound, displaced cardiac apex, jugular venous distension, hepatojugular reflux, rales, murmur, or peripheral edema.

▶ Any electrocardiographic (ECG) abnormality, radiographic evidence of pulmonary venous congestion, cardiomegaly, or pleural effusion

▶ Elevated B-type natriuretic peptide (BNP) or *N*-terminal pro-BNP levels

General Considerations

Increased survivorship after acute myocardial infarction (MI) and improved treatment of hypertension, valvular heart disease, and coronary artery disease (CAD) have led to a significant increase in the prevalence of heart failure in the United States. Overall prevalence of any heart failure diagnosis is estimated at 2.6% (2.7% in men; 1.7% in women) and increases with age. Asymptomatic left ventricular systolic dysfunction (LVSD) has been found to be as prevalent as symptomatic LVSD: 1.4% and 1.5%, respectively. In patients with clinical symptoms of heart failure, moderate or severe isolated diastolic dysfunction appears to be as common as systolic dysfunction, and systolic dysfunction appears to increase with the severity of diastolic dysfunction.

Pathogenesis

As defined by the American Heart Association (AHA) and the American College of Cardiology (ACC), heart failure is "a complex clinical syndrome that can result from any structural or functional cardiac disorder that impairs the ability of the ventricle to fill with or eject blood."As cardiac output decreases in response to the stresses placed on the myocardium (**Table 21-1**) activation of the sympathetic nervous and renin-angiotensin-aldosterone system occur. These neurohormonal adaptations help increase blood pressure for tissue perfusion and also increase blood volume to enhance preload, stroke volume, and cardiac output. These compensatory mechanisms, which increase afterload, also lead to further myocardial deterioration and worsening myocardial contractility.

Causes of Cardiac Failure

Coronary artery disease and diabetes mellitus are the leading causes of heart failure in the United States. It is estimated that 60–70% of patients having systolic heart failure have CAD as the underlying etiology. CAD is a substantial predictor of developing symptomatic heart failure with LVSD compared to asymptomatic LVSD. Heart failure is twice as common in diabetic patients and is one of the most significant factors for developing heart failure in women. This is likely due to the direct effect of diabetes in developing cardiomyopathy as well as the effects of CAD risk and progression. Poorly controlled hypertension and valvular heart disease also remain major precipitants of heart failure. Often overlooked risk factors in the development of heart failure are smoking, physical inactivity or obesity, and lower socioeconomic status. Tobacco is estimated to cause approximately 17% of heart failure cases in the United States, likely due to the enhanced CAD risk. Lower socioeconomic status may limit access to higher quality health care, resulting in decreased adherence to treatment of modifiable risk factors such as hypertension, diabetes mellitus, and CAD.

Table 21-1. Causes of heart failure.

Most common causes
Coronary artery disease
Diabetes
Hypertension
Idiopathic cardiomyopathy
Valvular heart disease

Less common causes
Arrhythmias (tachycardia, atrial fibrillation/flutter, bradycardia, heart block)
Collagen vascular disease (systemic lupus erythematosus, scleroderma)
Endocrine/metabolic disorders (thyroid disease, pheochromocytoma, other genetic disorders)
Hypertrophic cardiomyopathy
Myocarditis (including HIV)
Pericarditis
Postpartum cardiomyopathy
Restrictive cardiomyopathies (amyloidosis, hemochromatosis, sarcoidosis, other genetic disorders)
Stress-induced cardiomyopathy/Takotsubo cardiomyopathy
Toxic cardiomyopathy (alcohol, cocaine, heavy metals, chemotherapy, radiation)

Data from King M, Kingery J, Casey B. Diagnosis and evaluation of heart failure. *Am Fam Physician.* 2012;85(12):1161–1168; Institute for Clinical Systems Improvement (ICSI). *Heart Failure in Adults.* Bloomington, MN: Institute for Clinical Systems Improvement (ICSI); 2011.

Aurigemma GP, et al. Predictive value of systolic and diastolic function for incident congestive heart failure in the elderly: the Cardiovascular Health Study. *J Am Coll Cardiol.* 2001; 37:1042. [PMID: 11263606]

Bibbins-Domingo K, et al. Predictors of heart failure among women with coronary disease. *Circulation.* 2004;110:1424. [PMID: 15353499]

Gheorghiade M, Bonow RO. Chronic heart failure in the United States: a manifestation of coronary heart disease. *Circulation.* 1998; 97:282–289 (review).

He J, et al. Risk factors for congestive heart failure in US men and women: NHANES I epidemiologic follow-up study. *Arch Intern Med.* 2001; 161:996. [PMID: 11295963]

Classification & Prevention

The most important component to classifying heart failure is whether left ventricular ejection fraction (LVEF) is preserved or reduced (<50%). A reduced LVEF in heart failure is a powerful predictor of mortality. The American College of Cardiology (ACC)/American Heart Association (AHA) classified heart failure into stages emphasizing the progressive nature of the clinical syndrome. These stages more clearly define appropriate therapy at each level that can reduce morbidity and mortality and delay the onset of clinically evident disease (**Table 21-2**).

Patients in ACC/AHA stages A and B do not have clinical symptomatic heart failure but are at risk for developing heart failure. Stage A includes those at risk but not manifesting structural heart disease. Early identification and aggressive treatment of modifiable risk factors remain the best prevention for heart failure. Lifestyle modification, pharmacologic therapy, and counseling can improve or correct conditions such as CAD, hypertension, diabetes mellitus, hyperlipidemia, obesity, tobacco abuse, and alcohol or illicit substance abuse. Stage B represents patients who are asymptomatic but have structural heart disease or left ventricular systolic dysfunction. Stage C comprises the majority of patients with heart failure who have past or current symptoms and associated underlying structural heart disease, including left ventricular systolic dysfunction. Stage D includes refractory patients with heart failure who may need advanced and specialized treatment strategies.

The NYHA classification gauges the severity of symptoms for patients with stage C and D heart failure. The NYHA classification is a more subjective assessment that can change frequently, secondary to treatment response, but it is a well-established predictor of mortality.

▶ Clinical Findings

A high index of suspicion is necessary to diagnose the syndrome of heart failure early in its clinical presentation, because of nonspecific signs and symptoms. Patients are often elderly with comorbidity, symptoms may be mild, and routine clinical assessment lacks specificity. A prompt diagnosis allows for early treatment with therapies proven to delay the progression of heart failure and improve quality of life. Evaluation is directed at confirming the presence of heart failure, determining cause, identifying comorbid illness, establishing severity, and guiding response to therapy. Heart failure is a clinical diagnosis for which no single symptom, examination, or test can establish the presence or absence with certainty.

Hunt SA, et al. 2009 focused update incorporated into ACC/AHA 2005 guidelines for a report of the American College of Cardiology Foundation/; American Heart Association Task Force on Practice Guidelines. Developed in collaboration with the International Society for Heart and Lung Transplantation. *Circulation.* 2009; 119:e391–e479 (also available at http://circ.ahajournals.org/cgi/reprint/119/14/1977.pdf).

A. Symptoms and Signs

The most common manifestations of symptomatic heart failure are dyspnea and fatigue, but many conditions present with these symptoms. Limited exercise tolerance and fluid retention may eventually lead to pulmonary congestion and peripheral edema. Neither of these symptoms necessarily dominates the clinical picture at the same time. The absence of dyspnea on exertion is helpful to rule out the diagnosis

Table 21-2. Progression of heart failure and recommended evidence-based therapies.

	Progression of Heart Failure				
	At Risk for Heart Failure		**Heart Failure**		
NYHA classification	Not applicable	Class I: asymptomatic	Class II: symptoms with significant exertion	Class III: symptoms on minor exertion	Class IV: symptoms at rest
ACC/AHA stage	Stage A: high risk	Stage B: asymptomatic with cardiac structural abnormalities (MI, remodeling , reduced EF, valvular disease)	Stage C: cardiac structural abnormalities (reduced EF) and symptomatic or history of heart failure		Stage D: refractory end-stage heart failure
Treatments: beneficial, effective, recommended	*Goals:* disease management: Hypertension[a] Lipid disorders[a] Diabetes mellitus[c] Thyroid disease[c] Secondary prevention of atherosclerotic vascular disease[c] Behavior change[c] Smoking cessation Regular exercise Avoidance of alcohol and illicit drug use	*Goals:* stage A measures *Drugs* (in appropriate patients): ACEI[a] or ARB[b] β-blockers (history of MI[a]; no MI[c])	*Goals:* stage A/B measures, dietary sodium restriction[c] *Drugs/devices:* Routine use: Diuretics[c] (fluid retention) ACEI[a] or ARB[a] β-blockers[a] In selected patients: ARB[a] Aldosterone antagonists[a] Hydralazine or nitrates[a] Implantable cardioverter defibrillator[a]		*Goals:* stage A, B, and C measures Meticulous fluid retention control[b] Decision regarding appropriate level of care and referral to heart failure program[a] *Options:* End-of-life care or hospice[c] Extraordinary measures: heart transplantation[c]
Treatments: reasonably beneficial, probably recommended	*Drugs* (in appropriate patients): ACEI[a] or ARB[c] (in patients with vascular disease or diabetes mellitus)	–	*Drugs/devices (in selected patients):* Digitalis[b] Cardiac resynchronization therapy[b]		*Options:* extraordinary measures: permanent mechanical support[b]

[a]Level of evidence A (evidence from multiple randomized trials, meta-analysis).
[b]Level of evidence B (evidence from single randomized or nonrandomized trials).
[c]Level of evidence C (expert opinion, case studies, standard of care).
ACC/AHA, American College of Cardiology/American Heart Association ACEI, angiotensin-converting enzyme inhibitor;. ARB, angiotensin receptor blocker; NYHA, New York Heart Association.
Data from Hunt SA, et al. 2009 focused update incorporated into ACC/AHA 2005 guidelines for a report of the American College of Cardiology Foundation/American Heart Association Task Force on Practice Guidelines. Developed in collaboration with the International Society for Heart and Lung Transplantation. *Circulation.* 2009;119:e391–e479.

of heart failure with a sensitivity of 84%. Other symptoms that are helpful in diagnosing heart failure include orthopnea, paroxysmal nocturnal dyspnea (PND), and peripheral edema. PND has the highest specificity: 84% of any symptom for heart failure. It is important to remember that no single clinical symptom has been shown to be both sensitive and specific. A substantial portion of the population has asymptomatic left ventricular systolic dysfunction, and the history alone is insufficient to make the diagnosis of heart failure. However, a detailed history and review of symptoms

remain the best approach in identifying the cause of heart failure and assessing response to therapy.

B. Physical Examination

The clinical examination is helpful to assess the degree of reduced cardiac output, volume overload, and ventricular enlargement. It can also provide clues to noncardiac causes of dyspnea. A third heart sound, S_3 (ventricular filling gallop), on examination is specific for increased left ventricular end-diastolic pressure and decreased left ventricular ejection fraction. It has the best specificity of any exam finding for heart failure: 99%. Thus, a third audible sound along with a displaced cardiac apex are both very predictive and effectively rule in a diagnosis of left ventricular systolic dysfunction. Volume overload from heart failure can present with many signs on examination. The presence of jugular venous distention and a hepatojugular reflex can be present and moderately effective in diagnosing heart failure. Other signs such as pulmonary rales (crackles), a murmur, or peripheral edema have a smaller but helpful effective in diagnosing heart failure.

Other exam findings can assist in determining causes of heart failures or assess other differential diagnosis. Cardiac murmurs may be an indication of primary valvular disease. Asymmetric rales or rhonchi on the pulmonary examination may suggest pneumonia or chronic obstructive pulmonary disease (COPD). Dullness to percussion or auscultation of the lungs could indicate pleural effusion. Examination of the thyroid can exclude thyromegaly or goiter, which could cause abnormal thyroid function precipitating heart failure. Hepatomegaly can indicate passive hepatic congestion.

C. Laboratory Findings

Objective tests can aid in confirmation of heart failure by assessing the differential diagnosis and excluding other possible causes for the signs and symptoms. A complete blood count can rule out anemia as a cause of high-output failure. Electrolyte (including magnesium and calcium) analysis may reveal deficiencies that are commonplace with treatment and can render the patient prone to arrhythmias. Hyponatremia is a poor prognostic sign indicating significant activation of the renin-aldosterone-angiotensin system. Abnormalities on liver tests can indicate hepatic congestion. Thyroid function tests can detect hyper- or hypothyroidism. Fasting lipid profile, fasting glucose, and hemoglobin A_{1c} level can reveal comorbid conditions that may need to be better controlled. Iron studies can detect iron deficiency or overload. If the patient is malnourished or an alcoholic and presents with high-output failure, thiamine testing is indicated to rule out deficiency related to beriberi. Further testing to determine any other etiologic factors of heart failure should be based on historical findings.

1. B-type natriuretic peptide—B-type natriuretic peptide (BNP) and N-terminal pro-BNP levels can be effectively utilized to evaluate patients presenting with dyspnea for heart failure. BNP is a cardiac neurohormone secreted from the ventricles and, to some extent, the atrial myocardium in response to stretching and increased wall tension from volume and pressure overload. Circulating BNP levels are increased in patients with heart failure and have a rapid turnover; thus they vary as volume status changes. Factors to consider when interpreting BNP levels are that they increase with age, are higher in women and African-American

Table 21-3. Factors influencing B-type natriuretic peptide (BNP) levels.

Factors that Cause Elevated BNP (>100 pg/mL)	Factors that Lower BNP in the Setting of Heart Failure
Heart failure	Acute pulmonary edema
Advanced age	Stable NYHA class I disease with low ejection fraction
Renal failure[a]	Acute mitral regurgitation
Acute coronary syndromes	Mitral stenosis
Lung disease with cor pulmonale	Atrial myxoma
Acute large pulmonary embolism	
High-output cardiac states	

[a]Adjusted levels are based on glomerular filtration rate (GFR). GFR 60–89 mL/min: no adjustment in the 100 pg/mL threshold (see text). GFR 30–59 mL/min: BNP >201. GFR 15–29 mL/min: BNP >225. GFR <15 mL/min: unknown utility of BNP levels.
NYHA, New York Heart Association
Data from Wang CS, et al. Does this dyspneic patient in the emergency department have congestive heart failure? *JAMA.* 2005; 294:1944.

individuals, and can be elevated in renal failure. Overall, BNP appears to have better reliability than N-terminal pro-BNP, especially in older populations. Although no BNP threshold indicates the presence or absence of heart failure with 100% certainty, multiple systematic reviews have that shown normal or low BNP or N-terminal BNP levels can effectively rule out a heart failure diagnosis. The average BNP level for diagnosing heart failure in one review was 95 pg/ mL or an N-terminal pro-BNP level of 642 pg/ mL. Elevated BNP levels can assist in diagnosing heart failure, but the effect of this diagnostic tool is small at these cutoffs. As the levels increase, the specificity and likelihood of heart failure increases especially to differentiate between a pulmonary and cardiac cause of dyspnea (**Table 21-3**).

Recent studies have also shown that high BNP levels (>200 pg/mL) or N-terminal pro-BNP levels (>5180 pg/mL) during acute heart failure are a strong predictor of mortality and cardiovascular admissions events during the following 2–3 months. Some evidence also suggests that a 30–50% reduction in BNP at hospital discharge lead to improved survival and less frequent rehospitalization. Similarly, studies suggest that having improved outpatient BNP targets showed improvements in decompensations, hospitalizations, and mortality.

2. Electrocardiography (ECG)—The ECG helps identify possible causes of heart failure. Signs of ischemic heart disease, acute or previous myocardial infarction, left ventricular hypertrophy, left bundle branch block, or atrial fibrillation can be identified and lead to further cardiac evaluation and treatment options. A left bundle branch block with heart failure is a poor prognostic sign with an increased 1-year mortality rate from any cause, including sudden death. In terms of diagnostic value, a normal ECG (or only minor abnormalities) has a small effect on ruling out systolic heart failure. Similarly, the presence of atrial fibrillation, new T wave changes, or any abnormality has a small effect on the diagnostic probability of heart failure being present.

Balion C, Santaguida PL, Hill S, et al. Testing for BNP and NT-proBNP in the diagnosis and prognosis of heart failure. *Evid Rep Technol Assess.* 2006(142):1–147.
Chen W-C, Tran KD, Maisel AS. Biomarkers in heart failure. *Heart.* 2010;96(4):314–320.
Ewald B, et al. Meta-analysis of B type natriuretic peptide and N-terminal pro B natriuretic peptide in the diagnosis of clinical heart failure and population screening for left ventricular dysfunction. *Intern Med J.* 2008;38:101–113. [PMID: 18290826]
Madhok V, Falk G, Rogers A, et al. The accuracy of symptoms, signs and diagnostic tests in the diagnosis of left ventricular dysfunction in primary care: a diagnostic accuracy systematic review. *BMC Fam Practice.* 2008;9:56. [PMID: 2569936]

D. Imaging Studies

1. Chest radiography—The chest radiograph can provide valuable clues in patients presenting with acute dyspnea, especially to identify pulmonary causes such as pneumonia, chronic obstructive pulmonary disease, pneumothorax, or a mass. The presence of venous congestion and interstitial edema is more conclusive and effective in diagnosing heart failure (specificity levels 96% and 97%, respectively). Findings such as cardiomegaly and a pleural effusion are suggestive of heart failure but only slightly increase the likelihood of the diagnosis in dyspneic patients. Likewise, the absence of cardiomegaly or venous congestion only slightly decreases the probability of a diagnosis of heart failure.

2. Cardiac Doppler echocardiography—Echocardiography with Doppler imaging is the most important component in evaluation of suspected heart failure (**Table 21-4**). It identifies systolic dysfunction through assessment of left ventricular ejection fraction. Diastolic dysfunction can also be determined by assessing for elevated left atrial pressures as well as impaired left ventricular relaxation and decreased compliance.

Echocardiographic findings can also help differentiate among the various causes of heart failure, including ischemic heart disease (wall motion abnormalities), valvular heart disease or various cardiomyopathies such as dilated (idiopathic), hypertrophic, restrictive, or hypertensive cardiomyopathy

Table 21-4. Echocardiographic parameters useful in the diagnosis of heart failure.

Parameter	Information Provided
Left ventricular function (ejection fraction)	Normal value: ≥55–60% Abnormal value: <50% Significant systolic dysfunction value: ≤35–40%
Diastolic function	Elevated left atrial pressures Decreased left ventricular compliance Impaired left ventricular relaxation
Pulmonary artery pressure	Normal value: ≤30–35 mmHg

Data from Hunt SA, et al. 2009 focused update incorporated into ACC/AHA 2005 guidelines for a report of the American College of Cardiology Foundation/American Heart Association Task Force on Practice Guidelines. Developed in collaboration with the International Society for Heart and Lung Transplantation. *Circulation.* 2009;119:e391–e479; Vitarelli A, et al. The role of echocardiography in the diagnosis and management of heart failure. *Heart Fail Rev.* 2003;8:181.

(left ventricular hypertrophy). Other potential reversible etiologies of heart failure can be evaluated are pericardial disorders such as effusion or tamponade.

The routine reevaluation with echocardiography of clinically stable patients in whom no change in management is contemplated is not recommended. If the echocardiography results are inadequate or the body habitus of the patient makes it impractical, transesophageal echocardiography, radionuclide ventriculography, or cardiac catherization ventriculogram can be performed to assess left ventricular ejection fraction.

3. Cardiac catheterization—Coronary angiography is recommended for patients with new-onset heart failure of uncertain etiology, despite the absence of anginal symptoms or negative findings on exercise stress testing. Coronary angiography should be strongly considered for patients with LVSD and a strong suspicion of ischemic myocardium based on noninvasive testing (echocardiography or nuclear imaging).

As stated, heart failure remains a clinical diagnosis for which no single finding can establish its presence or absence with certainty. Historically, criteria's such as Framingham and Boston have been developed that utilize history, examination, and chest radiography to better determine a clinical diagnosis of heart failure. Ultimately, using a combination of history, examination, laboratory analysis (including BNP testing), chest radiography, and ECG provide the best information in suspected cases while proceeding to evaluate left ventricular function by echocardiography.

King M, Kingery J, Casey B. Diagnosis and evaluation of heart failure. *Am Fam Physician.* 2012;85(12):1161–1168.

Vitarelli A, et al. The role of echocardiography in the diagnosis and management of heart failure. *Heart Fail Rev.* 2003;8:181. [PMID: 12766498]

Wang CS, et al. Does this dyspneic patient in the emergency department have congestive heart failure? *JAMA.* 2005;294:1944. [PMID: 16234501]

▶ Differential Diagnosis

Because heart failure is estimated to be present in only ~30% of patients with dyspnea in the primary care setting, clinicians need to consider differential diagnoses for dyspnea such as asthma, COPD, infection, interstitial lung disease, pulmonary embolism, anemia, thyrotoxicosis, carbon monoxide poisoning, arrhythmia, anginal equivalent (CAD), valvular heart disease, cardiac shunt, obstructive sleep apnea, and severe obesity causing hypoventilation syndrome.

▶ Treatment

Most evidence-based treatment strategies have focused on patients with systolic rather than diastolic heart failure; hence, stage-specific outpatient management of patients with chronic systolic heart failure (left ventricular systolic dysfunction) is the focus of the discussion that follows. Although stages A–D of the ACC/AHA heart failure classification represent progressive cardiac risk and dysfunction, the treatment strategies recommended at earlier stages are applicable to and recommended for later stages (see Table 21-2).

A. Systolic Heart Failure

1. High risk for systolic heart failure (stage A)—Individuals with conditions and behaviors that place them at high risk for heart failure but who do not have structurally abnormal hearts are classified as ACC/AHA stage A and should be treated with therapies that can delay progression of cardiac dysfunction and development of heart failure. Optimizing hypertension treatment based on the current national guidelines, such as the Seventh Report of the Joint National Committee on Detection, Evaluation, and Treatment of High Blood Pressure (JNC VII) and JNC VIII panel members' recommendations can reduce new-onset heart failure by 50%. Therapies such as diuretics, β-blockers, angiotensin-converting enzyme inhibitors (ACEIs), and angiotensin II receptor blockers (ARBs) are proven to be more effective than calcium channel blockers and doxazosin in preventing heart failure. The use of hydroxymethylglutaryl coenzyme A (HMG CoA) reductase inhibitors or statin therapy in CAD patients based on current hyperlipidemia guidelines [the updated Adult Treatment Panel III (ATP III)] can also reduce the incidence of heart failure by 20%.

Evidence-based disease management strategies for diabetes mellitus, atherosclerotic vascular disease, and thyroid disease, as well as patient avoidance of tobacco, alcohol, cocaine, amphetamines, and other illicit drugs that can be cardiotoxic, are also important components of early risk modification for prevention of heart failure. In diabetic patients, both ACEIs and ARBs (specifically losartan and irbesartan) have been shown to reduce new-onset heart failure compared with placebo. In CAD or atherosclerotic vascular disease patients without heart failure, reviews of the EUROPA (European Trial on Reduction of Cardiac Events with Perindopril in Stable Coronary Artery Disease) and HOPE (Heart Outcomes Prevention Evaluation) results show a 23% reduction in heart failure with ACEI therapy as well as reduced mortality, MIs, and cardiac arrest.

ALLHAT Officers and Coordinators for the ALLHAT Collaborative Research Group. Major outcomes in high-risk hypertensive patients randomized to angiotensin-converting enzyme inhibitor or calcium channel blocker vs. diuretic: the Anti-hypertensive and Lipid-Lowering Treatment to Prevent Heart Attack Trial (ALLHAT). *JAMA.* 2002;288:2981. [PMID: 12479763]

Baker DW. Prevention of heart failure. *J Card Fail.* 2002; 8:333. [PMID: 12411985]

Brenner BM, et al. Effects of losartan on renal and cardiovascular outcomes in patients with type 2 diabetes and nephropathy. *N Engl J Med.* 2001;345:861. [PMID: 11565518]

Fox KM. Efficacy of perindopril in reduction of cardiovascular events among patients with stable coronary artery disease: randomized, double-blind, placebo-controlled, multicentre trial (the EUROPA study). *Lancet.* 2003;362:782. [PMID: 13678572]

Yusuf S, et al. Effects of an angiotensin-converting-enzyme inhibitor, ramipril, on cardiovascular events in high-risk patients. The Heart Outcomes Prevention Evaluation Study Investigators. *N Engl J Med.* 2000;342:145. [PMID: 10639539]

2. Asymptomatic with cardiac structural abnormalities or remodeling (stage B)—Patients who do not have clinical symptoms of heart failure but who have a structurally abnormal heart, such as a previous MI, evidence of left ventricular remodeling (left ventricular hypertrophy or low ejection fraction), or valvular disease, are at a substantial risk of developing symptomatic heart failure. Prevention of further progression in these at-risk patients is the goal, and appropriate therapies are dependent on the patient's cardiac condition.

In all patients with a recent or remote history of MI, regardless of ejection fraction, ACEIs and β-blockers are the mainstay of therapy. Both therapies have been demonstrated in randomized control trials to cause a significant reduction in cardiovascular death and symptomatic heart failure. These therapies are vital in post-MI patients, as is evidence-based management of an ST elevation MI and chronic stable angina, to help further achieve reduction in heart failure morbidity and mortality.

In asymptomatic patients who have not had an MI but have a reduced left ventricular ejection fraction (nonischemic cardiomyopathy), clinical trials reported an overall 37% reduction in symptomatic heart failure when treated with ACEI therapy. The SOLVD (Studies of Left Ventricular

Dysfunction) trial and a 12-year follow-up study confirmed the long-term benefit of ACEIs regarding the onset of symptomatic heart failure and mortality. A substudy of the SOLVD trial showed how enalapril attenuates progressive increases in left ventricular dilation and hypertrophy, thus inhibiting left ventricular remodeling. Despite a lack of evidence from randomized controlled trials, the ACC/AHA guidelines recommend β-blockers in patients with stage B heart failure, given the significant survival benefit that these agents provide in worsening stages of heart failure. The RACE (Ramipril Cardioprotective Evaluation) trial provided a clue as to why ACEIs are advantageous over β-blockers for nonischemic cardiomyopathy by demonstrating that ramipril is more effective than the β-blocker atenolol in reversing left ventricular hypertrophy in hypertensive patients.

There is no clear outcome evidence for the use of ARBs in asymptomatic patients with reduced left ventricular ejection fraction. ARB therapy is, however, a guideline recommended alternative in ACEI-intolerant patients. VALIANT (VALsartan In Acute myocardial iNfarcTion) was one trial that showed that the ARB valsartan was as effective as but not superior to captopril, an ACEI, in reducing cardiovascular morbidity and mortality in post-MI patients with heart failure or a reduced left ventricular ejection fraction. The combination of both therapies was no better than captopril alone.

Agabiti-Rosei E, et al. ACE inhibitor ramipril is more effective than the beta-blocker atenolol in reducing left ventricular mass in hypertension. Results of the RACE (ramipril cardioprotective evaluation) study on behalf of the RACE study group. *J Hypertens.* 1995; 13:1325. [PMID: 8984131]

Flather MD, et al. Long-term ACE-inhibitor therapy in patients with heart failure or left-ventricular dysfunction: a systematic overview of data from individual patients. ACE-Inhibitor Myocar-dial Infarction Collaborative Group. *Lancet.* 2000; 355:1575. [PMID: 10821360]

Greenberg B, et al. Effects of long-term enalapril therapy on cardiac structure and function in patients with left ventricular systolic dysfunction. Results of the SOLVD echocardiography substudy. *Circulation.* 1995; 91:2573. [PMID: 7743619]

Maggioni AP, Fabbri G. VALIANT (VALsartan In Acute myocar-dial iNfarcTion) trial. *Expert Opin Pharmacother.* 2005; 6:507. [PMID: 15794740]

3. Symptomatic systolic heart failure (stage C)—Patients with a clinical diagnosis of heart failure have current or prior symptoms of heart failure and structural heart disease with a reduced left ventricular ejection fraction comprise ACC/AHA stage C. This stage encompasses NYHA classes II, III, and IV, excluding patients who develop refractory end-stage heart failure (see Table 21-2). In patients with symptomatic heart failure and left ventricular dysfunction, neurohormonal activation creates deleterious effects on the heart, leading to pulmonary and peripheral edema, persistent increased afterload, pathologic cardiac remodeling, and a progressive decline in cardiac function. The overall goals

Table 21-5. Factors contributing to worsening heart failure.

Cardiovascular factors
Ischemia or infarction
New-onset or uncontrolled atrial fibrillation
Uncontrolled hypertension
Unrecognized or worsened valvular disease
Systemic factors
Anemia
Fluid retention from drugs (chemotherapy, COX1, 2 inhibitors, licorice, glitazones, glucocorticoids, androgens, estrogens)
Infection
Pregnancy
Pulmonary causes (pulmonary embolism, cor pulmonale, pulmonary hypertension)
Renal causes (renal failure, nephrotic syndrome, glomerulonephritis)
Sleep apnea
Thyroid dysfunction
Uncontrolled diabetes mellitus
Patient-related factors
Fluid overload (sodium intake, water intake, medication compliance)
Alcohol use
Substance abuse

Data from Colucci WS. Overview of the therapy of heart failure due to systolic dysfunction. In: Basow DS, ed. *UpToDate* Waltham, MA: 2013; King M, Kingery J, Casey B. Diagnosis and evaluation of heart failure. *Am Fam Physician.* 2012;85(12):1161–1168.

in this stage are to improve the patient's symptoms, slow or reverse the deterioration of cardiac functioning, and reduce the patient's long-term morbidity and mortality.

Accurate assessment of the cause and severity of heart failure; the incorporation of previous stage A and B treatment recommendations; and correction of any cardiovascular, systemic, and behavioral factors (**Table 21-5**) are important to achieve control in patients with symptomatic heart failure. Moderate dietary sodium restriction (3–4 g daily) with daily weight measurement further enhance volume control and allow for lower and safer doses of diuretic therapies. Exercise training is beneficial and should be encouraged to prevent physical deconditioning, which can contribute to exercise intolerance in patients with heart failure.

Patients with symptomatic heart failure should be routinely managed with a standard therapy of a diuretic, an ACEI (or ARB if intolerant), and a β-blocker (see Table 21-2). The addition of other pharmacologic therapies should be guided by the need for further symptom control versus the desire to enhance survival and long-term prognosis. A stepwise approach to therapy is presented in **Table 21-6** and expanded on later.

A. DIURETICS—Patients with heart failure who present with common congestive symptoms (pulmonary and peripheral

Table 21-6. Pharmacologic steps in symptomatic heart failure.[a]

Pharmacotherapy	Indications and Considerations
Standard therapy	
Loop diuretic	Titrate accordingly for fluid control and symptom relief (dyspnea, edema)
Angiotensin-converting enzyme inhibitor (ACEI)[b]	Initiate at low dose, titrating to target, during or after optimization of diuretic therapy for survival benefit
β-blocker	Initiate at low dose once stable on ADEI (or ARB) for survival benefit
	May initiate before achieving ACEI (or ARB) target doses and should be titrated to target doses unless symptoms become limiting
Additional therapies[c]	
Angiotensin II receptor blocker (ARB)	Used in ACEI-intolerant patients, as above, for survival benefit
	May be effective for persistent symptoms and survival (NYHA class II–IV)
Aldosterone antagonist	For worsening symptoms and survival in moderately severe to severe heart failure (NYHA class III with decompensations)
Digoxin	For persistent symptoms and to reduce hospitalizations
	Should be maintained at preferred serum digoxin concentration
Hydralazine plus isosorbide dinitrate	Effective for persistent symptoms and survival, particularly in African American

[a]Assessment of clinical response and tolerability should guide decision making and allow for variations.
[b]ARBs are recommended in patients who are intolerant to ACEIs.
[c]Decisions about whether to use additional therapy are guided by the need for symptom control versus mortality benefit.
NYHA, New York Heart Association
Data from Colluci WS. Overview of the therapy of heart failure due to systolic dysfunction. In: Basow DS, ed., .Waltham, MA: 2013; Hunt SA, et al. 2009 focused update incorporated into ACC/AHA 2005 guidelines for a report of the American College of Cardiology Foundation/ American Heart Association Task Force on Practice Guidelines. Developed in collaboration with the International Society for Heart and Lung Transplantation. *Circulation.* 2009;119:e391–e479.

edema) are given a diuretic to manage fluid retention and achieve and maintain a euvolemic state. Diuretic therapy is specifically aimed at treating the compensatory volume expansion driven by renal tubular sodium retention and activation of the renin-angiotensin-aldosterone system.

Loop diuretics are the treatment of choice because they increase sodium excretion by 20–25% and substantially enhance free water clearance. Furosemide is most commonly used, but patients may respond better to bumetanide or torsemide because of superior, more predictable absorptions and longer durations of action. To minimize the risk of over- or underdiuresis, the diuretic response should guide the dosage of loop diuretics (**Table 21-7**), with dose increases until a response is achieved. Frequency of dosing is guided by the time needed to maintain active diuresis and sustained volume and weight control.

Thiazide diuretics also have a role in heart failure, principally as antihypertensive therapy, but they can be used in combination with loop diuretics to provide a potentiated or synergistic diuresis. As a lone treatment, however, they increase sodium excretion by only 5–10% and tend to decrease free water clearance overall.

Symptom improvement with diuretics occurs within hours to days, as compared with weeks to months for other heart failure therapies. For long-term clinical stability, diuretics are not sufficient, and exacerbations can be greatly reduced when they are combined with ACEI and β-blocker therapies.

B. ACE INHIBITORS—ACEIs are prescribed to all patients with symptomatic heart failure unless contraindicated and have proven benefit in alleviating heart failure symptoms, reducing hospitalization, and improving survival. Current ACC/AHA guidelines recommend that all patients with left ventricular systolic dysfunction be started on low-dose ACEI therapy to avoid side effects and raised to a maintenance or target dose (see Table 21-7). There is, however, some uncertainty regarding target doses achieved in clinical trials, and whether these are more beneficial than lower doses. For ACEIs as a class, there does not appear to be any difference in agents in terms of effectiveness at improving heart failure outcomes.

C. β-BLOCKERS—In patients with NYHA class II or III heart failure, the β-blockers bisoprolol, metoprolol succinate (sustained release), and carvedilol have been shown to improve

Table 21-7. Medications used in treatment of symptomatic heart failure in patients with reduced left ventricular ejection fraction.

Drug Therapy	Initial Daily Dose	Target or Maximum Daily Dose
Loop Diuretics		
Bumetanide	0.5–1.0 mg/dose	10 mg/d
Furosemide	20–40 mg/dose	600 mg/d
Torsemide	5–10 mg/dose	200 mg/d
ACE Inhibitors		
Captopril	6.25 mg 3 times daily	50 mg 3 times daily
Enalapril	2.5 mg twice daily	10–20 mg twice daily
Fosinopril	5–10 mg once daily	20–40 mg once daily
Lisinopril	2.5–5 mg once daily	20–40 mg once daily
Perindopril	2 mg once daily	8–16 mg once daily
Quinapril	5 mg twice daily	20 mg twice daily
Ramipril	1.25–2.5 mg once daily	5 mg twice daily
Trandolapril	1 mg once daily	4 mg once daily
Angiotensin II Receptor Blockers		
Candesartan	4–8 mg once daily	32 mg once daily
Losartan	25–50 mg once daily	50–100 mg once daily
Valsartan	20–40 mg twice daily	160 mg twice daily
β-blockers		
Bisoprolol	1.25 mg once daily	10 mg once daily
Carvedilol	3.125 mg twice daily	25 mg twice daily [50 mg twice daily, if > 85 kg (187 lb)]
Metoprolol succinate, extended release (CR/XL)	12.5–25 mg once daily	200 mg once daily
Metoprolol tartrate, immediate release	12.5–25 mg twice daily	100 mg twice daily
Aldosterone Antagonists		
Eplerenone	25 mg once daily	50 mg once daily
Spironolactone	12.5–25 mg once daily	25 mg once or twice daily
Other Medication		
Digoxin	0.125–0.25 mg once daily	Serum concentration 0.5–1.1 ng/mL
Hydralazine plus isosorbide dinitrate	37.5 mg/20 mg 3 times daily	75 mg/40 mg 3 times daily

Data from Hunt SA, et al. 2009 focused update incorporated into ACC/AHA 2005 guidelines for a report of the American College of Cardiology Foundation/American Heart Association Task Force on Practice Guidelines. Developed in collaboration with the International Society for Heart and Lung Transplantation. *Circulation.* 2009;119:e391–e479.

mortality and event-free survival. These benefits are in addition to ACEI therapy and support the use of β-blockers as part of standard therapy in these patients. A similar survival benefit has been shown for patients with stable NYHA class IV heart failure.

β-blocker therapy should be initiated near the onset of a diagnosis of left ventricular systolic dysfunction and mild heart failure symptoms, given the added benefit on survival and disease progression. Titrating ACEI therapy to a target dose should not preclude the initiation of β-blocker therapy. Starting doses should be very low, given their effectiveness (see Table 21-7) but doubled at regular intervals, every 2–3 weeks as tolerated, toward target doses to achieve heart rate

reductions. Individual studies indicate that there might be a dose-dependent outcome improvement, but recent meta-analysis concluded that the magnitude of heart rate reduction (5 bpm reductions) was associated with an 18% reduction in the risk of death whereas the β-blocker dose was not.

Traditionally the negative inotropic effects of β-blockers were considered harmful in heart failure, but this impact is outweighed by the beneficial effect of inhibiting sympathetic nervous system activation. Current evidence suggests that these beneficial effects may not necessarily be equivalent among proven β-blockers. The COMET (Carvedilol or Metoprolol European Trial) findings showed that carvedilol (an α_1-, β_1-, and β_2-receptor inhibitor) is more effective than twice-daily dosed immediate-release metoprolol tartrate (a highly specific β_1-receptor inhibitor) in reducing heart failure mortality (40% vs 34%, respectively). Previous trials had investigated metoprolol succinate (sustained-release, once-daily dosing), but the COMET trial showed a mortality reduction even with metoprolol tartrate, a very cost-effective alternative. A recent systematic review and meta-analysis suggests, however, that the benefits may be a class effect with no superior agent over others.

Because β-blockers may cause a 4–10-week increase in symptoms before improvement is noted, therapy should be initiated when patients have no or minimal evidence of fluid retention. Relative contraindications include bradycardia, hypotension, hypoperfusion, severe peripheral vascular disease, a P-R interval of >0.24 seconds, second- or third-degree atrioventricular block, severe COPD, or a history of asthma. Race or gender differences in efficacy of β-blocker therapy have not been noted.

D. ANGIOTENSIN II RECEPTOR BLOCKERS—Certain ARBs (see Table 21-7) have been shown in clinical trials to be nearly as effective as, but not consistently as and not superior to, ACEIs as first-line therapy for symptomatic heart failure. The use of ARBs is recommended in ACEI-intolerant patients but not preferentially over ACEIs given the volume of evidence validating ACEIs. Despite unclear evidence, the ACC/AHA guidelines recommend that ARB therapy be considered in addition to ACEI and standard therapy for patients who have persistent symptoms of heart failure. A recent systematic review that analyzed the benefit of ARBs in heart failure found no mortality or morbidity benefit when compared to placebo or ACEI and no benefit to combination with an ACEI.

E. ALDOSTERONE ANTAGONISTS—For selected patients with moderately severe to severe symptoms who are difficult to control (NYHA class III with decompensations or class IV), additional treatment options include the aldosterone antagonists spironolactone and eplerenone (see Table 21-7) to improve mortality and reduce hospitalizations. A recent trial also proved the same outcome benefit of eplerenone in milder symptomatic heart failure, NYHA class II, and reduced ejection fraction of 35%.

The addition of aldosterone antagonist therapy can cause life-threatening hyperkalemia in patients with heart failure, who are often already at risk because of reduced left ventricular function and associated renal insufficiency. Current guidelines recommend careful monitoring to ensure that creatinine is <2.5 mg/dL in men or <2.0 mg/dL in women and that potassium is maintained below 5.0 mEq/L (levels >5.5 mEq/L should trigger discontinuation or dose reduction). Higher doses of aldosterone antagonists and ACEI therapy should also raise concern for possible hyperkalemia, and the use of nonsteroidal anti-inflammatory drugs (NSAIDs), cyclooxygenase-2 (COX2) inhibitors, and potassium supplements should be avoided if possible. If the clinical situation does not allow for proper monitoring, the risk of hyperkalemia may outweigh the benefit of aldosterone antagonist therapy.

F. DIGOXIN—Digoxin therapy is indicated only to reduce hospitalizations in patients with uncontrolled symptomatic heart failure or as a ventricular rate control agent if a patient has a known arrhythmia. The DIG (Digitalis Investigation Group) trial proved the benefit of digoxin added to diuretic and ACEI therapy in improving heart failure symptom control and decreasing the rate of hospitalization by 6%, but there was no overall mortality benefit. Subsequent retrospective subgroup analysis of the trial discovered some survival improvement at a serum digoxin concentration of 0.5–0.8 ng/mL in men. A similar but nonsignificant survival trend was also noted in women. Because survival is clearly worse when the serum digoxin concentration is >1.2 ng/mL, patients are best managed within the range noted to avoid potential adverse outcomes given the narrow risk/benefit ratio. Digoxin should be used cautiously in elderly patients, who may have impaired renal function that adversely affects drug levels.

G. HYDRALAZINE AND NITRATES—The combination of hydralazine and isosorbide dinitrate (H-I) is a reasonable treatment in patients, particularly African Americans, who have persistent heart failure symptoms with standard therapy. In V-HeFT I (Vasodilator Heart-Failure Trial), the mortality of African-American patients receiving H-I combination therapy was reduced, but mortality of white patients did not differ from that of the placebo group. In V-HeFT II, a reduction in mortality with the H-I combination was seen only in white patients who had been receiving enalapril therapy. No effect on hospitalization was found in either trial.

The A-HeFT (African-American Heart Failure Trial) findings further supported the benefit of a fixed dose H-I combination (see Table 21-7) by showing a reduction in mortality and heart failure hospitalization rates as well as improved quality-of-life scores in patients with moderate to severe heart failure (NYHA class III or IV) who self-identified as African-American. The H-I combination was in addition to standard therapies that included ACEIs or ARBs, β-blockers, and spironolactone.

H. ANTICOAGULATION—It is well established that patients with heart failure are at an increased risk of thrombosis from blood stasis in dilated hypokinetic cardiac chambers and peripheral blood vessels. Despite this known risk, the yearly incidence of thromboembolic events in patients with stable heart failure is between 1% and 3%, even in those with lower left ventricular ejection fractions and evidence of intracardiac thrombi. Such low rates limit the detectable benefit of warfarin therapy, and retrospective data analysis of warfarin with heart failure show conflicting results, especially given the major risk of bleeding. Warfarin therapy is indicated only in heart failure patients with a history of a thromboembolic event or those with paroxysmal or chronic atrial fibrillation or flutter. Likewise, the benefit of antiplatelet therapies, such as aspirin, has not been clearly proved, and these therapies could possibly be detrimental because of their known interaction with ACEIs. Aspirin can decrease ACEI effectiveness and potentially increase hospitalizations due to heart failure decompensation.

I. ADVERSE THERAPIES—Therapies that adversely affect the clinical status of patients with symptomatic heart failure should be avoided. Other than for control of hypertension, calcium channel blockers offer no morbidity or mortality benefit in heart failure. Nondihydropyridine calcium channel blockers (eg, diltiazem and verapamil) and older, short-acting dihydropyridines (eg, nicardipine and nisoldipine) can worsen symptoms of heart failure, especially in patients with moderate to severe heart failure. The newer long-acting dihydropyridine calcium channel blockers amlodipine and felodipine are safe but do not have a role in heart failure treatment and improving outcomes. NSAIDs can also exacerbate heart failure through peripheral vasoconstriction and by interfering with the renal effects of diuretics and the unloading effects of ACEIs. Most antiarrhythmic drugs (except amiodarone and dofetilide) have an adverse impact on heart failure and survival because of their negative inotropic activity and proarrhythmic effects. Phosphodiesterase inhibitors (cilostazol, sildenafil, vardenafil, and tadalafil) can cause hypotension and are potentially hazardous in patients with heart failure. Thiazolidinediones and metformin, both used in treatment of diabetes, can be detrimental in patients with heart failure because they increase the risk of excessive fluid retention and lactic acidosis, respectively.

J. IMPLANTABLE DEVICES—Nearly one-third of all heart failure deaths occur as a result of sudden cardiac death. The ACC/AHA recommendations include the use of implantable cardioverter-defibrillators (ICDs) for secondary prevention of sudden cardiac death in patients with symptomatic heart failure; a reduced left ventricular ejection fraction; and a history of cardiac arrest, ventricular fibrillation, or hemodynamically destabilizing ventricular tachycardia. ICDs are recommended for patients with NYHA class II or III heart failure, a left ventricular ejection fraction of <35%, and a reasonable 1-year survival with no recent MI (within 40 days).

As heart failure progresses, ventricular dyssynchrony can also occur. This is defined by a QRS duration of >0.12 ms in patients with a low left ventricular ejection fraction (usually <35%) and NYHA class III or IV heart failure. Clinical trials have shown that cardiac resynchronization therapy with biventricular pacing can improve quality of life, functional class, exercise capacity, exercise distance, left ventricular ejection fraction, and survival in these patients. Patients who meet criteria for cardiac resynchronization therapy and an ICD should receive a combined device, unless contraindicated.

Chatterjee S, Biondi-Zoccai G, Abbate A, et al. Benefits of beta blockers in patients with heart failure and reduced ejection fraction: network meta-analysis. *Br Med J.* 2013;346:f55.

Heran BS, Musini VM, Bassett K, Taylor RS, Wright JM. Angiotensin receptor blocker for heart failure. *Cochrane Database Syst Rev.* 2012;4:CD003040.

Jong P, et al. Angiotensin receptor blockers in heart failure: meta-analysis of randomized controlled trials. *J Am Coll Cardiol.* 2002; 39:463. [PMID: 11823085]

Jong P, et al. Effect of enalapril on 12-year survival and life expectancy in patients with left ventricular systolic dysfunction: a follow-up study. *Lancet.* 2003; 361:1843. [PMID: 12788569]

Juurlink DN, et al. Drug-drug interactions among elderly patients hospitalized for drug toxicity. *JAMA.* 2003; 289:1652. [PMID: 12672733]

McAlister FA, Wiebe N, Ezekowitz JA, Leung AA, Armstrong PW. Meta-analysis: beta-blocker dose, heart rate reduction, and death in patients with heart failure. *Ann Intern Med.* 2009;150(11):784–794.

Poole-Wilson PA, et al. Comparison of carvedilol and metoprolol on clinical outcomes in patients with chronic heart failure in the Carvedilol Or Metoprolol European Trial (COMET): randomised controlled trial. *Lancet.* 2003; 362:7. [PMID: 12853193]

Rochon PA, et al. Use of angiotensin-converting enzyme inhibitor therapy and dose-related outcomes in older adults with new heart failure in the community. *J Gen Intern Med.* 2004; 19:676. [PMID: 15209607]

Taylor AL, et al. Combination of isosorbide dinitrate and hydralazine in blacks with heart failure. *N Engl J Med.* 2004; 351:2049. [PMID: 15533851]

Yan AT, Yan RT, Liu PP. Narrative review: pharmacotherapy for chronic heart failure: evidence from recent clinical trials. *Ann Intern Med.* 2005;142(2):132–145.

Zannad F, McMurray JJ, Krum H, et al. Eplerenone in patients with systolic heart failure and mild symptoms. *N Engl J Med.* 2011;364(1):11–21.

4. REFRACTORY END-STAGE HEART FAILURE (STAGE D)—Despite optimal medical therapy, some patients deteriorate or do not improve and experience symptoms at rest (NYHA class IV). These patients can have rapid recurrence of symptoms, leading to frequent hospitalizations and a significant or permanent reduction in their activities of daily living. Before classifying patients as being refractory or having end-stage heart failure, providers should verify an accurate diagnosis, identify and treat contributing conditions that could be hindering improvement, and maximize medical therapy.

Control of fluid retention to improve symptoms is paramount in this stage, and referral to a program with expertise in refractory heart failure or referral for cardiac transplantation should be considered. Other specialized treatment strategies, such as mechanical circulatory support, continuous intravenous positive inotropic therapy, and other surgical management can be considered, but there is limited evidence in terms of morbidity and mortality to support the value of these therapies. Careful discussion of the prognosis and options for end-of-life care should also be initiated with patients and their families. In this scenario, patients with ICDs should receive information about the option to inactivate defibrillation.

B. Diastolic Heart Failure

Clinically, diastolic heart failure is as prevalent as LVSD, and the presentation of diastolic heart failure is indistinguishable from LVSD. Nearly 40–50% of patients with symptomatic heart failure experience diastolic failure. Patients with diastolic heart failure are more likely to be women, older, and have hypertension, atrial fibrillation, and left ventricular hypertrophy, but no history of CAD. Diastolic heart failure remains a diagnosis of exclusion in which a thorough differential of heart failure needs to be considered. Compared to systolic heart failure, the treatment of diastolic heart failure lacks validated evidence-based therapies. Management focuses on controlling systolic and diastolic blood pressure, ventricular rate, volume status, and reducing myocardial ischemia, because these entities are known to exert effects on ventricular relaxation. Diuretics are used to control symptoms of pulmonary congestion and peripheral edema, but care must be taken to avoid overdiuresis, which can cause decreased volume status and preload, manifesting as worsening heart failure.

King M, Kingery J, Casey B. Diagnosis and evaluation of heart failure. *Am Fam Physician*. 2012;85(12):1161–1168.

Prognosis

Despite favorable trends in survival and advances in treatment of heart failure and associated comorbidities, prognosis is poor, thus indicating the importance of appropriate diagnosis and treatment. Following diagnosis, survival is 90% at 1 month but declines to 78% at 1 year and only 58% at 5 years. Mortality increases in patients both with and without symptomatic heart failure as systolic function declines. There is also no difference in survival between diastolic and systolic heart failure.

Websites

American College of Cardiology clinical guidelines. http://www .cardiosource.org/science-and-quality/practice-guidelines-and-quality-standards.aspx

American Heart Association (AHA). http://www.americanheart.org.

AHA patient information. http://www.heart.org/HEARTORG/ Conditions/Conditions_UCM_001087_SubHomePage.jsp

National Heart, Lung, and Blood Institute patient information. http://www.nhlbi.nih.gov/health/health-topics/topics/hf/

Dyslipidemias

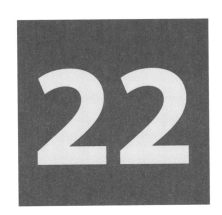

Brian V. Reamy, MD

▶ Serum cholesterol values greater than ideal for the prevention of atherosclerotic cardiovascular disease (ASCVD).

▶ Optimum values vary with the risk status of the individual patient.

General Considerations

The Framingham Heart Study firmly established an epidemiologic link between elevated serum cholesterol and an increased risk of morbidity and mortality from ASCVD. Although the benefits of lowering cholesterol were assumed for many years, not until 2001 had enough evidence accumulated to show unequivocal benefits from using lifestyle and pharmacologic therapy to lower serum cholesterol. Evidence in support of using statin agents is particularly strong and has revolutionized the treatment of dyslipidemias.

The efficacy of lipid reduction for the secondary prevention of ASCVD (reducing further disease-related morbidity in those with manifest disease) is supported by multiple trials and is appropriate in all patients with ASCVD. The efficacy of primary prevention (reducing the risk of disease occurrence in those without overt cardiovascular disease) is now supported even in patients at a low risk of ASCVD by the 10-year Framingham risk assessment (available at http://hp2010.nhlbihin.net/atpiii/calculator.asp).

The National Cholesterol Education Program (NCEP), Adult Treatment Panel (ATP) III released guidelines in 2001. New integrated guidelines for cardiovascular disease reduction were released at the end of 2013. These guidelines emphasize aggressive treatment of dyslipidemias and other cardiovascular risk factors with the intensity of treatment titrated to the patients risk status.

Pathogenesis

Serum cholesterol is carried by three major lipoproteins: high-density lipoprotein (HDL), low-density lipoprotein (LDL), and very-low-density lipoprotein (VLDL). Most clinical laboratories measure the total cholesterol, total triglycerides (TG), and the HDL fraction.

The triglyceride fraction, and to a lesser extent the HDL level, vary considerably depending on the fasting status of the patient. The NCEP/ATP III guidelines recommend that only fasting measurements including total cholesterol, triglycerides, HDL cholesterol, and a LDL cholesterol be used to guide management decisions.

Different populations have different median cholesterol values. For example, Asian populations tend to have total cholesterol values 20–30% lower than those of populations living in Europe or the United States. It is important to recognize that unlike a serum sodium electrolyte value, there is no normal cholesterol value. Instead, there are cholesterol values that predict higher morbidity and mortality from ASCVD if left untreated, and lower cholesterol values that correlate with less likelihood of cardiovascular disease.

Atherosclerosis is an inflammatory disease in which cells and mediators participate at every stage of atherogenesis from the earliest fatty streak to the most advanced fibrous lesion. Elevated glucose, increased blood pressure, and inhaled cigarette byproducts can trigger inflammation. However, one of the key factors triggering this inflammation is oxidized LDL. When LDL is taken up by macrophages, it triggers the release of inflammatory mediators, which can lead to thickening and/or rupture of plaque lining the arterial walls. Ruptured or unstable plaques are responsible for clinical events such as myocardial infarction and stroke. Lipid lowering, whether by diet or medication, can therefore be regarded as an anti-inflammatory and plaque stabilizing therapy.

▶ Clinical Findings

A. Symptoms and Signs

Most dyslipidemia patients have no signs or symptoms, of the disease, which is usually detected by routine laboratory screening in an asymptomatic individual. Rarely, patients with familial forms of hyperlipidemia may present with yellow xanthomas on the skin or in tendon bodies, especially the patellar tendon, Achilles tendon, and the extensor tendons of the hands.

A few associated conditions can cause a secondary hyperlipidemia (**Table 22-1**). These conditions should be considered before lipid-lowering therapy is begun or when the response to therapy is much less than predicted. In particular, poorly controlled diabetes and untreated hypothyroidism can lead to an elevation of serum lipids resistant to pharmacologic treatment.

B. Screening

The US Preventive Services Task Force (USPSTF) bases its screening recommendations on the age of the patient. It strongly recommends (rating A) routinely screening men aged ≥35 years and women aged ≥45 years for lipid disorders.

The USPSTF recommends (rating B) screening younger adults (men aged 20–35 years and women aged 20–45 years), if they have other risk factors for coronary disease.

They make no recommendation for or against screening in younger adults in the absence of known risk factors.

In contrast, the NCEP guidelines advise that screening should occur in adults aged ≥20 years with a fasting, lipid profile once every 5 years.

Screening children and adolescents is controversial. New Integrated guidelines released by the National Heart Lung and Blood Institute (NHLBI) in 2011 recommend universal screening of all 9–11-year-olds and gave this a grade B recommendation. Expert opinion recommends screening children from 2 to 8 years of age with significant family histories of hypercholesterolemia, premature ASCVD.

▶ Treatment

The current NCEP/ATP treatment guidelines are as rooted in evidence as possible. They are available online at www .nhlbi.nih.gov.

The 2001/2004 NCEP/ATP III guidelines follow a nine-step process (**Table 22-2**).

Step 1 begins after obtaining fasting lipoprotein levels. The profile is categorized according to the LDL, HDL, and total cholesterol values:

Table 22-1. Secondary causes of lipid abnormalities.

I. **Hypercholesterolemia**
    Hypothyroidism
    Nephrotic syndrome
    Obstructive liver disease
    Acute intermittent porphyria
    Diabetes mellitus
    Chronic renal insufficiency
    Cushing disease
    Drugs (oral contraceptives, diuretics)

II. **Hypertriglyceridemia**
    Diabetes mellitus
    Alcohol use
    Obesity
    Chronic renal insufficiency
    Drugs (estrogens, isotretinoin)

III. **Hypocholesterolemia**
    Malignancy
    Hyperthyroidism
    Cirrhosis

Table 22-2. Summary of nine steps in NCEP/ATP III guidelines.

Step 1	Determine lipoprotein levels after a 9–12-hour fast
Step 2	Identify the presence of coronary heart disease or equivalents (coronary artery disease, peripheral arterial disease, abdominal aortic aneurysm, diabetes mellitus)
Step 3	Determine the presence of major risk factors, other than LDL (smoking, hypertension, HDL <40 mg/dL, family history of premature coronary disease, men aged >45 years and women aged >55 years
Step 4	Assess level of risk; use Framingham risk tables if 2+ risk factors and no coronary heart disease (or equivalent) is present
Step 5	Determine risk category, LDL goal, and the threshold for drug treatment
Step 6	Initiate therapeutic lifestyle changes (TLC) if LDL is above goal
Step 7	Initiate drug therapy if LDL remains above goal
Step 8	Identify the presence of the metabolic syndrome and treat; determine the triglyceride and HDL goals of therapy
Step 9	Treat elevated triglycerides and reduced HDL with TLC and drug therapy to achieve goals

TLC, therapeutic lifestyle changes.

LDL cholesterol (mg/dL)

<100	Optimal
100–129	Near optimal
130–159	Borderline high
160–189	High
>190	Very high

HDL cholesterol (mg/dL)

<40	Low
>60	High

Total cholesterol (mg/dL)

<200	Desirable
200–239	Borderline high
>240	High

Step 2 focuses on determining the presence of clinical atherosclerotic disease such as coronary heart disease, peripheral arterial disease, or diabetes mellitus.

In **Step 3** the clinician should determine the presence of other major CAD risk factors, including smoking, age >45 years in men (>55 years in women), hypertension, HDL cholesterol <40 mg/dL, a family history of premature CHD in a male first-degree relative aged <55 years or a female first-degree relative aged <65 years of age. An HDL cholesterol of >60 mg/dL negates one risk factor.

Step 4 uses the Framingham coronary risk calculator to classify the patient into one of four risk categories: *high-risk*, having coronary artery disease or a 10-year risk of >20%; *moderately high risk*, having a 10-year risk of 10–20%; *moderate-risk*, having two or more risk factors but a 10-year risk of <10%; or *low-risk*, having zero to one risk factors. The Framingham risk calculator can be found at http://hp2010.nhlbihin.net/atpiii/calculator.asp.

Step 5 is the key step that determines the patient's suggested LDL cholesterol treatment goals. **Table 22-3** summarizes risk category determination and treatment goals.

A. Behavior Modification

Step 6 reviews the contents of therapeutic lifestyle changes (TLC). Saturated fat is limited to <7% of total calories; cholesterol intake to <200 mg/d. In addition, weight management and increased physical activity are encouraged. TLC also includes advice to increase the consumption of soluble fiber (10–25 gm/d) and the intake of plant sterols (sitostanol approximately 2 g/d). Several margarines (Benecol™, Take Control™) contain these plant sterols, and evidently they work in conjunction with cholesterol-lowering drugs. Excellent information sources of soluble fiber can be found at www.nhlbi.nih.gov/chd/tipsheets/solfiber.htm.

The cultural background of the patient will impact the choice of dietary recommendations. A skilled nutritional medicine consultant can easily adapt the fat/cholesterol intake recommendations to various culturally normative diets. Indeed, components of some cultures' diets that encourage the consumption of soluble fiber, plant sterols, soy protein, or fish oils have cholesterol-lowering effects. Dietary advice given without regard to a patient's culturally accepted diet is counterproductive.

B. Pharmacotherapy

Step 7 reviews the options for drug therapy if required (**Table 22-4**). Of note, NCEP/ATPIII now recommends the simultaneous use of TLC and drugs in patients at the highest risk. Medications should be added to TLC after 3 months if goal LDL levels are not reached in lower-risk patients. Given their proven efficacy, and enhanced patient compliance over other classes of medications, statin agents are the drugs of first choice. In particular, patients with diabetes or those in the highest-risk category derive special benefits from their use, due to their innate anti-inflammatory effects. Myopathy and increased liver enzymes are the main potential side

Table 22-3. Risk category determination and LDL cholesterol goals.

Risk Category	LDL Goal	LDL Level at Which to Begin Therapeutic Lifestyle Changes (TLC) (mg/dL)	LDL Level at Which to Consider Drug Treatment
High risk: CHD or equivalent (10-year risk >20%)	<100 mg/dL (<70 mg/dL optional)	>100	>100 mg/dL or <100 mg/dL
Moderately high risk: 10-year risk 10–20%	<130 mg/dL (<100 mg/dL optional)	> 130	> 130 mg/dL or (consider if 100–129 mg/dL)
Moderate risk: 2+ risk factors (10-year risk <10%)	<130 mg/dL	>130	>160 mg/dL
0-1 risk factor	<160 mg/dL	>160	>190 mg/dL (160–189 mg/dL drug use optional)

Data from 2001 NCEP/ATPIII Treatment Guidelines and 2004 update.

Table 22-4. Pharmacologic therapy of elevated cholesterol.

Drug Class	Drugs	Typical Effects[a]	Side Effects
Statins	Lovastatin, pravastatin, simvastatin, fluvastatin, atorvastatin,rosuvastatin	LDL: −20–60% HDL: +5–15% TG: −10–25%	Myopathy increased liver enzymes
Bile acid sequestrants	Cholestyramine, colestipol. colesevelam	LDL: −15% HDL: minimal TG: may increase 10%	GI distress, constipation, decreased absorption of other drugs
Nicotinic acid	Immediate-release, extended-release, sustained-release	LDL: −20% HDL: +20–35% TG: −20–50%	Flushing GI distress, hyperglycemia, hyperuricemia, hepatotoxicity
Fibrates	Gemfibrozil, fenofibrate	LDL: −5–15% HDL: +15% TG: −20–50%	GI distress,gallstones, myopathy
Cholesterol absorption inhibitors	Ezetimibe	LDL: −18% HDL: minimal TG: −8%	GI distress

[a]Lipid effects represent the average seen in most patients. Individual patients may display markedly different effects. This reinforces the need for dosage titration and close monitoring of lipid effects during drug initiation.

effects from statin agents. A reversible increase of serum aminotransferase levels to >3 times normal (ULN) occurs in 1% of patients taking high doses of statins. Discontinuation of the agent is required only if liver enzymes increase to >3 times ULN. Routine monitoring of liver function tests is no longer recommended by the FDA since hepatic side effects trigger symptoms that facilitate prompt discontinuation. Rhabdomyolysis occurs in <0.1% of cases. It can be prevented by the prompt discontinuation of the agent when muscle pain and elevated muscle enzymes occur. Unexplained pain in large muscle groups should prompt investigation for myopathy; however, routine monitoring of muscle enzymes is not supported by any evidence. Side effects from statins may not be class-specific. Therefore, a side effect with one agent should not prevent a trial with another statin agent. Prior concerns about statins causing cataracts or cancer have been alleviated by the release of several meta-analyses.

Statin agents can be combined with fibrates and nicotinic acid, but the potential for side effects is increased. When a statin is combined with a fibrate, the use of fenofibrate is preferred over gemfibrozil because the rate of rhabdomyolysis is much lower. Fibrate agents and nicotinic acid have special efficacy in patients with low HDL and elevated triglycerides, but to date there is limited evidence of improved cardiovascular outcomes despite favorable changes in lipid subfractions. Additionally, nicotinic acid can cause an increase in blood glucose, which can limit its use in diabetic patients.

The bile acid sequestrants cause gastrointestinal side effects and can lead to decreased absorption of other medications. Given their relatively low potency, they are useful mainly as adjuncts. Ezetimibe is a cholesterol absorption inhibitor that lowers LDL and is ideally used in combination with a statin agent. However, trials have not demonstrated benefits in improving cardiovascular outcomes.

C. Complementary and Alternative Therapies

Several complementary or alternative therapies are employed for cholesterol reduction, but the evidence supporting their use is variable. Several are harmless and some could lead to significant side effects. Oat bran (½ cup/d) is a soluble fiber that can reduce TC by 5 mg/dL and TG by 5%. Fish oil (1 g daily of unsaturated omega-3 fatty acids) can reduce triglycerides by ≤30% and raise HDL slightly with long-term use.

Garlic has few side effects, but several trials have shown that it changes lipids minimally. Soy can reduce LDL by ≤15%, with an intake of 25 g/d. This amount is unlikely to be achieved in a Western-style diet. Went yeast (*Monascus purpureus*) is the natural source for statin agents. As such, it is effective at lowering lipid values, but carries the same side effect profile as statins. Red wine can raise HDL' however, in amounts of >2 glasses per day, red wine will raise TG and potentially cause hepatic damage and other deleterious health effects. Several other supplements such as ginseng, chromium, and myrrh all have putative cholesterol-lowering effects but little patient-oriented clinical outcome evidence.

Step 8 of the NCEP/ATP III guidelines encourages clinicians to look for the "metabolic syndrome." The components of this syndrome are abdominal obesity, hypertriglyceridemia, low HDL, hypertension, and glucose intolerance. Aggressive treatment of inactivity, obesity, hypertension, and the use of low-dose aspirin are encouraged in these patients.

Step 9 is the final step of the algorithm. This step focuses on treating elevated triglycerides and low HDL as secondary endpoints of cholesterol therapy. Triglycerides are administered as follows:

The initial steps consist in employing TLC, (weight reduction, increased physical activity, dietary change) and then adding a fibrate or nicotinic acid to reach goal levels.

D. Treatment of Special Groups

The treatment of dyslipidemias in special groups presents problems because fewer trial data are available.

1. Women—Several statin trials included women, although they accounted for only 15–20% of the total enrolled patient population. Subset analysis and meta-analysis reveal that statins reduced coronary events by a similar proportion in women as in men.

2. Elderly—Given that ASCVD is more common in the elderly, it is expected that the benefits of cholesterol lowering would extend to this subgroup. Because of the increased frequency of ASCVD events in this population, the number needed to treat (NNT) is reduced from approximately 35:1, in patients aged 40–55 years, to just 4:1 in patients aged 65–75 years. The 2002 Prospective Study of Pravastatin in the Elderly at Risk (PROSPER) study and several others have confirmed the benefits of lipid lowering with statins for the primary and secondary prevention of ASCVD in patients aged 65–84 years.

3. Children—There are accumulating studies showing the safety of statins in adolescents. However, given concerns of interrupting cholesterol synthesis in the growing body, therapy is usually confined to the very high risk. Therapeutic lifestyle interventions are safe, and can have a profound impact on the long-term health of the child. Cholesterol levels should not be checked in children aged <2 years.

4. Patients aged <35 years—The Pathobiological Determinants of Atherosclerosis in Youth (PDAY) study has demonstrated the ability to correlate degrees of arterial intimal narrowing with the risk factors present in a patient across all age groups. The NCEP/ATP III guidelines specifically address this issue for patients aged 20–35 years. They state that although clinical CHD is rare in young adults, coronary atherosclerosis may progress rapidly, and young men who smoke and have an LDL 160–189 mg/dL may be candidates for drug therapy. In addition, drug therapy should be considered in young men and women with an LDL of >190 mg/d.

E. Indications for Referral

Patients who do not respond to combination therapy or have untoward side effects following therapy should be considered for specialty consultation. Combinations of multiple agents or lipid plasmapheresis may sometimes be required.

Anonymous. Statins for the primary prevention of cardiovascular disease. *Cochrane Database Syst Rev*. 2013;1:CD004816. [PMID: 23440795]

Anonymous. Drugs for lipids. Treatment guidelines from the *Medical Letter. Med Lett*. 2011;9(103):13–20.

Grundy SM, et al. Implications of recent clinical trials for the national cholesterol education program: adult treatment panel III guidelines. *Circulation*. 2004;110:227–239. [PMID: 15249516]

Third Report of the National Cholesterol Education Program (NCEP) Expert Panel on the Detection, Evaluation, and Treatment of High Blood Cholesterol in Adults (Adult Treatment Panel III). NIH/NHLBI, May 2001 (available at http://www.nhlbi.nih.gov).

Website

American Heart Association: www.americanheart.org (best peer-reviewed source for diet, exercise, and lifestyle information for physicians and patients).

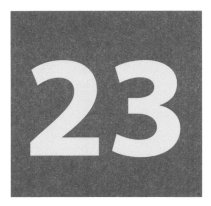

23

Urinary Tract Infections

Joe Kingery, DO

Urinary tract infections (UTIs) are among the most common bacterial infections encountered in medicine. Accurately estimating incidence is difficult because UTIs are not reportable, but estimates range from 650,000 to 7 million office visits per year.

A *UTI* is defined by urologists as any infection involving the urothelium, which includes urethral, bladder, prostate, and kidney infections. Some of these are diseases that have been clearly characterized (eg, cystitis and pyelonephritis), whereas others (eg, urethral and prostate infections) are not as well understood or described.

The terms *simple UTI* and *uncomplicated UTI* are often used to refer to cystitis. In this chapter *UTI* is used to refer to any infection of the urinary tract, and *cystitis* is used to specify a bladder infection. The generic term *complicated UTI* is often used to refer to cystitis occurring in a person with preexisting metabolic, immunologic, or urologic abnormalities, including kidney stones, diabetes, and AIDS, or caused by multidrug resistant organisms.

Asymptomatic bacteriuria, uncomplicated cystitis, complicated cystitis, two urethral syndromes, four prostatitis syndromes, and pyelonephritis are discussed in this chapter. Although separated into different diagnoses, differentiating among syndromes and deciding treatment is left to the clinician's discretion.

Antibiotic resistance is a topic that has been left mostly to the reader. General recommendations about specific antibiotics are inappropriate, given that antibiotic resistance differs from location to location. It is the responsibility of individual physicians to be familiar with local antibiotic resistances, and to determine the best first-line therapies for their practice. Always keep in mind that antibiotic use breeds resistance, and try to keep first-line drugs as simple and narrow-spectrum as possible.

Drekonja DM, Johnson JR. Urinary tract infections. *Prim Care.* 2008:35:345–367; vii. [PMID: 18486719]

ASYMPTOMATIC BACTERIURIA

 ESSENTIALS OF DIAGNOSIS

► Asymptomatic patient.
► Urine culture with more than 10^5 colony-forming units (CFUs); bacteria in spun urine; or urine dipstick analysis positive for leukocytes, nitrites, or both.

General Considerations

Asymptomatic bacteriuria is defined separately for men, women, and the type of specimen. For women, clean-catch voided specimens on two separate occasions must contain $>10^5$ CFU/mL of the same bacterial strain, or one catheterized specimen must contain $>10^2$ CFU/mL of bacteria. For men, a single clean-catch specimen with $>10^5$ CFU/mL of bacteria or one catheterized specimen with $>10^2$ CFU/mL of bacteria suffices for the diagnosis. By definition, the patient must be asymptomatic, that is, should not be experiencing dysuria, suprapubic pain, fever, urgency, frequency, or incontinence. Screening for bacteriuria does not need to be done in young, healthy, nonpregnant women; elderly healthy or institutionalized men or women; diabetic women; persons with spinal cord injury; or catheterized patients while the catheter remains in place. Pregnant women are now the only group that should be routinely screened and treated for asymptomatic bacteriuria. There are multiple guidelines recommending screening of this group of patients. Screening should occur between 12 and 16 weeks' gestation. The incidence is approximately 5–10% of pregnant women. There are numerous studies showing an association between asymptomatic bacteriuria and premature birth, low birth weight, and a high incidence of pyelonephritis. In the United States, screening is usually done by urine culture because dipstick screening can miss patients without pyuria or with unusual organisms.

Treatment

Treatment should be guided by local rates of resistance, keeping in mind safety of the antibiotic in pregnancy. The usual first-line treatment in the absence of significant resistance or penicillin allergy is a 7-day course of amoxicillin. Nitrofurantoin or a cephalosporin is suggested for penicillin-allergic pregnant patients, again for 7 days.

Guinto V, et al. Different antibiotic regiments for treating asymptomatic bacteriuria in pregnancy. *Cochrane Database Syst Rev.* 2010:CD007855. [PMID: 20824868]

Lin K, Fajardo K. Screening for asymptomatic bacteriuria in adults: evidence for the U.S. Preventive Services Task Force reaffirmation recommendation statement. *Ann Intern Med.* 2008;149:W20–W24. [PMID: 18591632]

Widmer M, et al. Duration of treatment for asymptomatic bacteriuria during pregnancy. *Cochrane Database Syst Rev.* 2011:CD000491. [PMID: 22161364]

UNCOMPLICATED BACTERIAL CYSTITIS

ESSENTIALS OF DIAGNOSIS

► Dysuria.

► Frequency, urgency, or both.

► Urine dipstick analysis positive for nitrites or leukocyte esterase.

► Positive urine culture (>10^4 organisms).

► No fever or flank pain.

General Considerations

Acute, uncomplicated cystitis is most common in women. Approximately one-third of all women have experienced at least one episode of cystitis by the age of 24 years, and nearly half will experience at least one episode during their lifetime. When a young woman presents to a health care provider with one or more symptoms, her probability of UTI is approximately 50%. Young women's risk factors include sexual activity, use of spermicidal condoms or diaphragm, and genetic factors such as blood type or maternal history of recurrent cystitis. Healthy, noninstitutionalized older women can also experience recurrent cystitis. Risk factors among these women include changes in the perineal epithelium and vaginal microflora after menopause, incontinence, diabetes, and history of cystitis before menopause.

Although men can also suffer from cystitis, it is rare (annual incidence: <0.01% of men aged 21–50 years) in men

aged <35 years who have normal urinary anatomy. Urethritis from sexually transmitted pathogens should always be considered in this age group, and prostatitis should always be ruled out in the older age group by a rectal examination. Any cystitis in a man is complicated, due to the presence of the prostate gland, and should be treated for 10–14 days to prevent a persistent prostatic infection.

Prevention

A. Young Women

Considering the frequency and morbidity of cystitis among young women, it is hardly surprising that the lay press and medical literature contain a host of ideas about how to prevent recurrent cystitis. These range from the suggestion that cotton underwear is "healthier" to wiping habits, voiding habits, and choice of beverage. Unfortunately, the vast majority of these preventive measures do not hold up to scientific study (**Table 23-1**).

Recent studies have shown no effect of back-to-front wiping, precoital voiding, tampon use, underwear fabric choice, or use of noncotton hose or tights. Behaviors that do appear to have an impact on frequency of cystitis in young women include sexual activity (four or more episodes per month in one study), delayed postcoital voiding, use of spermicidal condoms (several studies), use of unlubricated condoms (one study), use of diaphragms or cervical caps, and intake of cranberry juice.

It can be concluded from Table 23-1 that a few behaviorally oriented strategies can be offered to young women who suffer from recurrent cystitis. Recommending a change in contraception to oral contraceptive pills, intrauterine devices, or nonspermicidal, lubricated condoms may be helpful.

Table 23-1. UTI risk in young women.

Factors with No Evidence of Effect on Cystitis	Factors with Evidence of Effect on Cystitis	
	Promote	Prevent
Precoital voiding	Spermicide[a]	Cranberry juice
Underwear fabric	Diaphragm[a]	Prophylactic antibiotics
Wiping pattern	Cervical cap[a]	
Douching	Sexual activity	
Hot tub use	Genetic predisposition	
	Delayed postcoital voiding[a]	

[a]Drekonja DM, Johnson JR. Urinary tract infections. *Prim Care.* 2008;35:345–367, vii. [PMID: 18486719]

Cranberry juice and cranberry extract have long been proposed as a possible way to prevent UTIs. Cranberries supposedly contain a substance that changes the surface properties of *Escherichia coli* and prevents it from adhering to the bladder wall. A recent *Cochrane Review* identified 10 studies comparing the effects of cranberry products with placebo, juice, or water. There was evidence to show cranberries in the form of juice or capsules could prevent recurrent UTIs in women. A reasonable dose in capsule form is 300–400 mg twice daily. As for juice, 8 oz 3 times daily of unsweetened juice is recommended. It is unclear how long the duration should be.

Prophylactic antibiotics, either low-dose daily antibiotics or postcoital antibiotics, remain the mainstay of prevention of recurrent UTIs for young women and can reduce recurrence rates by ≤95%.

B. Postmenopausal Women

Risk factors for cystitis in older women include urologic factors such as incontinence, cystocele, and postvoid residual; hormonal factors resulting in a lack of protective lactobacillus colonization; and a prior history of cystitis. For the above mentioned risk factors, the most easily administered effective prevention is estrogen.

There are many possible ways to administer estrogen. These include traditional oral hormone replacement therapy, which is still considered indicative (after thorough discussion with the patient of risks and benefits) for menopausal symptoms, vaginal estrogen rings, or vaginal creams.

The only form of estrogen that has been proven to decrease recurrent UTIs in postmenopausal women is vaginal. The usual side effects of estrogen can be seen with vaginal use as well as oral. These include breast tenderness, vaginal bleeding, vaginal discharge, and vaginal irritation. Contraindications (as with oral estrogens) include a history of endometrial carcinoma, breast carcinoma, thromboembolic disorders, and liver disease. Patients' functional and cultural abilities should be considered before prescribing vaginal applications.

One study compared the effects of cranberry extract (500 mg daily) to trimethoprim for the prevention of recurrent UTIs in older women. There was only a slight advantage of the antibiotic over cranberry extract.

C. Young Men

The only studies focusing on prevention of UTI in young men have investigated infant circumcision; because the risk of UTI is so low in normal men, these studies are prohibitively expensive. In boys with recurrent UTI or high-grade ureteral reflux, the NNTs are 11 and 4, respectively. The complication rate of circumcision is 2–10%, with adverse sequelae ranging from minor transient bleeding (common) to amputation of the penis (extremely rare). It does appear to decrease the chance of UTI in boys and men. The risk of

UTI in normal boys hovers around 1% in the first 10 years of life, given that the number needed to treat (NNT) for circumcision is 111.

D. Future Trends in Prevention

Several investigations are ongoing in finding ways to prevent recurrent urinary tract infections, given the high prevalence and health burden that they impose. Vaginal vaccines are working their way through clinical trials and are not yet commercially available; whether they will prove to be more efficacious than prophylactic antibiotics is yet to be determined. Currently, a sublingual bacterial vaccine is also in development. This also looks promising, but needs more research.

▶ Clinical Findings

A. Symptoms and Signs

Symptoms include dysuria, ideally felt more internally than externally, and of sudden onset; suprapubic pain; cloudy, smelly urine; frequency; and urgency.

Physical examination in the afebrile, otherwise healthy patient with a classic history is done essentially to rule out other diagnoses and to ensure that red flags are not present. The examination might range from checking a temperature and percussing the costovertebral angles to a full pelvic examination, depending on where the history leads. There are no pathognomonic signs on physical examination for cystitis.

B. Laboratory Findings

Laboratory studies include dipstick test of urine, urinalysis, and urine culture. In some cases laboratory tests are not required to diagnose cystitis with high accuracy; however, they should probably be omitted only in settings where follow-up can be easily arranged in case of failure of treatment, which would, of course, indicate further workup. **Figure 23-1** provides a diagnostic algorithm for cystitis.

1. Urine dipstick testing—Dipstick findings are positive for leukocyte esterase or nitrite, or both. Several references now support treatment of simple, uncomplicated UTI in the young, nonpregnant woman on the grounds of clinical history alone, if that history leads to high suspicion for cystitis (and low suspicion of STD). For women with an equivocal clinical history, urine dipstick analysis may suffice to reassign the women to high or low suspicion and treat or not treat accordingly.

2. Urinalysis—Urinalysis will be positive for WBCs, with few or no epithelial cells. It should be noted, however, that urinalysis is more expensive than dipstick analysis and only minimally more accurate.

3. Urine culture—The gold standard of diagnosis is a culture growth of 100,000 (10^5) organisms in a midstream

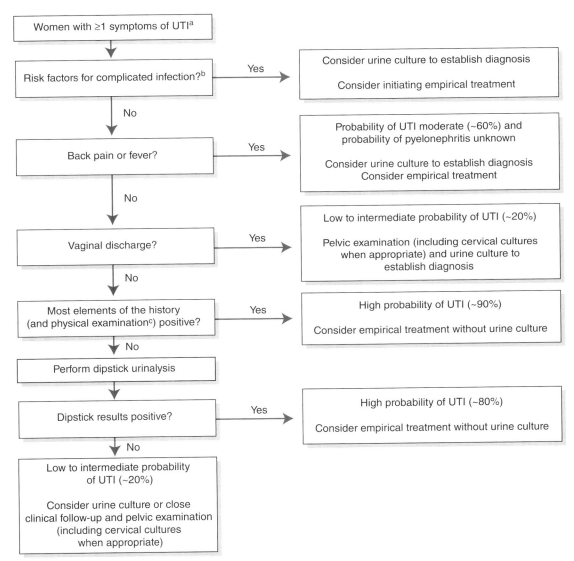

▲ **Figure 23-1.** Diagnostic algorithm for cystitis (STD, sexually transmitted disease; UTI, urinary tract infection).

Notations in the flowchart are as follows:
[a]In women who have risk factors for sexually transmitted diseases (STDs), consider testing for *Chlamydia*. The US Preventative Services Task Force recommends screening for *Chlamydia* for all women 25 years or younger and women of any age with more than one sex partner, a history of STD, or inconsistent use of condoms.
[b]For a definition of complicated UTI, see text.
[c]The only physical examination finding that increases the likelihood of UTI is costovertebral angle tenderness, and clinicians may consider not performing this test in patient with typical symptoms of acute uncomplicated UTI (as in telephone management). (Reproduced, with permission, from Bent S, et al. Does this woman have an acute uncomplicated urinary tract infection? *JAMA*. 2002;287:2701.)

clean-catch sample. However, some patients have classic clinical cases of UTI and only 100 (10^2) organisms on culture. Few laboratories are equipped to detect anything fewer than 10^4 organisms. Culture is strongly suggested if a relapsing UTI or pyelonephritis is suspected to ensure sensitivities and eradication (see Figure 23-1).

C. Imaging Studies

Imaging studies are seldom required for patients with simple uncomplicated UTIs.

D. Special Tests

These tests are generally required only for failures of treatment, symptoms suggesting a diagnosis other than cystitis, or complicated cystitis (see section on complicated cystitis, later).

▶ Differential Diagnosis

See **Table 23-2**.

▶ Complications

There are virtually no complications from repeated uncomplicated cystitis if it is recognized and treated. Delay in treatment may lead to ascending infection and pyelonephritis. In the case of infection with urea-splitting bacteria, "infection stones" of struvite with bacteria trapped in the interstices may be formed. These stones lead to persistent bacteriuria and must be completely removed to clear the infection. *Proteus mirabilis, Staphylococcus saprophyticus,* and *Klebsiella* bacteria can all split urea and lead to stones.

▶ Treatment

A. Acute Cystitis

There is ample evidence from randomized clinical trials to support the superiority of 3-day antibiotic therapy to 1-day treatment and, equivalently, of therapy for longer periods of time, with the exception of nitrofurantoin. This is true for treatment of older, noninstitutionalized women as well. Trimethoprim-sulfamethoxazole, in the absence of allergies to sulfa and local resistance rates of >10–20%, should be considered first-line therapy. Risk factors for trimethoprim-sulfamethoxazole resistance include recent antibiotic exposure, recent hospitalization, diabetes mellitus, three or more UTIs in the past year, and possibly use of oral contraceptive pills or estrogen replacement therapy. For patients who are allergic to sulfa drugs, a 5–7-day course of nitrofurantoin or a 3-day course of a fluoroquinolone (eg, ciprofloxacin) can be used. However, because of concern regarding fluoroquinolone resistance and frequency of cystitis, they should be used sparingly. β-Lactam antibiotics are not as effective as other classes of drugs against urinary pathogens and should not be used as first-line agents except in pregnant patients.

Table 23-2. Red-flag symptoms and differential diagnoses.

If Patient Has	Consider
Fever	Urosepsis, pyelonephritis, pelvic inflammatory disease (PID)
Vaginal discharge	Sexually transmitted disease (STD), PID
External burning pain	Vulvovaginitis, especially candidal vaginitis
Costovertebral angle tenderness	Pyelonephritis
Nausea/vomiting	Pyelonephritis, urosepsis, inability to tolerate oral medications
Recent UTI (<2 weeks)	Incompletely treated, resistant pathogen; urologic abnormality, including stones and unusual anatomy; interstitial cystitis
Dyspareunia	STD, PID, psychogenic causes
Recent trauma or instrumentation	Complicated UTI
Pregnancy	Antibiotic choice, treatment duration
Severe, colicky flank pain	UTI complicated by stones; preexisting or struvite stone caused by urea-splitting bacteria
Joint pains, sterile urine	Spondyloarthropathy (eg, Reiter or Behçet syndrome)
History of childhood infections, urologic surgery	Abnormal anatomy
History of kidney stones	Complicated UTI; bacterial persistence in stones
Diabetes	Complicated UTI
Immunosuppression	Complicated UTI

B. Acute Cystitis in the Pregnant Woman

Treatment with amoxicillin, a cephalosporin, nitrofurantoin, or another pregnancy-safe antibiotic for 7 days remains the standard. Asymptomatic bacteriuria, if found on cultures, is treated in pregnant women with the same antibiotics (see section on asymptomatic bacteriuria, earlier).

C. Prophylaxis for Recurrent Cystitis

Low-dose, prophylactic antibiotics have been shown to decrease recurrences by ≤95%. Most recommendations suggest starting prophylaxis after a patient has had more than

Table 23-3. Prophylactic antibiotics for recurrent UTI in women.

Regimen	Drug and Dose
Daily	Trimethoprim, 100 mg every day Trimethoprim-sulfamethoxazole, 80 mg/400 mg every day Nitrofurantoin, 50 mg every day[a] Nitrofurantoin macrocrystals, 100 mg every day Cranberry juice, 8 oz 3 times a day Cranberry tablets, 1:30 twice a day
Postcoital	One dose of any of the above antibiotics after coitus

[a]Preferred if patient could become pregnant. Trimethoprim should be avoided in the first trimester.

three documented UTIs in 1 year. Prophylactic antibiotics are usually administered for 6 months to 1 year but can be given for longer periods of time. Antibiotics can be taken daily at bedtime or used postcoitally by women whose infections are associated with intercourse (**Table 23-3**). Unfortunately, prophylaxis does not change the propensity of these women for recurrent UTIs; when prophylaxis is stopped, approximately 60% of women develop a UTI within 3–4 months. Prophylaxis should not start until cultures have shown no growth after treatment, to rule out bacterial persistence.

► **Prognosis**

Long-term prognosis in terms of kidney function is excellent; prognosis of arresting recurrent cystitis without permanent prophylaxis is not as good. New preventive treatments are currently being explored, and it is hoped that these will prove beneficial.

Drekonja DM, Johnson JR. Urinary tract infections. *Prim Care.* 2008:35:345–367, vii. [PMID: 18486719]

Guirguis-Blake J. Cranberry products for treatment of urinary tract infection. *Am Fam Physician.* 2008;78:332–333. [PMID: 18711947]

Jepson RG, Craig JC. Cranberries for preventing urinary tract infections. *Cochrane Database Syst Rev.* 2008;CD001321. [PMID: 18253990]

Lorenzo-Gomez MF, et al. Evaluation of a therapeutic vaccine for the prevention of recurrent urinary tract infections versus prophylactic treatment with antibiotics. *Int Urogynecol J.* 2013;24(1):127–134. [PMID: 22806485]

McMurdo ME, et al. Cranberry or trimethoprim for the prevention of recurrent urinary tract infections? A randomized controlled trial in older women. *J Antimicrob Chemother.* 2009;63: 389–395. [PMID: 19042940]

Nicolle LE. Short-term therapy for urinary tract infection: success and failure. *Int J Antimicrob Agents.* 2008;31(suppl 1):S40–S45. [PMID: 18023152]

Perrotta C, et al. Oestrogens for preventing recurrent urinary tract infection in postmenopausal women. *Cochrane Database Syst Rev.* 2008;CD005131. [PMID: 18425910]

COMPLICATED CYSTITIS & SPECIAL POPULATIONS

ESSENTIALS OF DIAGNOSIS

► Any cystitis not resolved after 3 days of appropriate antibiotic treatment.

► Any cystitis in a special population, such as a diabetic patient, a man, a patient with an abnormal urinary tract, or a patient with ureteral stones.

► Any cystitis involving multidrug resistant bacteria.

► **General Considerations**

The infections listed above warrant further workup by a physician or referral to an urologist. These infections should all be cultured to ensure that the antibiotics used are appropriate and that the organisms are sensitive to the chosen antibiotic.

► **Clinical Findings**

Special tests should include x-ray or computed tomography (CT) to evaluate for stones, intravenous pyelogram (IVP) to evaluate anatomy and stones, and cystoscopy and biopsy to rule out interstitial cystitis, cancer, or unusual pathogens.

► **Treatment**

Patients with complicated UTIs should be treated with long-course (≥10–14-day), appropriate antibiotics. Single-dose or 3-day regimens are not appropriate for this group of patients.

ACUTE URETHRAL SYNDROME

ESSENTIALS OF DIAGNOSIS

► Dysuria.

► Frequency and urgency.

► No vaginal discharge.

► Urine dipstick analysis may be negative or positive.

► Negative culture.

► **General Considerations**

Acute urethral syndrome is a term used by some to describe a young, healthy, sexually active woman who complains of recent-onset symptoms of cystitis but does not meet strict guidelines for diagnosis of cystitis (growth of $\leq 10^4$ or 10^5 organisms on culture). Some authors now feel that even 100 CFUs found on culture of a dysuric woman represent a true UTI. Because most laboratories are equipped to detect only $\geq 10^4$ organisms, these are patients in usual practice found to have "negative" cultures. They may have positive or negative urine dipstick analysis and positive or negative spun urine for bacteria, although bacteria and white blood cells (WBCs) in the urine are more convincing for cystitis than a completely negative workup.

Clinical Findings

Testing depends on the physician's assessment of the patient. In patients at low risk of acquiring a sexually transmitted disease (STD), no testing might be appropriate or maybe only after failure of empirical treatment for cystitis. In patients at higher risk of acquiring an STD, *Chlamydia* testing, by either cervical swab, urine polymerase chain reaction (PCR), or ligase chain reaction (LCR), might be appropriate.

Differential Diagnosis

This syndrome is not well defined. It is usually taken to represent an early cystitis, but it can also be an STD (*Chlamydia trachomatis* has been noted in women with the previously described symptoms).

Treatment

There is some evidence that the acute urethral syndrome will respond to antibiotics commonly used in the treatment of UTIs. Because the prevalence of *C. trachomatis* was found to be high in at least one study of women with these symptoms, use of antibiotics effective against STDs or *Chlamydia* testing for patients who do not respond completely to a course of antibiotics is highly recommended.

Leibovici L. Trimethoprim reduced dysuria in women with symptoms of urinary tract infection but negative urine dipstick test results. *Evid Based Med*. 2006;11:19. [PMID: 17213061]

Richards D, et al. Response to antibiotics of women with symptoms of urinary tract infection but negative dipstick urine test results: double blind randomized controlled trial. *Br Med J*. 2005;331:143. [PMID: 15972728]

URETHRITIS

ESSENTIALS OF DIAGNOSIS

▶ Pain or irritation on urination.

▶ No frequency or urgency.

▶ Discharge from the urethra (predominantly males).

▶ Vaginal discharge possible.

General Considerations

Isolated urethritis in men or women is almost always an STD, most often caused by *C. trachomatis*. This syndrome is differentiated from acute urethral syndrome by the time-course of symptoms; symptoms that have a gradual onset or persist without evolution into classic cystitis symptoms, including suprapubic symptoms such as pain, urgency, or frequency, are more indicative of urethritis than of acute urethral syndrome.

Clinical Findings

It can be very difficult to differentiate a symptomatic chlamydial infection from bacterial cystitis with coliform organisms, and testing for both may be required. The advent of *Chlamydia* urine PCR or LCR tests makes ruling out *Chlamydia* much easier than in the past, as the same urine sample can be sent for both tests.

Treatment

See Chapter 14 for current diagnosis and treatment of STDs such as *Chlamydia*.

ACUTE BACTERIAL PROSTATITIS

ESSENTIALS OF DIAGNOSIS

▶ Dysuria, frequency, urgency.

▶ Tender prostate.

▶ Leukocyte esterase or nitrite on urine dipstick analysis.

▶ Positive urine culture.

General Considerations

Prostatitis is a very common disease among men, with a prevalence and incidence among men ranging between 11% and 16%. There are apprximately 2 million office visits per year for prostatitis (1% of all primary care office visits), so it is useful for the primary care practitioner to be able to evaluate men for symptoms of prostatitis.

Previously, prostatitis was simply described as "acute," "chronic," or "nonbacterial." In 1995 the National Institutes of Health (NIH) revised the categorization of prostatitis, and the disease is now differentiated into four categories, as follows:

• Category I: acute bacterial prostatitis

• Category II: chronic bacterial prostatitis

• Category IIIA: inflammatory chronic pelvic pain syndrome

• Category IIIB: noninflammatory chronic pelvic pain syndrome

• Category IV: asymptomatic inflammatory prostatitis

Category IV is a diagnosis made incidentally, while working up other symptoms, and is not considered severe enough to require treatment. Discussion of category I, or acute bacterial prostatitis, follows. The other categories are discussed separately in this chapter.

Acute bacterial prostatitis is different from other types of prostatitis in that it is a well-defined entity with a relatively clear-cut etiology, diagnosis, and treatment. Acute bacterial prostatitis is caused by typical uropathogens and responds well to antibiotic treatment.

Prevention

There is no evidence for interventions that will prevent spontaneous prostatitis.

Clinical Findings

Symptoms and signs include dysuria, frequency, and urgency; low back, perineal, penile, or rectal pain; or tense or "boggy" tender prostate. Fever and chills may be present.

Laboratory findings include a urine dipstick analysis that is positive for leukocyte esterase or nitrites, or both, and urine culture that is positive for a single uropathogen. Imaging studies are rarely performed for acute uncomplicated prostatitis.

Prostatic massage is not generally performed in patients with acute bacterial prostatitis because it may lead to acute bacteremia.

Differential Diagnosis

Abnormal anatomy may include urethral strictures, polyps, diverticula, redundancies, or valves anywhere in the system from the penis to the kidneys (**Table 23-4**).

Complications

Complications of acute bacterial prostatitis may include ascending infection, infection-related stones, abscess, fistula, cysts, and acute urinary retention. In the case of acute urinary retention precipitated by prostatitis, a suprapubic catheter rather than a Foley catheter should be placed to avoid damage to the prostate.

Treatment

Treatment is determined by the severity of illness as well as local resistance rates. In cases of very ill patients, broad-spectrum parenteral antibiotics should be initiated. Typically, a penicillin or penicillin derivative and an aminoglycoside can be used. As the illness is treated, the patient can be transitioned to oral therapy with either a quinolone or trimethoprim-sulfamethoxazole for at least 3–4 weeks. Less ill patients can be started on oral therapy with a quinolone or trimethoprim-sulfamethoxazole, again for 3–4 weeks. An α-blocker can be considered for mild urinary retention. A urinary catheter should be considered for more severe retention.

Table 23-4. Differential diagnosis of dysuria in men.

If Patient Has	Consider
Acute, colicky flank pain or history of kidney stones	Kidney stone; complicated cystitis
Costovertebral angle tenderness, fevers	Pyelonephritis
Urethral discharge	Sexually transmitted disease
Diabetes/immunosuppression	Complicated cystitis, unusual pathogens
Testicular pain	Torsion; epididymo orchitis
Joint pains	Spondyloarthropathy (ie, Reiter or Behçet syndrome)
History of childhood UTI or urologic surgery	Abnormal anatomy; complicated cystitis
Recurrent symptoms after treatment	Abnormal anatomy; abscess; stone; chronic prostatitis; resistant organism; inadequate length of treatment; Munchausen syndrome; somatization disorder

Prognosis

The prognosis is very good for patients with acute uncomplicated bacterial prostatitis.

Benway BM, Moon TD. Bacterial prostatitis. *Urol Clin North Am.* 2008;35:23–32; v. [PMID: 18061021]
Murphy AB, et al. Chronic prostatitis: management strategies. *Drugs.* 2009;69:71–84. [PMID: 19192937]

CHRONIC BACTERIAL PROSTATITIS

 ESSENTIALS OF DIAGNOSIS

- ▶ Dysuria, frequency, urgency.
- ▶ Symptoms lasting more than 3 months.
- ▶ Urine dipstick analysis positive for leukocyte esterase or nitrites, or both.
- ▶ Pyuria on microscopy.
- ▶ Positive 4-glass or 2-glass test for prostatic origin.

General Consideration

Chronic bacterial prostatitis, or NIH category II prostatitis, is quite rare, and consequently very few studies have examined it. Bacterial disease represents only a small percentage of the cases of chronic prostatitis. It has been estimated that the percentage of both acute and chronic bacterial prostatitis cases constitute only 5–10 of all prostatitis diagnoses, and of the bacterial cases, the vast majority are acute.

► Prevention

Early and sufficient treatment of acute bacterial prostatitis is considered by some authors to prevent chronic prostatitis.

► Clinical Findings

A. Symptoms and Signs

Symptoms and signs include dysuria, frequency, and urgency; prostatic tenderness on examination; low back pain; and perineal, penile, or rectal pain. Symptoms are usually present for more than 3 months.

B. Laboratory and Imaging Findings

A urine dipstick analysis will be positive for leukocyte esterase or nitrites, or both. Additionally, a 4- or 2-glass test (discussed below) will be positive for prostatic origin. A transrectal prostatic ultrasound should be performed if an abscess or a stone is suspected.

C. Special Tests

1. 4-glass test—Not used by the majority of practitioners, this is a localization test for chronic prostatitis. The patient should not have been on antibiotics for a month, should not have ejaculated for 2 days, and needs a reasonably full bladder. Signs and symptoms of urethritis or cystitis should have been worked up previously and treated. To perform the test, the patient first cleans himself and carefully retracts the foreskin, then urinates the first 5–10 mL into a sterile container (VB_1). He then urinates 100–200 mL into the toilet, and a second 10–20-mL sample into a sterile container (VB_2). Prostatic massage is then done, milking secretions from the periphery to the center, and any expressed prostatic secretions (EPSs) are caught in a third sterile container. The patient then cleans himself again, and urinates a final 10–20 mL sample into a fourth container (VB_3).

All urine samples are examined microscopically and cultured. Expressed prostatic secretions are wet-mounted, examined, and cultured. The test is positive for prostatic localization if WBCs per high-power field (HPF) and colony counts in VB_3 are ≥ 10 times greater than in VB_1 or VB_2, or if there are 10 polymorphonuclear leukocytes (PMNL)/HPF in the wet mount. If there is a significant colony count in both VB_2 and VB_3, the patient should be treated for 3 days with nitrofurantoin, which does not penetrate the prostate, and the test should be repeated.

2. 2-glass test—A verified modification of the 4-glass test, this test requires an initial clean-catch urine sample,

prostatic massage, and a postmassage urine sample. It is functionally equivalent to the VB_2 and VB_3 portions of the 4-glass test and more often used in clinical practice.

► Differential Diagnosis

See Table 23-4.

► Complications

Complications of chronic bacterial prostatitis may include ascending infection, infection-related stones, abscess, fistula, cysts, and acute urinary retention.

► Treatment

Antibiotic treatment with quinolones has shown the best results. Therapy is with an oral quinolone for at least 4–6 weeks. Trimethoprim-sulfamethoxazole for 1–3 months can also be considered. α-blockers may provide some benefit to treatment as well.

► Prognosis

The prognosis for treatment of chronic bacterial prostatitis is not known. A clear differentiation of which patients will respond to antibiotics and which will not has not been obtained.

Nickel JC, Xiang J. Clinical significance of nontraditional bacterial uropathogens in the management of chronic prostatitis. *J Urol.* 2008:179:1391–1395. [PMID: 18289570]
Weidner W, et al. Acute bacterial prostatitis and chronic prostatitis/chronic pelvic pain syndrome: andrological implications. *Andrologia.* 2008:40:105–112. [PMID: 18336460]

CHRONIC ABACTERIAL PROSTATITIS/CHRONIC PELVIC PAIN SYNDROME

 ESSENTIALS OF DIAGNOSIS

Not very well characterized; most suggestive symptoms include the following:

► Perineal pain.
► Lower abdominal pain.
► Penile, especially penile tip, pain.
► Testicular pain.
► Ejaculatory discomfort or pain.
► STDs and UTI ruled out.

► General Considerations

Chronic abacterial prostatitis was renamed by the NIH in 1995. It is now called *chronic pelvic pain syndrome* and can be further subclassified into inflammatory, meaning with inflammatory cells isolated in tests, or noninflammatory. This change was made in an attempt to recognize that the pain syndrome that physicians have been referring to as "chronic abacterial prostatitis" or even "prostatodynia" in the absence of inflammatory cells on examination has never been proved to originate in the prostate.

The NIH further divided chronic prostatitis/chronic pelvic pain syndrome (CP/CPPS) into two categories: inflammatory (IIIA) and noninflammatory (IIIB). In category IIIA prostatitis, leukocytes are found in semen, in expressed prostatic secretions, or in a postprostatic massage urine sample. In category IIIB prostatitis, no leukocytes are found in secretions. Recent evidence suggests cytokines may play a role in diagnosis in the future. Current research efforts include the Chronic Prostatitis Clinical Research Network, founded in 1997 by the NIH to investigate the chronic pelvic pain syndrome. Their work is ongoing and not definitive at this time.

The etiology of chronic prostatitis remains unknown. Current theories include infection with unusual or fastidious organisms, lower urinary tract obstruction or dysfunctional voiding, intraprostatic ductal reflux and subsequent chemical irritation with urea from urine forced into the gland, immunologic or autoimmune processes, or neuromuscular causes, such as reflex sympathetic dystrophy. Although none of these theories has been proved, continued research, it is hoped, will increase our understanding of this problem.

Prevention

Trials of preventive measures for chronic prostatitis or chronic pelvic pain syndrome are lacking, and risk factors for prostatitis or chronic pelvic pain have not been investigated.

Clinical Findings

A. Symptoms and Signs

Symptoms include dysuria, frequency, urgency, other irritative voiding symptoms, and pain in the perineal area for >3 of the last 6 months.

B. Laboratory Findings

Laboratory testing shows no evidence of current cystitis or demonstrable bacterial infection. Patients with inflammatory-type chronic pelvic pain syndrome have leukocytes in expressed prostatic secretions or postprostatic massage urine.

C. Special Tests

If the patient has hematuria, urine cytology should be performed. The 2-glass test (first part of a clean-catch urine sample in one bottle; prostatic massage milking from periphery to center; second urine sample into a sterile container) has been shown to be as reliable as the more complicated 4-glass test

(discussed earlier) at distinguishing chronic bacterial prostatitis and inflammatory and noninflammatory prostatitis.

Differential Diagnosis

See Table 23-4.

Treatment

There is no clear-cut prescription for the treatment of chronic prostatitis of either the inflammatory or noninflammatory type. This treatment discussion therefore groups inflammatory and noninflammatory prostatitis into one entity for discussion.

Although CP/CPPS does not have a bacterial etiology, antimicrobials do improve symptoms in ≤50% of patients. Patients with a shorter duration of symptoms are more likely to respond. The antimicrobials utilized most include fluoroquinolones and trimethoprim/sulfamethoxazole for 4–6 weeks. α-blockers such as tamsulosin, terazosin, and doxazosin have shown some improvement in patients as well. Once again, the sooner treatment is started, the better the outcomes. At least 6 weeks of therapy are needed with α-blockers. A combination of antimicrobial and α-blocker shows slight improvement over monotherapy. Despite high use by providers, nonsteroidal anti-inflammatory drugs (NSAIDs) have shown only minimal effects. Unless the patient has concomitant benign prostatic hyperplasia (BPH), 5α-reductase inhibitors (eg, finasteride) have also demonstsrated only minimal effects.

There are several other modalities of treatment that need further review: (1) transurethral microwave thermotherapy (TUMT), (2) cooled transurethral microwave thermotherapy (cTUMT), (3) transurethral needle ablation (TUNA), (4) botulinum toxin A injections, (5) transurethral resection of the prostate (TURP), (6) electromagnetic therapy, and (7) electroacupuncture and application of capsaicin on the perineal area. Although none of these have been studied extensively, modalities 2 and 6 show promising results. A recent study also showed the efficacy of fluoxetine 20 mg/d for 3 months in treating symptoms of refractory chronic prostatitis/chronic pelvic pain syndrome.

Table 23-5 reviews controlled trials that have shown possible efficacy of treatments.

Prognosis

The prognosis for chronic prostatitis and chronic pelvic pain syndrome category III is not good. Prognosis appears to be worse for patients with previous episodes or more severe pain.

Kastner C. Update on minimally invasive therapy for chronic prostatitis/chronic pelvic pain syndrome. *Curr Urol Rep.* 2008;9:333–338. [PMID: 18765134]
Murphy AB, et al. Chronic prostatitis: management strategies. *Drugs.* 2009;69:71–84. [PMID: 19192937]

Table 23-5. Effective therapies for chronic abacterial prostatitis/chronic pelvic pain syndrome.

Therapy	Dose	Comments
Fluoroquinolone	Levofloxacin 500 mg every day Ciprofloxacin 500 mg twice a day	Although no infectious etiology in this disease, studies suggest that ~50% of patients can improve if treated early; treatment is for 6 weeks; currently considered a first-line therapy
α-blockers	Tamsulosin 0.4 mg every day[a] Doxazosin 4 mg every day 1 mg every day for 4 days 2 mg every day for 10 days 5 mg every day for 12 weeks	All considered first-line therapy; well tolerated; can be combined with fluoroquinolone for improved benefits Needs to be taken for ≥6 weeks[b–d] Studies have used ≥3 months of therapy[d]
Finasteride	5 mg every day	Minimal benefit.; not first-line therapy; mostly useful only if concomitant BPH; need to take for >1 year[b,c]
Pentosan polysulfate	100 mg 3 times a day for 6 months	Minimal improvement, with no statistical significance[b]
Thermotherapy		Still experimental, but some promising results[d]

[a]Ye ZQ, et al. Tamsulosin treatment of chronic non-bacterial prostatitis. *J Intern Med Res.* 2008:36:244–252. [PMID: 18380933]
[b]Murphy M, et al. Chronic prostatitis: management strategies. *Drugs.* 2009; 69:71–84. [PMID: 19192937]
[c]Nickel JC. Treatment of chronic prostatitis/chronic pelvic pain syndrome. *Int J Antimicrob Agents.* 2008;31(suppl 1):S112–S116. [PMID: 17954024]
[d]Kastner C. Update on minimally invasive therapy for chronic prostatitis/chronic pelvic pain syndrome. *Curr Urol Rep.* 2008; 9:333–338. [PMID: 18765134]

Nickel JC. Treatment of chronic prostatitis/chronic pelvic pain syndrome. *Int J Antimicrob Agents.* 2008;31(suppl 1):S112–S116. [PMID: 17954024]

Nickel JC, et al. Category III chronic prostatitis/chronic pelvic pain syndrome: insights from the National Institutes of Health Chronic Prostatitis Collaborative Research Network studies. *Curr Urol Rep.* 2008;9:320–327. [PMID: 18765132]

Xia D, et al. Fluoxetine ameliorates symptoms of refractory chronic prostatitis/chronic pelvic pain syndrome. *Chin Med J.* 2011;124:2158–2161. [PMID: 21933619]

Ye ZQ, et al. Tamsulosin treatment of chronic non-bacterial prostatitis. *J Int Med Res.* 2008;36:244–252. [PMID: 18380933]

PYELONEPHRITIS

ESSENTIALS OF DIAGNOSIS

► Fever.

► Chills.

► Flank pain.

► More than 100,000 CFUs on urine culture.

General Considerations

Pyelonephritis is an infection of the kidney parenchyma. It has been estimated to result in >100,000 hospitalizations per year. Information on outpatient visits is not readily available, but because many cases are now managed on an outpatient basis, it is likely to be seen by most primary care providers. Pyelonephritis usually results from upward spread of cystitis but can also result from hematogenous seeding of the kidney from another infectious source. The infection can be complicated by stones or renal scarring if untreated but usually resolves without sequelae in young, healthy people if treated promptly.

The most common bacteria involved are the same organisms that cause uncomplicated cystitis: *E. coli, S. saprophyticus, Klebsiella* species, and occasionally *Enterobacter*. As with simple cystitis, women with genetic predispositions are more commonly affected than other women.

Prevention

There are no recent studies on prevention of pyelonephritis. Prompt treatment of cystitis may prevent some cases of pyelonephritis, but this has not been demonstrated.

Clinical Findings

Symptoms and signs include fever, chills, malaise, dysuria, and flank pain. Nausea and vomiting may also occur.

Laboratory findings include a urine dipstick analysis that is positive for leukocyte esterase or nitrites and urine culture showing >100,000 CFUs.

Table 23-6. Differential diagnosis of pyelonephritis.

If Patient Has	Consider
Negative urine dipstick or culture	Pelvic inflammatory disease; stone obstructing ureter; lower-lobe pneumonia; herpes zoster
Guarding/rebound	Acute cholecystitis; acute appendicitis; perforated viscus
Recurrent infection	Kidney stone, spontaneous or infection-related; anatomic abnormality; resistant organism; inadequate treatment
Diabetes	Emphysematous pyelonephritis
History of childhood infections, urologic surgery	Abnormal anatomy
History of kidney stones	Pyelonephritis complicated by stones

Imaging studies are seldom required unless the patient is diabetic or there is suspicion that stones are complicating the infection, in which case a CT scan is the test of choice.

Differential Diagnosis

See **Table 23-6**.

Complications

Diabetic patients can experience emphysematous pyelonephritis. It is a severe necrotizing renal infection characterized by gas production within the renal parenchyma. This is diagnosed by CT scan or other imaging study showing gas in the renal collecting system or around the kidney. In a diabetic patient with emphysematous pyelonephritis, the definitive treatment is percutaneous drainage. If there is extensive, diffuse gas, nephrectomy is advised, as the mortality rate in diabetics approaches 75%. This condition rarely occurs in nondiabetic patients and is often related to obstruction. In some of these cases, relief of the obstruction and antibiotics may suffice.

Stones can complicate pyelonephritis by causing a partial or complete obstruction. These stones can be spontaneous or "infection" stones of struvite, caused by urea-splitting organisms. Stones complicating pyelonephritis must be removed before the infection can completely resolve.

People with a history of childhood pyelonephritis can experience renal scarring and recurrent infections. These scars are unusual in healthy adults with pyelonephritis. Young men with pyelonephritis should be investigated for a cause.

Patients who do not respond to 48 hours of appropriate antibiotics should be worked up for occult complicating factors or other diagnoses.

Treatment

The best drugs for treatment of pyelonephritis are bactericidal, with a broad spectrum to cover Gram-positive and Gram-negative bacteria, and concentrate well in urine and renal tissues. Aminoglycosides; aminopenicillins such as amoxicillin with clavulanic acid, ticarcillin, or piperacillin; cephalosporins; fluoroquinolones; or, in extreme cases, imipenem, are all appropriate. First-line outpatient treatment is usually a fluoroquinolone. Cure rates have been reported to approach 90% with a 10–14-day course of antibiotics. However, studies show similar cure rates with a 7-day course of ciprofloxacin.

Patients experiencing severe nausea and vomiting who are unable to tolerate oral agents may need to be hospitalized for parenteral therapy. Patients with severe illness, suspected bacteremia, or sepsis should also be admitted.

Prognosis

Prognosis after an acute episode of uncomplicated pyelonephritis in a previously healthy adult is excellent.

Colgan R, et al. Diagnosis and treatment of acute pyelonephritis in women. *Am Fam Physician*. 2011;84:519–26. [PMID: 21888302]

Pontin AR, Barnes RD. Current management of emphysematous pyelonephritis. *Nat Rev Urol*. 2009;6:272–279. [PMID: 19424175]

Sandberg T, et al. Ciprofloxacin for 7 days versus 14 days in women with acute pyelonephritis: a randomized, open-label and double-blind, placebo-controlled, non-inferiority trial. *Lancet*. 2012;380:484–490. [PMID: 22726802]

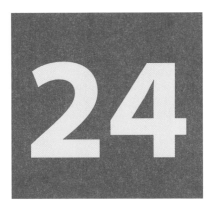

24

Arthritis: Osteoarthritis, Gout, & Rheumatoid Arthritis

Bruce E. Johnson, MD

Arthritis is a complaint and a disease afflicting many patients and accounting for >10% of appointments to a generalist practice. Arthritis is multifaceted and can be categorized in several different fashions. For simplicity, this chapter focuses on conditions affecting the anatomic joint composed of cartilage, synovium, and bone. Other discussions would include localized disorders of the periarticular region (eg, tendonitis and bursitis) and systemic disorders that have arthritic manifestations (eg, vasculitides, polymyalgia rheumatica, and fibromyalgia). The chapter discusses three prototypical types of arthritis: osteoarthritis, as an example of a cartilage disorder; gout, as an example of both a crystal-induced arthritis and an acute arthritis; and rheumatoid arthritis, as an example of an immune-mediated, systemic disease and a chronic deforming arthritis.

OSTEOARTHRITIS

 ESSENTIALS OF DIAGNOSIS

▶ Degenerative changes in the knee, hip, shoulder, spine, or virtually any other joint.

▶ Pain with movement that improves with rest.

▶ Joint deformity and mechanical alteration.

▶ Sclerosis, thickening, spur formation, warmth, and effusion in the joints.

▶ General Considerations

Arthritis is among the oldest identified conditions in humans. Anthropologists examining skeletal remains from antiquity deduce levels of physical activity and work by searching for the presence of the degenerative changes of osteoarthritis (OA). OA is more prevalent among people in occupations characterized by steady, physically demanding activity such as farming, construction, certain sports, and production-line work. Obesity is a significant risk factor for OA, especially of the knee. Heredity and gender play a role in a person's likelihood of developing OA, regardless of work or recreational activity.

▶ Pathogenesis

It is increasingly accepted that most OA results, at least in part, from altered mechanics within the joint. Certain metabolic conditions such as hemochromatosis and Gaucher disease involve a genetic defect in collagen/cartilage. Altered mechanics may occur from minor gait abnormalities or major traumas that, over a lifetime, result in repeated stress and damage to cartilage. Repeated trauma may result in microfracture of cartilage, with incomplete healing due to continuation of the altered mechanics. Disruption of the otherwise smooth cartilage surface allows differential pressure on remaining cartilage, as well as stress on the underlying bone. Debris from fractured cartilage acts as a foreign body, causing low-level inflammation within the synovial fluid. These multiple influences combine to alter intrinsic efforts at cartilage repair, leading to progressive cartilage destruction and bony joint change. Current thinking suggests that the process is not immutable, but any intervention would have to be made while the joint is still asymptomatic—an unlikely occurrence.

▶ Prevention

It is difficult to advise patients on measures to prevent osteoarthritis. Obese persons should lose weight, but few occupational or recreational precautions can be expected to alter the natural history of OA. Altered mechanics may be an important precipitating cause of arthritis, but recognizing minor changes, especially within the currently accepted range of normal, makes diagnosis and preventive steps unrealistic.

Brandt KD, Dieppe P, Radin E. Etiopathogenesis of osteoarthritis. *Med Clin North Am.* 2009;93:1–24. [PMID: 19059018]

► Clinical Findings

A. Symptoms and Signs

Symptomatic OA represents the culmination of damage to cartilage, usually over many years. OA typically progresses from symptomatic pain to physical findings to loss of function, but actually any of these can be first to present. OA can occur at any joint, but the most commonly involved joints are the knee, hip, thumb (carpometacarpal), ankle, foot, and spine. The strongly inherited spur formation at the distal interphalangeal joint (Heberden nodes) and proximal interphalangeal joint (Bouchard nodes) is often classified as OA, yet, although deforming, only infrequently causes pain or disability (**Figure 24-1**).

Cartilage has no pain fibers, so the pain of OA arises from other tissues. Osteoarthritic pain is typically associated with movement, meaning that at rest the patient may be relatively asymptomatic. Patient's awareness that at rest the joint is less painful can be maladaptive. A protective role played by surrounding muscle of both a normal and arthritic joint is that of a shock-absorber. Well-maintained muscle can actually reduce mechanical stress on cartilage and bone. However, if a patient learns to favor the involved joint, disuse of supporting muscle groups may result in relative muscle weakness. Such weakness may decrease the shock-absorber effect, hastening joint damage. This mechanism also may lead to the complaint that a joint "gives way," resulting in dropped items (if at the wrist) or falls (if at the knee). In joints with mild OA, pain and instability may counterintuitively improve with exercise or activity.

Advanced OA is characterized by bony destruction and alteration of joint architecture. Secondary spur formation with deformity, instability, or restricted motion is a common finding. Fingers, wrists, knees, and ankles appear abnormal and asymmetric. Warmth and effusion are seen in joints with advanced OA. At this stage, pain may be exacerbated by any movement, weight-bearing or otherwise.

B. Laboratory Findings

There are few laboratory studies of relevance to the diagnosis of OA. Rarely, the erythrocyte sedimentation rate (ESR) will be raised, but only if an inflammatory effusion is present (and even then an elevated ESR or C-reactive protein is more likely to be misleading than helpful). If an effusion is present, arthrocentesis can be helpful in ruling out other conditions (see discussion of laboratory findings in gout, later).

Osteoarthritis can be secondary to other conditions, and these diseases have their own laboratory evaluation. Examples include OA secondary to hemochromatosis (elevated iron and ferritin, liver enzyme abnormalities), Wilson disease (elevated copper), acromegaly (elevated growth hormone), and Paget disease (elevated alkaline phosphatase).

C. Imaging Studies

Radiographs are seldom needed for the early diagnosis of OA. Indeed, radiographs may be misleading. Plain films of joints afflicted with OA may show changes of sclerosis, thickening, spur formation, loss of cartilage with narrowing of the joint space, and malalignment (**Figure 24-2**). Such radiographic changes typically occur late in the disease process. Patients may complain of significant pain despite a relatively normal

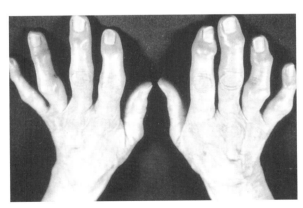

▲ **Figure 24-1.** Heberden nodes (distal interphalangeal joint) noted on all fingers and Bouchard nodes (proximal interphalangeal joint) noted on most fingers.

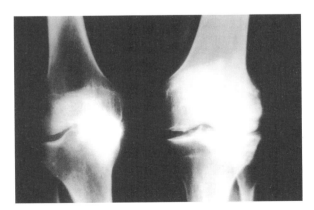

▲ **Figure 24-2.** Osteoarthritis of the knees showing loss of joint space with marked reactive sclerosis and probable malalignment.

appearance of the joint on plain films. Conversely, considerable radiographic damage may be seen with only modest symptoms. In addition, plain-film radiography does not provide useful information about cartilage, tendons, ligaments, or any soft tissue. Such findings may be crucial to explaining a patient complaint, especially if there is loss of function.

To see cartilage, ligaments, and tendons, magnetic resonance imaging (MRI) is important and, in many instances, essential. MRI can detect abnormalities of the meniscus or ligaments of the knee, cartilage, or femoral head deterioration at the hip; misalignment at the elbow; rupture of muscle and fascia at the shoulder; and a host of other abnormalities. Any of these findings may be incorrectly diagnosed as "OA" before MRI scanning.

Computed tomography (CT) and ultrasonography have lesser, more specialized uses. CT, especially with contrast, can detect structural abnormalities of large joints such as the knee or shoulder. Ultrasonography is an inexpensive means of detecting joint or periarticular fluid, or unusual collections of fluid such as a popliteal (Baker) cyst at the knee.

▶ Differential Diagnosis

In practice, it should not be difficult to differentiate among the three prototypical arthritides discussed in this chapter. **Table 24-1** suggests some key differential findings.

A common source of confusion and misdiagnosis occurs when a bursitis-tendinitis syndrome mimics the pain of OA. A common example is anserine bursitis. This bursitis, located medially at the tibial plateau, presents in a fashion similar to OA of the knee, but can be differentiated by a few simple questions and directed physical findings.

▶ Treatment

Typically, the early development of OA is silent. When pain occurs, and pain is almost always the presenting complaint,

the osteoarthritic process has already likely progressed to joint damage. Cartilage is damaged, bone reaction occurs, and debris mixes with synovial fluid. Consequently, when a diagnosis of OA is established, goals of therapy become control of pain, restoration of function, and reduction of disease progression. Although control of the patient's complaints is possible, and long periods of few or no symptoms may ensue, the patient permanently carries a diagnosis of OA.

Treatment of OA involves multiple modalities and is inadequate if only a prescription for anti-inflammatory drugs is written. Patient education, assessment for physical therapy and devices, and consideration of intraarticular injections are additional measures in the total management of the patient.

Hochberg MC, et al. American College of Rheumatology 2012 recommendations for the use of nonpharmacologic and pharmacologic therapies for osteoarthritis of the hand, hip and knee. *Arthritis Care Res.* 2012; 64(4):465.

A. Patient Education

Patient education is a crucial step. Patients must be made aware of the role they play in successful therapy. Many resources are available to assist the provider in patient education. Patient education pamphlets are widely available from government organizations, physician organizations (eg, American College of Rheumatology, American Academy of Family Physicians), insurance companies, pharmaceutical companies, or patient advocacy groups (eg, the Arthritis Foundation). Many communities have self-help or support groups that are rich sources of information, advice, and encouragement.

One of the most effective long-term measures to both improve symptoms and slow progression of disease is weight loss. Less weight carried by the hip, knee, ankle, or foot reduces stress on the involved arthritic joint, decreases the destructive processes, and probably slows progression of disease. Unfortunately, because of the pain and occasional limited

Table 24-1. Essentials of diagnosis.

	Osteoarthritis	Gout	Rheumatoid Arthritis
Key presenting symptoms	Pauciarticular; pain with movement, improving with rest; site of old injury (sport, trauma); obesity; occupation	Monoarticular; abrupt onset; pain at rest and movement; precipitating event (meal, physical stress); family history	Polyarticular; gradual, symmetric involvement; morning stiffness; hands and feet initially involved more than large joints; fatigue, poorly restorative sleep
Key physical findings	Infrequent warmth, effusion; crepitus; enlargement/spur formation; malalignment	Podagra; swelling, warmth; exquisite pain with movement; single joint (exceptions: plantar fascia, lumbar spine); tophi	Symmetric swelling, tenderness; MCP, MTP, wrist, ankle usually before larger, proximal joints; rheumatoid nodules
Key laboratory, x-ray findings	Few characteristic (early); loss of joint space, spur formation, malalignment (late)	Synovial fluid with uric acid crystals; elevated serum uric acid; 24-hour urine uric acid	Elevated ESR/CRP; rheumatoid factor; anemia of chronic disease; early erosions on x-ray, osteopenia at involved joints

CRP, C-reactive protein; ESR, erythrocyte sedimentation rate; MCP, metacarpophalangeal; MTP, metatarsophalangeal.

mobility of OA, exercise—an almost required component of weight loss regimens—is less likely to be utilized. On the other hand, exercise is a crucial modality that should not be overlooked. Evaluation for appropriate exercise focuses on two issues: overall fitness and correction of any joint-specific disuse atrophy. One must be flexible in the choice of exercise. Swimming is an excellent exercise that limits stress on the lower extremities. Many older persons are reluctant to learn to swim anew, yet they may be amenable to water aerobic exercises. These exercises encourage calorie expenditure, flexibility, and both upper and lower muscle strengthening in a supportive atmosphere. Stationary bicycle exercise is also accessible to most people, is easy to learn, and may be acceptable to those with arthritis of the hip, ankle, or foot. Advice from an occupational or recreational therapist can be most helpful.

B. Physical Therapy and Assistive Devices

The pain of OA can result in muscular disuse. The best example is quadriceps weakness resulting from OA of the knee. The patient who favors the involved joint loses quadriceps strength. This has two repercussions—both cushioning (shock-absorption) and stabilization are lost. The latter is usually the cause of the knee "giving way." Sudden buckling at the knee, often when descending stairs, is rarely due to the destruction of cartilage or bone but rather to inadequate strength in the quadriceps to handle the load required at the joint. Physical therapy with quadriceps strengthening is highly efficacious, resulting in improved mobility, increased patient confidence, and reduction in pain.

The physical therapist or physiatrist should also be consulted for advice regarding assistive devices. Advanced OA of lower extremity joints may cause instability and fear of falls that can be addressed by canes of various types. Altered posture or joint malalignment can be corrected by orthotics, which has the advantage, when used early, of slowing progression of OA. Braces can protect the truly unstable joint and permit continued ambulation.

Fransen M, et al. Land-based exercise for osteoarthritis of the knee: a metaanalysis of randomized controlled trials. *J Rheumatol.* 2009;36:1109.

C. Pharmacotherapy

The patient wants relief from pain. Despite the widespread promotion of nonsteroidal anti-inflammatory drugs (NSAIDs) for OA, there is no evidence that NSAIDs alter the course of the disease. Nevertheless, NSAIDs are used for their analgesic, rather than disease-modifying, effects. Although effective as analgesics, NSAIDs have significant side effects and are not necessarily first-line drugs.

Begin with adequate doses of acetaminophen. Acetaminophen should be prescribed in large doses, 3–4 g/d, and continued at this level until pain control is attained.

Once pain is controlled, dosage can be reduced if possible. Maintenance of adequate blood levels is essential and because acetaminophen has a relatively short half-life, frequent dosing is necessary (3 or 4 times a day). High doses of acetaminophen are generally well tolerated, although caution is important in patients with liver disease or in whom alcohol ingestion is heavy.

Administration of NSAIDs mixed as a cream or gel and rubbed onto joints has long been advocated for small- and even large-joint arthritis. There undoubtedly is less GI upset when delivered in this manner, but well-designed studies demonstrating prolonged effectiveness are lacking. There are two FDA-approved products on the US market (diclofenac, ketoprofen), although some compounding pharmacies apparently have more NSAIDs available.

Two main classes of NSAIDs are available, differentiated largely by half-life. NSAIDs with shorter half-lives (eg, diclofenac,, ibuprofen) need more frequent dosing than longer-acting agents (eg, naproxen, meloxicam). Several NSAIDs are available in generic or over-the-counter (OTC) form, which reduces cost. Despite differing pharmacology, there is little difference in efficacy, so a choice of medication should be based on individual patient issues such as dosing intervals, tolerance, toxicity, and cost. As with acetaminophen, adequate doses must be used for maximal effectiveness. For example, ibuprofen at doses of ≤800 mg 3 or 4 times a day should be maintained (if tolerated) before concluding that a different agent is necessary. Examples of NSAID dosing are given in **Table 24-2**.

Since such a major thrust of OA management is pain control, one must acknowledge the role played by narcotics. Narcotics should be confined to the patient with severe disease incompletely controlled by nonpharmacologic and nonnarcotic analgesics, and in whom joint replacement is not indicated. The narcotic medication should be additive to all other measures; for instance, full-dose acetaminophen or NSAIDs should be continued. The patient must be reminded of the fluctuating nature of OA symptoms and not expect complete elimination of pain. Once narcotics are started (in any patient for any cause), most generalist practices institute monitoring measures such as a "drug contract" or referral to a specialist pain management clinic.

Zhang W, et al. OARSI recommendations for the management of hip and knee arthritis, Part II: OARSI evidence-based, expert consensus guidelines. *Osteoarthr Cartilage.* 2008;16:137–162. [PMID: 18279766]

D. Intraarticular Injections

Hyaluronic acid (hyaluronan) is a constituent of both cartilage and synovial fluid. Injection of hyaluronic acid, usually in a series of several weekly intraarticular insertions, is purported to provide improvement in symptomatic OA for ≤6 months. It is unknown why hyaluronic acid helps; there is no

Table 24-2. Selected nonsteroidal anti-inflammatory drugs with usual and maximal doses.

Drug	Frequency of Administration	Usual Daily Dose (mg/d)	Maximal Dose (mg/d)
Oxaprozin (eg, Daypro)	Every day	1200	1800
Piroxicam (eg, Feldene)	Every day	10–20	20
Nabumetone (eg, Relafen)	1–2 times a day	1000–2000	2000
Sulindac (eg, Clinoril)	Twice a day	300–400	400
Naproxen (eg, Naprosyn)	Twice a day	500–1000	1500
Diclofenac (eg, Voltaren)	2–4 times a day	100–150	200
Ibuprofen (eg, Motrin)	3–4 times a day	600–1800	2400
Etodolac (eg, Lodine)	3–4 times a day	600–1200	1200
Ketoprofen (eg, Orudis)	3–4 times a day	150–300	300

evidence that hyaluronic acid is incorporated into cartilage, and it apparently does not slow the progression of OA. It is expensive, and the injection process is painful. Use of these agents (Synvisc, Artzal) is limited to patients who have failed other forms of OA therapy.

Intraarticular injection of corticosteroids has been both under- and overutilized in the past. There is little question that steroid injection rapidly reduces inflammation and eases symptoms. The best use is one in which the patient has an exacerbation of pain accompanied by signs of inflammation (warmth, effusion). The knee is most commonly implicated and is most easily approached. Most authorities recommend no more than two injections during one episode and limiting injections to no more than two or three episodes per year. Benefits of injection are often shorter in duration than similar injection for tendinitis or bursitis, but the symptomatic improvement buys time to reestablish therapy with oral agents, physical exercise, and assistive devices.

New therapeutic investigation and translational studies hold some promise for actual cartilage modification of damaged joints. Therapies involving strontium ranelate, platelet-rich plasma injections, and mesenchymal stem cells are currently in stages of development and may truly alter the otherwise somewhat relentless progression of this disease.

Arrich J. Intra-articular hyaluronic acid for the treatment of osteoarthritis of the knee: systematic review and meta-analysis. *Can Med Assoc J.* 2005;172:1039. [PMID: 15824412]

Reginster JY, et al. Efficacy and safety of strontium ranelate in the treatment of knee osteoarthritis: results of a double-blind, randomized placebo-controlled trial. *Ann Rheum Dis.* 2013;72:179.

E. Surgery

At one time, orthopedic surgeons performed arthroscopic surgery on osteoarthritic knees in an effort to remove accu-

mulated debris and to polish or débride frayed cartilage. However, a clinical trial using a sham-procedure methodology demonstrated that benefit from this practice could be explained by the placebo effect. Numbers of these procedures have reduced rather significantly, although there still remain some indications for performing this operation.

Joint replacement is a well-established option for treatment of OA, especially of the knee and hip. Pain is reduced or eliminated altogether. Mobility is improved, although infrequently to premorbid levels. Expenditures for total joint replacement have been increasing dramatically as the baby boomer generation reaches the age at which OA of large joints is more common. Indications for joint replacement (which also apply to other joints, including shoulder, elbow, and fingers) include pain poorly controlled with maximal therapy, malalignment, and decreased mobility. Improvement in pain relief and quality of life should be realized in ~90% of patients undergoing the procedure. Because complications of both the surgery and rehabilitation are increased by obesity, few orthopedic surgeons will consider hip or knee replacement without at least an attempt by the obese patient to lose weight. Patients need to be in adequate medical condition to undergo the operation and even more so to endure the often lengthy rehabilitation process. Some surgeons refer patients for "prehabilitation" or physical training prior to the operation. Counseling of patients should include the fact that there often is a 4–6-month recovery period involving intensive rehabilitation.

Moseley JB, et al. A controlled trial of arthroscopic surgery for osteoarthritis of the knee. *N Engl J Med.* 2002; 347:81. [PMID: 12110735]

F. Complementary and Alternative Therapies

Glucosamine, capsaicin, bee venom, acupuncture, and a host of other products have been promoted as alternative therapies for OA. Glucosamine and chondroitin sulfate are components of glycosaminoglycans, which make up cartilage; although some advocates might suggest otherwise, there is no evidence that orally ingested glucosamine or chondroitin sulfate is actually incorporated into cartilage. Studies suggest these agents are superior to placebo in symptomatic relief of mild OA. The onset of action is delayed, sometimes by weeks, but the effect may be prolonged after treatment is stopped. Glucosamine-chondroitin sulfate combinations are available over the counter and are generally well tolerated by patients.

Capsaicin, a topically applied extract of the chili pepper, relieves pain by depletion of substance P, a neuropeptide involved in pain sensation. Capsaicin is suggested for tendinitis or bursitis, but may be tried for OA of superficial joints such as the fingers. The cream should be applied 3 or 4 times a day for ≥2 weeks before reaching any conclusion regarding benefit.

Bee venom is promoted in complementary medicine circles. A mechanism for action in OA is unclear. Although anecdotal reports are available, comparison studies to other established treatments are difficult to find. Various vitamins (D, K) and minerals have been recommended for treatment of OA but are supported, if at all, by only poorly controlled studies.

Acupuncture can be useful in managing pain and improving function. There are more comparisons between acupuncture and conventional treatment for OA of the back and knee than for other joints. Generally, acupuncture is equivalent to oral treatments for mild symptoms at these two sites.

Prognosis

Restoring and rebuilding damaged cartilage is theoretically intriguing but not possible at this time. Investigations into regeneration of cartilage are proceeding as suggested earlier. Even so, reversal of the pathophysiologic process in OA is unlikely to be readily available anytime soon. With application of all modalities of treatment—adequate pain control, weight loss, appropriate exercise, orthotics and devices, and surgery—the successful management of osteoarthritis should be realized in most patients.

GOUT

ESSENTIALS OF DIAGNOSIS

▶ Podagra (intense inflammation of the first metatarsophalangeal joint).

▶ Inflammation of the overlying skin.

▶ Pain at rest and intense pain with movement.

▶ Swelling, warmth, redness, and effusion.

▶ Tophi (in long-established disease).

▶ Elevated serum uric acid level.

General Considerations

Gout, first described by Hippocrates in the fourth century BCE, has a colorful history, characterized as a disease of excesses, primarily gluttony. An association with diet is germane, as gout has a lower incidence in countries in which obesity is uncommon and the diet is relatively devoid of alcohol and reliance on meat and abdominal organs (liver, spleen). Gout is strongly hereditary as well, affecting as many as 25% of the men in some families.

Prevention

Despite the previously noted associations, it is difficult with any assurance to advise patients on measures to prevent gout. Even thin vegetarians develop gout, although at a markedly lower rate than obese, alcohol-drinking men. Gout has multiple etiologies, and no consistent preventive steps are available to patients.

Clinical Findings

A. Symptoms and Signs

Gout classically presents as an acute monoarthritis, perhaps best described by Thomas Sydenham in the seventeenth century. Podagra—abrupt, intense inflammation of the first metatarsophalangeal joint—remains the most common presentation (**Figure 24-3**). The first attack often occurs overnight, with intense pain awakening the patient. Any pressure, even a bed sheet on the toe, increases the agony. Walking is difficult. The overlying skin can be intensely inflamed. On questioning, an exacerbating event may be elicited. Common stories include an excess of alcohol, a heavy meal of abdominal organs, or a recent physiologic stress such as surgery or serious medical disease. Alcohol alters

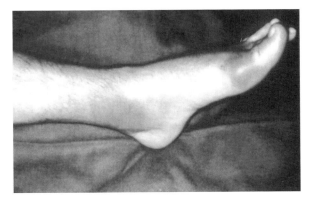

▲ **Figure 24-3.** Classic podagra involving the first metatarsophalangeal joint. In this photo, the ankle is also involved and the intense erythema could be mistaken for cellulitis.

Table 24-3. Inflammatory and noninflammatory causes of monoarthritis.

Inflammatory	Noninflammatory
Crystal-induced gout	Fracture or meniscal tear or other
Pseudogout (calcium pyrophosphate	trauma
deposition disease)	Osteoarthritis
Apatite (and others)	Tumors
Infectious	Osteochondroma
Bacteria	Osteoid osteoma
Fungi	Pigmented villonodular synovitis
Lyme disease or other spirochetes	Precancerous growths
Tuberculosis and other	Osteonecrosis
mycobacteria	Hemarthrosis
Viruses (eg, HIV, hepatitis B)	Cancers
Systemic diseases	
Psoriatic or other	
spondyloarthropathies	
Reactive (eg, inflammatory	
bowel, Reiter syndrome)	
Systemic lupus erythematosus	

Reproduced with permission from Schumacher HR. Signs and symptoms of musculoskeletal disorders. A Monoarticular joint disease. In: Klipper JH, ed. *Primer on the Rheumatic Diseases*, 11th ed. Arthritis Foundation, 1997:116.

renal excretion of uric acid, allowing rapid buildup of serum uric acid levels. Foods such as liver, sweetbread, anchovies, sardines, asparagus, salmon, and legumes contain relatively large quantities of purines that, when broken down, become uric acid.

Acute gout is not limited to the great toe; any joint may be affected, although lower extremity joints are more common. The abruptness of many gouty attacks and the single joint presentation (acute monoarthritis) at any joint other than the great toe may lead to diagnostic confusion (**Table 24-3**).

Gout in joints other than the great toe is often misdiagnosed. Atypical gout is not uncommon in older women and in men who have already experienced multiple previous episodes of podagra. Foot pain simulating plantar fasciitis is seen in older women. Gout of the ankle (with a positive Homans sign) can be mistaken for phlebitis.

The intense inflammation at some joints, especially smaller joints such as the ankle, can be impressive. The inflammation may appear to be spreading, encompassing an area greater than that assumed to be the joint. Such cases can be mistaken for cellulitis (see Figure 24-3) or superficial phlebitis. The subsequent lack of response to outpatient treatment of cellulitis can cascade to hospital admission and treatment with increasingly strong and expensive antibiotics.

Untreated, attacks of gout spontaneously resolve with the involved joint becoming progressively less symptomatic over 8–10 days. Longstanding gout is distinguished by the development of extraarticular manifestations. Tophi are deposits of urate crystals and are classically found as nodules in the ear helix or elsewhere; atypically placed tophi (eg, Heberden nodes, heart valves) serve as the source of colorful medical anecdotes. Chronic, untreated gout is a contributor to renal insufficiency (especially in association with heavy-metal lead exposure).

Physiologic stress is a common precipitating factor for an acute attack. Monoarthritis within days of a surgical procedure raises concern of infection (which it should!) but is just as likely due to crystal-induced gout or pseudogout. In some circumstances, prophylaxis in a person with known gout can prevent these attacks.

Approximately 10% of kidney stones include uric acid. A person with nephrolithiasis due to uric acid stones need not have attacks of gout, but patients with gout are at increased risk of developing uric acid stones. A prior history of nephrolithiasis is an important factor in choosing therapy in the patient with gout.

Gout is largely a disease of men, with a male-to-female ratio of 9:1. The first attack of podagra typically occurs in men in their 30s or 40s. One attack need not necessarily predict future attacks. In fact, in ≤20% of men who have one attack of gout, a second attack never follows. Even after a second attack, a sizable percentage (as many as 5%) do not progress to chronic, recurrent gout.

Premenopausal women rarely have gout; indeed, confirmed gout in a young woman might raise the question of an inborn error of metabolism. Diagnosis of gout in postmenopausal women is infrequent, less because it does not occur than because it is unsuspected. Gout is also more likely to have an atypical presentation in joints other than the great toe in women. A high index of suspicion must be practiced.

B. Laboratory Findings

The fundamental abnormality in gout is excess uric acid. In most first attacks of gout, serum uric acid is elevated. In longstanding disease, the uric acid value may be within the normal range yet symptoms still occur. It is important to note, however, that mild hyperuricemia has a rather high prevalence in the general population. Indeed, fewer than 25% of persons with elevated uric acid will ever have gout.

During acute attacks of gout, the white blood cell count may be slightly elevated and ESR increased, reflecting acute inflammation. Gout is not uncommon in chronic kidney disease, and measurement of blood urea nitrogen and creatinine is recommended following a first gout attack.

Gout usually results from either inappropriately low renal excretion of uric acid (implicated in 90% of patients) or abnormally high endogenous production of uric acid. Collecting a 24-hour urine sample for the evaluation of uric acid and creatinine clearance can be useful in therapy (discussed as follows).

A strong recommendation must be made to attempt arthrocentesis of the joint in suspected acute gout.

Table 24-4. Synovial fluid analysis in selected rheumatic diseases.

Disease	Fluid	WBC Count (in Fluid)	Differential	Glucose	Crystals
Gout	Clear/cloudy	10–100,000	>50% PMNs	Normal	Needle-shaped, negative birefringement
Pseudogout	Clear/cloudy	10–100,000	>50% PMNs	Normal	Rhomboid-shaped, positive birefringement
Infectious	Cloudy	>50,000	Often >95% PMNs	Decreased	None[a]
Osteoarthritis	Clear	2–10,000	<50% PMNs	Normal	None[a]
Rheumatoid arthritis	Clear	10–50,000	>50% PMNs	Normal or decreased	None[a]

[a]Debris in synovial fluid may be misleading on plain microscopy but only crystals respond to polarizing light.
PMNs, polymorphonuclear leukocytes; WBC, white blood cells.

First episodes of gout present as an acute monoarthritis, for which the differential diagnosis is noted in Table 24-3. Infectious arthritis is a medical emergency—the correct diagnosis must be made rapidly and appropriate antibiotic therapy begun to avoid destructive changes. Pseudogout is rarely distinguished from gout on the basis of symptoms alone. The settings of both pseudogout and gout can be similar (eg, immediately after surgery). Clinical features of many of the monoarthritides are not characteristic enough to ensure a correct diagnosis. However, finding negatively birefringent needle-shaped crystals in synovial fluid is diagnostic of gout. Features of synovial fluid in selected disease settings are highlighted in **Table 24-4**.

C. Imaging Studies

Radiographs are not needed for the diagnosis of gout. Other means of diagnosing gout (eg, arthrocentesis) are more useful. Characteristic erosions occur with longstanding gout but are rarely seen in first attacks.

▶ Differential Diagnosis

The first attack of gout must be distinguished from an acute monoarthritis. A review of Tables 24-1 and 24-3 is relevant.

▶ Treatment

The inflammation of acute gout is effectively managed with anti-inflammatory medications. Once recognized, most cases of gout can be controlled within days, occasionally within hours. Remaining as a challenge is the decision regarding long-term treatment.

Standard therapy for acute gout is a short course of NSAIDs at adequate levels. As one of the first NSAIDs developed, indomethacin (50 mg 3 or 4 times a day) is occasionally assumed to be somehow unique in the treatment of gout. In fact, all NSAIDs are probably equally effective, although many practitioners feel that response is faster with short-acting agents such as naproxen (375–500 mg 3 times a day) or ibuprofen (800 mg 3 or 4 times a day). Pain often decreases on the first day, with treatment indicated for not much more than 3–5 days.

A classic medication for acute gout is colchicine. Typically given orally, the instructions to the patient can sound bizarre. The drug is prescribed every 1–2 hours "until relief of pain or uncontrollable diarrhea." Most attacks actually respond to the first two or three pills, with a maximum of six pills in 24 hours as a prudent upper limit. Most patients develop diarrhea well before the sixth pill. Colchicine is then dosed 3 times daily and, as with NSAIDs, is seldom needed after 3–5 days. Unfortunately, in the United States, colchicine (which has been used for hundreds of years for gout) is no longer generic. It now can only be obtained as a branded product and is significantly more expensive than generic colchicine used to be.

On occasion, corticosteroids are used in acute gout. Oral prednisone (eg, ≥60 mg), methylprednisolone or triamcinolone (eg, 40–80 mg) intramuscularly, or intraarticular agents can be used. Indications include intense overlying skin involvement (mimicking cellulitis), polyarticular presentation of gout, and contraindication to NSAID or colchicine therapy. Intraarticular steroid use may be considered for ankle or knee gout, if infection is ruled out.

Decisions regarding long-term treatment of gout must factor in the natural history of attacks. The first attack, especially in young men with a clear precipitating event (such as an alcohol binge), may not be followed by a second attack for years, even decades. As stated earlier, as many as 20% of men will never have a second gouty attack. Data from the Framingham longitudinal study suggest that intervals of ≤12 years are common between first and second attacks. This is not always the case for young women with gout (who tend to have a uric acid metabolic abnormality) or for either men or women who have polyarticular gout.

But for many young men, a reasonable recommendation after a first episode is to watch expectantly but not necessarily to treat with uric acid–lowering drugs.

The physician and patient may even decide to withhold prophylactic medication after a second attack, but when episodes of gout become more frequent than one or two a year, both physician and patient are usually ready to consider long-term medication. The primary medications used at this point are probenecid and the xanthine oxidase inhibitors allopurinol and febuxostat (a recently marketed drug). Probenecid is a uric acid tubular reuptake inhibitor, which results in increased excretion of uric acid in the urine. Allopurinol and febuxostat inhibit the uric acid synthesis pathway, blocking the step at which xanthine is converted to uric acid. Xanthine is much more soluble than uric acid and is not implicated in acute arthritis, nephrolithiasis, or renal insufficiency.

Until recently, guidelines recommended obtaining 24-hour uric acid excretion levels. The patient found to have low excretion of uric acid (<600 mg/d) and normal renal function was often prescribed probenecid. Probenecid loses effectiveness when the creatinine clearance falls below 50 mL/min, so alternative therapy was necessary in patients with chronic kidney disease. If the patient had uric acid nephrolithiasis, probenecid was contraindicated to avoid increased delivery of uric acid to the stone-forming region.

Recent guidelines from the American College of Rheumatology have modified this approach. These guidelines now suggest that initial therapy can begin with a xanthine oxidase inhibitor, obviating the need to measure 24 hour uric acid excretion. The guidelines recommend treating to a serum uric acid level of ≤6 g/dL. If this goal cannot be reached with xanthine oxidase inhibitors alone (an infrequent occurrence), probenecid might then be added. This newer modification recognizes that both allopurinol and febuxostat are well tolerated with infrequent toxic side effects. An important difference, though, is that allopurinol is usually dosed lower in chronic kidney disease because of the potential for adverse effects while febuxostat does not seem to have such dosing requirements.

Xanthine oxidase inhibitors are especially indicated for treatment of tophaceous gout and for uric acid nephrolithiasis. These agents also are drugs of choice for those with uric acid metabolic abnormalities (often young women) and polyarticular gout. Caution must be used, however, when starting any uric acid–lowering drug for the first time. Rapid lowering of the serum uric acid causes instability of uric acid crystals within the synovial fluid and can actually precipitate an attack of gout. Consequently, prior establishment of either NSAID or colchicine therapy is recommended to obviate this complication.

Patients are occasionally seen who have been prescribed long-term therapy with colchicine. There is some conceptual attraction to this choice. Between attacks of gout (the "intercritical period"), examination of synovial fluid continues to show uric acid crystals. Using colchicine to prevent the spiral to inflammation seems to make sense. But this choice is deceptive. Colchicine does nothing to lower uric acid levels. Long-term use allows deposition of uric acid into destructive tophi or contributes to renal disease and kidney stones. Colchicine can be an effective prophylactic agent, however, if started prior to a surgical procedure in a patient with known gout who is not using allopurinol or probenecid. But use of this drug as a solo agent courts significant complications.

Prognosis

Gouty attacks can be both effectively treated and prevented. A clear diagnosis is important, and arthrocentesis is essential. Management is relatively straightforward, and no patient should have to endure tophi or repeated acute attacks.

Kanna D, et al. American College of Rheumatology guidelines for management of gout. Part 1: systemic nonpharmacologic and pharmacologic therapeutic approaches to hyperuricemia. *Arthritis Care Res.* 2012;64:1431.

Kanna D, et al. American College of Rheumatology guidelines for management of gout. Part 2: therapy and anti-inflammatory prophylaxis of acute gouty arthritis. *Arthritis Care Res.* 2012;64:1447.

RHEUMATOID ARTHRITIS

 ESSENTIALS OF DIAGNOSIS

▸ Arthritis of three or more joint areas.

▸ Arthritis in hands, feet, or both (bilateral joint involvement).

▸ Morning stiffness.

▸ Fatigue.

▸ Swelling, tenderness, warmth, and loss of function.

▸ Rheumatoid nodules.

▸ Elevated ESR and C-reactive protein.

▸ Positive test for rheumatoid factor.

General Considerations

Bony changes consistent with rheumatoid arthritis (RA) have been found in the body of a Native American who lived 3000 years ago. Differentiation of RA from other types of arthritis is more recent, delineated only in the late nineteenth century. RA is more frequently seen in women, with the ratio of premenopausal women to age-matched men approximately 4:1; after the age of menopause, the ratio of incident RA is closer to 1:1.

Pathogenesis

Although the etiology of RA is not known, the pathophysiology has been elucidated to a remarkable degree in recent decades. Important knowledge of all inflammatory processes has come from studies in RA. Early in the disease process, the synovium of joints is targeted by T cells (this is the feature that leads to the "autoimmune" moniker). Release of interleukins, lymphokines, cytokines, tissue necrosis factor, and other messengers attracts additional inflammatory cells to the synovium. Intense inflammation ensues, experienced by the patient as pain, warmth, swelling, and loss of function. Reactive cells move to the inflammatory synovium, attempting to repair damaged tissue. Without treatment, this intense reaction develops into the pathologic tissue called *pannus*, an exuberant growth of tissue engulfing the joint space and causing destruction itself. Cartilage becomes swept into the pathologic process, resulting in breakdown, deterioration, and eventual destruction. Periarticular bone responds to inflammation with resorption, seen as erosions on radiographs. All these changes clearly are maladaptive and responsible for deformity and disability.

Prevention

It is difficult with any assurance to advise patients on measures to prevent arthritis. RA has multiple etiologies, and no consistent preventive steps are available to patients. However, it is noted that RA may be more likely to occur in smokers, under the assumption that reaction in the trachea involving citrulline proteins promotes an inflammatory response to those proteins and that inflammatory response spills over to the synovium. While RA occurs in different frequencies in different ethnic groups, there are genetic similarities in each ethnic group that may differ from genetic patterns in other groups, pointing to the multiplicity of possible etiologies.

Clinical Findings

A. Symptoms and Signs

Rheumatoid arthritis is a systemic disease always involving joints but with inflammatory responses that include fatigue, rash, nodules, and even clinical depression as joints become increasingly stiff and inflamed. Most, but by no means all, of the initial symptoms are in the joints. There is inflammation, so the presence of swelling, warmth, and loss of function is imperative to the diagnosis. Joints of the hands (**Figure 24-4**) and feet are typically affected first, although larger joints can be involved at any time. The disease is classically symmetric with symptoms present bilaterally in hands, feet, or both. This mirroring is almost unique to RA; systemic lupus erythematosus, which is often confused with RA in its early stages, is not so consistently symmetric.

Fingers and wrists are stiff and sore in the mornings, requiring heat, rubbing, and movement to be functional

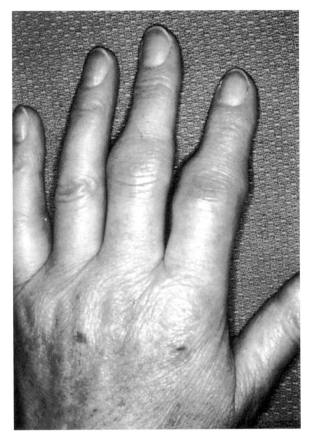

▲ **Figure 24-4.** Swelling of the proximal interphalangeal joints of the second and third fingers in rheumatoid arthritis. Symmetric swelling might be expected on the other hand.

("morning stiffness"). Stiffness after prolonged lack of movement ("gelling") is not uncommon in many joint disorders, but the morning stiffness of RA is so prolonged and characteristic that queries regarding this symptom are essential to the diagnosis.

The patient reports fatigue out of proportion to lack of sleep. Daytime naps are almost unavoidable, yet are not fully restorative. Anorexia, weight loss, or even low-grade fever, can be present. Along with musculoskeletal complaints, these somatic concerns may lead to mistaken diagnoses of fibromyalgia or even depression.

Rheumatoid arthritis can eventually involve almost any joint in the body. Selected important manifestations of RA in specific joints are listed in **Table 24-5**. The cause of any one manifestation may be unique to a particular joint and the surrounding periarticular structure. Common features include inflammation-induced stretching of tendons and

Table 24-5. Manifestations of rheumatoid arthritis in specific joints.

Joint	Complication
Hand	Ulnar deviation (hand points toward ulnar side), Swan neck deformity (extension of PIP joint), Boutonniere deformity (flexion at DIP)
Wrist	Swelling causing carpal tunnel syndrome
Elbow	Swelling causing compressive neuropathy Deformity preventing complete extension, loss of power
Shoulder	"Frozen shoulder" (loss of abduction, nighttime pain)
Neck	Subluxation of C_1-C_2 joint with danger of dislocation and spinal cord compression ("hangman's injury")
Foot	"Cockup" deformity and/or subluxation at MTP
Knee	Effusion leading to Baker cyst (evagination of synovial lining and fluid into popliteal space)

DIP, distal interphalangeal; MTP, metatarsophalangeal; PIP, proximal interphalangeal.

ligaments resulting in joint laxity, subconscious restriction of movement resulting in "frozen" joints, and consequences of inflammatory synovitis with cartilage destruction and periarticular bone erosion. An objective sign of destruction includes the high-pitched, "crunchy" sound of crepitus.

Extraarticular manifestations of RA can be seen at any stage of disease. Most common are rheumatoid nodules, found at some point in ≤50% of all patients with RA. These occur almost anywhere in the body, especially along pressure points (the typical olecranon site), along tendons, or in bursae. Vasculitis is an uncommon initial presentation of RA. Dry eyes and mouth are seen in the RA-associated sicca syndrome. Dyspnea, cough, or even chest pain may signal respiratory interstitial disease. Cardiac, gastrointestinal, and renal involvement in RA is not common. Peripheral nervous system symptoms are seen as compression neuropathies (eg, carpal or tarsal tunnel syndrome) and reflect not so much direct attack on nerves, but rather primarily as consequences of squeezing compression as nerves are forced into passages narrowed by nearby inflammation.

B. Laboratory Findings

In contrast to OA, the laboratory findings in RA can be significant and helpful. A normocytic anemia is common in active RA. This anemia is almost always the so-called anemia of chronic disease. The white blood cell count is normal or even slightly elevated; an exception is the rare Felty syndrome (leukopenia and splenomegaly in a patient with known RA).

Rheumatoid arthritis does not typically affect electrolytes and renal function. There is no pathophysiologic reason why transaminases, bilirubin, alkaline phosphatase, or other liver, pancreatic, or bone enzymes should be altered. Similarly, calcium, magnesium, and phosphate values should be unchanged. Most hormone measurements are normal, particularly thyroid and the adrenal axis. Any chronic inflammatory disease may alter the menstrual cycle, but measurement of luteinizing hormone and follicle-stimulating hormone is of little help.

An elevated ESR is almost ubiquitous in RA. C-reactive protein (CRP) is considered by many rheumatologists to be a more sensitive indicator of inflammation and might be increased in settings in which the ESR is either "normal" or minimally elevated. Although ESR is quite reliable, in some circumstances a false value may be reported (**Table 24-6**). For this reason, evaluation of C-reactive protein, although more expensive, is increasingly used by specialists.

The test most associated with RA is the rheumatoid factor (RF) blood test. RF is actually a family of antibodies, the most common of which is an immunoglobulin M (IgM) antibody directed against the Fc (fragment, crystallizable) portion of immunoglobulin G (IgG). There is no question this antibody is frequently present in RA, with RF-negative RA accounting for only ~5% of all patients with RA. The problem lies with the low specificity of the test. Surveys demonstrate that in a young population, 3–5% of "normal" individuals have a high RF titer (positive test) whereas in an older cohort the prevalence of positive RF reaches 25%. With the national prevalence of RA only 1%, it is clear that many people with an elevated RF titer do not have RA. In fact, a false-positive RF titer is a common reason for incorrect referral of patients to rheumatologists. Some of the conditions that are associated with a positive RF test are listed in **Table 24-7**.

Another frequent test useful for diagnosis of RA in the early stages is the anticyclic citrullinated peptide [anti-CCP; also called *anticitrullinated protein/peptide antibody* (ACPA)]. This test is positive in most patients with RA, and may precede the onset of clinically diagnosed RA by months or even years. When combined with the RF test, this test will confirm the diagnosis even in confusing settings.

Suarez-Almazor ME, et al. Utilization and predictive value of laboratory tests in patients referred to rheumatologists by primary care physicians. *J Rheumatol.* 1998;25:1980. [PMID: 9779854]

C. Imaging Studies

Radiographs are no longer needed for the initial diagnosis of rheumatoid arthritis. Other means of diagnosing RA are more useful. Nonetheless, RA is a disease of synovial tissue, and, because the synovium lies on and attaches to bone, inflammation can cause changes on plain film radiography. Small erosions, or lucencies, on the lateral portions of

Table 24-6. Nondisease factors that influence the ESR.

Increase ESR	Decrease ESR	No Effect on ESR
Aging	Leukocytosis (>25,000)	Obesity
Female	Polycythemia (Hgb >18)	Body temperature
Pregnancy	Red blood cell changes	
Anemia	Sickle cell	Recent meal
Macrocytosis	Anisocytosis	Aspirin
Congenital hyperfibrinogenemia	Microcytosis	NSAID
	Acanthocytosis	
Technical factors	Protein abnormalities	
Dilutional	Dysproteinemia with hyperviscosity	
Elevated specimen temperature	Hypofibrinogenemia	
	Hypogammaglobulinemia	
	Technical factors	
	Dilutional	
	Inadequate mixing	
	Vibration during test	
	Clotting of specimen	

ESR, erythrocyte sedimentation rate; Hgb, hemoglobin; NSAID, nonsteroidal anti-inflammatory drug.
Reproduced with permission from Brigden ML. Clinical utility of the erythrocyte sedimentation rate. Am Fam Physician 1999;60:1443.

phalanges are early indications of significant inflammation and should prompt immediate suppressive treatment.

Computed tomography and/or MRI have limited but useful supporting roles. An undesired complication of treatment of RA, aseptic necrosis (eg, of the femoral head), has a characteristic appearance on MRI. Scintigraphy is useful in detecting aseptic necrosis but, along with MRI, is better employed to differentiate the intense synovitis of RA from infection such as septic arthritis, overlying cellulitis, or adjacent osteomyelitis.

▶ **Differential Diagnosis**

In practice, it is should not be difficult to differentiate among the three prototypical arthritides discussed in this chapter (see Table 24-1). Relatively new (2010) criteria developed by subspecialty organizations give valuable guidelines to making an accurate diagnosis of RA (**Table 24-8**). Because treatment started early is generally successful, rheumatologists promote early referral—treating a new diagnosis of RA almost as a "medical emergency."

Table 24-7. Conditions associated with a positive rheumatoid factor test.

Normal aging
Chronic bacterial infections
  Subacute bacterial endocarditis
  Tuberculosis
  Lyme disease
  Others
Viral disease
  Cytomegalovirus
  Epstein-Barr virus
  Hepatitis B
Chronic inflammatory diseases
  Sarcoidosis
  Periodontal disease
  Chronic liver disease (especially viral)
  Sjögren syndrome
  Systemic lupus erythematosus
  Mixed cryoglobulinemia

Table 24-8. 1987 American College of Rheumatology diagnostic criteria for rheumatoid arthritis.

The diagnosis of rheumatoid arthritis is confirmed if the patient has had at least four of the seven following criteria, with criteria 1–6 present for ≥6 weeks:
1. Morning stiffness (≥1 hour)
2. Arthritis of three or more joint areas (areas are right or left of proximal interphalangeal joints, metacarpophalangeal, wrist, elbow, knee, ankle, and metatarsophalangeal)
3. Arthritis of hand joints (proximal interphalangeal joints or metacarpophalangeal joints)
4. Symmetric arthritis, by area
5. Subcutaneous rheumatoid nodules
6. Positive test for rheumatoid factor
7. Radiographic changes (hand and wrist radiography showing erosion of joints or unequivocal demineralization around joints)

Data from Arnett FC, et al. The American Rheumatism Association 1987 revised criteria for the classification of rheumatoid arthritis. *Arthritis Rheum.* 1988; 31:315.

Moreland LW, Bridges SL Jr. Early rheumatoid arthritis: a medical emergency? *Am J Med.* 2001;111:498. [PMID: 11690579]

Neil VP, et al. Benefit of very early referral and very early therapy with disease-modifying anti-rheumatic drugs in patients with early rheumatoid arthritis. *Rheumatology.* 2004;43:906.

► Complications

Serious extraarticular manifestations of RA are not infrequent. Some of these are life-threatening and require sophisticated management by physicians experienced in dealing with these crises. The responsibility often remains with the primary care physician to recognize these conditions and refer the patient appropriately. **Table 24-9** lists several of these complications with a brief description of the clinical presentation.

► Treatment

Therapy of RA has changed from managing inflammation to specific measures directed against the fundamental sources of the inflammation. In more recent decades, treatment of RA has undergone perhaps the most wholesale shift of any of the rheumatologic conditions. Therapy is now directed at fundamental processes and begins with aggressive, potentially toxic disease-modifying drugs. The outlook can be hopeful, with preservation of joints, activity, and lifestyle a realistic goal. RA need no longer be the "deforming arthritis" by which it was known just a short time ago.

Kremers HM, et al. Therapeutic strategies in rheumatoid arthritis over a 40-year period. *J Rheumatol.* 2004;31:2366. [PMID: 15570636]

A. Assessment of Prognostic Factors

One of the early steps in treating RA is to assess prognostic factors in the individual patient. Poor prognosis leads to the decision to start aggressive treatment earlier. Some prognostic features are demographic, such as female sex, age >50 years, low socioeconomic status, and a first-degree relative with RA. Clinical features associated with poor prognosis include a large number of affected joints, especially involvement of the flexor tendons of the wrist, with persistence of swelling at the fingers; rheumatoid nodules; high ESR or C-reactive protein and high titers of RF; presence of erosions on radiographs; and evidence of functional disability. Formal functional testing and disease activity questionnaires are frequently employed, not only in establishing stage of disease but also at interval visits. In practice, though, most rheumatologists urge their generalist colleagues to refer patients identified with new-onset RA early. Despite certain prognostic factors noted earlier, most patients are indicated for, and respond to, early therapeutic intervention.

Table 24-9. Extraarticular manifestations of rheumatoid arthritis.

Complication	Brief Comments
Rheumatoid nodules	Found over pressure points, classically olecranon; typically fade with disease-modifying antirheumatic drug (DMARD) therapy; also may be found in internal organs; if causing disability, may attempt intralesional steroids, or surgery
Popliteal cyst	Usually asymptomatic unless ruptures, then mimics calf thrombophlebitis; ultrasonography (and high index of suspicion) useful
Anemia	Usually "chronic disease" and, despite low measured iron, does not respond to oral iron therapy; improves with control of inflammatory disease
Scleritis/episcleritis	Inflammatory lesion of conjunctiva; more prolonged, intense, and uncomfortable than "simple" conjunctivitis; requires ophthalmologic management
Pulmonary disease	Ranges from simple pleuritis and pleural effusion (noted for low glucose) to severe bronchiolitis, interstitial fibrosis, nodulosis, and pulmonary vasculitis; may require high-dose steroid therapy once diagnosis established by bronchoscopy or even open-lung biopsy
Sjögren syndrome	Often occurring with RA, includes sicca syndrome with thickened respiratory secretions, dysphagia, vaginal atrophy, hyperglobulinemia, and distal renal tubule defects; treatment of sicca syndrome possible with muscarinic-receptor agonists; other manifestations more difficult
Felty syndrome	Constellation of RA, leukopenia, splenomegaly, and often anemia, thrombocytopenia; control underlying RA with DMARDs; may need granulocyte colony-stimulating factor, especially if infectious complications are frequent
Rheumatoid vasculitis	Spectrum from digital arteritis (with hemorrhage) to cutaneous ulceration to mononeuritis multiplex to severe, life-threatening multisystem arteritis involving heart, gastrointestinal tract, and other organs; resembles polyarteritis nodosum

Anderson J, et al. Rheumatoid arthritis disease activity measures: American College of Rheumatology recommendations for use in clinical practice. *Arthritis Care Res.* 2012;64:640.

B. Patient Education

Therapy begins with patient education, and again there are multiple sources of information from support and advocacy groups, professional organizations, government sources, and pharmaceutical companies. Patients should learn about the natural history of RA and the therapies available to interrupt the course. They should learn about joint protection and the likelihood that at least some activities need to be modified or discontinued. RA, especially before disease modification is established, is a fatiguing disorder. Patients should realize that rest is as important as appropriate types of activity. Of vital importance is the patient's acknowledgment that drug regimens about to be started are complex but that compliance is critical to successful outcomes. The patient should frankly be told that the drugs are toxic and may have adverse effects.

C. Pharmacotherapy

1. Pain relief—Pain in RA is caused by inflammation, and establishment of effective anti-inflammatory drugs is the first goal of RA intervention. This is a step often expected of generalist physicians if there is likely to be delay in referral of the newly diagnosed RA patient to the rheumatologist. NSAIDs, at doses recommended earlier (see Table 24-2), give the patient early relief. NSAIDs continue to be used throughout the course of treatment; it is not uncommon to switch from one to another as effectiveness falters. It should be noted, though, that NSAIDs will not alter the course of the disease, and the patient should not be deluded into thinking that early pain relief substitutes for comprehensive treatment.

However, the effective management of RA should limit uncontrolled pain. Indeed, the goal of any RA management is to find therapies that will limit pain. Consequently, both generalist and specialist physicians to the patient with RA should continuously seek treatment modifications rather than settle for a degree of uncontrolled pain that might prompt use of narcotics.

2. Complementary and alternative medicine—If the patient is reluctant to start drugs, fish oil supplementation may provide symptomatic relief. But the same caution mentioned earlier for pain relief applies to complementary and alternative therapies—these products do not alter the natural history of RA. Even with some degree of pain relief and anti-inflammatory efficacy, these products are no substitute for effective treatment.

Nevertheless, physicians regularly are asked for recommendations of alternative treatments. Both omega-3 and omega-6 fatty acids in fish oil modulate synthesis of highly inflammatory prostaglandin E_2 and leukotriene E_4. The fish oil chosen must contain high concentrations of the relevant fatty acids. A large number of capsules need to be taken, and palatability, diarrhea, and halitosis are frequent adverse effects. γ-linolenic acid interrupts the pathway of arachidonic acid, another component of the inflammatory cascades. Extracted from the oils of plant seeds such as linseed, sunflower seed, and flaxseed, γ-linolenic acid demonstrates some efficacy in short-term studies using large doses of the extract.

3. Anti-inflammatory medications—Rheumatoid arthritis is an inflammatory disease, and all treatments are directed, in one way or another, to the reduction or elimination of the inflammatory process. Patients with RA will be taking one form of anti-inflammatory medication throughout the course of the disease.

As noted earlier, NSAIDs, are almost continuously recommended, even with other effective treatments established. It is common to switch from one drug to another as efficacy wanes. It is important to modify use of NSAIDs if well-identified effects are noted. GI upset, even GI bleeding, is common; this may be ameliorated as well by use of H2-blockers such as ranitidine or proton-pump inhibitors such as omeprazole. NSAID use should be modified, if not discontinued, in advancing stages of chronic kidney disease.

Steroids are widely used in RA. Relatively high-dose oral or parenteral use of steroids can reduce inflammation in the early stages of RA or at times of RA flare. Certain manifestations of RA, such as vasculitis or pulmonary involvement, will require steroids for more prolonged periods of time. The use of steroids for intraarticular injection into symptomatic joints can enhance systemic anti-inflammatory medications. The well-known complications of high-dose steroids requires that these be used only for short periods of time if at all possible

Sulfasalazine, noted to have efficacy for RA although patients were being treated for another condition, is frequently used early in treatment of RA. The mechanism of action is not exactly anti-inflammatory, but the effect is. Similarly, another antibiotic, minocycline, seems to have anti-inflammatory effects presumably through inhibition of a metalloproteinease mechanism.

4. Disease-modifying antirheumatic drugs (DMARDs)—These agents are almost always the first line of intensive therapy for patients newly diagnosed with rheumatoid arthritis. Fortunately, a large number of patients can be maintained in disease remission with use of medications in this category. Depending on the classification used to describe RA therapy, there may be a limited number of DMARD agents available, or some of these may be used in combination with agents described under anti-inflammatories earlier. Nonetheless, almost all patients with RA will be prescribed agents in this class at some time during their therapy.

The prototypical DMARD agent is methotrexate. Methotrexate is effective at decreasing inflammation, lowering ESR, slowing bony erosions, and reducing destructive pannus. For most patients, there will be regular modification of the dose in an attempt to find the lowest effective dose. Methotrexate is generally given in weekly doses with beneficial results seen as early as 4–6 weeks. Treatment can be continued for years. Toxicity includes liver and hematologic changes and regular monitoring is essential. Other adverse effects are not infrequent and may require modification of dose.

Azathioprine and cyclosporine are occasionally used as DMARDs, although rarely concurrently with methotrexate. Complications from these drugs are well recognized, and patient counseling should be extensive before use. One use for these agents appears to be during therapy for complications such as vasculitis. Another antibiotic, the antimalarial drug hydroxychloroquine, is often given in conjunction with methotrexate. There is a rare, but unfortunate, adverse effect to the retina seen with use of hydroxychloroquine that requires periodic ophthalmologic visits. Leflunomide blocks protein synthesis by lymphocytes and has been shown to be almost as effective as methotrexate. However, its half-life is almost 2 weeks and liver toxicity is not infrequent. Also, leflunomide has been associated with birth defects, making effective contraception mandatory when used in women of reproductive age.

5. Tissue necrosis factor (TNF) inhibitors—Tissue necrosis factor is a messenger that attracts other inflammatory cells to a site. TNF is also involved in production of interferon and interleukins. Blockade of these TNF effects diminishes the inflammatory response, both decreasing patient symptoms and slowing disease progression. Etanercept, infliximab, and adalimumab are examples of frequently used TNF inhibitors in treatment of RA. Other TNF inhibitors are available and occasionally used in very specific circumstances. These drugs require subcutaneous or intravenous injection, as often as every other week. Yet, they are relatively well tolerated, and any hematologic toxicity responds to discontinuation. Although TNF inhibitors carry FDA indication for moderate to severe RA, they are often given with methotrexate or even as single agents.

A serious consideration relates to the role of TNF inhibitors in host defenses. In particular, patients on TNF inhibitors who have tuberculosis often have rapid extrapulmonary spread and poor response to treatment. Consequently, assurance of the absence of TB, either by the PPD test or even the blood-based test QuantiFERON, is indicated.

6. Interleukin (IL)-inhibitors—Currently at least two IL-inhibitors are used in conjunction with other modalities in treatment of RA. IL6-inhibitor (tocilizumab) and IL1-inhibitor (anakinra) block different steps in both immune response and acute-phase response. Both inhibitors can be used with methotrexate for added disease-modifying activity. Side effects are not uncommon, ranging from local injection inflammation to leukopenia, liver enzyme abnormalities, and even alterations in lipids. Also, interleukin inhibitors should not be used with TNF inhibitors as infectious complications are increased.

7. T cell blockade—Continuing the effort to block parts of the immune and/or inflammatory response, the T cell blocker abatacept functions by arresting activation of naïve T cells. When used in conjunction with other DMARDs, there can be a moderate improvement in response criteria

in a significant number of patients. This agent does carry an increased risk of infection. In addition, perhaps because of suppressed immune surveillance, there is concern for increased risk of neoplasia.

8. B cell depletion—The biologic agent rituximab is widely used in treatment of B cell lymphoma and has also been demonstrated to have efficacy in RA similar to that of abatacept. Rituximab works by blocking a signaling molecule from mature B cells, resulting in the depletion of B cells. Reduction of B cells reduces the inflammatory response in the synovium of the patient with RA. This agent, along with abatacept, may be used in patients with a poor response to TNF inhibitors.

9. Drug administration and precautions—While many of the anti-inflammatory and DMARD medications can be taken orally, most of the TNF inhibitors, the interleukin inhibitors, and the T and B cell blockers must be given either by injection (subcutaneous) or intravenous infusion. Since the frequency of administration, even once stabilized, ranges from weekly to monthly, it is clear that the patient will have frequent office visits to the rheumatologist. Unfortunately, local or systemic reaction to these agents is frequent and may require coadministration of other drugs (often steroids) to ameliorate the reactions.

As noted earlier, a frequent concern in use of biologics is increased infection. Patients are routinely tested for subclinical tuberculosis infection and are strongly advised to remain up-to-date with immunizations, including influenza and pneumococcal vaccines. A concern also alluded to above is the possibility of increased occurrence of neoplasm. Since the purpose of most of these products is to suppress the immune/inflammatory response, the very real concern is that neoplasia surveillance mechanisms are also suppressed. To date, while tumors have been reported during use of these agents, there does not seem to be a significant increase in incidence.

Singh JA, et al. 2012 Update of the 2008 American College of Rheumatology recommendations for the use of disease-modifying antirheumatic drugs and biologic agents in the treatment of rheumatoid arthritis. *Arthritis Care Res*. 2012;64:625.

Smolen JS, et al. EULAR recommendations for the management of rheumatoid arthritis with synthetic and biological disease-modifying antirheumatic drugs. *Ann Rheum Dis*. 2010;69:964.

D. Surgery

Joint instability and resultant disability are often due to a combination of joint destruction, a primary effect of synovial inflammation, and tendon or ligament laxity, a secondary effect or "innocent bystander." The innocent bystander effect notes that these connective tissues are stretched, weakened, or malaligned as a result of inflammation of the joints over which they cross but not the result of a direct attack on the tendon or ligament itself. Nonetheless, at some point joint destruction and connective tissue laxity combine to produce useless, and frequently painful, joints. At this point, the surgeon has much to offer. Joint stabilization, connective tissue reinsertion, and joint replacement of both small (interphalangeal) and large (hip, knee) joints provide return of function and reduction of pain. The timing of surgery is still an art and is most effective when close collaboration exists between the treating physician and surgeon.

Prognosis

Morbidity and mortality are increased in patients with RA over age-matched persons without RA. Correlated with active disease, there is a well-described increase in stroke and myocardial infarction. These manifestations may be due to a hypercoagulable state induced by the autoimmune process and circulating antibodies. There are suggestions that the increased rate of stroke and MI may be reduced by effective DMARD therapy. Even so, it is recommended that appropriate cardiovascular interventions be considered (eg, aspirin, lipid management). Even under conscientious treatment, complications from infection, pulmonary and renal disease, and gastrointestinal bleeding occur at rates higher than those in the general population. Many of the latter complications are related as much to the drugs used to control the disease as to the disease itself.

Myasoedova E, et al. Cardiovascular disease in rheumatoid arthritis: a step forward. *Curr Opin Rheumatol*. 2010;22:342.

Websites

American Academy of Family Physicians (Family Doctor-designed for patient information more than the academy website): www.familydoctor.org (accessed Feb., 2013).

American College of Physicians (for physicians; little of relevance for patients–nothing on OA, gout, or RA readily found–and much that requires sign-in by members): www.acponline.org (accessed Feb., 2013).

American College of Rheumatology (a section for patients, "Patient Resources," with appropriately written information is available without sign-in): www.rheumatology.org (accessed Feb., 2013).

Arthritis Foundation (user-friendly information for patients, written without medical jargon, somewhat superficial, strong community support): www.arthritis.org (accessed Feb., 2013).

National Center for Complementary and Alternative Medicine (NIH) (for physicians and patients; easy to use; comprehensive; balanced information on conventional and alternative treatments): www.nccam.nih.gov (accessed Feb., 2013).

National Guideline Clearinghouse (for physicians; functions as a search engine for guidelines on subject desired; links to publications, some of which require sign-in; comprehensive and international): www.guideline.gov (accessed Feb., 2013).

National Institute for Arthritis and Musculoskeletal and Skin Diseases (NIH) (for physicians and sophisticated patients; relatively easy to use; comprehensive, though technical, information): www.niams.nih.gov (accessed Feb., 2013).

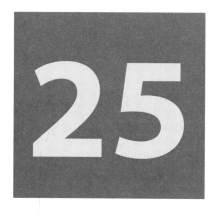

25

Low Back Pain in Primary Care: An Evidence-Based Approach

Charles W. Webb, DO

Francis G. O'Connor, MD, MPH

General Considerations

Low back pain (LBP), discomfort, tension, or stiffness below the costal margin and above the inferior gluteal folds, is one of the most common conditions encountered in primary care as an acute self-limited problem, second only to the common cold. LBP has an annual incidence of 5%, and a lifetime prevalence of 60–90%. It is the leading cause of disability in the United States for adults aged <45 years, is a leading cause of non–battle injury air evacuation from recent military deployments, and is responsible for one-third of workers' compensation costs and accounts for direct and indirect of nearly $90 billion per year. At any given time 1% of the US population is chronically disabled and another 1% temporarily disabled as a result of back pain. Numerous studies report a favorable natural history for acute and subacute LBP, with <90% of patients regaining function within 6–12 weeks with or without physician intervention. Recent evidence suggests that about one in five acute LBP patients will have persistent back pain resulting in limitations in activity at 1 year. Approximately 85% of back pain has no readily identifiable cause, and up to one-third of all patients will develop chronic low back pain. This chapter reviews a detailed evidence-based approach to the assessment, diagnosis, and management of the adult patient with acute, subacute, and chronic LBP.

Casazza BA. Diagnosis and treatment of acute low back pain. *Am Fam Physician.* 2012;85(4):343–350.

Dagenais S, Caro J, Haldeman S. A systematic review of low back pain cost of illness studies in the United States and internationally. *Spine J.* 2008;8:8–20.

Fourney DR, Andersson G, Arnold PM, et al. Chronic low back pain. *Spine.* 2011;36:S1–S9.

Goertz M, Thorson D, Bonsell J, et al. Institute for Clinical Systems Improvement: *Adult Acute and Subacute Low Back Pain*; updated Nov. 2012 (available at https://www.icsi.org/_asset/bjvqrj/LBP.pdf).

Hauret KG, Taylor BJ, Clemmons NS, et al. Frequency and causes of nonbattle injuries air evacuated from operations Iraqi freedom and enduring freedom, U.S. Army, 2001–2006. *Am J Prevent Med.* 2010; 38:S94–S107. [PMID: 20117605]

Last AR, Hulbert K. Chronic low back pain: evaluation and management. *Am Fam Physician.* 2009; 79(12):1067–1074.

Prevention

Low back pain is a heavy medical and financial burden to not only the patients who are experiencing the ailment but also society. The US Preventive Services Task Force produced a recommendation statement on primary care interventions to prevent low back pain in adults stating that currently there is insufficient evidence to support or rebuke the routine use of exercise to prevent low back pain. However, regular physical activity has been shown to be beneficial in the treatment and the limitation of recurrent episodes of chronic low back pain. Lumbar supports (back belts) and shoe inserts (orthotics) have not been found effective in the prevention of low back pain. Worksite interventions, including education on lifting techniques, have been shown to have some short-term effects, on decreasing lost time from work for patients with back pain.

Risk factor modifications may be the only way to truly prevent LBP. These risk factors can be classified as individual, psychosocial, occupational, and anatomic. **Table 25-1** lists the prominent risk factors for LBP.

Casazza BA. Diagnosis and treatment of acute low back pain. *Am Fam Physician.* 2012;85(4):343–350.

Dagenais S, Caro J, Haldeman S. A systematic review of low back pain cost of illness studies in the United States and internationally. *Spine J.* 2008;8:8–20.

Fourney DR, Andersson G, Arnold PM, et al. Chronic low back pain. *Spine.* 2011;36:S1–S9.

Last AR, Hulbert K. Chronic low back pain: evaluation and management. *Am Fam Physician.* 2009; 79(12):1067–1074.

Table 25-1. Risk Factors associated with LBP

Unchangeable Risk Factors	
Individual	**Anatomic**
Increasing age Birth defects of the spine High birth weight	Degenerative disk disease
Male gender	Osteoarthritis
Family history	Synovial cyst formation
Previous back injury	Lumbosacral transitional vertebra
Pregnancy	Schmorl nodes
History of spine surgery	Annular disruption
High birth weight	Spondylolysis Spondylolithesis History of birth defects (eg, spina bifida)

Modifiable Risk Factors			
Individual	**Psychosocial**	**Occupational**	**Others**
Sedentary lifestyle	Stress	Unemployment	Poor pain tolerance
Smoking	Depression	Perceived inadequate income	History of recurrent back pain
Overweight or obese	Decreased cognition	Monotonous tasks	Presence of sciatic
Poor posture and biomechanics	Somatization	Long periods of sitting or standing	Corticosteroid use
Education level	Fear/avoidance behaviors	Heavy lifting	Chronic illness that causes chronic cough (eg, COPD)
Poor general health	History of anxiety	Repetitive twisting, bending, squatting, pushing, pulling	Participation in strenuous or contact sports
	Neurotic personality disorder	Constant vibration Lack of recognition at work Poor job satisfaction Poor relations with employer, supervisor, and coworkers Low job control High pressure on time Unavailability of light duty Belief that job is dangerous for the lower back	

Lillios S, Young J. The effects of core and lower extremity strengthening on pregnancy-related low back and pelvic girdle pain: a systematic review. *J Women's Health Phys. Therapy.* 2012; 36(3):116–124.

Sahar T, Cohen MJ, Uval-Ne'eman V, et al. Insoles for prevention and treatment of back pain. *Spine.* 2009; 34(9):924–933.

Stoyer J, Jensen LD. The role of physical fitness as risk indicator of increased low back pain intensity among people working with physically and mentally disabled persons: a 30-month prospective study. *Spine.* 2008; 33(5):546–554.

▶ Clinical Findings

The key elements in the correct diagnosis and management of the issues surrounding the causes of LBP include an evaluation for serious health problems, screening for red and yellow flags (**Tables 25-2** and **25-3**), symptom control for acute and subacute LBP, and follow-up evaluation of patients whose condition worsen or fails to improve. The first step is the accurate and timely identification of clinical conditions for which low back pain is a symptom.

Table 25-2. Red flags and appropriate actions.

Condition	Red Flag	Action
Cancer	History of cancer Unexplained weight loss Age ≥50 years Failure to improve with therapy Pain ≥4–6 weeks; night/rest pain	If malignant disease of the spine is suspected, imaging is indicated and CBC and ESR should be considered Identification of possible primary malignancy should be investigated, eg, PSA, mammogram, UPEP/SPEP/IPEP
Infection	Fever History of intravenous drug use Recent bacterial infection: UTI, skin, pneumonia Immunocompromised states (steroid, organ transplants, diabetes, HIV) Rest pain	If infection in the spine is suspected, MRI, CBC, ESR and/or UA are indicated
Cauda equina syndrome	Urinary retention or incontinence Saddle anesthesia Anosphincter tone decrease/fecal incontinence Bilateral lower extremity weakness/numbness or progressive neurologic deficit	Request immediate surgical consultation
Fracture	Use of corticosteroids Age ≥70 or history of osteoporosis; recent significant trauma	Appropriate imaging and surgical consultation
Acute abdominal aneurysm	Abdominal pulsating mass Other atherosclerotic vascular disease; rest/night pain; age ≥ 60 years	Appropriate imaging (ultrasound) and surgical consultation
Significant herniated nucleus pulposus (HNP)	Major muscle weakness	Appropriate imaging and surgical consultation

CBC, complete blood count; ESR, erythrocyte sedimentation rate; HIV, human immunodeficiency virus; IBEP, immunoprotein electrophoresis; MRI, magnetic resonance imaging; PSA, prostate-specific antigen; SPEP, serum protein electrophoresis; UA, urinalysis; UPEP, urine protein electrophoresis; UTI, urinary tract infection.

A. Symptoms and Signs

A careful medical history and physical examination are critical in determining the presence of a more serious condition in the patient presenting with acute LBP. On examining the patient, the primary care provider must look for "red and yellow flags" that indicate the presence of a significant medical or psychological condition. If any red flags are identified, patients requiring emergent or urgent care should be given immediate consultation or referral to the appropriate specialist. Nonemergent patients with red flags should be scheduled for the appropriate diagnostic test to determine whether they have a condition that requires a referral. If any yellow flags are identified, this signifies the presence of psychological distress and strongly correlates to chronicity and poor patient outcomes in both pain control and disability. When yellow flags are identified early, an interdisciplinary approach should be considered.

1. History—The history should focus on the location of the pain, the mechanism of injury (to ascertain what the patient was doing when he/she first noticed the pain, whether it was insidious or whether there was a specific trauma or inciting activity), the character (mechanical, radicular, caludicant, or nonspecific), and duration of the pain (acute, <6 weeks; subacute, between 6 and 12 weeks; or chronic, >12 weeks). The provider must identify neurologic symptoms (bowel/bladder symptoms, weakness in the extremities, saddle anesthesia) suggestive of cauda equina syndrome (CES; a true neurosurgical emergency). The functional status of the patient should be noted as should any exacerbating or ameliorating factors. The presence of fever, weight loss, and night pain are particularly concerning as these could indicate a more serious disease, such as an underlying malignancy. The social history should include information about drug use/abuse, intravenous (IV) drug use, tobacco use, any physical demands at work, and the presence of psychosocial stressors. Past medical and surgical history should also be obtained, particularly a history of previous spinal surgery or immunosuppression (history of cancer, steroid use, HIV). A thorough history enables the primary care provider to identify

Table 25-3. Yellow flags in low back pain.

Attitudes and Beliefs	Comorbid Conditions
Fear/avoidance	Lack of or decreased sleep
Fear of movement, use of excessive rest	History of other disabling injuries or conditions
Catastrophizing	Lack of financial incentive to return to work
Excessive focus on pain	Pending litigation
Feeling out of control	Overprotective family
Passivity toward rehabilitation	
Affective factors	Waddell signs
Poor work history	Pain with axial loading of spine
Poor compliance with rehabilitation	Superficial tenderness to palpation (light touch)
Withdrawal from activities (ADLs, social)	Overreaction (pain out of proportion to physical findings)
History of substance abuse (self-medicating)	Straight leg raise test improves with distraction
Depression	Regional weakness
Anxiety	
Irritability	
History of psychological or physical abuse	
History of irregular or episodic physical activity	
Conflicting diagnosis from different providers	
Multiple medical providers	

any red and/or yellow flags that require a more extensive workup to rule out a potentially serious and disabling disease processes.

2. Physical examination—The physical examination supplements the information obtained in the history by helping to identify underlying serious medical conditions or possible serious neurologic compromise. The primary elements of the physical examination are inspection, palpation, observation (including range-of-motion testing), and a specialized neuromuscular evaluation. The examination should start with an evaluation of the spinal curvature and lumbar range of motion, specifically noting the amount of pain-free movement. Palpation should include the paraspinal muscles, the spinous processes, the sacroiliac joints, the piriformis muscles, and the position of the pelvic bones. Because the lumbar spine is kinetically linked to the pelvis (particularly the sacroiliac area), pain from the pelvis is often referred to the lumbar spine. Hip flexors and hamstring flexibility should also be assessed as a potential cause for the pain. The Waddell signs, which describe five physical signs (tenderness, simulation, distraction, regional numbness, and overreaction), are clinically useful in the identification of patients who have physical findings without a specific anatomic cause that would benefit from surgical intervention. If three or more of these tests are positive, psychological overlay

might be present, and this should be assessed with the yellow flags described earlier.

3. Neurologic evaluation—The neurologic evaluation should include Achilles (S_1) and patellar tendon (L_2-L_4) reflex testing, ankle and great toe dorsiflexion (L_4-L_5), and plantarflexion (S_1) strength, as well as the location of sensory complaints (dermatomes involved). Light touch testing for sensation in the medial (L_4), dorsal (L_5), and lateral (S_1) aspects of the foot should also be performed. In patients presenting with acute LBP and no specific limb complaints, a more elaborate neurologic examination is seldom necessary. A seated and supine straight leg raise test (SLR) evaluates for nerve root impingement. This abbreviated neurologic evaluation of the lower extremity allows detection of clinically significant nerve root compromise at the L_4-L_5 or L_5-S_1 levels. These two sites represent >90% of all significant radiculopathy secondary to lumbar disk herniation. Because this abbreviated examination may fail to diagnose some of the less common causes of LBP, any patient who has not improved in 4–6 weeks should return for further evaluation.

4. Risk stratification—All patients with acute LBP should be risk-stratified with an initial assessment attempting to identify red flags: responses or findings in the history and physical examination that indicate a potentially serious underlying condition, such as a fracture, tumor, infections, abdominal aneurysm, or CES that can lead to considerable patient morbidity and/or mortality. These clinical clues (red flags) include a history of major trauma, minor trauma in patients > 50 years, persistent fever, history of cancer, metabolic disorder, major muscle weakness, bladder or bowel dysfunction, saddle anesthesia, decreased sphincter tone, and unrelenting night pain. Red flags risk stratify the patient to an increased risk and should prompt an earlier clinical action, such as imaging or laboratory workup. See Table 25-2 for a listing of red flags and their related conditions.

Psychosocial factors also significantly affect pain and function in LBP patients. These psychosocial factors are known as "yellow flags" and are better predictors of treatment outcomes than physical factors in some patients. These yellow flags are listed in Table 25-3.

Casazza BA. Diagnosis and treatment of acute low back pain. *Am Fam Physician.* 2012;85(4):343–350. [PMID: 22335313]

Chapman R, Norvell C, Hermsmeyer T, et al. Evaluating common outcomes for measuring treatment success for chronic low back pain. *Spine.* 2011;36:S54–S68. [PMID: 21952190]

Chou R, et al. Diagnosis and treatment of low back pain: a joint practice guideline from the American College of Physicians and the American Pain Society [published correction appears in *Ann Intern Med.* 2008;148(3):247–248]. *Ann Intern Med.* 2007;147:478–491. [PMID: 17909209]

Fisher CG, Vaccaro AR, Mulpuri K, et al. Evidence-based recommendations for spine surgery. *Spine.* 2012;37(1):E3–E9. [PMID: 22751143]

Fourney DR, Andersson G, Arnold PM, et al. Chronic low back pain. *Spine.* 2011;36:S1–S9. [PMID: 21952181]

Goertz M, Thorson D, Bonsell J, et al. Institute for Clinical Systems Improvement. *Adult Acute and Subacute Low Back Pain*; updated Nov. 2012 (available at https://www.icsi.org/_asset/bjvqrj/LBP.pdf).

Last AR, Hulbert K, Chronic low back pain: evaluation and management. *Am Fam Physician.* 2009;79(12):1067–1074. [PMID: 19530637]

Sembrano JN, Reiley MA, Polly DW, et al. Diagnosis and treatment of sacroiliac joint pain. *Curr Orthop Practice.* 2011;22(4):344–350.

Waddell G, McCulloch JA, Kummel E, et al. Nonorganic physical signs in low back pain. *Spine.* 1980;5(2):117–125. [PMID: 6446157]

B. Imaging Studies

Diagnostic imaging is rarely indicated in the acute setting of LBP. Even though some studies have indicated greater patient satisfaction with lumbar radiography, the evidence demonstrates that it may not lead to greater improvement in outcomes. After the first 4–6 weeks of symptoms, the majority of patients will have regained function. However, if the patient is still limited by back symptoms, diagnostic imaging should be considered to look for conditions that present as low back pain. Patients for whom diagnostic imaging should be considered include children, patients aged >50 years with new-onset back pain, trauma patients, or patients for whom back pain fails to improve despite appropriate conservative treatment. Imaging studies must always be interpreted carefully since disk degeneration and protrusion has been noted in 20–25% of asymptomatic individuals. Therefore abnormal findings on diagnostic imaging may or may not represent the reason for the patient's pain.

Plain films remain the most widely available modality for imaging the lumbar spine and are rarely useful in evaluating or guiding treatment of adults with acute LBP in the absence of red flags. Plain lumbar x-rays are helpful in detecting spinal fractures, and evaluating tumor and/or infection. Anteroposterior (AP) and lateral views allow assessment of lumbar alignment, the intervertebral disc space, bone density, and a limited evaluation of the soft tissue. Oblique views should be used only when spondylolysis is suspected as they double the radiation exposure and add only minimal information. Sacroiliac views are used to evaluate ankylosing spondylitis, and again should be used only when this is suspected.

When the history or physical examination suggests an anatomic abnormality as a cause for the back pain with neurologic deficits, four imaging studies are commonly used: (1) plain myelography, (2) computed tomography (CT) scan, (3) magnetic resonance imaging (MRI) scan, and (4) CT myelography. These four tests are used in similar clinical situations and provide similar information. The objective of these studies is to define a medically or surgically remediable anatomic condition. These tests are not done routinely, and should be used only for patients who present with certain clinical findings, such as persistent radicular symptoms and clinically detectable nerve root compressive symptoms and signs (radiculopathy) severe enough to consider surgical intervention (major muscle weakness, progressive motor deficit, intractable pain, and persistent radicular pain beyond 6 weeks). For a listing of these and other special tests and tier indications and recommendations, see **Table 25-4**.

Diagnostic imaging plays a central role in diagnosing spinal infections. Plain films should be obtained but are often helpful only in the advanced stages of the infection. MRI is the imaging modality of choice in evaluating spinal infection.

Table 25-4. Special tests and indications/recommendations.

Special Test	Indications/Recommendations
Plain x-ray	Not recommended for routine evaluation of acute LBP unless red flags present Recommended for ruling out fractures Obliques are only recommended when findings are suggestive of spondylolisthesis or spondyloysis
Electrophysiological tests (EMG and SPEP)	Questionable nerve root dysfunction with leg symptoms ≥6 weeks Not recommended if radiculopathy is obvious
MRI or CT-myelography	Back-related leg symptoms and clinically detectable nerve root compromise History of neurogenic claudication suspicious for spinal stenosis Findings suggesting CES, fracture, infection, tumor
ESR	Suspected tumors, infection, inflammatory conditions, metabolic disorders
CBC	Suspected tumors, myelogenous conditions, infections
UA	Suspected UTI, pylonephritis, myeloma
IPEP	Suspected multiple myeloma
Chemistry profile to include TSH, calcium, and alkaline phosphatase	Suspected electrolyte disorders, thyroid dysfunction, metabolic dysfunction
Bone scan	Suspected occult pars interarticularis fracture, or metastatic disease Contraindicated in pregnant patient

CBC, complete blood count; CES, cauda equina syndrome; CT, computed tomography; EMG, electromyelogram; ESR, erythrocyte sedimentation rate; IPEP, immunoprotein electrophoresis; LBP, low back pain; MRI, magnetic resonance imaging; SPEP, serum protein electrophoresis; TSH, thyroid-stimulating hormone; UA, urinalysis; UTI, urinary tract infection.

When infection is identified or suspected, a spinal surgeon should be consulted immediately.

Casazza BA. Diagnosis and treatment of acute low back pain. *Am Fam Physician.* 2012;85(4):343–350.

Chapman R, Norvell C, Hermsmeyer T, et al. Evaluating common outcomes for measuring treatment success for chronic low back pain. *Spine.* 2011;36:S54–S68.

Chou R, et al. Diagnosis and treatment of low back pain: a joint practice guideline from the American College of Physicians and the American Pain Society [published correction appears in *Ann Intern Med.* 2008;148(3):247–248]. *Ann Intern Med.* 2007;147:478–491.

Fisher CG, Vaccaro AR, Mulpuri K, et al. Evidence-based recommendations for spine surgery. *Spine.* 2012;37(1):E3–E9.

Fourney DR, Andersson G, Arnold PM, et al. Chronic low back pain. *Spine.* 2011;36:S1–S9.

Goertz M, Thorson D, Bonsell J, et al. Institute for Clinical Systems Improvement: *Adult Acute and Subacute Low Back Pain*; updated Nov. 2012 (available at https://www.icsi.org/_asset/bjvqrj/LBP.pdf).

Sembrano JN, Reiley MA, Polly DW, et al. Diagnosis and treatment of sacroiliac joint pain. *Curr Orthop Practice.* 2011;22(4):344–350.

C. Laboratory Testing

Laboratory testing should be reserved for patients who seem to have conditions masquerading as simple LBP such as cancer or infection (**Table 25-5**). Laboratory tests that are recommended in the evaluating patients with a suspicious history for cancer include a complete blood count (CBC) with differential, and an erythrocyte sedimentation rate (ESR). An ESR of >50 mm/h is suggestive of malignancy, infection, or inflammatory disease. Blood urea nitrogen (BUN), creatinine (Cr), and urinalysis (UA) are helpful for identifying underlying renal or urinary tract disease. Serum calcium, phosphorus, and alkaline phosphatase should be checked in patients with osteopenia, osteolytic vertebral lesions, or vertebral body collapse. If prostate carcinoma is suspected, prostate-specific antigen and acid phosphatase levels should be checked. If multiple myeloma is suspected, a serum immunoelectrophoresis can help guide treatment.

Historical red flags such as IV drug abuse and immunocompromise, as well as fever, should raise concern for an underlying infection. An elevated white blood cell count (WBC) is a clue to an underlying infection, but can be within normal limits even in acute infection. The ESR and C-reactive protein (CRP) can be used to monitor the efficacy of treatment of spinal infections. Urinalysis and urine culture should be obtained because urinary tract infection (UTI) often precedes spinal infection. Blood cultures should be obtained as well. Although they are usually negative, positive cultures identify the infecting organism and provide antibiotic sensitivity to guide treatment.

Casazza BA. Diagnosis and treatment of acute low back pain. *Am Fam Physician.* 2012;85(4):343–350.

Table 25-5. Differential diagnosis of lower back pain.

System	Conditions
Vascular	Expanding aortic aneurysm
Gastrointestinal	Pancreatitis Peptic ulcers Cholecystitis Colonic cancer
Genitourinary	Endometriosis Tubal pregnancy Kidney stones Prostatitis Chronic pelvic inflammatory disease Perinephric abscess Pylonephritis
Endocrinologicmetabolic	Osteoporosis Osteomalacia Hyperparathyroidism Paget disease Acromegaly Cushing disease Ochronosis
Hematologic	Hemoglobinopathy Mylofibrosis Mastocytosis
Rheumatologic/inflammatory	Spondyloarthropathies Ankylosing spondylitis Reiter syndrome Psoriatic arthritis Enteropathic arthritis Bechet syndrome Familial mediterranean fever Whipple disease Diffuse idiopathic skeletal hyperostosis
Psychogenic	Affective disorder Conversion disorder Somatization disorder Malingering
Infection	Osteomyelitis Epidural/paraspinal abscess Disk space infection Pyogenic sacroiliitis
Neoplastic	Skeletal metastases Spinal cord tumors Leukemia Lymphoma Retroperitoneal tumors Primary lumbosacral tumors 　　Benign 　　Malignant
Miscellaneous	Sarcoidosis Subacute endocarditis Retroperitoneal fibrosis Herpes zoster Fat herniation of lumbar space Spinal stenosis

Chou R, et al. Diagnosis and treatment of low back pain: a joint practice guideline from the American College of Physicians and the American Pain Society [published correction appears in *Ann Intern Med*. 2008;148(3):247–248]. *Ann Intern Med*. 2007;147:478–491.

Fourney DR, Andersson G, Arnold PM, et al. Chronic low back pain. *Spine*. 2011;36:S1–S9.

Goertz M, Thorson D, Bonsell J, et al. Institute for Clinical Systems Improvement, *Adult Acute and Subacute Low Back Pain*; updated Nov. 2012 (available at https://www.icsi.org/_asset/bjvqrj/LBP.pdf).

▶ Differential Diagnosis

After potential red flags have been ruled out, the differential diagnosis for LBP remains extensive. Table 25-5 presents a list of conditions that can present as simple LBP.

▶ Treatment

If the patient has no red flags and the history and physical examination do not suggest an underlying cause, the diagnosis of mechanical LBP can be made, and treatment may be initiated. The patient should be reassured with a discussion of the natural history of mechanical low back pain, and treatment should then focus on pain control and improving individual function. Methods of symptom control should focus on providing comfort and keeping the patient as active as possible while awaiting spontaneous recovery. Evidence for the most common treatments currently used in the primary care setting is presented as follows. Depending on the patient, this treatment may include activity modification, bed rest (of short duration), conservative medications, progressive range of motion and exercise, manipulative treatment, and patient education. This line of treatment should be used for 4–6 weeks before ordering additional diagnostic test unless the history and physical examination identify a more concerning diagnosis.

A. Patient Education

Patient education is the cornerstone of effective treatment of LBP. Patients who present to the primary care clinic with acute LBP should be educated about expectations for recovery and the potential recurrence of symptoms. Management of patients' expectations of therapy and educating them about the management goals is an effective way to decrease apprehension and promote a quick recovery. Management goals focus on decreasing pain and improving overall function of the patient. Patients should be informed of safe and reasonable activity modifications, and be given information on how to limit the recurrence of low back problems through proper lifting techniques, treatment of obesity, and tobacco cessation. If medications are used, patients should be given information on their use and the potential side effects. Patients should be instructed to follow up in 1–3 weeks if they fail to improve with conservative treatment, develop bowel or bladder dysfunction, or experience worsening neurologic function.

B. Activity Modification

Patients with acute LBP may be more comfortable if they are able to temporarily limit or avoid specific activities that are known to increase mechanical stress on the spine. Prolonged unsupported sitting and heavy lifting, especially while bending or twisting, should be avoided. Activity recommendations for the employed patient with acute LBP should consider the patient's age, general health, and the physical demands of the job.

C. Bed Rest

A gradual return to normal activities is more effective than prolonged bed rest for the treatment of LBP. Bed rest for >4 days may lead to debilitating muscle atrophy and increased stiffness and therefore is not recommended. Most patients with acute or subacute LBP will not require bed rest. For patients with severe initial symptoms, however, limited bed rest for 2–4 days remains an option.

D. Medications

Oral medications [acetaminophen, nonsteroidal anti-inflammatory drugs (NSAIDs), muscle relaxants, and opioids] and injection treatments are available for the treatment of LBP. Most patients with chronic low back pain will self-medicate with an over-the-counter (OTC) pain relievers (acetaminophen and ibuprofen). Also, most are prescribed at least one medication to control pain and improve function. Currently there is good evidence supporting the use of NSAIDs and skeletal muscle relaxants for the management of acute LBP, but these agents are less effective when used as monotherapy. NSAIDs have both anti-inflammatory and analgesic properties, and are widely used for all kinds of LBP. However, they can cause gastrointestinal (GI), renal, and hepatic side effects, and have been linked to increased risk of cardiovascular events. Therefore all of these medications should be used with caution and at the lowest possible dose for the shortest duration. Because opioids are only slightly more effective in relieving low back symptoms than other analgesics (aspirin, acetaminophen), and because of their potential for other complications (dependence), opioid analgesics, if used, should be used only over a time-limited course. Oral corticosteroids are not recommended for the treatment of acute LBP.

There is limited evidence supporting the use of homeopathic and herbal remedies, such as devil's claw, willow bark, and capsicum for the treatment of acute episodes of chronic LBP.

Injection therapy for the treatment of low back symptoms includes acute pain management; trigger point; ligamentous, sclerosant, and facet joint; and epidural injections. Injections are an invasive treatment option that exposes patients to potentially serious complications. No conclusive studies have proved the efficacy of trigger point, sclerosant, ligamentous, or facet joint injections in the treatment of acute LBP. However, epidural and facet joint injections may benefit patients who fail conservative treatment as a means of avoiding surgery. A series of one to three epidural steroid injections may be beneficial for patients who have radiculopathy that has not improved after 4–6 weeks of conservative therapy.

E. Spinal Manipulation

There is some evidence supporting the use of manipulative therapy in the treatment of acute LBP. Spinal manipulation techniques attempt to restore joint and soft-tissue range of motion. Impaired motion of synovial joints has a detrimental effect on joint cartilage and vertebral disk metabolism leading to degenerative spinal changes. Manipulation is useful early after symptom onset for patients who have acute LBP without radiculopathy. If the patient's physical findings suggest progressive or severe neurologic deficit, aggressive manipulation should be postponed pending an appropriate diagnostic assessment.

F. Physical Agents and Modalities

Physical agents include ice and moist heat treatments. There is good evidence to support the use of superficial heat for muscle relaxation and analgesia. The evidence supporting cyrotherapy is limited at best. Self-administrated home programs using moist heat and cold are often used.

Transcutaneous electrical nerve stimulation (TENS) is thought to modify pain perception by counterstimulation of the nervous system. Currently there is insufficient evidence on the efficacy of the TENS to recommend its routine use.

Shoe insoles (or inserts) can vary from OTC foam, rubber inserts to custom orthotics. These devices aim to reduce back pain due to leg length discrepancies, or abnormal foot mechanics. There is limited evidence that shoe orthotics (either OTC or custom-made) may provide short-term benefit for patients with mild back pain, although there is no evidence supporting their long-term use or their use in prevention of back pain. The role of leg length discrepancies in LBP has not been established, and differences of <2 cm are unlikely to produce symptoms.

Lumbar support devices for low back problems include corsets, support belts, various types of braces, and molded jackets, and back rests for chairs and car seats. Lumbar corsets and support belts may be beneficial in preventing low back pain and time lost from work for individuals whose jobs require frequent lifting; however, the evidence is lacking. There is some recent evidence that lumbar belts in the setting of subacute low back pain can increase functional status and decrease both pain and medication use. Lumbar corsets have not been shown to be beneficial in the treatment of LBP.

A randomized control trial found that mattresses of medium firmness are beneficial in reducing pain symptoms and disability in patients with chronic low back pain.

Acupuncture and other dry needling techniques have not been found to be beneficial for treating acute or subacute LBP patients. However, recent evidence does suggest that traditional Chinese medical acupuncture and therapeutic massage is beneficial in the treatment of chronic low back pain. Acupuncture, when added to conventional therapies, improves function, sleep, and pain better than conventional therapy alone, and decreases medication use.

G. Exercise

Therapeutic exercises should be started early to control pain, avoid deconditioning, and restore function. Intensive therapeutic exercise can help decrease pain and improve function in patients with chronic LBP. No single treatment or exercise program has proved effective for all patients with LBP. Poor endurance and abnormal firing of the hip muscles have been noted in patients with both acute and chronic LBP. Various studies have shown that the occurrence of LBP may be reduced by strengthening the back, legs, and abdomen (core muscle groups) and by improving muscular stabilization. Initial exercises should focus on strengthening and stabilizing the spine and stretching the hip flexors. Lower extremity muscle tightness is common with LBP and must be corrected to allow normal range of motion of the lumbar spine.

Two recent studies have found that Iyengar yoga improves functional disability, pain intensity, and depression in patients with chronic low back pain. It was found to be cost-effective treatment by reducing office visits as well as medication use, with improved function at 6 months postintervention.

H. Behavioral Therapy

Multitudinous factors play a role in the patient's return to function and decreasing pain. Psychological stressors (yellow flags) have emerged as the strongest single baseline predictor of 4-year outcomes exceeding pain intensity. Fear/avoidance beliefs also have a strong influence on recovery. These factors highlight the importance of exercise as a management tool for low back pain. Exercise reduces fear/avoidance behavior and facilitates function despite ongoing pain. Graded behavior intervention reinforces the fact that pain does not necessarily mean harm. A patient may still have pain, but be able to function, and thereby improve his/her prognosis over time. Cognitive intervention and exercise programs have demonstrated similar results for improving disability as lumbar fusion, in patients with chronic back pain and disk degeneration.

I. Reevaluation

For those patients with LBP, whose condition worsens during the time of symptom control, reevaluation and consultation or referral to specialty care is recommended. Patients with LBP should always be reevaluated as indicated after 1–3 weeks to assess progress. This can be accomplished with either a follow-up phone call or an office visit. This empowers patients to take the initiative in their disease course. Patients must be advised to follow up sooner if their condition worsens. Any worsening of neurologic symptoms warrants a complete reevaluation.

Conservative treatment is warranted for 4–6 weeks from the initial evaluation. This follow-up visit is also the appropriate time to consider a work-related ergonomic evaluation. As the patient improves, there should be a gradual return to normal activity and a weaning of the medications.

J. Referral

Any patient who has LBP for >6 weeks despite an adequate course of conservative therapy should be reexamined in the office. A comprehensive reevaluation, including a psychosocial assessment and physical examination, should be performed. During follow-up visits, questions should be directed at identifying any detriments in the patient's condition, including new neurologic symptoms, increased pain, or increased medication use. If such problems are found, the patient should be reevaluated for other health problems, consultation, and/or imaging modalities.

For patients with pain that radiates below the knee, especially with a positive tension sign, the anatomy must be evaluated with an imaging study. If there are abnormal findings, then consultation with a neurosurgeon or spine surgeon is appropriate. If, however, the imaging study does not reveal anatomic pathology, then a nonsurgical back specialist may be necessary to help manage the patient. **Table 25-6** lists these specialists and indications for their referral. **Table 25-7** further identifies useful websites that can assist the provider in identifying resources for management and indications for referral.

If there are no abnormal findings on a comprehensive reassessment, including selected diagnostic tests, it is crucial to start patients on a program that will enable them to resume their usual activities. Management of the patient without structural pathology should be directed toward a physical conditioning program designed with exercise to progressively build activity tolerance and overcome individual limitations. This may include referral to behavior modification specialists, activity specific educators, or an organized multidisciplinary back rehabilitation program.

Antman EM, et al. Use of nonsteroidal anti-inflammatory drugs: an update for clinicians. A scientific statement from the American Heart Association. *Circulation*. 2007;115:1634–1642.

Baliki MN, Geha PY, Apkarian AV, et al. Beyond feeling: chronic pain hurts the brain, disrupting the default and thalamic gray matter density. *J Neurosci*. 2008;28:1398–1403. [PMID: 18256259]

Calmels P, Queneau P, Hamonet C, et al. Effectiveness of a lumbar belt in subacute low back pain: an open, multicentric, and randomized clinical study. *Spine*. 2009;34(3):215–220.

Table 25-6. Surgical back specialists.

Specialist	Indications
Physiatrist/physical medicine and rehabilitation	Chronic back pain >6 weeks Chronic sciatica >6 weeks Chronic pain syndrome Recurrent back pain
Neurology	Chronic sciatica for >6 weeks Atypical chronic leg pain (negative SLR) New or progressive neuromotor deficit
Occupational medicine	Difficult workers' compensation situations Disability/impairment ratings Return-to-work issues
Rheumatology	Rule out inflammatory arthropathy Rule out fibrositis/fibromyalgia Rule out metabolic bone disease (eg, osteoporosis)
Primary care sports medicine specialist	Chronic back pain for >6 weeks; chronic sciatica for >6 weeks Recurrent back pain

Casazza BA. Diagnosis and treatment of acute low back pain. *Am Fam Physician*. 2012;85(4):343–350.

Chapman R, Norvell C, Hermsmeyer T, et al. Evaluating common outcomes for measuring treatment success for chronic low back pain. *Spine*. 2011;36:S54–S68.

Chou D. Degenerative MRI changes in patients with chronic low back pain: a systematic review. *Spine*. 2011;36:S43–S53. [PMID: 21952189]

Chou R, et al. Diagnosis and treatment of low back pain: a joint practice guideline from the American College of Physicians and the American Pain Society [published correction appears in *Ann Intern Med*. 2008;148(3):247–248]. *Ann Intern Med*. 2007;147:478–491.

Chou R, Huffman LH. Medications for acute and chronic low back pain: a review of the evidence from an American Pain Society/American College of Physicians clinical practice guideline. *Ann Intern Med*. 2007;147:492–514.

Chuang LH, Soares MO, Tilbrook H, et al. A pragmatic multi-centered randomized controlled trial of yoga for chronic low back pain: economic evaluation. *Spine*. 2012;37(18):1593–1601. [PMID: 22433499]

Fisher CG, Vaccaro AR, Mulpuri K, et al. Evidence-based recommendations for spine surgery. *Spine*. 2012;37(1):E3–E9.

Fourney DR, Andersson G, Arnold PM, et al. Chronic low back pain. *Spine*. 2011;36:S1–S9.

Goertz M, Thorson D, Bonsell J, et al. Institute for Clinical Systems Improvement. *Adult Acute and Subacute Low Back Pain*; updated Nov. 2012 (available at https://www.icsi.org/_asset/bjvqrj/LBP.pdf).

Henschke N, Ostelo RWJG, van Tulder MW, et al. Behavioral treatment for chronic low-back pain. *Cochrane Database Syst Rev*. 2010 (7):CD002014. [PMID: 20614428]

Lillios S, Young J. The effects of core and lower extremity strengthening on pregnancy-related low back and pelvic girdle pain: a systematic review. *J Women's Health Phys Therapy*. 2012;36(3):116–124.

Table 25-7. Helpful websites.

Address	Information
http://www.ahcpr.gov/consumer	Agency for Healthcare Research and Quality
http://www.rheumatology.org/public/factsheets/backpain_new.asp?aud=pat	American College of Rheumatology, patient education on back pain
http://orthoinfo.aaos.org	American Academy of Orthopedic Surgeons information page
http://www.intelihealth.com/IH/ihtIH/WSAUS000/331/9519.html	Intelihealth back pain page
http://preventiveservices.ahrq.gov	US Preventative Services Task Force
http://www.icsi.org/knowledge/detail.asp?catID=29&itemID=149	Institute for Clinical Systems Improvement, low back pain guideline
http://www.medinfo.co.uk/conditions/lowbackpain.html	European Clinical Practice Guideline on the Treatment of Low Back Pain, including the pediatric population
http://www.chirobase.org/07Strategy/AHCPR/ahcprclinician.html	Quick reference to the US Agency for Health Care Policy and Research (1994) practice guideline
http://familydoctor.org/	Patient education handouts
http://www.ciap.health.nsw.gov.au/nswtag/publications/guidelines/LowBackPain4=12=02.pdf	Therapeutic assessment group, prescribing guidelines for LBP
http://www.guideline.gov/summary/summary.aspx?doc_id=4772&nbr=003451&string=LOW+AND+BACK+AND+PAIN	US Preventative Services Task Force recommendation statement on LBP, June 2005
http://www.fda.gov/cder/drug/infopage/cox2/NSAIDdecisionMemo.pdf	US Food and Drug Administration; analysis and recommendations for NSAIDs and cardiovascular risk
http://www.aafp.org/cmebulletin/lbp	CME bulletin, a peer-reviewed bulletin for the family physician The diagnosis and management of acute low back pain and caring for patients who have chronic low back pain
http://www.aafp.org/cmebulletin/lbp/yellowflags	CME bulletin, yellow-flag listing

Oleske DM, Lavender SA, Andersson GB, et al. Are back supports plus education more effective than educatioin alone in promoting recovery from low back pain? Results from a randomized clinical trial. *Spine.* 2007;32(19):2050–2057. [PMID: 17762804]

Pengel LHM, Refshauge KM, Maher CG, et al. Physiotherpist-directed exercise, advice, or both for subacute low back pain, a randomized trial. *Ann Intern Med.* 2007;146:787–796. [PMID: 17548410]

Prkachin KM, Schultz IZ, Hughes E. Pain behavior and the development of pain-related disability: the importance of guarding. *Clin J Pain.* 2007;23(3):270–277. [PMID: 17314588]

Roelofs PDDM, Deyo RA, Koes BW, Scholten RJPM, van Tulder MW. Non-steroidal anti-inflammatory drugs for low back pain. *Cochrane Database Syst Rev.* 2008;1:CD000396. [PMID: 182539776]

Sahar T, Cohen MJ, Uval-Ne'eman V, et al. Insoles for prevention and treatment of back pain. *Spine.* 2009;34(9):924–933. [PMID: 19359999]

Standaert C. Comparative effectiveness of exercise, acupuncture, and spinal manipulation for low back pain. *Spine.* 2011;36:S120–S130. [PMID: 21952184]

Stoyer J, Jensen LD. The role of physical fitness as risk indicator of increased low back pain intensity among people working with physically and mentally disabled persons: a 30-month prospective study. *Spine.* 2008;33(5):546–554. [PMID: 18317201]

Thomas KJ, MacPherson H, Thorpe L, et al. Randomized controlled trial of a short course of traditional acupuncture compared with usual care for persistent non-specific low back pain. *Br Med J.* 2006;333:623–626. [PMID: 16980316]

White AP. Pharmacologic management of chronic low back pain: synthesis of the evidence. *Spine.* 2011;36:S131–S143. [PMID: 21952185]

Williams K, Abildso C, Steinberg L, et al. Evaluation of the effectiveness and efficacy of Iyengar yoga therapy on chronic low back pain. *Spine.* 2009;34(19):2066–2076. [PMID: 19701112]

Witt CM, Ludtke R, Baur R, et al. Homeopathic treatment of patients with chronic low back pain: a prospective observational study with 2 years' follow-up. *Clin J Pain.* 2009;5(4):334–339. [PMID: 19590483]

▶ **Prognosis**

The long-term course of LBP is variable. Fortunately it does not develop into a chronic disabling condition for the majority. One recent review discovered that one in five patients report persistent low back pain after an acute episode

12 months after initial onset of symptoms. However, 90% of patients will regain function with decreasing pain after 6 weeks, despite physician intervention.

Baliki MN, Geha PY, Apkarian AV, et al. Beyond feeling: chronic pain hurts the brain, disrupting the default and thalamic gray matter density. *J Neurosci.* 2008;28:1398–1403.

Chapman R, Norvell C, Hermsmeyer T, et al. Evaluating common outcomes for measuring treatment success for chronic low back pain. *Spine.* 2011;36:S54–S68.

Dagenais S, Caro J, Haldeman S. A systematic review of low back pain cost of illness studies in the United States and internationally. *Spine J.* 2008;8:8–20. [PMID: 18164449]

Fourney DR, Andersson G, Arnold PM, et al. Chronic low back pain. *Spine.* 2011;36:S1–S9.

Prkachin KM, Schultz IZ, Hughes E. Pain behavior and the development of pain-related disability: the importance of guarding. *Clin J Pain.* 2007;23(3):270–277.

Neck Pain

26

Garry W. K. Ho, MD, CAQSM

Thomas M. Howard, MD, FASCM

General Considerations

Neck pain is a common clinical problem experienced by nearly two-thirds of people. Neck pain can be quite disabling, in some countries accounting for nearly as much disability as low back pain. Neck pain is also similar to low back pain in that the etiology is poorly understood and the clinical diagnoses can be vague. Compared to low back pain, however, neck pain has received limited study. The few available randomized controlled studies lack consistency in study design. This chapter reviews the epidemiology and anatomy of neck pain and provides an evidence-based guide for the evaluation, diagnosis, and management of this challenging disorder.

Neck pain is most prevalent in middle-aged adults; however, prevalence tends to vary with differing definitions and differing survey methodologies of neck pain. One study, found that the 1-year prevalence in adults ranged from 16.7% (youngest) to 75.1% (oldest). Almost 85% of neck pain may be attributed to chronic stress and strains or acute or repetitive injuries associated with poor posture, anxiety, depression, and occupational or sporting risks. The acceleration-deceleration of a whiplash injury may result in cervical sprains or strains, which, in turn, are common causes of neck pain. Radicular neck pain occurs later in life, with an estimated incidence of 10% among 25–29-year-olds, rising to 25–40% in those aged >45 years.

Occupational neck pain is ubiquitous and not limited to any particular work setting. Predictors for occupational neck pain include perception of little influence on the work situation, other work-related psychosocial factors, and perceived general tension. Predictors of occupational neck pain include prolonged sitting at work (>95% of the workday), especially with the neck forward-flexed ≥20° for >70% of the work time.

Fejer R et al. The prevalence of neck pain in the world population: a systematic critical review of the literature. *Eur Spine J.* 2006;15:834. [PMID: 15999284]

Pathogenesis & Functional Anatomy

The cervical spine is a highly mobile column that supports the 6–8-lb head, provides protection for the cervical spinal cord, and consists of 7 vertebrae intercalated by 5 intervertebral disks; 14 facet joints (zygapophyseal joints or Z-joints); 12 joints of Luschka (uncovertebral joints); and 14 paired anterior, lateral, and posterior muscles. The vertebrae can viewed as three major groups: the atlas (C_1), the axis (C_2), and the others (C_3-C_7). C_1 is a ring-shaped vertebra with two lateral masses articulating with the occiput and C_2. The C_2 consists of a large vertebral body (the largest in the cervical spine) with the anterior odontoid process (dens) articulating with C_1. This odontoid process has a precarious blood supply, placing it at risk for nonunion when fractured. The atlantooccipital articulation accounts for 50% of the flexion and extension neck range of motion (RoM), and the C_1-C_2 joints account for 50% of the rotational RoM of the neck. The remaining cervical vertebrae consists of an anterior body with a posterior projecting ring of the transverse and spinous processes that form the vertebral foramen for the spinal cord, as well as provide attachment sites for ligaments and muscles, which, in turn, can become sprained or strained. The most prominent palpable spinous processes are C_2 and C_7 (vertebral prominens). The joints of Luschka and the facet joints can be involved in degenerative and inflammatory processes. The most important ligaments are the anterior and posterior longitudinal ligaments (PLLs) along the vertebral bodies, the ligamentum nuchae along the spinous process, and the ligamentum flavum along the anterior surfaces of the laminae. The weaker PLLs stabilize the intervertebral disks posteriorly and are often damaged in disk herniation. Ligamentum flavum hypertrophy may contribute to spinal stenosis or nerve root impingement.

Eight cervical nerve roots exit posterolaterally through neuroforamina, each emerging through above the vertebra of its number (ie, the C_6 root arises between C_5 and C_6), with C_8 exiting between C_7 and T_1. The cervical cord also directly gives rise to nerves that innervate the neck, upper extremity, and diaphragm. Each intervertebral disk consists of a gelatinous center (nucleus pulposus) surrounded by a tougher, multilayered annulus fibrosis. Degenerative or acute disk injury may lead to herniation to the nucleus pulposus, which, in turn, can impinge on nearby cervical nerve roots, contributing to radiculopathy.

The musculature of the cervical spine includes flexors, extensors, lateral flexors, and rotators. Major flexors include the sternocleidomastoid, scalenes, and prevertebrals. Extensors include the posterior paravertebral muscles (splenius, semispinalis, capitis) and trapezius. Lateral flexors include the sternocleidomastoid, scalenes, and interspinous (between the transverse processes) muscles, and the rotators include the sternocleidomastoid and the interspinous muscles. The ability of the cervical spine to absorb and diffuse the energy from acute trauma is related to its lordotic curvature, the paraspinal muscles, and intervertebral disks. At 30° of forward flexion, the cervical spine is straight and most vulnerable to axial load–type injuries. The paraspinal muscles can be strained and become spastic. Occasionally, so-called trigger points—hyperirritable myo-nodules and taut muscle fiber bands—may develop. The combined motion of all the preceding structures gives a significant RoM to the neck, allowing the head to scan the environment with the eyes and ears. Flexion and extension are centered at C_5-C_6 and C_6-C_7, respectively; hence, degeneration and injury often occurs at these levels.

The mechanism of injury of the cervical spine can be classified in multiple ways: acute injuries—including a fall, blow to the head, or the whiplash injury—or chronic-repetitive injury—associated with recreational or occupational activities, or degenerative processes. Other classifications include the direction of the stress or force generating the injury: flexion, extension-hyperextension, axial load, lateral flexion, or rotation. Most chronic neck pain is associated with poor posture and ergonomics, anxiety or depression, neck strain, or occupational and sports-related injuries.

▶ **Prevention**

Prevention strategies for high-risk groups have been employed for both neck and lower back pain. A review of 27 investigations into educational efforts, exercises, ergonomics, and risk factor modification found sufficient evidence for only strengthening exercises as an effective prevention strategy. A more recent randomized controlled trial showed that specific resistance and all-around exercise programs were more effective than general health counseling in preventing occupation-related neck pain.

Anderson LL, et al. A randomized controlled intervention trial to relieve and prevent neck/shoulder pain. *Med Sci Sports Exerc.* 2008;40(6):983–990.

▶ **Clinical Findings**

A. Symptoms and Signs

In the evaluation of cervical spine problems it is critical to obtain a thorough history, ascertaining the mechanism of injury. In many cases, the mechanism of injury may identify the injury or guide the physical examination. A survey of prior injuries or problems with the cervical spine (eg, a history of prior surgery or degenerative arthritis) is helpful. Radicular or radiating symptoms in the upper extremity should be identified, including radiating pain, motor weakness, numbness, or paraesthesias of the extremities. Determining both the apparent origin and source of radiating symptoms is important. Occasionally, a myofascial trigger point may exhibit referral pain patterns mimicking those of radiculopathy, and often plays a role in chronic neck pain. Conversely, musculoskeletal neck pain can refer to the head playing a large role in cervicogenic headaches. The examiner should ask about any symptoms related to possible upper motor neuron pathology, including bowel or bladder dysfunction or gait disturbance.

Additional information should include the duration and course of symptoms, aggravating and alleviating motions or activities, and attempted prior treatments. Comorbid diseases such as inflammatory spondyloarthropathies, cardiac disease, or gastrointestinal problems should be identified, as well as a history of tobacco or alcohol abuse. Current occupational and recreational activities and requirements should be identified, as they may contribute to the underlying problem and identify the desired endpoint for recovery and return to activity.

B. Cervical Spine Examination

The cervical spine is examined in an organized and systematic way that includes adequate exposure of the neck, upper back, and shoulders for observation; palpation of bony and soft tissues; evaluation of RoM; tests for cervical radiculopathy (Spurling test, Lhermitte sign); upper extremity motor and sensory examination; and evaluation for upper motor neuron symptoms.

1. Observation—Observation should begin as the patient walks into the examination room, looking for the presence or absence of normal fluid motion of the neck and arm swing with walking. After exposure, the examiner may note the posture (look for a poor head-forward, rounded-shoulder posture contributing to chronic cervical muscular strain), shoulder position (looking for elevation from muscle spasm), evidence of atrophy, and any head tilt or rotation.

2. Palpation—Palpation of major bony prominences and the soft tissues should be performed. The spinous processes and the facet joints (~1 cm lateral and deep to the spinous process) should be gently palpated, noting (more than expected) tenderness. Palpation of the prevertebral and paravertebral muscles may reveal hypertonicity and pain. Common sites for trigger points include the levator scapulae (off the superior, medial margin of the scapula), upper trapezius, rhomboids, and upper paraspinals near the occiput. Palpation of trigger points may elicit tenderness, referred pain (which may mimic radicular symptoms), or a local twitch response.

3. Range of motion—Active RoM should be tested first with judicious use of passive motion as pain permits. Normal RoM includes extension of 70° (chin pointed straight up to the ceiling), flexion of 60° (chin on chest, or within 3 cm of chest), lateral flexion of approximately 45° (ear to shoulder), and rotation of approximately 80° (looking right and left). RoM should be tested in each of these planes and for both left and right sides, recording findings in degrees from the neutral position or as a percentage of the expected norm.

4. Spurling test—This test assesses for nerve root irritation, which can be related to spondylotic compression, discogenic compression, or the Stinger-Burner syndrome (a compression or stretch injury of the brachial plexus, commonly seen in sports injuries). To perform the Spurling test, the examiner extends, side-bends, and partially rotates the patient's head toward the side being tested. An axial load is then gently applied to the top of the head. A positive test is indicated by radiation of pain, generally into the posterior shoulder or arm on the ipsilateral side.

5. Lhermitte sign—The Lhermitte sign may also be used to test for cervical radiculopathy. Forward flexion of the neck that causes paraesthesias down the spine or extremities suggests cervical radiculopathy, spondylosis, myelopathy, or multiple sclerosis. Manual cervical distraction may reduce neck and limb symptoms in cervical radiculopathy.

6. Upper extremity motor examination—This includes manual muscle testing and deep tendon reflexes (DTRs; **Table 26-1**). A useful mnemonic to keep the upper extremity motor findings in order is *blocker > beggar > kisser > grabber > Spock* (**Figure 26-1**). The examiner systematically checks arm abduction (blocking position) for deltoid function, then resisted elbow flexion and extension (biceps and triceps), wrist extension and flexion, grip, and finger abduction (spread fingers). DTRs should be checked for the biceps (C_5), triceps (C_7), and brachioradialis (C_6). Sensory testing should focus on the dermatomes for the cervical roots, with focus on the lateral deltoid area (C_5), dorsal first web space (C_6), dorsal middle finger (C_7), small finger (C_8), and inner arm (T_1). Testing for thoracic outlet syndrome can be accomplished with the Adson test and Roo test. In the Adson test, the patient's neck is extended, with the head rotated toward the affected side and lungs in deep inspiration, while the examiner palpates the ipsilateral radial pulse. Decrease in the amplitude of the radial pulse with this maneuver is a positive test. The Roo test (also called the *elevated arm stress test*) is performed with both the patient's arms (shoulders) in an abducted and externally rotated position (90° each), and the elbow flexed to 90°. The patient then opens and closes both hands for 3 minutes. Inability to continue this maneuver for 3 minutes due to reproduction of symptoms suggests thoracic outlet syndrome. Reasonably low false-positive rates make the Roo test the preferred test.

7. Upper motor neuron symptoms—Upper motor neuron findings can be demonstrated by a Hoffman sign; with the third finger extended, a quick flexion-flick of the third distal interphalangeal joint is applied; an abnormal flexion reflex in the thumb or other fingers is a positive test (positive Hoffman sign). Lower extremity testing for upper motor neuron findings should be performed, including DTRs

Table 26-1. Upper extremity motor and sensory innervations.

Spinal Level	Motor	Reflex	Sensory	Peripheral Nerve
C_5	Deltoid (shoulder abduction) Biceps	Biceps	Lateral shoulder	Axillary
C_6	Biceps (elbow flexion) Wrist extensors	Brachioradialis	Lateral forearm Dorsal first web space	Musculocutaneous Radial
C_7	Triceps (elbow extension) Wrist flexion Finger extension	Triceps	Dorsal middle finger	Median
C_8	Finger flexors Thumb flexion/opposition	None	Ring finger Small finger Medial forearm	Ulnar Medial antebrachial cutaneous
T_1	Hand intrinsics (finger abduction/ adduction)	None	Medial arm axilla	Medial brachial cutaneous

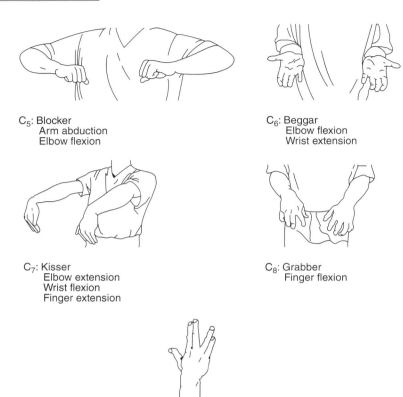

C₅: Blocker
   Arm abduction
   Elbow flexion

C₆: Beggar
   Elbow flexion
   Wrist extension

C₇: Kisser
   Elbow extension
   Wrist flexion
   Finger extension

C₈: Grabber
   Finger flexion

T₁: Spock
   Finger abduction

▲ **Figure 26-1.** Upper extremity motor evaluation.

(looking for hyperreflexia), assessment for ankle clonus, and testing for the Babinski reflex. The Babinski reflex may be elicited by firmly stroking the sole (plantar surface) of the foot. The reflex is present if the great toe dorsiflexes and the other toes fan out (abduct). This is normal in younger children, but abnormal after the age of 2 years.

C. Laboratory Findings

In cases with upper extremity weakness not improving with therapy, electromyography (EMG) and nerve conduction studies (NCSs) may be considered in evaluating upper extremity neurologic disorders and to help distinguish between peripheral (including brachial plexus) and nerve root injuries. EMG and NCS also distinguish between stable and active denervating and recovery processes. Testing may not be diagnostic until 3–4 weeks after an acute nerve injury, so this study should not be ordered in the acute setting. Routine follow-up EMG and NCS in patients with whiplash injuries may not contribute useful information to clinical and imaging findings. Other laboratory studies—including complete blood count, sedimentation rate, rheumatoid factor,

and others—should be reserved for the evaluation of spondyloarthropathies and play little role in the evaluation of most cases of isolated neck pain.

D. Imaging Studies

Potential imaging studies of the cervical spine can include plain radiographs, magnetic resonance imaging (MRI), computed tomography (CT), bone scan, and myelography. Bone scan does not significantly contribute to the evaluation of neck pain in most acute or chronic settings. Plain films include the basic three-view series (anteroposterior, lateral, open mouth), oblique, and lateral flexion-extension views. Indications for the use of imaging studies in the evaluation of neck pain can be divided into recommendations for acute (traumatic) or chronic neck pain.

In the acute trauma situation, the three-view radiograph is the basic study of choice, when CT is not available. CT or lateral flexion and extension views can be used to further evaluate nondiagnostic radiographs or cases of high clinical suspicion for injury. Cervical fractures may be ruled out on a clinical basis if the patient does not complain of neck pain when asked; does not have a history of loss of consciousness; does not have mental status change from trauma, drugs, or alcohol; does not have symptoms referable to the neck (paralysis or sensory change—present or resolved); does not have midline cervical tenderness to palpation; and does not have other distracting painful injuries. The American College of Radiology (ACR) appropriateness criteria for imaging of suspected cervical spine trauma recommend that thin-section CT, and not plain radiography, be the screening study of choice, and once a decision is made to scan the patient, the entire spine should be examined owing to the high incidence of noncontiguous multiple injuries. If CT scanning is not readily available, those with cervical tenderness should have, at a minimum, the basic three-view plain-film series. Patients who have upper or lower extremity paraesthesias (or other neurologic findings), are unconscious at the time of evaluation, have distracting injuries, or are in an altered mental state (due to alcohol or drugs) should undergo a CT scan of the cervical spine; MRI of the cervical spine may be considered, depending on the CT findings or in cases where myelopathy is suspected. Patients with neck pain and clinical findings suggestive of ligamentous injury, with normal radiographic and CT findings, may be considered for MRI of the cervical spine.

The ACR appropriateness criteria for imaging of chronic neck pain concluded that there are no existing evidence-based guidelines for the radiologic evaluation of the patient with chronic neck pain. The initial imaging study should be the three-view series. The most common findings include a loss of lordosis (straight cervical spine) or disk space narrowing with degenerative change at the C_5-C_6 and C_4-C_5 levels. When patients have chronic neck pain after hyperextension or flexion injury with normal radiographs

and persistent pain or evidence of neurologic injury, lateral flexion-extension views should be considered to rule out instability. Abnormal findings include >3.5-mm horizontal displacement or >11° of rotational difference to that of the adjacent vertebrae on resting or flexion-extension lateral radiographs. Oblique radiographs may be helpful to look for bony encroachment of the neuroforamina in the evaluation of radicular neck pain. MRI should be performed on all patients who have chronic neck pain with neurologic signs or symptoms. If there is a contraindication to MRI (ie, pacemaker, nonavailability, claustrophobia, or interfering hardware in the neck), CT myelography is recommended.

American College of Radiology (ACR), Expert Panel on Musculoskeletal Imaging. *Chronic Neck Pain in ACR Appropriateness Criteria*. ACR, 2010: 1–9.
American College of Radiology (ACR), Expert Panel on Musculoskeletal Imaging. *Suspected Spine Trauma in ACR Appropriateness Criteria*. ACR, 2012: 1–20.

▶ **Differential Diagnosis**

See **Table 26-2.**

▶ **Treatment**

Multiple treatment options are available, although there is limited evidence-based support for the efficacy of most of these. Early management focuses on proper initial evaluation, use of analgesics, early return to motion, and judicious use of physical modalities. Acupuncture and manual therapy may help reduce pain early. Chronic neck pain can be related to psychosocial factors at home and in the workplace and may be

Table 26-2. Differential diagnosis of neck pain.

Acute Injury	Noninflammatory Disease	Inflammatory Disease	Infectious Causes	Neoplasm	Referred Pain
Cervical sprain, strain, spasm, whiplash	Cervical osteoarthritis (spondylosis)	Rheumatoid arthritis	Meningitis	Primary	Temporomandibular joint
Cervical tendonitis, tendinosis	Discogenic neck pain	Spondyloarthropathies	Osteomyelitis	Myeloma	Cardiac
Cervical instability	Cervical spinal stenosis	Juvenile rheumatoid arthritis	Infectious discitis	Cord tumor	Diaphragmatic irritation
Fractures	Cervical myelopathy	Ankylosing spondylitis		Metastatic	Gastrointestinal
Vertebral body	Myofascial pain				Gastric ulcer
Teardrop	Trigger points				Gall bladder
Burst	Fibromyalgia				Pancreas
Chance	Reflex sympathetic dystrophy/ complex regional pain syndrome				Thoracic outlet syndrome
Compression					Shoulder disorders
Spinous process	Migraines (or variants)				Brachial plexus injuries
Transverse process	Torticollis				Occipital neuralgia
Facet					Peripheral nerve injury
Odontoid (C_2)					
Hangman (C_2)					
Jefferson (C_1)					
Stinger or Burner					

tied to litigation in whiplash-type injuries. Specialty consultation beyond physical therapy is rarely needed.

A. Initial Care

Initial management includes avoidance of aggravating factors at work or with recreational activities, as well as pain management, recognizing that most pain is self-limiting. Management should focus on early return to motion, isometric strengthening, and modification of occupational or recreational aggravating factors with return to activity with ergonomic precautions.

Absolute rest should be limited to a very short period of time (ie, <1–2 days). This includes the use of cervical collars. Early motion should be encouraged as soon as severe pain allows. Early mobilization after whiplash injury is associated with a better prognosis. Patients should focus on proper posture (neck centered and back over the shoulders) and gentle stretching of the neck for RoM. Each position should be held for 15–20 seconds. Proprioceptive neuromuscular facilitation or muscle energy techniques may be employed in a structured physical therapy program or home program with the goal to improve motion. This is done by having patients move their heads in a direction to the point of pain. Next, they attempt to move in the opposite direction against the resistance of their own hands on the chin for a count of 5, contracting the rehabilitating muscle throughout the entire maneuver. Then they attempt to further move in the original direction, usually with improved motion. This should be done in the six major RoM directions.

B. Pain Management

Pain management may take the form of ice, medications, physical modalities, or manual therapy techniques. Application of ice (15 minutes every 2 hours) is effective for acute pain after injury or for postactivity pain during the recovery process. Medications used in the management of acute and chronic neck pain include salicylates (aspirin), nonsteroidal anti-inflammatory drugs (NSAIDs; ibuprofen, naproxen, indomethacin, piroxicam, celecoxib), acetaminophen (500–1000 mg 4 times daily), muscle relaxants (diazepam, methocarbamol, cyclobenzaprine), narcotic medications (acetaminophen with codeine, acetaminophen with oxycodone, acetaminophen with hydrocodone, meperidine), and corticosteroids. For acute radicular symptoms, a short course of systemic corticosteroids may be considered to reduce inflammation associated with a herniated nucleus pulposus. Although there is no literature to support the use of ice or systemic steroids, anecdotal evidence suggests that they may be helpful in the acute setting.

For chronic neck pain (eg, lasting >30 days), tricyclic antidepressants (TCAs; nortriptyline, amitriptyline) or selective serotonin reuptake inhibitors (SSRIs; fluoxetine, sertraline) at bedtime may be used for chronic pain management and management of sleep disturbance that often accompanies chronic pain of any source. Side effects of TCAs include excessive drowsiness, dry mouth, urinary retention, and potential cardiac conduction problems. Side effects of SSRIs include insomnia, drowsiness, dry mouth, nausea, headache, and anorexia. The combination of SSRIs and TCAs may result in increased serum levels of the TCA and toxicity. Randomized controlled studies support the use of simple analgesics and NSAIDs in the management of acute pain but do not support the other treatment options.

C. Physical Modalities

Multiple physical modalities are available for pain management and to improve ROM, although there is little evidence of their effectiveness and few well-designed randomized controlled studies that support their use in management of acute or chronic neck pain. These modalities include the application of heat, cold, ultrasound, cervical traction, acupuncture, and electrical stimulation [including transcutaneous electrical nerve stimulation (TENS)]. However, evidence supporting the use of electrotherapy in neck disorders is limited and conflicting. Cervical traction can be effective for relief of spasm or in the management of radicular pain, and may be performed in a controlled setting at physical therapy or with the use of home traction units. Typical sessions in physical therapy are 2–3 days per week for 30 minutes per session. A typical home cervical traction regimen would start at 10 lb of longitudinal traction and increase by 5 lb every 1–2 days until a goal of 20–30 lb is reached. Home traction is used on a daily or alternate-day basis.

D. Acupuncture, Acupressure, and Needling

Acupuncture can be effective in the treatment of neck pain—although literature supporting its effectiveness beyond five treatment sessions for acute neck pain or 4 weeks of treatment for chronic neck pain—is limited. A home program of ischemic pressure (acupressure) with stretching can also be effective in the management of myofascial neck pain and trigger points. Although much of the evidence on trigger point injections has been conflicting, systematic reviews have reported that trigger point injections may be useful in relieving trigger point–related pain in chronic conditions lasting >3 months. Outcomes were not significantly different with regard to the injectant used, including dry needling. Intramuscular injections of botulinum toxin type A have been found to be no more efficacious than saline. However, the injection of a local anesthetic does seem to decrease discomfort related to the needling process.

E. Manual Therapy

Manual therapy (eg, osteopathic and chiropractic manipulation, or manual therapy techniques applied by a physical therapist) is commonly used in the management of chronic neck and lower back pain. For acute neck injuries, there is some evidence supporting the use of manual techniques involving passive neck motion aimed at restoring normal spinal RoM and function, excluding spinal manipulations. A study on the use of manual therapy in the treatment of neck and low back pain showed an average improvement of 53.8% in acute pain and 48.4% in chronic pain with 12 treatments over a 4-week period. A case report of a patient with persistent neck and arm pain—after failed cervical disk surgery with resolution after a program of manual therapy and rehabilitative exercises—further supports the use of manual therapy in the management of both myofascial and radicular neck pain. However, caution should be exercised, as one study reported that 30% of patients undergoing spinal manipulation had adverse effects, especially in those with severe neck pain or severe headache prior to treatment.

F. Therapeutic Exercise

There is some evidence to support the effectiveness of active RoM exercises for acute mechanical neck disorders. As patients recover, a program of strengthening should be instituted. Simple isometric exercises focusing on resisted forward flexion, extension, and right and left lateral flexion will improve pain and strength, contributing to recovery and long-term resistance to further injury. Attention to posture and an ergonomic survey are also important and can help in customizing a complete therapeutic exercise program for both treatment and prevention of neck pain. There is evidence to support the use of yoga in relieving chronic nonspecific neck pain.

G. Referral

Specialty referral may be considered at multiple points in the recovery process to aid in diagnosis or treatment of acute or chronic neck pain. Physical therapy may be used early in the process to incorporate physical modalities and initiate a strengthening program. *Physical medicine and rehabilitation* (PM&R) involvement may be considered for comanagement of chronic pain of any source and to obtain EMGs. The input of a neurologist may be considered to obtain EMGs or for consultation in patients with confusing neurologic conditions. Neurosurgery or orthopedic-spinal surgery should be considered for patients requiring operative management. Early referral should be considered for severe muscle weakness, fractures, and evidence of myelopathy (upper motor neuron signs). Success rates for surgery have been reported to be as high as 80–90% for radicular pain and 60–70% for myelopathy. There is insufficient evidence to compare conservative treatment with surgical management of patients who have neck pain and radiculopathy, and a recent systematic review found low-quality evidence that showed no overall differences between conservative and surgical management. For patients who have chronic radiating pain despite 9–12 weeks of conservative management, referral for chronic pain management at an anesthesiology, neurology, PM&R, or other pain management clinic should be considered for comanagement or consideration of epidural steroid (ESI), facet joint injections, or medial branch nerve procedures. Randomized controlled studies provide some evidence to support the use of ESI in chronic neck pain.

Cramer H, Lauche R, Hohmann C, et al. Randomized-controlled trial comparing yoga and home-based exercise for chronic neck pain. *Clin J Pain.* 2013;29(3):216–223. [PMID: 23249655]

Manchikanti L, Cash KA, Pampati V, Malla Y. Cervical epidural injections in chronic fluoroscopic cervical epidural injections in chronic axial or disc-related neck pain without disc herniation, facet joint pain, or radiculitis. *J Pain Res.* 2012;5:227–236. [PMID: 22826642]

Scott NA, Guo B, Barton PM, Gerwin RD. Trigger point injections for chronic non-malignant musculoskeletal pain: a systematic review. *Pain Med.* 2009;10(1):54–69. [PMID: 18992040]

Van Middelkoop M, Rubinstein SM, Ostelo R, et al. Surgery versus conservative care for neck pain: a systematic review. *Eur Spine J.* 2013:22:87–95. [PMID: 20949289]

▶ **Prognosis**

Neck pain usually resolves in days to weeks, but, like low back pain can become recurrent. High initial pain intensity is an important predictor of delayed functional recovery. The single best estimation of handicap due to whiplash injury was return of normal cervical RoM. Up to 40% of patients with whiplash injuries report symptoms for ≤15 years postinjury. These patients have a 3 times higher risk of neck pain in the next 7 years. A Swedish study showed that 55% of an exposed group and 29% of a control group had residual symptoms up to 17 years postinjury. The incidence of chronic standing neck pain is ~10%, and ~5% of people will experience severe disability. Patients who experience these symptoms for at least 6 months have a <50% chance of recovering even with aggressive therapy. Predictors of chronic neck pain include a prior history of neck pain or injury, motor vehicle collision, age of >60 years, female gender, number of children, poor self-assessed health, poor socioeconomic and psychological status (eg, excessive concerns about symptoms, unrealistic expectations of treatment, and psychosocial concerns), and history of low back pain.

Palmlöf L, Skillgate E, Alfredsson L, et al. Does income matter for troublesome neck pain? A population-based study on risk and prognosis. *J Epidemiol Community Health.* 2012;66:1063–1070.

Websites

The following are useful websites for patient education on topics such as home rehabilitation and correction of occupational and postural risk factors:

http://familydoctor.org/familydoctor/en/health-tools/search-by-symptom/neck-pain.html

http://www.nismat.org/services/orthopedic-surgery/therapeutic-exercise-programs/upper-extremity-and-neck-flexibility-program

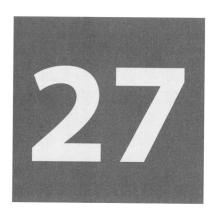

Cancer Screening in Women[1]

Nicole Powell-Dunford, MD, MPH, FAAFP

BREAST CANCER

ESSENTIALS OF DIAGNOSIS

▶ Lobular or ductal carcinoma *in situ* are localized breast cancers.

▶ Invasive breast cancer extends beyond the ducts and lobules and may present as a palpable mass.

▶ Inflammatory breast cancers can be mistaken for skin infection.

▶ Guidelines for early detection have evolved significantly.

General Considerations

Breast cancer is the second most common cancer in women after skin cancer. BRCA1 and BRCA2 tumor suppressor genes confer strong risk. Other risk factors include earlier age of menarche, later age of menopause, nulliparity, and late age of first birth, all reflecting higher total number of ovarian cycles. Obesity, alcohol use, older age, decreased physical activity, and other genetic and environmental factors have been linked to breast cancer. Recent studies challenge hormone replacement therapy (HRT) as a risk for breast cancer.

Prevention

Women positive for the heritable BCRA mutation may benefit from prophylactic tamoxifen and prophylactic total mastectomy. AAFP recommends that women whose family history is associated with an increased risk for BRCA mutation

be referred for genetic counseling and evaluation for BRCA testing (**Table 27-1**). Neither routine testing nor prophylactic medication is recommended for the general population. Smoking is a risk factor for cancer development, and cessation should be recommended in all current smokers.

Clinical Findings

Breast cancer most commonly presents as a painless, irregularly bordered mass. Other presentations may include local swelling, dimpling, breast pain, and skin and nipple changes as well as nipple discharge. Advanced clinical presentations may include pain and/or fracture from bony metastasis.

Differential Diagnosis

A. Clinically Evident Mass

A concerning breast mass can be further evaluated through diagnostic mammography, ultrasound with or without fine-needle aspiration, and/or ductal lavage and/or ductogram. Genetic and hormonal receptor testing further differentiates breast cancers.

B. Preclinical Detection

Screening guidelines for normal- and high-risk women have evolved considerably, balancing benefits of early detection against the anxiety, financial loss, and morbidity of false positive screening. **Table 27-2** outlines recommendations of several organizations.

Complications

Metastatic spread is often to lungs, liver, and bone.

Treatment

Treatment may include surgery, radiotherapy, chemotherapy, and/or hormone therapy. Breast conservation therapy,

---

[1]This publication does not reflect the views or opinions of the US Army or the Department of Defense.

Table 27-1. Indications for genetic referral for BRCA testing.

A first-degree relative with breast cancer before age 40
Two or more relatives with breast or ovarian cancer at any age
Three or more relatives with breast, ovarian, or colon cancer at any age

Data from Smith RA, Saslow D, Sawyer KA, Burke W. American Cancer Society guidelines for breast cancer screening: update 2003. *CA Cancer J Clin*. 2003; 53:141.

consisting of lumpectomy and radiation therapy, is standard treatment for early-stage cancer and is not associated with increased 20-year mortality compared to mastectomy. Hormonal therapy is often given for 5 years to prevent relapse in early-stage breast cancer. Invasive cancer is usually treated with both surgery and adjuvant systemic therapy. HER2-positive cancers are treated with a regimen that includes Herceptin. In premenopausal women, hormone receptor–positive cancers are treated with tamoxifen and ovarian ablation. In premenopausal women, hormonal receptor positive cancers are treated with anti-estrogen drugs other than tamoxifen and aromatase inhibitors. Treatment guidelines differ for men and pregnant women. The National Comprehensive Cancer Network updates detailed treatment guidelines for each population and breast cancer stage regularly. Second opinions are valuable. The National Cancer Institute can help enroll patients who wish to participate in ongoing clinical trials (**Table 27-3**).

▶ Prognosis

Five-year survival rates for women with stage 0 or stage 1 cancer are 93% and 88%, respectively, 74–81% for stage 2, 41–67% for stage 3, and 15% for stage 4. HER2 oncogene

Table 27-2. Breast cancer screening.

2012 Screening Recommendations	AAFP	ACOG	ACS	USPSTF	Other Guidance
Breast self-examination (BSE)	Recommend against	May be part of breast self-awareness	20+: BSE is optional; educate on benefits/limitations	Insufficient evidence	USPSTF, AAFP, ACS, and ACOG encourage breast self-awareness and/or early reporting of breast changes
Clinical breast examination	Insufficient evidence	40+: annual 20–39: every 1–3 years	40+: annual 20–39: every 1–3 years	Insufficient evidence	Use of fingerpads of the middle three fingers, overlapping dime-sized circular motions and sequential application of light, medium, and deep levels of pressure recommended
Mammography	40-49: individualize 50-74: biennial screening 75+, insufficient evidence	40+ offer annual 75+ individualize	40 through age of good health: offer annual	<50: individualize 50-74: biennial screening 75+, evidence lacking	Breast density influences ability to detect
MRI	Consider in high risk	Not for normal-risk screen	Not for normal-risk screen	Insufficient evidence for normal-risk screen	MRI may afford very high sensitivity in detecting small masses, but is expensive, associated with IV contrast risks, do not detect all breast cancers that mammography can and is not widely available with guided biopsy
High-risk women	Refer high-risk women by family history for genetic counseling and BRCA testing	Early enhanced screen	Annual mammogram + MRI for high-risk women 30+	Early enhanced screen	High risk considered to be BCRA-positive ± ≥20% risk on a valid prediction model

AAFP, American Association of Family Practitioners; ACOG, American College of Obstetricians and Gynecologists; ACS, American Cancer Society; USPSTF, US Preventive Services Task Force.

Table 27-3. Stages of breast cancer.

Stage	Description
Stage 0 (carcinoma *in situ*)	DCIS/ductal carcinoma *in situ* .... (noninvasive, may progress) LCIS/lobular carcinoma *in situ* .... (seldom invasive, but breast cancer risk) Paget's disease of nipple
Stage IA	Tumor </=2 cm... no LN involved Microscopic invasion possible but does not exceed 1 mm
Stage IB	No tumor .... LN cancer >0.2 mm but </= 2 mm Tumor </=2 cm...LN cancer >0.2 mm but </= 2 mm
Stage IIA	No tumor..1–3 axillary/sternal LN >2 mm Tumor </= 2 cm...1–3 axillary/sternal LN >2 mm Tumor is >2 cm but < 5 cm..no LN involved
Stage IIB	Tumor > 2 cm but </= 5 cm..LN (> 0.2 mm but </= 2 mm) Tumor > 2 cm but </= 5 cm..1–3 axillary/sternal LN Tumor > 5 cm ....No LN involved
Stage IIIA	No tumor or any size..4–9 axillary/sternal LNs Tumor > 5 cm...LN > 0.2 mm and </= 2 mm Tumor > 5 cm.. 1–3 axillary/sternal LN
Stage IIIB	No tumor or tumor of any size has spread to the chest wall and/or to the skin of the breast, causing swelling or an ulcer, with up to 9 axillary/sternal LNs May be inflammatory breast cancer
Stage IIIC	No tumor or tumor of any size; ≥10 axillary/sternal LNs; or LNs above or below the collarbone May be inflammatory breast cancer
Stage IV	The cancer has spread to other parts of the body, most often the bones, lungs, liver, or brain

expression is associated with higher risk for relapse and shorter survival. HER2 expression, hormonal receptors, biomarkers, and tumor gene signature are being used to predict disease outcome, recurrence risk, and/or response to specific medications.

Blichert-Toft M, Nielsen M, During M, et al. Long-term results of breast conserving surgery vs. mastectomy for early stage invasive breast cancer: 20-year follow-up of the Danish randomized DBCG-82TM protocol. *Acta Oncol.* 2008;47:672–681. [PMID: 18465335]

Breast Cancer–Clinical Preventive Services. *Recommendations, Resources & Policies* (available at American Association of Family Physicians. http://www.aafp.org/online/en/home/clinical/exam/breastcancer.html; accessed March 20, 2013).

Breastcancer.org. http://www.breastcancer.org/symptoms/diagnosis/staging#stage1 (last update May 1, 2013; accessed July 5, 2013).

Breast Cancer Survival by Stage (available at American Cancer Society. http://www.cancer.org/cancer/breastcancer/detailedguide/breast-cancer-survival-by-stage; updated Aug 23, 2012; accessed March 18, 2013).

Breast Cancer: Screening (available at US Preventive Services Task Force. http://www.uspreventiveservicestaskforce.org/uspstf/uspsbrca.htm; accessed March 20, 2013).

National Cancer Institute. http://www.cancer.gov/cancertopics/factsheet/Sites-Types/metastatic (accessed March 20, 2012).

National Cancer Institute. http://www.cancer.gov/cancertopics/pdq/treatment/breast/Patient/page2 (last update May 15, 2013; accessed July 2, 2013).

NCCN Guidelines Breast Cancer version 1. 2013. National Comprehensive Cancer Network. http://www.nccn.org/professionals/physician_gls/pdf/breast.pdf (updated March 11, 2013; accessed March 20, 2013).

Practice Bulletin no. 103: hereditary breast and ovarian cancer syndrome. *Obstet Gynecol.* 2009,113(4):957-966. [PMID: 19305347]

Practice Bulletin no. 122: breast cancer screening. *Obstet Gynecol.* 2011;118(2):372–382. [PMID: 21775869]

Recommendations for Early Breast Cancer Detection in Women without Breast Symptoms (available at American Cancer Society. http://www.cancer.org/cancer/breastcancer/moreinformation/breastcancerearlydetection/breast-cancer-early-detection-acs-recs; Aug. 30, 2012; accessed March 10, 2013).

Saslow D, Hannan J, Osuch J, et al. Clinical breast examination: practical recommendations for optimizing performance and reporting. *Canjclin.* 2004;54(6):327–344 (available at http://onlinelibrary.wiley.com/doi/10.3322/canjclin.54.6.327/full; accessed March 25, 2013).

Shapiro S, Farmer R, Stevenson J, et al. Does hormone replacement therapy (HRT) cause breast cancer? An application of causal principles to three studies. *J Fam Plann Reprod Health Care.* 2013;39(2):80–88. [PMID: 23493592]

Summary of Recommendations for Clinical Preventive Services; Oct. 2012 [available at AAFP. http://www.aafp.org/online/en/home/clinical/exam.html (paid subscription only); accessed March 30, 2013).

Tria TM. Breast cancer screening update. *Am Fam Physician.* 2013;87(4):274–278. [PMID: 23418799]

Weigel MT, Dowsett M. Current and emerging biomarkers in breast cancer: prognosis and prediction. *Endocrine-Related Cancer.* 2010:245–253. [PMID: 20647302]

CERVICAL CANCER

 ESSENTIALS OF DIAGNOSIS

▶ Cervical cancer often develops at the transition zone, making Pap smear screening useful in early diagnosis.

▶ HPV infections induce squamous cell and adenomatous cervical cancer. Cervical cancers of other histology are rare.

▶ Frequent spontaneous regression of HPV in young women as resulted in evolved screening guidelines.

General Considerations

Cervical cancer kills thousands of women each year in the United States, but mortality from this disease is largely preventable. High-risk HPV serotypes are known to trigger cervical cancer. Factors such as smoking, long-term OCP (oral contraceptive pill) use, immunosuppression, and parity influence either human papillomavirus (HPV) acquisition or natural history of disease progression.

Pathogenesis

The human papillomavirus triggers dysplastic changes.

Prevention

The CDC's Advisory Committee on Immunization Practices recommends routine vaccination of females aged 11 or 12 years with three doses of either HPV2 (Cervarix) or HPV4 (Gardasil) as early as 9 years old or as late as 26. The Centers for Disease Control and Prevention and the American Academy of Pediatrics also recommend vaccination of boys; it is unknown whether male immunization will further decrease transmission rates. Abstinence, monogamy, and use of barrier devices may reduce oncogenic viral transmission. Abstinence-only education programs may not reduce behaviors associated with HPV transmission. Smoking, family history of cervical cancer, high-risk sexual activity, personal history of vulvar/vaginal cancer, current use of OCPs, and immune suppression are other risk factors for cervical cancer.

Clinical Findings

Signs and symptoms often include heavy or irregular menstrual bleeding and/or postcoital bleeding. Advanced disease may manifest with pelvic pain.

Differential Diagnosis

A. Clinically Evident Disease

Abnormal vaginal bleeding/discharge and pelvic pain are initially evaluated through speculum and clinical pelvic examination in conjunction with infectious disease testing with or without colposcopy and focused biopsy, which may differentiate benign cysts, cervical infection/inflammation, and other noncancerous conditions from cervical cancer (**Figures 27-1–27-6**). Metastatic cancer can be further delineated through CT and/or MRI with or without PET and serological studies.

B. Preclinical Detection

Screening has dramatically lowered mortality rates. Precancerous cervical changes are identified through cytology. HPV testing guides further management of cytology results. Colposcopy examination and focused biopsy are used to evaluate concerning initial screening abnormalities. A biopsy result of CIN I (carcinoma in situ) is often associated with spontaneous disease remission in younger populations; CIN II and CIN III are precursors to invasive cancer, which entail closer follow-up. Certain diagnostic procedures such as biopsy and the loop electrosurgical excision procedure (LEEP)) may be simultaneously diagnostic and therapeutic. See **Table 27-4** for current screening and follow-up guidelines. Comprehensive guidelines, which include colposcopy follow-up recommendations, are regularly updated and published electronically by the American Society for Colposcopy and Cervical Pathology. Women with HIV positivity, organ transplant, and/or DES exposure should be considered for more frequent screening than low-risk women.

Complications

Bladder, bowel, and other pelvic organs may be locally invaded. Metastatic spread to the liver, lung, bones, and other distant organs may occur.

Treatment

Diagnosis of cervical cancer through LEEP and/or cone biopsy with negative margins may be therapeutic for early-stage carcinoma. Higher-grade cervical cancer is treated with surgery, brachytherapy, radiotherapy, and/or a chemotherapy regimen that includes cisplatin. Patients with recurrent nonoperative disease may be candidates for further cycles of chemotherapy, palliative care, or clinical trials.

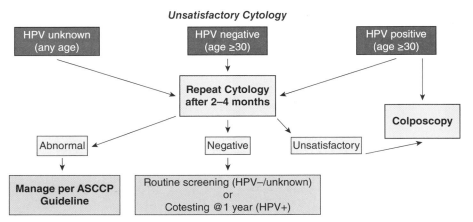

▲ **Figure 27-1.** Unsatisfactory cytology. (Reproduced with permission of American Society for Colposcopy and Cervical Pathology. Algorithms are updated consensus guidelines for managing abnormal cervical cancer screening test and cancer precursors, 2013.)

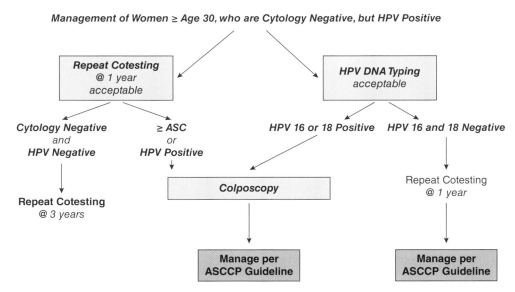

▲ **Figure 27-2.** Management of women aged ≥30 years who are cytology-negative, but HPV-positive. Acceptable meaning an acceptable strategy for further management. (Reproduced with permission of American Society for Colposcopy and Cervical Pathology. Algorithms are updated consensus guidelines for managing abnormal cervical cancer screening test and cancer precursors, 2013.)

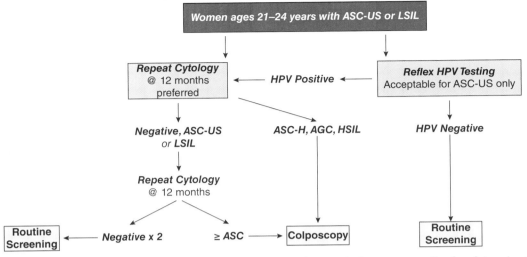

Management of Women Ages 21–24 years with either Atypical Squamous Cells of Undetermined Significance (ASC-US) or Low-grade Squamous Intraepithelial Lesion (LSIL)

▲ **Figure 27-3.** Management of women aged 21–24 years with either atypical squamous cells of undetermined significance or low-grade squamous intraepithelial lesion. (Reproduced with permission of American Society for Colposcopy and Cervical Pathology. Algorithms are updated consensus guidelines for managing abnormal cervical cancer screening test and cancer precursors, 2013.)

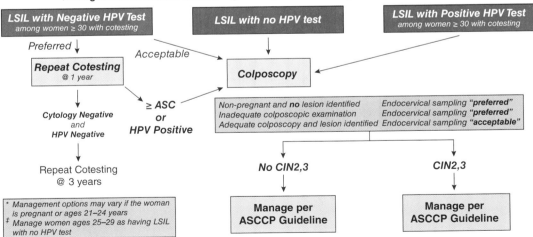

Management of Women with Low-grade Squamous Intraepithelial Lesions (LSIL)*‡

▲ **Figure 27-4.** Management of women with low-grade squamous intraepithelial lesions (variation in management options with pregnancy or aged 21–24 years). (Reproduced with permission of American Society for Colposcopy and Cervical Pathology. Algorithms are updated consensus guidelines for managing abnormal cervical cancer screening test and cancer precursors, 2013.)

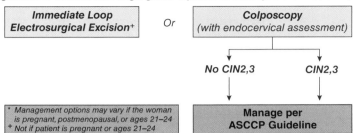

Management of Women with High-grade Squamous Intraepithelial Lesions (HSIL)*

▲ **Figure 27-5.** Management of high-grade squamous intraepithelial lesions (variation in management options with pregnancy or aged 21–24 years). (Reproduced with permission of American Society for Colposcopy and Cervical Pathology. Algorithms are updated consensus guidelines for managing abnormal cervical cancer screening test and cancer precursors, 2013.)

▶ **Prognosis**

Short-term disease-free survival is significantly shortened in women presenting with abnormal bleeding and/or pain compared to women identified through screening. The vast majority of invasive cancers identified through Pap smear screening are limited to nonmetastatic disease, with significantly increased rates of disease-free survival.

Brady M, Byington C, Davies H, et al. HPV vaccine recommendations; American Academy of Pediatrics Policy statement. *Pediatrics.* 2012;1(3):602-605. [PMID: 22371460]

Centers for Disease Control and Prevention. *HPV Vaccines* (available at http://www.cdc.gov/hpv/vaccine.html; updated Feb. 5, 2013; accessed July 2, 2013).

Hemminki K, Chen B. Familial risks for cervical tumors in full and half siblings: etiologic apportioning. *Cancer Epidemiol Biomarkers Prevent.* 2006;15(7):1413. [PMID: 16835346]

International Collaboration of Epidemiological Studies of Cervical Cancer, Appleby P, Beral V, et al. Cervical cancer and hormonal contraceptives: collaborative reanalysis of individual data for 16,573 women with cervical cancer and 35,509 women without cervical cancer from 24 epidemiological studies. *Lancet.* 2007;370(9599):1609. [PMID: 17993361]

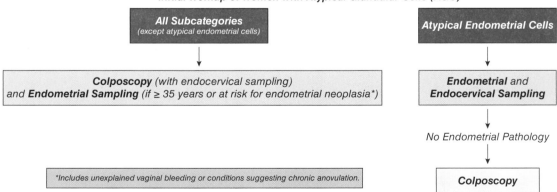

Initial Workup of Women with Atypical Glandular Cells (AGC)

▲ **Figure 27-6.** Initial workup of women with atypical glandular cells. (Reproduced with permission of American Society for Colposcopy and Cervical Pathology. Algorithms are updated consensus guidelines for managing abnormal cervical cancer screening test and cancer precursors, 2013.)

Table 27-4. Cervical cancer screening.

2012 Cytology Screening Recommendations	Initiation	Frequency[a]	Not Indicated
ACS/ASCCP/ASCP	Age 21 regardless of HPV immunization status	Every 3 years until age 29 Every 5 years with HPV cotesting is preferred over every 3 year screening for ages 30–65	Discontinue following hysterectomy for benign indication Discontinue < 65 with No CIN 2+ within past 20 years and with 3 negative Pap smears or 2 negative HPV tests within 10 years (most recent within 5 years)
USPSTF	Age 21 regardless of HPV immunization status	Every 3 years until age 29 Every 5 years with HPV cotesting or Pap alone every 3 years screening for ages 30–65 (no preference)	Discontinue following hysterectomy for benign indication Discontinue < 65 with No CIN 2+ within past 20 years and with 3 negative Pap smears or 2 negative HPV tests within 10 years (**most** recent within 5 years)

[a]Increased frequency for women with immunosuppression, HIV positivity, DES exposure.
ACS, American College of Surgeons; ASCCP, American Society for Colposcopy and Cervical Pathology; ASCP, American Society for Clinical Pathology.

Massad L, Einstein M, Huh W, et al. 2012 updated consensus guidelines for the management of abnormal cervical cancer screening tests and cancer precursors. *J Low Genit Tract Dis.* 2013;17(5 suppl 1):S1–S27. [PMID: 23519301]

Moyer VA. Screening for cervical cancer: US Preventive Services Task Force recommendation statement. *Ann Intern Med.* 2012;156(12):880–891. [PMID: 22711081]

National Cancer Institute. http://www.cancer.gov/cancertopics/factsheet/Sites-Types/metastatic (accessed March 20, 2012).

NCCN Guidelines Cervical Cancer version 2.2013. National Comprehensive Cancer Network. http://www.nccn.org/professionals/physician_gls/pdf/cervical.pdf; (subscription required) (updated Oct. 25, 2012; accessed March 9, 2013).

Saslow D, Solomon D, Lawson HW, et al. American Cancer Society, American Society for Colposcopy and Cervical Pathology, and American Society for Clinical Pathology screening guidelines for the prevention and early detection of cervical cancer. *CA Cancer J Clin.* 2012;62(3):147–172. [PMID: 22431528]

OVARIAN CANCER

 ESSENTIALS OF DIAGNOSIS

► Epithelial cell cancers represent the vast majority of ovarian cancers, usually affecting older women and having a poor prognosis.

► Germ cell, carcinosarcoma, borderline epithelial cell, and sex chord stromal cancers are rarer forms of ovarian cancer that affect younger women and have a better prognosis.

► Fallopian tube and primary peritoneal cancers are currently managed in a fashion similar to that for ovarian cancer.

► A gynecology oncologist should manage ovarian cancer.

► General Considerations

Epithelial ovarian cancer is the leading cause of gynecologic cancer death in the United States. Risk generally increases with age. Risk is reduced in women with early childbearing, breastfeeding, tubal ligation, or hysterectomy and/or OCP use, but is increased in women with endometriosis, infertility, or nulliparity and in women who delivered a first child at age ≥35 years.

Hormone replacement therapy has been associated with increased risk.

Women with family history of ovarian cancer are at higher risk, especially if BRCA-positive. Women with a history of breast, uterine, or colon cancer, as well as women of eastern European (Ashkenazi) Jewish descent, also have higher than average risk. Ovarian stimulation for IVF may increase risk for borderline epithelial cell cancer.

► Clinical Findings

Symptoms that are significantly associated with ovarian cancer are pelvic/abdominal pain, urinary urgency/frequency, increased abdominal size/bloating, and difficulty eating and feeling full (easily satiated) when these symptoms are present for <1 year and have occurred >12 days per month. Early symptoms are often missed because of their nonspecific nature. Advanced cancer may present acute symptoms of metastatic bowel obstruction or pleural effusion.

► Prevention

Prophylactic surgery and/or enhanced cancer screening in conjunction with genetic counseling may be beneficial in BRCA-positive women.

Differential Diagnosis

Ovarian cancer must be differentiated from other causes of abdominal mass and/or distension such as noncancerous ovarian conditions, gastrointestinal disease, lymphoma, and uterine or pancreatic cancers. Ultrasound with or without CT are used to further delineate the undiagnosed pelvic mass. Fine-needle aspiration of an ovarian mass should be avoided to prevent malignant seeding of the peritoneal cavity. Tumor markers and chest imaging are often obtained in the patient with a mass suspicious for ovarian cancer. Preclinical detection through CA-125 or other biomarker screening and/or ultrasound screening of asymptomatic women is not recommended.

Treatment

Select young women with very-early-stage ovarian cancer may be candidates for fertility-sparing surgery. Most cancers are treated with total abdominal hysterectomy and bilateral salpingo-oophorectomy in conjunction with staging laparotomy. Intraperitoneal therapy, debulking with cytoreduction surgery, and chemotherapy are used to treat advanced disease. Radiation therapy is used for palliative symptom control.

Complications

Complication of ovarian cancer include locally invasive disease and metastatic spread to the peritoneum, liver, and lungs.

Prognosis

Because most cancers are high-grade at the time of diagnosis, less than half of women with ovarian cancer are cured. However, for the small group of women diagnosed with isolated local disease, nonepithelial tumors, or borderline epithelial tumors, survival is very good.

Beral V. Million Women Study Collaborators, Bull D, Green J, et al. Ovarian cancer and hormone replacement therapy in the Million Women Study. *Lancet.* 2007; 369(9574):1703–1710. [PMID: 17512855]

Centers for Disease Control and Prevention. *Ovarian Cancer Risk Factors* (available at http://www.cdc.gov/cancer/ovarian/basic_info/risk_factors.htm; accessed March 29, 2013).

Colombo N, Peiretti M, Parma G, et al. Newly diagnosed and relapsed epithelial ovarian carcinoma: ESMO Clinical Practice Guidelines for diagnosis, treatment and follow-up. *Ann Oncol.* 2010; 21.S5:23–30. [PMID: 20555088]

Goff BA, Mandel LS, Drescher CW, et al. Development of an ovarian cancer symptom index: possibilities for earlier detection. *Cancer.* 2013; 109(2):221–7. [PMID: 17154394]

National Cancer Institute. http://www.cancer.gov/cancertopics/factsheet/Sites-Types/metastatic (accessed March 20, 2012).

NCCN Guidelines Ovarian Cancer version 1.2013. National Comprehensive Cancer. http://www.nccn.org/professionals/physician_gls/pdf/ovarian.pdf. (subscription required) (updated Oct. 12, 2012; accessed March 20, 2013).

van Leeuwen FE, Klip H, Mooij TM, et al. Risk of borderline and invasive ovarian tumours after ovarian stimulation for in vitro fertilization in a large Dutch cohort. *Hum Reprod.* 2011; 26(12):3456–3465. [PMID: 22031719]

UTERINE CANCER

ESSENTIALS OF DIAGNOSIS

- ▶ Cancers of the uterus include endometrial cancer and uterine sarcoma.
- ▶ Incidence increases with age.
- ▶ Commonly presents with abnormal vaginal bleeding.

General Considerations

Endometrial cancer is the most common gynecologic cancer in the United States; uterine sarcoma represents, 5% of all uterine cancers. Uterine cancer is more common in older women and typically presents with abnormal vaginal bleeding. Postmenopausal hormone replacement therapy, smoking, infertility/nulliparity and obesity, high-fat diet, and diabetes are risk factors. Tamoxifen, estrogen-secreting ovarian cancers, and polycystic ovary disease increase risk. Women with hereditary nonpolyposis colon cancer (HNPCC) syndrome have a ≤60% chance of endometrial cancer. A history of breast or ovarian cancer, or a history of pelvic radiation therapy, increases risk. Reduced number of lifetime menstrual cycles, pregnancy, OCP use, regular physical activity, and the use of nonhormonal IUDs also reduce the risk of endometrial cancer. Endometrial hyperplasia may progress to endometrial cancer.

Clinical Findings

Abnormal vaginal bleeding is the earliest sign of endometrial cancer, with advanced cancer potentially presenting as pelvic pain and/or mass.

Prevention

The American Cancer Society recommends educating women about risks and symptoms of endometrial cancer beginning at menopause. Total hysterectomy is preventive, but not indicated as a sole indication in low-risk women. Hysterectomy in conjunction with genetic counseling is considered for women with hereditary syndromes. There are no medications accepted for the prevention of uterine cancer.

Differential Diagnosis

A. Clinically Evident Disease

Abnormal vaginal bleeding may be caused by benign tumors such as polyps, benign hyperplasia, fibroids, infection, or other gynecological malignancy; endometrial biopsy is diagnostic. A negative office biopsy with clinical suspicion should be followed up by a dilation and curettage with or without hysteroscopy. Imaging can define extrauterine disease.

B. Preclinical Diagnosis

The American Cancer Society recommends offering annual endometrial biopsy beginning at age 35 to women with history of infertility, obesity, failure of ovulation, abnormal uterine bleeding, or use of estrogen therapy or tamoxifen. Women at high risk of endometrial cancer due to known or suspected hereditary nonpolyposis colorectal cancer (HNPCC)-associated genetic mutations should be routinely screened with endometrial biopsy beginning at age 35.

► Complications

Local invasion and metastatic spread to the liver, lungs, and peritoneum.

► Treatment

In premenopausal women with low-grade disease, ovary-sparing surgery is acceptable. Radiation therapy may afford symptom control and delay disease progression in inoperable patients. Postoperative symptoms of estrogen withdrawal may be treated with estrogen replacement, which does not

increase risk of relapse. Detailed current treatment guidelines are available through the National Comprehensive Cancer Network.

► Prognosis

Because of early presentation with abnormal bleeding, 75% of women diagnosed with endometrial cancer are diagnosed with noninvasive disease and have a good prognosis.

Beral V, Bull D, Reeves G, Million Women Study Collaborators. Endometrial cancer and hormone-replacement therapy in the Million Women Study. *Lancet.* 2005;365(9470):1543–1551.

Chronological History of ACS Recommendations for the Early Detection of Cancer in Asymptomatic People (available at American Cancer Society. http://www.cancer.org/healthy/findcancerearly/cancerscreeningguidelines/chronological history-of-acs-recommendations (accessed March 20, 2013).

Endometrial Cancer (available at American Cancer Society. http://www.cancer.org/cancer/endometrialcancer/detailedguide/endometrial-uterine-cancer-risk-factors (accessed March 29, 2013).

National Cancer Institute. http://www.cancer.gov/cancertopics/factsheet/Sites-Types/metastatic (accessed March 20, 2012).

NCCN Guidelines Uterine Neoplasms version 2.2013. National Comprehensive Cancer Network. http://www.nccn.org/professionals/physician_gls/pdf/uterine.pdf. (subscription required) (updated Feb. 21, 2013; accessed March 20, 2013).

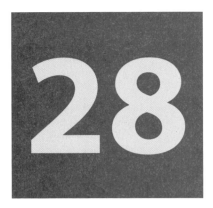

Respiratory Problems

Anja Dabelić, MD

Respiratory infections and chronic lung diseases are among the most common reasons why patients consult primary care physicians. Most respiratory problems encountered by primary care physicians are acute, with the majority comprising respiratory infections, exacerbations of asthma, chronic obstructive pulmonary diseases (COPDs), and pulmonary embolism (PE).

▼ UPPER RESPIRATORY TRACT INFECTIONS

COMMON COLDS/UPPER RESPIRATORY TRACT INFECTIONS

ESSENTIALS OF DIAGNOSIS

► Sore throat, congestion, low-grade fever, mild myalgias, and fatigue.

► Symptoms lasting for 12–14 days.

▶ General Considerations

Although colds are mild, self-limiting, and short in duration, they are a leading cause of sickness in industrial and school absenteeism. Each year, colds account for 170 million days of restricted activity, 23 million days of school absence, and 18 million days of work absence.

Most colds are caused by viruses. Rhinoviruses are the most common type of virus and are found in slightly more than half of all patients. Coronaviruses are the second most common cause. Rarely (0.05% of all cases) can bacteria be cultured from individuals with cold symptoms. It is not clear whether these bacteria cause the cold, are secondary infectious agents, or are simply colonizers. Bacterial pathogens

that have been identified include *Chlamydia pneumoniae,* *Haemophilus influenzae, Streptococcus pneumoniae*, and *Mycoplasma pneumoniae.*

▶ Prevention

The mechanisms of transmission suggest that colds can be spread through contact with inanimate surfaces, but the primary transmission appears to be via hand-to-hand contact. The beneficial effects of removing viruses from the hands are supported by observations that absences of children have been reduced through the use of antiseptic hand wipes throughout the day at school or daycare.

▶ Clinical Findings

Colds generally last 12–14 days. Reassurance and education to patients reduces misconceptions that symptoms lasting >1 week are abnormal. When the symptoms of congestion persist longer than 2 weeks, other causes of chronic congestion should be considered (**Table 28-1**).

Symptoms of colds include sore throat, congestion, low-grade fever, and mild myalgias and fatigue. In general, early in the development of a cold the discharge is clear. As more inflammation develops, the discharge takes on some coloration. A yellow, green, or brown-tinted nasal discharge is an indicator of inflammation, not secondary bacterial infection. Discolored nasal discharge raises the likelihood of sinusitis, but only if other predictors of sinusitis are present. Therefore education to patients and reassurance is needed, and not reflexive antibiotic prescriptions, which some patients ultimately desire.

▶ Complications

Primary complications from upper respiratory tract infection are otitis media and sinusitis. These complications develop from obstruction of the eustachian tube or sinus

Table 28-1. Differential diagnosis for congestion and rhinorrhea.

Common cold
Sinusitis
Viral
Allergic
Bacterial
Fungal
Seasonal allergic rhinitis
Vasomotor rhinitis
Rhinitis secondary to α-agonist withdrawal
Drug-induced rhinitis (eg, cocaine)
Nasal foreign body

ostia from nasal passage edema. Although treatment of these infections with antibiotics is common, the vast majority of infections clear without antibiotic therapy.

One misconception is that using antibiotics during the acute phase of a cold can prevent these complications. Evidence shows that taking antibiotics during a cold does not reduce the incidence of sinusitis or otitis media. Nor do antibiotics give a faster recovery than placebos.

▶ Differential Diagnosis

The differential diagnosis of colds includes complications of the cold such as sinusitis or otitis media, acute bronchitis, and noninfectious rhinitis. Influenza shares many of the symptoms of a common cold, but generally patients have a much higher fever, myalgias, and more intense fatigue.

▶ Treatment

Despite the widespread recognition that viruses cause common colds, several studies have shown that patients with the common cold who are seen in physicians' offices are often treated with antibiotics. The prescribing of antibiotics for colds occurs more often in adults than children. Although this practice appears to have declined in adults, the use of broad-spectrum antibiotics for colds is still common in children. The need to reduce the use of antibiotics for viral conditions has important ramifications on communitywide drug resistance; in areas in which prescribing antibiotics for respiratory infections has been curtailed, reversals in antibiotic drug resistance have been observed.

Currently, the most effective treatment is symptom reduction with over-the-counter (OTC) decongestants, the most popular of which include pseudoephedrine hydrochloride and topically applied vasoconstrictors. These agents produce short-term symptomatic relief. However, patients must be warned to use topical agents for a limited duration because prolonged use is associated with rebound edema of the nasal mucosa (rhinitis medicamentosa).

Several OTC medications contain a mix of decongestants, cough suppressants, and pain relievers. Again, the use of these preparations will not cure the common cold but will provide symptomatic reduction and relief.

Antihistamines, with a few exceptions, have not been shown to provide effective treatment. Zinc gluconate lozenges are available without a prescription, but a meta-analysis of 15 previous studies on zinc concluded that zinc lozenges were not effective in reducing the duration of cold symptoms.

Some herbal remedies are useful for treatment of the common cold. Echinacea, also known as the "American coneflower," has been purported to reduce the duration of the common cold by stimulating the immune system; however, evidence for its efficacy is mixed. Echinacea should be used for only 2–3 weeks to avoid liver damage and other possible side effects that have been reported during long-term use of this herb. Ephedra, also known as *ma huang*, has decongestant properties that make it similar to pseudoephedrine. Ephedra is more likely than pseudoephedrine to cause increased blood pressure tachyarrhythmia. This is especially true if used in conjunction with caffeine.

Linde K, et al. Echinacea for preventing and treating the common cold. *Cochrane Database Syst Rev.* 2006;(2):CD000530. [PMID: 16437427]

Mainous AG 3rd, et al. Trends in antimicrobial prescribing for bronchitis and upper respiratory infections among adults and children. *Am J Public Health.* 2003;93:1910. [PMID: 14600065]

SINUSITIS

 ESSENTIALS OF DIAGNOSIS

- ▶ "Double-sickening" phenomenon.
- ▶ Maxillary toothache and purulent rhinorrhea.
- ▶ Poor response to decongestants.
- ▶ History of discolored nasal discharge.
- ▶ Facial pain/pressure/fullness; increasing pain with bending forward
- ▶ Nasal congestion

▶ General Considerations

Sinusitis is most often a complication of an upper respiratory viral infection, so the incidence peaks in the winter cold season. Medical conditions that may increase the risk for sinusitis include cystic fibrosis, asthma, immunosuppression, and allergic rhinitis. Cigarette smoking may also increase the risk of bacterial sinusitis during a cold because of reduced mucociliary clearance.

Most cases of acute sinusitis are caused by viral infection. The inflammation associated with viral infection clears without additional therapy. Bacterial superinfection of upper respiratory infections (URIs) is rare and occurs in only 0.5–1% of colds. Fungal sinusitis is very rare and usually occurs in immunosuppressed individuals or those with diabetes mellitus.

► Clinical Findings

Acute sinusitis has considerable overlap in its constellation of signs and symptoms with URIs. One-half to two-thirds of patients with sinus symptoms seen in primary care are unlikely to have sinusitis. URIs are often precursors of sinusitis, and at some point symptoms from each condition may overlap. Sinus inflammation from a URI without bacterial infection is also common.

The signs and symptoms that increase the likelihood that the patient has acute sinusitis are a "double-sickening" phenomenon (whereby the patient seems to improve following the URI and then deteriorates), maxillary toothache, purulent nasal discharge, poor response to decongestants, and a history of discolored nasal discharge. Also on examination, patients will have tenderness to palpation of their sinuses and worsening pain with bending forward.

► Treatment

Nonsevere symptoms, such as mild pain and afebrile state of <7 days' duration should be treated with supportive care. Treatment would include analgesics, decongestants, and saline nasal irrigation. Narrow-spectrum antibiotics should be reserved for patients with no improvement in 7 days or worsening symptoms. No radiologic imaging is required. A rare complication of sinusitis to be aware of is orbital and/or intracranial bony involvement. If symptoms fail to improve with therapy course, consider referral to ENT. The effectiveness of antibiotics is unclear. Amoxicillin/clavulanate acid (ACA) is preferred over amoxicillin alone in treatment of children and adults, provided the patient is not allergic to the components. High doses of ACA at 90 mg/kgm daily in BID dosing is recommended for regions with >10% endemic rate of sinusitis, severe infection, children who attend daycare, a child <2 years old, an adult aged > 65 years, a recently hospitalized patient, any recent antibiotic use, or if a patient is immunocompromised. There are increasing rates of resistance to macrolides and septra and should not be used for empiric therapy. Alternatives if with allergy to ACA would be doxycycline, or levoflox/moxifloxacin. Treatment should be for 5–7 days for adults and 10–14 days for children on antibiotics for sinusitis.

Acute rhinosinusitis in adults. *Am Acad Fam Physicians.* 2011; 83(9):1057–1063.

Infectious Diseases Society of America (IDSA). IDSA clinical practice guideline for acute bacterial rhinosinusitis in children and adults. *Clin Infect Dis.* 2012 54(8):e72–e112.

American Academy of Pediatrics. Subcommittee on Management of Sinusitis and Committee on Quality Improvement: clinical practice guideline: management of sinusitis. *Pediatrics.* 2001;108:798. [PMID: 11533355]

Williams JW Jr., et al. Antibiotics for acute maxillary sinusitis. *Cochrane Database Syst Rev.* 2000;(2):CD000243. [PMID: 12804392]

INFLUENZA (ADULTS)

 ESSENTIALS OF DIAGNOSIS

► High fever.
► Extreme fatigue.
► Myalgias.

Diagnosis, treatment, and prevention of influenza in children are reviewed extensively in Chapter 5.

► General Considerations

Although most cases of the flu are mild and usually resolve without medical treatment within 2 weeks, some will develop complications. Currently, three types of viruses causing influenza have been identified in the United States: A, B, and C. Seasonal epidemics from influenza types A and B are seen every winter. Type C influenza usually causes a mild respiratory illness and is not responsible for epidemics. If a new strain emerges and infects a population, an influenza pandemic can result.

Influenza A is identified by two proteins on the virus surface: a hemagglutinin (H) and a neuraminidase (N). These proteins result in 16 different H subtypes and 9 different N subtypes. The A form of influenza can be further divided into strains. The two subtypes of influenza A found in humans currently are A(H1N1) and A(H3N2). In 2009, an influenza pandemic occurred when a very different strain of influenza A(N1H1) developed in humans. The influenza B is broken down by different strain, but not by subtypes.

► Prevention

Vaccination is the most effective prevention against influenza. The seasonal flu vaccination is a trivalent vaccine with each component selected to protect against one of the three main groups of influenza viruses circulating in humans. The influenza viruses in the seasonal flu vaccine are selected each year from surveillance-based forecasts about which viruses are most likely to cause illness in the upcoming season. The World Health Organization (WHO) recommends specific vaccine viruses for inclusion, but each country decides independently which strains should be included. The US Food and Drug Administration (FDA) determines which vaccine viruses will be used in US-licensed vaccines. Influenza vaccinations require annual dosing for adults and children aged >1 year. Therefore, the influenza vaccine does not cover all strains of the influenza virus, and patients who have received their annual vaccination can still develop influenza; this is an important education point for all patients. A complete listing of who should be immunized can be found on the Centers for Disease Control and Prevention's (CDC's) Advisory Committee on Immunization Practices (ACIP) website and others.

The spread of influenza is from person to person by sneezing or coughing. Therefore, everyday care to stay healthy can help prevent contracting the flu and/or spreading the flu to others. Simple steps, such as covering nose and mouth when sneezing or coughing with a tissue; avoiding touching mouth, nose, and eyes if sick; washing hands frequently with soap or germicide solution; and staying home if sick to avoid others, may help prevent the spread of influenza. Additionally, if a patient has been exposed to influenza by another, influenza antiviral prescription drugs can be used as chemoprophylaxis of influenza.

▶ Clinical Findings

The flu can last from 3 days to 2 weeks. Mild cases may be assumed to have the common cold and receive no medical treatment. Symptoms include high fever, extreme fatigue, and myalgias. Other symptoms associated with the flu include sore throat, rhinorrhea, cough, headache, and chills. Some people experience nausea, vomiting, and diarrhea. The diagnosis is most commonly clinical, but there are laboratory confirmation tests available with rapid influenza diagnostic tests (RIDTs), viral cultures, and immunoflourescence, and reverse transcription-PCR. Clinicians should realize that a negative RIDT result does not exclude a diagnosis of influenza, as sensitivities are 40–70%. When there is a clinical suspicion of influenza and antiviral treatment is indicated, the treatment should be started without waiting for results of additional influenza testing.

▶ Complications

Complications can lead to hospitalization and even death. These complications include, but are not limited to, otitis media, sinusitis, acute bronchitis, and pneumonia. Exacerbations of chronic illnesses such as asthma, congestive heart failure, and chronic obstructive lung disease are further complications of the flu.

▶ Differential Diagnosis

One must consider other viruses, such as the common cold viruses, which have many of the same symptoms in less severity.

Table 28-2. High-risk populations for flu-related complications.

- Children <5 years of age
- Adults >64 years of age
- Pregnant women
- Heart disease (heart failure, coronary artery disease, congenital heart disease, and others)
- Asthma
- Neurologic disorders (cerebral palsy, intellectual disability, developmental delay, spinal cord injury, epilepsy, muscular dystrophy, stroke, and others)
- Kidney diseases
- Liver diseases
- Blood disorders (sickle cell disease and others)
- Chronic lung disease (COPD, cystic fibrosis, and others)
- Endocrine diseases (diabetes mellitus and others)
- Metabolic disorders
- Immune deficiencies (people with cancer, HIV or AIDS, chronic steroid use, and others)
- Younger than 19 years on chronic aspirin therapy

▶ Treatment

People who develop flu symptoms should seek medical treatment as soon as possible, especially those in the high-risk group, as shown in **Table 28-2**. If treatment with antivirals is begun within 48 hours of the first signs or symptoms of illness, the patient gets the greatest benefit. These benefits include shortening the illness by at least 24 hours, preventing serious complications, and decreasing the likelihood of spreading the disease to others. Treatment with oseltamivir or zanamivir is effective against all forms of human influenza, including A (H1N1)/(H3N2), 2009 A(H1N1), and B. Two older medications, amantadine and rimantadine, remain susceptible to influenza A but not to B. The CDC recommends the use of oseltamivir or zanamivir at this time, due to the emergence of the new strain of A (N1H1). Treatment guidelines differ for age groups and high-risk groups. Therefore, it is important when considering treatment options to refer to the *Physician's Desk Reference* (PDR) to ensure that appropriate treatment is given. Symptomatic treatment can be given with an antipyretic for the fever and an anti-inflammatory for pain and myalgias.

Centers for Disease Control and Prevention (CDC). *2009 H1N1 Flu*; Feb. 12, 2010 (available at http://www.cdc.gov/h1n1flu/).

Centers for Disease Control and Prevention (CDC). *People at High Risk of Developing Flu-Related Complications*; Nov. 1, 2012 (available at http://www.cdc.gov/about/disease/high_risk.html).

Centers for Disease Control and Prevention (CDC). *Types of Influenza Viruses*; March 22, 2012 (available at http://www.cdc.gov/FLU/about/viruses/types.htm).

Centers for Disease Control and Prevention (CDC), Advisory Committee on Immunization Practices (ACIP). *Recommended Adult Immunization Schedule—United States 2011*; Jan. 28, 2011 (available at http://www.cdc.gov/vaccines/pubs/ACIP-list .htm).

Centers for Disease Control and Prevention [*MMWR, Recommendations and Reports* 60(1), Jan. 21, 2011]. *Antiviral Agents for the Treatment and Chemoprophylaxis of Influenza. Recommendations of the Advisory Committee on Immunization Practices (ACIP)* (available at www.cdc.gov/mmwr/pdf/rr/ rr6601.pdf).

▼ LOWER RESPIRATORY TRACT INFECTIONS

ACUTE BRONCHITIS

ESSENTIALS OF DIAGNOSIS

▶ Cough lasting >3 weeks.

▶ Fever, constitutional symptoms, and a productive cough.

▶ General Considerations

Viral infection is the primary cause of most episodes of acute bronchitis. A wide variety of viruses have been shown to cause acute bronchitis, including influenza, rhinovirus, adenovirus, coronavirus, parainfluenza, and respiratory syncytial virus. Nonviral pathogens, including M. *pneumoniae* and *Chlamydophila pneumoniae* (TWAR), have also been identified as causes.

The etiologic role of bacteria such as *H. influenzae* and *S. pneumoniae* in acute bronchitis is unclear because these bacteria are common upper respiratory tract flora. Sputum cultures for acute bronchitis are therefore difficult to evaluate because it is unclear whether the sputum has been contaminated by pathogens colonizing the nasopharynx.

▶ Clinical Findings

Patients with acute bronchitis may have a cough for a significant time. Although the duration of the condition is variable, one study showed that 50% of patients had a cough for >3 weeks and 25% for >4 weeks. Other causes of chronic cough are shown in **Table 28-3**.

Both acute bronchitis and pneumonia can present with fever, constitutional symptoms, and a productive cough. Although patients with pneumonia often have rales, this finding is neither sensitive nor specific for the illness. When pneumonia is suspected because of the presence of a high fever, constitutional symptoms, severe dyspnea, and certain

Table 28-3. Causes of chronic cough.

Pulmonary causes
Infectious
    Postobstructive pneumonia
    Tuberculosis
    Pneumocystis jiroveci (formerly, *Pneumocystis carinii*)
    Bronchiectasis
    Lung abscess
Noninfectious
    Asthma
    Chronic bronchitis
    Allergic aspergillosis
    Bronchogenic neoplasms
    Sarcoidosis
    Pulmonary fibrosis
    Chemical or smoke inhalation

Cardiovascular causes
Congestive heart failure/pulmonary edema
Enlargement of left atrium

Gastrointestinal tract
Reflux esophagitis

Other causes
Medications, especially angiotensin-converting enzyme (ACE) inhibitors
Psychogenic cough
Foreign-body aspiration

physical findings or risk factors, a chest radiograph should be obtained to confirm the diagnosis.

▶ Differential Diagnosis

Asthma and allergic bronchospastic disorders can mimic the productive cough of acute bronchitis. When obstructive symptoms are not obvious, mild asthma may be diagnosed as acute bronchitis. Further, because respiratory infections can trigger bronchospasm in asthma, patients with asthma that occurs only in the presence of respiratory infections resemble patients with acute bronchitis.

Finally, nonpulmonary causes of cough should enter the differential diagnosis. In older patients, congestive heart failure may cause cough, shortness of breath, and wheezing. Reflux esophagitis with chronic aspiration can cause bronchial inflammation with cough and wheezing. Bronchogenic tumors may produce a cough and obstructive symptoms.

▶ Treatment

Clinical trials of the effectiveness of antibiotics in treating acute bronchitis have had mixed results. Meta-analyses indicated that the benefits of antibiotics in a general population are marginal and should be weighed against the impact of excessive use of antibiotics on the development of antibiotic resistance as well as complications of developing *Clostridium difficile*.

Data from clinical trials suggest that bronchodilators may provide effective symptomatic relief to patients with acute bronchitis. Treatment with bronchodilators demonstrated significant relief of symptoms, including faster resolution of cough and return to work. The effect of albuterol in a population of patients with undifferentiated cough was evaluated, and no beneficial effect was found. Because various conditions present with cough, there may have been some misclassification in generalizing this finding to acute bronchitis.

Albert RH. Diagnosis and treatment of acute bronchitis. *Am Fam Physician.* 2010;82(11):1345–1350.

Bent S, et al. Antibiotics in acute bronchitis: a meta-analysis. *Am J Med.* 1999;107:62. [PMID: 10403354]

Braman SS. Chronic cough due to acute bronchitis. *Chest.* 2006; 129(1 suppl):95S–103S.

Smucny JJ, et al. Are antibiotics effective treatment for acute bronchitis? A meta-analysis. *J Fam Pract.* 1998;47:453. [PMID: 9866671]

COMMUNITY-ACQUIRED PNEUMONIA

 ESSENTIALS OF DIAGNOSIS

▶ Fever and cough (productive or nonproductive).

▶ Tachypnea.

▶ Rales or crackles.

▶ Positive chest radiograph.

General Considerations

Pneumonia is the cause of over 10 million visits to physicians annually, accounts for 3% of all hospitalizations, and is the eighth leading cause of death in the United States, per the American Lung Association. A variety of factors, including increasing age, increase the risk of pneumonia. Among the elderly, institutionalization and debilitation further increase the risk for acquiring pneumonia. Patients aged ≥55 years, smokers, and patients with chronic respiratory diseases are more likely to require hospitalization for pneumonia. Those with congestive heart failure, cerebrovascular diseases, cancer, diabetes mellitus, and poor nutritional status are more likely to die. Thus, age and comorbidities are important factors to consider when deciding whether to hospitalize a patient with pneumonia. These risk factors are summarized in **Table 28-4**.

Prevention

Pneumococcal pneumonia may be prevented through immunization with multivalent pneumococcal vaccine. There are currently two pneumococcal vaccines. The penumococal conjugate vaccine, PCV13, is currently recommended for all children aged <5 years and adults aged ≥19 years with certain medical conditions. The other is a 23-valent pneumococcal polysaccharide vaccine (PPSV23) and is indicated for all adults aged >65 years and children aged ≥2 years with high risk for disease (ie, diabetes mellitus, chronic pulmonary or cardiac disease, without a spleen, or with immunocompromise). The PPSV23 is also recommended for adults aged 19–64 years who smoke cigarettes or have asthma. Additionally, anyone who lives in a long-term care facility should be vaccinated. CDC recommends immunization of all patients with the following medical conditions: immunosuppressed patients, including those with human immunodeficiency virus (HIV) infection; alcoholism; cirrhosis; chronic renal failure; nephrotic syndrome; functional or anatomic asplenia (eg, sickle cell disease or splenectomy); cochlear implants; cerebrospinal fluid leaks; or multiple myeloma.

In addition to initial vaccination, clinicians should advise patients that the duration of protection is uncertain. For those at particularly high risk of mortality from pneumococcal pneumonia, such as patients with chronic pulmonary disease; lacking a spleen; or with chronic renal disease or nephrotic disease, functional or anatomic asplenia, or

Table 28-4. Risk factors associated with mortality in community-acquired pneumonia.

Category	Characteristics	Mortality	Location of Care
Very low risk	Age <60, no comorbidities	<1%	Outpatient
Low risk	Age >60, but healthy Age <60, mild comorbidity	3%	80% can be cared for as outpatient (depending on comorbidity)
Moderate risk	Age >60 with comorbidity	13–25%	Hospitalization
High risk	Serious compromise present on presentation (hypotension, respiratory distress, etc) regardless of age	50%	Intensive care unit

immunocompromising conditions, should receive a one-time revaccination after 5 years from their first vaccination. For patients aged >65 years, a one-time revaccination is also recommended if their last vaccination was earlier than 5 years ago or if they were <65 when they received their first vaccination.

Clinical Findings

The most common presenting complaints for patients with pneumonia are fever and a cough that may be either productive or nonproductive. As an example, in one study, 80% of patients with pneumonia had a fever. Other symptoms that may be suggestive of pneumonia include dyspnea and pleuritic chest pain. However, none of these symptoms is specific for pneumonia.

Symptoms of pneumonia may be nonspecific in older patients. Elderly individuals who suffer a general decline in their function, become confused or have worsening dementia, or experience more frequent falls should increase suspicion of infection. Elderly patients who have preexisting cognitive impairment or depend on someone else for support of their daily activities are at highest risk for not exhibiting typical symptoms of pneumonia.

The most consistent sign of pneumonia is tachypnea. In one study of elderly patients, tachypnea was observed to be present 3–4 days before the appearance of other physical findings of pneumonia. Rales or crackles are often considered the hallmark of pneumonia, but these may be heard in only 75–80% of patients. Other signs of pneumonia such as dullness to percussion or egophony, which are usually believed to be indicative of consolidation, occur in less than a third of patients with pneumonia.

Chest radiography is the standard for diagnosing pneumonia. In rare cases, the chest x-ray may be falsely negative. This generally occurs in patients exhibiting profound dehydration, early pneumonia (first 24 hours), infection with Pneumocystis, and severe neutropenia.

Microbiological testing for pneumonia is not very useful in relatively healthy patients with nonsevere pneumonia. Blood and sputum cultures are most likely to be beneficial in patients with risk factors for unusual organisms or who are very ill.

Differential Diagnosis

Other conditions such as postobstructive pneumonitis, pulmonary infarction from an embolism, radiation pneumonitis, and interstitial edema from congestive heart failure all may produce infiltrates that are indistinguishable from an infectious process.

Treatment

With the emergence of other pathogens causing pneumonia and the development of resistance to penicillin and other drugs in S. pneumoniae, treatment decisions have become more complex. The 2007 update to the Infectious

Table 28-5. Recommendations for empiric treatment of community-acquired pneumonia.

Treatment of patients not requiring hospitalization
No comorbidities or comorbidities but no recent antibiotic use: respiratory fluoroquinolone,[a] macrolide plus high-dose amoxicillin, or macrolide plus amoxicillin-clavulanic acid
With comorbidities and recent antibiotic use: respiratory fluoroquinolone, macrolide plus β-lactam (second- or third-generation cephalosporin or lactam-lactamase inhibitor)

Treatment of hospitalized patients not critically ill
β-lactam with or without a macrolide or respiratory fluoroquinolone

Treatment of critically-ill hospitalized patients
Pseudomonas *not suspected*: β-lactam with or without a macrolide or respiratory fluoroquinolone
Pseudomonas *possible*: antipseudomonal cephalosporin plus ciprofloxacin or antipseudomonal cephalosporin plus aminoglycoside plus respiratory fluoroquinolone

Other situations
Suspected aspiration: clindamycin or a β-lactam with β-lactamase inhibitor
Influenza superinfection: respiratory fluoroquinolone or β-lactam (second- or third-generation cephalosporin or lactam-lactamase inhibitor)

[a]Includes levofloxacin, sparfloxacin, and grepafloxacin.

Disease Society of America (ISDA) and American Thoracic Society (ATS) guidelines for the treatment of community-acquired pneumonia differ depending on the health and age of patients (ie, those aged ≥65 years), whether they have recently been treated with an antibiotic, and whether they are at risk for an aspiration pneumonia or influenza superinfection (**Table 28-5**). For patients with no serious comorbidities, the ISDA/ATS recommends a respiratory quinolone or an advanced macrolide plus high-dose amoxicillin [or amoxicillin-clavulanic acid (ACA)] as first-line therapy. If an antibiotic has been used recently, then either a respiratory quinolone or an advanced macrolide plus a second- or third-generation cephalosporin is a recommended option. If aspiration is suspected, the ISDA/ATS guidelines include a choice of ACA or clindamycin as initial treatment.

Suitable empiric antimicrobial regimens for inpatient pneumonia include an intravenous β-lactam antibiotic, such as cefuroxime, ceftriaxone sodium, or cefotaxime sodium, or a combination of ampicillin sodium and sulbactam sodium plus a macrolide. New fluoroquinolones with improved activity against S. pneumoniae can also be used to treat adults with community-acquired pneumonia. Vancomycin hydrochloride is not routinely indicated for the treatment of community-acquired pneumonia or pneumonia caused by drug-resistant S. pneumoniae.

Centers for Disease Control and Prevention (CDC). *Recommended Adult Immunization Schedule United States 2010*; Feb. 9, 2010 (available at http://www.cdc.gov/vaccines/pubs/ACIP-list .htm).

Ebell MH. Outpatient vs. inpatient treatment of community-acquired pneumonia. *Am Fam Physician.* 2006; 73:1425. [PMID: 16669565]

Mandell LA, et al. Infectious Diseases Society of America: update of practice guidelines for the management of community-acquired pneumonia in immunocompetent adults. *Clin Infect Dis.* 2003; 37:1405. [PMID: 14614663]

Ramanujam P, Rathlev NK. Blood cultures do not change management in hospitalized patients with community-acquired pneumonia. *Acad Emerg Med.* 2006; 13:740. [PMID: 16766742]

Vaccine Information Sheet (VIS) PCV13 from CDC dated 2/27/13; available at www.cdc.gov/vaccines/hcp/vis/vis-statements/pcv13.html

Vaccine Information Sheet (VIS) PPSV23 from CDC dated 10/06/09; available at www.cdc.gov/vaccines/hcp/vis/vis-statements/ppv.html

▼ NONINFECTIOUS RESPIRATORY PROBLEMS

ASTHMA

ESSENTIALS OF DIAGNOSIS

▶ Recurrent wheezing, shortness of breath, or cough.

▶ Histories of allergies in children.

▶ Increase in airway secretions.

▶ Airway constriction, obstruction, or both.

▶ Bronchospasm documented on spirometry.

▶ Dyspnea.

▶ General Considerations

Asthma is one of the most common illnesses in childhood. Risk factors for the development of asthma include living in poverty and being in a nonwhite racial group. Part of the difference in asthma rates noted among different races may be related to increased exposure to allergens and other irritants such as air pollution, cigarette smoke, dust mites, and cockroaches in less affluent families, but racial differences persist even after adjusting for socioeconomic status.

Allergy is an important factor in asthma development in children but does not appear to be as significant a factor in adults. Although as many as 80% of children with asthma also are atopic, 70% of adults aged <30 years and fewer than half of all adults aged 30 years have any evidence of allergy. Therefore, although an allergic component should be sought in adults, it is less commonly found than in children with asthma.

▶ Clinical Findings

In most cases, the diagnosis of asthma is based on symptoms of recurrent wheezing, shortness of breath, or cough.

Children with recurrent cases of "bronchitis" who experience nighttime cough or have difficulty with exercise tolerance should be suspected of having asthma. An additional history of allergies is useful, because 80% of childhood asthma is associated with atopy.

Formal spirometry testing can usually be accomplished in children as young as 5 years of age and can confirm the diagnosis of asthma. Both the forced expiratory volume in 1 second (FEV_1) and FEV_1 to forced vital capacity (FVC) ratio are useful in documenting obstruction to airway flow. Further confirmation is provided by improvement of the FEV_1 by ≥12% following the use of a short-acting bronchodilator. For a valid test, though, children should avoid using a long-acting β-agonist in the previous 24 hours or a short-acting β-agonist in the previous 6 hours.

In some patients with asthma, spirometry may be normal. When there is a high index of suspicion that asthma may still be present, provocative testing with methacholine may be necessary to make the diagnosis.

It is useful to stratify patients with asthma by the severity of their illness. The severity of asthma is based on the frequency, intensity, and duration of baseline symptoms; level of airflow obstruction; and the extent to which asthma interferes with daily activities. Stages of severity range from severe persistent (step 4), in which symptoms are chronic and limit activity, to mild intermittent (step 1), in which symptoms are present no more than twice a week and pulmonary function studies are normal between exacerbations (**Table 28-6**). Patients are classified as to severity on the basis of their worst symptom and frequency, regardless of whether they met all or the majority of the criteria in any category.

▶ Treatment

The approach to managing asthma relies on acute management of exacerbations, treatment of chronic airway inflammation, monitoring of respiratory function, and control of the factors that precipitate wheezing episodes. For all of these, patient and family education is vital.

Treatment of persistent asthma requires daily medication to prevent long-term airway remodeling. Mild, intermittent asthma may require therapy only during wheezing episodes. Guidelines for the management of asthma are based on the child's age (≤6 years) and are stratified by severity of illness. Guidelines for older children, adults, and younger children are provided in **Table 28-7**.

The treatment of exacerbations of asthma relies on fast-acting bronchodilators to produce rapid changes in airway resistance along with management of the late-phase changes that occur several hours after the initial symptoms are manifested. The failure to recognize the late-phase component of an acute exacerbation may lead to a rebound of symptoms several hours after the patient has left the office or emergency department. Corticosteroids are the mainstay for preventing the late-phase response.

Table 28-6. Classification of asthma severity.

Step	Symptoms	Nighttime Symptoms	Lung Function
Step 4 Severe persistent	Continual symptoms Limited physical activity Frequent exacerbations	Frequent	Forced expiratory volume in 1 second (FEV_1) or peak expiratory flow (PEF) & leq; 60% predicted PEF variability >30%
Step 3 Moderate persistent	Daily symptoms Daily use of inhaled short-acting β_2-agonist Exacerbations affect activity Exacerbations ≥2 times a week; may last days	>1 time a week	FEV_1 or PEF >60–<80% predicted PEF variability >30%
Step 2 Mild persistent	Symptoms >2 times a week but <1 time a day Exacerbations may affect activity	>2 times a month	FEV_1 or PEF ≥80% predicted PEF variability 20–30%
Step 1 Mild intermittent	Symptoms <2 times a week Asymptomatic and normal PEF between exacerbations Exacerbations are brief; variable intensity	≤2 times a month	FEV_1 or PEF ≥80% predicted PEF variability <20%

For patients with persistent symptoms (step 2 and higher), chronic therapy is required. The management of persistent asthma may include long-acting bronchodilators to control intermittent symptoms and nighttime cough, but also should provide chronic anti-inflammatory therapy to prevent long-term remodeling. Both inhaled steroids and nonsteroidal anti-inflammatory medications (ie, cromoglycates) can provide anti-inflammatory therapy. When symptoms are recurrent or large doses of anti-inflammatory agents are required, treatment with a leukotriene inhibitor can provide additional anti-inflammatory therapy and may allow a reduction in the dose of other anti-inflammatory agents such as steroids.

When drugs are selected for the treatment of asthma, the potential side effects of each agent need to be weighed against the potential benefits. For children, chronic use of inhaled steroids has been associated with a small decrease in total height attained. Although the difference in height attainment is small, it might be preferable to use nonsteroidal anti-inflammatory agents such as cromolyn and nedocromil in children.

In addition to pharmacologic management, patients with asthma should avoid known and possible airway irritants. These include cigarette smoke (including second-hand inhalation of smoke), environmental pollutants, suspected or known allergens, and cold air. Children who have difficulty participating in sports may benefit from the use of a short-acting β-agonist such as albuterol before participating in exertion to prevent wheezing or cough.

The monitoring of pulmonary function is an important component of asthma management for all patients with persistent disease. Children and adults should be provided with a peak-flow meter and instructed on how to use the device reliably. The use of a peak-flow meter can detect subtle changes in respiratory function that may not cause symptoms for several days. To use a peak-flow meter, patients must establish a "personal best," which represents the best reading that they can obtain when they are as asymptomatic as possible. Daily or periodic recordings of peak flows are compared with this personal best to gauge the current pulmonary function. Readings between 80% and 100% of the personal best indicate that the patient is doing well. Peak flows between 50% and 80% of an individual's personal best are cause for concern even if symptoms are mild. Patients should be instructed beforehand how to respond in these instances. If a repeat of the peak flow later in the day after appropriate measures have been taken does not show improvement, patients should seek further medical attention. Patients should be told that severe decreases in peak flow to <50% are cause for immediate medical attention.

For patients with allergic symptoms, the use of immunotherapy should be considered. However, although immunotherapy usually results in improvements in symptoms of allergic rhinitis, it seldom improves asthma symptoms.

Namazy JA, Schatz JM. Current guidelines for the management of asthma during pregnancy. *Immunol Allergy Clin North Am.* 2006; 26:93. [PMID: 16443415]

Siwik JP, et al. The evaluation and management of acute, severe asthma. *Med Clin North Am.* 2002; 86:1049. [PMID: 12428545]

CHRONIC OBSTRUCTIVE PULMONARY DISEASE

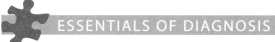 ESSENTIALS OF DIAGNOSIS

▶ Productive cough featuring sputum production for ≥3 months for 2 consecutive years.

▶ Chronic dyspnea.

▶ FEV_1 >80% predicted.

Table 28-7. Asthma drug therapy based on severity.

Step	Daily Medications	Quick Relief
	Ages 6 Years through Adulthood	
Step 4 Severe persistent	Choose all needed High-dose inhaled corticosteroid Long-acting bronchodilator A leukotriene modifier Oral corticosteroid	Short-acting bronchodilator Daily or increasing use of short-acting inhaled β_2-agonist indicates need for additional long-term control therapy
Step 3 Moderate persistent	Usually need two Either low- or medium-dose inhaled corticosteroid Long-acting bronchodilator	Short-acting bronchodilator Daily or increasing use of short-acting inhaled β_2-agonist indicates need for additional long-term control therapy
Step 2 Mild persistent	Choose one Low-dose inhaled corticosteroid cromolyn Sustained-release theophylline (to serum concentration of 5–15 µg/mL) A leukotriene modifier	Short-acting bronchodilator Daily or increasing use of short-acting inhaled β_2-agonist indicates need for additional long-term control therapy
Step 1 Intermittent	No daily medication needed	Short-acting bronchodilator Use of short-acting inhaled β_2-agonist >2 times per week indicates need for additional long-term control therapy
	Step Down	**Step Up**
	Review treatment every 1–6 months; a gradual stepwise reduction in treatment may be possible	If control is not maintained, consider step up; first, review patient medication technique, adherence, and environmental control (avoidance of allergens and/or other factors that contribute to asthma severity)
Step	**Daily Anti-inflammatory Medications**	**Quick Relief**
Step 4 Severe persistent	High-dose inhaled corticosteroid with spacer/holding chamber and facemask and, if needed, add systemic corticosteroids 2 mg/kg per day and reduce to lowest daily or alternate-day dose that stabilizes symptoms	Short-acting bronchodilator as needed for symptoms By nebulizer or metered-dose inhaler (MDI) with spacer/holding chamber and facemask or oral β_2-agonist Daily or increasing use of short-acting inhaled β_2-agonist indicates need for additional long-term control therapy
Step 3 Moderate persistent	Either medium-dose inhaled corticosteroid with spacer/holding chamber and facemask or low- to medium-dose inhaled corticosteroid and long-acting bronchodilator (theophylline)	Short-acting bronchodilator as needed for symptoms By nebulizer or MDI with spacer/holding chamber and facemask or oral β_2-agonist Daily or increasing use of short-acting inhaled β_2-agonist indicates need for additional long-term control therapy
Step 2 Mild	Young children usually begin with a trial of cromolyn or low-dose inhaled corticosteroid with spacer/holding chamber and facemask	Short-acting bronchodilator as needed for symptoms By nebulizer or MDI with spacer/holding chamber and facemask or oral β_2-agonist Daily or increasing use of short-acting inhaled β_2-agonist indicates need for additional long-term control therapy
Step 1 Intermittent	No daily medication	Short-acting bronchodilator as needed for symptoms <2 times a week By nebulizer or MDI with spacer/holding chamber and facemask or oral β_2-agonist Two times weekly or increasing use of short-acting inhaled β_2-agonist indicates need for additional long-term control therapy
	Step Down	**Step Up**
	Review treatment every 1–6 months; a gradual stepwise reduction in treatment may be possible	If control is not maintained, consider step up; first, review patient medication technique, adherence, and environmental control (avoidance of allergens and/or other factors that contribute to asthma severity)

General Considerations

Chronic airway disease is the second leading cause of disability in the United States after coronary artery disease. It is also fourth in the list of leading causes of death in the United States. Consistently more women died secondary to chronic obstructive pulmonary disease (COPD) than men. Symptoms of chronic bronchitis first develop when patients are between 30 and 40 years of age and become increasingly common as patients reach their 50s and 60s. The development of chronic bronchitis is associated with heavier cigarette use; those smoking over 25 cigarettes per day have a risk of chronic bronchitis that is 30 times higher than that for nonsmokers. Although chronic bronchitis affects both genders and all socioeconomic strata, it is more commonly observed in men and in those of lower socioeconomic classes. It is presumed that these populations may be at higher risk due to higher consumption of cigarettes observed in these groups.

In addition to smoking, air pollution may affect the development and exacerbation of symptoms in patients with chronic bronchitis. Patients with COPDs who live in industrialized areas with heavy levels of particulate air pollution may be at increased risk of recurrent disease and death.

Only 10–15% of smokers will develop COPD, so other factors must also play a role in the progression from acute to chronic lung damage. The development of chronic bronchitis is assumed to include both a predisposition to inflammatory damage and exposure to the proper stimuli that cause inflammation, such as cigarette smoke or pollutants. Genetic factors, prolonged heavy exposure to other inflammatory mediators such as environmental pollutants, preexisting lung impairment from other inflammatory processes such as recurrent infection or childhood passive smoke exposure, and other mechanisms may all predispose individuals to the development of chronic bronchitis from smoking.

α_1-antitrypsin deficiency is a rare genetic abnormality that causes panlobular emphysema in adults and is responsible for approximately 2–3% of cases of COPD. This trait is inherited in an autosomal-recessive pattern. Nonsmokers with this genetic defect develop emphysema at young ages. Those with this trait who smoke develop progressive emphysema at very early ages. Emphysema related to α_1-antitrypsin deficiency rarely shows up below age 25 and rarely in nonsmokers.

Clinical Findings

Chronic obstructive pulmonary disease includes both chronic bronchitis and emphysema, and these two often coexist. Chronic bronchitis is characterized by a productive cough featuring sputum production for ≥3 months for 2 consecutive years. Emphysema causes chronic dyspnea due to destruction of lung tissue, resulting in enlargement of airspace and reduced compliance. In most cases, chronic bronchitis and emphysema can be differentiated according to whether the predominant symptom is a chronic cough or dyspnea. In contrast to asthma, changes in COPD are relatively fixed and only partially reversible with bronchodilator use.

When suspected clinically, COPD can be confirmed with chest radiography and spirometry. Although chest radiographic findings occur much later in the course of the disease than alterations in pulmonary function testing, a chest x-ray may be useful in patients suspected of having COPD because it can detect several other clinical conditions often found in these patients.

Spirometry is generally used to diagnose COPD because it can detect small changes in lung function and is easy to quantify. Changes in the FEV_1 and the FVC can provide an estimate of the degree of airway obstruction in these patients. Symptoms of COPD usually develop when FEV_1 falls below 80% of the predicted rate. In addition, a peak expiratory flow rate (PEFR) of <350 L/min in adults is a sign that COPD is likely to be present.

Spirometry also is useful in gauging the severity of COPD. Decreases in FEV_1 on serial testing are associated with increased mortality rates (ie, patients with a faster decline in FEV_1 have a higher rate of death). The major risk factor associated with an accelerated rate of decline of FEV_1 is continued cigarette smoking. Smoking cessation in patients with early COPD improves lung function initially and slows the annual loss of FEV_1. Once FEV_1 falls below 1 L, 5-year survival is approximately 50%.

The United States Preventive Services Task Force (USPSTF) has recommended against the use of spirometry to screen asymptomatic adult patients for COPD, which carries a D recommendation.

Treatment

A. Nonpharmacologic Therapy

The first step in treating the patient with chronic bronchitis or COPD is to promote a healthy lifestyle. Regular exercise and weight control should be started and smoking stopped to maximize the patient's therapeutic options.

Smoking cessation is the first and most important treatment option in the management of chronic bronchitis or COPD. Several interventions to assist patients in smoking cessation are available. These include behavioral modification techniques as well as pharmacotherapy (see the next section). A combination of behavioral and pharmacologic approaches such as nicotine replacement appears to yield the best results. Even minimal counseling from the provider improves the effectiveness of the nicotine patch.

Once patients have stopped smoking, those who are hypoxemic with a Pao_2 (partial pressure of oxygen in arterial blood) of ≤55 mmHg or an O_2 saturation of ≤88% while sleeping should receive supplemental oxygen. Along with smoking cessation, home oxygen is the only therapy shown to reduce mortality in COPD. Continuous long-term oxygen therapy (LTOT) should be considered in those patients with stable chronic pulmonary disease with Pao_2 of <55 mmHg on room air, at rest, and awake. The presence of polycythemia, pulmonary hypertension, right heart failure, or hypercapnia (Pao_2 >45 mmHg) is also an indication for use of continuous LTOT.

Exercise and pulmonary rehabilitation may also be beneficial as adjunct therapies for patients whose symptoms are not adequately controlled with appropriate pharmacotherapy. Exercise and pulmonary rehabilitation are most useful for patients who are restricted in their activities and have decreased quality of life.

B. Pharmacotherapy

1. Smoking cessation pharmacotherapy—Multiple medications are available to assist with smoking cessation. Nicotine can be substituted 1 mg (1 cigarette) per milligram with the use of the patch, gum, or inhaler to help with symptoms of nicotine withdrawal. Patches and gum are both available over the counter as well as by prescription. Some evidence suggests that use of the patch and gum simultaneously enhances quit rates, but use of both is not approved by the Food and Drug Administration. Although all these products state that patients must not smoke while using nicotine replacement because of early case reports of myocardial infarction, more recent studies show that smoking is relatively safe when using nicotine replacement and may help reduce smoking before a patient actually quits. However, even at best, the cessation rate is only ~20–30% at 1 year.

Bupropion also is approved for smoking cessation as an adjunct to behavior modification. The main effect of bupropion is to reduce symptoms of nicotine withdrawal. Bupropion should be instituted for 2 weeks before the quitting target date. Then a nicotine substitute can be used in combination to maximize alleviation of symptoms of nicotine withdrawal. Because many patients with chronic bronchitis are already taking multiple medications, potential drug interactions and adverse effects must be considered before instituting therapy with bupropion.

A third agent to assist in smoking cessation is varenicline tartrate. Varenicline is a selective nicotine receptor partial agonist. The drug stimulates nicotine receptors to produce a nicotine replacement–type effect but also blocks the receptors from additional exogenous nicotine stimulation. Use of varenicline has been reported to achieve quit rates of 40% at 12 weeks and continuous quit rates of ~22% after 1 year, which was significantly more than either bupropion or nicotine replacement alone. Adverse effects of varenicline occur in 20–30% of patients and include nausea, insomnia, headache, and abnormal dreams but necessitated discontinuation of the drug in 2–3% of patients in clinical trials.

2. Bronchodilators—An anticholinergic agent such as ipratropium bromide is the drug of choice for patients with persistent symptoms of chronic bronchitis. Anticholinergic agents such as ipratropium bromide or tiotropium have fewer side effects and a better response than intermittent β-agonists. Although both of these agents have a delayed onset of action compared with short-acting β-agonists, the beneficial effects are prolonged. Ipratropium requires dosing several times a day; in contrast, tiotropium can be used once a day.

For patients with mild to moderately severe symptoms, intermittent use of a β-agonist inhaler such as albuterol is sometimes beneficial even without significant changes in their FEV_1. Adverse effects of β-agonist agents include tachycardia, nervousness, and tremor. Short-acting β-agonists may not last through the night; when nighttime symptoms develop, long-acting β-agonists such as salmeterol may be more useful. Levalbuterol, the active agent of racemic albuterol, has recently been studied and appears to have greater efficacy than albuterol with fewer side effects.

Combination inhalers of ipratropium bromide and albuterol have also been used in the treatment of patients with chronic bronchitis but have demonstrated only minimal changes in outcomes compared with single agents.

3. Antibiotics—Patients with acute exacerbations of chronic bronchitis pose a more difficult therapeutic dilemma. Many of these exacerbations are probably due to viral infections. However, a meta-analysis of studies using a wide range of antibiotics (ampicillin, sulfamethoxazole-trimethoprim, and tetracyclines) demonstrated some benefit from empiric use of antibiotics for exacerbations of chronic bronchitis.

4. Other agents—As symptoms increase, addition of inhaled β-agonists, theophylline, and corticosteroids may provide symptomatic relief of symptoms of chronic bronchitis. In a multicenter randomized placebo-controlled trial, patients who used inhaled fluticasone had improved peak expiratory flows, FEV_1, FVC, and midexpiratory flow. At the end of treatment, patients also showed increased exercise tolerance compared with the placebo group. Corticosteroids at a therapeutic dose of 60 mg/d for 5 days have been shown to provide some symptomatic relief for severe exacerbations.

Mucolytics have not been shown to be beneficial. Iodinated glycerol has not been shown to improve any objective outcome measurements.

Newer agents such as aerosolized surfactant also have been used to treat stable chronic bronchitis. A prospective randomized controlled trial showed a minimal but statistically significant improvement in spirometry and sputum clearance. However, the cost of such a treatment regimen is high and may not add any advantage to the underlying treatment.

For the treatment of cough, agents that may be of benefit for patients with chronic bronchitis include ipratropium bromide, guaimesal, dextromethorphan, and viminol.

Anabolic steroids have recently been used for patients who have severe malnutrition and in those in whom weight loss is a concern. These agents show some beneficial effects.

American Lung Association. *Chronic Obstructive Pulmonary Disease (COPD) Fact Sheet*; May 2014 (available at http://www.lungusa.org/lung-disease/copd/resources/facts-figures/COPD-Fact-Sheet.html).

Bach PB, et al. American College of Physicians—American Society of Internal Medicine; American College of Chest Physicians: management of acute exacerbations of chronic obstructive pulmonary disease: a summary and appraisal of published evidence. *Ann Intern Med*. 2001; 134:600. [PMID: 11281745]

Horsley L. Practice guidelines. ACCP guideline recommends diagnosis and management strategies for COPD. *Am Fam Physician*. 2008; 78(3).

Snow V, et al. Joint Expert Panel on Chronic Obstructive Pulmonary Disease of the American College of Chest Physicians and the American College of Physicians—American Society of Internal Medicine: evidence base for management of acute exacerbations of chronic obstructive pulmonary disease. *Ann Intern Med*. 2001;134:595. [PMID: 11281744]

Stephens MB, Yew KS. Diagnosis of chronic obstructive pulmonary disease. *Am Fam Physician*. 2008;78(1):87–92. [PMID: 18649615]

US Preventive Screening Task Force (USPSTF). *Screening for Chronic Obstructive Pulmonary Disease Using Spirometry*; March 2008 (available at http://www.ahrq.gov/clinic/uspstf08/copd/copdrs.htm).

EMBOLIC DISEASE

ESSENTIALS OF DIAGNOSIS

► Dyspnea.

► Hypoxia.

► Pleuritic pain.

General Considerations

Pulmonary embolism (PE) usually results from the mobilization of blood clots from thromboses in the lower extremities or pelvis. However, embolization of other materials, including air, fat, and amniotic fluid, also can obstruct the pulmonary vasculature. The symptoms of pulmonary embolism range from mild, intermittent shortness of breath or pleuritic chest pain to complete circulatory collapse and death.

The most common source of embolism is the disruption of thrombi formed in the deep veins. Mortality in untreated cases is 30% but can be reduced to 2% with prompt recognition and appropriate management. Recurrent pulmonary embolism carries a very high mortality in the range of 45–50%.

Strong risk factors for pulmonary embolism are leg or hip fracture, major general surgery, knee or hip replacement, spinal cord injury, and major trauma. Other risk factors include venous stasis, trauma, abnormalities in the deep veins, and hypercoagulable states. Hypercoagulability occurs with some cancers as well as with inherited conditions such as factor V Leiden mutation that results in resistance to the anticoagulant effects of protein C. Other congenital hypercoagulation disorders include protein C deficiency, protein S deficiency, and antithrombin III deficiency.

Hypercoagulation states also exist with the use of certain medications. Use of estrogens either as part of hormone replacement therapy or for contraception increases the risk by a factor of 3. The effects of these drugs are compounded in patients with factor V Leiden mutation. Pregnancy and postpartum states increase the risk of pulmonary embolism.

In addition, smoking appears to be an independent risk factor for deep-vein thrombosis (DVT) and pulmonary embolism. The presence of more than two of these risk factors places the patient at a synergistic increased risk for the development of venous thromboembolism.

Prevention

Because pulmonary emboli usually arise from lower extremity thromboses, prophylactic anticoagulation can be used to reduce the incidence of these thrombi in high-risk individuals. Both low-molecular-weight heparin products and unfractionated heparin are effective in preventing DVT. Selection of the agent and the dose is based on the risk. The decision to initiate VTE prophylaxis should be based on the patient's individual risk of thromboembolism and bleeding, and the balance of benefits versus harms. Risk factors for thromboembolism are inherited (eg, factor V Leiden mutation, prothrombin gene mutation, protein S or C deficiency, antithrombin deficiency) or are acquired (eg, surgery, cancer, immobilization, trauma, presence of a central venous catheter, pregnancy, medication use, congestive heart failure, chronic renal disease, antiphospholipid antibody syndrome, obesity, smoking, older age, history of thromboembolism). Although there are many tools for assessing thromboembolism risk, there is insufficient evidence to recommend one over the others. General evidence regarding risk factors also may be used to make decisions about the need for prophylaxis.

Heparin or a related drug can increase the risk of bleeding, especially in older patients; women; patients with diabetes mellitus, hypertension, cancer, alcoholism, liver disease, severe chronic kidney disease, peptic ulcer disease, anemia, poor treatment adherence, previous stroke or intracerebral hemorrhage, bleeding lesions, or bleeding disorder; and in patients taking certain concomitant medications.

Prophylaxis with heparin has been shown to significantly reduce pulmonary embolisms in hospitalized patients, although bleeding events were increased. In most patients, the clinical benefit of decreased pulmonary embolisms outweighs the risk of bleeding. Evidence is insufficient to conclude that these risks and benefits differ in patients with stroke, although prevention of recurrent stroke may be an added benefit in these patients.

The optimal duration of heparin therapy is unclear. The benefits and risks are not significantly different between low-molecular-weight heparin and unfractionated heparin, and fondaparinux (Arixtra) has not been directly compared with heparin. The choice of medication should be based on ease of use, adverse effect profile, and cost.

Use of graduated compression stockings was not shown to be effective in preventing VTE or reducing mortality, and can cause clinically important damage to the skin. Intermittent pneumatic compression may be a reasonable option if heparin is contraindicated, because evidence suggests that it is beneficial in patients undergoing surgery. However, the therapy has not been sufficiently evaluated as a standalone intervention in other patients.

In addition to preventing initial thrombi, the pulmonary embolism can be reduced through the use of a venacaval filter in patients with known thrombi and contraindications to long-term anticoagulation. The long-term impact of intravenacaval (IVC) filters has not been studied extensively. One study showed a complication rate, such as thrombi trapped in the filter or the filter tilting, malpositioning, or migrating, in nearly 50% of those who survived 3 years. However, given the high mortality rates from recurrent pulmonary embolism, the complication rates from long-term IVC filter insertion appear to be a worthwhile tradeoff in high-risk patients.

Clinical Findings

Patients with pulmonary emboli usually exhibit dyspnea and hypoxia, and often have pleuritic chest pain. However, other than hypoxia, most routine studies including chest radiographs may be normal. The clinical assessment of the patient should include the criteria in the Wells score looking at signs and symptoms consistent with DVT, different diagnosis less likely, a heart rate of >100 bpm, previous PE or DVT, surgery within the last 4 weeks or immobilization, current malignancy, and presence of hemoptysis. Scores placed patients in either a low, intermediate, or high probability of having a PE. The Christopher study (modified Wells study) further divided the scoring into PE likely or unlikely. Suspicious signs of embolism on a chest radiograph include a wedge-shaped infiltrate resulting from lobar infarction, new pleural effusion, or both. Confirmation of a pulmonary embolism is based on either demonstrating obstruction of vascular flow through pulmonary angiography, finding a mismatch of perfusion and ventilation, or visualization of a clot on spiral (helical) computed tomography (CT) scanning. Although pulmonary angiography is considered the gold standard, because of its invasiveness, spiral CT and ventilation-perfusion scan are usually employed to make the diagnosis. Of the noninvasive tests available, spiral CT has the best sensitivity for detecting pulmonary artery thrombi (95–100%), although it is not as useful in identifying subsegmental emboli.

D-dimer testing has been evaluated as a serum marker for pulmonary embolism or DVT. The presence of D-dimer is not specific for thrombotic disease because D-dimer also rises in other conditions such as recent surgery, congestive heart failure, myocardial infarction, and pneumonia. Although the presence of D-dimer is not useful in diagnosing thrombosis or embolism, the negative predictive value of the absence of D-dimer is very high (97–99%), so this test can be useful in ruling out embolism. Clinically predictive rules, such as the modified Wells, can be used together with the D-dimer test to identify those in the "PE unlikely" group who would not require further study. On the basis of these two tools, clinical assessment and laboratory test, those that fall into the "PE likely" category can be further evaluated with CT angiography or spiral CT.

Treatment

Options for management of patients with an acute pulmonary embolism include anticoagulation to prevent further embolism from occurring, clot lysis with thrombolytic agents, or surgical removal of the clot.

Patients without life-threatening embolism can be managed with acute anticoagulation with heparin followed by long-term maintenance on warfarin. Heparin may be administered as either unfractionated heparin or low-molecular-weight heparin. Unfractionated heparin is generally administered intravenously with the dosage rate titrated to produce a suitable anticoagulation state. The use of a weight-based nomogram for loading and maintenance dosing can improve the time to achieve adequate anticoagulation and reduce the risks of bleeding. The drawbacks of unfractionated heparin include the need for hospitalization to monitor coagulation status and administer the intravenous drug plus the possibility of thrombocytopenia associated with the use of this agent. Should bleeding occur as a complication of treatment with unfractionated heparin, stopping the heparin is the first step to stop further anticoagulation. If bleeding continues after stopping the heparin, protamine can be given to reverse the anticoagulation.

In contrast, low-molecular-weight heparin can be administered as a daily intramuscular dose without titration or frequent anticoagulation monitoring. As a result, low-molecular-weight heparin therapy usually can be provided in the patient's home.

To achieve long-term anticoagulation, warfarin should be started promptly at a dose of 5 mg/d. Starting with a higher dose of warfarin does not appear to achieve oral anticoagulation any faster or reduce the total number of days when heparin is needed. Heparin can be discontinued when a prothrombin time indicates that the international normalized ratio (INR) has reached 2.0–3.0. Should excessive anticoagulation resulting from administering warfarin and bleeding occur, vitamin K can be given to reverse the effect of warfarin.

The duration of anticoagulation for pulmonary embolism depends on whether the precipitating event is known and reversible or whether the cause is unknown. In situations in which the thrombosis and embolism are the result of an acute event such as an injury or surgery, treatment for 6 months is recommended. If the risk factor associated with the embolic event is not reversible, such as cancer or coagulation disorder, then lifetime anticoagulation is advisable. When a risk factor or event causing the embolism is not known, so-called idiopathic embolism, treatment with anticoagulants for 6 months is indicated.

The use of thrombolytic agents for pulmonary embolism is usually reserved for patients with extensive embolism who show hemodynamic instability. Thrombolytic agents available for use in this situation include urokinase, streptokinase, tissue plasminogen activator (tPA), and reteplase. Embolectomy is rarely performed and is reserved for patients in whom embolism is rapidly diagnosed and a very large embolism is suspected that completely occludes the pulmonary arteries. In most situations, this is treated as a "last ditch" effort to save the patient.

Geerts WH, Pineo GF, Heit JA, et al. Prevention of venous thromboembolism: the Seventh ACCP Conference on Antithrombotic and Thrombolytic Therapy. *Chest.* 2004; 126:338S–400S.

Gopinath A, Thomas R. *Pulmonary Embolism: Gildea of Cleveland Clinic Center for Continuing Education*; 2010 (available at http://www.clevelanclinicmeded.com/medicalpubs/diseasemanagement/pulmonary/pulmonary-embolism/).

Piazza G, Goldhaber SZ. Acute pulmonary embolism. Part I: epidemiology and diagnosis. *Circulation.* 2006;114:e28. [PMID: 16831989]

Piazza G, Goldhaber SZ. Acute pulmonary embolism. Part II: treatment and prophylaxis. *Circulation.* 2006;114:e42. [PMID: 16847156]

Qaseem A, Chou R, Humphrey LL, et al. Venous thromboembolism prophylaxis in hospitalized patients: a clinical practice guideline from the American College of Physicians. *Ann Intern Med.* 2011;155(9):625–632.

Takagi H, Umemoto T. An algorithm for managing suspected pulmonary embolism. *JAMA.* 2006;295:2603. [PMID: 16772621]

Evaluation & Management of Headache

29

C. Randall Clinch, DO, MS

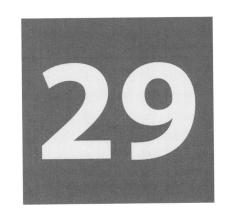

ESSENTIALS OF DIAGNOSIS

- ► Migraine.
  - ► Headache lasting 4–72 hours.
  - ► Unilateral onset often spreading bilaterally.
  - ► Pulsating quality and moderate or severe intensity of pain.
  - ► Aggravated by or inhibiting physical activity.
  - ► Nausea and photophobia.
  - ► May present with an aura.
- ► Cluster headache.
  - ► Strictly unilateral orbital, supraorbital, or temporal pain lasting 15–180 minutes.
  - ► Explosive excruciating pain.
  - ► One attack every other day to eight attacks per day.
- ► Tension-type headache.
  - ► Pressing or tightening (nonpulsating) pain.
  - ► Bilateral bandlike distribution of pain.
  - ► Not aggravated by routine physical activity.

General Considerations

Headache is among the most common pain syndromes presenting in primary care with a lifetime prevalence of >90% among adults. Population-based studies of US adults reveal that the prevalence of migraine and probable migraine is approximately 16%, with a female-to-male ratio of approximately 3:1. The prevalence among both genders is 31.2–38.3% for episodic and 2.2% for chronic tension-type headache. The main task before the primary care provider is to determine whether the patient has a potentially life-threatening headache

disorder and, if not, to provide appropriate management to limit disability from headache.

A distinction between primary headaches (benign, recurrent headaches having no organic disease as their cause) and secondary headaches (those caused by an underlying, organic disease) is practical in primary care. Over 90% of patients presenting to primary care providers have a primary headache disorder. These disorders include migraine (with and without aura), tension-type headache, and cluster headache. Secondary headache disorders constitute the minority of presentations; however, given that their underlying etiology may range from sinusitis to subarachnoid hemorrhage, these headache disorders often present the greatest diagnostic challenge to the practicing clinician. The International Headache Society provides a detailed classification of primary and secondary headache disorders on their website http://ihs-classification.org/en/02_klassifikation/.

Green MW. Secondary headaches. *Continuum.* 2012;18(4): 783–795. [22868541]

Kaniecki RG. Tension-type headache. *Continuum.* 2012;18(4): 823–834. [PMID: 22868544]

Sahler K. Epidemiology and cultural differences in tension-type headache. *Curr Pain Headache Rep.* 2012;16:525–532. [PMID: 22948318]

Smitherman TA, et al. The prevalence, impact, and treatment of migraine and severe headaches in the United States: a review of statistics from national surveillance studies. *Headache.* 2013;53(3):427–436. [PMID: 23470015]

Clinical Findings

A. Symptoms and Signs

1. History—The majority of patients presenting with headache have a normal neurologic and general physical examination; for this reason, the headache history is of utmost importance (**Table 29-1**). A key issue in the headache history is identifying patients presenting with "red flags"—diagnostic alarms

Table 29-1. Questions to ask when obtaining a headache history.

H:	How severe is your headache on a scale of 1–10 (1 = minimal pain, 10 = severe pain)? How did this headache start (gradually, suddenly, other)? How long have you had this headache?
E:	Ever had headaches before? Ever had a headache this bad before (first or worst headache)? Ever have headaches just like this one in the past?
A:	Any other symptoms noted before or during your headache? Any symptoms right now?
D:	Describe the quality of your pain (throbbing, stabbing, dull, other). Describe the location of your pain. Describe where your pain radiates. Describe any other medical problems you may have. Describe your use of medications (prescription and over-the-counter products). Describe any history of recent trauma or any medical or dental procedures.

that prompt greater concern for the presence of a secondary headache disorder and a greater potential need for additional laboratory evaluation and neuroimaging (**Table 29-2**).

The onset of primary headache disorders is usually between 20 and 40 years of age; however, they may occur at any age. Patients without a history of headaches who present with a new-onset headache outside this age range should be considered at higher risk for a secondary headache disorder. Additional testing or neuroimaging in these patients or those complaining of their "first or worst" headache should be seriously considered. Temporal (giant cell) arteritis should be a consideration in any patient aged ≥50 years with a new complaint of head, facial, or scalp pain, diplopia, or jaw claudication.

Symptoms suggesting a recurring, transient neurologic event, typically lasting 30–60 minutes and preceding headache onset, strongly suggest the presence of an aura and an associated migraine headache disorder. Migraine without aura, the most common form of migraine (formerly called *common migraine*), may present with unilateral pain in the head (cephalalgia) with subsequent generalization of pain to the entire head. Bilateral cephalalgia is present in a small percentage of migraineurs at the onset of their headache. Nausea accompanying a migraine may be debilitating and warrant specific treatment. After excluding secondary headache disorders, the combination of disability, nausea, and sensitivity to light has a positive predictive value of 0.93 for migraine headache among primary care patients.

Cluster headaches are strictly unilateral in location and are typically described as an explosive, deep, excruciating pain. They are associated with ipsilateral autonomic signs and symptoms, and have a much greater prevalence in men.

Tension-type headaches, the most prevalent form of primary headache disorder, often present with pericranial

Table 29-2. Red flags in the evaluation of acute headaches in adults.

Red Flag	Potential Etiologies	Possible Evaluation
Headache beginning at age >50 years	Temporal arteritis, tumor/mass	Erythrocyte sedimentation rate, CT with contrast vs MRI
Headache of sudden onset	Subarachnoid hemorrhage, pituitary hemorrhage, expansion or hemorrhage of ateriovenous malformation (AVM)	CT without contrast (to assess for acute bleed), lumbar puncture if computed tomography is negative
Headaches increasing in frequency and severity	Expansion of AVM or mass, subdural hematoma, medication overuse	CT with contrast vs MRI, urine drug screen
New-onset headache in immunocompromised patient (eg, HIV, cancer)	Meningitis, brain abscess, metastatic disease	CT with contrast vs MRI, lumbar puncture if neuroimaging is negative
Headache with signs of systemic illness (eg, fever, still neck, rash)	Meningitis, encephalitis, Lyme disease, systemic infection, collagen vascular disease	CT with contrast vs MRI, lumbar puncture, serology
Focal neurologic signs or symptoms (other than typical aura)	Mass/tumor, AVM, ischemic/hemorrhagic stroke, collagen vascular disease	CT with contrast vs MRI, serologic evaluation for collagen vascular disease evaluation
Papilledema	Mass/tumor, benign intracranial hypertension, meningitis	CT with contrast vs MRI, lumbar puncture
Posttraumatic headache	Intracranial hemorrhage, subdural hematoma, epidural hematoma, posttraumatic headache	CT vs MRI of brain, skull, and, possibly cervical spine

muscle tenderness and a description of a bilateral bandlike distribution of the pain.

Patients with chronic medical conditions have a greater possibility of having an organic cause of their headache (see Table 29-2). Patients with cancer, hypertension (with diastolic pressures >110 mmHg), or human immunodeficiency virus (HIV) infection may present with central nervous system (CNS) metastases, lymphoma, toxoplasmosis, or meningitis as the etiology of their headache. Numerous medications have headache as a reported adverse effect, and medication overuse headache (formerly drug-induced headache) may occur following frequent use of analgesics or any antiheadache medication, including the triptans (eg, sumatriptan). The duration and severity of withdrawal headache following discontinuation of the medication varies with the medication itself; withdrawal is shortest for triptans (4.1 days) compared with ergots (6.7 days) or analgesics (9.5 days), respectively. Medical or dental procedures (lumbar punctures, rhinoscopy, tooth extraction, etc) may be associated with postprocedure headaches. Any history of head trauma or loss of consciousness should prompt concern for an intracranial hemorrhage in addition to a postconcussive disorder.

2. Physical examination—Physical examination is performed to attempt to identify a secondary, organic cause for the patient's headache. Additionally, any red flags identified during the headache history (see Table 29-2) warrant special attention. A general physical examination should be performed, including vital signs; general appearance; and examinations of the head, eyes (including a funduscopic examination), ears, nose, throat, teeth, neck, and cardiovascular regions. Palpation of the head, face, and neck should also be a priority.

A detailed neurologic examination should be performed and the findings well documented. Assessment includes mental status testing; level of consciousness; pupillary responses; gait; coordination and cerebellar function; motor strength; sensory, deep tendon, and pathologic reflex testing; and cranial nerve tests. The presence or absence of meningeal irritation should be sought. Examinations such as evaluation for Kernig and Brudzinski signs should be documented; both signs may be absent, however, even in the presence of subarachnoid hemorrhage.

B. Laboratory Findings and Imaging Studies

Additional laboratory investigations should be driven by the history and any red flags that have been identified (see Table 29-2). The routine use of electroencephalography is not warranted in the evaluation of the patient with headache. Although various characteristics may lead to selection of either computed tomography (CT) or magnetic resonance imaging (MRI) (**Table 29-3**), routine use of neuroimaging is not cost-effective.

The US Headache Consortium has provided evidence-based guidelines on neuroimaging in the patient with nonacute

Table 29-3. Computerized tomographic scans versus magnetic resonance imaging in patients with headaches.

CT Scan	MRI
Need to identify an acute hemorrhage	Need to evaluate the posterior fossa
Generally more readily available at most medical centers	More sensitive at identifying pathologic intracranial processes[a]
Generally less expensive at most medical centers	

[a]Increased sensitivity may not correlate with an improved health outcome and may be associated with identifying more clinically insignificant findings.

headache. They revealed the prevalence of patients with a normal neurologic examination, and migraine having a significant abnormality (acute cerebral infarct, neoplastic disease, hydrocephalus, or vascular abnormalities, eg, aneurysm or arteriovenous malformation) on a neuroimaging test is 0.2%. Their recommendations are as follows:

- Neuroimaging should be considered in patients with nonacute headache and an unexplained abnormal finding on neurologic examination.

- Evidence is insufficient to make specific recommendations in the presence or absence of neurologic symptoms.

- Neuroimaging is seldom warranted for patients with migraine and normal neurologic examination. For patients with atypical headache features or patients who do not fulfill the strict definition of migraine (or have some additional risk factor), a lower threshold for neuroimaging may be applied.

- Data were insufficient to yield an evidence-based recommendation regarding the use of neuroimaging for tension-type headache.

- Data were insufficient to yield any evidence-based recommendations regarding the relative sensitivity of MRI compared with CT in the evaluation of migraine or other nonacute headache.

Although the US Headache Consortium based the preceding recommendations on a review of the best available evidence, clinicians must individualize management plans to meet a variety of needs, including addressing patient fears and medicolegal concerns.

Within the first 48 hours of acute headache, CT scanning without contrast medium followed, if negative, by lumbar puncture and cerebrospinal fluid (CSF) analysis, is the preferred approach to attempt to diagnose subarachnoid hemorrhage. Xanthochromia, a yellow discoloration detectable on spectrophotometry, may aid in diagnosis if the CT scan and CSF analysis are normal yet if suspicion of subarachnoid hemorrhage remains high. Xanthochromia may persist for ≤1 week following a subarachnoid hemorrhage.

In addition to CSF analysis, lumbar puncture is useful for documenting abnormalities of CSF pressure in the setting of headache. Headaches are associated with low CSF pressure (<90 mm H_2O as measured by a manometer) and elevated CSF pressure (>200–250 mm H_2O). Headaches related to CSF hypotension include those caused by post-traumatic leakage of CSF (ie, after lumbar puncture or CNS trauma). Headaches related to CSF hypertension include those associated with idiopathic intracranial hypertension and CNS space–occupying lesions (ie, tumor, infectious, mass, hemorrhage).

Abrams BM. Medication overuse headaches. *Med Clin North Am.* 2013;97(2):337–352. [PMID: 23419631]

Ashkenazi A, Schwedt T. Cluster headache–acute and prophylactic therapy. *Headache.* 2011;51(2):272–286. [PMID: 21284609]

Kaniecki RG. Tension-type headache. *Continuum.* 2012;18(4):823–834. [PMID: 22868544]

Langer-Gould AM, et al. The American Academy of Neurology's top five choosing wisely recommendations. *Neurology.* 2013;81(11):1004–1011. [PMID: 23430685]

Lester MS, Liu BP. Imaging in the evaluation of headache. *Med Clin North Am.* 2013;97(2):243–265. [PMID: 23419624]

Peng KP, Wang SJ. Migraine diagnosis: screening items, instruments, and scales. *Acta Anaesthesiol Taiwan.* 2012;50(2):69–73. [PMID: 22769861]

▶ Differential Diagnosis

In addition to migraine, tension-type, and cluster headaches, the differential diagnosis for acute headaches in adults is presented in Table 29-2.

▶ Treatment

Treatment of headache is best individualized with respect to a thorough history, physical examination, and the interpretation of appropriate ancillary testing. Secondary headaches require accurate diagnosis and therapy directed at the underlying etiology (see Tables 29-2 and 29-3). Nonpharmacologic measures and cognitive behavioral therapy (CBT) are worth consideration in most patients with primary headache disorders. CBT may have a prophylactic effect in migraine similar to propranolol (an approximate 50% reduction). Cluster headache, chronic tension-type headache, and medication overuse headache respond poorly to CBT as monotherapy. The evidence for a benefit of acupuncture in preventive migraine and tension-type headache treatment now reveals it to be an effective prophylactic option. A systematic review [six total randomized controlled trials (RCTs)] revealed no positive effect of various manual therapies in the treatment of tension-type headache.

A. Migraine

The US Headache Consortium lists the following general management guidelines for treatment of migraine patients:

- Educate migraine sufferers about their condition and its treatment, and encourage them to participate in their own management.

- Use migraine-specific agents [triptans, dihydroergotamine (DHE), ergotamine, etc] in patients with more severe migraine and in those whose headaches respond poorly to nonsteroidal anti-inflammatory drugs (NSAIDs) or combination analgesics such as aspirin plus acetaminophen plus caffeine.

- Select a nonoral route of administration for patients whose migraines present early with nausea or vomiting as a significant component of the symptom complex.

- Consider a self-administered rescue medication for patients with severe migraine who do not respond well to (or fail) other treatments.

- Guard against medication overuse headache (the terms *rebound headache* and *drug-induced headache* are sometimes used interchangeably with *medication overuse headache*; however, the latter is the recommended terminology).

Pharmacologic treatment options are numerous in the management of migraine headache. Effective acute/abortive treatment options include an oral, intranasal, or subcutaneous triptan (eg, sumatriptan), intravenous (DHE 45), or intranasal (Migranal) DHE, and intravenous antiemetics (eg, prochlorperazine, metoclopramide, promethazine). On the basis of available evidence, first-line use of these agents is preferred over the commonly used meperidine (or other narcotic analgesics) or ketorolac in abortive migraine treatment. A meta-analysis of seven RCTs (pooled data on 742 patients) of the addition of dexamethasone to standard acute migraine treatment in the emergency department (ED) setting revealed a moderate benefit [relative risk (RR) = 0.87, 95% confidence interval (CI) = 0.80—0.95] to reducing the risk of having a moderate or severe migraine headache at 24–72 hours after ED evaluation.

The goal of therapy in migraine prophylaxis is a reduction in the severity and frequency of headache by ≥50%. The strongest evidence surrounds the use of amitriptyline, propranolol, timolol, and divalproex sodium for migraine prevention. Topiramate also has proven prophylactic effects in migraine treatment. Botulinum toxin A has been found to lead to a reduction in headache days for chronic migraines and chronic daily headaches but not for episodic migraine.

B. Tension-Type Headache

Initial medical therapy of episodic tension-type headache often includes aspirin, acetaminophen, or NSAIDs. Avoidance of habituating, caffeine-containing over-the-counter (OTC) or prescription drugs as well as butalbital-, codeine-, or ergotamine-containing preparations (including combination products) is recommended given the significant risk of developing drug dependence or medication overuse headache.

Similar general management principles for treatment of migraine headaches can be applied to the treatment of chronic tension-type headaches. In a randomized placebo-controlled trial of tricyclic antidepressant use (amitriptyline hydrochloride, ≤ 100 mg/d or nortriptyline hydrochloride ≤ 75 mg/d) and stress management (eg, relaxation, cognitive coping) therapy, combined therapy produced a statistically and clinically greater reduction ($\geq 50\%$) in headache activity. A meta-analysis of antidepressant treatment (eg, tricyclic antidepressants, serotonin antagonists, and selective serotonin reuptake inhibitors) of chronic headache (eg, migraine, tension-type, or both) revealed that treated study participants were twice as likely to report headache improvement and consumed less analgesic medication than nontreated patients. Other considerations for prophylaxis of chronic tension-type headaches include calcium channel blockers and β-blockers. Botulinum toxin A use is not associated with an improvement in the frequency of either chronic or episodic tension-type headaches.

C. Cluster Headache

Acute management of cluster headache includes the use of sumatriptan in either its subcutaneous (FDA-approved indication), intranasal, or oral forms (the latter two are less effective), intranasal zolmitriptan, 100% oxygen at 7–10 L/min via face mask, and intranasal lidocaine. Verapamil, lithium, divalproex sodium, gabapentin, lithium, melatonin (possibly), topiramate (possibly), methysergide, and prednisone may be considered for prophylaxis. Because of side effects related to chronic use, methysergide and prednisone should be used with caution.

D. Referral

Referral to a headache specialist should be considered for patients whose findings are difficult to classify into a primary or secondary headache disorder. Additionally, referral is often warranted in cases of daily or intractable headache, drug rebound, habituation, or medication overuse headache, or in any scenario in which the primary care provider feels uncomfortable in making a diagnosis or offering appropriate treatment. Patients who request referral, who do not respond to treatment, or whose condition continues to worsen should be considered for referral.

Ashkenazi A, Schwedt T. Cluster headache–acute and prophylactic therapy. *Headache.* 2011;51(2):272–286. [PMID: 21284609]

Chaibi A, Russell MB. Manual therapies for cervicogenic headache: a systematic review. *J Headache Pain.* 2012;13(5): 351–359. [PMID: 22460941]

Haghshenas SM, et al. High-flow oxygen for treatment of cluster headache: a randomized trial. *JAMA.* 2009;302(22):2451–2457. [PMID: 19996400]

Jackson JL, et al. Botulinum toxin A for prophylactic treatment of migraine and tension headaches in adults: a meta-analysis. *JAMA.* 2012;307(16):1736–1745. [PMID: 22535858]

Kelly NE, Tepper DE. Rescue therapy for acute migraine, part 3: opoids, NSAIDs, steroids, and post-discharge medications. *Headache.* 2012;52(3):467–482. [PMID: 22404708]

Linde K, et al. Acupuncture for migraine prophylaxis. *Cochrane Database Syst Rev.* 2009;(1):CD001218. [PMID: 19160193]

Linde K, et al. Acupuncture for tension-type headache. *Cochrane Database Syst Rev.* 2009;(1):CD007587. [PMID: 19160338]

Linde K, et al. Topiramate for the prophylaxis of episodic migraine in adults. *Cochrane Database Syst Rev.* 2013;(6):CD010610. [PMID: 23797676]

Mauskop A. Nonmedication, alternative, and complementary treatments for migraine. *Continuum.* 2012;18(4):796–806. [PMID: 22868542]

Mulleners WM, Chronicle EP. Anticonvulsants in migraine prophylaxis: a Cochrane review. *Cephalalgia.* 2008;28(6):585–597. [PMID 18454787]

Singh A, et al. Does the addition of dexamethasone to standard therapy for acute migraine headache decrease the incidence of recurrent headache for patients treated in the emergency department? A meta-analysis and systematic review of the literature. *Acad Emerg Med.* 2008;15:1223. [PMID: 18976336]

Osteoporosis

Jeannette E. South-Paul, MD

General Considerations

Osteoporosis is a public health problem affecting more than 40 million people, one-third of postmenopausal women and a substantial portion of the elderly in the United States and almost as many in Europe and Japan. An additional 54% of postmenopausal women have low bone density measured at the hip, spine, or wrist. Osteoporosis results in approximately 1,500,000 fractures annually in women in the United States alone, as well as in men. At least 90% of all hip and spine fractures among elderly women are a consequence of osteoporosis. The direct expenditures for osteoporotic fractures have increased during the past decade from $5 billion to almost $15 billion per year. The number of women experiencing osteoporotic fractures annually exceeds the number diagnosed with heart attack, stroke, and breast cancer combined. Thus, family physicians and other primary care providers will (1) frequently care for patients with subclinical osteoporosis, (2) recognize the implications of those who present with osteoporosis-related fractures, and (3) determine when to implement prevention for younger people.

The female-to-male fracture ratios are reported to be 7:1 for vertebral fractures, 1.5:1 for distal forearm fractures, and 2:1 for hip fractures. Approximately 30% of hip fractures in persons aged ≥65 years occur in men. Osteoporosis-related fractures in older men are associated with lower femoral neck bone mineral density (BMD), quadriceps weakness, higher body sway, lower body weight, and decreased stature. Osteoporotic fractures are more common in whites and Asians than in African Americans and Hispanics, and more common in women than in men. Little is known regarding the influence of ethnicity on bone turnover as a possible cause of the variance in bone density and fracture rates among different ethnic groups. Significant differences in bone turnover in premenopausal and early perimenopausal women can be documented. The bone turnover differences do not appear to parallel the patterns of BMD. Other factors, such as differences in bone accretion, are likely responsible for much of the ethnic variation in adult BMD.

Finkelstein JS, et al. Ethnic variation in bone turnover in pre- and early perimenopausal women: effects of anthropometric and lifestyle factors. *J Clin Endocrinol Metab*. 2002;87:3051. [PMID: 12107200]

Watts NB, et al. *Endocr Practice*. 2010;16 (Suppl 3):1–37.

Pathogenesis

Osteoporosis is characterized by microarchitectural deterioration of bone tissue that leads to decreased bone mass and bone fragility. The major processes responsible for osteoporosis are accelerated bone loss during the perimenopausal period (mid-50s to the sixth decade in women and the seventh decade in men) and beyond and, to a lesser extent, poor bone mass acquisition during adolescence. Both processes are regulated by genetic and environmental factors. Reduced bone mass, in turn, is the result of varying combinations of hormone deficiencies, inadequate nutrition, decreased physical activity, comorbidity, and the effects of drugs used to treat various medical conditions.

The term *primary osteoporosis* is now used less frequently than in the past and signifies deterioration of bone mass not associated with other chronic illness—usually related to increasing age and decreasing gonadal function. Therefore, early menopause or premenopausal estrogen deficiency states may hasten its development. Prolonged periods of inadequate calcium intake, a sedentary lifestyle, and tobacco and alcohol abuse also contribute to primary osteoporosis.

Secondary osteoporosis results from chronic conditions that contribute significantly to accelerated bone loss. These include endogenous and exogenous thyroxine excess, hyperparathyroidism, cancer, gastrointestinal diseases, medications, renal failure, and connective tissue diseases. Secondary forms of osteoporosis are listed in **Table 30-1**. If secondary

Table 30-1. Conditions, diseases, and medications that contribute to osteoporosis or fractures.

Lifestyle factors		
Alcohol abuse	High salt intake	Falling
Low calcium intake	Inadequate physical activity	Excessive thinness
Vitamin D insufficiency	Immobilization	
Excess vitamin A	Smoking (active or passive)	
Genetic factors		
Cystic fibrosis	Homocystinuria	Osteogenesis imperfecta
Ehlers-Danlos syndrome	Hypophosphatasia	Parental history of hip fracture
Gaucher's disease	Idiopathic hypercalciuria	Porphyria
Glycogen storage diseases	Marfan syndrome	Riley-Day syndrome
Hemochromatosis	Menkes steely hair syndrome	
Hypogonadal states		
Androgen insensitivity	Hyperprolactinemia	Premature ovarian failure
Anorexia nervosa and bulimia	Premature menopause	Athletic amenorrhea
Turner's & Klinefelter's syndromes	Panhypopituitarism	
Endocrine disorders		
Adrenal insufficiency	Cushing's syndrome	Central adiposity
Diabetes mellitus (types 1 & 2)	Hyperparathyroidism	Thyrotoxicosis
Gastrointestinal disorders		
Celiac disease	Inflammatory bowel disease	Primary biliary cirrhosis
Gastric bypass	Malabsorption	
GI surgery	Pancreatic disease	
Hematologic disorders		
Multiple myeloma	Monoclonal gammopathies	Sickle cell disease
Hemophilia	Leukemia and lymphomas	Systemic mastocytosis
Thalassemia		
Rheumatologic and autoimmune diseases		
Ankylosing spondylitis	Lupus	Rheumatoid arthritis
Other rheumatic and autoimmune diseases		
Central nervous system disorders		
Epilepsy	Parkinson's disease	Stroke
Multiple sclerosis	Spinal cord injury	

(Continued)

Table 30-1. Conditions, diseases, and medications that contribute to osteoporosis or fractures. (*Continued*)

Miscellaneous conditions and diseases		
AIDS/HIV	Congestive heart failure	Muscular dystrophy
Alcoholism	Depression	Posttransplant bone disease
Amyloidosis	End-stage renal disease	Sarcoidosis
Chronic metabolic acidosis	Hypercalciuria	Weight loss
Chronic obstructive lung disease	Idiopathic scoliosis	
Medications		
Aluminum (in antacids)	Cyclosporine A and tacrolimus	Proton pump inhibitors
Anticoagulants (heparin)	Medroxyprogesterone (Depo) (premenopausal contraception)	Selective serotonin reuptake inhibitors
Anticonvulsants	Glucocorticoids (≥ 5 mg/d prednisone or equivalent for ≥ 3 months)	Tamoxifen (premenopausal u e)
Aromatase inhibitors	GnRH (gonadotropin-releasing hormone) antagonists and agonists	Thiazolidinediones (such as Actos and Avandia)
Barbiturates	Lithium	Thyroid hormones (in excess)
Cancer chemotherapeutic drugs	Methotrexate	Parenteral nutrition

Data from Office of the Surgeon General (US). *Bone Health and Osteoporosis: A Report of the Surgeon General.* Rockville, MD: Office of the Surgeon General (US); 2004 (available at http://www.ncbi.nlm.nih.gov/books/NBK45513/; accessed March 2014); *2013 Clinicians's Guide to Prevention and Treatment of Osteoporosis* 2013: 14–15 (available at www.nof.org).

osteoporosis is suspected, appropriate diagnostic workup may identify a different management course.

Kelman A, Lane NE. The management of secondary osteoporosis. *Best Pract Res Clin Rheumatol.* 2005;19(6):1021-1037. [PMID: 16301195]

Kok C, Sambrook PN. Secondary osteoporosis in patients with osteoporotic fracture. *Best Pract Res Clin Rheumatol.* 2009; 23:769–779. [PMID: 19945688]

▶ Prevention

A. Nutrition

Bone mineralization is dependent on adequate nutritional status in childhood and adolescence. Therefore, measures to prevent osteoporosis should begin with increasing the milk intake of adolescents to improve bone mineralization. Nutrients other than calcium are also essential for bone health. Adolescents must, therefore, maintain a balance in calcium intake, protein intake, other calorie sources, and phosphorus. Substituting phosphorus-laden soft drinks for calcium-rich dairy products and juices compromises calcium uptake by bone and promotes decreased bone mass.

Eating disorders are nutritional conditions that affect BMD. Inability to maintain normal body mass promotes bone loss. The body weight history of women with anorexia nervosa has been found to be an important predictor of the presence of osteoporosis as well as the likelihood of recovery. The BMD of these patients does not increase to a normal range, even several years after recovery from the disorder, and all persons with a history of an eating disorder remain at high risk for osteoporosis in the future.

Major demands for calcium are placed on the mother by the fetus during pregnancy and lactation. The axial spine and hip show losses of BMD during the first 6 months of lactation, but this bone mineral loss appears to be completely restored 6–12 months after weaning. Risk factors for osteoporosis are summarized in **Table 30-2**.

B. Lifestyle

Sedentary lifestyle or immobility (confinement to bed or a wheelchair) increases the incidence of osteoporosis. Low body weight and cigarette smoking negatively influence bone mass. Excessive alcohol consumption has been shown to depress osteoblast function and, thus, to decrease

Table 30-2. Risk factors for osteoporosis.

Female gender
Petite body frame
White or Asian race
Sedentary lifestyle/immobilization
Nulliparity
Increasing age
High caffeine intake
Renal disease
Lifelong low calcium intake
Smoking
Excessive alcohol use
Long-term use of certain drugs
Postmenopausal status
Low body weight
Impaired calcium absorption

bone formation. Those at risk for low BMD should avoid drugs that negatively affect BMD (see Table 30-1).

C. Behavioral Measures

Behavioral measures that decrease the risk of bone loss include eliminating tobacco use and excessive consumption of alcohol and caffeine. A balanced diet with adequate calcium and vitamin D intake and a regular exercise program (see discussion below) retard bone loss. Medications, such as glucocorticoids, that decrease bone mass should be avoided if possible. The importance of maintaining estrogen levels in women should be emphasized. Measurement of bone density should be considered in the patient who presents with risk factors, but additional evidence is needed before instituting preventive measures.

D. Exercise

Regular physical exercise can reduce the risk of osteoporosis and delay the physiologic decrease of BMD. Short- and long-term exercise training (measured up to 12 months; eg, walking, jogging, stair climbing) in healthy, sedentary, postmenopausal women results in improved bone mineral content. Bone mineral content increases more than 5% above baseline after short-term, weight-bearing exercise training. With reduced weight-bearing exercise, bone mass reverts to baseline levels. Similar increases in BMD have been seen in women who participate in strength training. In the elderly, progressive strength training has been demonstrated to be a safe and effective form of exercise that reduces risk factors for falling and may also enhance BMD.

Estrogen deficiency results in diminished bone density in younger women as well as in older women. Athletes who exercise much more intensely and consistently than the average person usually have above-average bone mass.

However, the positive effect of exercise on the bones of young women is dependent on normal levels of endogenous estrogen. The low estrogen state of exercise-induced amenorrhea outweighs the positive effects of exercise and results in diminished bone density. When mechanical stress or gravitational force on the skeleton is removed, as in bed rest, space flight, immobilization of limbs, or paralysis, bone loss is rapid and extensive. Weight-bearing exercise can significantly increase the BMD of menopausal women. Furthermore, weight-bearing exercise and estrogen replacement therapy have independent and additive effects on the BMD of the limb, spine, and Ward triangle (hip).

There have been no randomized prospective studies systematically comparing the effect of various activities on bone mass. Recommended activities include walking and jogging, weight training, aerobics, stair climbing, field sports, racquet sports, court sports, and dancing. Swimming is of questionable value to bone density (because it is not a weight-bearing activity), and there are no data on cycling, skating, or skiing. It should be kept in mind that any increase in physical activity may have a positive effect on bone mass for women who have been very sedentary. To be beneficial, the duration of exercise should be between 30 and 60 minutes and the frequency should be 3–4 times per week.

Cadogan J, et al. Milk intake and bone mineral acquisition in adolescent girls: randomised, controlled intervention trial. *Br Med J.* 1997;315:1255. [PMID: 9390050]

Ernst E. Exercise for female osteoporosis. A systematic review of randomised clinical trials. *Sports Med.* 1998;25:359. [PMID: 9680658]

Rantalainen T, Nikander R, Heinonen A, et al. Differential effects of exercise on tibial shaft marrow density in young female athletes. *J Clin Endocrinol Metab.* 2013;98(5):2037–2044. [PMID: 23616150]

▶ Clinical Findings

A. Symptoms and Signs

The history and physical examination are neither sensitive enough nor sufficient for diagnosing primary osteoporosis. However, they are important in screening for secondary forms of osteoporosis and directing the evaluation. The goals of the evaluation should be to: (1) establish the diagnosis of osteoporosis by assessing bone mass, (2) determine fracture risk, and (3) determine whether intervention is needed. A medical history provides valuable clues to the presence of chronic conditions, behaviors, physical fitness, and the use of long-term medications that could influence bone density. Those already affected by complications of osteoporosis may complain of upper or midthoracic back pain associated with activity, aggravated by long periods of sitting or standing, and easily relieved by rest in a recumbent position. The history should also assess the likelihood of fracture. Other indicators of increased fracture risk are low bone density, a propensity to fall, taller stature, and the presence of prior fractures.

The physical examination should be thorough for the same reasons. For example, lid lag and enlargement or nodularity of the thyroid suggests hyperthyroidism. Moon facies, thin skin, and a "buffalo hump" (dorsocervical fat pad) suggest hypercortisolism. Cachexia mandates screening for an eating disorder or cancer. A pelvic examination is one aspect of the total evaluation of hormonal status in women and a necessary part of the physical examination in women. Osteoporotic fractures are a late physical manifestation. Common fracture sites are the vertebrae, forearm, femoral neck, and proximal humerus. The presence of a "dowager hump" in elderly patients suggests multiple vertebral fractures and decreased bone volume.

Studies completed under the auspices of the World Health Organization Collaborating Centre for Metabolic Bone Diseases were used to create a 10-year probability model for a more accurate assessment of fracture risk. The fracture risk assessment tool (FRAX) that was developed identifies and accounts for clinical risk factors for fracture—age, low body mass index, parental history of hip fracture, current smoking, alcohol intake of >3 units daily, rheumatoid arthritis or other secondary causes of osteoporosis, oral glucocorticoids, and previous fragility fracture. Primary data were used from nine large patient cohorts in North America, Europe, Asia, and Australia representing over 1 million patient-years. The primary data are used to accurately evaluate the interaction of each risk factor, rather than being limited to the potential bias of published data. Additional secondary causes of osteoporosis include untreated hypogonadism, inflammatory bowel disease, prolonged immobility, organ transplantation, type 1 diabetes, thyroid disorders, and chronic obstructive pulmonary disease. This tool estimates the 10-year, patient-specific absolute risk of hip or major osteoporotic fracture (hip, spine, shoulder, or wrist), taking account of death from all causes and death hazards (eg, smoking). The tool may be used alone employing individual clinical risk factors, with or without BMD, and is easily accessed online.

Kanis JA et al. European guidance for the diagnosis and management of osteoporosis in postmenopausal women. *Osteoporos Int.* 2008;19:399-428. [PMID: 18266020]

Kanis JA et al. FRAX and the assessment of fracture probability in men and women from the UK. *Osteoporos Int* 2008; 19: 385–397. [PMID: 18292978]

Watts NB et al. *J Bone Miner Res.* 2009; 24:975–979.

B. Laboratory Findings

Basic chemical analysis of serum is indicated when the history suggests other clinical conditions influencing bone density. The tests presented in **Tables 30-3** and **30-4** are appropriate for excluding secondary causes of osteoporosis.

Table 30-3. Exclusion of causes of secondary osteoporosis.

Consider the following diagnostic studies for causes of secondary osteoporosis:
Blood or serum
  Complete blood count (CBC)
  Chemistry levels (calcium, renal function, phosphorus, and magnesium)
  Liver function tests
  Thyroid-stimulating hormone (TSH) level
  Serum 25(OH)D level
  Parathyroid hormone (PTH)
  Total testosterone and gonadotropin levels in younger men
  Consider in selected patients:
  Serum protein electrophoresis (SPEP), serum immunofixation, serum-free light chains
  Tissue transglutaminase antibodies
  Iron and ferritin levels
  Homocysteine in select cases
  Tryptase
Urine
  24-hour urinary calcium
  Consider in selected patients:
  Protein electrophoresis (UPEP)
  Urinary free cortisol level
  Urinary histamine

Modified with permission from Harper KD, Weber TJ. Secondary osteoporosis. Diagnostic considerations. *Endocrinol Metab Clin North Am.* 1998;27(2):325-348.

These tests provide clues to serious illnesses that may otherwise have gone undetected and that, if treated, could result in resolution or modification of the bone loss. Specific biochemical markers (human osteocalcin, bone alkaline phosphatase, immunoassays for pyridinoline crosslinks and type 1 collagen–related peptides in urine) that reflect the overall rate of bone formation and bone resorption are now available. These markers are primarily of research interest and are not recommended as part of the basic workup for osteoporosis. They suffer from substantial biological variability and diurnal variation and do not differentiate causes of altered bone metabolism. For example, measures of bone turnover increase and remain elevated after menopause but do not necessarily provide information that can direct management.

C. Imaging Studies

Plain radiographs are not sensitive enough to diagnose osteoporosis until total bone density has decreased by 50%, but bone densitometry is useful for measuring bone density and monitoring the course of therapy (**Table 30-5**). Single- or dual-photon absorptiometry (SPA, DPA) has been used in the past but provides poorer resolution, less accurate analysis, and more radiation exposure than

Table 30-4. Directed laboratory assessment for secondary osteoporosis.

Hypogonadism	↓Testosterone in men ↓Estrogen in women ↑Gonadotropins (LH and FSH)
Hyperthyroidism	↓TSH ↑T_4
Hyperparathyroidism	↑PTH ↑Serum calcium ↑1,25(OH)D
Vitamin D deficiency	↓25-Hydroxycalciferol
Hemochromatosis	Serum iron Ferritin
Cushing syndrome	24-hour urine free cortisol excretion Overnight dexamethasone suppression test
Multiple myeloma	Serum protein electrophoresis—spike and Bence-Jones proteinuria ↑ESR Anemia Hypercalcemia ↓PTH

ESR, erythrocyte sedimentation rate; FSH, follicle-stimulating hormone; LH, luteinizing hormone; PTH, parathyroid hormone; TSH, thyroid-stimulating hormone; T_4, thyroxine; 1,25(OH)D, 1,25-hydroxyvitamin D; ↑, increased; ↓, decreased.
Modified with permission from Harper KD, Weber TJ. Secondary osteoporosis. Diagnostic considerations. *Endocrinol Metab Clin North Am.* 1998; 27:325.

x-ray absorptiometry. The most widely used techniques for assessing BMD are dual-energy x-ray absorptiometry (DXA) and quantitative computerized tomography (CT). These methods have errors in precision of 0.5–2%. Quantitative CT is most sensitive, but results in substantially greater radiation exposure than DXA. For this reason, DXA is the diagnostic measure of choice. Vertebral fracture assessment is now available through imaging completed with the

Table 30-5. Indications for measuring bone density.

Concerned perimenopausal women willing to start therapy
Radiographic evidence of bone loss
Patient on long-term glucocorticoid therapy (≥1 month at 7.5 mg of prednisone per day)
Asymptomatic hyperparathyroidism where osteoporosis would suggest parathyroidectomy
Monitoring therapeutic response in women undergoing treatment for osteoporosis if the result of the test would affect the clinical decision

DXA assessment and provides more accurate assessment of the patient's bone density.

Smaller, less expensive systems for assessing the peripheral skeleton are now available. These include DXA scans of the distal forearm and the middle phalanx of the nondominant hand and a variety of devices for performing quantitative ultrasound (QUS) measurements on bone. Prospective studies using QUS of the heel have predicted hip fracture and all nonvertebral fractures nearly as well as DXA at the femoral neck. Both of these methods provide information regarding fracture risk and predict hip fracture better than DXA at the lumbar spine. Clinical trials of pharmacologic agents have used DXA rather than QUS, so it is unclear whether the results of these trials can be generalized to patients identified by QUS to have high risk of fracture.

Bone densitometry reports provide a *T* score (the number of standard deviations above or below the mean BMD for sex and race matched to young controls) or *Z* score (comparing the patient with a population adjusted for age as well as for sex and race). The BMD result enables the classification of patients into three categories: normal, osteopenic, and osteoporotic. Normal patients receive no further therapy; osteopenic patients are counseled, treated, and followed so that no further bone loss develops; osteoporotic patients receive active therapy aimed at increasing bone density and decreasing fracture risk. Osteoporosis is indicated by a *T* score of >2.5 standard deviations below the sex-adjusted mean for normal young adults at peak bone mass. *Z* scores are of little value to the practicing clinician.

There is little evidence from controlled trials that women who receive bone density screening have better outcomes (improved bone density or fewer falls) than women who are not screened. The US Preventive Services Task Force (USPSTF) suggests that the primary argument for screening is that postmenopausal women with low bone density are at increased risk for subsequent fractures of the hip, vertebrae, and wrist, and that interventions can slow the decline in bone density after menopause. The presence of multiple risk factors (eg, age ≥80 years, poor health, limited physical activity, poor vision, prior postmenopausal fracture, psychotropic drug use) seems to be a stronger predictor of hip fracture than low bone density. The patient who is not asymptomatic but may have only one or two risk factors can benefit from BMD screening. Indications for BMD screening are outlined in Table 30-5.

Davison KS, et al. Assessing fracture risk and effects of osteoporosis drugs: bone mineral density and beyond. *Am J Med.* 2009; 122:992–997. [PMID: 19854322]

NIH Consensus Statement. March 27–29, 2000; 17(1):1–45. Osteoporosis prevention, diagnosis, and therapy. [No authors listed] [PMID: 11525451]

Lewiecki EM, Watts NB, McClung MR, et al. International Society for Clinical Densitometry. Official positions of the international society for clinical densitometry. *J Clin Endocrinol Metab.* 2004; 89(8):3651–3655.

▶ Differential Diagnosis & Screening

The approach to the patient is governed by the presentation. The greatest challenge for clinicians is to identify which asymptomatic patients would benefit from screening for osteoporosis, rather than determining a treatment regimen for those with known disease (see Table 30-2). All women and girls should be counseled about appropriate calcium intake and physical activity. Assessment of osteoporosis risk is also important when following a patient for a chronic disease known to cause secondary osteoporosis (see Table 30-1). **Figure 30-1** presents an algorithm to assist in the evaluation. Preventive measures are always the first step in therapy.

Should there be a suspicion of osteoporosis in a man or evidence of a pathologic fracture in a man or a woman, assessment of risk via medical history and determination of BMD should be completed. BMD measurement and laboratory evaluation are necessary to document the extent of bone loss and to rule out secondary causes of osteoporosis. Should there be clinical evidence of a particular condition, the evaluation can focus on the suspected condition when the basic laboratory work has been completed as described in Table 30-3 and Figure 30-1.

Recognizing the variety of conditions conferring risk of osteoporosis, the National Osteoporosis Foundation makes the following recommendations to physicians:

Universal recommendations:

- Counsel on the risk of osteoporosis and related fractures.
- Advise on a diet rich in fruits and vegetables and that includes adequate amounts of total calcium intake (1000 mg per day for men aged 50–70 years; 1200 mg per day for women aged ≥51 years and men ≥71 years).
- Advise on vitamin D intake (800-1000 IU per day), including supplements if necessary for individuals aged ≥50 years.
- Recommend regular weight-bearing and muscle-strengthening exercise to improve agility, strength, posture, and balance and reduce the risk of falls and fractures.
- Assess risk factors for falls and offer appropriate modifications (eg, home safety assessment, balance training exercises, correction of vitamin D insufficiency, avoidance of certain medications, and bifocals use when appropriate).
- Advise on cessation of tobacco smoking and avoidance of excessive alcohol intake.
- Measure height annually, preferably with a wall-mounted stadiometer.

Diagnostic assessment:

- In women aged ≥65 years and men aged ≥70, recommend bone mineral density (BMD) testing.
- In postmenopausal women and men aged 50–69 years, recommend BMD testing based on risk factor profile.
  - Recommend BMD testing and vertebral imaging to those who have had a fracture, to determine degree of disease severity.
  - BMD testing should be performed at DXA facilities using accepted quality assurance measures.
- Vertebral imaging should be performed
  - In all women aged ≥70 years and all men aged ≥80 years.
  - In women aged 65–69 and men aged 75–79 years if BMD *T*, score is ≤1.5.
  - In postmenopausal women aged 50-64 and men aged 50-69 years with specific risk factors:
    - Low trauma fracture
    - Historical height loss of ≥1.5 inches (4 cm)
    - Prospective height loss of ≥0.8 inch (2 cm)
    - Recent or ongoing long-term glucocorticoid treatment
- Check for causes of secondary osteoporosis.

When monitoring patients who have the diagnosis of osteoporosis, perform BMD testing 1–2 years after initiating therapy to reduce fracture risk and every 2 years thereafter. In certain clinical situations more frequent testing may be indicated. Likewise, the interval for repeat screening may be longer if the initial *T* score is in the normal or upper low bone mass range or the patient is without major risk factors.

National Osteoporosis Foundation. Available at http://www .nof.org/files/nof/public/content/resource/913/files/580.pdf (accessed May 16, 2013).

▶ Treatment

Decisions to intervene when osteoporosis is diagnosed reflect a desire to prevent early or continuing bone loss, a belief that there can be an immediate impact on the patient's well-being, and a willingness to comply with the patient's desires. Bone densitometry can assist in the decision-making process if the patient's age confers risk, there are no manifestations of disease, and if the decision point is prevention rather than treatment. BMD measurements can also assist in therapy when there are relative contraindications to a specific agent, and demonstrating efficacy could encourage continuation of therapy. Medicare currently reimburses costs of bone densitometry according to the conditions outlined in **Table 30-6**. The decision to intervene with pharmacologic therapy involves clinical judgment based on a global assessment, rather than BMD measurement alone. All currently approved therapeutic agents for

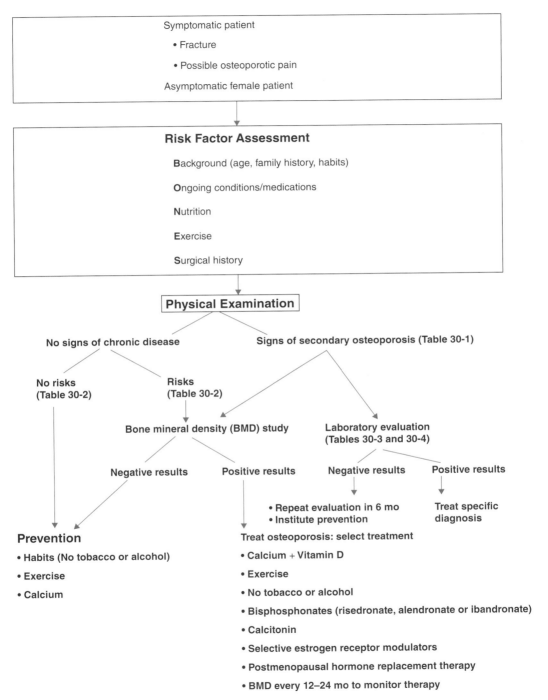

▲ **Figure 30-1.** Protocol for approaching osteoporosis.

Table 30-6. Conditions qualifying for Medicare coverage of densitometry.

Estrogen-deficient woman at clinical risk for osteoporosis
Individual with vertebral abnormalities (eg, osteopenia, vertebral fractures, osteoporosis)
Individual receiving long-term (>3 months) glucocorticoid therapy
Primary hyperparathyroidism
Individual monitored to assess response to osteoporosis drug therapy

the prevention and treatment of osteoporosis work by inhibiting or decreasing bone resorption.

A. Estrogen

Adequate estrogen levels remain the single most important therapy for maintaining adequate bone density in women. Prior to 2003, estrogen replacement therapy was considered for all women with decreased bone density, absent contraindications. However, in July 2002, the Women's Health Initiative randomized controlled primary prevention trial was stopped at a mean 5.2 years of follow-up by the Data and Safety Monitoring Board because the test statistic for invasive breast cancer exceeded the stopping boundary for the adverse effect of estrogen and progesterone versus placebo. Estimated hazard ratios were excessive for coronary heart disease, breast cancer, and strokes, but were <1.0 for colorectal cancer, endometrial cancer, and hip fracture. Therefore, careful risk assessment is needed for each patient to determine whether the improvement of risk for hip fracture (0.66) balances the risk for cardiovascular and breast disease. Contraindications to estrogen replacement therapy are listed in **Table 30-7**.

Table 30-7. Contraindications to estrogen replacement therapy.

Absolute
History of breast cancer
Estrogen-dependent neoplasia
Undiagnosed or abnormal genital bleeding
History of or active thromboembolic disorder
Relative
Migraine
History of thromboembolism
Familial hypertriglyceridemia
Uterine leiomyomas
Uterine cancer
Gallbladder disease
Strong family history of breast cancer
Chronic hepatic dysfunction
Endometriosis

Data from Scientific Advisory Board, Osteoporosis Society of Canada. Clinical practice guidelines for the diagnosis and management of osteoporosis. *Can Med Assoc J.* 1996; 155:1113.

Studies have been done to determine the effect of the timing of initiation and the duration of postmenopausal estrogen therapy on BMD. Current users who started estrogen therapy at menopause had the highest BMD levels, which were significantly higher than those of women who never used estrogen therapy or past users who started at menopause (with a duration of use of ≥10 years). BMD was similar for women using unopposed estrogen or estrogen plus progestin, and for current smokers or nonsmokers. Current users who started estrogen within 5 years of menopause had a decreased risk of hip, wrist, and all nonspinal fractures compared with those who never used estrogen. Long-term users who initiated therapy 5 years after menopause had no significant reduction in risk for all nonspinal fractures, despite an average duration of use of 16 years. Therefore, early initiation of estrogen with respect to menopause may be more important than the total duration of use. Estrogen initiated early in the menopausal period and continued into late life appears to be associated with the highest bone density.

As more and more women utilize estrogen therapy, there has been increasing concern regarding its impact on breast cancer risk. The relation between the use of hormones and the risk of breast cancer in postmenopausal women was assessed in a follow-up survey of participants in the Nurses' Health Study in 1992. The risk of breast cancer was significantly increased among women who were currently using estrogen alone or estrogen plus progestin, as compared with postmenopausal women who had never used hormones. Women currently taking hormones who had used such therapy for 5-9 years had an adjusted relative risk (RR) of breast cancer of 1.46, as did those currently using hormones who had done so for a total of 10 or more years (RR = 1.46). The addition of progestins to estrogen therapy does not reduce the risk of breast cancer among postmenopausal women.

The only randomized trial of estrogen-progesterone therapy describes secondary prevention of coronary heart disease in postmenopausal women [Heart and Estrogen/progestin Replacement Study (HERS)] and included only women who had a prior history of cardiovascular disease. Women received either estrogen alone or estrogen plus progesterone. There was an excessive number of deaths from coronary heart disease and a threefold excess risk of venous thrombosis during the first year of the trial in women on estrogen and a small risk of stroke in women on estrogen and progesterone. Recommendations at the conclusion of the trial included not starting women who already have clinical cardiovascular disease on estrogen and progesterone therapy (ie, secondary prevention).

B. Calcium and Vitamin D

Calcium supplementation produces small beneficial effects on bone mass throughout postmenopausal life and may reduce fracture rates by more than the change in BMD

Table 30-8. Calcium-rich foods.[a]

Milk (skim, lowfat, or whole), 8 oz
Plain yogurt, 8 oz
Frozen yogurt, fruit, 8 oz
Swiss cheese, 1 oz
Ricotta cheese, part skim, 4 oz
Sardines, canned, 3 oz
Cooked greens, collards, or mustard, 8 oz
Firm cheeses (Edam, brick, cheddar, Gouda, Colby, mozzarella), 1 oz
Calcium-fortified orange juice, 8 oz

[a]Approximately 300 mg.

would predict—possibly as much as 50%. Postmenopausal women receiving supplemental calcium over a 3-year period in a placebo-controlled, randomized clinical trial had stable total body calcium and BMD in the lumbar spine, femoral neck, and trochanter compared with the placebo group.

Vitamin D increases calcium absorption in the gastrointestinal tract, so that more calcium is available in the circulation and is subsequently reabsorbed in the renal proximal tubules. There is now evidence of significant reductions in nonvertebral fracture rates from physiologic replacement of vitamin D in the elderly. Vitamin D supplementation is important in those of all ages with limited exposure to sunlight.

Dietary calcium augmentation should be recommended to maintain lifetime calcium levels and to help prevent early postmenopausal bone loss (**Table 30-8**). Adults should ingest 1200 mg of elemental calcium per day for optimal bone health. Teenagers, pregnant or lactating women, women aged >50 years taking estrogen replacement therapy, and everyone aged >65 years should ingest 1500 mg of elemental calcium per day for optimal bone health. If this cannot be achieved by diet alone, calcium supplementation is recommended. Calcium preparations should be compared relative to elemental calcium content. Therefore, attention to which form the patient is ingesting is important.

C. Calcitonin

Calcitonin, a hormone directly inhibiting osteoclastic bone resorption, is an alternative for patients with established osteoporosis in whom estrogen replacement therapy is not recommended. A unique characteristic of calcitonin is that it produces an analgesic effect with respect to bone pain and, thus, is often prescribed for patients who have suffered an acute osteoporotic fracture. The American College of Rheumatology recommends treatment until the pain is controlled, followed by tapering of medication over 4–6 weeks. Calcitonin decreases further bone loss at vertebral and femoral sites in patients with documented osteoporosis but has a questionable effect on fracture frequency. Calcitonin has been shown to prevent trabecular bone loss during the first few years of menopause, but it is unclear whether it has

any impact on cortical bone. Calcitonin is also thought to be effective in decreasing the fracture rate of vertebrae and peripheral bones.

For reasons that are poorly understood, the increase in BMD associated with administration of calcitonin may be transient, or there may be the development of resistance. Therefore, calcitonin should be prescribed more acutely and other medications used for chronic management. Calcitonin can be provided in two forms. Nasal congestion and rhinitis are the most significant side effects of the nasal form. The injectable formulation has gastrointestinal side effects and is less convenient than the nasal preparation. The increase in bone density observed by this therapy is significantly less than that achieved by bisphosphonates or estrogen and may be limited to the spine, but it still has recognized value in reducing risk of fracture.

The FDA is currently reviewing prescribing recommendations for calcitonin and new guidelines are forthcoming in the near future.

http://www.nof.org/files/nof/public/content/resource/913/ files/580.pdf (accessed June 8, 2013).

D. Bisphosphonates

Bisphosphonates are antiresorptive agents and effective for preventing bone loss associated with estrogen deficiency, glucocorticoid treatment, and immobilization. Antiresorptive agents improve the quality of bone by preserving trabecular architecture. They may increase bone strength by methods other than by increasing BMD. All bisphosphonates act similarly on bone in binding permanently to mineralized surfaces and inhibiting osteoclastic activity. Thus, less bone is degraded during the remodeling cycle. First-, second-, and third-generation bisphosphonates are now available (alendronate, risedronate, and ibandronate). Because food and liquids can reduce the absorption of bisphosphonates, they should be given with a glass of plain water 30 minutes before the first meal or beverage of the day. Patients should not lie down for at least 30 minutes to lessen the chance of esophageal irritation. In addition, patients should consider taking supplemental calcium and vitamin D if their dietary intake is inadequate.

Bisphosphonates are of comparable efficacy to hormone replacement therapy in preventing bone loss and have a demonstrated positive effect on symptomatic and asymptomatic vertebral fracture rate as well as on nonvertebral fracture rate (forearm and hip). More than 4 years of treatment would be needed in women with low bone density (T score ≥ -2.0), but without preexisting fractures, to substantially reduce the risk of clinical fracture.

In clinical trials, alendronate was generally well tolerated and no significant clinical or biological adverse experiences were observed. Alendronate appears to be effective at doses of 5 mg daily in preventing osteoporosis induced by long-term glucocorticoid therapy. In placebo-controlled studies of men and women (aged 17–83) who were receiving glucocorticoid therapy, femoral neck bone density and the bone density of the trochanter and total body increased significantly in patients treated with alendronate.

Alendronate appears to be a safe, well-tolerated, and lower-cost agent for the osteoporosis and is a good first-line treatment. Some small-scale studies suggest an additional benefit of adding alendronate to hormone replacement therapy, and ongoing studies should provide additional information. However, all of the bisphosphonates accumulate over time in bone, and further research is needed to determine their long-term impact as well as their potential for use in premenopausal women and men.

Risedronate is a pyridinyl bisphosphonate approved as treatment for several metabolic bone diseases in 2000. In doses of 5 mg daily, risedronate reduces the incidence of vertebral fractures in women with two or more fractures by rapidly increasing BMD at sites of cortical and trabecular bone. In a randomized trial of 2458 postmenopausal women with diagnosed osteoporosis, participants were treated with either 2.5 mg or 5 mg of risedronate or placebo as well as calcium supplementation and cholecalciferol if they had low baseline 25-hydroxyvitamin D levels. The 2.5-mg dose was found to be ineffective in other trials and was discontinued. After 3 years of treatment, the 5-mg risedronate group showed a 41% reduction in risk of new vertebral fractures and a 39% reduction in incidence of nonvertebral fractures.

In a large, prospective, hip fracture prevention trial of elderly women, risedronate was shown to significantly reduce the risk of hip fracture in women with osteoporosis. Bisphosphonates should be prescribed for 3–4 years in women with osteoporosis and low bone density.

Ibandronate is currently approved by the Food and Drug Administration (FDA) for the treatment and prevention of osteoporosis in postmenopausal women. Over a 3-year period, ibandronate was shown to decrease the incidence of new vertebral fractures by 52% and to increase BMD at the spine by 5%. It can be administered daily or once a month.

Zoledronic acid was approved by the FDA in 2011 and is marketed as Reclast. A single annual intramuscular dose of 5 mg was studied in 1367 patients. Femoral neck BMD increased by 3.7% above placebo 3 years after a single dose of zoledronic acid. Clinical fracture rates were reduced by 32% in patients receiving single infusions and 34% in those receiving three infusions over a 3-year period. There is no general agreement regarding how long to wait before repeating the injection.

Strontium ranelate is approved and used in the European Union and is effective in treating osteoporosis in both men and women.

Reid IR, Black DM, Eastell R, et al. Reduction in the risk of clinical fractures after a single dose of zoledronic acid 5 milligrams. *J Clin Endocrinol Metab.* 2013;98(2):557–563.

More than 150 million bisphosphonate scripts were dispensed between 2005 and 2009. Postmarketing surveillance reports atypical femoral fracture, jaw osteonecrosis, and esophageal cancer. FDA reviews of alendronate, residronate, and zoledronic acid reveal rare side effects of 1 in 1000 to 10,000 users. Little additional benefit in fracture prevention is seen after 3–5 years of use, except for vertebral fractures.

Compston J, Bowring C, Cooper A, et al. Diagnosis and management of osteoporosis in postmenopausal women and older men in the UK: National Osteoporosis Guideline Group (NOGG) update 2013; Maturitas (2013) (available at http://dx.doi.org/10.1016/j.maturitas.2013.05.013).

Whitaker M, Guo J, Kehoe T, et al. Bisphosphonates for osteoporosis—where do we go from here? *N Engl J Med.* 2012;366: 2048–2051.

E. Selective Estrogen Receptor Modulators

Raloxifene was the first drug to be studied from a new class of drugs termed *selective estrogen receptor modulators*. This drug has a mixed agonist-antagonist action on estrogen receptors: specifically, estrogen agonist effects on bone and antagonist effects on breast and endometrium. Its discovery evolved from a structural rearrangement of the antiestrogen tamoxifen, although it is structurally very different. It blocks estrogen in a manner similar to tamoxifen, while also binding and stimulating other tissue receptors to act like estrogen. Raloxifene inhibits trabecular and vertebral bone loss in a manner similar, but not identical, to estrogen (ie, by blocking the activity of cytokines that stimulate bone resorption).

Raloxifene therapy results in decreased serum total and low-density lipoprotein (LDL) cholesterol without any beneficial effects on serum total high-density lipoprotein (HDL) cholesterol or triglycerides. Reported side effects of raloxifene are vaginitis and hot flashes. Investigators in the Multiple Outcomes of Raloxifene (MORE) trial of >7000 postmenopausal, osteoporotic women over 3 years showed a decreased risk of breast cancer in those already at low risk for the disease. The study results were analyzed separately for women presenting with preexisting fracture. Although treatment effectiveness was similar in both groups, the absolute risk of fractures in the group with preexisting fractures was 4.5 times greater than in the group with osteoporosis, but no preexisting fracture (21% vs 4.5%). Thus, it is important to identify and treat patients at higher risk. Studies of women at higher risk for breast cancer are currently under way.

A summary of overall treatment strategies is given in **Table 30-9,** and guidelines for dosing the pharmacologic agents are given in **Table 30-10. Table 30-11** summarizes the risks and benefits of osteoporosis therapy.

F. Other Modalities

Fluoride increases bone formation by stimulating osteoblasts and increasing cancellous bone formation in patients

Table 30-9. Treatment strategies.

Overall

Calcium-rich diet ± vitamin D supplements

Weight-bearing exercise

Avoidance of alcohol, tobacco products, excess caffeine, and drugs

Estrogen replacement within 5 years of menopause, and used for ≥10 years

Antiresorptives—bisphosphonates and denosumab

Anabolics

Estrogen agonists/antagonists

For patients on glucocorticoids

Lowest dose of a short-acting glucocorticoid or topical preparations whenever possible

Maintain a well-balanced, 2–3-g sodium diet

Weight-bearing and isometric exercise to prevent proximal muscle weakness

Calcium intake of 1500 mg/d and vitamin D intake of 400–800 IU/d after hypercalciuria is controlled

Gonadal hormones in all postmenopausal women, premenopausal women with low levels of estradiol, and in men who have low levels of testosterone (unless contraindicated)

Thiazide diuretic to control hypercalciuria

Measure bone mineral density at baseline and every 6–12 months during the first 2 years of therapy to assess treatment efficacy

If bone loss occurs during treatment or hormone replacement therapy is contraindicated, treat with calcitonin or bisphosphonate

Data from Lane NE, Lukert B. The science and therapy of glucocorticoid induced bone loss. *Endocrinol Metab Clin North Am*. 1998; 27:465.

with osteoporosis. However, the bone is formed only in the spine and is abnormal—irregularly fibrous and woven with lacunae of low mineral density. Cessation of therapy resulted in rapid loss of much of the bone formed during treatment. The major side effect of fluoride therapy is gastric distress, an effect that is thought to be related to the direct effect of hydrofluoric acid on the gastric mucosa. Fluoride is also associated with joint pain and swelling. For these reasons, sodium fluoride is not routinely used for treatment of osteoporosis and does not have FDA labeling for this indication.

Anabolic therapy produces some increase in bone mass. Teriparatide (PTH 1-34), marketed under the trade name Forteo, or recombinant parathyroid hormone, is FDA-approved for the treatment of osteoporosis in perimenopausal women who are at high risk for fracture. Teriparatide also has FDA labeling for increasing bone mass in men with primary or hypogonadal osteoporosis who are at high risk for fracture. Unlike antiresorptive agents, teriparatide stimulates new bone formation. There are some concerns regarding extended use of teriparatide because of the long-term effects on multiple organ systems (ie, significant hepatotoxicity, reduced HDL, and elevated LDL cholesterol).

Teriparatide is the first approved agent for the treatment of osteoporosis that stimulates new bone formation. It is administered once a day by injection (20 μg/d) in the thigh or abdomen. Patients treated with 20 μg/d of teriparatide, along with calcium and vitamin D supplementation, had

Table 30-10. Pharmacologic doses.

Medication	Dosage	Route
Estradiol patch	0.05 mg every week	Topical
Conjugated estrogens	0.625–1.25 mg/d	Oral
Elemental calcium	1200–1500 mg/d	Oral
Calcitonin	200 IU/d 50–100 IU/d	Intranasal Subcutaneous or intramuscular
Vitamin D	800–2000 IU/d For repletion – 50,000 IU orally once per week for 8 weeks, then return to maintenance	Oral
Alendronate	5 mg/d (prevention) 10 mg/d (Rx) 35 mg every week	Oral Oral
Risedronate	35 mg every week or 150 mg every month	Oral
Ibandronate	2.5 mg/d or 150 mg every month	Oral
Raloxifene	60 mg/d	Oral
Zoledronic acid	5 mg annually	IV
Denusomab	60 mg every 6 months + oral Ca + vitamin D	SC

Table 30–11. Risks and benefits of osteoporosis therapy.

	Antiresorptives					Anabolics	Estrogen Agonist/Antagonist	Estrogen	Others – Non-FDA, but available overseas	
	Alendronate	Risedronate	Ibandronate	Zoledronic acid	Denosumab	Teriparatide (PTH)	Raloxifene (formerly known as SERM)	Estrogen	Strontium	Sodium Fluoride*
Reduction of vertebral fracture	Yes	Yes	Yes	Yes	Yes	Yes	Yes	Yes	Yes	
Reduction of non-vertebral fracture	Yes	Yes	Yes	Yes	Yes	Yes	No	Yes	Yes	No
Experience with long-term use	RCT 4 y in length	RCT 3 y in length	RCT 3 y in length			2 y maximum Rx	RCT 3 y in length	Large epidemiologic studies over decades	No	No
Administration	Once daily in morning, 30 min before eating, with water while upright; or weekly	Once daily (or weekly) in morning, 30–60 minutes before eating, with water, while upright	Orally: once monthly in morning, 30–60 min before eating, with water, while upright, or IV every 3 mo	IV over at least 15 min once yearly (rx) and every 2 y (prevention)	SC injection every 6 mo	Daily SC injections	Orally: once daily any time or weekly	Orally once daily anytime		
Adverse effects	Dyspepsia; esophagitis; avoid in patients with esophageal disorders	Dyspepsia	Dyspepsia	To decrease risk, acute-phase reaction (arthralgias, headaches, myalgia, fever) pretreat with acetaminophen	Hypocalcemia, cellulitis, ONJ	Leg cramps, nausea, dizziness	Increased risk of venous thrombosis, hot flashes, leg cramps	Breast tenderness, vagina bleeding, thromboembolic disorders		

(Continued)

Table 30–11. Risks and benefits of osteoporosis therapy. *(Continued)*

	Antiresorptives			Anabolics	Estrogen Agonist/ Antagonist	Estrogen	Others – Non-FDA, but available overseas	
Effect on CV mortality	None	None	No data	No data	No final outcome data	Increased in those with preexisting CV disease	Unclear	Unclear
Breast cancer	None	None	No data	No data	Possibly protective	Increased	No data	

Notes:

- Osteonecrosis of jaw (ONJ)–risk in use of all bisphosphonates, especially high-dose IV treatments.
- Limited evidence of efficacy beyond 5 years for all medications listed above.
- Estrogen agonist/antagonists were formerly known as *selective estrogen receptor modulators* (SERMs).
- Calcitonin recommendations currently under review by the FDA and changes in prescribing are anticipated. Not recommended as first-line therapy.
- Others (rightmost column)–currently not FDA approved in the United States, but are used overseas.

Data from *Managing Osteoporosis—Part 3: Prevention and Treatment of Postmenopausal Osteoporosis.* AMA CME Program, 2000 and Khosla S, Burr D, Cauley J, et al. Bisphosphonate-associated osteonecrosis of the jaw: report of a task force of the American Society for Bone and Mineral Research. *J Bone Miner Res.* 2007;22(10):1470-1491 (available at www.nof .org/files/nof/pubic/content/resource/913/files/580.pdf; accessed May 18, 2013).

statistically significant increases in BMD at the spine and hip when compared with patients receiving only calcium and vitamin D supplementation. Clinical trials also demonstrated that teriparatide reduced the risk of vertebral and nonvertebral fractures in postmenopausal women. The effects of teriparatide on fracture risk have not been studied in men.

Of note, osteosarcoma developed in animals in early studies, and the possibility that humans treated with teriparatide may face an increased risk of developing this cancer cannot be ruled out. This safety issue is highlighted in a black box warning in the drug label for health professionals and explained in a brochure for patients. Children and adolescents with growing bones and patients with Paget disease of the bone have a higher risk for developing osteosarcoma and should not be treated with this agent. Because the effects of long-term treatment with teriparatide are not known, therapy for >2 years is not recommended.

Testosterone replacement is acceptable therapy for many of the causes of hypogonadism in men [eg, Klinefelter syndrome, isolated gonadotropin deficiency (Kallmann syndrome)].

Denosumab, a fully human, monoclonal antibody that inhibits Rank Ligand—a key modulator of osteoclast formation, function, and survival—was approved by the FDA in 2012. The FREEDOM study of 7808 postmenopausal women with osteoporosis compared 60 mg of denosumab with placebo given every 6 months for 36 months. DXA and quantitative CT scans were used for monitoring. Denosumab significantly increased BMD (bone mineral content) and does not appear to delay fracture healing. Denosumab usage warrants caution in the presence of hypocalcemia; serious side effects include skin infections, osteonecrosis of the jaw, and suppression of bone turnover, which could include atypical femoral fracture after long-term use.

Adami S. *J Bone Joint Surg Am.* 2012;94:2113–2119.
Simon JA, Recknor C, Moffett AH, et al. Impact of denosumab on the peripheral skeleton of postmenopausal women with osteoporosis. *Menopause.* 2013;20(2):130–137.
The European Medicines Agency recommends limiting long term use of calcitonin medicines (information is available at http://www.ema.europa.eu/ema/index.jsp?cur/pages/medicines/human/public_health_alerts/2012/07/human_pha_detail_000065.jsp&mid=wc0b01ac058001d126; accessed Oct. 17, 2012).

G. Complementary and Alternative Therapies

Nutraceuticals are now being used more frequently by patients to promote bone health. There is a paucity of data confirming the benefit of these products, but likewise no evidence of harm. The most common nutraceuticals used for bone health are phytoestrogens (isoflavones, lignins, and coumestans), vitamin A, the B vitamins [B_2 (folate) and B_{12}], vitamin K, magnesium, and omega-3 fatty acids.

Evidence from animal studies suggests a beneficial effect of phytoestrogens on bone, but long-term human studies are lacking. Epidemiologic evidence that Asian women have a lower fracture rate than white women, even though the bone density of Asian women is less than that of African-American women, promotes consideration of the impact of nutrition. It is possible that high soy intake contributes to improved bone quality in Asian women. A comparison study of a soy protein and high isoflavone diet versus a milk protein diet or medium isoflavone and soy protein diet demonstrated that only those receiving the higher isoflavone preparation were protected against trabecular (vertebral) bone loss.

A topical form of natural progesterone derived from diosgenin in either soybeans or Mexican wild yam has been promoted as a treatment for osteoporosis, hot flashes, and premenstrual syndrome, and a prophylactic against breast cancer. However, eating or applying wild yam extract or diosgenin does not produce increased progesterone levels in humans because humans cannot convert diosgenin to progesterone.

All patients should be encouraged to maintain a bone-healthy diet. This includes reducing soft drink and sodium consumption, eating potassium-rich foods, encouraging iron and folate supplementation in adolescent females and women of childbearing age, and vitamin B_{12} supplementation in persons aged 50 years and vitamin D supplementation in the elderly, in dark-skinned people, and in those with low UVB exposure.

Nieves J. Nutraceuticals: effects on bone metabolism. Talk presented at 8th International Symposium on Osteoporosis Meeting, Washington, DC, April 1–5, 2009.
Weaver C. Nutrition an osteoporosis. Talk presented at 8th International Symposium on Osteoporosis Meeting. Washington, DC, April 1–5, 2009.

H. Glucocorticoid-Induced Osteoporosis

Glucocorticoids are widely used in the treatment of many chronic diseases, particularly asthma, chronic lung disease, and inflammatory and rheumatologic disorders, and in those who have undergone organ transplantation. The risk that oral steroid therapy poses to bone mineral density, among other side effects, has been known for some time. As a result, clinicians have eagerly substituted inhaled steroids in an endeavor to protect the patient from unwanted negative steroid effects. Recent evaluations of the effects of inhaled glucocorticoids on bone density in premenopausal women demonstrated a dose-related decline in bone density at both the total hip and the trochanter. Women with asthma were enrolled and were divided into three groups: those using no inhaled steroids, those using four to eight puffs per day, and those using more than eight puffs per day at 100 μg per puff. No dose-related effect was noted at the femoral neck or the spine. Serum and urinary markers of bone turnover or adrenal function did not predict the degree of bone loss. To achieve the best possible outcome for the patient, given the potentially devastating effects of systemic steroids, therapy to combat the steroids should begin as soon as the steroids are begun. See Table 30-9 for specific guidelines.

American College of Rheumatology recommendations are to initiate bisphosphonate use in glucocorticoid-induced osteoporosis and to initiate therapy if: (1) the glucocorticoid use will equal or exceed 3 months, (2) if the patient has a *T* score of less than –1, or (3) if the patients receiving long-term glucocorticoid therapy have had fractures on, or cannot tolerate hormone replacement therapy.

ACR Ad Hoc Committee on GIO. *Arthritis Rheum.* 2001;44: 1496-1503

Col NF, et al. Patient-specific decisions about hormone replacement therapy in postmenopausal women. *JAMA.* 1997;277:1140. [PMID: 9087469]

Ettinger B, et al. Reduction of vertebral fracture risk in postmenopausal women with osteoporosis treated with raloxifene: results from a 3-year randomized clinical trial. Multiple Outcomes of Raloxifene Evaluation (MORE) Investigators. *JAMA.* 1999; 282:637. [PMID: 10517716]

Harris ST, et al. Effects of risedronate treatment on vertebral and nonvertebral fractures in women with postmenopausal osteoporosis: a randomized controlled trial. Vertebral Efficacy with Risedronate Therapy (VERT) Study Group. *JAMA.* 1999;282: 1344. [PMID: 10527181]

Israel E, et al. Effects of inhaled glucocorticoids on bone density in premenopausal women. *New Engl J Med.* 2001; 345:941. [PMID: 11575285]

Potter SM, et al. Soy protein and isoflavones: their effects on blood lipids and bone density in postmenopausal women. *Am J Clin Nutr.* 1998; 68:(suppl):1375S. [PMID: 9848502]

Rossouw JE, et al. Risks and benefits of estrogen plus progestin in healthy postmenopausal women: principal results from the Women's Health Initiative randomized controlled trial. *JAMA.* 2002; 288:321. [PMID: 12117397]

Saag KG, et al. Alendronate for the prevention and treatment of glucocorticoid-induced osteoporosis: glucocorticoid-Induced Osteoporosis Intervention Study Group. *N Engl J Med.* 1998; 339:292. [PMID: 9682041]

Summary recommendations for postmenopausal women and men aged ≥50 years are to: (1) counsel on the risk of osteoporosis and fractures, (2) check for secondary causes, (3) advise on adequate calcium and vitamin D, (4) recommend regular exercise, and (5) advise on avoidance of tobacco and alcohol intake. In women aged ≥65 years and men aged ≥70 years, recommend BMD testing. In postmenopausal women between the ages of 50 and 69, recommend BMD testing based on the risk factor profile. Furthermore, when a patient has already experienced a fracture, recommend BMD to determine the severity of the disease.

Websites

Food and Drug Administration. http://www.accessdata.fda.gov/scripts/cder/drugsatfda; http://www.ama-cmeonline.com/osteo_mgmt (accessed Jan.10, 2010); http://www.fda.gov/bbs/topics/ANSWERS/2002/ANS01176

The National Osteoporosis Foundation. http:/www.nof.org (accessed June 9, 2013).

Osteoporosis management, American Medical Association CME On-Line. http://www.ama-cmeonline.com/osteo_mgmt (accessed Nov. 26, 2010).

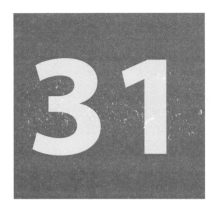

Abdominal Pain

Cindy M. Barter, MD, MPH, IBCLC, CTTS, FAAFP

Laura Dunne, MD, CAQSM, FAAFP

Carla Jardim, MD

General Considerations

Abdominal pain is the chief complaint for 5–10% of patients presenting to emergency departments and one of the top 10 complaints in the office. Because of the wide differential diagnoses, accurate diagnosis can be difficult. Detailed history, thorough physical examination, and often, diagnostic testing, are necessary.

Clinical Findings

A. History

ESSENTIALS OF DIAGNOSIS

▶ Acuity, onset, and duration of symptoms.

▶ Quality, location, and radiation of pain.

▶ Associated symptoms.

History is the most important component of evaluating abdominal pain. Effective communication is necessary for a thorough, accurate history. Enough time should be allowed for open-ended history using the method "engage, empathize, educate, enlist."

1. Onset—Determining onset of pain can help determine the cause of abdominal pain as well as the need for emergent referral. Abdominal pain is categorized as acute, subacute, or chronic. Symptoms lasting more than 3 months are considered chronic. Acute pain is often associated with peritoneal irritation, such as appendicitis, and abdominal organ rupture and may require emergency management and consultation with a surgeon. Many patients present to the office with more gradual onset or chronic abdominal pain (**Table 31-1**).

2. Quality of pain—A patient's description of the quality of the pain provides clues to etiology. Pain can be sharp, stabbing, burning, dull, gnawing, colicky, crampy, gassy, focal, migrating, or radiating. Pressure like pain ("there's an elephant sitting on me") suggests cardiac ischemia. Focal symptoms help determine location and diagnosis.

3. Location—Location and radiation of pain are important. The abdomen is separated into four quadrants—right upper (RUQ), left upper (LUQ), right lower (RLQ), and left lower (LLQ)—or as midepigastric or suprapubic. Some causes of abdominal pain have classic patterns of location and radiation. Pain from the lower esophagus may be referred higher in the chest and confused with pain associated with cardiac conditions.

4. Frequency and timing—Frequency and pattern of pain are particularly useful in identifying the cause of chronic pain. Symptoms may be associated with eating, types of food, defecation, body position, or movement. Peritoneal irritation may be eased by lack of movement. Visceral pain may trigger a patient to move more to try to find a more comfortable position. Pain caused by colonic pathology may be relieved by defecation.

5. Other diagnostic clues and symptoms—Physicians should determine whether other symptoms are present such as nausea, vomiting, diarrhea, constipation melena, mucus, or hematochezia. Fever and chills suggest an infectious etiology. Feculent emesis correlates with bowel obstruction. The presence of blood or melena in the stool requires evaluation for gastrointestinal (GI) bleeding. A patient's age may be a factor in both cause and perception of pain. The elderly may not present with classic symptoms of serious conditions and complain of vague or mild pain because of a 10–20% reduction in pain perception for each decade of age over 60 years. Emotional stress can trigger symptoms of functional bowel disease. Organic diseases also may be exacerbated by emotional stress.

Table 31-1. Common causes of abdominal pain by location.

Localized
  Midepigastric
    Dyspepsia
    GERD
    Pancreatitis
    PUD
  RUQ
    Gallbladder diseases
    Hepatitis
    Hepatomegaly
  RLQ
    Appendicitis
    Crohn disease
    GYN-related diseases
      Ruptured ovarian cyst
      Ectopic pregnancy
      PID
      Pregnancy
    Meckel diverticulitis
  LUQ
    MI
    Pneumonia
    Sickle cell crisis
    Lymphoma
    Splenomegaly—EBV
    Gastritis
  LLQ
    Diverticulitis
    Bowel obstruction
    Ischemic colitis
    Ulcerative colitis
    Urinary calculi
  Suprapubic
    Cystitis
    Prostatitis
    Urinary retention
Generalized
  Abdominal wall pain—multiple causes
  Celiac disease
  Constipation
  Chronic diarrhea
  IBS
  Gastroenteritis/infectious diarrhea
  Mesenteric lymphadenitis
  Perforated colon
  Ruptured aortic aneurysm
  Trauma

EBV, Epstein–Barr virus; GERD, gastroesophageal reflux disease; GYN, gynecologic; IBS, inflammatory bowel disease; LLQ, left lower quadrant; LUQ, left upper quadrant; MI, myocardial infarction; PID, pelvic inflammatory disease; PUD, peptic ulcer disease; RLQ, right lower quadrant; RUQ, right upper quadrant.

Past medical history provides important clues to the etiology of pain. Previous abdominal surgery increases the risk for bowel obstruction secondary to adhesions, strangulation, or hernia. Patients with cardiovascular diseases are at greater risk for bowel infarction. Tobacco, alcohol, or medications such as nonsteroidal anti-inflammatory drugs (NSAIDs) are associated with increased incidence of gastroesophageal reflux disease (GERD) and peptic ulcer disease (PUD). Alcohol abuse is a common cause of pancreatitis. Multiparity, obesity, and diabetes mellitus increase risk of gallbladder disease. Tubal ligation or pelvic inflammatory disease (PID) history indicate a greater risk for an ectopic pregnancy.

Medication history should include use of prescription and over-the-counter (OTC) medications and herbal supplements. Aspirin and other platelet aggregation inhibitors, steroids and nonsteroidal anti-inflammatory drugs (NSAIDs), and antidepressants increase the risk of gastrointestinal bleeding. Antibiotics can cause nausea, diarrhea, or both.

B. Physical Examination

ESSENTIALS OF DIAGNOSIS

▶ Inspect, auscultate, palpate, and percuss abdomen.
▶ Palpate for tenderness and rebound tenderness.
▶ Assess bowel sounds

1. Inspection—Position the patient supine with knees slightly bent. Inspect for distention, discoloration, scars, and striae. Distention suggests ascites, obstruction, or other masses. Discoloration from bruising associated with hemoperitoneum is found in the central portion of the abdomen, especially following abdominal trauma. The location of scars helps clarify and confirm past history. Striae suggest rapid growth of the abdomen. New striae or those related to endocrine abnormalities tend to be purplish or dark pink. Striae may appear as darkening of the skin in darker-skinned persons. The abdomen should be inspected for hernias with the patient in an upright position.

2. Auscultation—Auscultation is performed prior to palpation. Bowel sounds may be normal, hypoactive, hyperactive, or high-pitched. Hypoactive or hyperactive bowel sounds can be present with partial bowel obstruction, or ileus. Bruits over the aorta, renal arteries, and femoral arteries suggest aneurysms. Gentle palpation while auscultating decreases the likelihood that a patient will guard, embellish, or magnify symptoms.

3. Palpation—Palpation of the abdomen begins with light touch away from the area of greatest pain. Assess for rigidity, tenderness, masses, and organ size. Increased rigidity may indicate an acute abdomen and need for emergent intervention. A Murphy sign is the sudden cessation of a patient's inspiratory effort during deep palpation of the RUQ and suggests acute cholecystitis.

Pain from visceral organs may radiate because of shared nerve innervation. Pain from pancreatitis often radiates to the back. Abdominal pain radiating to the left shoulder (Kehr sign) indicates splenic rupture, renal calculi, or ectopic pregnancy. Radiation of pain may be caused by inflammation of surrounding tissues.

The iliopsoas muscle test, performed by having the patient flex the right hip while lying supine and applying pressure to the leg, can be used to evaluate the deep muscles of the abdomen. Inflammation of the psoas muscle may indicate inflammation of nearby structures as seen with appendicitis or retroperitoneal dissection.

Rebound tenderness indicates peritoneal irritation and can occur with gastrointestinal perforation or non-GI sources such as a ruptured ovarian cyst and PID. Peritoneal irritation is often associated with guarding. Voluntary guarding occurs when a patient anticipates the pain. Patients who close their eyes as the examiner approaches ("closed-eye sign") are more likely to have underlying psychosocial factors contributing to pain. Involuntary guarding is caused by flexion of the abdominal wall muscle as the body attempts to protect internal organs. The Carnett test, performed by having the patient flex the abdominal wall as the point of greatest tenderness is palpated, may help differentiate visceral pain from abdominal wall or psychogenic pain. Pain less severe with palpation of the flexed abdomen wall has a higher probability of being visceral than pain from abdominal wall pathology or nonorganic causes.

Two approaches may help examine a ticklish patient: use of a stethoscope for light palpation by curling fingers past the edge of the stethoscope to create a less sensitive touch; and placement of hands over the patient's hand to palpate.

Evaluate liver and spleen by having the patient take a deep breath and exhale while palpating the organ's border. The normal liver span at the midclavicular line is 6–12 cm depending on the height and gender of the patient. Assessing the midsternal liver size can be helpful. The normal span is 4–8 cm. A span of >8 cm is considered enlarged. The tip of the spleen may not be palpable.

Examine for masses that may be seen with colon cancer, kidney abnormalities, and non-GI tumors. A palpated mass should be examined for location, size, shape, consistency, pulsations, mobility, and movement with respiration.

4. Percussion—Percussion can help determine the size of organs and other abdominal pathology. A change in the character of the sound indicates a solid organ. The examiner should percuss both liver edges. The upper border usually sits at the fifth to seventh intercostal space. Inferior displacement suggests emphysema or other pulmonary diseases. The span of the spleen is evaluated in the left midaxillary line and usually extends from the sixth to the tenth ribs. The scratch

test is another form of percussion. It is performed by placing the stethoscope over the liver and gently scratching the surface of the skin beginning above the upper border of the liver and progressing to below the lower border of the liver. The quality of the sound changes as the examiner's scratch travels from the lung field to liver and abdomen. Changes in sound help identify the liver borders.

Increased tympany should be present over the stomach in the area of the left lower border of the rib cage and left epigastrium because of the gastric air bubble. Increased tympany throughout the rest of the abdomen suggests dilation or perforation of the bowel. Dullness can be stationary, as with solid masses, or shifting, as with mobile fluid. Shifting dullness generally is present with significant ascites.

5. Pelvic exam—A pelvic examination may be indicated in female patients with abdominal pain.

C. Laboratory Findings

ESSENTIALS OF DIAGNOSIS

▶ CBC, electrolytes, BUN, creatinine, and glucose are useful in most patients.

▶ All women of childbearing age should have a pregnancy test.

▶ Consider iron studies for adults aged >50 years.

Testing should include complete blood cell count (CBC), electrolytes, blood urea nitrogen (BUN), creatinine, and glucose. Alkaline phosphatase and liver function tests can be helpful. Normal hemoglobin and hematocrit in the setting of acute rapid blood loss can be misleading and should be rechecked after the patient is fluid-resuscitated. Anemia, especially in those aged >50 years, should prompt iron studies, including ferritin level. Hypothyroidism in the elderly may present with vague abdominal pain, so a thyroid-stimulating hormone level may be helpful.

Right upper quadrant pain should be evaluated with bilirubin, lipase, amylase, trypsin, and liver function tests. Hepatitis panels may be useful. Amylase is elevated in pancreatitis and many other abdominal problems. Therefore, lipase and trypsin level are more specific for pancreatitis.

Stool studies may be indicated when the patient presents with abdominal pain and diarrhea. Stool testing should be done for dehydration, for blood in the stool, or with immunocompromised patients. Stool white blood cell count (WBC), hemoccult testing, ova and parasite, culture for enteric pathogens, and *Clostridium difficile* toxin level, are indicated for chronic or bloody diarrhea. Erythrocyte sedimentation rate (ESR) and C-reactive protein (CRP) should be checked if inflammatory bowel disease is suspected, especially if WBCs are found in stool. Intermittent symptoms suggesting celiac disease may warrant laboratory tests for antiendomysial antibody.

Women of childbearing age should have a pregnancy test regardless of history of tubal ligation. Patients with lower abdominal pain may need a urinalysis (UA), although other intraabdominal problems can cause changes in UA similar to urinary tract infection. Consider vaginal testing for sexually transmitted infections, including gonorrhea and *Chlamydia*. Cardiac studies should be considered for at-risk patients. Studies including magnesium, calcium, and vitamin D levels may be indicated for nonspecific complaints.

D. Imaging Studies

ESSENTIALS OF DIAGNOSIS

▶ A CT scan is the test of choice for acute abdominal pain.

▶ An ultrasound (US) is the test of choice for RUQ pain.

▶ Colonoscopy should be considered for abdominal pain in all patients aged >50 years.

Plain films of the abdomen are low-cost, widely available, and safe initial diagnostic tests. Upright and lateral decubitus films of the abdomen can show dilated small bowel loops (suggestive of obstruction), free air (perforated organ), mass (tumor or other obstructing cause), or stones (biliary or renal). Small bowel follow-through may show ulcer or mass. Barium enema can be useful for evaluation of constipation.

Computerized tomography (CT) of the abdomen and pelvis is the test of choice for many acute and nonacute causes of abdominal pain. Protocols for specific problems limit radiation exposure while providing accurate information. Spiral CT for appendicitis and renal calculus has been shown to be fast, safe, effective, and cost-effective. Other problems well visualized by CT scan include diverticulitis, bowel obstruction, pancreatitis, abdominal aortic aneurysm, pneumoperitoneum, soft-tissue tumors, and radiopaque renal and biliary stones.

Ultrasonography (US) is the most reliable imaging study for the biliary system and pelvic organs, the test of choice for most RUQ pain, and can identify hernias. The lack of contrast material and radiation makes it useful for pregnant patients. Children may tolerate US better than CT scan because the exam time is shorter and there is less need to remain completely still. The accuracy of US is more operator-dependent and is limited by obesity.

Direct visualization of the GI tract is often needed for chronic pain. Upper endoscopy is used for evaluation of dyspepsia, ulcers, and other upper gastric abnormalities. This imaging modality allows for visualization, biopsy of mucosal lesions, and treatment of bleeding. Colonoscopy or sigmoidoscopy is indicated for most patients aged >50 years or with other risk factors for cancer. Direct visualization of the colonic mucosa can help in diagnosis of diverticulosis, cancer, diarrhea, and inflammatory bowel disease.

Other modalities available for imaging of the abdomen include magnetic resonance imaging (MRI). Imaging modalities for urinary system problems are discussed elsewhere.

DYSPEPSIA

▶ General Considerations

The term *dyspepsia* was first used in the early eighteenth century to describe a person's ill humor, indigestion, or disgruntlement. The term now describes a set of symptoms encompassing different diseases and the etiologies associated with them. Chronic or recurrent discomfort centered in the upper abdomen commonly describes dyspepsia and can be associated with heartburn, belching, bloating, nausea, or vomiting. Common etiologies include PUD and GERD. Rare causes include gastric and pancreatic cancers.

Dyspepsia is reported to affect 40% of the world's adult population and accounts for 2–3% of all visits to primary care providers. Only ~10% of affected adults seek medical advice. No specific etiology is found for 50–60% of patients presenting with epigastric pain. *Nonulcer dyspepsia* or *functional dyspepsia* applies to patients with symptoms lasting >3 months without a clear etiology. Other infrequent etiologies include gastric, esophageal, and pancreatic cancer; biliary tract disease; gastroparesis; pancreatitis; carbohydrate malabsorption; medication-induced symptoms; hepatoma; intestinal parasites, non-GI diseases such as sarcoidosis, diabetes, thyroid, and parathyroid conditions; and metabolic disturbances such as hypercalcemia and hyperkalemia. Studies have shown that symptoms and degree of symptoms do not correlate with findings on endoscopy.

Dyspepsia is caused by PUD in 15–25% and GERD in 5–15% of cases. Abdominal exam may be unremarkable unless an ulcer perforates, causing signs of peritonitis. Treatment for dyspepsia depends on the etiology and is discussed in sections on PUD, GERD, and nonulcer dyspepsia.

Hungin AP, et al. Systmatic review: frequency and reasons for consultation for gastro-oesophageal reflux disease and dyspepsia. *Aliment Pharmacol Ther.* 2009; 30:331–342. [PMID: 19660016]

Leong RW. Differences in peptic ulcer between the East and the West. *Gastroenterol Clin North Am.* 2009; 38(2):363–379. [PMID: 19446264]

Peptic Ulcer Disease

▶ General Considerations

The four major causes of ulcers are *Helicobacter pylori*–induced ulcers, NSAIDs, acid hypersecretory conditions, and idiopathic ulcers. Clear evidence supports eradication of *H. pylori* in patients with documented ulcers. Since the early 1990s, the association of *H. pylori* with peptic ulcers has decreased from 90% to as low as 15–20% in some countries. This decrease is related to increased treatment of *H. pylori* infections, which are commonly associated with low income, low educational levels, and overcrowded living conditions. African Americans and Hispanics have about a one-third higher rate of infection than white Americans. In the United States, 40% of adults are infected with *H. pylori* by the age of 50, compared with only 5% of children aged 6–12 years. In developing countries, children commonly are infected at a younger age and there is a higher incidence of infection in the entire population.

Pathogenesis

In the past, infection with *H. pylori* was the leading cause of peptic ulcers and NSAID use was second. Now NSAID use and idiopathic ulcers are the most common causes. In the United States, one in seven individuals uses NSAIDs. Of long-term NSAID users undergoing upper endoscopy, 5–20% are found to have an ulcer. Risk factors for developing ulcers due to NSAID use are a personal history of ulcer, age >65 years, current steroid use, use of anticoagulants, history of cardiovascular disease, and impairment of another major organ. NSAIDs are prescribed to nearly 40% of all persons aged >65 years. Elderly patients treated with a course of with NSAIDs have a 1–8% chance of being hospitalized within the first year of therapy for GI complications. Patients who are *H. pylori*–positive and take NSAIDs have a higher risk of complications.

Prevention

Eradication of *H. pylori* infection before starting a course of treatment with NSAIDs reduces the risk of developing an ulcer early in the treatment, particularly with duodenal ulcers. Treatment with PPI is standard for secondary prevention of gastoduodenal ulcers.

Clinical Findings

Factors suggesting PUD include gnawing pain with the sensation of hunger, prior personal or family history of ulcers, tobacco use, and a report of melena. The most accurate diagnostic test is esophagogastroduodenoscopy (EGD). It allows both visualization and biopsy of an ulcer as well as testing for *H. pylori*. Good evidence supports a "test and treat" approach. The most cost-effective noninvasive test is the monoclonal stool antigen test. Breath urea testing is noninvasive but more expensive and may not be as accurate. Serology testing is used mainly for research or surveillance but may be indicated for actively bleeding ulcers, complicating performance of an EGD.

Complications

Elderly patients (aged ≥80 years) with ulcers who take aspirin or have *H. pylori* infection have a much higher incidence of complications. A hypersecretory condition, such as Zollinger-Ellison syndrome, caused by a gastrin-producing tumor should be suspected in patients with multiple ulcers. The incidence of GI bleeding from the upper GI tract has decreased. This may be related to the increased treatment of *H. pylori*.

Treatment

Treatment of PUD requires initial eradication of *H. pylori* if present, reducing or discontinuing NSAID use, and treatment with a proton pump inhibitor (PPI). The Food and Drug Administration (FDA)-approved regimens for treatment of *H. pylori* include concomitant or sequential treatment with two or three antibiotics plus a PPI. Refer to Centers for Disease Control and Prevention (CDC) and local guidelines. Treatment of *H. pylori* facilitates healing of ulcers and decreases rate of recurrence in the first year from 75% to 10%. Increased effectiveness of medical treatment for PUD has decreased the need for surgical intervention. Surgery, when performed, is commonly laparoscopic.

Calvet X, et al. Accuracy of diagnostic tests for *Helicobacter pylori*: a reappraisal. *Clin Infect Dis*. 2009;48:1385–1391. [PMID: 19368506]

McMoll K. *Helicobacter pylori* infection. *N Engl J Med*. 2010; 362:1597.

Venerito M, et al. Interaction of *helicobactoer pylori* infection and nonsteroidal anti-inflammatory drugs in gastric and duodenal ulcers. *Helicobacter*. 2010;15:239–250

Wu DC, et al. Sequential and concomitant therapy with four drugs is equally effective for eradication of H pylori infection. *Clin Gastoenterol Hepatol*. 2010;8:36

Gastroesophageal Reflux Disease

Clinical Findings

Heartburn is the single most common symptom of GERD. Ten percent of the US population experience heartburn at least once a day, and almost 50% experience symptoms once a month. Other common symptoms include regurgitation, belching, and dysphagia. GERD can be associated with extraesophageal symptoms and conditions. Pulmonary conditions include asthma, chronic bronchitis, aspiration pneumonia, sleep apnea, atelectasis, and interstitial pulmonary fibrosis. Ear, nose, and throat manifestations of GERD include chronic cough, sore throat, hoarseness, halitosis, enamel erosion, subglottic stenosis, vocal cord inflammation, granuloma, and, possibly, cancer. Noncardiac chest pain, chronic hiccups, and nausea may be associated with GERD. Changes in body position such as lying down or bending forward may exacerbate symptoms of GERD.

The esophagus has three mechanisms in place to prevent mucosal injury. The lower esophageal sphincter (LES) creates a barrier to acid reflux. Peristalsis, gravity, and saliva provide acid clearance mechanisms. Epithelial cells provide resistance.

Diagnosis is based on the medical history and response to treatment with H_2-receptor antagonists, prokinetic agents, or PPIs. Symptomatic improvement following treatment can indicate GERD. Diagnosis may be suggested by use of symptom questionnaires, catheter and wireless pH-metry, and impedance-pH monitoring. Upper endoscopy fails to reveal 36–50% of patients diagnosed via esophageal pH monitoring. Patients with typical symptoms and response to PPIs do not need further evaluation. Endoscopy should be performed if alarming symptoms are present, such as bleeding, weight loss, dysphagia, or persistence of symptoms after treatment with a PPI, especially in elderly patients. Complications of GERD include Barrett esophagus, esophageal strictures, ulceration, hemorrhage, and rarely, perforation. Barrett esophagus is found in 8–20% of patients who undergo upper endoscopy for GERD.

Treatment

Lifestyle modifications with the greatest impact on reducing symptoms of GERD include weight loss in overweight and obese patients, cessation of smoking, moderation of alcohol, consumption , and reduction of dietary fat intake. Limiting foods that decrease LES pressure (chocolate), stimulate acid secretion (coffee, tea, and cola beverages), or produce symptoms by their acidity (orange or tomato juice) may be helpful. Elevating the head of the bed by 6 inches, avoiding bedtime snacks, and reducing meal size, particularly in the evening, may help ameliorate symptoms.

Medication treatment options decrease acid or help with other defense mechanisms. Commonly used over-the-counter (OTC) medications include antacids, simethicone, and H_2-blockers. Prescription medications include prescription-strength H_2-blockers, PPIs, prokinetic agents, bethanechol, and sucralfate. Agents that irritate the mucosa (eg, aspirin and NSAIDs) should be avoided. Other agents to avoid include α-adrenergic antagonists, anticholinergics, β-adrenergic agonists, calcium channel blockers, diazepam, narcotics, progesterone, and theophylline.

If a patient's symptoms resolve or significantly improve with treatment, no further evaluation is needed. If the symptoms do not improve with an 8-week course of PPIs, endoscopy is indicated. Risks of developing long-term complications remain even when symptoms improve. Patients with Barrett esophagus need close monitoring because of a 50–100-fold increased risk of developing esophageal cancer.

Gaude GS. Pulmonary manifestations of gastroesophageal reflux disease. *Ann Thorac Med.* 2009;4(3):115–123. [PMID: 19641641]

Katz P, et al. Guidelines for the diagnosis and management of gastroesophageal reflux disease. *Am J Gastroenterol.* 2013; 108:308–328.

Sifrim D, et al. Utility of non-endoscopic investigations in the practical management of oesophageal disorders. *Best Practice Res Clin Gastroenterol.* 2009; 23:369–386. [PMID: 19505665]

Nonulcer Dyspepsia

 ESSENTIALS OF DIAGNOSIS

► Persistent or recurrent dyspepsia present for the past 3 months, onset at least 6 months prior to diagnosis, without evidence of organic disease.

► Diagnosis made by excluding other causes of dyspepsia.

► No diagnostic gold standard; consider EGD to rule out other causes if no response to PPIs and "test and treat" for *H. pylori.*

General Considerations

Nonulcer dyspepsia, also called *idiopathic* or *functional dyspepsia,* is defined as persistent or recurrent dyspepsia without evidence of organic disease present for 3 months with onset more than 6 months prior to diagnosis, not relieved by defecation, and not associated with the onset of change in stool frequency or form. Nonulcer dyspepsia is divided into at least two distinct subgroups: postprandial distress syndrome, which features postprandial fullness and early satiety; and epigastric pain syndrome, which features more constant and less meal-related symptoms.

Nonerosive reflux disease (NERD) is defined as having typical symptoms of GERD but absence of visible esophageal mucosal injury when EGD is performed. Nonulcer dyspepsia and NERD may represent different aspects of the same disease entity.

Pathogenesis

The pathophysiology of nonulcer dyspepsia is not entirely clear and is probably multifactorial. Suggested causes include changes in gastric physiology, nociception, motor dysfunction, central nervous system (CNS) dysfunction, and psychological and environmental factors. *H. pylori* and its effects on nonulcer dyspepsia are highly controversial. A percentage of patients with nonulcer dyspepsia and *H. pylori* have significant improvement in their symptoms after using eradication therapy, yet improvement cannot be guaranteed. Approximately 50% of patients with nonulcer dyspepsia are *H. pylori*–positive.

Clinical Findings

Nonulcer dyspepsia is diagnosed by excluding other causes of dyspepsia. Endoscopy is negative with nonulcer dyspepsia and

NERD. A therapeutic trial of PPIs and/or "test and treat" for *H. pylori* are common practices supported in the literature. Cost-effectiveness data indicate that testing and treating patients for *H. pylori* decreases the number of EGDs performed by about one-third.

Treatment

Management of nonulcer dyspepsia is multifactorial. Early diagnosis and explanation of the relevant physiology is helpful to patients. Physicians should avoid excessive investigation, although patients with previous diagnosis of nonulcer dyspepsia should be investigated whenever alarm symptoms are present or a new objective symptom arises. Alarm symptoms are highlighted by the mnemonic **VBAD**: **v**omiting, **e**vidence of **b**leeding or anemia, presence of **a**bdominal mass or weight loss, and **d**ysphagia. The prevalence of *H. pylori* in the community may factor into the decision to "test and treat" or perform other investigations. Physicians should determine why the patient with chronic symptoms presented at this particular time.

Psychosocial factors exacerbate symptoms. Physicians should address these issues and offer counseling. Postevaluation reassurance is a mainstay of management. Patients should be told to avoid foods or substances that exacerbate symptoms (NSAIDs, alcohol, tobacco, and certain foods). Not all patients want or need prescription medications and may prefer to explore other treatment options. Eating six small meals per day may alleviate symptoms of bloating or postprandial fullness.

Numerous medications have been used in studies of nonulcer dyspepsia. Results are confounded by different study definitions of the disorder and the lack of differentiation of symptom types. Medications include antacids, H_2-blockers, PPIs, bismuth, and sucralfate. PPIs appear to benefit ulcer like dyspepsia but not dysmotility like dyspepsia. Prokinetic agents such as metoclopramide have been poorly studied. Cisapride, which was taken off the market, showed a twofold decrease in symptoms compared to placebo. Domperidone has been shown to be superior to placebo and does not cross the blood-brain barrier to cause CNS side effects but is not available in the United States. Peppermint and caraway oils produced similar results when compared to cisapride. Motilin agonists such as erythromycin increase the rate of gastric emptying. Visceral analgesics such as fedotozine reduce gastric hypersensitivity. Buspirone and $5HT_1$ agonists such as sumatriptan have shown promise. Antispasmodics such as dicyclomine have not been shown to be more effective than placebo in patients with dyspepsia. Antinausea agents such as ondansetron and perchlorperazine have been shown to modestly improve symptoms. Perchlorperazine had more side effects. Antihistamines such as dimenhydrinate and cyclizine decrease gastric dysrhythmias. Promethazine has been used to treat mild nausea. Tricyclic antidepressants have been the most extensively studied antidepressant treatment of functional dyspepsia. Selective serotonin reuptake inhibitors have shown promising results with other functional bowel diseases [eg, irritable bowel syndrome (IBS)].

Other treatment approaches include acupuncture, acupressure, and gastric electrical stimulation. No randomized, double-blind controlled trials have been performed to evaluate their effectiveness. Follow-up appointments are important to assess patient function and response to treatment.

Keohane J, Quigley MM. Functional dyspepsia and nonerosive reflux disease: clinical interactions and their implications. *MedGenMed*. 2007; 9(3):31. [PMID: 18092037]

Nakajima S. Stepwise diagnosis and treatment from uninvestigated dyspepsia to functional dyspepsia in clinical practice in Japan: proposal of a 4-step algorithm. *Digestion*. 2009; 79(suppl 1): 19–25. [PMID: 19153486]

DISEASES OF THE GALLBLADDER & PANCREAS

The four main causes of abdominal pain related to the gallbladder and pancreas are biliary colic, gallstones, cholecystitis, and pancreatitis. Gallbladder-related pain usually is located in the midepigastric region with radiation to the right shoulder, right scapula, right clavicular area, or back. Pancreatitis often produces pain throughout the entire upper abdomen with frequent radiation to the back. See Chapter 33 for a detailed discussion of these and other diseases of the biliary tract and pancreas.

IRRITABLE BOWEL SYNDROME

General Considerations

Estimates indicate that symptoms consistent with a diagnosis of IBS are present in 3–20% of adults in the Western world. Although IBS occurs worldwide, cultural and social factors affect its presentation. Women in Western countries have a higher incidence of IBS and are more likely to consult a physician. In India and Sri Lanka, men have a higher incidence. IBS symptoms are common in South Africans who live in urban zones and unusual in people who live in rural areas. In the United States, prevalence is similar in blacks and whites. Some studies show lower prevalence in Hispanics from Texas and Asians from California.

Up to 50% of individuals with symptoms consistent with IBS do not seek physician care. Many who seek care had a major life event such as a death in the family or loss of job before presenting. Primary care providers see more of these patients than GI specialists.

Pathogenesis

Physiologic changes contributing to symptoms of IBS have not been elucidated. Many theories exist, including disturbance in motility, postinfectious changes, altered perception either locally in the GI tract or in the central nervous system, visceral hypersensitivity, mucosal inflammation, autonomic nerve dysfunction, and psychological disturbance. A study using positron emission tomography (PET) scan examined the activity of the brain when GI symptoms were induced. Patients with IBS did not activate the anterior cingulate cortex associated with opiate binding but activated the prefrontal cortex associated with hypervigilance and anxiety. Studies to determine whether patients with IBS have a lower threshold of pain with colonic distention are inconclusive. Studies have not clarified whether symptoms of IBS are a normal perception of an abnormal function or an abnormal perception of a normal function.

▶ Clinical Findings

A. Symptoms and Signs

Irritable bowel syndrome is a functional bowel disorder, without identified organic cause, in which abdominal discomfort or pain is associated with defecation or change in bowel habits and with features of disordered defecation. Diagnostic criteria developed by the Rome Consensus Committee for IBS are at least 3 days per month for the past 3 months with onset at least 6 months prior to diagnosis of abdominal discomfort or pain characterized by two of the following three features: (1) relieved with defecation, (2) onset associated with a change in frequency of stool, and (3) onset associated with change in form or appearance of the stool.

The Bristol Stool Form Scale describes seven types of stool forms. Other symptoms supporting the diagnosis of IBS include abnormal stool frequency (more than three per day or fewer than three per week), abnormal stool form (lumpy/hard or loose/watery), abnormal stool passage (straining, urgency, or feeling of incomplete evacuation), passage of mucus, and sensation of bloating or feeling of abdominal distention. Stool form has been demonstrated to reflect GI transit time. Using the Bristol Stool Form Scale and frequency of bowel movements is more precise and useful than using the imprecise terms *diarrhea* and *constipation*, since these terms have different meanings to different patients. Patients may complain of feeling constipated because of a feeling of incomplete evacuation despite having just passed soft or watery stool.

B. History

Patient history is the single most useful tool in diagnosing IBS. Continuity of care and a well-established rapport contribute significantly to obtaining accurate and complete history. A positive physician-patient interaction, psychosocial history, precipitating factors, and discussion of diagnosis and treatment with patients result in fewer return visits for IBS and lower utilization of health care resources. Chronic or recurrent abdominal pain indicates a need to assess quality of life. In a study of undergraduate students with

IBS, quality-of-life scores similar to those of patients with congestive heart failure, indicated the significant impact of IBS symptoms. As noted earlier, stressful life events often precede onset of symptoms of IBS. Although stressful life events may not be the cause of IBS, they may factor into the decision by patients to seek care. The decision of women with IBS symptoms of to seek care has been shown to have a significant and positive correlation between daily stress levels and daily symptoms.

A history of abuse should be sought in patients with chronic abdominal pain. A study at a tertiary care gastroenterology clinic revealed that 60% of the overall study population reported a history of physical or sexual abuse. All were women. Self-reported history of abuse was highest for those with functional bowel disease (≤84%) and lowest for those with organic bowel disease, such as ulcerative colitis (38%).Treatment success can be affected by exploring a patient's psychosocial stressors. Physicians should assess for abuse when considering referral to a gastroenterologist. Family physicians are uniquely positioned to assess and address issues associated with abuse.

Patients with IBS have not been demonstrated to have a higher incidence of psychiatric diagnosis such as depression, anxiety, somatization, stress, lack of social support, or abnormal illness behavior compared with other patients presenting with abdominal pain of organic origin. However, patients presenting with abdominal pain do have more psychosocial concerns than control subjects without abdominal pain. Psychosocial factors have not been shown to help in differentiating between organic and functional abdominal disease, but do help in understanding some health-seeking behaviors.

Signs or symptoms of an anatomic disease should be absent. These include fever, GI bleeding, unintentional weight loss, anemia, and abdominal mass. Laxative use should be assessed as laxatives may cause IBS-like symptoms. Patients with IBS may have had surgery, particularly appendectomy, hysterectomy, or ovarian surgery. The most common discharge diagnosis for patients hospitalized for abdominal pain is "nonspecific abdominal pain." A study of patients discharged with this diagnosis showed that 37% of women and 19% of men met the criteria for IBS 1–2 years after discharge. Of these patients, 70% had prior attacks of abdominal pain. Only 6% of charts listed IBS in the differential diagnosis on the initial admission. Of patients presenting with acute pain of <1 week's duration, 50% had symptoms of IBS at time of admission. Assessing for diagnostic criteria of IBS symptoms may reduce length of hospitalization, extent of testing, and cost of treatment for patients presenting with acute abdominal pain who do not need immediate surgical intervention.

C. Physical Examination

Physical examination is often unremarkable except for abdominal tenderness and an increased likelihood of abdominal scars.

D. Special Tests

No specific testing is required for diagnosis of IBS, although normal CBC and ESR may be reassuring. Patients with criteria for colon cancer screening should be examined by flexible sigmoidoscopy or colonoscopy. Other studies may include *Clostridium difficile* toxin if the patient has recently taken antibiotics, testing for giardiasis in endemic areas, evaluation for lactose intolerance, and serologic testing or gluten elimination diet for celiac disease.

▶ Treatment

A. Therapeutic Relationship

A therapeutic relationship is critical to the effective management of IBS. The therapeutic relationship is achieved by a nondirective, patient-centered, nonjudgmental history, eliciting the patient's understanding of the illness and his/her concerns, identifying and responding realistically to the patient's expectation for improvement, setting consistent limits, and involving the patient in the treatment approach. The most effective treatment option is explanation and reassurance. A confident diagnosis based on previously outlined clinical criteria helps convey the lack of association with a higher risk of other diseases such as cancer and chronic nature of symptoms. Patients' reasons for seeking care and possible contributing psychosocial issues should be assessed. Counseling regarding psychosocial stressors may not resolve all the symptoms of IBS, but may help patients cope better with symptoms.

B. Diet and Exercise

Many different dietary approaches have been tried. Patients in whom gas-forming vegetables, lactose, caffeine, or alcohol exacerbate symptoms should be counseled to minimize exposure; however, food intolerance and elimination diets have not proved effective. Dietary fiber has been shown to improve symptoms of constipation, hard stools, and straining, particularly if 30 g of soluble fiber is consumed each day. Patients often need to gradually increase the amount of fiber to improve adherence, as a sudden increase can increase symptoms of bloating and gas. The most common reason for failure of a high-fiber diet is insufficient dose. Fiber is safe and inexpensive, and should be routinely recommended, particularly to patients for whom constipation is a predominant symptom. Nondietary bulking agents have not been found more effective than placebo. Probiotics are live organisms that may benefit. Probiotics have been found to provide global improvement in IBS symptoms and abdominal pain. The exact mechanism contributing to the improvement in symptoms is not completely understood and can vary between strains and dose used. There is insufficient evidence to recommend the use of one particular strain or dose. Patients should be encouraged to consume probiotic-rich fermented foods such as yogurt, kefir, miso, tempeh, and sauerkraut. Increased physical activity has shown

improvement in severity of IBS symptoms and significantly lower likelihood of worsening of symptoms. Given the multiple benefits of increased physical activity, it should be routinely recommended.

C. Complementary and Alternative Therapies

A meta-analysis of five double-blind, placebo-controlled randomized trials of peppermint oil given as a monopreparation in a dosage range of 0.2–0.4 mL suggested a significant ($P < .001$) positive effect compared with placebo. Randomized controlled trials of Chinese herbal medicine indicated that both a standardized herbal formulation (Tong Xie Yao Fang is a commonly used formula) as well as individualized Chinese herbal medicine treatment improved symptoms of IBS compared with placebo. Padma Lax, a Tibetan herbal digestive formula, has been used and studied in Europe and shown global improvement in symptoms. Acupuncture has been shown to be more beneficial than some antispasmodic medications. Moxibustion has been shown to be helpful compared to placebo treatments.

D. Psychological Therapies

Various psychological therapies have been studied in randomized, controlled trials comparing control therapy and a physician's "usual management." Psychological therapies studied include hypnotherapy, relaxation training, multicomponent psychological therapy, dynamic psychotherapy, cognitive-behavioral therapy (CBT), stress management, and self-administered CBT. Dramatic improvements in a high proportion of patients with poorly controlled IBS symptoms were seen for both individual and group hypnotherapy. Therapeutic audiotapes are an easy, low-cost alternative but may be somewhat inferior to hypnotherapy. Psychotherapy effectiveness relies on the relationship between therapist and patient, making it difficult to study in randomized, controlled trials. The quality of the data is not as strong as that for pharmacotherapy, but the number needed to treat with psychological therapies to prevent IBS symptom persistence for one patient is four. The number needed to treat with antidepressants to prevent persistent symptoms also is four. Patients with IBS are more likely to have coexisting mood disorders and anxiety. Psychological interventions should be considered.

E. Pharmacotherapy

A meta-analysis that concluded that smooth-muscle relaxants and anticholinergics were better than placebo has been criticized for methodologic inadequacies. Common GI complaints and the drugs most frequently used to treat them are as follows:

Constipation: psyllium, methylcellulose, calcium polycarbophil, lactulose, 70% sorbitol, and polyethylene glycol (PEG) solution. A partial $5HT_4$ agonist (tegaserod) was removed from the market secondary to cardiovascular side effects. Lubiprostone and linaclotide are newer agents requiring further evaluation.

Diarrhea: loperamide, cholestyramine. Alosetron for female patients with diarrhea-predominant IBS symptoms was removed from the market secondary to risk of ischemic colitis and severe constipation but is now available again with warnings.

Gas, bloating, or flatus: simethicone, α-galactosidase (Beano), probiotic, antibiotics. Rifaximin is expensive and not recommended for long-term treatment.

Abdominal pain: anticholinergics and antispasmodics (dicyclomine, hyoscine, cimetropium, and pinaverium).

Chronic pain: tricyclic antidepressants, selective serotonin reuptake inhibitors.

A positive therapeutic relationship and regular visits to a family physician can prevent a continual and costly quest by patients for a "miracle" cure.

Ford AC, et al. Efficacy of antidepressants and psychological therapies in irritable bowel syndrome: systematic review and meta-analysis. *Gut.* 2009; 58(3):367–378. [PMID: 19001059]

Hoveyda N, et al. A systematic review and meta-analysis: probiotics in the treatment of irritable bowel syndrome. *BMC Gastroenterol.* 2009;9:15. [PMID: 19220890]

Johannesson E, et al. Physical activity improves symptoms in irritable bowel syndrome: a randomized controlled trial. *Am J Gastroenterol.* 2011; 106:915.

Lewis SJ, Heaton KW. Stool Form Scale as a useful guide to intestinal transit time. *Scand J Gastroenterol.* 1997;32:920. [PMID: 9299672]

Manheimer E, et al. Acupuncture for treatment of irritable bowel syndrome. *Cochrane Database Syst Rev.* 2012;5:CD005111.

Ruepert L, et al. Bulking agents, antispasmodics and antidepressants for the treatment of irritable bowel syndrome. *Cochrane Database Syst Rev.* 2011: CD003460.

CELIAC DISEASE

ESSENTIALS OF DIAGNOSIS

▶ Abdominal pain due to autoimmune destruction of mucosa.

▶ Testing for IgA endomysial antibodies and IgA tissue transglutaminase.

▶ Confirm with small bowel biopsy.

▶ Confirm with resolution of symptoms on gluten-free diet.

▶ General Considerations

Celiac disease may cause chronic abdominal pain. It is present in 0.5–1% of the US population. It is commonly associated with other autoimmune disorders, a known family history of celiac disease, and Down's syndrome. Because of the low prevalence of disease, general screening may result in false-positive results.

▶ Clincal Findings

Symptoms of clinical disease (or celiac sprue) include abdominal pain, diarrhea, and weight loss. It can be associated with liver enzyme abnormalities, skin problems, osteoporosis, iron deficiency anemia, flatulence, and neurologic dysfunction. Severe deficiency of vitamin D, vitamin K, or iron may be present. This may result in failure to thrive or short stature.

Mechanism of illness is an autoimmune process causing destruction of the small bowel mucosa, infiltration of mucosa with lymphatic T cells, and enlargement of crypts after repeated exposure to gluten proteins such as are found in wheat, rye, and barley.

▶ Diagnosis

Serum immunoglobulin A (IgA) endomysial antibodies and IgA tissue transglutaminase (tTG) antibodies should be tested while patients consume a diet containing gluten. Positive results should be confirmed with endoscopic small bowel biopsy in four locations. Testing is more accurate in higher-risk populations such as those with family history, other autoimmune disorders, or iron deficiency anemia. Testing for IgA deficiency maybe helpful if clinical suspicion is high despite negative endoscopy.

▶ Treatment

Treatment is a strict gluten-free diet. Patients should be referred to a knowledgeable nutritionist. Most patients' symptoms will improve significantly in 3 months and have improved absorption and decreased blood loss. Risk of gastrointestinal adenoma is considerably higher in this population. Strict adherence to diet may help decrease risk.

Barker JM, Liu E. Celiac disease: pathophysiology, clinical manifestations, and associated autoimmune conditions. *Adv Pediatr.* 2008; 55:349–365.

Presutti RJ, Cangemi JR, Cassidy HD, Hill DA. Celiac disease. *Am Fam Physician.* 2007; 76(12):1795–1802.

Schuppan D, Junker Y, Barisani D. Celiac disease: from pathogenesis to novel therapies. *Gastroenterology.* 2009; 137(6):1912–1933.

CONSTIPATION

ESSENTIALS OF DIAGNOSIS

▶ Best treated with lifestyle modification.

▶ Laboratory studies and imaging rarely needed.

▶ Caution if red flags present, including bleeding or weight loss.

General Considerations

Constipation can cause abdominal pain. Causes should be sought. Causes of constipation often can be addressed without laboratory studies or imaging studies.

History

History includes infrequent stooling (<3 times per week), straining in >25% of attempts, need for maneuvers to help facilitate defication such as digital evacuation, support of pelvic floor, or rare loose stools without use of laxatives. Evaluation for underlying disorders should be explored if warning signs are present. Red flags include bleeding, anemia, change in stool caliper, unintended weight loss of ≥10 lb, or abnormal findings on exam.

Physical Examination

Examination should include abdominal and rectal exam. The rectal exam should evaluate anal wink, integrity and strength of anal sphincter, presence of impacted stool, pain with palpation, presence of fissures or hemorrhoids, and presence of blood.

Diagnostic Studies

Laboratory or imaging studies are occasionally needed. Endoscopy should be performed in patients aged >50 years without prior colon cancer screening, patients with evidence of bleeding, rectal prolapse, change in stool caliper, and patients with weight loss. Simple radiologic studies can demonstrate the presence of large amounts of stool in the rectum and large bowel. Laboratory testing includes complete blood count, complete metabolic panel, and screening for hypothyroidism. A vitamin D level may be useful in some circumstances. Constipation can be evaluated further with defecography and colon transit testing. Pelvic floor dysfunction testing, including radiography, anal manometry, and electromyography, may be helpful in patients not responsive to initial treatment attempts.

Treatment

The most effective initial treatment is lifestyle modification. Modifications include increased physical activity, increased dietary fiber, and increased fluid intake. Biofeedback techniques can be used for pelvic floor dysfunction. Secondary treatment includes consistent intake of osmotic agents such as magnesium hydroxide or lactulose.

Treatment with polyethylene glycol (Miralax) may be tried. Other laxatives have shown variable effectiveness in clinical trials. These include senna, bisacodyl, methylcellulose, docusate, psyllium, and other bulking agents. Studies on probiotics and prebiotics show mixed results. Most studies were done in patients with constipation-dominant irritable bowel syndrome rather than isolated constipation. The use of some probiotics seems to improve transit time and stool consistency. Stimulants such as $5HT_4$ agonists should be reserved for patients after further evaluation from a gastrointestinal specialist.

Chatoor D, Emmnauel A. Constipation and evacuation disorders. *Best Practice Res Clin Gastroenterol.* 2009; 23(4):517–530.

Cohn A. Stool withholding . *J Pediatr Neurol.* 2009; 8(1):29–30.

Emmanuel AV, Tack J, Quigley EM, Talley NJ. Pharmacological management of constipation. *Neurogastroenterol Motil.* 2009: 21:41–54.

Jamshed N, Lee ZE, Olden KW. Diagnostic approach to chronic constipation in adults. *Am Fam Physician.* 2011; 84(3):299–306.

McCallum IJD, Ong S, Mercer-Jones M. Chronic constipation in adults. *Br Med J.* 2009; 338:b831.

Walia R, Mahajan L, Steffen R. Recent advances in chronic constipation. *Curr Opin Pediatr.* October 2009; 21(5):661–666.

APPENDICITIS

 ESSENTIALS OF DIAGNOSIS

▶ History of periumbilical pain migrating to RLQ with anorexia, nausea, and vomiting is often diagnostic.

▶ CT scan is test of choice for most suspected cases that need confirmation.

▶ Urgent surgical consult is needed.

▶ Left shift of elevated WBC count 7000–19,000 is helpful in diagnosis.

General Considerations

Appendicitis occurs in >250,000 people per year in the United States alone. Appendicitis occurs in people of any age, but is most common in later childhood through young adulthood. The presentation of appendicitis in young children and the elderly is often atypical. There is no race or gender predilection. Diagnosis in female patients can be more difficult, although males are more likely to have a perforated appendix.

Pathogenesis

The appendix is a long diverticulum extending from the cecum. Appendicitis results when the long lumen is occluded. Proliferation of lymphoid tissue, associated with viral infections, Epstein-Barr virus, upper respiratory infection, or gastroenteritis, is the most common cause of obstruction and appendicitis in young adults. Other causes of occlusion include tumors, foreign bodies, fecaliths, parasites, and complications of Crohn's disease.

Clinical Findings

A. Symptoms and Signs

History is the most important component of diagnosis. Missed diagnosis of appendicitis can have severe sequelae. The presence of the following historical indicators should be elicited: abdominal pain, usually RLQ pain often preceded by periumbilical pain (~100% of patients); anorexia (~100%); nausea (90%), with vomiting (75%); progression of abdominal pain from periumbilical to RLQ (50%); and classic progression from vague abdominal pain to anorexia, nausea, vomiting, RLQ pain, and low-grade fever (50%).

B. Physical Examination

Careful abdominal examination with inspection, palpation, and percussion often identifies the cause of abdominal pain. Peritoneal signs, including rigidity, rebound tenderness, and guarding, and a low-grade fever [38°C (100.4°F)], are characteristic findings. Rebound tenderness and sharp pain on palpation of the McBurney point is usually elicited 2 inches from the anterior superior iliac spine on a line drawn from this process through the umbilicus. However, the size of the appendix and the location of pain with palpation may vary, so pain may occur at a remote distance from the classic McBurney point.

Pelvic examination should be performed in all women who present with RLQ pain to rule out gynecologic causes. Thorough respiratory and genitourinary examination is often helpful. Rectal examination is useful when the diagnosis remains unclear.

There is debate about the use of analgesics during the evaluation of possible appendicitis. Traditional practice suggested that the use of pain medication may mask important signs or symptoms. Studies showed mixed results, although more recent one have shown that the use of opiate medications alleviate pain without compromising, and possibly enhancing, the examination. Recent studies have shown increased pain relief on treatment when nonsteroidal anti-inflammatory pain medication is used. This contrasts with results of prior studies. Additional studies suggest that informed consent is compromised by not using adequate pain medication. Observational units and sequential examines can be helpful.

C. Laboratory Findings

Many laboratory studies are performed routinely on patients with abdominal pain. Few, if any, are truly helpful and can be misleading. Studies suggest the WBC count is seldom helpful diagnostically, although if the WBC count is <7000/mm³, appendicitis is unlikely. A WBC count of >19,000/mm³ is associated with an 80% probability of appendicitis. The presence of neutrophilia makes the diagnosis of appendicitis more likely but is not diagnostic. Increased WBCs with neutrophilia generally is accompanied by increased C-reactive protein levels. The presence of all three is not diagnostic, but the absence of all three rules out appendicitis.

Routine use of a chemistry examination is helpful to determine the level of dehydration. Urinalysis commonly shows leukocytosis and increased red blood cells and thus may be misleading. All women of childbearing age should have a pregnancy test. Urine markers of acute pediatric appendicitis may help improve diagnostic accuracy in children.

D. Imaging Studies

Imaging studies can delay treatment, increase cost, and increase radiation exposure. When the diagnosis is clear from the history and physical (H&P), rapid surgical consult should be obtained prior to imaging studies. Studies are helpful in less clear cases and may decrease rate of removal of normal appendices. Current rate of negative pathology is ~3%. CT scan is the single best test for diagnosing appendicitis. It is cost-efficient and fast, and provides low radiation exposure when specific protocols are used. Complete adominal radiographs can be misleading, are not diagnostic in most cases, and cost about the same as CT scan. CT scan can be done without contrast yet without loss of accuracy. Use of oral contrast is difficult and unnecessary in cases of suspected appendicitis. Ultrasound is less invasive than CT, is cost-efficient, and can be useful in situations when CT scan is not possible. Findings are considered "normal" only if a normal appendix is seen. An appendix located retroperitoneally or in the pelvis can be difficult to visualize. Ultrasound may be useful for gynecologic abnormalities and in evaluation of pregnant patients. It also is a good choice for children because of lack of contrast and patient compliance. Focused spiral CT without contrast can be performed in less than an hour and is very sensitive and specific for appendicitis. Use of contrast may be helpful in certain cases, especially in patients who are thin or older, and those with unclear etiology.

Treatment

Treatment consists of surgical removal of inflamed appendix via laparotomy or laparoscopy. Laparotomy is faster, simpler, and less expensive, and has a lower rate of complications. Laparoscopy allows visualization of other possible causes of pain. Recent advances in surgical technology have shown other benefits of laparoscopic procedures: faster recovery, shorter hospital stay, and decreased postoperative pain. Choice of surgical options should be done on an individual basis and based on surgical experience and opinion at time of surgery. A few small studies suggest that treatment with antibiotics and observation can result in temporary resolution of symptoms but generally result in high reoccurrence rates. This may be an option for medically unstable patients or where surgery is not readily available.

Armstrong C. ACEP releases guidelines on evaluation of suspected acute appendicitis. *Am Fam Physician.* 2010; 81(8):1043–1044.

Cartwright SL, Knudson MP. Evaluation of acute abdominal pain in adults. *Am Fam Physician.* 2008; 77(7):971–978. [PMID: 18441863]

Ebell MH. Diagnosis of appendicitis part II: laboratory and imaging tests. *Am Fam Physician* 2008 April 15; 77(8):1153–1155. [PMID: 18481565]

Frei SP, et al. Is early analgesia associated with delayed treatment of appendicitis? *Am J Emerg Med.* 2008; 26(2):176–180. [PMID: 18272097]

Hlibczuk V, Dattaro JA, Jin Z, Falzon L, Brown MD. Diagnostic accuracy of noncontrast computer tomography for appendicitis in adults: a systematic review. *Ann Emerg Med.* 2010; 55(1):51–59.

Kentsis A, Lin YY, et al. Discovery and validation of urine markers of acute pediatric appendicitis using high-accuracy mass spectrometry. *Ann Emerg Med.* 2010; 55(1):62–70.

Rybkin AV, Thoeni RF. Current concepts in imaging of appendicitis. *Radiol Clin North Am.* 2007; 45(3):411–422, vii. [PMID: 17601500]

Sonanvane S. Sonography of the surgical abdomen in children (includes images). *Ultrasound Clin.* 2008; 3(1);67–82.

INFLAMMATORY BOWEL DISEASE

 ESSENTIALS OF DIAGNOSIS

▶ Inflammatory bowel disease should be considered in patients with abdominal pain associated with blood in stool or elevated sedimentation rate.

▶ CT scan remains helpful; colonoscopy is essential only after control of acute attack.

▶ Current medical management is changing rapidly.

▶ General Considerations

Inflammatory bowel disease (IBD) is a broad category encompassing several disease subtypes. The most common are ulcerative colitis (UC) and Crohn's disease (CD). Other inflammatory bowel conditions, including acute infectious colitis and gastroenteritis, are addressed elsewhere. The Human Genome Project has shown a clear genetic predisposition to both UC and CD. Prevalence of CD is much higher in Caucasians, especially in those of Jewish descent. Onset of IBD is most commonly seen at ages 15–30 years. Specific gene loci have been identified showing a correlation with susceptibility to either CD or UC. This susceptibility seems to be affected by environmental factors such as smoking and microflora of the gut. There appears to be an inappropriate inflammatory response to normal intestinal microbiology.

Environmental factors may make IBD more prevalent in people who work indoors and less prevalent in manual laborers who work outdoors. There is a 20–50% increase in the prevalence of IBD in first-degree relatives and a 50–100-fold increase in the offspring of patients with IBD. Risk factors, including work environment and diet, differ among subtypes of IBD. Smoking appears to decrease the risk of UC but increases risk and severity of CD. Birth control pills seem to increase the risk of CD. Both diseases are more prevalent in urban areas, suggesting environmental factors such as pollution, chemical exposure, and sun exposure. Patients with IBD have a higher incidence of ankylosing spondylosis, cholangitis, and psoriasis.

▶ Pathogenesis

Increased knowledge of genetic susceptibility has increased the understanding of pathogenesis. Environmental factors seem to allow for altered immunologic responses to normal intestinal flora and destruction within the mucosa of the GI tract. CD appears to be related to altered macrophage function. UC is more likely related to a pathologic inflammatory response to normal intestinal microflora. Decreased bifidobacteria and lactobacilli levels are noted in patients with active CD compared with those in remission and healthy controls. *Fusobacterium varium* may be a factor in pathogenesis of UC. Changes within the microflora, combined with the immune response, result in altered mucosal barriers, luminal antigens, and macrophage function.

▶ Clinical Findings

A. Symptoms and Signs

Inflammatory bowel diseases usually present with abdominal pain, bleeding, vomiting, diarrhea, abdominal cramping, muscle spasm, weight loss, and anemia. Abdominal pain is more common in patients with CD. Patients with UC almost always present with perirectal pain and bloody diarrhea. CD can be more difficult to differentiate from other diseases based on history and physical examination alone. CD can present anywhere from mouth to anus (skip lesions). UC is focused at the rectum and colon. RLQ pain is present in most patients with CD, reflecting involvement of the terminal ileum in 85% of cases. Only the mucosa is affected in UC. CD can affect the entire bowel wall, resulting in more destructive lesions causing fistula, bowel obstruction, and extraintestinal lesions. CD can be associated with liver, skin, joint, and ocular lesions.

B. Physical Examination

Physical examination findings are not specific. Evaluation of the rectum for evidence of fissures, ulceration, or abscess can be helpful. Fullness or a palpable mass suggests abscess. Examination often reveals nonspecific generalized tenderness, with focal findings dependent on extent and activity of disease. Skin examination may be useful. CD is associated with erythema nodosa and aphthous stomatitis. UC is associated with pyoderma gangrenosa. Growth retardation and delayed sexual maturation can occur from disease process and medications used to treat disease.

C. Laboratory Findings

Recommended laboratory tests include ESR; C-reactive protein; CBC; liver function tests (LFTs); albumin and prealbumin; electrolytes; stool studies; and vitamin B_{12}, folate, and vitamin D levels. ESR is elevated in 80% of patients with CD and 40% of patients with UC. Elevated C-reactive protein is present in 95% of symptomatic patients with CD. Anemia from iron deficiency and blood loss is common. Leukocytosis with increased eosinophilia is noted often. Liver involvement in patients with CD (eg, sclerosing cholangitis, autoimmune hepatitis, and cirrhosis) may affect LFTs. Albumin and prealbumin are indicators of malnutrition from malabsorption. Stool studies rule out infectious etiologies of colitis. Perinuclear antineutrophil antibody (pANCA) titer is useful to differentiate between CD and UC. pANCA is present in ~6% of patients with CD and 70% of patients with UC. *Saccharomyces cervisiae* (ASCA) is found in ~50% of individuals with CD and correlates closely with involvement of small bowel, stenosing lesions, and perforation.

D. Imaging Studies

Colonoscopy is the most accurate diagnostic test, allows direct visualization of mucosa, and biopsy. It is not recommended in acute active disease because of the risk of perforation. Histological variances help differentiate CD from UC. Visualizaion of skip lesions, cobblestoning, and strictures suggest CD. Colonoscopy with ileoscopy, capsule endoscopy, CT scan, and small bowel follow-through help evaluate all areas of disease. Capsule endoscopy, when combined with other testing, improves sensitivity to >90% and improves specificity. Capsule endoscopy is contraindicated in patients with known or suspected stricture. MRI and ultrasound help identify extraintestinal areas and complications of disease. Plain films are most helpful identifying toxic megacolon, and the "thumbprinting" sign (seen with bowel wall edema) and may identify strictures, skip lesions, and perforation. The classic string sign is seen on barium enema. Abdominal CT is helpful in identifying abscess, fistula, bowel wall thickening, and fat striation.

▶ Treatment

Management of IBD includes medical therapy, nutritional support, psychological support, and surveillance for cancer. Familial and genetic counseling is important to help family members cope with exacerbations of the disease and because of the strong pattern of inheritance.

Mesalamine products are used for mild to moderate disease and believed to have anti-inflammatory and immunosuppressive properties and include mesalamine, balsalazide, olsalazine, and sulfasalazine. All can cause nausea, headache, and abdominal pain. Antibiotics, including metronidazole and ciprofloxacin, are widely used, and have anti-inflammatory as well as anti-infectious properties. Mild cases can improve with use of budesonide. Moderate to severe cases may be treated with prednisone. Severe cases are treated with azathioprine and 6-mercaptopurine. Immune modulating medications are used for long-term maintenance of remission in combination with steroids or anti-TNF preparations such as infliximab, adalimamab, and certolizumab pegol. Methotrexate use can enable the practitioner to wean the patient from steroids but may cause bone marrow suppression, leukopenia, hepatic fibrosis, and pneumonitis.

Patients with severe disease require hospital admission for bowel rest, parenteral nutritional support, and corticosteroids. Increased use of immunomodulators has allowed for less use of systemic steroids.

Nutritional therapy is helpful to maintain remission and decrease likelihood of nutritional deficiency due to malabsorption, especially in children. Research suggests that the use of fecal basteriotherapy, helminthic therapy, and other biologics may have a role in treatment by altering the bacterial flora of the gut.

Surgical therapy is often required. Approximately 85% of patients with persistent elevation of C-reactive protein and frequent liquid stools require total colectomy. Strictures and abscess formation may necessitate surgical excision of small segments of bowel or strictureplasty. Surgery is used for intractable bleeding, abscess, or fistula formation. Patients with limited resection have fewer stools, and better anorectal function.

Risk of adenocarcinoma is increased in patients with chronic colon disease. Risk of cancer development in UC is equivalent to CD with colon involvement. Biannual colonoscopy and biopsy is recommended for disease present for ≥10 years. Risk of other cancers, such as adenocarcinoma of the jejunum and ileum (when involved), lymphoma, and squamous cell carcinoma of the vulva and rectum, is increased in CD.

Abraham C, Cho J. Inflammatory bowel disease. *N Engl J Med*. 2009;361:2066–2078.

Borody TJ, Torres M, Campbell J, et al. Reversal of inflammatory bowel disease (IBD) with recurrent fecal microbiota transplants (FMT). *Am J Gastroenterol*. 2011; 106:352.

Centers for Disease Control and Prevention. www.cdc.gov/ibd/

Feller M, Huwiler K, Schoepfer A, et al. Long-term antibiotic treatment for Crohn's disease: systematic review and meta-analysis of placebo-controlled trials. *Clin Infect Dis*. 2010; 50(4): 473–480.

Larsen S, Bendtzen K, Nielsen OH. Extraintestinal manifestations of inflammatory bowel disease: epidemiology, diagnosis, and management. *Ann Med.* 2010;42(2):97–114.

Marrero F. Severe complications of inflammatory bowel disease. *Med Clin North Am.* 2008; 92(3):671–686. [PMID: 18387381]

Peyrin-Biroulet L, Loftus EV Jr, Colombel JF, Sandborn WJ. The natural history of adult Crohn's disease in population-based cohorts. *Am J Gastroenterol.* 2010; 105(2):289–297.

Tamboli CP. Current medical therapy for chronic inflammatory bowel diseases. *Surg Clin North Am.* 2007; 87(3):697–725. [PMID: 17560421]

Wilkins T, Jarvis K, Patel J. Diagnosis and management of Crohn's disease. *Am Fam Physician.* 2011;84(12):1365–1375.

DIVERTICULITIS

 ESSENTIALS OF DIAGNOSIS

▶ More than 3 days of abdominal pain with low-grade fever.

▶ Commonly left-sided pain (right-sided pain more common in people of Asian descent).

▶ CT scan test of choice.

▶ Early antibiotic treatment, bowel rest, hydration.

General Considerations

Diverticulitis occurs in 10–25% of patients with diverticulosis. In the twentieth century, the incidence of diverticulosis increased as fiber intake decreased. In addition to insufficient fiber, age is the single greatest risk factor. Typically, diverticulosis is seen in patients aged ≥60 years, is uncommon before age 40, and is present in 50% of people aged >90 years. Patients of western European descent have increased prevalence of left-sided diverticula. Patients of Asian descent have increased prevalence of right-sided diverticula.

Pathogenesis

The pathology of diverticulitis is directly related to the anatomy of the bowel wall. True diverticula consists of outpouching of all three layers of the wall: mucosa, submucosa, and muscular layer. Most cases of diverticulitis involve pseudodiverticula with herniation of the mucosa and submucosa through the muscular layer. Diverticula tend to form in rows between mesenteric and lateral teniae. The area of penetration of the vasa recta has the greatest muscular weakness and is therefore the most common site of herniation.

Lack of dietary fiber contributes to the development of diverticula. As fiber content of the stool decreases, colonic pressure increases and transit time decreases. As we age, increased cross-fibers within the collagen and elastin render the bowel wall less compliant, resulting in high pressure in the colon, and essentially blowing out areas of weakness in the colon wall. Previous recommendation to avoid seeds, nuts, and corn were based on the misconception that these foods caused aggravation of diverticulitis. Recent studies do not support avoiding these foods and suggest that higher intakes of corn and nuts could help decrease the incidence of diverticulitis, at least in men.

Diverticulitis occurs when infection is associated with one or more of these diverticula. Micro- or macroperforations of diverticula may occur, resulting in bowel contents contacting the peritoneum and infecting the pericolonic fat, mesentery, and associated organs. This can localize and result in the development of an abscess, peritonitis, or fistula. A fistula can form between the colon and an abdominal organ. A colovesical fistula, connecting the colon and urinary bladder, is most common.

Clinical Findings

A. Symptoms and Signs

Left lower quadrant (LLQ) pain occurs in 93–100% of patients. Pain may be right-sided, especially in patients of Asian descent. A duration of ≥3 days of RLQ pain is suggestive of diverticulitis rather than appendicitis. Patients commonly have nausea, vomiting, constipation, or diarrhea. Dysuria and urinary frequency may be present. Complicated diverticulitis, as with a colovesical fistula, can present with recurrent urinary tract infections. In macroperforation, diffuse abdominal pain is present.

B. Physical Examination

Abnormal vital signs, including tachycardia and temperature of ≥38.1°C (≥100.7°F), give supporting evidence for the diagnosis of diverticulitis. Fever is present in most patients. Examination should include complete abdominal examination. Signs suggestive of diverticulitis include tender LLQ or less frequently RLQ tenderness, signs of peritoneal irritation such as guarding or tenderness to percussion, and occasional presence of a tender mass, suggesting the presence of an abscess. Rectal examination may demonstrate rectal tenderness or mass.

C. Laboratory Findings

Patients suspected of having diverticulitis should undergo a CBC and urinalysis. The WBC count is increased in more than two-thirds of patients, with a high prevalence of polymorphonuclear leukocytes, Anemia may be noted if there is associated diverticular bleeding. Urinalysis can show evidence of inflammation if there is irritation of the peritoneum surrounding the bladder or evidence of infection if a fistula is present.

D. Imaging Studies

Flat and upright abdominal films, or CT of the abdomen and pelvis if the diagnosis is unclear, should be obtained. Abdominal films can show evidence of free air, ileus, or mass. CT scan shows a thickened colonic wall and allows insertion of percutaneous drainage if an abscess is present, allowing for delay in surgical intervention. Similar findings can be seen on ultrasound, but CT best confirms diverticulitis by revealing the presence and location of an abscess and allowing for identification of other pathologic processes such as cancer, Crohn's disease, and appendicitis. Ureteral obstruction, fistula, or air in the bladder can be seen. Colonoscopy should be done 4–6 weeks after resolution of diverticulitis to evaluate for concomitant cancerous lesions, and if IBD is suspected.

▶ Treatment

Treatment depends on severity of disease and the health of the patient. Outpatient treatment includes clear liquid diet and oral broad-spectrum antibiotics, although research does not show clear benefit with the use of antibiotics. Current recommendations include ciprofloxacin and metronidazole for 7–10 days, but CDC or Sanford antibiotic guidelines should be followed because of changing antibiotic resistance. Medications such as morphine increase colonic pressure and should be avoided. Meperidine is the best choice for pain control because it decreases colonic pressure. Steroids and NSAIDs should be avoided because of the increased risk of GI bleeding and perforation.

Patients with signs and symptoms of inflammation, such as fever and leukocytosis, require hospitalization. Treatment includes complete bowel rest, intravenous fluids, and intravenous broad-spectrum antibiotics. A nasogastric tube is not needed unless there is significant ileus or obstruction. Most patients improve in 48–72 hours, at which time they can resume their regular diet, receive oral antibiotics, and be discharged home with close follow-up. A high-fiber diet is recommended for all patients after recovery. Surgical resection is recommended for perforation or uncontrolled bleeding.

Surgery is seldom recommended after a first attack, given a recurrence rate of 20–30%. However, this rate increases with each subsequent attack, as does the risk of associated morbidity. Therefore, surgery should be considered after the second or third attack. Surgical intervention can be considered with a first attack for immunocompromised patients because of their increased risk of morbidity and mortality. Surgical intervention is done on a case-by-case basis for complicated diverticulitis. Allowing decreased inflammation of the bowel wall prior to resection and anastomosis by use of percutaneous drainage and antibiotic treatment improves outcome. Morbidity and mortality rates are improved when primary anastomosis can be performed, rather than a two-stage approach with colostomy. Patients aged <40 years at the first attack have an increased lifelong risk, due to the increased life expectancy, although risk with each attack is not increased. These cases are determined on an individual bases based on frequency and severity of attacks.

de Korte N, Unlü C, Boermeester MA, et al. Use of antibiotics in uncomplicated diverticulitis. *Br J Surg.* 2011;98(6):761–767.

Nelson RS, et al. Clinical outcomes of complicated diverticulitis managed nonoperatively. *Am J Surg.* 2008; 196(6):969-972; discussion 973–974. [PMID: 19095117]

Touzios JG, Dozois EJ. Diverticulosis and acute diverticulitis. *Gastroenterol Clin North Am.* 2009; 38(3):513–525. [PMID: 19699411]

Weisberger L, Jamieson B. Clinical inquiries: How can you help prevent a recurrence of diverticulitis? *J Fam Practice.* 2009; 58(7): 381–382.

Meckel's Diverticulum

Meckel's diverticulum is a congenital anomaly of the GI tract in which an outpouching portion of intestine, derived from the fetal yolk stalk, contains gastric or pancreatic tissue. Patients can present with abdominal pain, nausea, vomiting, or intestinal bleeding. Complications include diverticulitis, intussusception, perforation, and obstruction. The best diagnosistic test is the technetium-99m pertechnetate scan. Treatment is surgical.

Marinella MA, Mustafa M. Acute diverticulitis in patients 40 years of age and younger. *Am J Emerg Med.* 2000; 18:140. [PMID: 10750916]

Salzman H, Lillie D. Diverticular disease: diagnosis and treatment. *Am Fam Physician.* 2005; 72:1229. [PMID: 16225025]

ABDOMINAL WALL PAIN

There are many presentations of abdominal wall pain because of the multiple different causes of abdominal wall pain. Causes include hernias, herpes zoster, neuromas, hematomas of the abdominal wall or rectus sheath, desmoid tumor, endometriosis, myofascial tears, intraabdominal adhesions, neuropathies, slipping rib syndrome, and general myofascial pain. Examination findings suggesting abdominal wall pain include lack of evidence for an intraabdominal process; pain unrelated to meals or bowel function; pain related to posture, a trigger point; and a positive Carnett sign. This is elicited by having the patient tense the abdominal muscles. Areas of tenderness after tensing are considered positive and suggest abdominal wall rather than visceral pain.

Hernias

Types of hernias include inguinal, femoral, umbilical, epigastric, spigelian, and Richter hernias. Hernias are more commonly identified by exam rather than history. History can be confusing with herniation of bowel wall or omentum. Bowel herniation causes visceral pain and obstruction. Omentum herniation causes visceral pain without signs of obstruction. A history of prior surgery, especially laparoscopic surgery, increases the likelihood of a hernia.

Men more typically develop inguinal hernias. Women tend to develop femoral hernias. Umbilical and epigastric hernias are more common in obese or gravid patients. Spigelian hernias, a hernia along the border of the arcuate ligament, is most common in athletes.

Richter hernia is defined by the pathology rather than the location of the hernia. The side of the bowel wall herniates, rather than the entire bowel segment. Often the hernia produces a slight bulge that may be confused with adenopathy or fat. Because this type of hernia results in subtle findings, there often is a delay in diagnosis and a higher fatality rate. Richter hernia is generally found in women aged >50 years, but the incidence is increasing in young men, due to the increased frequency of laparoscopic procedures. Because the instruments used for laparoscopy are so small, the abdominal wall defect remaining after surgery may allow only a portion of the bowel wall to herniate. The resultant tight hernia causes strangulation of the tissue passing through. Prior surgical sites must be examined. Erythema at these sites can be a sign of local infection, fistula formation, or an inflammatory process at the site of scarring.

Although a CT scan can identify hernias, they are often overlooked unless the radiologist is focused on thorough examination of the abdominal wall.

Hernias are best treated surgically. If surgery is contraindicated, hernias causing pain or posing risk of bowel obstruction can be treated with a truss or other restrictive garment.

Rectus Sheath Hematoma

Rectus sheath hematomas can be difficult to diagnose. They tend to occur more commonly in elderly or pregnant patients. The epigastric vessels are sheared, resulting in intramuscular bleeding. Shearing can occur from trauma or twisting motions. History is the most important factor in directing the clinician. A history of unilateral midabdominal pain, use of anticoagulants such as aspirin or warfarin, and abdominal trauma are all important risk factors. Pain is unilateral and worse when patients tense their abdominal muscles. There is often a palpable mass within the rectus sheath.

Coagulation studies and blood count are the most useful laboratory studies. Helpful imaging studies include CT, ultrasound, and MRI. Ultrasound is the cheapest and most useful study if the diagnosis is highly suspected. CT is more useful for identifying other possible causes. MRI sometimes helps if the diagnosis remains unclear. Treatment is generally expectant, but severe cases may warrant reversal of coagulation abnormalities, administration of fluids, or surgical evacuation and ligation or coagulation of vessels.

Herpes Zoster

Herpes zoster should be suspected when there is an abrupt onset of severe abdominal wall pain. Pain associated with zoster can precede the rash by >1 week, although more commonly by 2–4 days. Zoster occurs most frequently in patients aged >50 years. Postherpetic neuralgia (PHN) causes persistant pain, especially in patients aged >60 years. Thorough history and close follow-up are the best measures to establish the diagnosis. Varicella vaccine may help prevent zoster. Treatment of acute zoster with acyclovir, valacyclovir, or famciclovir in combination with a prednisone taper seems to decrease incidence and severity of PHN. Treatment of PHN has proved difficult. Many modalities have been tried with minor success, incuding analgesics, narcotics, nerve stimulation, antidepressants, capsaicin, biofeedback, and nerve blocks.

Other Causes of Abdominal Wall Pain

Surgical scars are the location of many causes of abdominal wall pain. Hernias and endometriosis can occur at these site. Neuromas often form at the border of scars. Other unusual causes include desmoid tumors, myofascial tears, and intraabdominal adhesions. Desmoid tumors are dysplastic tumors of the connective tissue, tend to form in young adults, and can be identified only after surgical removal. Myofascial tears and intraabdominal adhesions occur most frequently in athletes.

▶ Treatment

Trigger points often reproduce abdominal wall pain. Finding this point can help both diagnosis and treatment. Trigger points are often found along the lateral border of the rectus abdominis muscle, where nerve roots become stretched, compressed, and irritated. Points are also found at areas of tight-fitting clothing or at insertion points of muscles. The Carnett sign, described earlier, is useful for diagnosis of trigger points. Relief of many causes of abdominal wall pain can be achieved by injection of lidocaine or its equivalent into the point of most tenderness. This treatment can be diagnostic and therapeutic. Insertion of the needle into the correct point elicits intense pain, which improves dramatically after injection. Areas requiring more than one injection can be injected with a small amount of steroids. Steroids should be avoided in areas near hernias or into fascia, as they can cause hernia formation. Dry needling has proved useful, but initial treatment may cause more pain.. Patients with severe needle aversion may benefit from a therapeutic trial of a transcutaneous lidocaine patch. Pain clinics may help in more difficult cases.

Management of this type of pain can be difficult. Patient education and reassurance are important. Preventing further unnecessary testing can be avoided by decreasing patients' concerns about the pain. Tricyclic antidepressants can be useful at low doses.

Suleiman S, Johnston DE. The abdominal wall: an overlooked source of pain. *Am Fam Physician*. 2001; 64:431. [PMID: 11515832]

GYNECOLOGIC CAUSES OF ABDOMINAL PAIN

Gynecologic causes of abdominal pain can be separated into three categories: acute causes in nonpregnant patients, chronic problems in nonpregnant patients, and acute causes in pregnant patients. Acute causes include PID, adnexal torsion, ruptured ovarian cyst, hemorrhagic corpus luteum cyst, endometriosis, and tuboovarian abscess. Chronic causes in nonpregnant patients include dysmenorrhea, mittelschmerz, endometriosis, obstructive müllerian duct abnormalities, leiomyomas, cancer, and pelvic congestion syndrome. Causes in pregnant patients include ectopic pregnancy, retained products of conception, septic abortion, and ovarian torsion. Psychological factors greatly contribute to abdominal and pelvic pain. Patients can present with acute pain after a sexual assault.

A wide differential, careful history, and pregnancy test should be considered when evaluating women and girls with abdominal pain. History includes last menstrual period, detailed menstrual history, sexual history including possible assault, and family history. Physical examination includes careful abdominal, pelvic, and rectovaginal examinations. Laboratory evaluation is based on findings from the physical examination. LFTs can help identify Fitz-Hughes and Curtis syndromes, especially in the presence of RUQ pain.

Pelvic inflammatory disease occurs in 11% of US women of reproductive age, although it is rare in pregnancy. Numerous biological factors contribute to a higher incidence of PID in adolescents, including lower prevalence of protective chlamydial antibodies, more penetrable cervical mucus, and larger zones of cervical ectopy with more vulnerable columnar cells. Other risk factors increasing the likelihood of PID include early age at first sexual intercourse, higher number of lifetime partners, or a new partner within the last 30–60 days. Diagnosis of PID requires the presence of abdominal pain, adnexal pain, cervical motion tenderness, and at least one of the following: temperature of >38.3°C (>101°F), vaginal discharge, leukocytosis with a cell count of >10,500/mm^3, positive cervical cultures, intracellular diplococci, or WBCs on vaginal smear. Treatment depends on whether the patient requires inpatient or outpatient treatment. Inpatient treatment is required for surgical emergencies, pregnancy, no response to outpatient therapy in 72 hours, nausea and vomiting, or immunodeficiency.

Endometriosis is found in 15–32% of women undergoing laparoscopic evaluation of abdominopelvic pain. The pain is generally cyclical but can present acutely with ruptured ovarian endometrioma. A retroverted, fixed uterus with ash spots on the cervix suggests endometriosis. Conservative treatment includes NSAIDs and oral contraceptive use.

Most gynecologic causes of abdominal pain can be evaluated by ultrasound. Laparoscopy may be needed and can be therapeutic as in ovarian torsion. CT may help delineate unclear ultrasound findings. Consultation with a gynecologist often is warranted.

Baines PA, Allen GM. Pelvic pain and menstrual related illnesses. *Emerg Med Clin North Am* 2001; 19:763. [PMID: 11554286]

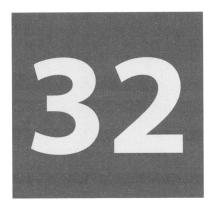

Anemia

Brian A. Primack, MD, PhD, EdM, MS

Kiame J. Mahaniah, MD

► General Considerations

A. Adults

Anemia is defined as an abnormally low circulating red blood cell (RBC) mass, reflected by low serum hemoglobin (Hb). However, the normal range of Hb varies among different populations. For menstruating women, anemia is present if the Hb level is ≤11.6–12.3 g/dL. In men and postmenopausal women, anemia is present if the Hb level is ≤13.0-14.0 g/dL. Other factors, such as age, race, altitude, and exposure to tobacco smoke, can also alter Hb levels.

Anemia is usually classified by cell size (**Table 32-1**). Microcytic anemias, mean corpuscular volume (MCV) < 80 fL, are usually due to iron deficiency, chronic inflammation, or thalassemia. Macrocytic anemias, MCV > 100 fL, are classified as megaloblastic or nonmegaloblastic. Megaloblasts are seen with vitamin B_{12} deficiency and folic acid deficiency. Nonmegaloblastic causes of macrocytosis include alcoholism, hypothyroidism, and chronic liver disease. Causes of normocytic anemia (MCV between 80 and 100 fL) are classified as either hemolytic or nonhemolytic.

B. Children

Normal Hb levels vary with age. At birth, mean Hb is ~16.5 g/dL. This level increases to 18.5 g/dL during the first week of life, followed by a drop to 11.5 g/dL by 1–2 months of age. This physiologic anemia of infancy is mediated by changes in erythropoietin levels. By 1–2 years of age, the Hb level begins to rise, to 14 g/dL in adolescent girls and 15 g/dL in adolescent boys. Thus, laboratory values in children should always be compared with age-appropriate norms.

Many inherited causes of anemia are discovered in infancy and childhood. It is therefore important to obtain a careful family history in an anemic child, especially if the episodes of anemia are intermittent. Sickle cell anemia, thalassemia, glucose-6-phosphate dehydrogenase (G6PD) deficiency, and spherocytosis are examples of inherited forms of anemia.

Other elements of the history are also important when evaluating a child for anemia. Because infants with anemia can exhibit poor feeding, irritability, and tachycardia rather than classic adult symptoms and signs, these atypical features should be explored with the family. Nutrition should be evaluated carefully, with attention to dietary sources of vitamin B_{12}, folic acid, and iron. Potential sources of lead poisoning must also be considered. Finally, adolescents often require additional support and explanation. For instance, adolescent girls may not know what constitutes a normal menstrual period, so the specific number of tampons and pads used should be obtained.

Beutler E, Waalen J. The definition of anemia: what is the lower limit of normal of the blood hemoglobin concentration? *Blood.* 2006;107(5):1747–1750.

Gabrilove J. Anemia and the elderly: clinical considerations. *Baillieres Clin Haematol.* 2005;18:417. [PMID: 15792915]

Little DR. Ambulatory management of common forms of anemia. *Am Fam Physician.* 1999;59:1598. [PMID: 10193599]

Mehta BC. Approach to a patient with anemia. *Indian J Med Sci.* 2004;58:26. [PMID: 14960799]

Onega T. Sorting out the common anemias. *J Am Acad Physician Assist.* 2000;13:30. [PMID: 11521621]

Rodgers GM, et al. Cancer- and chemotherapy-induced anemia. *J Natl Compreh Cancer Netw.* 2008;6:536. [PMID: 18597709]

Ruiz-Arguelles GJ, et al. Altitude above sea level as a variable for definition of anemia. *Blood.* 2006;108(6):2131–2132. [PMID: 16956960]

Scott S, et al. Clinical inquiries. How should we follow up a positive screen for anemia in a 1-year old? *J Fam Practice.* 2005;54:272. [PMID: 15755383]

Smith DL. Anemia in the elderly. *Am Fam Physician,* 2000;62:1565. [PMID: 11037074]

Woodman R, et al. Anemia in older adults. *Curr Opin Hematol.* 2005;12:123. [PMID: 15725902]

Table 32-1. Anemia classification by cell size.

Microcytic	Macrocytic
Iron deficiency	Megaloblastic
Anemia of chronic disease	Vitamin B_{12} deficiency
Thalassemias	Folic acid deficiency
Sideroblastic anemia	Drug-related
	Nonmegaloblastic
	Hypothyroidism
	Liver disease
	Alcoholism
	Myelodysplastic syndromes

Normocytic

Hemolytic	Nonhemolytic
Intrinsic	Acute blood loss
Membrane defects (spherocytosis)	Aplastic anemia
Enzyme deficiencies (G6PD deficiency)	Anemia of chronic disease
Hemoglobinopathies (sickle cell disease)	Chronic renal insufficiency
Extrinsic	Myelophthisis
Autoimmune	
Warm antibody–mediated (chronic	
lymphocytic leukemia, systemic	
lupus erythematosus, idiopathic)	
Cold antibody–mediated (*Mycoplasma*,	
idiopathic)	
Alloimmune	
Nonimmune	
Splenomegaly	
Physical trauma (thrombotic thrombocyto	
penic purpura, disseminated	
intravascular coagulation, burns)	
Infections (malaria)	

G6PD, glucose-6-phosphate dehydrogenase.

▼ MICROCYTIC ANEMIA

IRON-DEFICIENCY ANEMIA

ESSENTIALS OF DIAGNOSIS

▶ Low iron and serum ferritin levels, and elevated total iron-binding capacity (TIBC).

▶ Response to therapeutic trial of iron.

▶ In adults, nearly always due to blood loss.

▶ Can also be due to poor iron intake or poor absorption.

▶ General Considerations

Iron deficiency is the most common cause of anemia. Approximately 2% of women and 1% of men develop anemia due to the deficiency.

The average adult has 2–4 g of stored iron. About 65% of this reserve is located in the RBCs, with the remainder in the bone marrow, liver, spleen, and other body tissues. Iron deficiency occurs when there is a net imbalance resulting from either excessive loss or poor intake.

Toddlers aged 1–3 years are vulnerable to iron-deficiency anemia. National surveys report rates as high as 15% in this age group.

▶ Pathogenesis

Extracorporeal blood loss is the most common cause of iron-deficiency anemia. When RBCs are destroyed within the body, the reticuloendothelial system usually adequately recycles iron into the next generation of RBCs. Poor iron uptake, due to either poor nutrition or inadequate absorption, is a less common cause of iron-deficiency anemia.

Women develop iron deficiency more readily than men because of increased potential for iron loss. On average, women lose an additional 1 mg of iron each day in menstruation. Pregnancy, lactation, and delivery additionally cost a woman an average of 1000 mg of iron each.

In infancy, risk factors for iron deficiency are primarily dietary and include exclusive breastfeeding beyond 6 months without iron supplementation, prolonged bottle-feeding, and excessive cow's milk consumption. However, other risk factors for iron deficiency in childhood include Hispanic ethnicity, poverty, and being overweight.

▶ Prevention

The US Preventive Services Task Force (USPSTF) recommends primary prevention of iron-deficiency anemia by encouraging parents to breastfeed their infants and to include iron-enriched foods in the diet of infants and young children.

Although there is insufficient evidence to recommend for or against the routine use of iron supplements for healthy infants or pregnant women, the USPSTF does currently recommend screening for iron-deficiency anemia—using Hb or hematocrit—for both asymptomatic pregnant women and high-risk infants (B recommendation).

▶ Clinical Findings

A. Symptoms and Signs

Iron deficiency can be asymptomatic, especially in the early stages. However, patients can present with varying degrees of any of the common symptoms associated with anemia, such as weakness, fatigue, dizziness, headaches, exercise intolerance, or palpitations. Possible signs on physical examination include tachycardia, tachypnea, and pallor, especially of the palpebral conjunctivae.

One symptom associated with iron deficiency in particular is pica—the craving for ice, clay, or other unusual substances that may or may not contain iron. Rare symptoms include koilonychia ("spoon nails"), blue sclerae, and atrophic glossitis. In childhood, iron-deficiency anemia has been associated with cognitive and motor delays.

▶ B. Laboratory Findings

Hemoglobin levels can be normal in early iron deficiency. Mild deficiency yields Hb levels of 9–11 g/dL, whereas in severe deficiency levels can fall as low as 5 g/dL.

Serum iron levels below 60 µg/dL indicate iron deficiency. As iron stores are depleted, serum ferritin falls below 30 ng/dL. TIBC therefore rises above 400 µg/dL. Percent iron saturation, which is inversely proportional to TIBC, falls below ~15%.

Although serum ferritin levels are the most accurate measure of iron deficiency, it should be noted that ferritin is an acute-phase reactant that can be elevated during acute illnesses, chronic inflammatory states, or cancer.

The gold standard of iron deficiency is bone marrow examination, which shows absent iron reserves in affected patients.

▶ Treatment

Iron can be increased in the diet. Foods particularly rich in iron include meats (especially liver) and fish. Whole grains, green leafy vegetables, nuts, seeds, and dried fruit also contain iron. Toddlers' multivitamins commonly contain iron. Cooking with iron pots and pans also increases iron intake.

Oral iron therapy is available in the form of iron salts. One 300-mg tablet of iron sulfate, for example, delivers 60 mg of elemental iron. One 300-mg tablet of iron gluconate delivers 34 mg of elemental iron and may be better tolerated by some patients. Up to 180 mg of elemental iron can be given each day, depending on the degree of deficiency. Absorption of oral iron is dependent on many environmental factors. An acidic environment increases absorption; thus iron tablets are often given with ascorbic acid. For this same reason, antacids should be avoided within several hours of iron ingestion. Other substances that impair the absorption of iron include calcium, soy protein, tannins (found in tea), and phytate (found in bran). Side effects of oral iron therapy include gastrointestinal distress and constipation. For this reason, some physicians routinely prescribe an as-necessary stool softener along with each iron prescription.

Iron can be given intramuscularly or intravenously to patients who cannot tolerate oral iron because of gastrointestinal upset. This route may also be convenient for patients who have concurrent gastrointestinal malabsorption or ongoing blood loss, such as those with severe inflammatory bowel disease. Phlebitis, muscle breakdown, anaphylaxis, and fever are possible side effects of parenteral iron.

Specialist consensus is that efficacy of treatment should be tracked with a CBC and differential every 3 months for a year.

Brotanek JM, et al. Iron deficiency in early childhood in the United States: risk factors and racial/ethnic disparities. *Pediatrics.* 2007;120(3):568–575. [PMID: 17766530]

Leung AK, Chan KW. Iron deficiency anemia. *Adv Pediatr.* 2001;48:385. [PMID: 11480764]

Screening for iron deficiency anemia, Topic Page, May 2006. US Preventive Services Task Force; Agency for Healthcare Research and Quality, Rockville, MD (available at http://www.ahrq.gov/clinic/uspstf/uspsiron.htm; accessed July 30 2010).

Short M. Iron deficiency anemia, evaluation and treatment. *Am Fam Physician.* 2013;87(2):98–104.

Third Report on Nutrition Monitoring in the US. Bethesda, MD: Federation of American Societies for Experimental Biology, Life Sciences Research Office; 1995: 2.

ANEMIA OF CHRONIC DISEASE

 ESSENTIALS OF DIAGNOSIS

- ▶ Presence of a chronic disease or chronic inflammation.
- ▶ Shortened RBC survival but poor compensatory erythropoiesis.
- ▶ High or normal serum ferritin level and low TIBC.

▶ General Considerations

Many chronic diseases—such as cancer, collagen vascular disease, chronic infections, diabetes mellitus, and coronary artery disease—can be associated with anemia (**Table 32-2**).

Table 32-2. Selected chronic diseases or disorders as causes of anemia.

Chronic infections
Abscesses
Subacute bacterial endocarditis
Tuberculosis
Collagen vascular disease
Rheumatoid arthritis
Systemic lupus erythematosus
Temporal arteritis
Neoplasia
Hodgkin and non-Hodgkin lymphomas
Adenocarcinoma
Squamous cell carcinoma

Pathogenesis

In spite of shortened RBC survival, bone marrow RBC production is low. This is thought to be due to (1) trapping of iron stores in the reticuloendothelial system, (2) a mild decrease in erythropoietin production, and (3) impaired response of the bone marrow to erythropoietin.

Clinical Findings

A. Symptoms and Signs

The anemia of chronic disease (ACD) is often mild and therefore general anemic symptoms, such as fatigue, dizziness, and palpitations, can be mild or nonexistent. Signs such as pallor of the palpebral conjunctivae are only sometimes present. The condition must therefore be suspected and investigated in patients known to have underlying conditions such as collagen vascular diseases, cancers, or chronic infections. The condition is often diagnosed incidentally on laboratory reports.

B. Laboratory Findings

Hemoglobin levels are generally mildly decreased (10–11 g/dL), but levels can occasionally be <8 g/dL. RBCs are often hypochromic. MCV can be either normal (80–100 fL) or low (<80 fL). Because RBC production is poor, the absolute reticulocyte count is often low (<25,000/μL). Acute-phase reactants such as erythrocyte sedimentation rate (ESR), platelets, and fibrinogen can be elevated.

Because ACD is associated with decreased production of transferrin, serum iron level and TIBC are often both low. Calculated percent saturation, however, remains normal. This is to be distinguished from iron-deficiency anemia, in which TIBC is often high, resulting in low-percent saturation. Serum ferritin level is high or normal in ACD but low in iron- deficiency anemia.

Treatment

Treatment of ACD should be aimed at the underlying condition. Symptomatic patients or heart patients often require packed transfusions of RBCs, especially if the HBG count is <10 mg/dL. Erythropoietin is also used to correct anemia associated with certain chronic diseases, especially cancer.

Corwin HL. Anemia and blood transfusion in the critically ill patient: role of erythropoietin. *Crit Care* (London). 2004;8 (suppl 2):S42. [PMID: 15196323]
Fink MP. Pathophysiology of intensive care unit–acquired anemia. *Crit Care* (London). 2004;8(suppl 2):S9. [PMID: 15196314]
Knight K, et al. Prevalence and outcomes of anemia in cancer: a systematic review of the literature. *Am J Med.* 2004;116(suppl 7A):11S. [PMID: 15050883]

Thomas C, Thomas L. Anemia of chronic disease: pathophysiology and laboratory diagnosis. *Lab Hematol.* 2005;11:14. [PMID: 15790548]
Weiss G, Goodnough LT. Anemia of chronic disease. *N Engl J Med.* 2005;352:1011. [PMID: 15758012]

THALASSEMIA

 ESSENTIALS OF DIAGNOSIS

- ▶ Elevated RBC count despite decreased Hb level.
- ▶ Exaggerated microcytosis.
- ▶ Positive family history.
- ▶ Mediterranean or African heritage.
- ▶ Pattern of inheritance.

General Considerations

A normal adult Hb molecule, also known as HbA, consists of two α Hb chains and two β Hb chains. The thalassemias are the diverse group of genetic diseases resulting from abnormal Hb, classified as α-thalassemias or β-thalassemias, based on the abnormal gene.

Other Hb chains exist, such as γ and δ chains. Fetal Hb consists of two α chains and two γ chains ($\alpha_2\gamma_2$), and HbA$_2$ consists of two α chains and two δ chains ($\alpha_2\delta_2$). Although ordinarily these lesser types of Hb constitute ≤5% of the total amount of Hb, the thalassemias are characterized by increased proportions of non-A Hb because of defective α or β chains.

Thalassemia traits are more common in those of Mediterranean, African, and South Asian ancestry. This is due at least in part to the fact that these parts of the world are inhabited by *Plasmodium* species, and heterozygous thalassemic traits confer survival advantage to those afflicted with malaria.

Pathogenesis

Because there are four α Hb genes per individual (two on each copy of chromosome 16), there are four major types of α-thalassemia. If only one α Hb gene is damaged, the result is called *α-thalassemia minima*, an essentially asymptomatic condition. Damage to two different α Hb genes results in α-thalassemia minor, which has only mild clinical significance. Three damaged α Hb genes can lead to a relative abundance of α Hb, causing an abundance of Hb β$_4$, also known as HbH. This disorder, also called *hemoglobin H disease*, is characterized by severe clinical manifestations of chronic hemolysis, hospitalizations, and decreased lifespan. Absence of normal α Hb chains causes Hb Barts disease and is fatal *in utero*.

The two β Hb genes are found on chromosome 11. If one is damaged, β-thalassemia minor results, with few clinical effects. Infants with two damaged copies of β Hb will be phenotypically normal at birth because of the predominance of fetal Hb ($\alpha_2\gamma_2$). Affected infants become severely symptomatic in the first year of life: 80% of patients die in the first 5 years of life as a result of severe anemia, high-output congestive heart failure, or infection.

▶ Clinical Findings

A. Symptoms and Signs

α-thalassemia minima is almost always asymptomatic. α-thalassemia minor can be accompanied by occasional mild symptoms of anemia, including headaches, fatigue, and dizziness. Patients with HbH disease, however, often exhibit severe clinical manifestations of chronic hemolytic anemia, including hepatosplenomegaly and cholelithiasis. These patients often require chronic transfusions, usually beginning in late childhood and adolescence. The clinical appearance of β-thalassemia minor often mimics that of mild or moderate iron deficiency, and often laboratory findings are necessary to distinguish the two. β-thalassemia major, however, results in a severe phenotype. Widespread hemolysis in these patients causes pallor, irritability, jaundice, and hepatosplenomegaly.

B. Laboratory Findings

As with iron deficiency, Hb levels and MCV are often low with the thalassemias. In contrast to iron deficiency, however, thalassemias are usually characterized by an *elevated* RBC count. Furthermore, the decrease in MCV is often more exaggerated in the thalassemias; levels as low as 50–60 fL are not unusual. The red cell distribution width (RDW) can also be used to distinguish the two conditions. With iron deficiency, the RDW is elevated due to a variety of cell sizes, whereas the RDW is usually normal in thalassemic patients because RBCs are uniformly small.

Hemoglobin electrophoresis should be conducted on any patient with suspected thalassemia. Although some patients with α-thalassemia minima or media can have normal electrophoresis patterns, abnormalities are often seen in other thalassemic patients. In β-thalassemia minor, for example, relative proportions of fetal Hb ($\alpha_2\gamma_2$) and HbA$_2$ are increased.

▶ Treatment

Patients with α-thalassemia minor, α-thalassemia minima, and β-thalassemia minor are generally asymptomatic and should be treated only if necessary. These patients may require blood transfusions under certain conditions, such as after vaginal delivery or surgery.

Patients with β-thalassemia major and HbH disease, however, require the care of a hematologist. These patients may require frequent transfusions, splenectomy, or both. Iron overload is a frequent complication in these patients, those both with and without transfusion therapy. Chelation therapy is often required to avoid end-organ damage in the heart, endocrine organs, and liver. Patients with a personal or family history of thalassemia should be offered genetic counseling when planning a family.

Schrier SL. Pathophysiology of thalassemia. *Curr Opin Hematol.* 2002;9:123. [PMID: 11844995]
Shine JW. Microcytic anemia. *Am Fam Physician.* 1997;55:2455. [PMID: 9166144]

▼ MACROCYTIC ANEMIA

VITAMIN B$_{12}$ DEFICIENCY

 ESSENTIALS OF DIAGNOSIS

▶ Macrocytosis.

▶ Serum vitamin B$_{12}$ level <100 pg/mL.

▶ Hypersegmented neutrophils.

▶ General Considerations

Vitamin B$_{12}$ (cobalamin) is involved in two important enzymatic reactions: the conversion of methylmalonylcoenzyme A (CoA) to succinyl-CoA and the methylation of homocysteine to methionine. This latter reaction is required for synthesis of thymidine, a component of DNA.

Because vitamin B$_{12}$ is present in all animal products, only people with unusual diets (vegans, fad dieters) receive inadequate intake. These individuals should receive vitamin B$_{12}$ supplementation. Some special populations, such as pregnant women and those who have had bariatric surgery, may require increased levels of vitamin B$_{12}$.

▶ Pathogenesis

When vitamin B$_{12}$ deficiency is not due to inadequate dietary intake, it usually reflects a defect in the B$_{12}$ absorption and transport chain. Vitamin B$_{12}$ is transported from the stomach to the jejunum by the intrinsic factor (IF), a protein produced in gastric parietal cells. Pernicious anemia occurs when autoantibodies against parietal cells are produced, resulting in a lack of intrinsic factor and inadequate uptake of vitamin B$_{12}$.

▶ Clinical Findings

A. Symptoms and Signs

Many clinical features are common to all megaloblastic anemias: anemia, pallor, weight loss, fatigue, glossitis, lightheadedness, jaundice, and abdominal symptoms. Neurologic symptoms are specific to vitamin B$_{12}$ deficiency, however, beginning with paresthesias in the hands and feet. Disturbances in vision, taste, smell, proprioception, and vibratory sense can also occur. Untreated, vitamin B$_{12}$ deficiency can lead to posterior spinal column demyelination, resulting in spastic ataxia and dementia mimicking that of Alzheimer disease. These changes are often irreversible. Vitamin B$_{12}$ deficiency can also lead to psychotic depression and paranoid schizophrenia.

B. Laboratory Findings

The MCV is usually >100 fL, and vitamin B$_{12}$ levels are usually <100 pg/mL. The higher the MCV, the more likely the diagnosis. Lactate dehydrogenase and indirect bilirubin can be modestly elevated because of increased RBC destruction. The reticulocyte count can be depressed. Because DNA synthesis affects all cell lines, pancytopenia can occur. Peripheral blood smear can show markedly abnormal RBCs along with hypersegmented neutrophils, which are pathognomonic for megaloblastic anemia.

The presence of anti–intrinsic factor (IF) antibodies confirms the diagnosis of pernicious anemia. There is evidence suggesting that early or asymptomatic vitamin B$_{12}$ deficiency can be diagnosed by elevated levels of methylmalonic acid (as sensitive as but more specific than serum homocysteine). Increased levels of methylmalonic acid confirm B$_{12}$ deficiency.

The Schilling test, although rarely used today, has historically been used to confirm the diagnosis of pernicious anemia. It involves following the percentage absorption of radiolabeled vitamin B$_{12}$, with and without the administration of IF.

▶ Treatment

Historically, treatment required monthly parenteral treatment of vitamin B$_{12}$ in doses of 100–1000 μg, usually administered daily or every other day for the first few weeks, followed by maintenance doses every 1–3 months. Once vitamin B$_{12}$ levels have been reestablished, oral therapy (1 mg/d) would be substituted. Recent evidence shows that oral therapy alone, 1–2 mg daily for 90–120 days is equivalent to IM treatment. Treatment often also consists of concurrent administration of folate, 1–5 mg each day.

Carmel R. How I treat cobalamin (vitamin B12) deficiency. *Blood.* 2008;112(6):2214–2221. [PMID: 18606874]

Langan R, Zawitoski K. Update on vitamin B12 deficiency. *Am Fam Physician.* 2011;12:1425–1430.

Oh R, Brown DL. Vitamin B$_{12}$ deficiency. *Am Fam Physician.* 2003;67:979. [PMID: 12643357]

Spoelhof GD. Reliability of serum B$_{12}$ levels in the diagnosis of B$_{12}$ deficiency. *Am Fam Physician.* 1996;54:465. [PMID: 8701832]

FOLIC ACID DEFICIENCY

 ESSENTIALS OF DIAGNOSIS

▶ Reduced RBC or serum folate levels.

▶ Macrocytic anemia.

▶ Normal vitamin B$_{12}$ levels.

▶ Hypersegmented neutrophils.

▶ General Considerations

In contrast to vitamin B$_{12}$ reserves, which can last 3–5 years, folate reserves last only 4–5 months. The human body requires ~75–100 μg/d of folic acid, which is present in leafy green vegetables, fruits, nuts, beans, wheat germ, and liver. Like vitamin B$_{12}$, folate is involved in the synthesis of thymidine.

▶ Pathogenesis

Folic acid deficiency can occur as a result of decreased intake, especially in alcoholics and patients with atypical diets. Malabsorption can also affect intake of folate. Because small intestine microvilli convert the ingested complex folic acid molecule into an absorbable one, diseases of the small intestine, such as gluten enteropathy and Crohn disease, can cause deficiency. Drugs such as anticonvulsants and oral contraceptives also predispose to folate malabsorption. Other medications (eg, antineoplastic agents, trimethoprim, and certain antimalarial drugs) inhibit the enzyme necessary for the replenishment of intracellular folate and can affect folate levels.

Folate deficiency can also result if increased requirements are not met. Pregnancy, for instance, increases folate requirements 5–10-fold by the third trimester. Patients with hemolytic anemia and exfoliative skin diseases also have increased requirements and should receive supplementation. Because folate is dialyzable, patients on dialysis can suffer from folate deficiency if they do not receive supplementation.

Folate deficiency is common among alcoholics for several reasons. First, although some folic acid is present in beer, alcoholics tend to consume less of other foods rich in folic acid, such as leafy green vegetables. Alcohol can also adversely affect intracellular processing of folate. Finally, alcohol may suppress bone marrow function.

▶ Clinical Findings

A. Symptoms and Signs

Patients with mild folate deficiency often present with anemia on a routine blood screening. Those with more severe disease can present with pallor, weight loss, fatigue, glossitis, lightheadedness, jaundice, or abdominal symptoms, as in vitamin B_{12} deficiency. In contrast to vitamin B_{12} deficiency, however, neurologic symptoms are absent.

B. Laboratory Findings

Many laboratory findings are similar to those of vitamin B_{12} deficiency: Hb levels can be variably depressed, pancytopenia can occur, and hypersegmented neutrophils can be seen on the peripheral blood smear. Also as with vitamin B_{12} deficiency, examination of the bone marrow can show erythroid hyperplasia and marked asynchrony in maturation between cytoplasmic components and nuclear material.

With folate deficiency, however, serum and RBC folate levels are low, whereas vitamin B_{12} levels are normal. RBC folate—which is low at <150 pg/L—is considered to be a more precise indicator of chronic folate deficiency than serum folate. In cases where diagnosis remains in doubt, an elevated homocysteine level, despite a normal methylmalonic acid level, suggests folate deficiency.

▶ Treatment

Foods rich in folic acid should be consumed, which include leafy green vegetables, fruits, nuts, beans, wheat germ, and liver. Supplementation with oral folic acid—ranging from 1 to 5 mg daily—is used to treat deficiency. Total correction often occurs within 6–8 weeks. Patients with increased folate requirements, such as pregnant women, should receive supplementation. Some authorities recommend treating all patients with macrocytic anemia, regardless of cause, with empirical addition of folic acid.

Abramson SD, Abramson N. "Common" uncommon anemias. *Am Fam Physician.* 1999;59:851. [PMID: 10068709]

Barney-Stallings RA, Heslop SD. What is the clinical utility of obtaining a folate level in patients with macrocytosis or anemia? *J Fam Practice.* 2001;50:544. [PMID: 11401743]

Davenport J. Macrocytic anemia. *Am Fam Physician.* 1996;53:155. [PMID: 8546042]

Hebert PC et al. Physiologic aspects of anemia. *Crit Care Clin.* 2004;20:187. [PMID: 15135460]

▼ NORMOCYTIC ANEMIA

HEMOLYTIC ANEMIA

Hereditary Spherocytosis

ESSENTIALS OF DIAGNOSIS

- ▶ Autosomal-dominant inheritance pattern (in most cases).
- ▶ Spherocytes on peripheral blood smear.
- ▶ Hemolysis.

▶ General Considerations & Pathogenesis

Hereditary spherocytosis (HS) is the most common inherited defect of the RBC membrane. Patients with this condition inherit one of a series of mutations of the structural proteins of the RBC membrane,. The resulting decreased membrane elasticity causes loss of the normal biconcave shape of the RBC. These deformed, spherical RBCs are then detained and phagocytosed in the narrow fenestrations of the splenic cords. Less common related defects also exist, including hereditary elliptocytosis and hereditary stomatocytosis.

▶ Clinical Findings

A. Symptoms and Signs

Hereditary spherocytosis can be classified as mild, moderate, or severe. Individuals with mild disease rarely manifest symptoms and signs. Increased erythropoietin levels compensate for early destruction of RBCs. Individuals with moderate disease represent 60–75% of HS patients and can develop intermittent episodes of jaundice, dark urine, abdominal pain, and splenomegaly in infancy or early childhood. Individuals with severe disease have more marked jaundice and splenomegaly.

If bilirubin levels are chronically elevated, bilirubin gallstones can form, leading to right upper quadrant abdominal pain and tenderness, nausea, and a positive Murphy sign.

B. Laboratory Findings

Patients with moderate and severe disease often have low Hb, reticulocyte counts between 5% and 20%, and elevated serum bilirubin level.

The mean corpuscular Hb concentration (MCHC) is a useful test in diagnosing HS. It is generally elevated to 36 g/dL in patients with HS, reflecting decreased membrane surface area and increased Hb concentration in the RBC.

The peripheral blood smear of a patient with HS shows characteristic spherocytes—small RBCs that have lost their central pallor. Special tests can also be used to evaluate patients for HS. The osmotic fragility test involves suspending a patient's RBCs in increasingly dilute salt solutions and observing for cell lysis. RBCs from patients with HS will be more sensitive to hypotonic solutions because of membrane instability. The newer acidified glycerol lysis test is also used.

▶ Treatment

Patients with moderate disease may need blood transfusions; however, for patients with severe disease, regular transfusions are essentially unavoidable. Folic acid supplementation is useful for patients with this and other hemolytic diseases.

The definitive treatment is splenectomy, which leads to significantly increased RBC lifespan. For patients who have had a splenectomy, immunization against *Pneumococcus* and *Meningococcus* is recommended for secondary prevention of sepsis.

An X, Mohandas N. Disorders of red cell membrane. *Br J Haematol.* 2008;141:367. [PMID: 18341630]

Glucose-6-Phosphate Dehydrogenase Deficiency

 ESSENTIALS OF DIAGNOSIS

- ▶ X-linked inheritance pattern.
- ▶ African or Mediterranean heritage.
- ▶ Recent exposure to oxidizing substances such as primaquine, sulfa drugs, naphthalene (mothballs), or fava beans.

▶ General Considerations

The World Health Organization (WHO) classifies glucose-6-phosphate dehydrogenase (G6PD) deficiency into five variants, from class I (the most severe enzyme deficiency) to class V (no clinical significance). The deficiency is most common in people of African and Mediterranean heritage. Although it is seen primarily in men, as are most X-linked disorders, women who carry the defective gene can also manifest symptoms, due to inactivation of their normal X chromosomes.

Overall, G6PD deficiency is the most common enzymatic disorder of RBCs in humans and affects 200–400 million people. Less common enzymatic deficiencies also exist. Pyruvate kinase deficiency, for example, has a similar clinical presentation.

The most common variants are G6PD A and G6PD Mediterranean. G6PD A is a variant in which patients have 10–60% of the normal level of G6PD and therefore experience intermittent hemolysis, generally associated with infections or drugs. G6PD Mediterranean also generally manifests with intermittent hemolysis, but the enzyme deficiency is usually more severe (eg, ~10% of normal enzymatic activity).

▶ Pathogenesis

Glucose-6-phosphate dehydrogenase is a cytoplasmic enzyme that prevents oxidative damage to RBCs by reducing nicotinamide adenine dinucleotide phosphate (NADP) to NADPH. Individuals who are deficient in this enzyme are more susceptible to damage from oxidative substances such as superoxide anion (O_2^-) and hydrogen peroxide. In addition to being normal byproducts of cell metabolism, these substances are produced by certain drugs, household chemicals, and foods.

▶ Clinical Findings

Persons affected with G6PD deficiency are often asymptomatic. However, a spectrum of clinical manifestations can occur, from infrequent mild episodic hemolysis to severe chronic hemolysis.

A. Symptoms and Signs

The most common clinical manifestations are jaundice, dark urine, pallor, abdominal pain, and back pain. These symptoms usually occur hours to days after an oxidative insult, which can be caused by a number of different agents. Chemicals that can cause such an insult include primaquine, sulfa drugs, dapsone, nitrofurantoin, and naphthalene (found in mothballs). Antimalarials, aspirin, and acetaminophen can precipitate hemolysis in certain individuals as well. Attacks can also be associated with infections (such as pneumonia, viral hepatitis, and *Salmonella*) and diabetic ketoacidosis. Finally, foods such as fava beans have been implicated. These beans are common in the Mediterranean and are harvested in late spring.

Infants with G6PD deficiency can also present with jaundice. Again a spectrum of disease exists, from mild transient jaundice to severe jaundice, kernicterus, and death. Those with class I G6PD deficiency can have lifelong, life-threatening chronic hemolysis.

B. Laboratory Findings

Hemoglobin levels mirror the severity of disease. During periods of active hemolysis, other laboratory measures can be abnormal. The absolute reticulocyte count is elevated above 2–3%, and sometimes above 10–15%. Haptoglobin levels are often depressed below 50 mg/dL, as this plasma protein binds Hb released from fragmented RBCs.

The peripheral blood smear in G6PD deficiency shows characteristic Heinz bodies, which represent masses of denatured, damaged Hb. "Bite cells," which appear as RBCs with a small semicircular defect, can also be seen. The definitive test for G6PD deficiency is an enzymatic assay that measures *in vitro* production of NADPH.

▶ Treatment

Individuals with mild disease require no treatment except for avoidance, whenever possible, of oxidative triggers. Individuals with more severe disease may require inpatient treatment of acute exacerbations with transfusion, intravenous fluid support, and monitoring of renal function. Although vitamin E and splenectomy have been advocated as possible treatments in more severe cases, neither has provided consistent benefit.

Glader BE. Hereditary hemolytic anemias due to red blood cell enzyme disorders. In: Lee GR, et al, eds: *Wintrobe's Clinical Hematology*, 12th ed. Baltimore, MD: Williams & Wilkins; 2009: 933–955.

Sickle Cell Anemia

 ESSENTIALS OF DIAGNOSIS

- ▶ African, Mediterranean, or Asian heritage.
- ▶ Family history.
- ▶ Autosomal-recessive inheritance.
- ▶ Characteristic pattern on Hb electrophoresis.

▶ General Considerations

Sickle cell anemia (SCA) is a common genetic disorder. Traits that lead to SCA are common in those with African and South Asian heritage. The gene frequency for SCA in African Americans is approximately 4%.

A spectrum of other sickle cell syndromes exists. HbC results from a different mutation in the β Hb chain. Patients with HbSC disease have one of each mutation and generally experience a milder phenotype than those with homozygous sickle cell anemia (HbSS). Patients with the HbSA genotype have one sickle cell gene and one regular gene. They tend to have mild, if any, clinical manifestations of disease. Other permutations of abnormal Hb genes can cause similar syndromes. Patients with one sickle cell gene and one β-thalassemia gene, for example, can have significant clinical manifestations of hemoglobinopathy.

▶ Pathogenesis

Patients with SCA are homozygous for a mutation in the β Hb chain. The resulting HbS, which consists of two normal α Hb chains and two abnormal β Hb chains, is poorly soluble when deoxygenated. The polymerization of HbS into elongated fibers within the RBC leads to the characteristic "sickle" shape. These abnormal RBCs occlude capillary beds and lead to the many clinical manifestations of SCA.

▶ Prevention

Newborn screening for HbSS, HbSA, and HbSC is highly recommended and required by law throughout the United States. Several prophylactic measures can reduce the likelihood of pain crises and other manifestations of disease in patients with SCA (ie, secondary prevention). First,

adequate hydration and oxygenation reduce the risk of Hb polymerization and subsequent vasoocclusive crises. Folic acid should be supplemented, 1 mg orally every day. Some physicians recommend hydroxyurea, which seems to reduce the likelihood of RBC sickling by stimulating production of fetal Hb. Infectious complications can be reduced by immunization against *Streptococcus pneumoniae*, *Haemophilus influenzae* type B, hepatitis B, and influenza. Daily oral penicillin prophylaxis should be given until age 5 years. Use of penicillin prophylaxis, along with intensive medical care, has reduced the mortality of SCA from 25% to 3% during the first 5 years of life.

▶ Clinical Findings

A. Symptoms and Signs

Patients with homozygous SCA manifest disease early. Approximately 30% of patients are discovered by 1 year of age and >90% by 6 years of age. Acute pain episodes are the most common presentations; they can occur in the extremities, abdomen, back, or chest. Although generally no inciting factor is found, stresses such as cold, infection, and dehydration can precipitate attacks. Fever, joint swelling, vomiting, and tachypnea can accompany pain episodes.

Most patients experience autoinfarction of the spleen by early childhood due to occlusion of splenic capillary beds. For this and other reasons, patients with SCA are significantly vulnerable to infection, especially from encapsulated pathogens such as *S. pneumoniae* and *H. influenzae*. Pneumonia, meningitis, osteomyelitis, and bacteremia are causes of significant morbidity and mortality in these patients.

Pulmonary complications are the most common causes of death in patients with SCA. RBCs in the pulmonary system are particularly vulnerable to sickling because of its low PO_2 and relatively low blood pressure. *Acute chest syndrome* refers to the clinical triad of chest pain, pulmonary infiltrate on x-ray, and fever, which can be due to pulmonary infarction, pneumonia, or both.

Sickled RBCs can occlude vasculature and cause infarction of nearly any tissue in the body. Therefore, other serious manifestations of SCA include stroke, myocardial infarction, bone infarction, retinopathy, leg ulcers, and priapism. Depression, low self-esteem, and social withdrawal are common, especially when adequate coping mechanisms are not in place.

B. Laboratory Findings

Laboratory findings often reflect the chronic hemolysis that accompanies SCA. Classically the patient has a reticulocyte count increased to 3–15%, Hb mildly or moderately decreased to 7–11 g/dL, elevated direct bilirubin and lactate dehydrogenase, and a depressed haptoglobin level.

The peripheral blood smear shows sickling of half of the RBCs. Howell-Jolly bodies and target cells are also present on the smear, indicating hyposplenism. The white blood cell count can be elevated at 12,000–15,000/mm³, even in the absence of infection.

Treatment

Despite the preventive measures discussed earlier, most patients with SCA require frequent hospitalization for acute painful vasoocclusive crises or infectious complications. During acute exacerbations, patients often require hydration and oxygenation, analgesia with nonnarcotic or narcotic medications, antibiotics if appropriate, and blood transfusions.

American Academy of Pediatrics; Section on Hematology/ Oncology. Health supervision for children with sickle cell disease. *Pediatrics*. 2002;109:526. [PMID: 11875155]

Kaye CI. Newborn screening fact sheets. *Pediatrics*. 2006;118:e934. [PMID: 16950973]

US Preventive Services Task Force. Screening for sickle cell disease in newborns: recommendation statement. *Am Fam Physician*. 2008;77:1300. [PMID: 18540496]

Vichinsky E et al. Newborn screening for sickle cell disease: effect on mortality. *Pediatrics*. 1988;81:749. [PMID: 3368274]

Wethers D. Sickle cell disease in childhood: part II. *Am Fam Physician*. 2000;15:1309–1314.

Autoimmune Hemolytic Anemia

 ESSENTIALS OF DIAGNOSIS

▶ Positive direct Coombs test.

▶ Elevated indirect bilirubin and decreased serum haptoglobin.

▶ Inciting factor such as medication or illness.

General Considerations

Autoimmune hemolytic anemia (AIHA) results when a patient produces antibodies directed against the body's RBCs AIHA can be classified by the temperature at which the antibodies are most reactive. "Warm" autoantibodies bind most strongly near 37°C (98.6°F), whereas "cold" autoantibodies bind RBCs near 0–4°C (32–39.2°F). Occasionally, a mixture of both types of autoantibodies is present.

Pathogenesis

Although the production of autoantibodies is idiopathic in nearly 50% of cases, at other times an inciting factor can be found. Lymphoproliferative disorders such as chronic lymphoblastic leukemia and autoimmune disorders such as rheumatoid arthritis, for example, can induce production of either warm or cold autoantibodies. Infections such as *Mycoplasma* and syphilis have been implicated, primarily in cold AIHA. Transfusion reactions are mediated by a similar process.

Medications can induce a warm antibody autoimmune reaction. Some drugs, such as methyldopa, alter RBC antigens so that they become targets of the host immune system. Other drugs bind with RBC antigens to form immunogenic complexes. This "hapten" reaction can occur with penicillin as well as a variety of other drugs.

Prevention

Any patient who receives a splenectomy should also receive secondary prevention in the form of immunizations against *Pneumococcus*, *Haemophilus*, and *Meningococcus*.

Clinical Findings

A. Symptoms and Signs

Overall, a wide spectrum of possible manifestations exists. A typical patient with AIHA presents with pallor, fatigue, or headaches due to loss of circulating RBCs. Jaundice may also be present, due to elevation of indirect bilirubin resulting from the release and breakdown of RBC heme. A patient may also have splenomegaly due to increased sequestration of damaged RBCs within the splenic cords of Billroth. In some cases, hemoglobinuria can lead to renal failure. The rate of disease progression depends on the underlying cause of hemolysis. Although clinical manifestations progress slowly in some patients, in others severe symptoms can develop in a matter of hours.

B. Laboratory Findings

A positive direct Coombs test helps diagnose AIHA.

Other laboratory findings reflect the general hemolytic process. Levels of bilirubin and lactate dehydrogenase are increased, haptoglobin levels tend to decrease, and the corrected reticulocyte count is increased. Other appropriate laboratory investigations specific to underlying causes—such as collagen vascular diseases, cancer, and infections—may be warranted.

Treatment

Although further hemolysis can result, blood transfusion should be given when the Hb level is significantly low (5–7 g/dL). Corticosteroids are often considered the treatment of choice, especially when autoantibodies are warm. Those who need long-term treatment and cannot take steroids can use other immunomodulating agents such as azathioprine, cyclosporine, and rituximab. Intravenous immunoglobulin is advocated for the acute treatment of adults with AIHA, but it is not as effective in children. Exchange transfusion, which not only delivers new RBCs but also removes destructive autoantibodies and complement, can also be useful. Splenectomy should be considered in refractory cases; as previously noted, any patient who receives a splenectomy should also receive immunizations against *Pneumococcus*, *Haemophilus*, and *Meningococcus*. Finally, underlying disorders should be treated as appropriate.

Brill JR, Baumgardner DJ. Normocytic anemia. *Am Fam Physician*. 2000;62:2255. [PMID: 11126852]

Gehrs BC, Friedberg RC. Autoimmune hemolytic anemia. *Am J Hematol*. 2002;69:258. [PMID: 11921020]

Extrinsic Nonimmune Hemolytic Anemia

ESSENTIALS OF DIAGNOSIS

▶ Negative Coombs test.

▶ Negative family history.

▶ Known mechanical trauma to RBCs, hemolytic infection, or drug or toxin exposure.

There are many causes of extrinsic hemolysis not related to immunity (**Table 32-3**). The first group of conditions results from mechanical damage to RBCs. Any process that enlarges the spleen, for instance, can lead to an acquired hemolytic process because the spleen is the major organ recycling RBCs. Mechanical damage can also occur as RBCs rush past

Table 32-3. Nonimmune causes of hemolysis.

Hypersplenism
Microangiopathy
Disseminated intravascular coagulation
Thrombotic thrombocytopenic purpura
Physical destruction
Prosthetic valve
March hemoglobinuria
Burns
Infection
Malaria, babesiosis
Leishmaniasis
Medications
Primaquine
Dapsone
Nitrates
Toxins
Lead, copper
Arsine gas
Snake, spider venom

a prosthetic valve or other internal machinery. Disseminated intravascular coagulation and thrombotic thrombocytopenic purpura can result in hemolysis of RBCs that flow through areas of intravascular coagulation. Mechanical destruction of RBCs can also be due to exposure to heat, burns, or even repeated trauma such as that encountered in the feet while marching long distances.

Infectious diseases such as malaria, babesiosis, and leishmaniasis can also cause an acquired hemolysis. This is due to both to direct parasitic action and increased activity of macrophages within the spleen.

Finally, drugs and toxins can lead to hemolysis. Medications such as primaquine, dapsone, nitrites, and even topical anesthesia can induce oxidative stress, damaging RBCs. This can occur even in patients without G6PD deficiency. Toxins such as lead, copper, and arsine gas, as well as venom from snakes, insects, and spiders, can also cause hemolysis.

Symptoms and signs, laboratory findings, and treatments will be based on the specific diagnosis. Rather than a specific disorder, extrinsic nonimmune hemolytic anemia is a general categorization of heterogeneous disease processes.

Brill JR, Baumgardner DJ. Normocytic anemia. *Am Fam Physician*. 2000;62:2255. [PMID: 11126852]

NONHEMOLYTIC ANEMIA

Aplastic Anemia

ESSENTIALS OF DIAGNOSIS

▶ Pancytopenia.

▶ Hypocellular bone marrow.

▶ Normal hematopoietic cells.

▶ General Considerations

Aplastic anemia is characterized by the suppression of all bone marrow lines—erythroid, granulocytic, and megakaryocytic—leading to pancytopenia. Most commonly the disorder is idiopathic. However, drugs, toxins, radiation, infections (eg, hepatitis, parvovirus), and pregnancy can all induce aplastic anemia. Although it is uncommon—affecting only two to four persons per million per year—it is often an important consideration for differential diagnoses for undiagnosed anemias.

▶ Pathogenesis

The etiology is unclear. Although some causative agents have been shown to be directly toxic to the bone marrow, others seem to induce an autoimmune process. The specific etiology plays a role in prognosis; drug-induced aplastic anemia carries a more favorable prognosis than idiopathic aplastic anemia. The more severe the pancytopenia, the worse is the prognosis.

Clinical Findings

A. Symptoms and Signs

Anemia leads to pallor, fatigue, and weakness. Neutropenia increases susceptibility to bacterial infections. Thrombocytopenia can present as mucosal bleeding, easy bruising, or petechiae. Splenomegaly is common in advanced disease.

B. Laboratory Findings

Pancytopenia is the hallmark of aplastic anemia. The associated anemia can be severe and is generally normocytic. The reticulocyte count is often low. The white blood cell count can be lower than 1500/mm^3, and the platelet count is generally <150,000/mL. Bone marrow aspirate, which reveals marrow hypocellularity, is essential to the diagnosis of aplastic anemia and important in distinguishing it from other causes of pancytopenia.

Treatment

Fever or other signs of infection should be aggressively investigated. Often, empiric broad-spectrum antibiotics should be used. Other means of decreasing risk of infection include the use of stool softeners and antiseptic soaps. Menstrual blood loss can be suppressed with oral contraceptive pills. Although replacement of blood products is often necessary, it should be used as little as possible, to avoid sensitizing potential candidates for bone marrow transplantation. Hematopoietic growth factors (erythropoietin and granulocyte colony-stimulating factor) are seldom used, due to transient or nil effect.

In a patient aged <50 years with a human leukocyte antigen (HLA)-matched sibling, immediate bone marrow transplantation is the treatment of choice. The toxicity associated with treatment increases with age, along with the risk of graft-versus-host disease. If successful, transplantation is curative. The 5-year survival rate is approximately 70%.

In those lacking matched siblings or those aged >50 years, treatment consists of immunosuppression with antithymocyte globulin, augmented with high-dose cyclosporine. Most patients relapse, but remission rates with additional antithymocyte globulin treatments are encouraging. Survival at 5 years is ~75%.

Young NS. Acquired aplastic anemia. *Ann Intern Med.* 2002; 136:534.

Young NS, Maciejewski J. The pathophysiology of acquired aplastic anemia. *N Engl J Med.* 1997;336:1365. [PMID: 9134878]

Anemia of Chronic Renal Insufficiency

ESSENTIALS OF DIAGNOSIS

▶ Elevated serum creatinine level.

▶ Clinical presentation consistent with renal insufficiency.

General Considerations

Although anemia of chronic renal insufficiency (CRI) commonly occurs in patients with a creatinine clearance of 30 mL/min per ≤1.73 m^2, it can appear in patients with serum creatinine as low as 2 mg/dL.

Clinical Findings

A. Symptoms and Signs

Patients may exhibit bleeding or bruising due to thrombocytopenia and platelet dysfunction. Pallor and fatigue are also common. Early symptoms of uremia include nausea, vomiting, weight loss, malaise, and headache. As the blood urea nitrogen (BUN) level rises, paresthesias, decreased urine output, and waning level of consciousness can be seen. Other signs and symptoms depend on the etiology of the patient's renal insufficiency.

B. Laboratory Findings

Blood urea nitrogen and serum creatinine are generally both elevated, above 30 and 3.0 mg/dL, respectively. The anemia tends to be normocytic and normochromic, but in some cases it can be microcytic. Hyperphosphatemia, hypocalcemia, and hyperkalemia can occur, as can metabolic acidosis. Reticulocyte count tends to be normal or decreased. Bone marrow is inappropriately normal for the degree of anemia.

Treatment

Treatment involves erythropoietin replacement. Erythropoietin or darbepoetin is indicated when the Hb level is ≤10 g/dL. Darbepoetin has a longer half-life and more predictable bioavailability. Prior to initiation of therapy, the patient should be screened and treated for deficiency of iron, folate, and vitamin B$_{12}$ as well as for occult blood loss.

Erythropoietin is given at 80–120 U/kg per week. The most common side effect of erythropoietin therapy is hypertension. The target Hb level is 11–12 g/dL.

Brill JR, Baumgardner DJ. Normocytic anemia. *Am Fam Physician.* 2000;62:2255. [PMID: 11126852]

Rao M et al. Management of anemia. *Contrib Nephrol.* 2004;145:69. [PMID: 15496793]

Anemia Associated with Marrow Infiltration

ESSENTIALS OF DIAGNOSIS

▶ Anemia with abnormally shaped RBCs on peripheral smear, along with abnormalities of other cell lines.

▶ Bone marrow study showing infiltration or a "dry tap."

▶ Underlying neoplastic, inflammatory, or metabolic disease with nonspecific systemic signs and symptoms.

▶ General Considerations

The bone marrow can tolerate fairly extensive infiltration. When marrow infiltration causes anemia or pancytopenia, however, it is referred to as *myelophthisic anemia*. The most common cause of myelophthisic is metastatic carcinoma of the lung, breast, or prostate. Other causes include hematologic malignancies (leukemia, lymphoma), infections (tuberculosis, fungi), and metabolic diseases (Gaucher disease, Niemann-Pick disease).

▶ Clinical Findings

A. Symptoms and Signs

Anemia is most commonly manifested by pallor or fatigue. Thrombocytopenia can cause petechiae, bleeding, or bruising. Neutropenia can lead to frequent or atypical infections. Fractures, bony pain, bony tenderness, hepatomegaly, and splenomegaly may occur. Other presenting signs and symptoms are usually related to the underlying cause of marrow infiltration.

B. Laboratory Findings

The anemia tends to be normocytic and mild to moderate. White blood cells and platelets may also be decreased. Because of the hypocellular marrow, aspirate often yields few cells ("dry tap").

▶ Treatment

Treatment targets the underlying disease. Successful treatment of the malignancy, through radiation, chemotherapy, or bone marrow transplantation, can resolve the anemia. Erythropoietin or blood transfusion may be used to augment the RBC count. Platelet transfusions may be needed. The prognosis in patients with marrow metastases is generally poor.

Corwin HL. Anemia and blood transfusion in the critically ill patient: role of erythropoietin. *Crit Care* (London). 2004; 8(Suppl 2):S42. [PMID: 15196323]

Hellstrom-Lindberg E. Management of anemia associated with myelodysplastic syndrome. *Semin Hematol.* 2005;42(Suppl 1):S10. [PMID: 15846579]

Waltzman RJ. Treatment of chemotherapy-related anemia with erythropoietic agents: current approaches and new paradigms. *Semin Hematol.* 2004;41(Suppl 7):9. [PMID: 15768474]

Hepatobiliary Disorders

Samuel C. Matheny, MD, MPH
Kristin Long, MD
J. Scott Roth, MD, FACS

BILIARY DISEASES

Kristin Long, MD
J. Scott Roth, MD, FACS

GENERAL CONSIDERATIONS

Approximately 10–20% of the population has gallstones, making biliary pathology an increasing consideration in a patient with abdominal pain. Females are twice as likely to have gallstones. Gallstones are more frequently seen with increasing age and obesity, and are more common in Caucasians and Native Americans than African Americans. Most patients with cholelithiasis remain asymptomatic and never require surgery, but the sequelae of biliary disease remains significant: symptomatic cholelithiasis, gallstone pancreatitis, acute cholecystitis, chronic cholecystitis, choledocholithiasis, and ascending cholangitis. Understanding the basic pathophysiology of each of these conditions is essential to appropriately diagnose and treat patients with biliary disease.

A basic understanding of biliary disease requires a vocabulary of terms used in describing them. Many have similar sounding names and can be confusing. A summary of the definitions can be found in **Table 33-1**. Although the treatment of most biliary diseases ultimately requires cholecystectomy, each condition must be evaluated and treated in a unique fashion.

OPERATIVE PROCEDURES & COMPLICATIONS

Laparoscopic Cholecystectomy

Laparoscopic cholecystectomy has replaced the open operation as the gold standard for removing the gallbladder. Many studies have documented an improved recovery time, decreased postoperative ileus, and decreased pain along with improved aesthetics associated with laparoscopy.

Although associated with less morbidity, laparoscopic cholecystectomy does require pneumoperitoneum (insufflation of carbon dioxide gas into the abdomen) and may not be feasible in patients with other severe comorbid conditions (eg, the morbidly obese, severe congestive heart failure, advanced pulmonary disease, uncontrolled coagulopathy). If operation is required, open cholecystectomy remains the only viable option for these patients.

Advanced Laparoscopic & Robotic Cholecystectomy

In carefully selected patients, both single-incision laparoscopic cholecystectomy (SILC) and robotic cholecystectomy have been shown to be feasible and safe approaches in institutions with available technology. Although both techniques have been noted to have slightly longer operative times (mean difference of 18.5 minutes), a steep learning curve is observed and no increase in overall complication rates has been reported.

Postoperative Complications

The most feared complication of laparoscopic cholecystectomy is injury to the common bile duct. The reported incidence of bile duct injuries varies from 0% to 3% depending on the underlying pathology necessitating cholecystectomy. Minor biliary injuries include cystic duct leaks and biliary leaks from the hepatic parenchyma. These injuries may be managed with percutaneous drain placement or endoscopic retrograde cholangiopancreatography (ERCP) to facilitate drainage into the duodenum.

Major biliary injuries include clipping or transection of the common hepatic or common bile duct. When identified intraoperatively, these injuries are best managed with immediate repair, requiring open operation and a skilled surgeon. Those biliary injuries identified in the postoperative setting

Table 33-1. Basic definitions.

Term	Definition
Cholelithiasis	Presence of stones in the gallbladder
Cholecystitis	Inflammation of the gallbladder
Choledocholithiasis	Presence of gallstones in the common bile duct
Cholangitis	Inflammation (most commonly due to infection) of the bile ducts ascending into the liver
Cholecystectomy	Surgical removal of the gallbladder
Cholecystic	Relating to the gallbladder
Calculous	Related to the presence of gallstones
Acalculous	In absence of gallstones
ERCP	Endoscopic retrograde cholangiopancreatography

are best treated with externalization of the bile flow (percutaneous transhepatic biliary drainage) and a definitive repair at a later date, often 2–3 months following the initial injury. In most circumstances, a Roux-en-Y hepaticojejunostomy is required to reconstruct the biliary tree.

Patients who present with jaundice after elective cholecystectomy should be evaluated for retained common bile duct stones or a biliary injury. Presence of common bile duct dilatation on abdominal ultrasound should prompt immediate ERCP for both diagnosis and treatment. Patients undergoing elective cholecystectomy should be aware that ≤12% of those undergoing surgery may experience postcholecystectomy syndromes, including diarrhea (usually responsive to dietary measures), continued abdominal pain, or dyspepsia. Late sequelae of cholecystectomy can include bile duct strictures or recurrent bile duct stones. Patients suspected of these diagnoses should be promptly referred back to the operating surgeon.

Gurusamy KS, Davidson BR. Surgical treatment of gallstones. *Gastroenterol Clin North Am.* 2010;39(2):229–244.
Song T, Liao B, Cheng N. Single-incision versus conventional laparoscopic cholecystectomy: a systematic review of available data. *Surg Laparosc Endosc Percutan Tech.* 2012;22(4):190–196.

CHOLELITHIASIS

Asymptomatic Cholelithiasis

A landmark study from the University of Michigan followed the course of 123 faculty members identified as having asymptomatic gallstones during a routine health examination. After >2 decades of follow-up, 14 (11%)

patients went on to develop complications requiring surgery. Subsequent studies have not demonstrated a survival advantage with prophylactic cholecystectomy, and as a result, cholecystectomy for asymptomatic cholelithiasis is rarely indicated. Hemolytic conditions such as hereditary spherocytosis remain one indication to consider prophylactic cholecystectomy during other abdominal operations such as splenectomy.

Symptomatic Cholelithiasis

 ESSENTIALS OF DIAGNOSIS

► Episodic right upper quadrant (RUQ) pain.
► Ultrasound evidence of gallstones.

Unlike asymptomatic cholelithiasis, symptomatic cholelithiasis will generally necessitate operative intervention. The typical patient presentation will include RUQ abdominal pain, usually following a fatty meal and frequently associated with nausea (biliary colic). The pain can be severe and debilitating, and a trip to the emergency room is not an infrequent occurrence. Symptoms are related to transient obstruction of the gallbladder neck or infundibulum by stones or biliary sludge. As the gallbladder attempts to contract in response to cholecystokinin secretion, the obstructed cystic duct prevents the egress of bile from the gallbladder into the biliary system, resulting in acute RUQ pain. In addition to RUQ pain, the character of biliary colic is often described as a colicky or crampy pain that may radiate to the back or shoulder. The pain is generally postprandial in nature and typically resolves within 1–2 hours. Persistence of pain beyond this time should prompt the clinician to suspect acute cholecystitis or other disorders discussed later.

In most circumstances, there will be no abnormalities in the liver function tests or complete blood counts of patients with symptomatic cholelithiasis. An abdominal ultrasound will reveal the presence of cholelithiasis without gallbladder wall thickening or pericholecystic fluid. The treatment of symptomatic cholelithiasis remains elective cholecystectomy in patients suitable to undergo a general anesthetic. Following cholecystectomy, most patients (95%) with symptomatic cholelithiasis will have no further sequela of biliary diseases.

Chronic Cholecystitis

The term *chronic cholecystitis* is often used synonymously with *symptomatic cholelithiasis*. It may also be a result of multiple episodes of untreated acute cholecystitis. The gallbladder will become scarred from multiple episodes of inflammation. Pathological examination will demonstrate

Rokitansky-Aschoff sinuses. The patient will usually describe multiple episodes of biliary colic. Ultrasound will demonstrate cholelithiasis and occasionally gallbladder wall thickening (from the scarring).

The treatment of chronic cholecystitis is cholecystectomy. Following cholecystectomy, most patients recover with no adverse effects.

Gracie WA, Ransohoff DF. The natural history of silent gallstones: the innocent gallstone is not a myth. *New Engl J Med.* 1982;307:798–800.

Z'Graggen K et al. Complications of laparoscopic cholecystectomy in Switzerland. A prospective study of 10,174 patients. Swiss Association of Laparoscopic and Thoracoscopic Surgery. *Surg Endosc.* 1998;12:1301–1310.

ACUTE CHOLECYSTITIS

 ESSENTIALS OF DIAGNOSIS

► Persistent severe RUQ pain (>4–6 hours).

► RUQ tenderness.

► Fever, leukocytosis.

► Ultrasound evidence of gallstones.

Acute cholecystitis is caused most commonly by obstruction of the cystic duct, resulting in localized edema and inflammation. Biliary cultures of most patients reveal bacteria. Women are 3 times more likely to develop acute cholecystitis than men. Over 90% of cases of acute cholecystitis are related to gallstones causing obstruction (calculous cholecystitis). The remaining cases are classified as acalculous cholecystitis, in which other comorbid conditions result in gallbladder wall ischemia or biliary stasis.

Acute cholecystitis is defined by the triad of RUQ pain, fever, and leukocytosis. Abdominal ultrasound will demonstrate gallbladder wall thickening (> 3 mm) with pericholecystic fluid. Symptoms typically begin after a meal. The pain is similar to, but far more severe than, that of symptomatic cholelithiasis. In cases where acalculous cholecystitis is suspected or when ultrasound is inconclusive, radionucleotide scanning [ie, hepatobiliary iminodiacetic acid (HIDA)] may be used. Presence of radionucleotide in the extrahepatic biliary tree without filling the gallbladder is diagnostic of acute cholecystitis.

The treatment of acute cholecystitis is cholecystectomy. The timing of the operation is a controversial subject matter for general surgeons. Localized edema and subsequent scar formation after an episode of acute cholecystitis can make laparoscopic cholecystectomy difficult. Traditional teaching has been that cholecystectomy should be performed within 3 days of onset of symptoms—before myoepthelial changes can occur in the right upper quadrant. The localized edema associated with acute cholecystitis aides with dissection of tissue planes and facilitates cholecystectomy. Compared to delayed cholecystectomy (after 7 days of symptoms), this approach is associated with a decreased conversion rate to open operation (2% vs 30%) and decreased recovery time (12 vs 28 days). Many patients present, however, outside the initial 72-hour window. Most current recommendations extend the period for safely performing laparoscopic cholecystectomy during acute cholecystitis to within one week of symptom onset. If outside of this 7-day window, many surgeons advocate a course of intravenous and (later) oral antibiotics with a plan to perform cholecystectomy in a delayed fashion at least 6 weeks later. This delay will allow the scarring in the right upper quadrant to subside, allowing for safer and easier dissection during laparoscopy. If the patient has continued pain or recurrence of cholecystitis during this waiting period, laparoscopic cholecystectomy should be attempted immediately. The patient should be counseled on the high probability of conversion to an open operation. For patients who are not operative candidates, percutaneous tube cholecystotomy remains a viable option to drain the infected bile as a bridge to elective cholecystectomy when the patient has stabilized.

Untreated cholecystitis can lead to gallbladder ischemia, necrosis, or perforation, resulting in biliary leak or fistula formation to the surrounding structures. Those undergoing successful immediate cholecystectomy will generally have no further sequel of biliary disease. The potential for choledocholithiasis and common bile duct injury must be considered in patients presenting with jaundice after cholecystectomy.

Gurusamy K, Samraj K, Gluud C, Wilson E, Davidson BR. Meta-analysis of randomized controlled trials on the safety and effectiveness of early versus delayed laparoscopic cholecystectomy for acute cholecystitis. *Br J Surg.* 2010;97(2):141–150.

Meyers WC et al. A prospective analysis of 1518 laparoscopic cholecystectomies. *N Engl J Med.*1991;324:1073–1078

Choledocholithiasis

Choledocholithiasis, or common bile duct stones, are present in ≤10% of patients undergoing cholecystectomy. The treatment is cholecystectomy with evaluation of the biliary tree and clearance of all stones within the ductal system. Choledocholithiasis should be suspected in any patient with biliary ductal dilatation seen on imaging, elevated bilirubin levels (conjugated), elevated alkaline phosphatase levels, or elevated amylase and lipase levels. Patients presenting with choledocholithiasis may develop symptoms related to obstruction of the bile duct, pancreatic duct, or both.

Gallstone Pancreatitis

ESSENTIALS OF DIAGNOSIS

▶ RUQ or epigastric pain.

▶ Elevated serum amylase and lipase.

▶ Ultrasound evidence of gallstones.

Gallstones small enough to pass through the biliary tree may enter the pancreatic duct and potentially obstruct at the level of the ampulla of Vater. These stones will then cause obstruction of the pancreatic ductal system, resulting in pancreatitis. Gallstones are associated with approximately 45–50% of all cases of pancreatitis in the United States.

Patients presenting with pancreatitis typically have varying degrees of abdominal pain—usually located in the epigastrium or right upper quadrant. The pain may radiate to the back or shoulders. Nausea and vomiting are common. Laboratory studies will reveal elevation of lipase and (occasionally) amylase. If gallstones remain in the biliary tree, then liver transaminases and bilirubin may also be elevated. Although ultrasound is useful to confirm presence of gallstones, CT scanning is useful in delineating the severity of pancreatitis.

The treatment of gallstone pancreatitis is eventual cholecystectomy. As the gallbladder is the source of the stones, cholecystectomy will prevent subsequent episodes of pancreatitis. Cholecystectomy should not be attempted until the resolution of pancreatitis. Treatment for pancreatitis involves bowel rest with intravenous hydration. Severe cases of pancreatitis may require ICU admission with cardiovascular and respiratory support. Regardless of the patient's condition, cholecystectomy should be postponed until after the pancreatitis has resolved. It has been suggested that morbidity and mortality is improved if these patients undergo ERCP within 2 days of onset of symptoms. ERCP may be able to remove an impacted stone and thus allow for pancreatic decompression. This approach is generally considered in patients with moderate or severe pancreatitis.

The presence or absence of a persistent bile duct stone should be determined prior to proceeding with cholecystectomy. In most circumstances, normalization of serum lipase, amylase, and liver function tests (if originally elevated) occurs rapidly. In these circumstances, no imaging of the biliary tree is required because of the low probability of a persistent bile duct stone. However, patients with persistent abnormalities of their liver functions, amylase, or lipase should be evaluated for the presence of common bile duct stones. Biliary imaging may be obtained by means of intraoperative cholangiography at the time of cholecystectomy, perioperative ERCP, or magnetic resonance cholangiopancreatography (MRCP). MRCP is the least invasive modality but is only diagnostic. ERCP allows for both visualization and extraction of stones of diameter ≤1.5 cm. ERCP may be utilized to extract common bile duct stones either antecedent or subsequent to cholecystectomy. Common bile duct stones not amenable to endoscopic removal are removed operatively by performing a common bile duct exploration.

The overall long-term outcome of patients is related to the severity of the pancreatitis. Localized morbidity includes pancreatic necrosis, splenic vein thrombosis with gastric varices, hemorrhagic pancreatitis, and pancreatic abscesss formation. Systemic morbidity can result in multisystem organ failure or even death.

Behrns KE et al. Early ERCP for gallstone pancreatitis: for whom and when? *J Gastrointest Surg.* 2008;12:629–633.

Kaw M et al. Management of gallstone pancreatitis: cholecystectomy, or ERCP and endoscopic sphincterotomy. *Gastroinest Endosc.* 2002;56:61–65.

Tse F, Yuan Y. Early routine endoscopic retrograde cholangiopancreatography strategy versus early conservative management strategy in acute gallstone pancreatitis. *Cochrane Database Syst Rev.* 2012;16:5.

Cholangitis

ESSENTIALS OF DIAGNOSIS

▶ Persistent RUQ pain.

▶ Jaundice.

▶ Fever.

▶ Hypotension, mental status changes (acute suppurative cholangitis).

Cholangitis is defined as inflammation of the biliary system. It is most commonly caused by an impacted gallstone at the ampulla of Vater preventing bile drainage into the duodenum, although other etiologies such as extrinsic compression from an adjacent mass, inflammatory process, or a primary tumor of the ampulla, duodenum, or bile duct should also be considered. Cholangitis is considered a medical emergency.

Patients with cholangitis may present with Charcot's triad (fever, RUQ pain, and jaundice) or with Reynold's pentad (the addition of hypotension or mental status changes). Laboratory studies will show hyperbilirubinemia and leukocytosis. Ultrasound will likely show biliary ductal dilatation.

With clinical suspicion of cholangitis, patients should be immediately resuscitated and given broad-spectrum antibiotics. Biliary decompression should be urgently performed by ERCP. If ERCP fails to resolve the obstruction or is not available, percutaneous transhepatic cholangiography (PTC) with drainage may be performed. In the presence of stones, once biliary decompression has been performed, cholecystectomy should be performed electively following resolution of the cholangitis. In rare circumstances in which percutaneous or endoscopic biliary drainage is not possible, urgent cholecystectomy with common bile duct exploration should be performed.

The mortality associated with cholangitis varies widely and is related to the underlying etiology of the cholangitis. Cholangitis secondary to stones is associated with a low overall mortality provided the patient can be successfully supported through the infectious period. Cholangitis related to an underlying periampullary malignancy requires careful oncologic consideration prior to surgical intervention. This may require a more involved oncologic resection (such as a pancreaticoduodenectomy or extrahepatic biliary resection) or palliative care depending on the extent of the malignancy. In the event of an unresectable periampullary tumor, a biliary bypass (hepaticojejunostomy) may be considered. Most periampullary cancers are associated with very poor 5-year survival even with complete extirpation of the tumor.

Lai EC et al. Endoscopic biliary drainage for severe acute cholangitis. N Engl J Med. 1992;326:1582–1586.
Lee JG. Diagnosis and management of acute cholangitis. Nat Rev Gastroenterol Hepatol. 2009; 6(9):533–541.
Sugiyama M, Atomi Y. Treatment of acute cholangitis due to choledocholithiasis in elderly and younger patients. Arch Surg. 1997; 132:1129–1133.

Biliary Dyskinesia

A small group of patients will present with RUQ abdominal pain and symptoms that follow the pattern of biliary disease but will have essentially negative imaging for biliary pathology. One key factor in ascertaining whether the gallbladder is contributing to their pain would be to perform a HIDA scan with cholecystokinin (CCK) injection. Likewise, measurement of gallbladder ejection fraction (EF) during this scan can further identify patients with biliary pathology. Ejection fractions of <35% are considered pathophysiologic and warrant evaluation for cholecystectomy. Reproduction of pain with CCK injection is diagnostic for biliary dyskinesia, and these patients benefit from referral for cholecystectomy. Laparoscopic cholecystectomy has been reported to alleviate pain in ≤94% of patients with biliary dyskinesia. Patients with the highest success rate were those presenting with complaints of nausea, pain, or with EF <15% by HIDA scan. Patients with vague abdominal complaints should be cautioned that laparoscopic cholecystectomy is not guaranteed to alleviate their symptoms, and the decision to proceed with surgical intervention should be made carefully on a case-by-case basis.

Bingener J, Sirinek KR, et al. Laparoscopic cholecystectomy for biliary dyskinesia. Surg Endosc. 2004;18:802–806.

Yost F, Murayama K. Cholecystectomy is an effective treatment for biliary dyskinesia. Am J Surg. 1999;178(6):462–465.

BILIARY MALIGNANCIES

Gallbladder Polyps

Gallbladder polyps are present in ~5% of the population and are usually found incidentally during abdominal ultrasonography. The different types of polyps include cholesterolosis, adenomyomatosis, hyperplastic cholecystosis, and adenocarcinomatosis. The goal of surgical management is to identify which polyps are cancerous (adenocarcinoma) or at risk of developing cancer (adenomyomatosis) and select these patients for cholecystectomy.

Unfortunately, short of cholecystectomy, there is currently no way to distinguish among the different types of gallbladder polyps. With the relative safety of laparoscopic cholecystectomy, some advocate surgery immediately after discovering polyps. Patients who have polyps with gallstones or are aged >50 years should be referred for cholecystectomy. Further imaging techniques, including endoscopic ultrasound (EUS), have been advocated for small polyps. Recent recommendations include removing polyps of diameter ≥6 mm because of an increased likelihood of malignancy. If cancer is present in the surgical specimen, the depth of invasion dictates the next course of therapy.

Gallahan WC, Conway JD. Diagnosis and management of gallbladder polyps. Gastroenterol Clin North Am. 2010;39(2):359–367.

Gallbladder Cancer

Patients with gallbladder cancer have presentations similar to those with symptomatic cholelithiasis or chronic cholecystitis. Presentation is often late, and with advanced disease, systemic complaints such as gradual weight loss and loss of appetite also appear. Since presentation is often assumed to be related to gallstone disease, ultrasound is usually the initial diagnostic modality used. Ultrasound findings of a mass >1 cm, calcified gallbladder wall, discontinuity of gallbladder wall layers, and loss of interface between the gallbladder wall and the liver should raise suspicion of gallbladder cancer. Computed tomography is useful in these circumstances to delineate anatomic structures for resectability, as well as evidence of metastatic disease.

The presence of paraaortic or peripancreatic lymphadenopathy is deemed unresectable disease. This can be confirmed with endoscopic ultrasound with biopsies. Cancers that are limited to the mucosa or muscular layer of the gallbladder can be treated with cholecystectomy with negative margins alone. Tumors that invade the pericholecystic connective tissue require resection of the gallbladder fossa with en bloc cholecystectomy. Tumors that invade the liver require formal resection of the involved segments. Unfortunately, 15–50% of tumors that penetrate the muscular wall of the gallbladder have nodal disease that will render them unresectable. Gallbladder cancer may also be found incidentally in cholecystectomy specimens. If it is invasive, additional resection of involved hepatic margins will be necessary. The 5-year survival of early tumors (those confined to the muscular or mucosal layer) is excellent (90–100%). The survival for more advanced tumors is measured in terms of weeks or months.

Bartlett DL et al. Long-term results after resection for gallbladder cancer: implications for staging and management. *Ann Surg.* 1996;224:639–646.

Fong Y et al. Gallbladder cancer: comparison of patients presenting initially for definitive operation with those presenting after prior noncurative intervention. *Ann Surg.* 2000;232:557–569.

Choledochal Cyst

Classically, a choledochal cyst is described as a palpable RUQ mass in a young female with jaundice. Most choledochal cysts are described in Asian populations but are increasingly seen in the United States, males, and older patients. Choledochal cysts are classified by their anatomic location; most involve solitary fusiform dilatation of the extrahepatic biliary tree. Their presentation in Western series is similar to that of symptomatic cholelithiasis. They can be easily seen on ultrasound—provided the ultrasonographer evaluates the biliary tree in addition to the gallbladder.

Choledochal cysts are associated with a 70-fold increased incidence of cholangiocarcinoma, so surgical resection is indicated when discovered. Operative treatment involves resection of the entire extrahepatic biliary tree, cholecystectomy, and reconstruction with a Roux-en-Y hepaticojejunostomy. Surgical resection is considered curative; Edil et al. (2008) reported no subsequent malignancy over 30 years in patients without cancer at the time of cyst excision.

Edil BH et al. Choledochal cyst disease in children and adults: a 30-year single institution experience. *J Am Coll Surg.* 2008; 206:1000–1005.

Cholangiocarcinoma

For various reasons, cholangiocarcinomas along with other RUQ malignancies are associated with very poor survival: (1) these lesions often present late and are not amenable to resection; (2) their biological activity is not well understood, and systemic therapy offers little benefit; and (3) operative resection is technically difficult, and patients need to be seen in specialized centers.

The vast majority of cholangiocarcinomas present with jaundice, sometimes in the setting of cholangitis. Ultrasound will often show a dilated proximal biliary tree. ERCP and endoscopic ultrasound are useful to delineate the tumor. Preoperative endoscopic brushings are often nondiagnostic and should not be aggressively pursued in patients with resectable disease on cross-sectional imaging. While most proximal cholangiocarcinomas (70%) are not amenable to resection, approximately half of distal tumors may be resected. Resection involves pancreaticoduodenectomy for distal tumors and extrahepatic biliary resection with Roux-en-Y hepaticojejunostomy for proximal disease. The 5-year survival rate remains poor even after complete resection (20–25%). For patients with unresectable disease, survival is again measured in weeks or months.

Fong Y et al. Outcome of treatment for distal bile duct cancer. *Br J Surg.* 1996;83:1712–1715.

Jarnigan WR et al. Staging, resectability and outcome in 225 patients with hilar cholangiocarcinoma. *Ann Surg.* 2001;234:507–517.

LeFemina J, Jarnagin WR. Surgical management of proximal bile duct cancers. *Langenbecks Arch Surg.* 2012;397(6):869–879.

▼ LIVER DISEASE

Samuel C. Matheny, MD, MPH

VIRAL HEPATITIS

 ### ESSENTIALS OF DIAGNOSIS

► Variable prodromal signs and symptoms.

► Positive specific viral hepatitis tests.

► Elevation of serum aspartate aminotransferase (AST) and alanine aminotransferase (ALT).

Acute viral hepatitis is a worldwide problem, and in the United States alone there are probably between 200,000 and 700,000 cases per year according to the Centers for Disease Control and Prevention (CDC). Over 32% of cases are caused by hepatitis A virus (HAV), 43% by hepatitis B virus (HBV), 21% by hepatitis C virus (HCV), and the remainder are not identified. Although few deaths (~250) due to acute hepatitis are reported annually, considerable morbidity can result from chronic hepatitis caused by HBV and HCV infections, and mortality from complications can be pronounced for years to come.

Hepatitis A

► General Considerations

Hepatitis A virus (HAV), first identified in 1973, is the prototype for the former diagnosis of *infectious hepatitis.* Over the past several decades, the incidence of HAV infection has varied considerably, and a high number of cases have gone unreported. HAV is a very small viral particle that is its own unique genus (hepatovirus).

Most individuals infected worldwide are children. In general, there are four patterns of HAV distribution (high, moderate, low, and very low), which roughly correspond to differing socioeconomic and hygienic conditions. Countries with poor sanitation have the highest rates of infection. Most children aged <9 years in these countries manifest evidence of HAV infection. Countries with moderate rates of infection have the highest incidence in later childhood; food- and waterborne outbreaks are more common. In countries with low endemicity, the peak age of infection is likely to be at early adulthood, and, in very low endemic countries, outbreaks are uncommon.

Hepatitis A is usually transmitted by ingestion of contaminated fecal material of an infected person by a susceptible individual. Contaminated food or water can be the source of infection, but occasionally infection can occur by contamination of different types of raw shellfish from areas contaminated by sewage. The virus can survive for 3–10 months in water. Other cases of infection by blood exposures have been reported but are less common. The incubation period for HAV averages 30 days, with a range of 15–50 days.

In countries of low endemicity, persons at greatest risk for infection include travelers to intermediate and high-HAV-endemic countries, men who have sex with men (MSMs), intravenous drug users, and persons with chronic liver disease, including those who have received transplants. In areas of high endemicity, all young children are at increased risk.

Prevention

Currently in the United States, the CDC recommends that certain populations at increased risk be considered for pre-exposure vaccination; these include the groups listed earlier. In addition, the CDC now recommends universal immunization for all children aged >1 year. The immunization schedule consists of three doses for children and adolescents, and two for adults. In groups with the potential for high risk of exposure, including any adult aged >40 years, prevaccination testing for prior exposure may be cost-effective. The appropriate test is the total anti-HAV. Travelers aged <40 years who receive the vaccine may assume to be protected after receiving the first dose, although the second dose is desired for long-term protection. For certain travelers (older adults and those with underlying medical conditions), immunoglobulin (Ig) may be given in a different site for additional protection within 2 weeks of travel. A combination vaccine with HBV is available for persons aged >18 years who are immunocompetent and is used on the same three-dose schedule as HBV.

Immunoglobulin or hepatitis A vaccine (if previously unvaccinated) may also be used for postexposure prophylaxis in healthy patients between 12 months and 40 years of age, if given within 14 days, and would most often be used for household or intimate contacts of an infected person, in some institutional settings, or if a common source is identified. For persons with chronic illness, or those aged <12 months or >40 years, Ig is preferred.

Clinical Findings

A, Symptoms and Signs

The symptoms and signs of acute viral hepatitis are quite similar regardless of type and are difficult to distinguish on the basis of clinical findings. The prodrome for viral hepatitis is variable and may be manifested by anorexia, including changes in olfaction and taste, as well as nausea and vomiting, fatigue, malaise, myalgias, headache, photophobia, pharyngitis, cough, coryza, and fever. Dark urine and clay-colored stools may be noticed 1–5 days before jaundice.

Clinical jaundice varies considerably and may range from an anicteric state to rare hepatic coma. In acute HAV infection, jaundice is usually more pronounced in older age groups (ie, 70–80% in those aged 14 years) and rare in children aged <6 years (<10%). Weight loss may also be present, as well as an enlarged liver (70%) and splenomegaly (20%). Spider angiomata may be present without acute liver failure. Patients may also report a loss of desire for cigarette smoking or alcohol.

B. Laboratory Findings

Usually, the onset of symptoms coincides with the first evidence of abnormal laboratory values. Acute elevations of ALT and AST are seen, with levels as high as 4000 units or more in some patients. The ALT level is usually higher than the AST. When the bilirubin level is >2.5, jaundice may be obvious. Bilirubin levels may go from 5 to 20, usually with an equal elevation of conjugated and unconjugated forms. The prothrombin time is usually normal. If significantly elevated, it may signal a poor prognosis. The complete blood count may demonstrate a relative neutropenia, lymphopenia, or atypical lymphocytosis. Urobilinogen may be present in urine in the late preicteric stage.

Serum IgM antibody (anti-HAV) is present in the acute phase and usually disappears within 3 months, although occasionally it persists longer. IgG anti-HAV is used to detect previous exposure and persists for the lifetime of the patient. The more commonly available test for IgG anti-HAV is the total anti-HAV.

Treatment

Treatment for the most part is symptomatic, with many clinicians prohibiting only alcohol during the acute illness phase. Most patients can be treated at home.

Prognosis

In the vast majority of patients with HAV, the disease resolves uneventfully within 3–6 months. Rarely, fulminant hepatitis may develop, with acute liver failure and high mortality rates. Rare cases of cholestatic hepatitis, with persistent bilirubin elevations, have also been reported. Some patients develop relapsing hepatitis, in which HAV is reactivated and shed in the stool. Affected patients demonstrate liver function test abnormalities, but virtually all recover completely. HAV does not progress to chronic hepatitis.

Hepatitis B

General Considerations

Hepatitis B virus (HBV) is a double-shelled DNA virus. The outer shell contains the hepatitis B surface (HBsAg). The inner core contains several other particles, including hepatitis core antigen (HBcAg) and HBeAg. These antigens and their subsequent antibodies are described in more detail later.

Worldwide, over 400 million people are infected with HBV, but the distribution is quite varied. More than 45% of the global population live in areas of high incidence (infections in >8% of population). There, the lifetime risk of infection is over 60%, and early childhood infections are very common. Intermediate-risk areas (infections in 2–7% of the population) represent 43% of the global population. The lifetime risk of infection in these areas is between 20% and 60%, and infections occur in various age groups. In low-risk areas (infections in <2%), which represent ~12% of the global population, the lifetime risk of infection is <20% and is usually limited to specific adult risk groups.

In the United States, HBV is normally a disease of young adults. The largest numbers of cases are reported in adults aged 20–39 years, but many cases in younger age groups may be asymptomatic and go unreported. Of the specific risk groups in the United States, over 50% in recent studies are those with sexual risk factors (more than one sex partner in the past 6 months, sexual relations with an infected person, or MSM transmission). Over 15% had a history of injection drug use, and 4% had other risk factors such as a household contact with HBV or a healthcare exposure. The mode of transmission can thus be sexual, parenteral, or perinatal, through contact of the infant's mucous membranes with maternal infected blood at delivery.

Body fluids with the highest degree of concentration of HBV are blood, serum, and wound exudates. Moderate concentrations are found in semen, vaginal fluid, and saliva, and low or nondetectable amounts are found in urine, feces, sweat, tears, or breast milk. Saliva can be implicated in transmission through bites, but not by kissing.

The average incubation period for HBV is between 60 and 90 days, with a range of 45–180 days. Although the incidence of jaundice increases with age (<10% of children <5 years demonstrate icterus compared with 30–50% of those aged >35 years), the likelihood of chronic infection with HBV is greater when infection is contracted at a younger age. Between 30% and 90% of all children who contract HBV before the age of 5 years develop chronic disease, compared with 2–10% of those aged >35 years.

Prevention

Current immunization recommendations in the United States call for routine immunization of all infants, children, adolescents, and adults in high-risk groups, including all diabetic patients aged 19–58 years, and all patients with chronic liver disease. Acknowledgment of a specific risk factor is not a requirement for immunizations. These recommendations include immunizing all children at birth, 1, and 6 months. Additionally, all high-risk groups should be screened, as well as all pregnant women. Prevaccination testing of patients in low-risk groups is probably not necessary, but in high-risk groups, this may be cost-effective. As illustrated in the first test scenario of **Table 33-2**, a negative HBsAg titer and a negative anti-HBs titer are evidence of susceptibility to HBV.

Table 33-2. Interpretation of the hepatitis B panel.

Tests	Results	Interpretation
HBsAg Anti-HBc Anti-HBs	Negative Negative Negative	Susceptible
HBsAg Anti-HBc Anti-HBs	Negative Positive Positive	Immune because of natural factors
HBsAg Anti-HBc Anti-HBs	Negative Negative Positive	Immune because of hepatitis B vaccination
HBsAg Anti-HBc IgM anti-HBc Anti-HBs	Positive Positive Positive Negative	Acutely infected
HBsAg Anti-HBc IgM anti-HBc Anti-HBs	Positive Positive Negative Negative	Chronically infected
HBsAg Anti-HBc Anti-HBs	Negative Positive Negative	Four interpretations possible[a]

[a]May be (1) recovering from acute HBV infection, (2) distantly immune and the test is not sensitive enough to detect very low levels of anti-HBs in serum, (3) susceptible with a false-positive anti-HB, or. (4) an undetectable level of HBsAg is present in the serum and the person is actually a carrier.

The vaccine contains components of HBsAg. Pretesting with anti-HB core antibody (anti-HBc) is probably the single best test, because it would identify those who are infected and those who have been exposed. Posttesting for vaccine is seldom recommended, except for individuals who may have difficulty mounting an immune response (eg, immunocompromised patients). In these patients, the HB surface antibody (anti-HBs) would be the appropriate test. Some authorities recommend revaccinating high-risk individuals if titer levels have fallen below 10 IU/L after 5–10 years, or if they have failed to mount an appropriate immune response with the standard dosing and schedule.

Children born to women of unknown hepatitis B status should receive a first dose of hepatitis B vaccine at birth and hepatitis B immune globulin (HBIG) within 7 days of birth if maternal blood is positive. Repeat testing of all infants born to HBV-infected mothers should be performed at 9–18 months with HBsAg and anti-HBs. Infants born to HBV-infected mothers should receive both the first dose of hepatitis B vaccine at birth as well as 0.5 mL of HBIG in separate sites within 12 hours after birth. Recommendations for postexposure prophylaxis of HBV can be reviewed in the current CDC recommendations.

Clinical Findings

Acute infection may range from an asymptomatic infection to cholestatic hepatitis to fulminant hepatic failure. HBsAg and other markers usually become positive about 6 weeks after infection and remain positive into the clinical signs of illness. Other biochemical abnormalities begin to show abnormalities in the prodromal phase and may persist several months, even with a resolving disease process. Anti-HB core IgM becomes positive early, with onset of symptoms, and both anti-HB core IGM and anti-HB core IgG may persist for many months or years. Anti-HBs is the last antibody to appear and may indicate resolving infection. The presence of HBeAg indicates active viral replication and increased infectivity (**Figure 33-1**). Liver function tests should be obtained early in the course of infection, and evidence of prolonged prothrombin time (>1.5 INR) should raise concern for hepatic failure. Patients who remain chronically infected may demonstrate HBsAg and HBeAg for at least 6 months, with a usual trend in liver function tests toward normal levels, although results may remain persistently elevated (**Figure 33-2**). Extrahepatic manifestations of HBV infection may occur and include serum sickness, polyarteritis nodosa, and membranoproliferative glomerulonephritis.

Complications

Complications of chronic infection may include progression to cirrhosis and hepatocellular carcinoma (HCC). Patients with active viral replication are at highest risk of chronic disease, with 15–20% developing progressive disease over a 5-year period. Continued positivity for HBeAg is associated with an increased risk of HCC. Most patients who are chronically infected remain HBsAg-positive for their lifetime. There is no general agreement concerning the appropriate screening for patients with chronic infection for HCC. Some experts would not screen carriers if all laboratory tests are normal but would screen with ultrasonography and α-fetoprotein for evidence of chronic active hepatitis every 2–3 years, and more frequently in patients with cirrhosis.

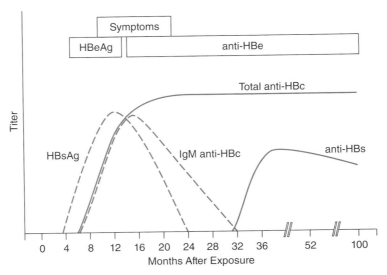

▲ **Figure 33-1.** Acute hepatitis B virus infection with recovery.

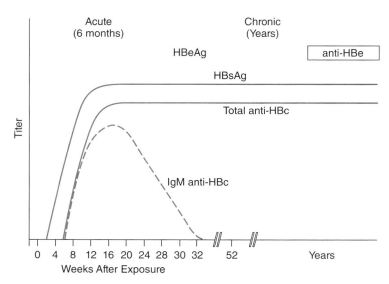

▲ **Figure 33-2.** Progression to chronic hepatitis B virus infection.

It appears that the incidence of progression of disease is greater in countries with high endemicity, and clinicians in these countries screen as frequently as every 6 months.

▶ Treatment

Treatment for chronic disease depends on evidence of viral activity, HBeAg status, HIV and HCV comorbidity, histologic evidence of liver injury, and elevated liver function tests. Currently approved treatment modalities include interferon alfa, pegylated interferon, lamivudine, telbivudine, adefovir, tenofovir, and entecavir. Other new antiviral agents are currently being tested. Sensitive tests for determination of response to therapy, such as covalently closed circular DNA (cccDNA), may be more readily available in the future.

Hepatitis C

▶ General Considerations

Hepatitis C virus (HCV) has become the most common bloodborne infection as well as the leading cause of chronic liver disease and subsequently, liver transplantation in the United States. Worldwide, more than 180 million people are infected, but the infection rates vary considerably. In the United States, it is estimated that approximately 4 million people may be infected with HCV; it is the main cause of death from liver disease. The responsible virus is an RNA virus of the Flaviviridae family. Six major genotypes, numbered 1 through 6, are known, with additional subtypes. There are varying distributions of these genotypes, and they

may affect the progression of disease and the response to treatment regimens.

Hepatitis C is spread primarily through percutaneous exposure to blood. Since 1992, all donated blood has been screened for HCV. Injection drug use is responsible for >50% of new cases. Within 1–3 months after a first incident of needle sharing, 50–60% of intravenous drug users are infected. Other risk factors include use of intranasal cocaine, hemodialysis, tattooing (debatable), and vertical transmission, which is rare. Breastfeeding carries a low risk of transmission. Sexual transmission is uncertain but is probably 1–3% over the lifetime of a monogamous couple, one of whom is infected. Healthcare workers are at particular risk following a percutaneous exposure (1.8% average incidence).

One-time screening of all individuals born between 1945 and 1965 has been recommended by the CDC, along with screening of patients with known risk factors.

▶ Prevention

No immunizations are currently available for HCV infections. Prevention consists mainly of reduction of risk factors, including screening of blood and blood products, caution to prevent percutaneous injuries, and reduction in intravenous drug use.

▶ Clinical Findings

A. Symptoms and Signs

1. Acute hepatitis—The incubation period for HCV varies between 2 and 26 weeks, but most commonly is 6–7 weeks.

Most patients with HCV are asymptomatic at the time of infection. However, >20% of all recognized cases of acute hepatitis in the United States are caused by HCV, and as many as 30% of adults who are infected may present with jaundice. Acute, fulminant hepatic failure is rare.

2. Chronic hepatitis—In contrast to HAV and HBV, most people infected with HCV (85%) develop a chronic infection. The incidence of significant liver disease is 20–30% for cirrhosis and 4% for liver failure; over 1–4% of patients with chronic infection develop HCC annually, or 11–19% over 4–11 years in one study. It appears that certain risk factors increase the likelihood of progression to serious disease. These include increased alcohol intake, age >40 years, HIV coinfection, and possibly male gender and other liver coinfections.

Extrahepatic manifestations of chronic infection are fairly common and are similar to those of HBV, including autoimmune conditions and renal conditions such as membranous glomerulonephritis.

B. Laboratory Findings

Patients in a high-risk category for HCV should be tested with both an approved HCV antibody test such as the OraQuick HCV Rapid Antibody test or other approved tests and a confirmatory test by nucleic acid testing (NAT) to detect HCV RNA if positive. All patients with HCV infection should have quantitative NAT as well as HCV genotyping prior to therapy in order to predict a therapeutic response as well as duration of therapy. The appropriate role of liver biopsy in decisions concerning therapy is in a state of flux, particuarly regarding threatment for genotype 1 patients. Consultation with a liver specialist should be considered to ascertain the value of this additional information that a liver biopsy would provide.

▶ Treatment

Treatment for both acute and chronic HCV has undergone significant strides in more recent years. A recent study documents the conversion of a significant number of patients to negative serology when treated in the acute phase of infection. Chronic HCV genotype 1 is treated with either a combination of direct acting antibody drugs (DAA) such as simeprevir and sofosbuvir with or without an interferon regimen and/or ribavirin. Treatment recommendations are rapidly changing. The other genotypes are less sensitive to therapy with the protease inhibitors and are usually managed with only interferon and rivavirin. Other new treatments are currently under investigation.

It is important to immunize patients with chronic HCV infection for HAV, because the incidence of fulminant hepatitis A has been shown to be significantly increased in this population. Patients infected with HCV should also abstain from alcohol. It has also been recommended that HCV-infected individuals be vaccinated for HBV, owing to the poor prognosis of coinfected individuals. Chronic hepatitis C can also progress to cirrhosis and HCC, and appropriate screening measures as discussed under Hepatitis B apply to hepatitis C-infected patients as well.

Other Types of Infectious Hepatitis

Over 97% of the viral hepatitis in the United States is either A, B, or C. Other types of viral hepatitis occur much less frequently, although worldwide, they may be more important.

Hepatitis D

Hepatitis D virus (HDV) can replicate only in the presence of HBV infection. HDV infection can occur either as a coinfection with HBV or as a superinfection in a chronically infected individual with HBV. Although coinfection can produce more severe acute disease, a superinfection poses the risk of more significant chronic disease, with 70–80% of patients developing cirrhosis. The mode of transfmission is most commonly percutaneous. The only tests commercially available in the United States are IgG–anti-HDV. Prevention of HDV depends on prevention HBV. There are no products currently available to prevent HDV infection in patients infected with HBV.

Hepatitis E

Hepatitis E virus (HEV) is the most common cause of enterically transmitted non-A, non-B hepatitis. Acute HEV infection is similar to other forms of viral hepatitis; no chronic form is known. Severity of illness increases with age, and for reasons that are unclear, case fatality rates are particularly high in pregnant women. Most cases of HEV reported in the United States have occurred in travelers returning from areas of high endemicity. In certain areas of the world (Mexico, North Africa, the Middle East, and Asia), epidemics of HEV may be common. Prevention includes avoidance of drinking water and other beverages of unknown purity, uncooked shellfish, and uncooked vegetables and fruits. No vaccines are currently available, although one recently developed has proven to be highly effective.

Acute Hepatitis: A Cost-Effective Approach

Because the vast majority of viral hepatitis cases are caused by HAV, HBV, or HCV, tests to determine the precise etiology are necessary for appropriate primary and secondary prevention for the patient, as well as potential for therapy. **Figure 33-3** outlines one cost-effective approach. If these tests fail to indicate a diagnosis, the etiology may be due to less frequent causes of viral hepatitis such as Epstein-Barr virus, in which jaundice rarely accompanies infectious mononucleosis; cytomegalovirus or herpesvirus in immunocompromised patients; or other nonviral etiologies, such

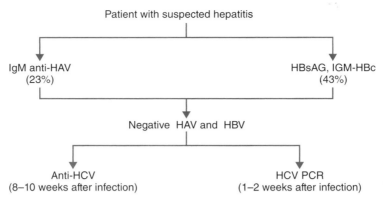

Patient with suspected hepatitis

IgM anti-HAV
(23%)

HBsAG, IGM-HBc
(43%)

Negative HAV and HBV

Anti-HCV
(8–10 weeks after infection)

HCV PCR
(1–2 weeks after infection)

▲ **Figure 33-3.** Cost-effective workup for acute viral hepatitis. (Reproduced, with permission, from Ahmed A, Keefe EB. Cost-effective evaluation of acute viral hepatitis. *West J Med.* 2000;172:29-32.)

as alcoholic hepatitis, drug toxicity, Wilson disease, or an autoimmune hepatitis.

Ahmed A, Keefe E. Cost-effective evaluation of acute viral hepatitis. *West J Med.* 2000;(179):29.[PMID 10695442]

Belongia EA et al. NIH consensus development conference on management of hepatitis B. *NIH Consens State Sci Statements.* 2008;25(2). [PMID: 18949020]

Centers for Disease Control and Prevention: Testing for HCV Infection: an update of guidance for clinicans and laboratorians. *MMWR.* 2013;62(18):362–365.

Ghany MG, Nelson DR, Strader DB, Thomas DL, Seeff LB. An update on treatment of genotype 1 chronic hepatitis C virus infection: 2011 practice guideline by the American Association for the Study of Liver Diseases. *Hepatology.* 2011;54:1433–1444.

Matheny S, Kingery J. Hepatitis A. *Am Fam Physician.* 2012; 86(11);1027–1034. [PMID 231998670]

US Public Health Service. Updated US Public Health Service guidelines for the management of occupational exposures to HBV, HCV, and HIV and recommendations for postexposure prophylaxis. *MMWR* (CDC *Morbidity & Mortality Weekly Report*)2001;50(RR-11):1. [PMID 11442229]

Websites

American Association for the Study of Liver Diseases. Ghany MG, Strader DB, Thomas DL Seelf LB. *Diagnosis, Management, and Treatment of Hepatitis C: Update 2009* (available at http://www.aasld.org/practiceguidelines/Documents/Bookmarked%20Practice%20Guidelines/Chronic_Hep_B_Update_2009%208_24_2009.pdf).

American Association for the Study of Liver Diseases. Lok ASF, McMahan BJ. *Chronic Hepatitis B: Update 2009* (available at http://www.aasld.org/practiceguidelines/Documents/Bookmarked%20Practice%20Guidelines/Chronic_Hep_B_Update_2009%208_24_2009.pdf).

American Liver Foundation. *Liver Update: Function and Disease* (excellent survey of issues pertaining to hepatitis): http://www.liverfoundation.org.

Centers for Disease Control and Prevention, hepatitis information (references for immunization and testing, as well as patient information in several languages). http://www.cdc.gov/hepatitis/

ALCOHOLIC LIVER DISEASE

 ESSENTIALS OF DIAGNOSIS

▶ History of alcohol use.

▶ Mildly elevated serum ALT and AST.

▶ Variable clinical signs (may include jaundice, hepatomegaly).

▶ General Considerations

Alcoholic liver disease includes several different disease entities, spanning a large clinical spectrum. These diseases range from the syndrome of acute fatty liver to severe liver damage as manifested by cirrhosis. *Fatty liver* is usually asymptomatic except for occasional hepatomegaly and is the histologic result of excessive use of alcohol over a several-day period. In *perivenular fibrosis*, fibrous tissue is deposited in the central areas of the liver, particularly the central veins; this indicates that the individual may then rapidly progress to more severe forms of liver disease. Patients can progress from this stage directly to cirrhosis. *Alcoholic hepatitis* is a condition in which necrosis of hepatic cells occurs as part of an inflammatory response, which includes polymorphonuclear cells, along with evidence of fibrosis. *Cirrhosis* may result from continued progression of disease from alcoholic hepatitis or may occur without evidence of prior alcoholic hepatitis. Cirrhosis is characterized by distortion of the liver structure, with bands of connective tissue forming between portal and central zones. Changes in hepatic blood circulation may also occur, resulting in portal hypertension. Additionally, evidence of abnormal fat metabolism, inflammation, and cholestasis may be seen. Progression to *hepatocellular carcinoma* (HCC) may also occur, although the exact risk of cirrhosis itself in the progression to HCC is not clear.

It is known that women are more likely than men to develop alcoholic liver disease, although the reasons for this phenomenon are only now being clarified. There may be additional genetic factors, most notably in specific enzyme systems, such as the metabolism of tumor necrosis factor (TNF) and alcohol-metabolizing systems, which affect the development of disease. Concomitant disease, such as HCV infection, is also a risk factor. Other factors (eg, obesity) may also play a role in the progression of disease.

▶ Clinical Findings

A. Symptoms and Signs

A history of drinking alcohol in excess of 80 g/day (six to eight drinks) is seen with the development of more advanced forms of the disease, although there is considerable individual variation. Numerous questionnaires have been designed for detection of excessive drinking, but the CAGE questionnaire (**c**ut down, **a**nnoyed by criticism, **g**uilty about drinking, **e**ye-opener drinks) is probably the most useful.

Clinical findings may be limited at this stage to occasional hepatomegaly. Patients with alcoholic hepatitis may present with classic signs and symptoms of acute hepatitis, including weight loss, anorexia, fatigue, nausea, and vomiting. Hepatomegaly may be evident, as well as other signs of more advanced disease, such as cirrhosis, because the development of cirrhosis may occur concomitant with a new episode of alcoholic hepatitis. These signs include jaundice, splenomegaly, ascites, spider angiomas, and signs of other organ damage secondary to alcoholism (eg, dementia, cardiomyopathy, or peripheral neuropathy).

▶ B. Laboratory Findings

Various commercially available laboratory tests have been used to detect excessive alcohol intake in the early stages. The sensitivity and specificity of these tests vary. Liver function tests for elevations of AST, ALT, and GGT are frequently used. Elevation of mean corpuscular volume (MCV) has also been noted in patients with early-stage disease.

Transaminase levels are usually only mildly elevated in pure alcoholic hepatitis unless other disease processes, such as concomitant viral hepatitis, or acetaminophen ingestion are present; AST is usually elevated to $\leq$200 IU/L; and AST, to $\leq$500 IU/L. AST elevation is usually greater than that of ALT. Elevated prothrombin time and bilirubin levels have a significant negative prognostic indication. *The presence of jaundice may have special significance in any actively drinking person and should be carefully evaluated.* Several instruments have been used for evaluation of severity, but the most common is the Maddrey discriminant function (MDF):

$$MDF = 4.6 \times (\text{prothrombin time in seconds} - \text{control}) + \text{serum bilirubin (mg/dL)}$$

A score > 32 is indicative of high risk of death.

▶ Treatment

Abstinence from alcohol is essential, and is probably the most important of all therapies. Recovery from the acute episode is associated with an 80% 7-year survival rate in patients who can abstain from alcohol versus 50% survival in those who continue drinking. The use of naltrexone or acamprosate in conjunction with counseling and support groups to prevent recidivism should be considered.

Initial treatment of the acutely ill patient centers on ensuring adequate volume replacement, with concern for the ability to handle normal saline. Diuretics should be avoided. Patients should be assessed for protein-calorie malnutrition and vitamin and mineral deficiencies. Adequate nutrition should be given to patients with severe disease, parenterally if necessary. There is no indication that avoidance of protein is helpful in patients with encephalopathy. Broad-spectrum antibiotics should be considered early in the treatment course. Many patients develop spontaneous peritonitis, pneumonia, or cellulitis, which should be treated aggressively. Corticosteroids have been suggested as beneficial, but considerable debate still ensues as to whether there is any benefit to survival, although current recommendations are that patients with severe disease (MDF $\geq$32) with or without encephalopathy and without contraindications for steroid use should be considered for a 4-week course of prednisone followed by a 2-week taper. Pentoxifylline, which modifies tumor necrosis factor alpha (TNFα), may also be considered, especially if steroids are contraindicated.

Liver transplantation may be an option. Alcoholic liver disease is currently the second most common reason for liver transplantation in the United States. To be considered for transplantation, patients should not have active alcoholic hepatitis, should have remained sober for more than 6 months, and should have had addictive treatment. The prognosis is excellent if relapse from drinking can be avoided. Relapse occurs in 15–30% of patients.

Other treatment methodologies in various stages of testing include other TNFα modifiers; antioxidant therapy with agents such as *S*-adenosyl-l-methionine (SAM-e), silymarin, or vitamin E; antifibrotics such as polyenylphosphatidylcholine (PPC); or other medications such as colchicine. Further studies are needed before these therapies can be recommended.

Maher J. Advances in liver disease: alcoholic hepatitis, non-cirrhotic portal fibrosis, and complications of cirrhosis. Treatment of alcoholic hepatitis. *J Gastroenterol Hepatol.* 2002; 17:448. [PMID: 11987726]

O'Shea R, et al. Alcoholic liver disease. *Am J Gastroenterol.* 2010; 105:14–32. [PMID: 19904248]

Yeung E, Wong FS. The management of cirrhotic ascites. *Medscape Gen Med.* 2002;4(4) (available at http://www.medscape.com/viewarticle/44236454).

OTHER LIVER DISEASES

Nonalcoholic Fatty Liver Disease

A relatively new condition described around 1980, nonalcoholic fatty liver disease (NAFLD), encompasses a wide clinical spectrum of patients whose liver histology is similar to those of patients with alcohol-induced hepatitis, but without the requisite history. Women are affected more frequently than men. Many of these patients progress to cirrhosis. NAFLD is now the most common liver disease in the United States, occurring in ≤20% of the population in some studies. This condition is common in obese patients, as well as in patients with type 2 diabetes mellitus. It may be a part of the syndrome X, which includes obesity, diabetes mellitus, dyslipidemia, and hypertension. Clinical features include hepatomegaly (75%) and splenomegaly (25%), but no pathognomonic laboratory markers. Elevations of ALT and AST may be ≤5 times normal, with an AST:ALT ratio of <1. Evidence of steatosis can be seen on hepatic ultrasonography. Treatment includes weight reduction, treatment of diabetes, and treatment of lipid disorders. There is no current evidence of the efficacy of specific pharmacologic therapy.

Wilson Disease

Wilson disease, which is characterized by hepatolenticular degeneration, is caused by abnormal metabolism of copper. It is inherited in an autosomal-recessive pattern and has a prevalence in the general population of approximately 1 in 30,000. Although patients in asymptomatic stages may manifest only transaminasemia or Kayser-Fleischer rings (golden-greenish granular deposits in the limbus), hepatomegaly or splenomegaly may already be present. In most symptomatic patients (96%), the serum ceruloplasmin level is <20 mg/dL. In patients with more advanced disease, symptoms of acute hepatitis or cirrhosis may be present. Neurologic signs include dysarthria, tremors, abnormal movements, and psychological disturbances. HCC may occur in patients with advanced disease. Treatment includes penicillamine, trientine, or zinc salts.

Hemochromatosis

An inborn error of iron metabolism leading to increased iron absorption from the diet, hemochromatosis is associated with diabetes, bronze skin pigmentation, hepatomegaly, loss of libido, and arthropathy. Patients may also show signs of cardiac or endocrine disorders. Symptoms usually first manifest between 40 and 60 years of age, and men are 10 times more likely than women to be affected. Hemochromatosis is the most common inherited liver disease in people of European descent. Physical signs include hepatomegaly (95% of symptomatic patients), which precedes abnormal liver function tests. Cardiac involvement includes congestive heart failure and arrhythmias. Many patients have cirrhosis by the time they are symptomatic (50–70%), 20% have fibrosis, and 10–20% have neither. HCC is common in patients with cirrhosis (30%) and is now the most common cause of death. Laboratory findings include elevated serum iron concentration, serum ferritin, and transferrin saturation. Therapy involves treatment of the complications of hemochromatosis, removal of excess iron by phlebotomy, and, in patients with cirrhosis, surveillance for HCC and treatment of hepatic and cardiac failure.

Autoimmune Hepatitis

Autoimmune hepatitis is a hepatocellular inflammatory disease of unknown etiology. Diagnosis is based on histologic examination, hypergammaglobulinemia, and presence of serum autoantibodies. The condition may be difficult to discern from other causes of chronic liver disease, which need to be excluded before diagnosis. Immunoserologic tests that are essential for diagnosis are assays for antinuclear antibodies (ANAs), smooth-muscle antibodies (SMAs), antibodies to liver and kidney microsome type 1 (anti-LKM1), and anti-liver cytosol type 1 (anti-LCI), as well as perinuclear antineutrophil cytoplasmic antibodies (aANCAs). Treatment, when indicated, is usually immunosuppressive with either prednisone, azathioprine, or both.

Drug-Induced Liver Disease

More than 600 drugs or other medicinals have been implicated in liver disease. Worldwide, drug-induced liver disease represents approximately 3% of all adverse drug reactions; in the United States, more than 20% of cases of jaundice in the elderly are caused by drugs. Acetaminophen and other drugs account for 25–40% of fulminant hepatic failure. Diagnosis is based on the discovery of abnormalities in hepatic enzymes or the development of a hepatitis like syndrome or jaundice. Most cases occur within 1 week to 3 months of exposure, and symptoms rapidly subside after cessation of the drug, returning to normal within 4 weeks of acute hepatocellular injury. Hepatic damage may manifest as acute hepatocellular injury (isoniazid, acetaminophen), cholestatic injury (contraceptive steroids, chlorpromazine), granulomatous hepatitis (allopurinol, phenylbutazone), chronic hepatitis (methotrexate), vascular injury (herbal tea preparations with toxic plant alkaloids), or neoplastic lesions (oral contraceptive steroids).

Statins, on the other hand, are widely used and can commonly cause mild liver enzyme elevations, but mild elevations of ALT or AST (<3 times the upper limit of normal) do not appear to contribute to liver toxicity.

Primary Biliary Cirrhosis

This autoimmune disease of uncertain etiology is manifested by inflammation and destruction of interlobular and septal bile ducts, which can cause chronic cholestasis and biliary cirrhosis. It is predominantly a disease of middle-aged women (female-to-male ratio of 9:1) and is particularly prevalent in northern Europe. The condition may be diagnosed on routine testing or be suspected in women with symptoms of fatigue or pruritus, or in susceptible individuals with elevated serum alkaline phosphatase, cholesterol, and IgM levels. Antimitochondrial antibodies are frequently found. Ursodeoxycholic acid is the only therapy currently available, although some patients may benefit from liver transplantation.

Hepatic Tumors & Cysts

Hepatocellular carcinoma is the most common malignant tumor of the liver; it is the fifth most common cancer in men and the eighth most common in women. Incidence increases with age, but the mean age in ethnic Chinese and African populations is lower. Signs of worsening cirrhosis may alert the clinician to consider HCC, but, in many cases, the onset is subtle. There are no specific hepatic function tests to detect HCC, but elevated serum tumor markers, most notably α-fetoprotein, are useful. Ultrasonography can detect the majority of HCC but may not distinguish it from other solid lesions. CT and MRI are also helpful in making the diagnosis. Risk factors for HCC include HBV, HCV, all etiologic forms of cirrhosis, ingestion of foods with aflatoxin B_1, and smoking. In these patients, ultrasonography and α-fetoprotein measurements every 4–6 months are recommended. In moderate-risk patients (ie, with later-onset HBV), measurement of α-fetoprotein every 6 months and annual ultrasound study are suggested.

Benign Tumors

Benign tumors include hepatocellular adenomas, which have become more common with the use of oral contraceptive steroids, and cavernous hemangiomas, which may occur with pregnancy or oral contraceptive steroid use and are the most common benign tumor of the liver.

Liver Abscesses

Liver abscesses can be the result of infections of the biliary tract or can have an extrahepatic source such as diverticulitis or inflammatory bowel disease. In ~40% of cases, no source of infection is found. The most common organisms are *Escherichia coli*, *Klebsiella*, *Proteus*, *Pseudomonas*, and *Streptococcus* species. Amebic liver abscesses are the most common extraintestinal manifestation of amebiasis, which occurs in >10% of the world's population and is most prevalent in the United States in young Hispanic adults. Amebic abscesses may have an acute presentation, with symptoms present for several weeks; few patients report typical intestinal symptoms such as diarrhea. Ultrasonography or CT scans with serologic tests such as enzyme-linked immunosorbent assay (ELISA) or indirect fluorescent antibody tests help confirm the diagnosis.

Chan HL, et al. How should we manage patients with non-alcoholic fatty liver disease in 2007? *J Gastroenterol Hepatol*. 2007;22: 801–808. [PMID: 17565632]

Lewis JH. Drug-induced liver disease. *Med Clin North Am*. 2000;84:1275. [PMID 11026929]

Manns MP, Czaja AJ, Gorham JD, et al. Diagnosis and management of autoimmune hepatitis. *Hepatology*. 2010;51(6): 2103–2213.

Onusko E. Statins and elevated liver tests: what's the fuss? *J Fam Practice*. 2009;67(7):449–452. [PMID: 18625167]

Powell LW, Yapp TR. Hemochromatosis. *Clin Liver Dis*. 2000; 4;211. [PMID 11232185]

PANCREATIC DISEASE

Samuel C. Matheny, MD, MPH

ACUTE PANCREATITIS

 ESSENTIALS OF DIAGNOSIS

► Sudden, severe, abdominal pain in epigastric area, with frequent radiation to the back.

► Elevated serum amylase and lipase.

► Elevated ALT (biliary pancreatitis).

► Evidence of etiology on ultrasound (biliary causes) or CT and MRI (other causes).

General Considerations

Hospital admissions for acute pancreatitis are fairly frequent, and the most common causes vary with the age and sex of the patient. In the United States, gallstones and alcohol abuse are the most frequent etiologies (20–30%), but infectious causes such as mumps virus or parasitic disease should be considered, as well as medications, tumors, trauma, and metabolic conditions. Approximately 20% of cases are idiopathic. It is important to determine the etiology of pancreatitis, as early recognition of acute biliary pancreatitis in particular may be important in selecting the appropriate therapeutic approach.

A more detailed discussion of gallstone pancreatitis appears earlier in this chapter.

▶ Clinical Findings

A. Symptoms and Signs

Abdominal pain—usually epigastric, which may radiate to the back—is an common presenting sign. However, the pain may not be significant, and some cases of acute pancreatitis are missed or diagnosed after more significant complications have occurred. Abdominal tenderness ranging from rigidity to mild tenderness may be present. Lack of a specific diagnostic test may affect the accuracy of an early diagnosis.

B. Laboratory Findings

Useful laboratory tests include serum amylase (elevated 3–5 times above normal), serum lipase (more than twice normal), and, for determining the etiology, liver function tests, especially ALT. Serum amylases that are significantly elevated in the presence of epigastric pain are strong indicators of pancreatitis. However, amylase clears rapidly from the blood, and levels may be normal even in patients with severe pancreatitis. A urine dipstick test for trypsinogen-2 may also be useful. The triglyceride levels should be checked, as well as calcium in an attempt to identify pancreatitis associated with hyperlipemia and hyperparathyroidism.

C. Prognostic Tests

Over 20% of patients have a severe case of pancreatitis, and of these a significant number die. It is therefore important to accurately stage the severity of the illness and treat accordingly. Attempts to quantify severity of disease have lead to certain scoring criteria, such as the Acute Physiology and Chronic Health Evaluation (APACHE) II score (>7 on admission is indicative of severe illness), or the Ranson or Glasgow scores. All are complicated and have varying degrees of sensitivity and specificity. A simplified scoring test, the Bedside Index of Severity in Acute Pancreatitis (BISAP), has recently been introduced, and utilitzes two additional components of risk assessment—a rise in blood urea nitrogen (BUN) and the systemic inflammatory response syndrome (SIRS) as well as age, presence of pleural effusion, and mental status. Peritoneal lavage has also been used, but it is difficult to justify in patients with mild symptoms. C-reactive protein scores of >150 mg/L in the first 48 hours, interleukin-6 values of >400 pg/mL, and interleukin-8 values of >100 pg/mL on admission have also been suggested as indicators of severe pancreatitis. Other prognostic tests that may indicate severe illness are described in the following paragraphs, but their usefulness in clinical practice is still under review.

D. Imaging Studies

Ultrasonography of the right upper quadrant is helpful in identifying the etiology of pancreatitis, and is usually the initial imaging study of choice However, it has limited value in staging the severity of disease. (See the discussion earlier in the chapter on gallstone pancreatitis). Contrast-enhanced CT is the most common currently available imaging technique for staging the severity of pancreatitis and can determine the presence of glandular enlargement, intra- and extrapancreatic fluid collections, inflammation, necrosis, and abscesses. This study may not be necessary for patients with mild disease. MRCP may be just as accurate and has some advantages over contrast-enhanced CT in certain patients. Magnetic resonance imaging (MRI) is an alternative when CT is not helpful or feasible.

▶ Complications

Complications include organ failure, cardiovascular collapse, and fluid collections around the pancreas. The latter may be asymptomatic or they may enlarge, causing pain, fever, and infection. Extrapancreatic infections, either bacteremia or pneumonia, have recently been shown to complicate the management of acute pancreatitis in a significant number of patients, usually within the first 2 weeks. Pancreatic pseudocysts may occur in patients with very high amylase levels and obstruction of the pancreatic duct. Pancreatic necrosis may also occur and can be fatal. Infection of necrotic tissue should be suspected in patients with unexpected deterioration, fever, and leukocytosis, and confirmed by CT scan and fine-needle aspiration. Sterile necrosis should probably be managed nonoperatively unless progressive deterioration occurs. Septic necrosis usually requires surgical débridement.

▶ Treatment

Patients who have the potential to develop severe pancreatitis, or who already have severe pain, dehydration, or vomiting, should be hospitalized and their hydration needs monitored closely. These patients should receive nothing by mouth and should be given intravenous pain medication. Patients should be monitored carefully to assess adequate renal function, because renal failure is a major cause of morbidity and mortality. Signs of worsening condition include rising hematocrit, tachycardia, and lack of symptom improvement in 48 hours.

Nutritional treatment has evolved in recent years, but areas of controversy remain. Increasing evidence indicates that in cases of mild pancreatitis, there is no benefit to nasogastric suction, and patients who are not vomiting may continue on oral fluids or resume oral fluids after the first week. There is also growing evidence that in severe pancreatitis, early enteral feeding within the first week may lower endotoxin absorption and reduce other complications. If patients cannot absorb adequate quantities via the enteric route, then parenteral feeding may be necessary.

The use of antibiotics is also controversial. Prophylactic antibiotics have been used in severe pancreatitis, but there is some concern that they may predispose patients to fungal infections. The general consensus is to use antibiotics, preferably broad-spectrum agents, for severe pancreatitis and for as brief a period as possible (ie, <7 days).

Neeraj A, Park JH, Wu BU. Modern management of acute pancreatits. *Gastroenterol Clin North Am.* 2012;41(1):1–8.

Pezzilli R, et al. Diagnosis and treatment of acute pancreatitis: the position statement of the Italian Association for the Study of the Pancreas. *Dig Liver Dis.* 2008;40:803-808. [PMID: 18387862]

Rettally CA, et al. The usefulness of laboratory tests in the early assessment of severity of acute pancreatitis. *Crit Rev Clin Lab Sci.* 2003;40:117. [PMID: 12755453]

Whitcomb D. Clinical practice. Acute pancreatitis. *N Engl J Med.* 2006;354:2142. [PMID: 16707751]

Yousaf M, et al. Management of severe acute pancreatitis. *Br J Surg.* 2003;90:407. [PMID: 12673741]

PANCREATIC CANCER

 ESSENTIALS OF DIAGNOSIS

- ▶ Anorexia, jaundice, weight loss, epigastric pain radiating to back, dark urine, and light stools.
- ▶ Spiral CT of the abdomen or endoscopic ultrasonography showing evidence of tumor.
- ▶ CA 19-9 serum tumor marker.

General Considerations

Although pancreatic cancer is diagnosed in only 30,000 patients each year in the United States, it is the fourth most common cause of death from cancer and the second most common gastrointestinal malignancy. Pancreatic cancer has a very poor prognosis: >80% of patients die within the first year, and the 5-year survival rate is <4%. In the vast majority of patients, the cancer is discovered at too late a stage to benefit from resection, and the response to chemotherapy is very poor. Over 90% of pancreatic cancers are ductal adenocarcinoma.

Cigarette smoking is the major risk factor established to date. Diet may also be a factor, with high intake of fat or meat and obesity associated with an increased risk; fruits, vegetables, and exercise help protect against pancreatic cancer. Likewise, a history of chronic pancreatitis is considered a risk factor, along with surgery for peptic ulcer disease, hereditary pancreatitis, and some genetic mutations (eg, *BRAC2*, associated with hereditary breast cancer). No guidelines currently exist regarding screening of the general population for pancreatic cancer, although some experts feel that patients with a family history of hereditary pancreatitis should be screened.

Clinical Findings

A. Symptoms and Signs

The clinical presentation of pancreatic cancer can vary widely; tumors that occur in the head of the pancreas (two-thirds of all pancreatic cancer) may produce early signs of obstructive jaundice. Tumors in the body and tail of the pancreas may grow quite large and cause fewer signs of obstruction. Symptoms more likely to be associated with pancreatic cancer include abdominal pain, jaundice, dark urine, light-colored stools, and weight loss. Pain may be worse when the patient is lying flat or eating. Other physical signs associated with pancreatic cancer include Courvoisier sign (palpable, nontender gallbladder in a patient with jaundice).

B. Laboratory Findings

Laboratory evaluation should include liver function tests. The serum tumor antigen CA 19-9 may be useful in confirming a diagnosis but is not an appropriate screening tool. Other markers are under consideration.

C. Imaging Studies

There is some debate as to the best imaging study. Dual-phase spiral CT with a pancreatic protocol has a high rate of sensitivity and can also assist in staging of the tumor, which is important for clinical management. Endoscopic ultrasonography may become the most accurate test for diagnosis. If patients have jaundice, then transabdominal ultrasound may be the first imaging test performed.

Treatment

Because the only hope for a cure is surgical resection, staging of pancreatic tumors is important for management. The difficulty lies in identifying the small fraction of patients who will benefit from surgery from those who will not—patients with metastatic disease who would otherwise be subjected to unnecessary invasive procedures and the resultant increased morbidity and mortality.

For patients with metastatic disease, chemotherapy and palliative care should be offered; surgery is avoided. Patients with advanced local disease but no metastases may benefit from radiotherapy and chemotherapy, and those without invasion or metastases may be candidates for resection. Even with resection, the outlook is poor (5-year survival rates of <25%). Radiation therapy may be useful in some patients with localized but nonresectable tumors, and chemotherapy (5-fluorouracil and gemcitabine) has some limited success.

Pain management can be a significant problem, and various modalities may need to be utilized. Biliary decompression may be required for jaundice.

Vincent A, Herman J, Schulick R, Hruban RH, Goggins M. Pancreatic cancer. *Lancet.* 2011;13:378(9791):607–620. [PMID: 21620466]

Vaginal Bleeding

Patricia Evans, MD, MA

ESSENTIALS OF DIAGNOSIS

▶ A clinical history of a menstrual cycle pattern outside the normal parameters.

▶ The normal menstrual cycle is generally 21–35 days in length with a menstrual flow lasting 2–7 days and a total menstrual blood loss of 20–60 mL.

General Considerations

Abnormal bleeding affects ≤30% of women at some time during their lives. Common terminology and the bleeding patterns associated with each term are listed in **Table 34-1**. ACOG recently adopted a classification system known by the acronym PALM–COEIN (polyp, adenomyosis, leiomyoma, malignancy and hyperplasia, coagulopathy, ovulatory dysfunction, endometrial, iatrogenic, and not yet classified). The recommendation of ACOG is to classify abnormal uterine bleeding (AUB) as heavy menstrual bleeding (HMB) or intermenstrual bleeding (IMB) in addition to a letter denoting the cause in order to achieve uniformity in nomenclature and eliminate the terminology of dysfunctional uterine bleeding (DUB).

Committee on Practice Bulletins—Gynecology. Diagnosis of abnormal uterine bleeding in reproductive-aged women. *Obstet Gynecol.* 2012;120(1):197–206. [PMID: 22914421]

Clinical Findings

A. Symptoms and Signs

1. History—The physician should try to establish whether the patient's pattern is cyclic or anovulatory. If the patient menstruates every 21–35 days, her cycle is consistent with an ovulatory pattern of bleeding. To confirm ovulation, patients can check their basal body temperature, cervical mucus, and luteinizing hormone (LH) levels. Basal body temperature can be checked using a basal body temperature thermometer, which allows for a precise measurement of the patient's temperature within a narrower range than a standard thermometer. After ovulation the ovary secretes an increased amount of progesterone, causing an increase in temperature of approximately 0.5°F over the baseline temperature in the follicular phase. The luteal phase is often accompanied by an elevation of temperature that lasts 10 days. Patients can also be taught to check the consistency of their cervical mucus, watching for a change from the sticky, whitish cervical mucus of the follicular phase to the clear, stretching mucus of ovulation. Finally, the patient can use an enzyme-linked immunosorbent assay (ELISA) testing kit to check for the elevation of LH over baseline that occurs with ovulation. The patient should be asked to describe the current vaginal bleeding in terms of onset, frequency, duration, and severity. Age, parity, sexual history, previous gynecological disease, and obstetrical history will further assist the physician in focusing the evaluation of the women with vaginal bleeding. The physician should ask about medications, including contraceptives, prescription medications, and over-the-counter (OTC) medications and supplements. The patient should be asked about any OTC preparations she might be taking. Patients may not be aware that herbal preparations may contribute to vaginal bleeding. Ginseng, which has estrogenic properties, can cause vaginal bleeding, and St John's Wort can interact with oral contraceptives to cause breakthrough bleeding. A review of symptoms should include questions regarding fever, fatigue, abdominal pain, hirsutism, galactorrhea, changes in bowel movements, and heat/cold intolerance. A careful family history will aid in identifying patients with a predisposition to polycystic ovarian syndrome (PCOS), congenital adrenal hyperplasia, thyroid disease, premature ovarian failure, fibroids, and cancer.

Table 34-1. Patterns of vaginal bleeding.

Descriptive Term	Bleeding Pattern
Menorrhagia	Regular cycles, prolonged duration, excessive flow
Metrorrhagia	Irregular cycles
Menometrorrhagia	Irregular cycles, prolonged duration, excessive flow
Hypermenorrhea	Regular cycles, normal duration, excessive flow
Polymenorrhea	Frequent cycles
Oligomenorrhea	Infrequent cycles

2. Physical examination—The physical examination for women complaining of vaginal bleeding should begin with an evaluation of the patient's vital signs, weight, thyroid gland, and hair distribution for hirsutism. The pelvic examination will aid in identifying many causes of bleeding, including anatomic abnormalities, infections, pregnancy, and signs of fibroids.

B. Evaluation

The evaluation of patients presenting with vaginal bleeding includes a combination of laboratory testing, imaging studies, and sampling techniques. The evaluation is directed by both patient presentation and a risk evaluation for endometrial cancer.

C. Laboratory Findings

Most patients presenting with vaginal bleeding should be evaluated with a complete blood count. In addition, every woman of reproductive age should have a urine or serum pregnancy test. A thyroid-stimulating hormone (TSH) should be drawn on women presenting with symptoms consistent with hypo- or hyperthyroidism or in women presenting with a change from a normal menstrual pattern. Adolescents presenting with menorrhagia at menarche should have an evaluation for coagulopathies, including a prothrombin time (PT), partial thromboplastin time (PTT), and bleeding time. In patients with symptoms suggestive of PCOS it is reasonable to check for elevated LH, testosterone, and androstenedione. These may be elevated in patients with PCOS, but because of the large variation among individual women, these tests are not definitive. Therefore, the physician needs to interpret test results in conjunction with the clinical picture to make a diagnosis of PCOS.

Overall, the incidence of adult-onset congenital adrenal hyperplasia (CAH) is ~2% in women with hyperandrogenic symptoms. The incidence is higher in individuals of Italian, Ashkenazi Jewish, and Yugoslav heritage. The decision on screening for adult-onset CAH should be based on the patient's clinical presentation and ethnic background. A basal 17-hydroxyprogesterone (17-HP) should be drawn in the early morning to screen for adult-onset CAH. Patients with an abnormal result can have another 17-HP level drawn after receiving a dose of adrenocorticotropic hormone (ACTH).

D. Imaging Studies

1. Pelvic ultrasound—A pelvic ultrasound can be used to evaluate the ovaries, uterus, and endometrial lining for abnormalities. An evaluation of the ovaries can assist in the diagnosis of PCOS as many women with PCOS will have enlarged ovaries with multiple, small follicles. A pelvic ultrasound is also useful for evaluating an enlarged uterus for the presence of fibroids. Fibroids will appear as hypoechoic, solid masses seen within the borders of the uterus. Subserosal fibroids can be pedunculated and therefore can be seen outside the borders of the uterus. An endovaginal ultrasound can be used to evaluate the thickness of the endometrial stripe. The results need to be interpreted according to whether a patient is pre- or postmenopausal. An endovaginal ultrasound is a sensitive test for patients with postmenopausal bleeding regardless of whether they are using hormone replacement therapy (HRT). Therefore, postmenopausal patients with an endometrial stripe thicker than 4–5 mm should have a histological biopsy. Hormone replacement therapy can cause proliferation of a patient's endometrium, rendering an endovaginal evaluation less specific. An endovaginal ultrasound is also useful in evaluating the endometrial stripe in premenopausal or perimenopausal patients. Whereas the normal endometrial stripe is thicker in the premenopausal patient than in the postmenopausal patient, the median thickness of an abnormal endometrium is similar for both. The endovaginal ultrasound examination is less likely to detect myomas and polyps.

2. Sonohysterography—In a patient who has an endometrial stripe thicker than 5 mm, a saline infusion sonohysterography (SIS) may be helpful in delineating the cause. SIS involves performing a transvaginal ultrasound following installation of saline into the uterus. This study, which is performed after an abnormal vaginal ultrasound, is most useful in differentiating focal from diffuse endometrial abnormalities. Detection of a focal abnormality indicates evaluation by hysteroscopy, and detection of an endometrial abnormality indicates the need to perform an endometrial biopsy or dilation and curettage (D&C). This can be considered as a study of first choice in premenopausal women with abnormal uterine bleeding.

3. Magnetic resonance imaging—Magnetic resonance imaging (MRI) can be used to evaluate the uterine structure. The endometrium can be evaluated with an MRI, but the endometrial area seen on MRI does not correspond exactly to the endometrial stripe measured with ultrasound. In most situations, a transvaginal ultrasound is the preferred imaging modality, but if the patient cannot tolerate the procedure MRI does provide an option for evaluation. MRI is better than ultrasound in distinguishing adenomyosis from fibroids, so if the history and examination suggests adenomyosis, an MRI may be the best first choice. MRI is also sometimes used to evaluate fibroids prior to uterine artery embolization or to map multiple myomas.

E. Special Examinations: Endometrial Sampling

The workup for endometrial cancer should be pursued most aggressively with patients at greatest risk for the disease, such as postmenopausal patients who present with vaginal bleeding. In patients aged <40 years, endometrial cancer is usually seen in obese patients and/or patients who are chronically anovulatory. Therefore, a patient who presents with an anovulatory pattern of bleeding for >1 year should be evaluated for hyperplasia and neoplasm with an endometrial sample. In addition, ACOG recommends the evaluation of women aged >45 years presenting with new-onset menorrhagia with endometrial sampling since the incidence of endometrial cancer increases with age.

1. Dilation and curettage—Dilation and curettage (D&C) provides a blind sampling of the endometrium. The D&C generally will provide sampling of less than half of the uterine cavity. The D&C is useful in patients with cervical stenosis or other anatomic factors that prevent an adequate endometrial biopsy.

2. Endometrial biopsy—An endometrial biopsy is an adequate method of sampling the endometrial lining to identify histological abnormalities. The rates of obtaining an adequate endometrial sample depend on the age of the patient. Many postmenopausal women will have an atrophic endometrium, so sampling in this group will more often result in an inadequate endometrial specimen for examination. In this situation, the clinician must use additional diagnostic studies to fully evaluate the cause of the vaginal bleeding.

3. Diagnostic hysteroscopy—Direct exploration of the uterus is useful in identifying structural abnormalities such as fibroids and endometrial polyps. Small-caliber hysteroscopes allow the endometrium to be evaluated without the need for cervical dilatation. These instruments are limited by the fact that instruments cannot be passed through the endoscope and by their limited field of view. Larger-diameter hysteroscopes do allow for specific biopsy of lesions. In general, the diagnostic hysteroscopy is combined with a D&C or endometrial biopsy to maximize identification of abnormalities.

Goldstein S. Sonography in postmenopausal bleeding. *J Ultrasound Med.* 2012;31:333–336. [PMID: 22298878]

McLucas B. Diagnosis, imaging and anatomical classification of uterine fibroids. *Best Practice Res Clin Obstet Gynaecol.* 2008;22:627–642. [PMID: 18328787]
Svirsky R, et al. Can we rely on endometrial biopsy for detection of focal intrauterine pathology? *Am J Obstet Gynecol.* 2008; 199:115. [PMID 18456238]

▶ Differential Diagnosis

The differential diagnosis of vaginal bleeding, excluding pregnancy related bleeding, encompasses a wide range of possible etiologies. (**Table 34-2**).

A. Bleeding Secondary to Hormone Medications

1. Contraception—Vaginal bleeding is a common side effect of many forms of contraception. Many women starting oral contraceptive pills (OCPs) experience breakthrough bleeding in the initial months. Lower-dose oral contraceptive pills have higher rates of spotting and breakthrough bleeding. Possible causes of vaginal bleeding in patients taking OCPs include inadequate estrogenic or progestogenic stimulation of the endometrium, skipped pills, or altered absorption and metabolism of the pills. Breakthrough bleeding is common among users of extended contraceptive regimens. Having the patient institute a 3-day hormone-free interval at the onset of breakthrough bleeding is an effective treatment for this side effect.

Vaginal bleeding is also frequent with Depo-Provera (medroxyprogesterone), and is the most commonly cited reason why women discontinue taking it as well as OCPs. After the initial dose of Depo-Provera, half of women will experience irregular bleeding or spotting. After a year this decreases to 25%.

2. Hormone replacement therapy—Bleeding is common with hormone replacement therapy (HRT), and can occur with both the continuous and sequential regimens. Approximately 40% of women starting continuous regimens will experience bleeding in the first 4–6 months after starting treatment.

B. Anatomic Causes

1. Fibroids—Fibroids or leiomyomas are benign uterine tumors that are often asymptomatic. The most common symptoms associated with fibroid tumors are pelvic discomfort and abnormal uterine bleeding. Most commonly, women with symptomatic fibroids experience either heavy or prolonged periods.

2. Adenomyosis—*Adenomyosis* is defined as the presence of endometrial glands within the myometrium. This is usually asymptomatic, but women can present with heavy or prolonged menstrual bleeding as well as dysmenorrhea. The dysmenorrhea can be severe and begin ≤1 week prior

Table 34-2. Differential diagnosis of vaginal bleeding.

Diagnosis	Clinical Presentation	Most Commonly Associated Bleeding Pattern
Contraception	Known OCP/Depo use	OCP: spotting Depo: irregular or continuous bleeding
HRT	Known HRT use	Sequential: menorrhagia or spotting Continuous: irregular spotting
Fibroids	Asymptomatic, pelvic pain, and/or dysmenorrhea	Menorrhagia
Adenomyosis	Dysmenorrhea	Menorrhagia
Endometrial polyps	Asymptomatic	Intermenstrual spotting, metrorrhagia and/or menorrhagia
Cervical polyps	Asymptomatic	Intermenstrual and/or postcoital bleeding
PID	High-risk sexual behavior, fever, pelvic pain, tenderness	Menorrhagia and/or metrorrhagia
PCOS, adult-onset CAH	Hirsutism, acne, central obesity, or asymptomatic	Oligomenorrhea, menometrorrhagia
Hyperthyroidism	Nervousness, heat intolerance, diarrhea, palpitations, weight loss	Oligomenorrhea, amenorrhea, polymenorrhea, or menorrhagia
Hypothyroidism	Fatigue, cold intolerance, dry skin, hair loss, constipation, weight gain	Menorrhagia, polymenorrhea, oligomenorrhea, amenorrhea
Bleeding disorder	Asymptomatic mucocutaneous bleeding, easy bruising	Menorrhagia
Endometrial hyperplasia	Asymptomatic	Menorrhagia and/or metrorrhagia
Endometrial cancer	Asymptomatic	Postmenopausal: irregular spotting Perimenopausal: menometrorrhagia
Cervical cancer	Asymptomatic	Irregular spotting, postcoital bleeding

CAH, congenital adrenal hyperplasia; HRT, hormone replacement therapy; OCP, oral contraceptive pill; PCOS, polycystic ovarian syndrome; PID, pelvic inflammatory disease.

to menstruation. The appearance of symptoms usually occurs after age 40.

3. Endometrial and cervical polyps—Endometrial polyps can cause intermenstrual spotting, irregular bleeding, and/or menorrhagia. Cervical polyps usually cause intermenstrual spotting or postcoital bleeding.

C. Infectious Causes

Pelvic inflammatory disease (PID) in its classic form presents with fever, pelvic discomfort, cervical motion tenderness, and adnexal tenderness. Patients can present atypically with merely a change in their bleeding pattern. Cervical inflammation from trichomonas and gonorrheal and chlamydial cervicitis can cause intermenstrual spotting and postcoital bleeding.

D. Anovulatory Bleeding

There are multiple causes of anovulation, including physiological and pathological etiologies. During the first year following menarche, anovulation is a normal result of an immature hypothalamic-pituitary-gonadal axis. Irregular ovulation also is a normal physiological result of declining ovarian function during the perimenopausal years, and the hormonal changes associated with lactation. Hyperandrogenic causes of anovulation include PCOS, adult-onset CAH, and androgen-producing tumors. Confirming the diagnosis of PCOS involves the evaluation of clinical features and endocrine abnormalities, and the exclusion of other etiologies. Women with PCOS can present with oligomenorrhea or abnormal uterine bleeding from prolonged anovulation. In addition, these women can have hirsutism, acne, and central obesity. Endocrinologically, they can have increased testosterone activity, elevated luteinizing hormone concentration with a normal follicle-stimulating hormone level, and hyperinsulinemia due to insulin resistance. PCOS usually begins during puberty, and so these women often report a long history of irregular periods.

Adult-onset CAH results from an enzyme defect in the adrenal gland, most commonly a deficiency of 21-hydroxylase.

Phenotypically, women can present in a variety of ways: with PCOS symptoms, with hirsutism alone, or with hyperandrogenic laboratory work but no hyperandrogenic symptoms. Typically patients will present at or after puberty. As a result, these women will also report a long history of irregular periods.

E. Endocrine Abnormalities

Both hyper- and hypothyroidism can cause changes in a woman's menstrual cycle. Oligomenorrhea is seen more commonly in patients with hyperthyroidism. A patient with hypothyroidism may experience changes in her menstrual cycle, including amenorrhea, oligomenorrhea, polymenorrhea, or menorrhagia. Menstrual abnormalities occur more frequently with severe than with mild hypothyroidism.

F. Bleeding Disorders

Formation of a platelet plug is the first step of homeostasis during menstruation. Patients with disorders that interfere with the formation of a normal platelet plug can experience menorrhagia. The two most common disorders are von Willebrand disease and thrombocytopenia. Bleeding can be particularly severe at menarche, due to the dominant estrogen stimulation causing increased vascularity. Cases of menorrhagia in women with coagulation deficiencies have been reported, but these deficiencies are more common in men.

G. Endometrial Hyperplasia

Endometrial hyperplasia is an overgrowth of the glandular epithelium of the endometrial lining. This usually occurs when a patient is exposed to unopposed estrogen, either estrogenically or because of anovulation. The rate of neoplasms found with simple hyperplasia is 1%, and the rate with complex hyperplasia reaches almost 30% when atypia is present. Patients having hyperplasia with atypia should have a hysterectomy because of the high incidence of subsequent endometrial cancer. Most patients without atypia will respond to high-dose progestin treatment for 21 days. Endometrial ablation may also play a role in the treatment of hyperplasia.

H. Neoplasms

Uterine cancer is the fourth most common cancer in women. Risk factors for endometrial cancer include nulliparity, late menopause (after age 52), obesity, diabetes, unopposed estrogen therapy, tamoxifen, and a history of atypical endometrial hyperplasia. Endometrial cancer most often presents as postmenopausal bleeding in the sixth and seventh decades, although investigations have revealed that only 10% of patients with postmenopausal bleeding will have endometrial cancer. In the perimenopausal period endometrial cancer can present as menometrorrhagia. Vaginal bleeding

is the most common symptom in patients with cervical cancer. The increased cervical friability associated with cervical cancer usually results in postcoital bleeding, but also can appear as irregular or postmenopausal bleeding.

Furness S, Roberts H, Marjoribanks J, Lethaby A. Hormone therapy in postmenopausal women and risk of endometrial hyperplasia. *Cochrane Database Syst Rev.* 2012;8:CD000402.

Lacey JV, Chia VM. Endometrial hyperplasia and the risk of progression to carcinoma. *Maturitas.* 2009;63:39–44. [PMID: 19285814]

Plastina KA, Sulak PJ. New forms of contraception 2008. *Obstet Gynecol Clin North Am.* 35:185–197.

Soresky JI. Endometrial cancer. *Obstet Gynecol.* 2008;111:436–447. [PMID: 18238985]

Sweet MG, Schmidt-Dalton TA, Weiss PM, et al. Evaluation and management of abnormal uterine bleeding in premenopausal women. *Am Fam Physician.* 2012;85:35–43. [PMID: 22230306]

Teede H, Deeks A, Moran L. Polycystic ovary syndrome: a complex condition with psychological, reproductive and metabolic manifestations that impacts on health across the lifespan. *BMC Med.* 2010;8:41.[PMID: 20591140]

▶ Treatment

The treatment for vaginal bleeding should be directed at the underlying disease once it is identified.

A. Bleeding from Contraception

Physicians often change formulations of OCPs to try to decrease the incidence of intermenstrual bleeding. All formulations share the characteristic of a higher incidence of intermenstrual bleeding during the first cycle of use. Therefore, one of the most important things physicians can do is to reassure the patient and encourage continued use. The physician can try adding exogenous estrogen daily for 7–10 days to control prolonged intermenstrual bleeding. Physiologically, this approach makes sense, as OCPs cause endometrial atrophy.

Similarly, bleeding is common with Depo-Provera, especially early during the treatment. Reassurance and patience should be the initial treatment of any bleeding. With continued bleeding, physicians can consider the unstudied practice of adding low-dose estrogen supplementation for 1–3 months.

B. Fibroids

Medical management of fibroids is limited. Oral contraceptives have not been found to effectively treat fibroid symptoms. In selected patients, there is evidence that the levonorgestrel intrauterine device can effectively reduce fibroid symptoms. Recently there has been some evidence that depot medroxyprogesterone acetate may significantly improve menorrhagia attributed to fibroids. Mifepristone and selective estrogen receptor modulator (SERM) have been studied and may be available as treatment options after further study. Administration of a gonadotropin-releasing hormone (GnRH) agonist can greatly reduce the volume of a patient's fibroids. As this effect is temporary, this treatment is largely reserved for preoperative therapy to facilitate the removal of the uterus or fibroid. Pretreatment can also improve the patient's hematologic parameters by decreasing vaginal bleeding prior to surgery. Treatment with nonsteroidal anti-inflammatory drugs (NSAIDs) may be effective in decreasing abnormal uterine bleeding, but there is a lack of randomized trials examining this treatment. Ibuprofen at doses of 1200 mg daily effectively reduces bleeding in patients with primary menorrhagia, but this may not be as effective in women with fibroids. If patients fail these ambulatory approaches surgical options include a myomectomy, hysterectomy, or uterine embolization. Myomectomy is a good option for the patient who does not want her uterus removed or who desires future childbearing. The risk exists for the growth of new fibroids and the growth of fibroids too small for removal at the time of surgery. Women undergoing hysterectomies may have the option of an abdominal or vaginal hysterectomy. Vaginal hysterectomies involve fewer complications and shorter hospital stays. The size of the uterus at the time of surgery determines the feasibility of this approach, as the surgeon must be able to remove the uterus completely through a vaginal incision.

Women wanting to avoid hysterectomy have the option of uterine fibroid embolization. In this procedure an interventional radiologist injects tiny poly (vinyl alcohol) particles into the uterine arteries. Because the hypervascular fibroids have no collateral vascular supply, they undergo ischemic necrosis. Women with pedunculated or subserosal fibroids are not considered ideal candidates for this procedure. In addition, because the effects of uterine artery embolization on childbearing are not well known, the procedure is generally not done on women desiring future fertility.

C. Anovulatory Bleeding

Medical management is the preferred treatment for anovulatory bleeding. Treatment goals should include alleviation of any acute bleeding, prevention of future noncyclic bleeding, a decrease in the patient's future risk of long-term health problems secondary to anovulation, and improvement in the patient's quality of life. Treatment options include prostaglandin synthetase inhibitors, estrogen (for acute bleeding episodes), contraceptive methods, and cyclic progesterones. Those failing medical management have surgical options, including hysterectomy and endometrial ablation. Blood loss can be reduced by 50% in women treated with prostaglandin synthetase inhibitors, including mefenamic acid, ibuprofen, and naproxen. Because many of the studies evaluating the role of prostaglandin synthetase inhibitors were completed in women with ovulatory cycles, the results cannot be directly applied to women with anovulatory bleeding. In addition, this treatment does not address the issues of future noncyclic bleeding and decreasing future health risks due to anovulation. Estrogen alone is generally used to treat an acute episode of heavy uterine bleeding. Premarin used intravenously will temporarily stop most uterine bleeding, regardless of the cause. The dose commonly used is 25 mg of conjugated estrogen every 4 hours. Nausea limits using high doses of estrogen orally, but lower doses can be used in a patient with acute heavy bleeding who is hemodynamically stable. One suggested regimen is 2.5 mg of conjugated estrogen every 4–6 hours. After acute bleeding is controlled, the physician should add a progestin to the treatment regimen to induce withdrawal bleeding. A combination of estrogen and progesterone is given for 7–10 days and then stopped, inducing a withdrawal bleed. To decrease the risk of future hyperplasia and/or endometrial cancer, a progestin is continued for 10–14 days each cycle. Traditionally, treatment has been with medroxyprogesterone acetate (Provera) 10 mg. Other progestational agents include norethindrone acetate (Aygestin), norethindrone (Micronor), norgestrel (Ovrette), and micronized progesterone (Prometrium, Crinone). The micronized progesterones are natural progesterones modified to ensure a prolonged half-life and less destruction in the gastrointestinal tract. OCPs provide an option for treatment of both the acute episode of bleeding and future episodes of bleeding as well as prevention of long-term health problems from anovulation. Acutely, one option to control bleeding is to administer a 50-µg estrogen OCP 4 times a day until bleeding ceases, then continue the OCP for a week. Long-term OCPs are effective in treating all patterns of abnormal uterine bleeding related to anovulation. Patients with a history of thromboembolism, cerebrovascular disease, coronary artery disease, estrogen-dependent neoplasias, or liver disease should not be started on an oral contraceptive. Relative contraindications include migraine headaches, hypertension, diabetes, age >35 years in a smoking patient, and active gallbladder disease. Other methods of combined hormone treatment can be considered, including the transdermal contraceptive patch, the vaginal contraceptive ring, and the levonorgestrel intrauterine device (IUD). Menstrual blood loss is significantly reduced with the use of the levonorgestrel IUD and may represent a better option than cyclic progesterone for the treatment of menorrhagia. The FDA approved an oral form of transexamic acid for use in the United States. Transexamic acid has been used for the treatment of heavy menstrual bleeding outside the United States for several decades. It is taken the first 5 days of menses and should be avoided in women with risks for thromboembolic disease or renal disease.

Patients who are unable to tolerate hormonal management can consider endometrial ablation. Initially used exclusively in patients with menorrhagia, these treatments are now also used in women with anovulatory bleeding.

Because endometrial glands often persist after ablative treatment, few women will experience long-term amenorrhea after treatment. The risk of endometrial cancer is not eliminated after treatment, so women at risk for endometrial cancer from long-term unopposed estrogen exposure still need preventive treatment. As pregnancies have occurred after endometrial ablation, some form of contraception may be needed after the procedure.

Casablanca Y. Management of dysfunctional uterine bleeding. *Obstet Gynecol Clin North Am.* 2008;35:219–234.

Damlo S. ACOG guidelines on endometrial ablation. *Am Fam Physician.* 2008;77:545–549.

Munro M. Uterine leiomyomas, current concepts: pathogenesis, impact on reproductive health, and medical, procedural, and surgical management. *Obstet Gynecol Clin North Am.* 2011;38:703–731. [PMID: 22134018]

Tsai MC, Goldstein SR. Office diagnosis and management of abnormal bleeding. *Clin Obstet Gynecol.* 2012;55:635–650. [PMID: 22828096]

Hypertension

Maureen O'Hara Padden, MD, MPH

Kevin M. Bernstein, MD, MMS

▶ General Considerations

Approximately 76.4 million people aged ≥20 years in the United States have *hypertension*, defined as an average systolic blood pressure of ≥140 mmHg, a diastolic blood pressure of ≥90 mmHg, the current use of blood pressure–lowering medication, and/or being informed twice of the diagnosis by a health care professional. This translates to one in three adults and more than half of those aged >60 years. The incidence of hypertension increases with age. If an individual is normotensive at age 55, the lifetime risk for hypertension is 90%. High blood pressure resulted in the death of 61,005 Americans in 2008. From 1998 to 2008, the death rate from hypertension rose by 20.2% and the actual number of deaths rose by 49.7%. Of persons with high blood pressure, 81% are aware of their diagnosis. Of this group, 72% are under treatment, while only 50% are well controlled. A higher percentage of men than women have hypertension until the age of 45. From the age of 45 to 64, the percentage of men and women affected by hypertension is similar. Above the age of 65, a higher percentage of women than men have hypertension. Although the true incidence of hypertension in children is unknown, the number of hospitalizations for children with hypertension between 1997 and 2006 doubled from 12,661 to 24,602. Hypertension is most prevalent

among the African-American population, affecting about 42% of them. Non-Hispanic Afro Americans and Mexican Americans are also more likely to suffer from high blood pressure than non-Hispanic whites. In 2010, the economic cost of hypertensive disease was estimated at $76.6 billion. Nearly 90% of the US adults with uncontrolled hypertension have a usual source of health care and insurance.

The National High Blood Pressure Education Program (NHBPEP), which is coordinated by the National heart, Lung, and Blood Institute (NHBLI) of the National Institutes of Health, was established in 1972. The program was designed to increase awareness, prevention, treatment, and control of hypertension. Data from the National Health and Nutrition Examination Survey (NHANES), conducted between 1976 and 2008, revealed that of patients aware of their high blood pressure and under treatment, the number who had achieved control of their high blood pressure had increased. Coincident with these positive changes was a dramatic reduction in morbidity and mortality (40–60%), including stroke and myocardial infarction (MI) secondary to hypertension. However, the most recent series of NHANES surveys conducted between 2007 and 2008 continue to show a leveling off of improvement.

High blood pressure is easily detected and usually controlled with appropriate intervention. Of the patients with high blood pressure, 81% are aware of their diagnosis. Among this group, 72% are under treatment, 50% are well controlled, and 50% are not. In addition, the incidence of end-stage renal disease and the prevalence of heart failure continue to increase. Both conditions have been linked to uncontrolled hypertension.

In 2003, the *Seventh Report of the Joint National Committee on Prevention, Detection, Evaluation, and Treatment of High Blood Pressure* (JNC VII) was released. It provided updated recommendations based on recent studies, including more concise clinical guidelines and a simplified blood pressure

Table 35-A

Deaths/100,000 individuals	Race/gender
50.3	African American/male
16.5	Caucasian/male
38.6	African American/female
14.5	Caucasian/female

classification (**Table 35-1**). The eighth edition was released in 2013.

Centers for Disease Control and Prevention (CDC). Vital signs: awareness and treatment of uncontrolled hypertension among adults—United States, 2003–2010. *MMWR.* 2012;61(35):703–709. [PMID: 22951452]

Chobanian AV et al. Seventh Report of the Joint National Committee on Prevention, Detection, Evaluation, and Treatment of High Blood Pressure: The JNC 7 report. *JAMA.* 2003; 289:2560. [PMID: 12748199]

Roger VL, Go AS, Lloyd-Jones DM, et al. Heart disease and stroke statistics: 2012 update: a report from the American Heart Association. *Circulation.* 2012;125(1):e2–e220. [PMID: 22179539]

Tran CL, Ehrmann BJ, Messer KL, et al. Recent trends in healthcare utilization among children and adolescents in the United States. *Hypertension.* 2012;60(2):296–302. [PMID: 22710648]

Viera AJ, Hinderliter, AL. Evaluation and management of the patient with difficult-to-control or resistant hypertension. *Am Fam Physician.* 2009;79(10):863–869. [PMID: 19496385]

▶ Pathogenesis

A. Primary or Essential Hypertension

In 90–95% of cases of hypertension, no cause can be identified. A role for genetics has been implicated in the development of high blood pressure (eg, hypertension is more prevalent in some families and in African Americans). Additional risk factors include increased salt intake, excess alcohol intake, obesity, sedentary lifestyle, dyslipidemia, depression, vitamin D deficiency, and certain personality traits, including aggressiveness and poor stress coping skills.

B. Secondary Hypertension

It is reasonable to look for an underlying cause in patients diagnosed with hypertension even though a specific condition can be found in only 2–10% of cases. History or physical examination may suggest an underlying etiology, or the first clue may come later when patients fail to respond appropriately to standard drug therapy. In addition, secondary hypertension should be considered in those with sudden-onset hypertension, in those with suddenly uncontrolled blood pressure that had previously been well controlled, and in patients aged <30 years without a family history of hypertension.

Etiologies of secondary hypertension that must be considered in the appropriate patient include use of certain medications such as oral contraceptives, sympathomimetics, decongestants, nonsteroidal anti-inflammatory drugs (NSAIDs), appetite suppressants, antidepressants, adrenal steroids, cyclosporine, and erythropoietin. All of these medications can contribute to an elevation in blood pressure.

Table 35-1. Classification and management of blood pressure in adults.[a]

BP Classification	SBP[a] (mmHg)	DBP[a] (mmHg)	Lifestyle Modification	Initial Drug Therapy	
				Without Compelling Indication	**With Compelling Indication** (see Table 34-5)
Normal	< 120	and <80	Encourage	No antihypertensive drug indicated	Drug(s) for compelling indications[b]
Prehypertension	120–139	or 80–90	Yes		
Stage 1 hypertension	140–159	or 90–99	Yes	No specific medication is recommended as first line—most important is to control blood pressure; start with ACE inhibitors for most; also, thiazide-type diuretics, ARB, β-blocker, calcium channel blocker, or combination	Drug(s) for compelling indications;[c] other antihypertensive drugs (diuretics, ACE inhibitors, β-blockers, calcium channel blockers) as needed
Stage 2 hypertension	≥160	or ≥100	Yes	Two-drug combination for most[c] (usually ACE inhibitor and calcium channel blocker; or thiazide-type diuretic or ARB or β-blocker)	

[a]Treatment determined by highest BP category.
[b]Treat patients with chronic kidney disease or diabetes to BP goal of <130/80 mmHg.
[c]Initial combined therapy should be used cautiously in those at risk for orthostatic hypotension.
ACE, angiotensin-converting enzyme; ARB, angiotensin II receptor blocker; BP, blood pressure; DBP, diastolic blood pressure; SBP, systolic blood pressure.
Data from *Seventh Report of the Joint National Committee on Prevention, Detection, Evaluation, and Treatment of High Blood Pressure.* NIH Publication 03-5233. US Department of Health and Human Services, 2003; Jamerson K. Weber MA. Bakris GL, et al. Benazepril plus amlodipine or hydrochlorothiazide for hypertension in high-risk patients: avoiding cardiovascular events in combination therapy with systolic hypertension (ACCOMPLISH) trial. *N Engl J Med.* 2008;359(23):2417. [PMID: 19052124]

Drug interactions, particularly between monoamine oxidase inhibitors with tricyclic antidepressants, antihistamines, or tyramine-containing food, can also cause an elevation in blood pressure. Additionally, hypertension can be related to excessive use of caffeine, nicotine, decongestants containing ephedrine, alcohol, excessive ingestion of black licorice, or use of illicit drugs such as cocaine or amphetamines. Other over-the-counter (OTC) formulations including weight-loss products, energy drinks, anabolic steroids and other body-building supplements should also be considered.

Hypertension can also occur secondary to acute and chronic kidney disease, which might be suggested by flank mass, elevated creatinine level, or abnormal findings such as proteinuria, hematuria, or casts on routine urinalysis. Rarely, hypertension may be related to renal artery stenosis, particularly if onset occurs at age <20 or >50 years. Abdominal bruits with radiation to the renal area may be heard. Other causes to consider in the differential diagnosis include white coat hypertension, postoperative hypertension, hypo- or hyperthyroidism, hyperparathyroidism, primary hyperaldosteronism, Cushing syndrome, coarctation of the aorta, vasculitis, collagen vascular disease, CNS trauma, spinal cord disorders, pheochromocytoma, pregnancy-induced hypertension, and sleep apnea syndrome in the appropriate clinical presentation. When such causes are entertained, appropriate evaluation should be undertaken.

▶ Prevention

A healthy lifestyle is hailed as both prevention and initial therapy for hypertension (**Table 35-2**). Clinical trials assessing both prevention (Trials of Hypertension Prevention–phase II, TONE) and nonpharmacologic treatment of mild hypertension (TOMHS, DAH, low-sodium DASH, PREMIER) support the positive impact of maintaining optimal weight; a regular aerobic exercise program; strength training with either dynamic or isometric exercise; and a diet low in sodium, saturated fat, and total fats and rich in fruits and vegetables. Excessive alcohol intake should be reduced and smoking cessation encouraged.

▶ Clinical Findings

Before patients with hypertension can be offered adequate treatment, they must be properly diagnosed. Because patients are often asymptomatic, the risk factors for hypertension must be understood and appropriate patients screened. In addition to the modifiable risk factors noted earlier, there are nonmodifiable factors, including African American race, family history of hypertension, and increasing age.

▶ A. Symptoms and Signs

There are usually no physical findings early in the course of hypertension. In some patients, the presence of hypertension may be signaled by early-morning headaches or, in those with severe hypertension, by signs or symptoms associated with target organ damage. Such symptoms might include nausea, vomiting, visual disturbance, chest pain, or confusion. More typically, the first indication is an elevated blood pressure measurement taken with a sphygmomanometer

Table 35-2. Lifestyle modifications to manage hypertension.[a]

Modification	Recommendation[b]	Approximate SBP Reduction (Range)
Weight reduction	Maintain normal body weight (BMI 18.5–24.9 kg/m^2)	5–20 mmHg/10 kg weight loss
Adopt DASH eating plan	Consume a diet rich in fruits, vegetables, and low-fat dairy products with a reduced content of saturated and total fat	8–14 mmHg
Dietary sodium reduction	Reduce dietary sodium intake to ≤100 mmol/d (2.4 g sodium or 6 g sodium chloride)	2–8 mmHg
Physical activity	Engage in regular aerobic physical activity such as brisk walking (≥30 min/d, most days of the week)	4–9 mmHg
Moderation of alcohol consumption	Limit consumption to ≤2 drinks (1 oz or 30 mL ethanol; eg, 24 oz beer, 10 oz wine, or 3 oz 80-proof whiskey) per day in most men and to ≤1 drink per day in women and lighter-weight persons	2–4 mmHg

[a]For overall cardiovascular risk reduction, stop smoking.
[b]The effects of implementing these modifications are dose- and time-dependent, and could be greater for some individuals.
BMI, body mass index; DASH, dietary approaches to stop hypertension; SBP, systolic blood pressure.
Data from *Seventh Report of the Joint National Committee on Prevention, Detection, Evaluation, and Treatment of High Blood Pressure.* NIH Publication 03-5233. US Department of Health and Human Services, 2003.

during a routine visit to a medical provider or after the patient has had a stroke or MI.

For proper measurement of blood pressure, the patient should be seated in a chair with the back supported and the arm bared and supported at heart level. Caffeine and tobacco should be avoided in the 30 minutes preceding measurement, and measurement should begin after 5 minutes of rest. The cuff size should be appropriate for the patient's arm, defined by a cuff bladder that encircles 80% of the arm. It is important that the diagnosis be made after the elevation of blood pressure is documented with three separate readings, on three different occasions, unless the elevation is severe or is associated with symptoms requiring immediate attention (hypertensive urgency or emergency). Transient elevation of blood pressure secondary to pain or anxiety, as experienced by some patients when they enter a physician's office ("white coat syndrome"), does not require treatment. In cases in which the diagnosis is in question, properly taken home blood pressure measurements can be useful.

2. Classification of blood pressure—A goal of JNC VII was to simplify blood pressure classification when making the diagnosis of hypertension (see Table 35-1). A new category, designated *prehypertension*, was added, and stages 2 and 3 from JNC VI were combined to form a single category (stage 2). These classifications are based on the average of two or more provider-obtained blood pressure measurements from a seated patient.

2. Self-monitoring—Patients should be encouraged to self-monitor their blood pressure at home. Many easy-to-use blood pressure monitors are commercially available at reasonable cost for use at home. Validated electronic devices are recommended, and independent reviews of available devices, such as that published by Consumer Reports, are available to assist the consumer. These devices should be periodically checked for accuracy. Self-measurement can be helpful, not only in establishing the diagnosis of hypertension but also in assessing response to medical therapy, and in encouraging patient compliance with therapy by providing regular feedback on therapy response.

B. Evaluation

Patients with documented hypertension must undergo a thorough evaluation that includes objectives advanced by JNC VII: assessment of lifestyle and identification of cardiovascular risk factors, identification of comorbidities that would guide therapy, and surveillance for identifiable causes of high blood pressure, and to establish whether the patient already manifests evidence of target end-organ damage.

1. History—A thorough history should be obtained. Any prior history of hypertension should be elicited, as well as response and side effects to any previous hypertension therapy. It is important to inquire about any history or symptoms suggestive of coronary artery disease or other significant comorbidities, including diabetes mellitus, heart failure, dyslipidemia, renal disease, and peripheral vascular disease. The family history should also be reviewed, with special attention to the presence/absence of hypertension, premature coronary artery disease, diabetes, renal disease, dyslipidemia, or stroke. Use of tobacco, alcohol, or illicit drugs should be documented, as well as dietary intake of sodium, saturated fat, and caffeine. Recent changes in weight and exercise level should be queried. Current medications used by the patient should be reviewed, including OTC medications, supplements, and herbal formulations.

2. Physical examination—The initial physical examination should be comprehensive, with careful attention to the areas outlined in **Table 35-3**.

C. Laboratory and Diagnostic Studies

The Joint National Committee (JNC VII) specifically recommends that the following tests be performed: electrocardiogram (ECG), urinalysis, fasting blood glucose level, potassium level, creatinine level, calcium level, and fasting

Table 35-3. Physical examination: hypertension.

Component of Examination	Assessment Focus
General	Baseline height, weight, and waist circumference Upper and lower extremity blood pressure measurement to assess for coarctation of the aorta Features of Cushing syndrome
Eyes	Funduscopic examination for signs of hypertensive retinopathy (eg, arteriolar narrowing, focal arteriolar constriction, atrioventricular nicking, hemorrhages, exudates)
Neck	Carotid bruits Neck vein distention or thyroid gland enlargement
Heart	Abnormalities in rate, rhythm, murmurs, or extra heart sounds
Lungs	Rales, rhonchi, or wheezes
Abdomen	Abdominal bruits suggestive of renal artery stenosis Enlargement of kidneys (mass) or aortic pulsation suggesting aneurysm
Extremities	Diminished or absent peripheral arterial pulsations Edema Signs of vascular compromise
Neurologic	Neurologic deficits

lipid panel. Urinalysis should be assessed for evidence of hematuria, proteinuria, or casts suggestive of intrinsic renal disease. The complete blood count is helpful to rule out anemia or polycythemia. Potassium levels help assess for hyperaldosteronism, and creatinine levels reflect renal function. The fasting blood glucose level is used to asses for diabetes mellitus, and the lipid profile is an indicator of cardiovascular risk. Further testing is warranted if blood pressure control is not achieved. Additional tests to consider include hemoglobin A_{1C}, thyroid-stimulating hormone, urine microalbumin, creatinine clearance, and 24-hour urine for protein. Echocardiograms and chest x-rays are not routinely recommended for evaluation of hypertensive patients. In certain cases, however, an echocardiogram may prove useful in guiding therapy when baseline abnormalities are found on the ECG (eg, left ventricular hypertrophy or signs of previous silent MI). A chest radiograph may be useful if there are abnormal findings on physical examination. Tests that evaluate for rare causes of hypertension, such as renal artery stenosis (renal ultrasound) or pheochromocytoma (24-hour urine for catecholamines), should be ordered only in patients whose history and physical examination findings raise suspicion.

▶ **Treatment**

A. Cardiovascular Risk Stratification

In treating hypertension, the public health goal is reduction of cardiovascular and renal morbidity and mortality. Hypertension is clearly important, but it is not the only risk factor. JNC VII defines specific components of cardiovascular risk and recommends evaluation of patients for evidence of target organ damage in performing risk stratification and in considering recommendations for therapy (**Table 35-4**).

The JNC VII guidelines include an algorithm for use when considering initial therapy for patients with hypertension (**Figure 35-1**). It is recognized that most patients, especially those aged ≥50 years, will reach their diastolic blood pressure goal once the systolic blood pressure goal is reached. Lifestyle modification may be used initially if blood pressure is in the prehypertensive range (<140/90 mmHg). When no risk factors, no target organ damage, and no evidence of cardiovascular disease are identified in a patient, the target blood pressure for treatment is <140/90 mmHg. Recent data regarding blood pressure control in patients with mild hypertension (<150/90 mmHg) and no preexisting cardiovascular disease are unproven. Blood pressure control in the elderly has also sparked controversy. If diabetes mellitus or renal disease is present, the blood pressure target for treatment is <130/80 mmHg.

When lifestyle modification is used as initial therapy but successful control is not achieved, drug therapy should be initiated (see section on pharmacotherapy, later). Further reassessments should consider optimization or titration of

Table 35-4. Components of cardiovascular risk stratification in patients with hypertension.

Major risk factors
  Hypertension[a]
  Age (>55 years for men, 65 years for women)[b]
  Diabetes mellitus[a]
  Elevated LDL (or total) cholesterol, or low HDL cholesterol[a]
  Estimated GFR <60 mL/min
  Family history of premature CVD (men aged <55 years or women aged <65 years)
  Microalbuminuria
  Obesity[a] (BMI ≥30 kg/m^2)
  Physical inactivity
  Tobacco usage, particularly cigarettes
Target organ damage
  Heart
    Left ventricular hypertrophy
    Angina or prior myocardial infarction
    Prior coronary revascularization
    Heart failure
  Brain
    Stroke or transient ischemic attack
    Dementia
  Chronic kidney disease
  Peripheral arterial disease
  Retinopathy

[a]Components of the metabolic syndrome. Reduced HDL, elevated triglycerides, and abdominal obesity also are components of the metabolic syndrome.
[b]Increased risk begins at ~55 and 65 years of age for men and women, respectively. Adult Treatment Panel III used earlier age cut-off points to suggest the need for earlier action
BMI, body mass index; CVD, cardiovascular disease; GFR, glomerular filtration rate; HDL, high-density lipoprotein; LDL, low-density lipoprotein.
Data from *Seventh Report of the Joint National Committee on Prevention, Detection, Evaluation, and Treatment of High Blood Pressure.* NIH Publication 03-5233. US Department of Health and Human Services, 2003.

the drug regimen in terms of dosage or combinations, as well as reinforcing adherence to lifestyle modification. Follow-up visits should occur at approximately monthly intervals until the blood pressure goal is reached, or more frequently in patients with significant comorbidities. Once patients reach their goal, 3–6-month intervals for visits are appropriate.

If the blood pressure goal is not achieved with triple-drug therapy (ie, agents from different classes, including a diuretic), further investigation must ensue. A lack of motivation on the patient's part can undo the most effective regimen; however, this outcome can be minimized through positive experiences with the clinician to address misunderstandings about the condition and treatment. Poor response to therapy by patients receiving a triple regimen of

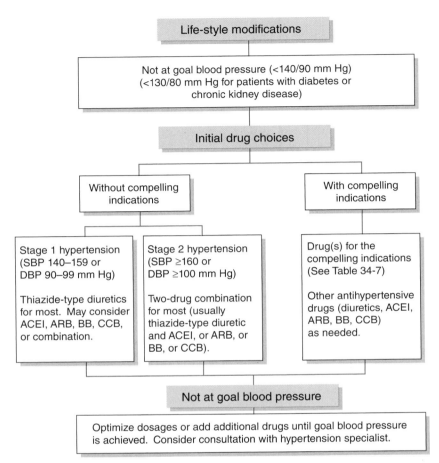

▲ **Figure 35-1.** Algorithm for treatment of hypertension (ACE, angiotensin-converting enzyme; ARB, angiotensin II receptor blocker; BB, β-blocker; CCB, calcium channel blocker; DBP, diastolic blood pressure; SBP, systolic blood pressure). (From the *Seventh Report of the Joint National Committee on Prevention, Detection, Evaluation, and Treatment of High Blood Pressure.* NIH Publication 03-5233. US Department of Health and Human Services, 2003.)

antihypertensive drugs should also prompt consideration of referral to a hypertension specialist for evaluation and recommendations concerning treatment.

B. Lifestyle Modification

The Joint National Committee (JNC VII) cites the adoption of lifestyle modification as critical, not only for the prevention of hypertension but also in the treatment thereof. Major recommendations include encouraging the overweight patient to lose weight. Even small amounts of weight loss [10 lb (4.5 kg)] can improve blood pressure control and reduce cardiovascular risk. Weight loss can be facilitated through dietary changes and increased exercise. Patients should be encouraged to set their weekly aerobic exercise goal of ≥150 minutes of moderate intensity physical activity, or 75 minutes of vigorous intensity as outlined by *Healthy People 2020*. Adoption of the *dietary approaches to stop hypertension* (DASH) eating plan is also recommended. This plan promotes potassium and calcium intake, reduced sodium and fat intake, exercise, and moderation of alcohol consumption. The blood pressure reduction gained is roughly equivalent to that of single-drug therapy. However, patients taking angiotensin-converting enzyme inhibitors (ACEIs) or angiotensin II receptor blockers (ARBs) should be cautioned regarding potassium intake, because these medications can result in potassium retention. Any use of tobacco should be discouraged, and patients currently using tobacco should be counseled to quit, as this may help lower blood pressure.

C. Pharmacotherapy

Many medications are available to treat hypertension. Medication should be initiated at a low dose and titrated slowly to achieve desired blood pressure control. When available, formulations available in once-daily dosing are preferred because of increased patient compliance. Also useful are the many combination formulations now available that incorporate two different classes of drugs. Good clinical outcomes and trial data exist demonstrating reduction in complications of hypertension with blood pressure lowering by β-blockers, calcium channel blockers, thiazide diuretics, ACE inhibitors, and angiotensin II blockers. When selecting a medication, side effect profile and patient comorbidities should help guide choice as well as the possible out-of-pocket cost that the patient may have to incur as a result of varying economic status and insurance coverage, depending on the patient population being treated (please refer to **Table 35-5** for price comparisons).

Table 35-5. Pricing chart of drugs.

Class	Drug	Price[a]
Diuretic (thiazide)	Chlorthalidone	$$
	HCTZ	$
	Indapamide	$
	Metolazone	$$
Diuretic (loop)	Furosemide	$
	Torsemide	$
	Bumetanide	$
Diuretic (potassium-sparing) ACEI	Triamterene	$$
	Amiloride	$$
	Ramipril	$$
	Captopril	$
	Lisinopril	$
	Enalapril	$
	Benazepril	$
	Fosinopril	$$
	Quinopril	$
ARB	Candesartan	$$
	Olmesartan	$$
	Irbesartan	$$$
	Losartan	$$$
	Telmisartan	$$$
	Valsartan	$$$
β-Blocker	Atenolol	$
	Labetalol	$$
	Propranolol	$
	Metoprolol	$
	Timolol	$$
α_2-Agonist (central)	Clonidine	$
	Methyldopa	$

Table 35-5. Pricing chart of drugs. (*Continued*)

Class	Drug	Price[a]
α_1 - Blocker (peripheral)	Doxazosin	$
	Prazosin	$
	Terazosin	$
CCB (dihydropyridine)	Nifedipine	$$
	Felodipine	$$
	Amlodipine	$
	Isradipine	$$$
	Nisoldipine	$$$$
CCB (nondihydropyridine)	Verapamil	$
	Diltiazem	$
Aldosterone antagonist	Spironolactone	$
	Eplenerone	$$$
Renin inhibitor	Aliskiren	$$$
Vasodilator	Hydralazine	$
	Minoxidil	$$
Combination[b]		

[a]Values based on estimates from Epocrates and are only for a brief comparison of common generic medicines used within separate classes. They are intended to provide a crude idea of price when prescribing various medications and are in no way a reflection of efficacy, side effect profile, or current treatment recommendations. Key: $, <$30/90–100 tablets; $$, $30–$70/90–100 tablets; $$$, $70–$200/90–100 tablets; $$$$, >$200/90–100 tablets.
[b]Combination tablets exist between most of the classes listed above, vary in pricing, and offer convenience for patients on multiple medications. They also may enhance compliance and prevent medication errors, especially in the elderly and in patients with polypharmacy.

Favorable effects of selective antihypertensive agents may increase interest in their use. Thiazide diuretics slow demineralization in osteoporosis. β-Blockers are useful for atrial arrhythmias and fibrillation, migraine headache prophylaxis, thyrotoxicosis, and essential tremor. Calcium channel blockers are useful in Raynaud syndrome and some arrhythmias, and α-blockers are helpful in prostatism.

Unfavorable effects include cautions for the use of thiazide diuretics in patients with gout or a history of hyponatremia. β-Blockers should be avoided in patients with asthma or with second- or third-degree heath block. ACE inhibitors and ARBs have the potential to cause birth defects and thus should be avoided in women likely to become pregnant and discontinued in those who do become pregnant. Hyperkalemia may be caused by aldosterone antagonists and potassium-sparing diuretics.

Ethnic differences have been noted in the blood pressure response to monotherapy. African Americans, who have increased prevalence and severity of hypertension, have demonstrated blunted response to monotherapy, such as β-blockers and ACE inhibitors versus diuretics or calcium channel blockers. This effect is eliminated by combination therapy.

Given the large number of major trials with conflicting data, there is no overall consensus for initial single-drug therapy, and treatment decisions should be individually based. In fact, according to the American Heart Association and the 2010 European Society of Hypertension/European Society of Cardiology guidelines on the management of hypertension, the amount of blood pressure reduction is more important than the choice of antihypertensive drug in the appropriate patient population. A number of recent trials (CAPPP, STOP-Hypertension-2, NORDIL, CAMELOT, UKPDS, INSIGHT) also found little to no difference in outcomes between older and newer antihypertensive drugs. Typically, monotherapy for hypertension will consist of an ACE inhibitor/ARB, calcium channel blocker, or thiazide diuretic.

If a single drug does not achieve control, a second drug from a different class should be added. If the blood pressure remains >20/10 mmHg above goal or initially presents as >20/10 mmHg above goal, two-drug therapy should be considered. Effective and timely control for most patients will be accomplished with at least two antihypertensive medications. The clinician should advise patients—especially

those who are diabetic, have autonomic dysfunction, or are elderly—of the risk for orthostatic hypotension.

The recommendations that follow are summarized in **Table 35-6** and are based on a number of major trials, including JNC VII and the Avoiding Cardiovascular Events in Combination Therapy with Systolic Hypertension (ACCOMPLISH) trial.

1. ACE inhibitors—The ACE inhibitors stimulate vasodilation by blocking the renin-angiotensin-aldosterone system and inhibiting degradation of bradykinin. In several randomized, controlled clinical trials, these agents have been shown to reduce cardiovascular events in hypertensive patients (CAPPP trial), including particular subgroups [high-risk patients aged >55 years (HOPE study), older men (ANBP study), and diabetic patients (FACET and ACAPP trials)]. Compelling indications exist for ACE inhibitor use in patients with diabetes mellitus, congestive heart failure, and chronic kidney disease, and in patients who have had a MI with systolic dysfunction. ACE inhibitors have been shown to reduce progression of renal disease in African Americans (AASK trial) and diabetics but may increase the risk of stroke when used as monotherapy in African Americans (ALLHAT trial). These agents have also been shown to be more effective in promoting regression of left ventricular hypertrophy than diuretics, β-blockers, or calcium

Table 35-6. Clinical trial guideline basis for compelling indications for individual drug classes.

Compelling Indication[a]	Recommended Drugs						Clinical Trial Basis[b]
	D	BB	ACEI	ARB	CCB	Aldo ANT	
Heart failure	•	•	•	•		•	ACC/AHA Heart Failure Guideline, MERIT-HF, COPERNICUS, CIBIS, SOLVD, AIRE, TRACE, ValHEFT, RALES, ACCOMPLISH
Post-MI		•	•			•	ACC/AHA Post-MI Guideline, BHAT, SAVE, Capricorn, EPHESUS
High coronary disease risk	•	•	•		•		ALLHAT, HOPE, ANBP2, LIFE, CONVINCE, ACCOMPLISH
Diabetes mellitus	•	•	•	•	•		NKF-ADA Guideline, UKPDS, ALLHAT, ACCOMPLISH
Chronic kidney disease			•	•			NKF Guideline, Captopril Trial, RENAAL, IDNT, REIN, AASK
Recurrent stroke prevention	•		•				PROGRESS

ACEI, angiotensin-converting enzyme inhibitor; Aldo ANT, aldosterone antagonist; ARB, angiotensin II receptor blocker; CCB, calcium channel blocker; D, diuretic; BB, β-blocker.
[a]Compelling indications for antihypertensive drugs are based on benefits from outcome studies or existing clinical guidelines; the compelling indication is managed in parallel with the blood pressure.
[b]Conditions for which clinical trials demonstrate benefit of specific classes of antihypertensive drugs.
Data from *Seventh Report of the Joint National Committee on Prevention, Detection, Evaluation, and Treatment of High Blood Pressure.* NIH Publication No. 03-5233. US Department of Health and Human Services, 2003.

channel blockers. Left ventricular hypertrophy is considered one of the best predictors of cardiovascular events in patients with hypertension.

Angiotensin-converting enzyme inhibitors have relatively few side effects and are well tolerated by most patients. A dry cough may be reported in as many as 25% of patients. Because hyperkalemia may occur, particularly in patients who are also receiving potassium-sparing diuretics, periodic monitoring of electrolytes and serum creatinine should be performed.

Angiotensin-converting enzyme inhibitors must be used cautiously in patients with known renovascular disease and, when used, may need dose adjustment because of reduced drug clearance. When creatinine elevations exceed 30% above baseline, temporary cessation or reduction of dose is warranted. These agents should be used with extreme caution, if at all, in patients whose serum creatinine level exceeds 3.0 mg/mL. Fosinopril is a good option in patients with renovascular disease as it is the only ACE inhibitor that is excreted by both the liver and the kidney.

However, ACE inhibitors should not be used in patients with bilateral renal artery stenosis. Angioedema may occur with these agents, and this complication is 2–4 times more frequent in African Americans.

2. Calcium channel blockers—There are two classes of calcium channel blockers: (1) the dihydropryidine calcium channel blockers, which vasodilate (nifedipine, amlodipine, felodipine), and (2) the rate-lowering calcium channel blockers (verapamil, diltiazem). They have relatively few side effects but may cause headache, nausea, rash, or flushing in some patients. Calcium channel blockers are not recommended as first-line therapy by JNC VII, although the guidelines suggest use of long-acting dihydropyridine calcium channel blockers as an alternative to β-blockers in patients with stable angina in ischemic heart disease; and in diabetics, nondihydropyridines, with their negative inotropic and chronotropic actions, have a beneficial role in atrial fibrillation and supraventricular tachyarrhythmias. Data for the use of calcium channel blockers in the elderly are mixed. The Systolic Hypertension in Europe (SYSEUR) trial, released in 1997, randomized 5000 elderly patients with isolated systolic hypertension to treatment with either placebo or the long-acting dihydropyridine calcium channel blocker nitrendipine. In 2 years of follow-up there was significant reduction in stroke and cardiovascular events. Similar benefits were reported in elderly patients with hypertension and diabetes using nitrendipine, although the findings were not superior to other antihypertensive agents. In African Americans, response to monotherapy using β-blockers, ACE inhibitors, and ARBs in blunted. This is not the case when using calcium channel blockers or diuretics. Use of combination regimens with a diuretic eliminates these differential responses.

The ACCOMPLISH trial combined benazepril with amlodipine and showed a substantial advantage over combination therapy consisting of benazepril with hydrochlorothiazide, thereby making amlodipine a highly recommended first-line add-on therapy to ACE inhibitors for combination therapy as well as making amlodipine a viable first-line monotherapy option. The ASCOT trial found a decrease in cardiovascular disease and death with amlodipine (calcium channel blocker) versus atenolol (β-blocker). The VALUE trial comparing amlodipine versus valsartan (ARB) found better outcomes with blood pressure control but no difference in rates of cardiovascular events.

3. Diuretics—JNC VII recommends initially treating uncomplicated hypertension with diuretics, in the absence of a compelling reason to use another agent. This strong recommendation is based on the many randomized controlled trials that have demonstrated a superior response for diuretics in reduction of morbidity—including stroke, coronary artery disease, and congestive heart failure—and total mortality. ALLHAT (Antihypertensive and Lipid-Lowering treatment to prevent Heart Attack Trial) was one of the largest such trials. It compared diuretics, calcium channel blockers, and ACE inhibitors as initial therapies in a population with a large number of African American participants. The authors concluded that regardless of age, sex, or race, the use of diuretics in hypertensive, high-cardiovascular-risk patients was associated with similar risk of cardiovascular events equivalent to that of calcium channel blockers and ACE inhibitors, but was superior in performance in patients with underlying heart conditions including heart failure. ACCOMPLISH compared combination therapy in patients at high risk for cardiovascular events with benazepril plus either amlodipine or hydrochlorothiazide and was terminated early because of a substantial disadvantage in combination therapy with hydrochlorothiazide. Because of this large, well-designed study along with a number of other well-designed studies showing similar efficacy across different antihypertensive classes, initial monotherapy with a specific agent, specifically a diuretic, became controversial and has led to a difference in opinion in regards to the use of a specific agent for monotherapy.

Diuretics should be used cautiously in patients with gout, as worsening hyperuricemia can result. They may also cause muscle cramps or impotence in some individuals. Diuretics may be effective at lower doses in patients with dyslipidemia and diabetes mellitus, but patients placed on higher doses must be observed closely for worsening hyperglycemia or hyperlipidema. The thiazide diuretics are most commonly used in the treatment of hypertension, because loop diuretics are more likely to lead to electrolyte abnormalities such as hypokalemia and to have a shorter duration of action. However, loop diuretics can sometimes be useful in the treatment of hypertension in patients with chronic renal disease and a serum creatinine level of >2.5 mg/dL. The loop diuretics have found most utility in the treatment of congestive heart failure.

ALLHAT Officers Coordinating for the ALLHAT Collaborative Research Group. Major outcomes in high-risk hypertensive patients randomized to angiotensin-converting enzyme inhibitor or calcium channel blocker vs diuretic: the Antihypertensive and Lipid-Lowering treatment to prevent Heart Attack Trial (ALLHAT). *JAMA.* 2002;288:2981. [PMID: 12479763]

Jamerson K, Weber MA, Bakris GL, et al. Benazepril plus amlodipine or hydrochlorothiazide for hypertension in high-risk patients: the Avoiding Cardiovascular Events in Combination Therapy with Systolic Hypertension (ACCOMPLISH) trial. *N Engl J Med.* 2008;359(23):2417. [PMID: 19052124]

4. β-blockers—Whether used as first-line agents in the case of compelling indications or in a drug therapy combination, β-blockers have favorable effects on migraine headache, hyperthyroidism, and anxiety. Patients should be informed that β-blockers may cause sexual dysfunction. These agents should be used with caution, if at all, in patients with a history of depression, asthma or reactive airway disease, second- or third-degree heart block, or peripheral vascular disease. In patients with mild to moderate reactive airway disease, β-blockers do not produce adverse effects in the short term. The United Kingdom Prospective Diabetes Study (UKPDS) demonstrated that β-blockers can be used safely and effectively for type 2 diabetes mellitus, although there is concern that hypoglycemic episodes might be masked. Any patient with diabetes mellitus placed on a β-blocker should, therefore, be carefully monitored. Although previously not recommended, patients with congestive heart failure are now being successfully treated with β-blockers lacking intrinsic sympathomimetic activity, including two of the most studied agents, carvedilol and metoprolol. Careful use of these agents has shown promise in reducing mortality and improving ejection fraction in patients with New York Heart Association class II or III congestive heart failure.

5. Angiotensin II receptor blockers (ARBs)—ARBs selectively block angiotensin II activation of AT1 receptors, which are responsible for mediating vasoconstriction, salt and water retention, and central and sympathetic activation, among others. Angiotensin II is still able to activate AT_2-blockers, facilitating vasodilation and production of bradykinin, which aids in reduction of blood pressure. This class of medication is well tolerated and has a favorable side effect profile. ARBs are a good alternative for patients who cannot tolerate ACEI-associated cough, but should be avoided in patients with ACEI-associated angioedema. JNC VII does not recommend that ARBs be used for initial therapy in treatment of hypertension; however, compelling indications for use include heart failure, diabetes mellitus, and chronic kidney disease. ARBs have been shown to be more effective than β-blockers in preventing cardiovascular events in hypertensive patients with left ventricular hypertrophy, both with and without diabetes (LIFE trial). Renal protective effects of ARBs have been shown clinically to reduce the progression of nephropathy in diabetic hypertensive patients (RENAAL trial) and to reduce the incidence of new-onset diabetes (VALUE trial). Recently, it has been demonstrated that ARBs reduce subsequent events in patients with acute ischemic stroke (ACCESS study).

6. Other drug—Other drugs, including α_2-agonists and direct vasodilators, are used to treat hypertension, although less commonly than the other classes of drugs. They are typically used as second- or third-line agents because of increased side effects. The ALLHAT trial suggested that α_2-agonists and direct vasodilators such as doxazosin may increase the risk of stroke and congestive heart failure when used in the treatment of hypertension, resulting in discontinuation of that arm of the trial. Eplenerone (Inspra), a selective aldosterone receptor antagonist, was recently approved for the treatment of hypertension. Interest is focused on its use in patients with congestive heart failure or in combination with other antihypertensives; however, data on morbidity and mortality are not yet available. Aliskiren, a renin inhibitor, works by blinding renin to block the conversion of angiotensinogen to angiotensin I, the rate-limiting step of the renin-angiotensin-aldosterone system (RAAS). It is the only renin inhibitor available on the market and is typically used in patients who do not tolerate ACE inhibitors or ARBs. They can also be used in conjunction with these medications, although evidence regarding safety in patients with diabetes and renal disease is worrisome. For this reason, the FDA suggests avoiding multiple RAAS agents in the setting of diabetes or kidney insufficiency. A combination tablet with hydrochlorothiazide is approved and currently in use.

7. Combination therapy—It is important to also consider the recent developments in combination therapy that allow patients who are on a multidrug regiment to take fewer pills overall. This has been done with various antihypertensive classes such as combining an ACEI and a calcium-channel blocker (ACCOMPLISH). Many patients will eventually require a multidrug regiment and by ingestion of fewer pills, compliance can be improved. Studies have examined the value in combining medications especially in the elderly, who often take many pills per day. One study showed favorable outcomes with an ACEI-diuretic combination in the elderly over the course of 1 year. The drug was well tolerated, and compliance was improved.

These medications tend to be more expensive for patients, so it is important to weigh cost and compliance issues to maximize the likelihood of successful treatment. This is where the family physician's role is crucial to the overall care of the patient. More research still needs to be conducted to see the long-term efficacy of various combination therapies.

D. Special Considerations

The drug selections noted in Table 35-6 are based on favorable outcome data from clinical trials and should be considered in light of current medications, tolerability, and blood pressure target goal.

1. Ischemic heart disease—β-Blockers are the first-line drug for patients with stable angina; alternatively, long-acting calcium channel blockers may be considered. ACE inhibitors should be added in patients with acute coronary syndromes, and administration of aldosterone antagonists post-MI should be considered.

2. Heart failure—ACE inhibitors and β-blockers are recommended for asymptomatic patients with ventricular dysfunction. Symptomatic or end-stage heart disease should be treated with ACE inhibitors, β-blockers, ARBs, aldosterone blockers, and loop diuretics.

3. Diabetes mellitus—All classes of antihypertensive medications have proved beneficial in reducing the incidence of cardiovascular disease and stroke in diabetic patients. The progression of diabetic nephropathy is reduced with ACE inhibitors or ARBs.

4. Chronic kidney disease—Goals for these patients include slowing deterioration of renal function and preventing cardiovascular disease. Typically a combination of three drugs is needed to accomplish aggressive blood pressure management. ACE inhibitors and ARBs should be used and may be continued in patients with an increase in serum creatinine clearance of 35% above baselines, unless hyperkalemia develops. Increasing doses of loop diuretics are usually needed once the creatinine level reaches 2.5–3.0 mg/dL.

5. Cerebrovascular disease—The combination of an ACE inhibitor and thiazide diuretic has been shown to lower recurrent stroke rates.

6. Pregnancy—Chronic hypertension occurs in ≤5% of pregnant women. It may result in perinatal morbidity and mortality for both mother and baby. It is important to differentiate chronic hypertension from other pregnancy-related conditions, including pregnancy-induced hypertension (PIH) and preeclampsia because the management and treatments differ. According to the American College of Obstetrics and Gynecology (ACOG), *chronic* hypertension in pregnancy is defined as the use of antihypertensive medication before pregnancy, onset of elevated blood pressures prior to gestation week 20, or the persistence of high blood pressure beyond the "usual" postpartum period. *Mild* hypertension in considered SBP ≥140 mmHg and/or DBP >90 mmHg. *Severe* is considered SBP greater than, or equal to, 180 mmHg, and DBP above 110 mm Hg. Women with mild hypertension who are doing well generally do not need medication. Current evidence has yet to show whether antihypertensive therapy at this level improves perinatal outcomes. Studies have shown that outcomes are improved and thus medications are indicated when necessary to keep blood pressure under 160/110 mmHg.

Classically, methyldopa and labetalol have been used to control severe hypertension in pregnancy with demonstrated improvement in outcomes. There is little difference in outcome when comparing these medications. The use of β-blockers has been associated with a higher rate of babies that are small for gestational age. Calcium channel blockers, such as nifedipine, have proved neither beneficial nor detrimental to the health of either mother or baby in the long term. According to the National High Blood Pressure Education Program Working Group on High Blood Pressure in Pregnancy, diuretics can potentiate the positive effects of other antihypertensives and are not contraindicated unless uteroplacental perfusion is already present as a result of another issue such as preeclampsia or intrauterine growth restriction (IUGR). ACE inhibitors are considered category D. This class is contraindicated in the second and third trimesters because of an association with teratogenic effects, including severely underdeveloped clavarial bone, renal failure, oligohydramnios, anuria, renal dysgenesis, and others, including death.

7. Children and adolescents—Although the true incidence and prevalence of hypertension in children and adolescents is unknown, there is a growing concern for identifying, diagnosing, and treating hypertension in this population given the growing amount of evidence showing an early development of cardiovascular disease within this population. In this population, hypertension diagnosis is based on percentiles for gender, age, and height. Patients who are below the 90th percentile of systolic and diastolic blood pressure are considered in the normal range, patients between the 90th and 95th percentiles or at >120/80 mmHg are considered prehypertensive, those in the 95th–99th percentiles plus 5 mmHg are considered stage I, and those who are above the 99th percentile plus 5 mmHg are stage II. Among children who are obese, ≤30% will have hypertension. Given that hypertension in this population is uncommon, secondary causes of hypertension should be higher on the differential versus the adult population when performing a diagnostic workup on a child or adolescent with hypertension. These children should be tested for CBC, BUN and creatinine levels, urinalysis, and renal ultrasound within their initial hypertension workup. Additionally, children and adolescents with hypertension should also be screened for hyperlipidemia and diabetes mellitus. Lifestyle modifications in this population are first-line treatment for hypertension. However, in children and adolescents with symptomatic hypertension, secondary hypertension, evidence of end-organ damage, diabetes, or persistent hypertension despite nonpharmacological measures, antihypertensive medication should be initiated. Goals for treatment vary. In children with primary, uncomplicated hypertension, goal blood pressure is below the 95th percentile. In children with chronic renal disease, diabetes, or evidence of target organ damage, the blood pressure goal is below the 90th percentile. There is currently no consensus for a specific initial drug of choice for monotherapy. Initial therapy should factor in the child's concurrent medical conditions as most are well tolerated and achieve similar goals. Titration and addition of additional agents are similar to that of adults and typically dosed according to the child's weight. Pregnancy status, testing, and counseling in adolescent females should also be factored in when initiating pharmacotherapy (see section on pharmacotherapy in pregnancy, above).

Riley M, Bluhm B. High blood pressure in children and adolescents. *Am Fam Physician.* 2012;85(7):693–700.

E. Hypertensive Urgency and Emergency

Hypertensive urgencies are situations in which the blood pressure must be lowered within several hours, because of either (1) an asymptomatic, severely elevated blood pressure (>200/130 mmHg) or (2) a moderately elevated blood pressure (> 200/120 mmHg) with associated symptoms, including angina, headache, and congestive heart failure. When such symptoms are present, even lower blood pressures may warrant more urgent treatment. Oral therapy can often be utilized with good response.

Hypertensive emergencies require treatment of elevated blood pressures within 1 hour to avoid significant morbidity and mortality. The symptomatology with which the patient presents warrants the immediate attention, not the actual blood pressure value itself. Such patients show evidence of end-organ damage from the elevated blood pressure, including encephalopathy (headache, irritability, confusion, coma), renal failure, pulmonary edema, unstable angina, MI, aortic dissection, and intracranial hemorrhage. Hypertensive emergency is an indication for hospital admission, and such patients typically require intravenous therapy with antihypertensives.

The goal of therapy is reduction of systolic pressure by 20–40 mmHg and diastolic pressure by 10–20 mmHg. The initial blood pressure target is a systolic blood pressure in the range of 180–200 mmHg and a diastolic blood pressure in the range of 110–120 mmHg. Blood pressure should not be lowered too quickly, because doing so can result in hypoperfusion of the brain and myocardium. Once initial treatment goals are achieved, blood pressure can subsequently be reduced gradually to more appropriate levels.

Nitroprusside is the preferred agent in emergencies such as hypertensive encephalopathy, because the infusion can be titrated easily to effect. When myocardial ischemia is present, intravenous nitroglycerin or intravenous β-blockers such as labetalol or esmolol are preferred. Once blood pressure has been brought under control using intravenous therapy, oral agents should be initiated slowly as intravenous therapy is gradually withdrawn. Whether a patient is being treated for hypertensive urgency, hypertensive emergency, or benign hypertension, long-term therapy and lifestyle modification are essential. Patients must receive regular follow-up and meet the treatment goals established by JNC VII to prevent unnecessary morbidity and mortality.

Diabetes Mellitus

36

Belinda Vail, MD, MS, FAAFP

ESSENTIALS OF DIAGNOSIS

▶ Random plasma glucose ≥200 mg/dL with polydipsia, polyuria, polyphagia, and/or weight loss.

▶ Fasting plasma glucose ≥126 mg/dL (require confirmatory test).

▶ Two-hour oral glucose tolerance test ≥200 mg/dL after a 75-g glucose load (require confirmatory test).

▶ A1C ≥ 6.5% [by labwork using a method that is certified by the National Glycohemoglobin Standardization Program (NGSP) and standardized to the DCCT assay] (require confirmatory test).

General Considerations

The age-adjusted prevalence of diabetes has doubled in the United States since the late 1990s. The adoption of a Western diet and the resulting worldwide explosion of obesity have led to an epidemic of diabetes with >347 million people worldwide afflicted. It is a major cause of blindness, renal failure, lower extremity amputations, cardiovascular disease, and congenital malformations. Rates are disproportionately high in African Americans, Native Americans, Pacific Islanders, Hispanics, and Asians. With 90% of patients receiving their care from primary care physicians, diabetes is the epitome of a chronic disease requiring a multidisciplinary management approach.

Centers for Disease Control diabetes fact sheet: http://www.cdc .gov/diabetes/pubs/factsheet11.htm.
World Health Organization diabetes fact sheet: http://www.who .int/mediacentre/factsheets/fs312/en/.

Pathogenesis

Type 1 diabetes is the result of an autoimmune destruction of the pancreatic β cells with an inability of the body to produce insulin. Type 2 diabetes develops from an increasing cellular resistance to insulin; a process accelerated by obesity and inactivity, and is becoming increasingly common in adolescents and children. A small percentage of patients will develop a more insidious onset of autoimmune diabetes, latent autoimmune diabetes of adulthood (LADA), that may respond for a short period of time to oral medications.

Prevention

Patients with metabolic syndrome or a hemoglobin A_{1c} (HbA$_{1c}$) of 5.7–6.4% should be targeted for intensive lifestyle intervention. Conversion to a Mediterranean style diet, a reduction in screen time, and at least 150 minutes of moderate intensity exercise weekly, leading to weight loss as well as smoking cessation, have been shown to delay the onset of diabetes more effectively than medications. In women, exercise (of at least moderate intensity) decreases the risk of developing type 2 diabetes, and more exercise creates a greater risk reduction. Motivation for lifestyle change is difficult, but more cost-effective and safer medications, and these changes will also improve blood pressure and lipids, leading to greater reductions in cardiovascular risk.

Medications that may also slow progression to diabetes include metformin (cheapest and fewest side effects), acarbose, and a thiazolidinedione. Tight control of hyperglycemia and blood pressure reduce the complications of diabetes, and a sustained reduction in A_{1c} is associated with significant cost savings within 1–2 years.

Burnet DL, et al. Can diabetes prevention programs be translated effectively into Section of General Internal Medicine, Department of Medicine. Diabetes Research and Training Center, The University of Chicago, Chicago, IL, USA real-world settings and still deliver improved outcomes? A synthesis of evidence. *Diabet Med.* 2013; 30(1):3-15. [PMID: PMC3555428]

Screening

Fasting glucose is the preferred screening method, although a random glucose or A_{1c} is acceptable. The American

Diabetes Association (ADA) recommends universal screening every 3 years beginning at age 45 or any adults with a BMI of ≥25 kg/m² and one of the following:

- Physical inactivity
- First-degree relative with diabetes
- High-risk race/ethnicity (Native Americans, African Americans, Asians, Hispanics, or Pacific Islanders)
- Previous gestational diabetes or a baby weighing >9 lb
- Hypertension (≥140/90 mmHg)
- HDL cholesterol <35 mg/dL and/or triglycerides >250 mg/dL
- Polycystic ovary syndrome
- A1c ≥ 5.7%, or impaired fasting glucose or glucose tolerance
- Signs of insulin resistance (acanthosis nigricans)
- History of cardiovascular disease

The US Preventive Services Task Force has updated its recommendations to more closely follow those of the ADA.

A consensus panel has recommended screening of overweight children [weight >120% of ideal or a body mass index (BMI) >85th percentile] every 2 years beginning at age 10 or onset of puberty with two of the following risk factors:

- Family history of diabetes in first- or second-degree relative
- High-risk racial or ethnic group (same as above)
- Signs of, or conditions associated with, insulin resistance (eg. acanthosis nigricans, hypertension, dyslipidemia, and polycystic ovarian syndrome)
- History of high birth weight or maternal gestational diabetes during pregnancy

Screening for gestational diabetes in pregnancy is common, but there are no clear data on screening those at low risk. **Table 36-1** lists the diagnostic criteria in pregnancy. Women with diabetes prior to pregnancy are at risk for miscarriage and congenital abnormalities. The most common complication of gestational diabetes is macrosomia.

US Preventive Services Task Force. *Screening for Type 2 Diabetes Mellitus in Adults.* Agency for Healthcare Research and Quality (available at http://www.ahrq.gov; accessed March 23, 2013).

▶ Clinical Findings

A. Signs and Symptoms

The classic symptoms of diabetes are polyuria, polydypsia, and polyphagia, but the first signs may be subtle and nonspecific. Patients with type 1 diabetes exhibit fatigue, malaise, nausea and vomiting, irritability abdominal pain, and weight loss. They present early in the disease process, but usually

Table 36-1. Diabetes in pregnancy.

Risk factors
  Age >25 years
  High-risk racial or ethnic group
  Body mass index ≥25
  History of abnormal glucose tolerance test
  Previous history of adverse pregnancy outcomes usually
    associated with gestational diabetes
  Diabetes in a first-degree relative

Criteria for diagnosis
  Initial screen: 1-hour glucose tolerance test (GTT)[a]
    50-g glucose load between 10 and 28 weeks' gestation
    Positive screen ≥135–140 mg/dL
  Diagnosis: 3-hour GTT with a 100-g glucose load
    After an overnight fast with two abnormal values
      Fasting ≥95 mg/dL
      1 hour ≥190 mg/dL
      2 hours ≥165 mg/dL
      3 hours ≥140 mg/dL

[a]ADA now recommends initial 2-hour GTT:
Fasting ≥ 92 mg/dL
1 hour ≥ 180 mg/dL
2 hours ≥ 153 mg/dL
Only one abnormal value represents a diagnosis of gestational diabetes.

are quite ill at presentation, arguably ~25% with ketoacidosis. Signs and symptoms of ketoacidosis include tachypnea, labored respirations with the classic "fruity" breath, abdominal pain, confusion, and those associated with dehydration (dry skin and mucous membranes, decreased skin turgor, tachycardia, and hypotension),

Signs of type 2 diabetes are seen well after onset of the disease and may be due to complications. The classic symptoms are still prominent, but patients may also complain of fatigue, irritability, and drowsiness; blurred vision; numbness or tingling in the extremities; slow wound healing; and frequent infections of the skin, gums, or urinary tract infections.

B. History and Physical Examination

A personal or family history of autoimmune disorders may aid in the diagnosis. Type 1 usually occurs in children and adolescents, while type 2 becomes more common as individuals age. A BMI of <25 is more frequently seen in type 1 and LADA while BMI > 30 are usually indicative of type 2; however, neither age nor BMI should be used as criteria for diagnosis. Hypertension is commonly found at presentation. Retinal changes of cotton-wool spots and hemorrhages, decreased sensation in the extremities, and evidence of cardiovascular disease may also be found in type 2 diabetes.

C. Laboratory Findings

Serum glucose and A_{1c} levels are elevated, usually higher in type 2 as the development is more insidious. Serum glucose is often in the 400–600 mg/dL range. Sodium levels are low as a result of dilution as water follows glucose into the extracellular fluid. A dyslipidemia with low HDL and high triglyceride content is common in type 2. Increased albumin in the urine represents damage to the glomerular endothelium, and serum creatinine may be elevated.

For diagnosis, C-terminal peptide (C-peptide), the cleaved end of native insulin, is high in type 2 as the body increases insulin production to overcome resistance. It is extremely low in type 1 as insulin levels fall, and is usually low to low-normal in LADA. Antibody testing is useful in diagnosing type 1. Glutamic acid decarboxylase antibody (GAD 65) is most commonly used, also islet cell antibodies (ICAs) and insulin antibodies. Insulinoma-associated antigen (IA-2) is more predictive but less frequently found. Antibodies against zinc transporter 8 may also be useful.

In ketoacidosis (usually in type 1) serum glucose is > 250 mg/dL (commonly 500–800 mg/dL). Blood pH is <7.30 with an increased anion gap (>10). Bicarbonate is <18 mEq/L. Serum and urine ketones are high, but high β-hydroxybutyrate is a more accurate evaluation of the degree of ketosis.

Patients who present with hyperosmolar hyperglycemic state (usually in type 2) have very high serum glucose levels (600–1200 mg/dL), but do not have metabolic acidosis (pH >7.30 and serum bicarbonate (>15 mEq/L). Serum osmolality is >320 mOsm/kg.

▶ Complications

Preventing and delaying progression of all complications in patients with diabetes is dependent on lifestyle modification, tight control of blood glucose and blood pressure, and smoking cessation. The ACCORD trial, however, found that intensive glycemic control (HgbA$_{1c}$ ≤6%) did not lower the incidence of adverse microvascular outcomes.

A. Cardiovascular Disease

Heart disease is the leading cause of death in patients with diabetes. Men have double and women 4–5 times the risk for myocardial infarction (MI) as well as a higher incidence of diffuse, multivessel disease, plaque rupture, superimposed thrombosis, and in-hospital mortality. Five-year survival following angioplasty or coronary artery bypass graft (CABG) is lower in patients with diabetes, but survival rates are higher with CABG. Aspirin therapy at 81 mg/d is indicated for men aged >50 years and women aged >60 years with one additional cardiovascular risk factor. Smoking cessation must be emphasized. There are no specific guidelines for cardiac evaluation. An ECG and stress echocardiogram are recommended for symptoms and may be considered with the onset of microalbuminuria as the onset of those two entities often correspond.

Peripheral vascular disease is quite common in diabetes and 80% more common in Hispanic Americans. Treatment focuses on slowing progression as well as symptom

improvement. Besides smoking cessation and regular exercise, cilostazol (Pletal) can improve blood flow. Other choices include pentoxifylline (Trental) and gingko biloba.

1. Hypertension—ACE inhibitors are the first-line choice of treatment in diabetic patients producing a significant decrease in stroke, MI, cardiac death, post-MI mortality, and ischemic events following revascularization procedures. In the HOPE trial the use of ACE inhibitors correlated with a 34% reduction in the onset of new cases of diabetes and a mild improvement in lipid profiles. They may be used in all diabetic patients with systolic blood pressure of >100 mmHg or with hypertension and signs of insulin resistance. There is no specific creatinine level at which they must be stopped, but they are limited by rising potassium levels. The most troublesome side effect is a bradykinin-induced dry cough, and they are contraindicated in pregnancy. Angiotensin receptor blockers (ARBs) have similar data for cardiovascular risk reduction, and they are better tolerated than ACE inhibitors.

Thiazide diuretics and β-blockers are effective in lowering blood pressure and have been shown to reduce cardiovascular morbidity and mortality. Although they can have some effect on glucose control, they are acceptable for use in diabetes if used judiciously.

2. Hyperlipidemias—Patients with type 2 diabetes often have a distinct triad of elevated triglyceride and LDL (low-density lipoprotein) levels with decreased HDL levels. Each of these abnormalities has been shown to be an independent factor in atherogenesis. Current recommendations are to maintain total cholesterol below 200 mg/dL, triglycerides below 150 mg/dL, and LDL cholesterol of <100 mg/dL or below 70 mg/dL in the presence of cardiovascular disease, but JNC-8 abandoned specific goals and recommends moderate dose statin therapy (or high dose statins if 10-year ASCVD risk is ≥ 7.5%).

3. Hydroxymethylglutaryl coenzyme A (HMG-CoA)—HMG-CoA reductase inhibitors (statins) are the drugs of choice in treating hyperlipidemia in diabetic patients. Most outcome studies on lipid management have excluded patients with diabetes, but subgroup analysis shows a reduction in cardiovascular events of 25–37% with the use of statins to improve the lipid profile. The JUPITER study suggests an increased incidence in diabetes in patients taking statins, but the outcomes are still improved. Statins are contraindicated in pregnancy and must be used with caution in adolescents. Fish oil is helpful for reducing triglycerides, but fibrates are sometimes needed as well. Gemfibrozil will raise levels of simvastatin and increase risk of muscle injury.

B. Microvascular Complications

1. Nephropathy—Diabetic nephropathy is the most common cause of end-stage renal disease (ESRD) in the United States, and the rates are highest in Asian and African Americans. The incidence is much higher in type 1 diabetes, but the prevalence is higher in type 2. Glomerular hyperfiltration is an early indication of impending deterioration. All patients should be screened yearly with a microalbumin or microalbumin/creatinine ratio. Microalbuminuria is defined as 30–300 mg protein in a 24-hour urine collection, a more accurate but cumbersome test. More than 300 mg/24 hour constitutes macroalbuminuria or nephropathy.

Angiotensin-converting enzyme inhibitors are the drugs of choice for treatment of microalbuminuria. Ramipril has been shown to reduce ESRD and death by 41% and proteinuria by 20% compared with amlodipine. ARBs have comparable efficacy and should be used when the use of ACE inhibitors is limited. There is no advantage in using both simultaneously.

2. Retinopathy—Approximately 20% of patients with type 2 diabetes show signs of retinopathy at the time of diagnosis. Progression is orderly from mild abnormalities (small retinal hemorrhages) to proliferative retinopathy with growth of new vessels on the retina and into the vitreous culminating in vision loss. The risk of retinopathy increases with increasing A_{1c} and duration of the disease, but African Americans develop retinopathy at lower levels of A_{1c}. In the ACCORD trial, intensive therapy lowered retinopathy but not ultimate vision loss. Patients with type 1 diabetes may begin yearly ophthalmology visits 5 years after diagnosis, but patients with type 2 should begin yearly office visits with diagnosis. Laser photocoagulation therapy is the only treatment option once the disease progresses.

3. Neuropaathy—*Peripheral neuropathy* leads to a loss of sensation and pain in the extremities and is the major cause of foot problems in diabetic individuals. Treatment of peripheral neuropathy remains symptomatic. Pregabalin (Lyrica) and duloxetine (Cymbalta) are indicated for its treatment, but other treatment options that have proved effective include antidepressants (amitriptyline, nortriptyline, venlafaxine), and anticonvulsants (gabapentin, carbamazepine), topical capsaicin cream, and lidocaine patches. Opioids, tramadol, transcutaneous electrical nerve stimulation, and alternative therapies (relaxation therapy, biofeedback, α-lipoic acid, and evening primrose oil) may also be effective.

Autonomic neuropathy is common, and patients should be asked about symptoms of nausea, diarrhea or constipation, lightheadedness, incontinence, impotence, and heat intolerance. It is also important to check for any of the following: resting tachycardia, orthostatic hypotension, dependent edema (to assess impaired venoarteriolar reflex), and decreased diameter of dark-adapted pupil. Gastrointestinal motility may be improved with metoclopramide or erythromycin.

C. Ketoacidosis

Ketoacidosis occurs when there is insufficient insulin to meet the body's needs, leading to increased gluconeogenesis, fatty acid oxidation, and ketogenesis, and resulting in metabolic acidosis, osmotic diuresis, and dehydration. It is a leading cause of death in children and the incidence is highest for children with poor control, inadequate insurance, or psychiatric disorders.

Treatment involves rehydration with normal saline and an IV insulin infusion. Potassium is replaced as it starts to fall near the upper limits of normal. Glucose is added to fluids when serum glucose approaches 250 mg/dL. Patient should be in a monitored bed and labs should initially be drawn hourly. The insulin infusion is continued until acidosis is resolved and ketones are cleared. Subcutaneous insulin is started prior to stopping the insulin drip.

D. Infections

Patients with diabetes are at greater risk for infections, including community-acquired pneumonia (particularly pneumococcal), influenza, cholecystitis, urinary tract infections, and pyelonephritis. Persistent fever and flank pain for more than 3–4 days despite appropriate antibiotic treatment should elicit an evaluation (preferably by CT) for a perinephric abscess. Fungal infections are frequently seen, especially vaginal candidiasis, but also eye and skin infections. Foot infections include cellulitis, osteomyelitis, plantar abscesses, and necrotizing fasciitis.

E. Diabetic Foot

Diabetes is the leading nontraumatic cause of foot amputation and Charcot foot in the United States, due to the combination of neuropathy, altered foot structure, and vasculopathy. Overall, 15% of diabetics will have a foot ulcer, and 20% of these will lead to amputation. Native Americans have the highest rates of foot infection. Feet should be examined at every office visit and patients instructed in good foot care. Medicare will pay for special shoes and the fitting of these shoes by a podiatrist or orthotist; however, careful attention to foot care by primary providers was found to be more effective at preventing ulcers than special shoes or inserts.

Treatment of diabetic foot ulcers requires removing pressure on the ulcer and good wound care with deep debridement and appropriate dressings. The best indication of ability to heal is an intact pulse, and revascularization may be necessary if pulses are absent. Antibiotics should be used only if infection is clearly present as they have been shown to retard healing in the noninfected foot. Wound cultures almost always yield multiple organisms, and are not helpful unless taken from the bone in osteomyelitis. The test of choice for diagnosis of osteomyelitis is MRI, although bone scans are an alternative. Treatment efficacy can be followed by monitoring the sedimentation rate.

Vinik AI, Caselini CM. Guidelines in the management of diabetic nerve pain: clinical utility of pregabalin. *Diabetes Metab Syndr Obes.* 2013;6:57-78. [PMID: 23467255]

Westerberg DP. Diabetic ketoacidosis: evaluation and treatment, *Am Fam Physician.* 2013;87(5):337-346.

▶ Treatment

Management goals should be individualized according to the patient's age, life expectancy, and comorbid conditions. ADA recommendations are to maintain fasting glucose levels of 80–100 mg/dL and HgbA$_{1c}$ levels <7%; the American College of Endocrinology recommends a 2-hour postprandial glucose <140 mg/dL and has set a goal for HgbA$_{1c}$ at <6.5%. Blood pressure should be maintained below 130/80 mmHg, but the ADA has recently liberalized the systolic goal to 140, and JNC-8 recommends < 140/90 mmHg.

The initial and ongoing evaluation for diabetes includes counseling regarding lifestyle and self-management including smoking cessation, goals and motivation, psychosocial issues, and compliance, family support, and self-image.

Every visit should include the following:

Weight and BMI

Blood pressure measurement

Funduscopic examination

Basic physical exam concentrating on cardiovascular evaluation

Brief skin examination

Visual examination of feet

Regular screening and laboratory measurements include the following:

A$_{1c}$ level every 3 months (every 6 months if usually well controlled)

Verbal or written screen for depression

Yearly dilated retinal exam to screen for retinopathy

Yearly microalbumin to screen for nephropathy

Yearly foot exam including monofilament, vibratory, and evaluation of pulses

Yearly fasting lipid profile

Yearly electrolytes, BUN, creatinine, and urinalysis

Immunizations should be updated:

Influenza yearly

Pneumococcus (Pneumovax) once and repeat at age 65

Tdap

Hepatitis B (most evidence for those aged <60)

Use of guidelines, electronic health records, patient management systems, checklists and questionnaires, standing orders (**Table 36-2**), and a team approach can increase efficiency and provide more comprehensive care for patients with diabetes.

CDC Recommendations for Hepatitis B Vaccination among Adults with Diabetes: Grading of Scientific Evidence in Support of Key Recommendations (last update Aug. 6, 2012; available at http://www.cdc.gov/vaccines/acip/recs/GRADE/hepB-vac-adults-diabetes.html).

Table 36-2. Standing orders for diabetic patients.

1. Update the electronic record or place an updated flowsheet in the patient's chart.
2. Monitor and record blood pressure in the same arm at each visit.
3. Measure and record the patient's weight.
4. If HbA$_{1c}$ has not been evaluated in the past 6 months, order.
5. If urinalysis and microalbumin testing have not been done in the past year:
   a. Perform a urine dipstick and record the results on the flowsheet.
   b. Order a urine microalbumin test.
6. If a lipid profile has not been obtained in the past year, order.
7. If a dilated eye examination has not been performed in the past year, complete a referral for an ophthalmology examination.
8. Ask the patient to remove his/her shoes and socks.
   a. Palpate dorsalis pedis and posterior tibial pulses.
   b. Inspect the skin for any skin breakdown.
   c. Record the findings on the patient's flowsheet.
9. Check to see if patient has received a pneumococcal vaccine, a dT or Tdap vaccine in the last 10 years, a flu shot for the current season, and completed a hepatitis B series. If patient has not received the flu shot, administer following standard clinic protocol.

Physician Signature: _____ Date: _____

A. Education

Education and ownership are imperative for self-management, and include lifestyle changes, smoking cessation, home monitoring, management of blood pressure and lipids, medication effects and side effects, and skin and foot care. This education may require multiple formats, including the following:

- Multidisciplinary clinician education
- Group visits
- Reading materials
- Internet sites
- Self-tests

B. Nutrition

Individualization of nutrition therapy is necessary to achieve glucose and lipid goals, health, and well-being. A Mediterranean-style diet is recommended with limited alcohol, decreased fat and overall calorie intake, leading to a modest weight loss of 10–15%. When combined with abstinence from tobacco, it can lower mortality by 50%. Individuals receiving fixed daily doses of insulin should try to maintain a consistent daily caloric intake. Those on intensive insulin therapy should adjust their insulin according to the carbohydrate content of their meals.

C. Exercise

Exercise increases strength and endurance, HDL cholesterol, and insulin sensitivity; reduces stress; improves circulation, digestion, sleep, energy levels, and self-esteem; controls appetite and reduces weight; and lowers heart rate, blood pressure, lipid levels, and blood glucose, thereby delaying the onset of diabetes and reducing the risk of cardiovascular disease. Prescribe a regular exercise program adapted to complications for all patients including moderate aerobic or physical activity for 20–60 minutes most days with resistance training twice a week. Older patients and those at increased risk of coronary artery disease should have a careful physical examination and an exercise stress test prior to beginning or significantly advancing an exercise program and should avoid sudden strenuous exercise. Recommendations for children include at least 1 hour of daily exercise and no more than 2 hours of non-school-related screen time daily. Athletes with type 1 diabetes may not participate in strenuous exercise when their blood glucose is >300 mg/dL or >250 mg/dL with urine ketones.

D. Home Glucose Monitoring

The American Diabetes Association (ADA) has recommended that all patients with diabetes perform home glucose monitoring. Overall, 84% of patients who monitor their blood glucose are within 20% of their target range. Glucose monitors now feature memory and download capabilities, but because of cost and discomfort, monitoring should be limited when glucose levels are stable. Patients who are using insulin, sulfonylureas, or corticosteroids; are ill; or are changing therapy should monitor frequently.

E. Pharmacologic Therapy

In most cases, therapy is begun with one medication and dosage is increased before adding a second, but two may be synergistic. Efficacy is variable between drugs and individuals, but expected lowering of HgbA$_{1c}$ is 0.5–2.0%. Choices of medication should be made to maximize efficacy and minimize side effects (**Table 36-3**). When patients with type 2 diabetes present with A$_{1c}$ > 9%, insulin can be used initially in combination with an oral medication to lower glucose levels to a manageable level.

1. Biguanides—Metformin is the initial choice in type 2 diabetes (especially with obesity), and it should be continued if possible when insulin is added. It is weight-neutral and reduces cardiovascular deaths and all-cause mortality. It is used in metabolic syndrome to delay the onset of diabetes and is the only approved oral hypoglycemic for children. Because it is associated with lactic acidosis (mortality 50%), metformin cannot be used in patients with renal insufficiency or when using IV contrast material. It is a category B in pregnancy and can be used in children but not while breastfeeding. Metformin may induce vitamin B$_{12}$ malabsorption, so regular B$_{12}$ monitoring is advised.

2. Sulfonylureas—The oldest oral medications for diabetes, they can be used in patients with hepatic or renal insufficiency and cautiously in the elderly. They should be

taken 1 hour before meals to induce insulin secretion or at bedtime where they limit hepatic glucose production. Approximately 20% of patients will not respond, and sulfonylureas lose efficacy over time. Glyburide has the greatest potential for hypoglycemia and cannot be used in renal failure, but it is a category B in pregnancy. Glimepiride has a more rapid onset and longer duration of action but induces less hypoglycemia, and may be the best choice in patients with known coronary disease.

3. Meglitinides—These rapid-acting medications are taken only with meals and are useful in patients whose fasting glucose levels are well controlled but who have high postprandial values or for patients who eat few or irregular meals. Nateglinide has a more rapid onset and shorter duration of action than repaglinide.

4. Thiazolidinediones—These agents are useful as an adjunct medication or with marked insulin resistance. Pioglitazone decreases triglyceride levels by 33% and increases HDL cholesterol, but improvement in outcomes has not been shown. It may take 12 weeks for the medication to reach its maximum potential, so dosage should be increased only after several weeks. They are teratogenic in rats, and are not recommended for use in pregnancy or in children. Pioglitazone has been shown to increase the risk of bladder cancer and of distal limb fractures in women.

5. α-Glucosidase inhibitors—Taken only with meals, they blunt postprandial hyperglycemia. Therapy should be initiated at a low dose and increased slowly to minimize side effects. If they are used with a sulfonylurea or insulin, and hypoglycemia occurs, treatment must utilize simple sugars (glucose or lactose), not sucrose. Efficacy is altered with digestive enzymes, antacids, or cholestyramine. Serum transaminase levels must be followed every 3 months for the first year, and they must be stopped when the serum creatinine reaches 2 mg/dL. They have been linked to pancreatitis

6. DPP4 inhibitors—Glucagon like peptide 1 (GLP1) stimulates insulin secretion and biosynthesis and inhibits glucagon secretion and gastric emptying. It is degraded by dipeptidyl peptidase-4 (DPP4). These inhibitors of DPP4 effectively increase GLP1 and decrease postprandial glucose levels. They are well tolerated with once-daily dosing, but they do carry a risk for pancreatitis.

7. Incretin mimetics—These synthetic incretins are given by subcutaneous injection and carry the same warning for pancreatitis. They also increase the risk of T-cell thyroid tumors. Exenatide is a GLP1 analog derived from Gila monster saliva and is given prior to morning and evening meals. A 70 μg dose can be given once weekly. It is used as an adjunct to metformin, sulfonylureas, or thiazolidinediones. Pramlintide is an analog of human amylin, given with insulin prior to meals, and liraglutide is given once daily.

Table 36-3. Medications for the treatment of diabetes.

Drug	Dosage Range (mg/d)	Mechanism of Action	Advantages	Side Effects and Precautions	Cost
Biguanides Metformin (Glucophage) Metformin XR (Glucophage XR)	Daily or BID 500–2500 500–2000	↓ gluconeogenesis in liver ↑ insulin sensitivity	Decreases mortality No hypoglycemia Lowers insulin levels Possible weight loss Improves lipids and endothelial function	Nausea and diarrhea Hold before and after IV contrast Stop if creatinine >1.5 Caution with CHF and hepatic dysfunction	Generic $
Sulfonylureas Glipizide (Glucotrol) Glipizide XL (Glucotrol XL) Glyburide (DiaBeta, Micronase) Glyburide, micronized (Glynase) Glimeperide (Amaryl)	Daily or BID 5–40 2.5–20 2.5–20 1–8 1–6	Induce insulin secretion from pancreatic β cells	Can be used in renal (except glyburide) or hepatic failure	Hypoglycemia Weight gain	Generic $
Meglitinides Repaglinide (Prandin) Nateglinide (Starlix)	TID dosing 1.5–16 180–360	Induce secretion of insulin from pancreatic β cells	Rapid onset and short half-life; can use in renal insufficiency	Caution in hepatic insufficiency	$$
Thiazolodinedione Pioglitazone (Actos) Rosiglitzone (Avandia)	Daily dosing 15–45 4–5	Insulin sensitizers in muscle and adipose tissue		Do not use in class III or IV heart failure; monitor LFTs	$$$
SGLT2 inhibitor Canagliflozin (Invokana) Dapagliflozin (Farxiga) Empaglifloin (jardiance)	Daily dosing 100–300 5–10	Block renal reabsorption of glucose, causing urinary excretion		Orthostatic hypotension, urinary tract and vaginal yeast infections	$$$
α-Glucosidase inhibitors Acarbose (Precose) Miglitol (Glyset)	TID dosing 75–300 75–300	Inhibit breakdown of disaccha- rides and delay carbohydrate absorption in brush border of small intestine	No hypoglycemia	Flatulence Cannot use with GI disorders, cirrhosis, Cr >2 mg/dL	$$
DPP4 inhibitor Sitagliptin (Januvia) Saxagliptin (Onglyza) Linagliptin (Tradjenta) Alogliptin (Nesina)	Daily dosing 100 (25–50 renal impairment) 2.5–5 5 (long half-life) 25–400	Block the breakdown of natural incretins	No hypoglycemia Lowers postprandial glucose	Nausea and vomiting Must decrease dose in renal impairment	$$$
Incretin mimetics Exenatide (Byetta) Liraglutide (Victoza) Pramlintide (Symlin) Albiglutide (Tanzeum) Dulaglutide	SC 5–10 μg (70 /wk) 0.6–1.8 μg 15–120 μg 30–50 mg/wk 0.75–15 mg/k	Enhance glucose-dependent insulin secretion Suppress inappropriate glucagon secretion and slow gastric emptying	Early satiety and weight loss	Nausea and vomiting Exenatide associated with hemorrhagic or necrotiz- ing pancreatitis	$$$

Albiglutide and dulaglutide are available for once weekly dosing. They all increase insulin in response to glucose at meals, promote satiety, slow gastric emptying, and may lead to significant weight loss.

8. SGLT-2 inhibitors—Sodium-glucose cotransporter 2 inhibitors reduce the reabsorption of filtered glucose in the kidney and lower the reabsorption concentration at the proximal tubule causing more excretion of glucose

Table 36-4. Available insulins.

Drug	Onset of Action	Peak (hours)	Duration (hours)	Cost
Rapid-acting				
Lispro (Humalog)	15 minutes	0.5–1.5	2–4	
Aspart (NovoLog)	15 minutes	1–3	3–5	$$
Glulisine (Apidra)	15 minutes	1–1.5	5	$$$
Inhaled insulin (Afrezza)	12–15 minutes	< 1	2–5	
Short-acting				
Regular (Humulin)	30 minutes	2–4	5.8	$
Intermediate				
NPH (Novolin)	1–3 hours	5–7	16–18	$
Long-acting				
Glargine (Lantus)	1 hour	None	24	$$$
Detemir (Levemir)	1 hour	None	20	$$$

in the urine. They also induce weight reduction and lower systolic blood pressure. They reduce intravascular volume and may induce postural hypotension as well as increasing urinary tract infections and vaginal mycotic infections.

9. Combination therapy—Combining drugs with different mechanisms of action is most efficacious, but caution must be exercised in combining drugs with similar side effects (TZDs and α-glucosidase inhibitors are both hepatotoxic). Metformin can be combined with any of the other medications, and there are now multiple commercial combinations of metformin, thiazolidinediones, sulfonylureas, and DPP4 inhibitors.

10. Insulin—The United Kingdom Prospective Diabetes Study (UKPDS) trial did not show any increase in cardiovascular disease due to the use of insulin but did demonstrate a significant improvement in all complications of diabetes with tight control. A long-acting insulin provides a basal rate that minimizes hepatic glucose production. A rapid-acting insulin is used with meals to minimize the postprandial insulin peak.

The new synthetic insulins, lispro, aspart, and glulisine, have a short onset, rapid peak, and 2–4 hour duration of action more closely mimicking the pharmacokinetics of human insulin *in vivo* (**Table 36-4**). They are preferred over regular insulin with its slower onset and longer duration of action, necessitating regular snacking. Inhaled insulin, with pharmacokinetics similar to the rapid-acting insulins, has returned to the market. The long-acting insulin analogs glargine and detemir are peakless insulins with a consistent 24-hour duration. They are less soluble in subcutaneous tissue, prolong absorption, and can be used with oral medications or with any of the short-acting insulins (but not mixed in the same syringe). They are usually taken once a day but may be divided into two doses (especially helpful when giving >100 units). Neutral protamine hagedorn (NPH) insulin has

a duration of <24 hours, necessitating twice-daily dosing with peaks occurring in the afternoon and early morning. Dosage changes are made based on fingersticks taken ~8 hours following the dose. Its primary utility lies in its low cost.

When initiating insulin therapy in type 1 diabetics, the total insulin requirement for 24 hours should be estimated. Half of this amount may be given as a long-acting insulin and the other half as a rapid-acting insulin. Adjustments in the long-acting insulin dosage are based primarily on fasting glucose levels. The rapid-acting portion can be divided with 40% given before breakfast, 40% before dinner, and the remaining 20% prior to lunch. It should then be adjusted according to caloric intake and resulting postprandial fingerstick glucose levels.

Bioavailability with insulin changes with the site of injection with the abdomen the fastest. It is recommended that injections be rotated within the same area.

11. Insulin pump—Current insulin pumps weigh ~4 oz and are about the size of a beeper, allowing for continuous use of short-acting insulin with a more consistent absorption rate. Half of the insulin is given continuously as a basal dose, and the other half is divided into mealtime boluses. Patients must monitor their blood glucose ≥3 times a day and count carbohydrates at meals. When compliant, patients can achieve tighter control with the pump while gaining more flexibility in eating habits and a more normal lifestyle with fewer episodes of severe hypoglycemia, a reduction of total insulin usage, and less weight gain. Particularly good candidates for insulin pump therapy are patients who are difficult to control or have wide glucose swings, have erratic schedules, or have a significant dawn phenomenon; pregnant women and teenagers with poor control and/or frequent episodes of ketoacidosis are also good candidates.

F. Bariatric Surgery

As the popularity of bariatric surgery increases, it is being recognized as an effective treatment for diabetes. In observational studies, it has been shown to decrease the incidence of diabetes, with ≤75% of patients reverting to a normal A_{1c}. Either Lap Band [laparoscopic adjustable gastric banding (LAGB)] or Roux-n-Y surgery is effective. Because of its malabsorptive component, the latter surgery is more effective but requires much more monitoring for complications.

Dixon JB, et al. Bariatric surgery: an IDF statement for obese type 2 diabetes. *Diabetic Med.* 2011; 28(6):628-642. [PMCID: PMC3123702]

Gropler RJ. Lost in translation: modulation of the metabolic-functional relation in the diabetic human heart. *Circulation.* 2009;119:2020-2022.

Kooy A, et al. Long-term effects of metformin on metabolism and microvascular and macrovasculaar disease in patients with type 2 diabetes mellitus. *Arch Intern Med.* 2009;169:616-625. [PMID: 19307526]

▶ Prognosis

The risk of premature death in patients with diabetes is twice that of the general population. Overall, 15% of patients with type 1 diabetes will die before age 40, which is 20 times the rate of the general population. Patients with type 1 diabetes die from ketoacidosis, renal failure, and coronary artery disease. Patients who develop type 2 diabetes after age 40 have a decreased life expectancy of 5–10 years, and 80% of all patients with type 2 diabetes die from cardiovascular causes. The prognosis improves with significant lifestyle change, control of blood sugar and blood pressure, and smoking cessation.

Websites

American Diabetes Association (ADA): http://www.diabetes.org/
Centers for Disease Control and Prevention (CDC), Division of Diabetes: http://www.cdc.gov.diabetes/
Joslin Diabetes Center: http://www.joslin.org/
National Diabetes Education Program: http://www.ndep.nih.gov/
National Institute of Diabetes and Digestive and Kidney Diseases: http://www2.niddk.nih.gov/

Endocrine Disorders

Pamela Allweiss, MD, MSPH

William J. Hueston, MD

Peter J. Carek, MD, MS

▼ THYROID DISORDERS

Thyroid disorders affect 1 in 200 adults but are more common in women and with advancing age. The incidence of hypothyroidism, for instance, is 0.3–5 cases per 1000 individuals per year, including 7% of women and 3% of men aged 60–89 years. Hypothyroidism is much more common than hyperthyroidism, nodular disease, or thyroid cancer. Thyroid nodules occur in 4–8% of all individuals and, like other thyroid problems, increase in incidence with age.

Thyroid disease is more common in people who have conditions such as diabetes or other autoimmune diseases (eg, lupus); in those with a family history of thyroid disease or a history of head and neck irradiation; and in patients who use certain medications, including amiodarone and lithium. Recent guidelines from the American Thyroid Association suggest that all adults have their serum thyroid-stimulating hormone (TSH) concentrations measured, beginning at age 35 and every 5 years thereafter.

HYPOTHYROIDISM

▶ General Considerations

Causes of hypothyroidism are outlined in **Table 37-1**. The most common noniatrogenic condition causing hypothyroidism in the United States is Hashimoto thyroiditis. Other common causes are post–Graves disease, thyroid irradiation, and surgical removal of the thyroid. Hypothyroidism may also occur secondary to hypothalamic or pituitary dysfunction, most commonly in patients who have received intracranial irradiation or surgical removal of a pituitary adenoma. In addition, some patients may have mild elevations of TSH despite normal thyroxine levels, a condition termed *subclinical hypothyroidism*.

▶ Clinical Findings

A. Symptoms and Signs

Patients with hypothyroidism present with a constellation of symptoms that can involve every organ system. Symptoms include lethargy, weight gain, hair loss, dry skin, slowed mentation or forgetfulness, depressed affect, cold intolerance, constipation, hair loss, muscle weakness, abnormal menstrual periods (or infertility), and fluid retention. Because of the range of symptoms seen in hypothyroidism, clinicians must have a high index of suspicion, especially in high-risk populations. In older patients, hypothyroidism can be confused with Alzheimer disease or other conditions that cause dementia. In women, hypothyroidism is often confused with depression.

Physical findings that can occur with hypothyroidism include low blood pressure, bradycardia, nonpitting edema, generalized hair thinning along with hair loss in the outer third of the eyebrows, skin drying, and a diminished relaxation phase of reflexes. The thyroid gland in a patient with chronic thyroiditis may be enlarged, atrophic, or of normal size. Thyroid nodules are common in patients with Hashimoto thyroiditis.

B. Laboratory Findings

The most valuable test for hypothyroidism is the sensitive TSH assay. Measurement of the free thyroxine (T_4) level may also be helpful. TSH is elevated and free T_4 decreased in overt hypothyroidism (**Table 37-2**). Other laboratory findings may include hyperlipidemia and hyponatremia. Hashimoto thyroiditis, an autoimmune condition, is one of the most common causes of hypothyroidism. Testing for thyroid autoantibodies (antiperoxidase, antithyroglobulin) is positive in 95% of patients with Hashimoto thyroiditis.

Patients with associated subclinical hypothyroidism have a high TSH level (usually in the 5–10 µIU/mL range) in

Table 37-1. Causes of hypothyroidism.

Primary hypothyroidism (95% of cases)
  Idiopathic hypothyroidism (probably old Hashimoto thyroiditis)
  Hashimoto thyroiditis
  Postthyroid irradiation
  Postsurgical
  Late-stage invasive fibrous thyroiditis
  Iodine deficiency
  Drugs (lithium, interferon)
  Infiltrative diseases (sarcoidosis, amyloid, scleroderma,
      hemochromatosis)
Secondary Hypothyroidism (5% of cases)
  Pituitary or hypothalamic neoplasms
  Congenital hypopituitarism
  Pituitary necrosis (Sheehan syndrome)

conjunction with normal free T_4 level. Between 3% and 20% of these patients will eventually develop overt hypothyroidism. Patients who test positive for thyroid antibodies are at increased risk.

▶ Treatment

In patients with primary hypothyroidism, therapy should begin with thyroid hormone replacement. In patients with secondary hypothyroidism, further investigation with provocative testing of the pituitary can be performed to determine whether the cause is a hypothalamic or pituitary problem.

Most healthy adult patients with hypothyroidism require ~1.6 µg/kg of thyroid replacement, with requirements falling to 1 µg/kg for the elderly. The initial dosage may range from 12.5 µg to a full replacement dose of 100–150 µg of levothyroxine (0.10–0.15 mg/d). Doses will vary depending on age, weight, cardiac status, duration, and severity of the hypothyroidism. Therapy should be titrated after at least 6 weeks

following any change in levothyroxine dose. The serum TSH level is the most important measure to gauge the dose.

Treatment of subclinical hypothyroidism remains controversial. Subclinical hypothyroidism is characterized by a serum TSH above the upper reference limit in combination with a normal free thyroxine (T_4) at a time when thyroid function has been stable for several weeks, the hypothalamic-pituitary-thyroid axis is normal, and there is no recent or ongoing severe illness The prevalence of subclinical hypothyroidism is ~5–10%, more common in white older women. The American Association of Clinical Endocrinologists (AACE) guidelines suggest treating patients with TSH levels of >10 µIU/mL as well as those with TSH levels between 5 and 10 µIU/mL in conjunction with goiter or positive antithyroid peroxidase antibodies, or both (level of evidence for American Thyroid Association recommendations: level 3 or 4, clinical consensus based on the literature). Others base any therapeutic intervention on the individual situation (pregnancy status, cardiovascular risk factors, etc).

Once the TSH level reaches the normal range, the frequency of testing can be decreased. Each patient's regimen must be individualized, but the usual follow-up after TSH is stable is at 6 months; the history and physical examination should be repeated on a routine basis thereafter.

Thyroid hormone absorption can be affected by malabsorption, age, and concomitant medications such as cholestyramine, ferrous sulfate, sucralfate, calcium, and some antacids containing aluminum hydroxide. Drugs such as anticonvulsants affect thyroid hormone binding, whereas others such as rifampin and sertraline hydrochloride may accelerate levothyroxine metabolism, necessitating a higher replacement dose. The thyroid dose may also need to be adjusted during pregnancy. There has been some interest in using a combination of T_4 and triiodothyronine (T_3) or natural thyroid preparations in pregnant women with hypothyroidism, but studies to date have been small and findings inconsistent.

Table 37-2. Laboratory changes in hypothyroidism.

TSH	Free T$_4$	Free T$_3$	Likely Diagnosis
High	Low	Low	Primary hypothyroidism
High (>10 µIU/mL)	Normal	Normal	Not consistent with the AACE guideline mentioned previously; subclinical hypothyroidism with high risk for future development of overt hypothyroidism
High (6–10 µIU/mL)	Normal	Normal	Subclinical hypothyroidism with low risk for future development of overt hypothyroidism
High	High	Low	Congenital absence of T_4–T_3-converting enzyme or amiodarone effect
High	High	High	Peripheral thyroid hormone resistance
Low	Low	Low	Pituitary thyroid deficiency or recent withdrawal of thyroid replacement after excessive replacement

TSH, thyroid-stimulating hormone; T_3, triiodothyronine; T_4, thyroxine.

Pregnant women with thyroid dysfunction need close attention. Overt maternal hypothyroidism is known to have serious adverse effects on the fetus. The Endocrine Society has developed practice guidelines that address the management of thyroid dysfunction during pregnancy and postpartum.

Abalovich M, Amino N, Barbour LA, et al. Management of thyroid dysfunction during pregnancy and postpartum. *J Clin Endocrinol Metab.* 2007;92(8 Suppl):S1–S47.

American Association of Clinical Endocrinologists and American Thyroid Association. Clinical practice guidelines for hypothyroidism in adults. *Endocr Practice.* 2012;18:989–1027.

American Thyroid Association. Guidelines for the treatment of hypothyroidism. *Thyroid Journal* (ahead of print) http://www.thyroid.org/thyroid-guidelines/hypothyroidism 2014.

Bunevicius R, et al. Effects of thyroxine as compared with thyroxine plus triiodothyronine in patients with hypothyroidism. *N Engl J Med.* 1999;340:424. [PMID: 9971866]

De Groot L, Abalovich M, Alexander E, Amino N, Barbour L, et al. Management of thyroid dysfunction during pregnancy and postpartum: an Endocrine Society clinical practice guideline. *J Clin Endocrinol Metab.* 2012;97:2543–2565.

Franklyn J. The thyroid—too much and too little across the ages. *Clin Endocrinol.* 2013;78(1):1–8.

Gussekloo J, et al. Thyroid status, disability and cognitive function, and survival in old age. *JAMA.* 2004;292:2591. [PMID: 15572717]

Haddow JE, et al. Maternal thyroid deficiency during pregnancy and subsequent neuropsychological development of the child. *N Engl J Med.* 1999;341:549. [PMID: 10451459]

Johnson J, Duick D. Diabetes and thyroid disease: a likely combination. *Diabetes Spectrum.* 2002;15:140–142.

Kritz-Silverstein D, et al. The association of thyroid stimulating hormone levels with cognitive function and depressed mood: the Rancho Bernardo study. *J Nutr Health Aging.* 2009;13(4):317–321. [PMID: 19300866]

National Endocrine and Metabolic Diseases Information Service: www.endocrine.niddk.nih.gov/pubs/thyroidtests/index.aspx

Surks MI, Ortiz E, Daniels GH, et al. Subclinical thyroid disease: scientific review and guidelines for diagnosis and management. *JAMA.* 2004;291:228–238.

Tan Z, et al. Thyroid function and the risk of Alzheimer disease: the Framingham study. *Arch Intern Med.* 2008;168 (14):1514–1520. [PMID: 18663163]

HYPERTHYROIDISM

General Considerations

Hyperthyroidism has several causes. The most common is toxic diffuse goiter (Graves disease), an autoimmune disorder caused by immunoglobulin G (IgG) antibodies that bind to TSH receptors, initiating the production and release of thyroid hormone. Other causes include toxic adenoma; toxic multinodular goiter (Plummer disease); painful subacute thyroiditis; silent thyroiditis, including lymphocytic and postpartum thyroiditis; iodine-induced hyperthyroidism (eg, related to amiodarone therapy); oversecretion of

pituitary TSH; trophoblastic disease (very rare); and excess exogenous thyroid hormone secretion.

Clinical Findings

A. Symptoms and Signs

Patients with hyperthyroidism usually present with progressive nervousness, tremor, palpitations, weight loss, dyspnea on exertion, fatigue, difficulty concentrating, heat intolerance, and frequent bowel movements or diarrhea. Physical findings include a rapid pulse and elevated blood pressure, with the systolic pressure increasing to a greater extent than the diastolic pressure, creating a wide pulse-pressure hypertension. Exophthalmos (in patients with Graves disease), muscle weakness, sudden paralysis, dependent low extremity edema, or pretibial myxedema may also be present. Cardiac arrhythmias such as atrial fibrillation may be evident on physical examination or electrocardiogram, and a resting tremor may be noted on physical examination.

In patients with subacute thyroiditis, symptoms of hyperthyroidism are generally transient and resolve in a matter of weeks. There may be a recent history of a head and neck infection, fever, and severe neck tenderness. Postpartum thyroiditis may occur in the first few months after delivery. Both types of thyroiditis may have a transient hyperthyroid phase, a euthyroid phase, and occasionally a later hypothyroid phase.

B. Laboratory and Imaging Evaluation

Hyperthyroidism is detected by a decreased sensitive TSH assay and confirmed, if necessary, by the finding of an elevated free T_4 level. Testing for thyroid autoantibodies, including TSH receptor antibodies (TRAb) or thyroid-stimulating immunoglobulins (TSI), may be done as necessary. Once hyperthyroidism is identified, radionucleotide uptake and scanning of the thyroid, preferably with iodine-123, is useful to determine whether hyperthyroidism is secondary to Graves disease, an autonomous nodule, or thyroiditis (ie, by showing activity and anatomy of the thyroid). In scans of patients with Graves disease, there is increased uptake on radionucleotide imaging with diffuse hyperactivity. In contrast, nodules demonstrate limited areas of uptake with surrounding hypoactivity, and in subacute thyroiditis, uptake is patchy and decreased overall.

Complications

Thyroid storm represents an acute hypermetabolic state associated with the sudden release of large amounts of thyroid hormone. This occurs most often in Graves disease but can occur in acute thyroiditis. Individuals with thyroid storm present with confusion, fever, restlessness, and sometimes with psychosislike symptoms. Physical examination shows tachycardia, elevated blood pressure, and sometimes fever. Cardiac dysrhythmias may be present or develop. Patients will have other signs of high-output heart failure (dyspnea on exertion, peripheral vasoconstriction) and may exhibit signs of cardiac or cerebral ischemia. Thyroid storm is a medical crisis requiring prompt attention and reversal of the metabolic demands from the acute hyperthyroidism.

Treatment

A. Radioactive Iodine

Radioactive iodine is the treatment of choice for Graves disease (GD) in adult patients who are not pregnant. Pretreatment with methimazole prior to radioactive iodine therapy for GD should be considered in patients who are at increased risk for complications due to worsening of hyperthyroidism (ie, those who are extremely symptomatic or have free T_4 estimated at 2–3 times the upper limit of normal). Treatment with β-adrenergic blockers should be done prior to radioactive iodine therapy in patients with GD who are at increased risk for complications due to worsening of hyperthyroidism (ie, those who are extremely symptomatic or have free T_4 estimates 2–3 times the upper limit of normal). Iodine-131 has also been used on an individual basis in patients aged <20 years. To date, studies have shown no evidence of adverse effects on fertility, congenital malformations, or increased risk of cancer in women who were treated with radioactive iodine during their childbearing years or in their offspring. Patients should be advised to postpone pregnancy for at least 6 months postablation therapy.

Radioactive iodine should not be used in breastfeeding mothers. There is also concern that the administration of radioactive iodine in patients with active ophthalmopathy may accelerate progression of eye disease. For this reason, some experts initially treat Graves disease with oral suppressive therapy until the ophthalmologic disease has stabilized.

B. Pharmacotherapy

Antithyroid drugs are well tolerated and successful at blocking the production and release of thyroid hormone in patients with Graves disease. These drugs work by blocking the organification of iodine. Methimazole is the drug of choice in patients who choose antithyroid drug therapy for GD, except during the first trimester of pregnancy when propylthiouracil is preferred. Methimazole is administered once a day, and is associated with a reduced risk of major side effects such as agranulocytosis and hepatic injury compared to propylthiouracil (PTU). Patients need a baseline complete blood count, including white count with differential, and a liver profile including bilirubin and transaminases before starting antithyroid drug therapy for GD.

β-adrenergic blockade should be given to elderly patients with symptomatic thyrotoxicosis and to other thyrotoxic patients with resting heart rates of >90 bpm or coexistent cardiovascular if there are no relative contraindications such as bronchospasm.

C. Surgical Intervention

Surgery is reserved for patients in whom medication and radioactive iodine ablation are not acceptable treatment strategies or in whom a large goiter is present that compresses nearby structures or is disfiguring.

D. Treatment of Thyroid Storm

For patients with thyroid storm, aggressive initial therapy is essential to prevent complications. Treatment should include the administration of high doses of PTU (100 mg every 6 hours) to quickly block thyroid release and reduce peripheral conversion of T_4 to T_3. In addition, high doses of β-blockers (propranolol, 1–5 mg intravenously or 20–80 mg orally every 4 hours) can be used to control tachycardia and other peripheral symptoms of thyrotoxicosis. Hydrocortisone (200–300 mg/d) is used to prevent possible adrenal crisis.

E. Postablation Follow-up

Follow-up is necessary to evaluate possible hypothyroidism postablation. Follow-up can begin 6 weeks after therapy and continue on a regular basis until there is evidence of early hypothyroidism, as confirmed by an elevated TSH level. Therapy should then be started as described earlier in the discussion of hypothyroidism.

American Association of Clinical Endocrinologists and American Thyroid Association. Hyperthyroidism and other causes of thyrotoxicosis. *Endocr Practice.* 2011;17:456–520.
Cappola A, et al. Thyroid status, cardiovascular risk, and mortality in older adults. *JAMA.* 2006;295:1033–1041. [PMID: 16507804]

THYROID NODULES

General Considerations

Thyroid nodules are a common clinical finding, reported in 37% of patients on the basis of palpation. The prevalence of diagnosed thyroid nodules has increased dramatically since the early 1990s because of the widespread use of ultrasonography for the evaluation of thyroid and nonthyroid neck conditions. Autopsy data indicate that thyroid nodules may be present in 50% of the population. Thyroid nodules are more common in women, the elderly, patients with a history of head and neck irradiation, and those with a history of iodine deficiency.

Pathogenesis

Thyroid nodules may be associated with benign or malignant conditions. Benign causes include multinodular goiter, Hashimoto thyroiditis, simple or hemorrhagic cysts, follicular adenomas, and subacute thyroiditis. Malignant causes include carcinoma (papillary, follicular, Hürthle cell, medullary, or anaplastic), primary thyroid lymphoma, and metastatic malignant lesion.

Clinical Findings

A. Symptoms and Signs

Many patients with thyroid nodules are asymptomatic. Often the nodule is discovered incidentally on physical examination or by imaging studies ordered for unrelated reasons. Evaluation is needed to rule out malignancy. A thorough history should be obtained, including any history of benign or malignant thyroid disease (see sections on hyper- and hypothyroidism, earlier) and head or neck irradiation. Patients should be asked about recent pregnancy, characteristics of the nodule, and any neck symptoms (eg, pain, rate of swelling, hoarseness, swelling of lymph nodes).

Several features of the history are associated with an increased risk of malignancy in a thyroid nodule. These include prior head and neck irradiation, family history of medullary carcinoma or multiple endocrine neoplasia syndrome type 2, age <20 years or >70 years, male gender, and rapid growth of a nodule. Physical findings that should raise clinical suspicion of malignancy include firm consistency, cervical adenopathy, and symptoms such as persistent hoarseness, dysphonia, dysphagia, or dyspnea.

B. Laboratory and Diagnostic Findings

Laboratory and diagnostic evaluation relies on ultrasound, measurement of TSH level, and fine-needle aspiration (FNA). Ultrasound is not useful as a universal screening tool but can be helpful in screening patients whose history places them at high risk for developing thyroid cancer (see section on symptoms and signs, earlier).

1. Workup of a palpable thyroid nodule—If the nodule is palpable, TSH assay and ultrasonography of the thyroid should be performed. These two modalities will help guide clinical decision making. If the nodule appears suspicious on ultrasound (on the basis of position, shape, size, margins, or echogenic pattern), FNA should be performed irrespective of whether the patient's TSH level is elevated, normal, or suppressed. For instance, it has been reported that nodules in patients with Graves disease may be malignant in 9% of the cases. If the nodule does not appear suspicious on ultrasound, the clinician can proceed with workup of the abnormal TSH level. For example, if the TSH level is suppressed, the patient may have hyperthyroidism caused by either a single autonomous nodule or a multinodular goiter. The patient would then be evaluated for hyperthyroidism and therapy initiated, as appropriate.

In patients with an elevated TSH level suggestive of hypothyroidism, the next steps would be based on the ultrasound findings. If the nodule does not appear suspicious, thyroid

peroxidase antibodies (useful for diagnosing Hashimoto thyroiditis) can be measured and treatment of hypothyroidism initiated (ie, using levothyroxine therapy). If the nodule appears suspicious, FNA should be performed.

2. Workup of an "incidental" thyroid nodule—If the thyroid nodule is found incidentally by ultrasonography, the next step is to obtain a TSH level. If the TSH level is normal, the nodule is <10 mm, the patient does not have risk factors for thyroid malignancy, and the ultrasound findings do not appear suspicious, clinical follow-up is performed. If the nodule is >10 mm or the patient has risk factors for thyroid malignancy, FNA should be performed.

Approximately 70% of FNA specimens are classified as benign, 5% are malignant, 10% are suspicious, and 10–20% are nondiagnostic. If FNA reveals malignant cells, surgical intervention is indicated and further treatment will be based on the characteristics noted at surgery (pathologic findings, positive lymph nodes, etc).

Treatment

Patients with malignant thyroid nodules should be referred to surgical and medical oncologists familiar with the management of these tumors. The remainder of this discussion focuses on follow-up and management of patients with FNA-negative thyroid nodules.

Use of exogenous levothyroxine therapy in a euthyroid patient in an effort to "suppress the TSH" (ie, decrease TSH level to <0.1 IU/mL) and "shrink" the nodule is of benefit in only a few patients with palpable nodules. The side effects of exogenous thyroid therapy (cardiac arrhythmias, osteoporosis, etc) must be considered, especially in older patients and in postmenopausal women; its use in these populations is thus relatively contraindicated.

Patients with very large nodules may require surgery, especially if symptoms secondary to the size (eg, dysphagia) are present. If there is a change in size of the nodule, a repeat FNA should be performed.

Ultrasound-guided percutaneous ethanol injection (PEI) is a therapeutic option for patients with benign nodules that have a large fluid component (thyroid cysts). Aspiration (eg, during FNA) itself may drain a cyst and shrink the size, but recurrences are common. Surgery is sometimes needed if the cyst is very large. Some data show that PEI is more effective in decreasing the size of a nodule than aspiration alone.

AACE/AME Task Force on Thyroid Nodules. American Association of Clinical Endocrinologists and Associazione Medici Endocriniologi guidelines for clinical practice for the diagnosis and management of thyroid nodules. *Endocr Practice*. 2006;12:63 [updated *Endocr Practice*. 2010;16 (Suppl 1)].

Bilezikian JP, et al. Guidelines for the management of asymptomatic primary hyperparathyroidism: summary statement from the third international workshop. *J Clin Endocrinol Metab*. 2009; 94(2):335–339.

Regalbuto C, Frasca F, Pellegriti G, et al. Update on thyroid cancer treatment. *Future Oncol.* 2012;8(10):1331–1348.

Sebo T. What are the keys to successful thyroid FNA interpretation? *Clin Endocrinol.* 2012;77(1):13–17.

▼ ADRENAL DISORDERS

ADRENAL INSUFFICIENCY

▶ General Considerations

The most common cause of primary adrenal insufficiency is autoimmune adrenalitis (Addison disease). Other possible causes include AIDS and the antiphospholipid syndrome. Secondary adrenal insufficiency may result from pituitary or hypothalamic disease. Iatrogenic tertiary adrenal insufficiency caused by suppression of hypothalamic-pituitary-adrenal function secondary to glucocorticoid administration is a more common secondary cause of adrenal insufficiency (**Table 37-3**).

▶ Clinical Findings

A. Symptoms and Signs

Adrenal insufficiency presents with a wide range of symptoms and signs, including weakness, malaise, anorexia, hyperpigmentation (especially of the gingival mucosa, scars, and skin creases), vitiligo, postural hypotension, abdominal pain, nausea and vomiting, diarrhea, constipation, myalgia, and arthralgia. The most specific sign of primary adrenal insufficiency is hyperpigmentation of the skin and mucosal surfaces. Another specific symptom of adrenal insufficiency is a craving for salt. Autoimmune adrenal disease can be accompanied by other autoimmune endocrine deficiencies, such as thyroid disease, diabetes mellitus, pernicious anemia, hypoparathyroidism, and ovarian failure.

In acute adrenal failure, adrenal crisis occurs. Adrenal crisis is characterized by hypotension, bradycardia, fever, hypoglycemia, and a progressive deterioration in mental status. Abdominal pain, vomiting, and diarrhea also may be present. In the patient with spontaneous adrenal insufficiency, acute adrenal hemorrhage and adrenal-vein thrombosis should be considered.

B. Laboratory Findings

Laboratory abnormalities occur in nearly all patients and include hyponatremia, hyperkalemia, acidosis, slightly elevated plasma creatinine concentrations, hypoglycemia, hypercalcemia, mild normocytic anemia, lymphocytosis, and mild eosinophilia. The diagnosis of adrenal insufficiency relies on a finding of inadequate cortisol production. Plasma cortisol concentration fluctuates throughout the day in a diurnal pattern that is normally high in the early morning and low in the late afternoon. Cortisol levels also increase with stress. A low plasma cortisol level of <3 μ/dL (<83 nmol/L) either in the morning or at a time of stress provides presumptive evidence of adrenal insufficiency. Conversely, a level of ≥20 μg/dL (≥550 nmol/L) rules out adrenal insufficiency. An intermediate plasma cortisol level of 3–19 μg/dL (83–525 nmol/L) is not diagnostic.

For most patients in whom adrenal insufficiency is considered, a short adrenocorticotropic hormone (ACTH) stimulation test should be performed. In this test, a low dose of ACTH (1 g or 0.5 g/1.73 m² surface area) is given and the patient's blood is tested 30 and 60 minutes later to confirm a corresponding increase in plasma cortisol. A rise in plasma cortisol concentration after 30 or 60 minutes to a peak of ≥20 μg/dL (≥55 nmol/L) is considered normal. No increase in serum cortisol or a blunted response after ACTH administration confirms adrenal insufficiency. If the test is slightly abnormal, an insulin or a metyrapone test using 30 mg/kg of metyrapone with a snack at midnight should be performed.

C. Imaging Studies

In patients with adrenal insufficiency, radiologic studies may be indicated. In patients having headaches and visual disturbances, a magnetic resonance imaging (MRI) scan should be performed to investigate for a possible pituitary or hypothalamic tumor. In patients with suspected primary

Table 37-3. Causes of adrenal insufficiency.

Primary
Autoimmune adrenalitis
Tuberculosis
Adrenomyeloneuropathy
Systemic fungal infections
AIDS
Metastatic carcinoma
Isolated glucocorticoid deficiency
Adrenal hemorrhage, necrosis, or thrombosis
Secondary
Pituitary or metastatic tumor
Craniopharyngioma
Pituitary surgery or radiation
Lymphocytic hypophysitis
Sarcoidosis
Histiocytosis
Empty-sella syndrome
Hypothalamic tumors
Long-term glucocorticoid therapy
Postpartum pituitary necrosis (Sheehan syndrome)
Necrosis or bleeding into pituitary macroadenoma
Head trauma, lesions of the pituitary stalk
Pituitary or adrenal surgery for Cushing syndrome

Reproduced, with permission, from Oelkers W. Adrenal insufficiency. *N Engl J Med.* 1996;335:1206.

adrenal insufficiency, a computed tomography (CT) scan of the adrenal glands should be performed to rule out hemorrhage, adrenal vein thrombosis, or metastatic disease as the cause of the adrenal dysfunction.

Treatment

For patients with symptomatic adrenal insufficiency, fluid management, correction of other metabolic abnormalities such as hypoglycemia and hyperkalemia, and the administration of corticosteroids are primary concerns. An approach to managing this condition is shown in **Table 37-4.**

While providing fluid resuscitation and addressing other metabolic emergencies, the practitioner should administer emergency doses of hydrocortisone. Once the patient is stabilized, corticosteroid maintenance should be provided in divided doses early in the morning and afternoon to simulate the diurnal release of cortisol by the adrenal gland. The smallest dose that relieves the patient's symptoms should be used to minimize weight gain and risk of osteoporosis. During febrile illnesses, acute injury, or other periods of physiologic stress, the dose of hydrocortisone should be doubled or tripled temporarily. Patients with primary adrenal insufficiency should also receive fludrocortisone as a substitute for aldosterone.

August GP. Treatment of adrenocortical insufficiency. *Pediatr Rev.* 1997;18:59. [PMID: 9029933]
Malchoff CD, Carey RM. Adrenal insufficiency. *Curr Ther Endocrinol Metab.* 1997;6:142. [PMID: 9174724]

Ten S, New M, Maclaren N. Addison's disease 2001. *J Clin Endocrinol Metab.* 2001;86: 2909–2922.

CUSHING SYNDROME

General Considerations

Cushing syndrome refers to overproduction of cortisol due to any cause (eg, adrenal hyperplasia, exogenous steroid use). *Cushing disease* is a more specific term that refers to excessive cortisol resulting from excessive ACTH produced by pituitary corticotrophic tumors. ACTH-producing tumors account for 80% of cases of Cushing syndrome. The remaining 20% are caused by adrenal tumors, such as adenomas, carcinomas, and micronodular and macronodular hyperplasia, associated with autonomous production of glucocorticoids.

Cushing syndrome is rare, with a prevalence estimated at approximately 10 per 1 million persons. Cushing disease is 4–6 times more prevalent in women than in men, whereas ectopic ACTH secretion is more common in men, largely due to the higher incidence in men of bronchogenic lung cancers that produce ACTH.

Clinical Findings

A. Symptoms and Signs

The most common signs of Cushing syndrome are sudden onset of central weight gain, often accompanied by thickening of the facial fat, which rounds the facial contour ("moon facies"), and a florid complexion due to telangiectasia. Other

Table 37-4. Approach to treating acute adrenal insufficiency.

1. Stabilize blood pressure and replace fluids	Administer bolus with normal saline (500 mL/m^2) over 1 hour, then adequate fluids to maintain sufficient urine output
2. Correct other metabolic problems a. Hypoglycemia b. Hyperkalemia	 Give 25% glucose if hypoglycemia Treat with polystyrene sulfonate (Kayexalate) oral suspension every 3–4 hours; give 10% calcium gluconate for dangerously high potassium levels, monitoring heart rate for bradycardia
3. Emergency corticosteroid replacement therapy a. Hydrocortisone	 Adults: 100 mg bolus dose followed by infusion of 100–200 mg/24 hours Children: 25–50 mg/m^2 per 24 hour-period
4. Chronic corticosteroid replacement a. Hydrocortisone b. Cortisone	 Adults: 25 mg (divided into doses of 15 and 10 mg) Children: 25 mg/m^2 daily in 3 divided doses Adults: 37.5 mg (divided into doses of 25 and 12.5 mg) Children: 32 mg/m^2 daily TID
5. Evaluate for mineralocorticoid deficiency and replace if needed a. Fludrocortisone (substitute for aldosterone)	 Adults: 50–200 μg (single daily dose) Children: 50–150 μg (single daily dose)

Adapted, with permission, from August GP. Treatment of adrenocortical insufficiency. *Pediatr Rev.* 1997; 18:59.

Table 37-5. Clinical symptoms and signs of Cushing syndrome.

General
Central obesity
Proximal muscle weakness
Hypertension
Headaches
Psychiatric disorders
Skin
Wide (>1 cm), purple striae
Spontaneous ecchymoses
Facial plethora
Hyperpigmentation
Acne
Hirsutism
Fungal skin infections
Endocrine and metabolic derangements
Hypokalemic alkalosis
Osteopenia
Delayed bone age in children
Menstrual disorders, decreased libido, impotence
Glucose intolerence, diabetes mellitus
Kidney stones
Polyuria
Elevated white blood cell count

Data from Meier CA, Biller BM. Clinical and biochemical evaluation of Cushing's syndrome. *Endocrinol Metab Clin North Am.* 1997; 26:741.

concomitant signs include an enlarged fat pad ("buffalo hump"), hypertension, glucose intolerance, oligomenorrhea or amenorrhea in premenopausal women, decreased libido in men, and spontaneous ecchymoses (**Table 37-5**).

B. Laboratory Findings

The evaluation of suspected excessive glucocorticoid production includes screening and confirmatory tests for the diagnosis and localization of the source of hormone excess. The Endocrine Society recommends the initial use of one test with high diagnostic accuracy (urine cortisol, late-night salivary cortisol, 1 mg overnight, or 2 mg 48-hour dexamethasone suppression test). Those patients with an abnormal result should undergo a second test, either one of the above or, in some cases, a serum midnight cortisol or dexamethasone-CRH test.

Affective psychiatric disorders (eg, major depression) and alcoholism can be associated with the biochemical features of Cushing syndrome and, therefore, may decrease the reliability of test results.

C. Imaging Studies

Following confirmation of Cushing syndrome, imaging studies should be performed to look for adenomas (MRI scan) or adrenal tumors (CT scan). If both of these studies are negative, chest radiography or CT scanning should be performed to look for ectopic sources of ACTH production.

▶ Treatment

For patients with a pituitary adenoma (Cushing disease) in whom a circumscribed microadenoma can be identified and resected, the treatment of choice is transsphenoidal microadenomectomy. If an adenoma cannot be clearly identified, patients should undergo a subtotal (85–90%) resection of the anterior pituitary gland. Patients who wish to preserve pituitary function (ie, in order to have children) should be treated with pituitary irradiation. If radiation does not decrease exogenous ACTH production, bilateral total adrenalectomy is a final treatment option. For adult patients not cured by transsphenoidal surgery, pituitary irradiation is the most appropriate choice for the next treatment.

Patients who have a nonpituitary tumor that secretes ACTH are cured by resection of the tumor. Unfortunately, nonpituitary tumors that secrete ACTH are seldom amenable to resection. In these cases, cortisol excess can be controlled with adrenal enzyme inhibitors, alone or in combination, with the proper dose determined by measurements of plasma and urinary cortisol.

For patients with adrenal hyperplasia, bilateral total adrenalectomy is required. Patients with an adrenal adenoma or carcinoma can be managed with unilateral adrenalectomy. Patients with hyperplasia or adenomas almost invariably have recurrences that are not amenable to either radiation or chemotherapy.

Patients who are taking corticosteroids for prolonged periods of time may exhibit signs or symptoms of Cushing syndrome. Once the primary problem for which steroids are being prescribed is controlled, patients should be withdrawn from their corticosteroid treatment slowly to avoid symptoms from adrenal suppression. There are few studies evaluating methods of withdrawal from chronic steroid use, however. Clinicians should be guided by the severity of the underlying condition, the duration that steroids have been used, and the dosage of steroids in determining how quickly dosages of steroids should be reduced.

Endocrine Society. Diagnosis of Cushing's syndrome. *J Clin Endocrinol Metab.* 2008; 93(5):1526–1540.
Newell-Price J, et al. Cushing's syndrome. *Lancet.* 2006;367:1605. [PMID: 16698415]
Nieman LK, Ilias I. Evaluation and treatment of Cushing's syndrome. *Am J Med.* 2005;118:1340. [PMID: 16378774]

HYPERALDOSTERONISM

▶ General Considerations

Primary hyperaldosteronism accounts for 70–80% of all cases of hyperaldosteronism and is usually caused by a solitary unilateral adrenal adenoma. Other causes of hyperaldosteronism include bilateral adrenal hyperplasia, so-called idiopathic hyperaldosteronism, and glucocorticoid-remediable hyperaldosteronism. Adrenal carcinoma and unilateral adrenal hyperplasia are rare causes.

▶ Clinical Findings

A. Symptoms and Signs

Patients with hyperaldosteronism present with hypertension and hypokalemia. Other complaints include headaches, muscular weakness or flaccid paralysis caused by hypokalemia, or polyuria. Inappropriate hypersecretion of aldosterone is an uncommon cause of hypertension, accounting for <1% of cases. Any patient presenting with hypertension and unprovoked hypokalemia should be considered for the evaluation of hyperaldosteronism. Hypertension may be severe, although malignant hypertension is rare. The peak incidence occurs between 30 and 50 years of age, and most patients are women.

B. Laboratory Findings

Initially, laboratory evaluation is used to document hyperaldosteronemia and suppressed renin activity. Further diagnostic tests, including imaging procedures, are used to determine whether the etiology is amenable to surgical intervention or requires medical management.

Screening aldosterone measurements can be performed on plasma or 24-hour urine collection. Plasma aldosterone is usually measured after 4 hours of upright posture. Plasma renin activity should be measured in the same sample. A ratio of plasma aldosterone concentration to plasma renin activity of >20:25 is very suspicious for hyperaldosteronism.

In the hypertensive patient with hypokalemia or kaliuresis or with an elevated plasma aldosterone/renin ratio, the diagnosis of hyperaldosteronism is confirmed by demonstrating failure of normal suppression of plasma aldosterone. Urine aldosterone excretion of >30 nmol (>14 μg)/d after oral sodium loading over 3 days establishes the diagnosis.

The intravenous saline suppression test is also widely used to confirm hyperaldosteronism. In this test, isotonic saline is infused intravenously at a rate of 300–500 mL/h for 4 hours, after which plasma aldosterone and renin activity are measured. Aldosterone levels normally fall to <0.28 nmol/L (<10 ng/dL), and renin activity is suppressed. Failure to suppress normally identifies patients with aldosterone-producing adenomas, because most patients with secondary forms of hyperaldosteronism suppress normally. False-negative results are most often seen in patients with bilateral hyperplasia.

Once the diagnosis is established, it is necessary to distinguish between aldosterone-producing adrenal adenoma and bilateral adrenal hyperplasia. A widely used test is based on the less complete suppression of renin activity in

hyperaldosteronism caused by bilateral hyperplasia. Plasma renin activity rises slightly and aldosterone concentration increases significantly after the stimulation of 2–4 hours of upright posturing in these patients. In contrast, renin remains suppressed and aldosterone does not rise in patients with adenomas, in whom plasma aldosterone level may fall.

C. Imaging Studies

Imaging procedures can assist in differentiating causes of hyperaldosteronism and lateralizing adenomas. The diagnostic accuracy of high-resolution CT scans is only ~70% for aldosterone-producing adenomas, largely because of the occurrence of nonfunctioning adenomas. MRI is no better than CT in differentiating aldosterone-secreting tumors from other adrenal tumors. Scintigraphic imaging with ^{131}I-labeled cholesterol derivatives during dexamethasone suppression provides an image based on functional properties of the adrenal gland. Asymmetric uptake after 48 hours indicates an adenoma, whereas symmetric uptake after 72 hours indicates bilateral hyperplasia. Diagnostic accuracy is 72%. However, if the adrenal CT scan is normal, iodocholesterol scanning is unlikely to be helpful.

▶ Treatment

For adrenal adenoma, total unilateral adrenalectomy is the treatment of choice and provides a cure in most cases. Although some patients with primary bilateral hyperplasia may benefit from subtotal adrenalectomy, these patients cannot be accurately identified preoperatively. Following surgery, the electrolyte imbalances usually correct rapidly, whereas blood pressure control may take several weeks to months.

Medical therapy is indicated for most patients with bilateral adrenal hyperplasia or for patients with adrenal adenomas who are unable to undergo adrenalectomy. Spironolactone controls the hyperkalemia, although it is not a very potent antihypertensive agent. Amiloride and calcium channel blockers are often used to control blood pressure.

Bravo EL. Primary aldosteronism. Issues in diagnosis and management. *Endocrinol Metab Clin North Am.* 1994;23:271. [PMID: 8070422]

Endocrine Society. Endocrine Society clinical practice guideline, case detection, diagnosis and treatment of patients with primary aldosteronism. *J Clin Endocrinol Metab.* 2008;93(9):3266–3281.

▼ PARATHYROID DISORDERS

HYPERPARATHYROIDISM

▶ General Considerations

Hyperparathyroidism refers to excessive production of parathyroid hormone (PTH). *Primary* hyperparathyroidism is the overproduction of PTH in an inappropriate fashion, usually resulting in hypercalcemia. Primary hyperparathyroidism is more common in postmenopausal women. The most common cause is a benign solitary parathyroid adenoma (80% of all cases). Another 15% of patients have diffuse hyperplasia of the parathyroid glands, a condition that tends to be familial. Carcinoma of the parathyroid occurs in <1% of cases.

In secondary hyperparathyroidism, patients have appropriate additional production of PTH because of hypocalcemia related to other metabolic conditions such as renal failure, calcium absorption problems, or vitamin D deficiency.

Clinical Findings

A. Symptoms and Signs

Most patients have nonspecific complaints that may include aches and pains, constipation, muscle fatigue, generalized weakness, psychiatric disturbances, polydipsia, and polyuria. The hypercalcemia can cause nausea and vomiting, thirst, and anorexia. A history of peptic ulcer disease or hypertension may be present, as well as accompanying constipation, anemia, and weight loss. Precipitation of calcium in the corneas may produce a band keratopathy, and patients may also experience recurrent pancreatitis. Finally, skeletal problems can result in pathologic fractures.

B. Laboratory Findings

Hypercalcemia (serum calcium level >10.5 mg/dL when corrected for serum albumin level) is the most important clue to the diagnosis. In patients who have an elevated calcium level with no apparent cause, serum PTH should be determined using a two-site immunometric assay. An elevated PTH level in the presence of hypercalcemia confirms the diagnosis of primary hyperparathyroidism.

Other findings may include a low serum phosphate level (<2.5 mg/dL) with excessive phosphaturia. Urine calcium excretion may be high or normal. Alkaline phosphatase levels are elevated only in the presence of bone disease, and elevated plasma chloride and uric acid levels may be seen.

C. Imaging Studies

With chronic hyperparathyroidism, diffuse bone demineralization, loss of the dental lamina dura, and subperiosteal resorption of bone (particularly in the radial aspects of the fingers) may be apparent on x-rays. Cysts may be noted throughout the skeleton, and "salt-and-pepper" appearance of the skull may be seen. Pathologic fractures can occur, and renal calculi and soft-tissue calcification may be visualized.

Imaging studies are usually reserved for patients with resistant or recurrent disease. In these cases, ultrasonography, CT scanning, MRI, and thallium-201–technetium-99m (^{201}Tl–^{99m}Tc) scanning may help locate ectopic parathyroid tissue.

Treatment

Treatment of severe hypercalcemia and parathyroidectomy are the mainstays for therapy. When hypercalcemia is severe, treatment includes aggressive hydration. Correction of any underlying hyponatremia and hypokalemia should be initiated, along with administration of a loop diuretic to accelerate calcium clearance. Other medications that can be effective in reducing hypercalcemia include etidronate, plicamycin, and calcitonin. Any medications or other products that increase calcium levels, such as estrogens, thiazides, vitamins A and D, and milk, should be avoided.

In addition to management of acute hypercalcemia, surgical removal of parathyroid tissue should be undertaken. Surgical resection provides the most rapid and effective method of reducing serum calcium in these patients. Hyperplasia of all glands requires removal of three glands along with subtotal resection of the fourth. Surgical success is directly related to the experience and expertise of the operating surgeon.

For mild cases and poor surgical candidates, conservative therapy with adequate hydration and long-term pharmacologic therapy is recommended. Patients should avoid drugs and products that elevate calcium and should have their serum calcium monitored closely.

American Association of Clinical Endocrinologists and American Association of Endocrine Surgeons. Position statement on the diagnosis and management of hyperparathyroidism. *Endocr Practice.* 2005;11:49–54.

HYPOPARATHYROIDISM

General Considerations

Hypoparathyroidism results from underproduction of PTH. The most common cause is the removal of the parathyroid glands during a thyroidectomy or following surgery for primary hyperparathyroidism. Less commonly, hypoparathyroidism is idiopathic, familial, or the result of a congenital absence of the parathyroid glands (DiGeorge syndrome). Patients with idiopathic hypoparathyroidism often have antibodies against parathyroid and other tissues, and an autoimmune component may play a role. Other unusual causes of hypoparathyroidism include previous neck irradiation, magnesium deficiency, metastatic cancer, and infiltrative diseases.

Clinical Findings

A. Symptoms and Signs

The lack of PTH results in hypocalcemia, which produces most of the symptoms associated with hypoparathyroidism. Symptoms associated with hypocalcemia include tetany, carpopedal spasms, paresthesias of the lips and hands, and a positive Chvostek sign or Trousseau sign. Patients may also exhibit less specific symptoms such as anxiety, depression, or fatigue. Additionally, hyperventilation, respiratory alkalosis with or without respiratory compromise, laryngospasm, hypotension, and seizures may occur with severe hypocalcemia.

B. Laboratory Findings

On laboratory evaluation, patients with hypoparathyroidism have low serum calcium and elevated serum phosphate levels, with a normal alkaline phosphatase level. Urinary levels of calcium and phosphate are decreased. The key finding is a low to absent PTH value.

▶ Treatment

Acute hypocalcemia with tetany requires aggressive therapy with multiple drugs. Therapy should be started with calcium gluconate administered intravenously in a 10% solution. The infusion is given slowly until tetany resolves. Oral calcium along with vitamin D supplementation should be given after the acute crisis has resolved. Hypomagnesemia should be corrected with intravenous magnesium sulfate administered at a dose of 1–2 g every 6 hours. Chronic replacement of magnesium can be accomplished using 600-mg magnesium oxide tablets once or twice daily.

For the maintenance of normal calcium, vitamin D supplementation along with oral calcium should be given. Calcium in the form of calcium carbonate (40% elemental calcium) is the drug of choice, administered in a dose of 1–2 g of calcium per day. Serial calcium levels should be obtained regularly (every 3–6 months), and "spot" urine calcium levels should be maintained below 30 mg/dL.

Acute Musculoskeletal Complaints

38

Jeanne Doperak, DO
Kelley Anderson, DO

ROTATOR CUFF IMPINGEMENT

ESSENTIALS OF DIAGNOSIS

- ▶ Anterior shoulder pain that is often atraumatic.
- ▶ Discomfort frequently worse with repetitive or overhead activities.
- ▶ Strength often maintained on exam.

▶ General Considerations

The term subacromial *impingement syndrome* defines any entity that compromises the subacromial space and irritates the enclosed rotator cuff tendons. It is not clearly or consistently defined and may represent a variety of disorders from subacromial bursitis to calcific tendinosis. Often these entities arise in a similar fashion and may be difficult to differentiate. Diagnosis is based on a meticulous history and physical exam and appropriate imaging.

▶ Clinical Findings

A. Symptoms and Signs

Diagnosis of subacromial impingement is primarily clinical. The patient complains of dull shoulder pain of insidious onset over weeks to months. Less often, these symptoms arise following trauma. Pain is typically localized to the anterolateral acromion and radiates to the lateral deltoid. Pain is often aggravated by repetitive overhead activities, such as a carpenter swinging a hammer or a baseball player throwing a ball. Individuals often complain of pain when

they roll onto the shoulder at night and will awaken with symptoms if the arm is positioned over the head.

Physical exam usually reveals normal range of motion, although the patient may experience pain on reaching the maximum forward flexion and abduction. Muscular weakness can be seen but is often secondary to pain and not secondary to loss of function. In other words, a patient who is coached to try to resist on manual muscle testing despite pain will often exhibit near-full strength. The maintenance of strength can help differentiate between inflammation and a high-grade cuff tear.

B. Imaging Studies

Radiographs that may aid in diagnosis include anteroposterior (AP), outlet, and axillary views of the affected shoulder. The outlet view provides visualization of acromial morphology exhibiting curvature or spurs that may contribute to the underlying pathology. Plain films may also provide evidence of tendon calcification, underlying degenerative disease, and cystic changes in the humeral head. MRI can confirm the diagnosis but seldom changes the treatment plan.

C. Special Tests

Provocative testing includes the Neer test and the Hawkins test. The Neer test involves passive elevation of an internally rotated, forward-flexed arm. In the Hawkins test the arm is positioned in 90° of forward flexion and is internally rotated with a bent elbow. These motions cause "impingement" of the supraspinatous tendon against the acromion. Pain with either maneuver is considered a positive test; however, these tests may also be positive in patients with other pathology.

▶ Differential Diagnosis

Differential diagnosis includes acromioclavicular joint arthritis, rotator cuff tear, glenohumeral instability, arthritis, supraspinatus nerve entrapment, and cervical disk disease.

Treatment

Nonsurgical management of shoulder impingement continues to be successful in most patients. Evidence supports early initiation of physical therapy aimed at eccentric strengthening of the shoulder complex, including the scapular stabilizers for restoration of function and improvement of symptoms. A subacromial steroid injection can be used to help control pain initially if discomfort is a barrier to starting manual exercise therapy. Addition of NSAIDs can aid in pain control when necessary. Modification of offending activities may be needed for a period of time; for instance, swimmers may need a kickboard in the pool, or a pitcher may need to modify pitch counts. Surgical intervention is considered only after failure of conservative treatment.

Crawshaw DP, Helliwell PS, Hensor EMA, et al. Exercise therapy after corticosteroid injection for moderate to severe shoulder pain: large pragmatic randomized trial. *Br Med J.* 2010; 340:c3037.

Harrison AK, Flatow EL. Subacromial impingement syndrome. *J Am Acad Orthop Surg.* 2011; 19(11):701–708.

Holmgren T, Hallgren HB, Oberg B, Adolfsson L, Johnson K. Effect of specific exercise strategy on need for surgery in patients with subacromial impingement syndrome: randomized controlled study. *Br Med J.* 2012; 344:e787.

Papadonikolakis A, McKenna M, Warme W, Martin BI, Matsen FA. Published evidence relevant to the diagnosis of impingement syndrome of the shoulder. *J Bone Joint Surg Am.* 2011; 93:1827–1832.

ROTATOR CUFF TEARS

ESSENTIALS OF DIAGNOSIS

▶ Frequently traumatic shoulder pain in a middle-aged individual.

▶ Significant loss of function in affected arm especially overhead.

▶ Pain often radiates to lateral deltoid.

▶ Rare in young athletes.

General Considerations

Rotator cuff tears are often patients' perceived source of shoulder pain. In reality, this pathology is exceedingly rare in young athletes and often asymptomatic in older adults with several studies illustrating cuff tears in >50% of individuals aged >60 years. This epidemiology leads to challenges in treatment plans that are often individualized.

The rotator cuff complex contains four muscles (the SITS muscles): the subscapularis, infraspinatous, teres minor, and supraspinatus. Biomechanically the cuff assists in abduction and internal and external rotation of the humerus, and together the muscles facilitate stabilization of the humeral head in the glenoid. Disruption of any part of this complex can result in shoulder dysfunction and pain.

Clinical Findings

A. Signs and Symptoms

Many rotator cuff tears are asymptomatic, especially in older individuals. If symptoms are present, a careful history will often reveal a single event such as a fall onto an outstretched arm or picking up a large bag, resulting in an audible pop and sudden pain. This pain is often located in the front of the shoulder or over the lateral deltoid. Weakness and stiffness are frequently described, especially with overhead motion or internal rotation of shoulder. Patients will complain of difficulty brushing their hair or fastening a bra strap and/or seat belt.

Careful examination may demonstrate subtle atrophy of the shoulder musculature, which suggests a chronic problem. Patients will have limitations in active range of motion and pain as the arm is raised over 90° in flexion, in abduction, and sometimes in internal rotation when the subscapularis tendon is involved. The affected arm can be passively taken through a full range of motion suggesting an extraarticular process. Manual muscle testing will typically display pronounced weakness in the plane of the torn tendon.

B. Imaging Studies

Plain films can be useful to rule out other causes of shoulder pain such as osteoarthritis or fracture. Changes seen on plain films that may be consistent with rotator cuff tears can include loss of space between the humeral head and acromion and cystic changes in the greater tuberosity. Ultrasound can diagnose a rotator cuff tear if performed and read by an experienced individual, but the MRI arthrogram is considered the gold standard in the diagnostic imaging of rotator cuff disease. The injection of dye at the time of MRI increases the sensitivity and specificity of the test significantly.

C. Special Tests

Testing for the most commonly torn rotator cuff tendon, the supraspinatus, includes the empty-can test. The examiner positions the patient's arm in 70° abduction, 30° forward flexion, and internally rotates it so that the thumb points down (as if emptying a held can). The examiner then pushes down against resistance. Pain and weakness are considered a positive test.

The lift-off test evaluates the subscapularis. The patient rotates the arm behind the back at approximately the midlumbar level and attempts to push the examiner's hand away from the back. As with the empty-can test, weakness and pain indicate a positive test.

Treatment

Treatment focuses on eliminating pain and restoring function. In light of the age-related epidemiologic data presented earlier, treatment is not a one-size-fits-all algorithm. If a rotator cuff tear has been confirmed in an individual aged <60 years, in most all cases, a timely referral to an orthopedic surgeon should be made.

In contrast, older, less active individuals should pursue surgical options only as a last resort. Initial treatment for most of those aged >60 years should include physical therapy, anti-inflammatories, and perhaps a corticosteroid injection. The challenge is that in an increasingly active aging population, more individuals may need to be considered for surgical consultation if unable to restore preinjury function. This becomes the "art of medicine," and as primary care providers, highlights the importance of knowing your patients and their pre- and postinjury expectations.

Longo UG, Berton A, Ahrens PM, Maffulli N, Denaro V. Clinical tests for the diagnosis of rotator cuff disease. *Sports Med Arthrosc Rev.* 2011; 19(3):266–278.

Pergreffi F, Paladini P, Campi F, Porcellini G. Conservative management of rotator cuff tear. *Sports Med Arthrosc Rev.* 2011; 19(4):348–353.

Seida JC, LeBlanc C, Schouten JR, et al. Systematic review: non-operative and operative treatments for rotator cuff tears. *Ann Intern Med.* 2010; 153(4):246–256.

ACROMIOCLAVICULAR JOINT SPRAIN

ESSENTIALS OF DIAGNOSIS

▶ Pain and deformity over top of shoulder.

▶ Pain usually occurs after a fall onto the lateral shoulder with patient's arm at the side.

General Considerations

The acromioclavicular (AC) joint is the articulation between the distal clavicle and scapula. This is a common injury in young active individuals after a fall onto the lateral aspect of their shoulder with the arm at the side. Classification of the injury is based on the extent of soft-tissue injury. In type 1 sprain, the joint remains intact and there is no clavicle displacement on shoulder inspection or radiographically. Type 2 injury involves the AC ligaments that are torn. In a type 2 injury the distal clavicle is slightly widened on radiograph but there is no vertical displacement on inspection as the coracoclavicular (CC) ligaments are maintained. Type 3 injury involves both the AC and CC ligaments and results in elevation of the distal clavicle that can be enough to tent the skin. Type 4–6 injuries are extremely rare and always surgical.

Clinical Findings

A. Symptoms and Signs

Patients with AC joint injuries will present with pain that localizes to the top of the shoulder. Based on the extent of injury there may be notable asymmetry when compared to the unaffected side. Pain is often worse with overhead or crossbody shoulder motions. This discomfort will often lead to limited range of motion (RoM) and weakness on exam.

B. Imaging Studies

Plain radiographs are sufficient to view and evaluate the AC joint. The Zanca view is the most accurate. It is helpful to get bilateral Zanca views on the same cassette to compare one side to the other.

C. Special Tests

The cross-arm adduction test evaluates the AC joint. The involved arm is brought across the body in the horizontal plane so that the elbow points forward. Pain at the AC joint in this position is a positive test.

Treatment

Type 1–3 injuries are typically treated nonsurgically. A brief period of sling immobilization for comfort should be followed by early initiation of RoM exercises. NSAIDs may be used for early pain control. Return to play for athletes is based on restoration of strength, motion, and function. Rarely are type 3 injuries surgical, and there is no evidence of any difference in strength at 2-year follow-up when comparing surgical and nonsurgical groups. Type 4–6 injuries should be referred urgently to an orthopedic surgeon.

Bontempo NA, Mazzocca AD. Biomechanics and treatment of acromioclavicular and sternoclavicular joint injuries. *Br J Sports Med.* 2010; 44:361–369.

RUPTURE OF BICEPS TENDON

ESSENTIALS OF DIAGNOSIS

▶ Associated with eccentric load and reported "pop."

▶ Proximal lesion with residual "popeye" muscle deformity.

▶ Distal lesion with elbow swelling and ecchymosis.

General Considerations

The biceps muscle of the arm functions to flex and supinate at the elbow. Injury to the biceps tendons can occur at either the distal attachment at the radial tuberosity or at the proximal attachment where the long head of the biceps tendon inserts at the supraglenoid tubercle. These injuries are both associated with a sudden eccentric load and occur most commonly in middle-aged men. Smoking and corticosteroid use are risk factors.

Clinical Findings

A. Symptoms and Signs

Patients with distal ruptures will present with variable pain patterns. Some individuals complain of anterior shoulder pain, while others will be pain-free. Nearly all distal ruptures will exhibit bunching of the biceps muscle in the distal arm—a "popeye" muscle.

Patients with proximal ruptures will present with pain, swelling, and ecchymosis at the elbow. Often there is weakness with manual muscle testing, and a positive hook test will be present (see special tests, eg, hook test, discussed below).

B. Imaging Studies

Plain radiographs of the shoulder and elbow would be necessary only to rule out concurrent injury. MRI will confirm the diagnosis either proximally or distally.

C. Special Tests

The hook test is performed to evaluate for a distal biceps tendon rupture. The patient actively supinates the flexed elbow. An intact hook test permits the examiner to hook her or his finger under the intact biceps tendon from the lateral side. With an avulsion there is no cordlike structure to palpate or hook. Absence of the tendon is a positive test.

Treatment

A proximal biceps tendon rupture is usually treated nonsurgically with a period of activity modification and physical therapy. Anti-inflammatories can be used for pain control if needed. Patients do not have persistent strength deficits as the short head of the muscle remains attached. Keep in mind that, relative to the location of the tear and mechanism of injury, there may be overlapping pathology (cuff/labral tear) that may need to be considered if the patient does not improve as expected over time.

A distal biceps tendon rupture is nearly always operative as the patient will loose >50% strength with flexion and supination over time. This injury should be referred to an orthopedic surgeon in a timely manner for best results.

Branch GL. Biceps rupture. *Medscape Reference* (available at http://emedicine.medscape.com/article/327119-overview; published Jan. 18, 2012; accessed March 19, 2013).

Wheeless CR III, ed. Distal biceps tendon rupture. In: *Wheeless' Textbook of Orthopaedics* (available at http://www.wheelessonline.com/ortho/distal_biceps_tendon_rupture; published July 27, 2012; accessed March 19, 2013).

SHOULDER INSTABILITY

 ESSENTIALS OF DIAGNOSIS

► Encompasses large continuum of disorders with traumatic, congenital, and biomechanical causes.

► Patient reports feeling of looseness or slipping of shoulder.

► Excessive motion can be subtle to gross with complete disarticulation of the humeral head at the glenoid.

General Considerations

Shoulder instability can be viewed as any condition in which the balance of various stabilizing structures in the shoulder are disrupted, resulting in increased humeral head translation. This excessive motion at the humeral head can be partial as in a subluxation or grossly unstable with complete disarticulation of the humeral head at the glenoid. By far, most complete dislocations are anterior, but they can be posterior and on rare occasions inferior. In younger patients instability can be due to trauma, congenital laxity, weakness, poor biomechanics, or a combination of each of these entities. In older patients instability is most often caused by trauma, specifically falls.

Clinical Findings:

A. Symptoms and Signs

Patients with acute anterior dislocations that have not self-reduced will present with shoulder pain, an unwillingness to move the affected arm and a tendency to cradle the arm. Inspection will reveal a bulge (due to the displaced humeral head) as well as dimpling inferior to the acromion where the humeral head should be.

If a patient is not dislocated at the time of the exam but reports a recent dislocation, the exam usually reveals limited RoM, weakness, and global pain complaints. If the patient has more subtle instability with no true dislocation, the exam will often reveal hypermobility with an increased arc of motion and retained strength. Special tests as described below will help with the diagnosis.

B. Imaging Studies

Radiographs will confirm a shoulder dislocation but will often be normal with more subtle chronic subluxations. AP and outlet views are standard, but an axillary view shows the relationship of the humeral head to the glenoid fossa and is more accurate when assessing for joint congruency. Occasionally a bony defect is seen in the posterolateral portion of the humeral head, called a *Hill-Sachs lesion*. The axillary view will also allow the examiner to assess for any glenoid fractures after a dislocation; these fractures are called *Bankart lesions*.

Magnetic resonance imaging is often warranted to assess for cuff pathology in older individuals and labral pathology in younger patients. An MRI arthrogram is the gold standard.

C. Special Tests

The apprehension test helps determine anterior shoulder instability. The patient is placed supine with the arm in 90° of abduction. The examiner then applies a external rotation stress. Patient apprehension due to subluxation of the humeral head is considered a positive test. Posterior pressure on the proximal humeral head can provide relief of symptoms if shoulder instability is the cause of the pain (relocation test).

▶ Treatment

In episodes of acute dislocation the initial treatment is to reduce the shoulder pain and swelling. Once reduced, the patient may be placed in a sling for comfort, but there is no evidence that immobilization in internal rotation prevents recurrent instability. Anti-inflammatories can be given for pain control, and early rehab should focus on RoM, cuff strength, and scapular stabilization. Return to play for athletes is when full function (strength and ROM) is regained.

In episodes of more subtle chronic instability without frank dislocation, a trial of physical therapy should be the initial treatment. If the patient has recurrent episodes of dislocation or ongoing pain/dysfunction after physical therapy, more aggressive surgical options should be pursued. Younger patients (<25 years) are known to have greater incidence of recurrence; therefore the practitioner's threshold for surgical opinions should be much lower.

Abrams GD, Safran MR. Diagnosis and management of superior labrum anterior posterior lesions in overhead athletes. *Br J Sports Med.* 2010; 44:311–318.

Boone JL, Arciero RA. First time shoulder dislocations: has the standard changed?. *Br J Sports Med.* 2010; 44:355–360.

Kuhn JE. A new classification system for shoulder instability. *Br J Sports Med.* 2010; 44:341–346.

LATERAL & MEDIAL EPICONDYLITIS

ESSENTIALS OF DIAGNOSIS

▶ Gradual onset of elbow pain often related to repetitive stress.

▶ Pain localizes to the epicondyles of the humerus and is worse with flexion/extension of the wrist, based on medial or lateral pathology

▶ General Considerations

For many years epicondylitis was attributed to inflammation at the tendon origin; however, recent evidence shows that it is actually due to a breakdown of collagen from aging, microtrauma, or vascular compromise. Although properly termed *tendinosis*, the condition is referred to by its long-standing, more common name "epicondylitis" throughout this discussion to avoid confusion. Lateral and medial epicondylitis occur at the elbow and are primarily overuse or repetitive stress disorders.

▶ Clinical Findings

A. Signs and Symptoms

Lateral epicondylytis is a tendinosis at the origin of the extensor tendons on the lateral epicondyle of the humerus. It is commonly known as "tennis elbow" because it is seen in activities that involve repetitive wrist extension (such as a backhand stroke in tennis). Patients complain of pain over the lateral elbow that may radiate down the forearm. There is tenderness to palpation over the origin of the extensor carpi radialis brevis tendon, which is anterior and distal to the lateral epicondyle. Pain is aggravated with wrist extension or forearm supination.

Medial epicondylitis, also known as "golfer's elbow," is seen after repetitive use of the flexor and pronator muscles of the wrist and hand (as occurs when playing golf, using a screwdriver, or hitting an overhand tennis stroke). Pain is insidious at the medial elbow and worsens with resisted forearm pronation and wrist flexion. Patients may complain of a weak grasp. Tenderness to palpation occurs just distal and anterior to the medial epicondyle.

B. Imaging Studies

Radiographs will confirm that there is no other overlapping pathology such as degenerative joint disease. However, imaging is not necessary to make this diagnosis.

▶ Treatment

While epicondylitis is not challenging to diagnose, it can be very difficult to treat. Conservative treatment is the mainstay of treatment, and the natural history of this problem shows that 70–80% of patients will improve in 1 year even in the absence of treatment. Few patients like to wait that long, and there are interventions that may help speed recovery. Activity modification with reduction of the offending activity is key in improvement. NSAIDs can help with early pain management, and a rehabilitation program focusing on eccentric exercises will promote healing. Corticosteroid injections are often requested by patients as they provide short-term relief, but studies have shown that after 6 weeks, those receiving injections had higher recurrence of symptoms.

Forearm bands can be worn in order to relieve tension at the tendon insertion. While patients will report relief with the orthoses, there is not evidence to support their efficacy. Nitroglycerine patches are used topically and applied over the painful area to act as a local and systemic vasodilator. Limited studies have shown improved outcomes in the first 6 months but not longer-term. The prescriber should be aware that patches must be used "off label," cut into smaller doses, and can cause significant side effects, especially in older individuals. Patch treatment should be reserved for a very specific patient population. Autologous platelet-rich plasma (PRP) injections are the newest in treatment options and remain controversial. PRP injections involve drawing blood from the patient, centrifuging the sample, and then injecting the PRP layer at the site of injury. There is mixed evidence regarding this newer treatment, which can be quite expensive, making it typically not a first-line therapy. Surgery should be considered only in those who have failed a sustained period of conservative treatment.

Behrens SB, Deren ME, Matson AP, Bruce B, Green A. A review of modern management of lateral epicondylitis. *Physician Sportsmed*. 2012;40(1):34–40.

Orchard J, Kountouris A. The management of tennis elbow. *Br Med J*. 2011;342:d2687.

Snyder KR, Evans TA. Effectiveness of cortiocosteriods in the treatment of lateral epicondylosis. *J Sports Rehab*. 2012;21:83–88.

DE QUERVAIN TENOSYNOVITIS

ESSENTIALS OF DIAGNOSIS

▶ Atraumatic pain at first dorsal compartment of wrist radiating into thumb and forearm.

▶ Often caused by repetitive activity.

▶ General Considerations

De Quervain tenosynovitis involves the abductor pollicis longus and the extensor pollicis brevis of the thumb. Although this was once assumed to be an inflammatory condition, recent evidence has shown that degeneration of the tendon is present. The condition can arise with repetitive activity that requires grasping or repetitive thumb use.

▶ Clinical Findings

A. Symptoms and Signs

Diagnosis is largely clinical. Patients may complain of difficulty gripping items and often rub the area over the radial

styloid. Pain is located on the radial side of the wrist and thumb and occasionally radiates proximally or distally.

There is tenderness to palpation just distal to the radial styloid. Pain can also be reproduced with resisted thumb abduction and extension, or with thumb adduction into a closed fist and passive ulnar deviation (Finkelstein test). Pain over the tendons represents a positive test; however, other conditions can cause a positive test such as arthritis of the first carpometacarpal joint.

B. Imaging Studies

Radiographs are not necessary for diagnosis but can be useful to rule other other pathology such as osteoarthritis or a fracture.

▶ Treatment

The goals of treatment are to decrease inflammation, prevent adhesion formation, and prevent recurrent tendonitis. Brief periods of icing and use of NSAIDs are helpful initially, and the patient should be placed in a thumb-restricting splint (thumb spica splint). If pain continues, a corticosteroid injection may be considered. In most patients symptoms resolve after a single steroid injection. Steroid injection may be repeated after 8–12 weeks if symptoms are not 50% improved. If no improvement occurs after two injections within the year, a referral for surgical consultation should be obtained.

Shehab R, Mirabilli MH. Evaluation and diagnosis of wrist pain: a case-based approach. *Am Fam Physician*. 2013; 87(8):568–573.

ULNAR COLLATERAL LIGAMENT INJURY OF THE THUMB

ESSENTIALS OF DIAGNOSIS

▶ Pain at medial aspect of metacarpophalangeal (MCP) joint of thumb.

▶ History of valgus force to thumb.

▶ General Considerations

The collateral ligaments of the MCP joint of the thumb stabilize the joint to both valgus- and volar-directed forces. Injury to the medial collateral ligament is extremely common and reported to be 86% of all injuries to the base of the thumb. The term "gamekeeper's thumb" was initially applied to this pathology as a result of Scottish gamekeepers with ligament rupture due to chronic valgus stresses. These days the injury is more accurately described as "skier's thumb" as it typically occurs secondary to a fall onto an outstretched hand with an abducted thumb receiving a valgus force (as would occur when falling holding a ski pole). However, it is important to recognize that this injury occurs in many other sports and settings. Identification of the injury and timely treatment will result in more favorable outcomes.

▶ Clinical Findings

A. Symptoms and Signs

The patient with an acute UCL tear typically describes a specific event of a valgus-directed force onto an abducted thumb. This results in pain, swelling and occasionally ecchymosis over the ulnar aspect of the MCP joint of the thumb. A mass or lump can occasionally be palpated at the site of tenderness, which might suggest a Stener lesion. A Stener lesion occurs then the ruptured ligament displaces in such a manner that the adductor aponeurosis becomes interposed between the ligament and bone. This prevents healing and typically requires surgical repair.

The gold standard for testing the UCL has been to compare laxity at the joint to that at the contralateral side. The thumb should be held proximal and distal to the MCP joint and a gentle valgus force applied at both 30° joint flexion and full extension. If laxity is seen only at 30° of MCP joint flexion, partial tear is suggested. When there is laxity at both 30° flexion and full extension, a complete rupture is likely.

B. Imaging Studies

Although diagnosis of UCL injury of the thumb is based largely on history and physical exam, radiograph should be obtained to rule out other coexisting pathology. Plain films of the thumb in the anteroposterior and lateral planes can be evaluated for fracture. An MRI of the thumb may be ordered to confirm the diagnosis.

▶ Treatment

If the MCP joint is stable on exam and only a partial tear is suspected, nonsurgical management is often successful. The injured thumb should be immobilized in a hand-based thumb spica splint for 4 weeks. After this period of immobilization physical therapy can help the patient regain thumb function. If the MCP joint is not stable on exam and a complete rupture is diagnosed, the patient should be referred to an orthopedic surgeon for surgical repair. If this injury is left untreated, chronic instability will lead to arthritic changes of the MCP joint, which in most cases are irreversible.

Ritting AW, Baldwin PC, Rodner CM. Ulnar collateral ligament injury of the thumb metacarpophalangeal joint. *Clin J Sport Med.* 2010;20(2):106–112.

PATELLAR TENDINOPATHY

 ### ESSENTIALS OF DIAGNOSIS

- ▶ Pain at inferior pole of patella.
- ▶ Results from overuse/overloading the patella tendon.
- ▶ Initially occurs after activity, but can progress over time.

▶ General Considerations

The patellar tendon is an extension of the quadriceps femoris tendon and traverses from the inferior pole of the patella to its anchor point at the tibial tuberosity. *Patellar tendinopathy*, sometimes referred to as "jumper's knee," causes pain at the inferior pole of the patella and usually results from recurrent overload of the knee during running, jumping, or lunging. Historically this process was thought to be a result of inflammation. However, as with most tendinopathy, we now know that the pain results from strain and microtearing. Diagnosis is made clinically through history and physical exam.

▶ Clinical Findings

A. Symptoms and Signs

Clinically, patellar tendinopathy presents with the insidious onset of well-localized anterior knee pain, focused at the inferior pole of the patella. Pain is often exacerbated by activities such as jumping, lunging, ascending/descending stairs, and kneeling. Onset of pain typically begins after exertion but can progress over time to encompass the entire activity.

On physical exam, the most consistent finding is tenderness to palpation over the tendon at the inferior pole of the patella and pain with resisted knee extension. As an extraarticular process, this diagnosis should not cause a knee effusion or mechanical symptoms. Range of motion is typically preserved but can be painful at endpoints.

In adolescents, overloading the patellar tendon can lead to Osgood-Schlatter disease (epiphysitis resulting in fragmentation of the tibial tubercle) or Sinding-Larsen-Johansson yndrome (epiphysitis involving fragmentation of the inferior pole of the patella), both of which will have open growth plates on plain radiographs.

B. Imaging Studies

Standard knee radiographs including anteroposterior (AP), PA weight bearing with 45° flexion, lateral, and merchant. These are helpful to assess for tendon calcification, underlying degenerative changes, or other bony pathology. MRI is confirmatory, but will unlikely change the treatment plan.

Differential Diagnosis

Differential diagnosis includes patellofemoral pain syndrome, fat pad impingement, Osgood-Schlatter disease, Sinding-Larsen-Johansson syndrome, chondromalacia, patellar subluxation/dislocation, and patellar tendon rupture.

Treatment

Previously tendon pain was treated with rest and anti-inflammatories. More recent evidence has changed our approach to address the underlying degenerative, microtearing pathology. Initial treatment should include a rehab program focused on hip and quadriceps strengthening (specifically eccentric exercises). Activities should be modified to offload the anterior knee, and biomechanical abnormalities should be addressed. Although limited evidence exists, patients may experience pain relief wearing a patellar tendon strap. Corticosteroid injections should be avoided in weight-bearing tendons secondary to risk of rupture. Some clinicians are utilizing platelet-rich plasma and nitroglycerine patch therapy to treat this difficult diagnosis. However, both are off-label uses of the product, and scientific evidence is still limited. Recovery can be prolonged, but after 6 months of failed conservative treatment, surgical options can be considered. It is important to educate patients that the literature shows similar outcomes in surgical and conservative treatment groups.

Childress MA, Beutler A. Management of chronic tendon injuries. *Am Fam Physician.* 2013; 87(7):486–490. [PMID: 23547590]
Mautner MD et al. Outcomes after ultrasound-guided Platelet-rich plasma injections for chronic tendinopathy: a multicenter, retrospective review. *Am Acad Phys Med Rehab.*2013;5:169–175.
Rodriguez-Merchan EC. The treatment of patellar tendinopathy. *J Orthopaed Traumatol.* 2013; 14(2):77–81.

PATELLOFEMORAL PAIN SYNDROME

 ESSENTIALS OF DIAGNOSIS

▶ Overuse injury presents with anterior knee pain.
▶ Often occurs after a recent change in activity type, intensity, and frequency.

General Considerations

Patellofemoral pain syndrome (PFPS) is the most common conditiion that prompts active people to seek treatment for anterior knee pain. The pain is typically described under the patella and/or at the anterior medial aspect of the knee.

The patella articulates with the femur in the trochlear groove. It is stabilized by its attachments with the quadriceps femoris, vastus lateralis, vastus medialis, and the medial and lateral retinacula. Weakness of these supporting structures can lead to biomechanical changes in patellar alignment, resulting in lateral tracking and causing irritation to the chondral surfaces.

Three major contributing factors have been evaluated in relation to PFPS: malalignment of the lower extremity, muscular imbalances within the quadriceps, and overactivity. Lower extremity alignment factors associated with PFPS include torsion of the femur or tibia, genu valgum, genu recurvatum, increased Q angle, femoral anteversion, and foot pronation. Each of these factors has the potential to draw the patella laterally and contribute to abnormal patellar tracking.

Clinical Findings

A. Symptoms and Signs

Historically, patients with PFPS present with an insidious onset of diffuse, aching, anterior knee pain often described as around and/or behind the patella. Pain can be bilateral and is aggravated by climbing stairs, ascending hills, squatting, or sitting for a prolonged period of time ("theater" sign). The patient sometimes reports a sensation of popping or grinding with activity.

Although the extent of their contributions is unclear, alignment, gait, and stance should be assessed and gross abnormalities addressed. On exam, there is often tenderness with palpation of the posteromedial or posterolateral patellar facets, as well as a positive "patellar grind" or Clarke sign (pain with slight compression of the patella that is exacerbated by quadriceps contraction). Although not typically in end-stage disease, a knee effusion can be present with mechanical symptoms.

B. Imaging Studies

Radiographs are seldom indicated unless pain is prolonged or associated with trauma, or if bony pathology is suspected. A typical knee series includes a bilateral standing AP view, a lateral view, a bilateral posteroanterior (PA) flexion weight-bearing or tunnel view (45° of flexion), and a patellar profile (Merchant or skyline) view. The images are used to evaluate patella height, joint space narrowing, lateral patella deviation, or other bony abnormality such as a tumor.

Differential Diagnosis

Differential diagnosis includes patellar tendinopathy, patellofemoral osteoarthritis, osteochondral defect of the trochlear or patellar surface, iliotibial band syndrome, anterior fat pad inflammation, synovial plica, retinacular strain, and epiphysitis. (*Note*: It is important to rule out referred pain from hip pathology in children.)

Treatment

Treatment is directed at correcting patellar maltracking and biomechanical factors and modifying activities that cause symptoms. Exercises designed to strengthen the medial quadriceps and hip muscles and stretch the hamstrings and iliotibial bands have shown success in restoring normal function. The use of foot orthotics can be considered for those with pes planus, pes cavus, and significant hind foot eversion. Patients often perceive relief with bracing or taping, which helps guide the patella medially, especially during activities. Limited evidence exists for the effectiveness of NSAIDs, and their utility is questioned in patients with this disorder. Viscosupplementation has been found to provide pain relief in patients with more advanced disease and significant chondral damage from chronic maltracking. Surgery is reserved for patients with significant damage to the chondral surface and for those who have failed prolonged conservative therapy.

Barton CJ, Webster KE, Hylton BM. Evaluation of the scope and quality of systematic reviews on nonpharmacological conservative treatment for patellofemoral pain syndrome. *J Orthop Sports Phys Ther*. 2008;38(9):529–541.

LIGAMENTOUS INJURIES OF THE KNEE

The knee is a modified hinge joint that is stabilized by the anterior cruciate ligament (ACL), posterior cruciate ligament (PCL), medial collateral ligament (MCL), lateral collateral ligament (LCL), menisci, capsule, and surrounding musculature. Injury to one or more of these ligaments can lead to knee joint instability.

Anterior Cruciate Ligament Injury

 ESSENTIALS OF DIAGNOSIS

▶ Acute trauma resulting in immediate joint effusion and pain.

▶ Positive Lachman test.

General Considerations

An intact ACL prevents anterior translation of the tibia on the femur and creates rotational stability. Injury to the ACL commonly results when there is an abrupt deceleration combined with a twisting mechanism, typically during cutting or pivoting after the foot is planted. Less commonly it can occur after forced hyperextension.

Clinical Findings

A. Symptoms and Signs

This injury typically occurs with a sudden change in direction and 70% of the time without contact. The patient often hears or feels a "pop." Swelling is usually rapid (minutes to hours) as a large hemarthrosis develops within the joint along with pain and decreased range of motion. Without the restraint of an intact ACL, the tibia displaces anteriorly as the patient ambulates and causes a sensation of instability or giving way, particularly with pivoting motions.

An acute ACL injury can often be diagnosed immediately; however, the majority of patients present a day or more after the injury. By that time, muscle spasm and pain may limit the examination and make clinical diagnosis difficult. In the setting of an acute knee injury with effusion, the Lachman test is the most sensitive test to rule in or out an ACL tear.

B. Imaging Studies

Although radiographs are of limited value in diagnosing ACL tears, a *standard knee series* is recommended to rule out other bony pathology. A fracture of the lateral tibial plateau (Segond fracture) is pathognomonic of an ACL tear. MRI is the imaging modality of choice to confirm a clinically suspected ACL tear. The typical bone bruise pattern occurs in the medial femoral condyle and lateral tibial plateau. There may be associated articular cartilage damage, meniscus pathology, and multiple ligament injuries.

C. Special Tests

With either of the following tests, significant anterior translation of the tibia or lack of a discrete endpoint indicates a positive test; the injured knee must always be compared to the uninjured side as the patient may have some inherent laxity:

Lachman test: With the patient supine and the knee relaxed in 30° of flexion with just slight external rotation of the hip, the examiner stabilizes the distal femur with one hand, grasps the proximal tibia with the other, and attempts to sublux the tibia anteriorly.

Anterior drawer test: Less sensitive than the Lachman test, the anterior drawer test is performed with the patient supine and the knee flexed to 90°. The examiner stabilizes the relaxed leg by sitting on the patient's foot, grasps the tibial plateau with both thumbs on the tibial tubercle, and applies an anteriorly directed force.

Treatment

Initial treatment includes a hinged knee brace, protected weight bearing for comfort, cryotherapy, early RoM exercises, quadriceps sets, and straight leg raises. The majority of active individuals should be referred for surgical consultation. In a very specific subset of patients nonsurgical treatment is a viable option. These patients are typically older and not active in "cutting" sports. They have to accept some degree of chronic instability and the potential for further meniscal and articular surface injuries.

Posterior Cruciate Ligament Injury

ESSENTIALS OF DIAGNOSIS

▶ Posterior force on flexed knee.

▶ Positive posterior drawer and "sag" sign.

▶ General Considerations

The PCL limits posterior displacement of the tibia on the femur. PCL tears are less common than ACL tears and often go undetected. The usual mechanism of injury is a posteriorly directed force on the proximal tibia typically in hyperflexion as when a flexed knee strikes a dashboard in a vehicle accident. When seen actually in the emergency department, 95% of PCL injuries are found in combination with other pathology.

▶ Clinical Findings

A. Symptoms and Signs

Unlike the scenario with ACL tears, patients rarely report a "pop." The initial trauma may be subtle, and subsequent symptoms can be vague. Patients present with knee pain, effusion, and difficulty with the final 10°–20° of flexion. Unsteadiness may be a complaint, but significant instability is more likely to be reported with combined ligamentous injuries. The posterior drawer test is the most accurate test for assessing PCL integrity.

B. Imaging Studies

Imaging preferences are the same as with suspected ACL injuries, and MRI is ≤100% sensitive and specific in determining complete PCL tear. A typical bone bruise pattern is found in the anterior tibia. It is imperative that a careful vascular exam be completed, given possible injury to the popliteal artery with PCL tears.

C. Special Tests

The posterior drawer is performed with the patient supine with the knee flexed to 90°. The examiner stabilizes the relaxed leg by sitting on the patient's foot, grasps the tibial plateau with both thumbs on the tibial tubercle, and applies a posterior-directed force. If significant posterior translation of the tibia or lack of a discrete endpoint is greater than that of the unaffected limb, the test is positive.

▶ Treatment

Nonsurgical management is acceptable for chronic and/or isolated, low-grade, acute PCL tears. The PCL has greater healing potential than the ACL and can heal over time. Initial treatment for a low-grade PCL injury involves early range of motion and emphasizes quadriceps strengthening and partial weight bearing with protection against posterior sag (a brace can be useful and locked in extension for 1–2 weeks). A complete tear is treated initially with 2–4 weeks of immobilization in full extension. Indications for expeditious surgical referral include combined ligamentous injury (eg, posterolateral corner), significant laxity, and avulsion fractures. Guidelines for conservative versus surgical management of PCL injuries are still being debated.

Injuries of the Medial Collateral & Lateral Collateral Ligaments

ESSENTIALS OF DIAGNOSIS

▶ MCL tear results from valgus force causes medial knee pain, laxity.

▶ LCL tear results from varus force causing lateral knee pain, laxity.

▶ If effusion is present, consider combined pathology.

▶ General Considerations

The MCL is the most commonly injured stabilizing ligament of the knee. A medially directed or valgus force is the most common cause of MCL disruption. Isolated LCL disruption is relatively rare and occurs with a blow to the anteromedial knee with a varus force.

Clinical Findings

A. Symptoms and Signs

Patients with an isolated collateral ligament tear generally present with a classic mechanism of injury and may report the sensation of a "pop." Patients complain of localized pain and tenderness over the damaged ligament but rarely report significant instability or locking. Localized swelling may be seen with isolated tears, but a significant effusion is uncommon.

B. Imaging Studies

Radiographs are helpful in ruling out other bony pathology but are seldom necessary for diagnosis of isolated tears of the MCL or LCL. X-ray findings may reveal calcification, more commonly in the proximal origin, with chronic injury (Pellegrini-Stieda lesion). MRI is the gold standard for diagnosis and is useful when examination findings are equivocal and can also show associated posterior oblique ligament involvement, bone bruising, or trabecular microfractures that can be found in lateral femoral condyle or lateral tibial plateau, which typically resolve spontaneously by 4 months.

C. Special Tests

Valgus and varus stress testing, to evaluate the MCL and LCL respectively, is performed at full extension (0°) and 30°. Laxity that is apparent only at 30° of flexion suggests an isolated MCL or LCL injury (1st or 2nd degree). Additional laxity in full extension (3rd degree) suggests concomitant soft-tissue injury (ACL or PCL).

▶ Treatment

Treatment of isolated collateral ligament tears is primarily conservative. Ice and use of a compression wrap help to control local swelling. Achieving stability using a hinged knee brace locked in extension is appropriate in a 2nd-degree injury for 1–2 weeks and 3–6 weeks for 3rd -degree injury. However, regardless of severity, the patient must be encouraged to gradually increase weight bearing as soon as possible. Prior to full return to sports, athletes should have achieved full nonpainful RoM and strength and completed a functional rehabilitation program. Platelet-rich plasma injections for this injury are still being investigated but have promising early results. Recovery may vary from days to weeks, but nonsurgical management is routinely favored. Surgical fixation is reserved for failed conservative therapy in isolated injuries, which are typically tibial-sided injuries.

Fabrican MD, Peter, et al. Reconstruction of the anterior cruciate ligament in the skeletally immature athlete: a review of current concepts: AAOS exhibit selection. *J Bone Joint Surg.* 2013; 95(5):e28, 1–13.

Kocher MS, Shore B, Nasreddine A, Heyworth BE.. Treatement of posterior cruciate ligament injuries in pediatric and adolescent patients. *J Pediatr Orthop.* 2012; 32(6):553–560.

Lee MC, et al. Rupture of posterior cruciate ligament: diagnosis and treatment principles. *Knee Surg Relat Res.* 2011; 23(3): 135–141.

Levine JW et al. Clinically relevant injury patterns after an anterior cruciate ligament injury provide insight into injury mechanisms. *Am J Sports Med.* 2013; 41:385–394.

Muyamoto RG, Bosco JA, Sherman OH. Treatment of medial collateral ligament injuries. *J Am Acad Orthop Surg.* 2009;17: 152–161.

Pierce CM et al. Posterior cruciate ligament tears: functional and postoperative rehabilitation. *Knee Surg Sports Traumatol Arthrosc.* 2012;.

MENISCAL TEARS

ESSENTIALS OF DIAGNOSIS

▶ Mechanism of Injury is typically a pivoting motion with the foot planted.

▶ Swelling is likely to occur and pain can be palpated along the joint line.

▶ Patient may describe a clicking or locking sensation in the knee.

▶ General Considerations

The lateral and medial menisci are C-shaped wedges of cartilage that act as shock absorbers between the femur and the tibia. They attach at the anterior and posterior aspects of the tibial plateau and help with load bearing and distribution. In addition, they contribute to overall joint stability and proprioception. The medial meniscus sustains more force during weight bearing and is fused with the MCL, which renders it much less mobile than the lateral meniscus and therefore more susceptible to tearing. Active patients are more prone to acute tears and often have associated ligamentous injuries that occur with sudden twists or turns during activity. As one ages, the meniscus thins and weakens, which can lead to degenerative tears that require less force.

▶ Clinical Findings

A. Symptoms and Signs

Acute, isolated meniscal tears result primarily from shearing forces during a twisting or hyperflexion injury with the foot planted. Patients describe a "pop" and pain initially. An effusion will likely develop over 24–48 hours. Patients often complain of pain with squatting, mechanical symptoms such as locking or catching, and instability.

Occasionally, a fragment with break off or a large bucket-handle tear will displace the joint and become lodged within it, preventing full extension and creating a "locked knee." This presentation requires early surgical referral.

Patients with degenerative tears tend to present with an insidious onset of pain, mechanical symptoms, and only mild intermittent swelling. These patients have a more arthritic presentation.

Exam should focus on range of motion to ensure that there is no loss of extension or flexion. Joint line tenderness over the affected meniscus is the best clinical indicator of a meniscal tear. Several provocative maneuvers have been developed to re-create impingement of the torn fragment. Examples are the McMurray and Apley tests, which are helpful but only marginally sensitive or specific.

B. Imaging Studies

Although radiographs cannot confirm the diagnosis of a meniscal tear, a standard knee series (see section on anterior cruciate ligament injury, earlier) is obtained to rule out additional bony pathology and to examine for joint space narrowing. It is important to be aware that the amount of joint space narrowing and degenerative change will direct treatment in older individuals. MRI is the confirmatory imaging modality of choice and may show increased uptake within the meniscus and possible extrusion.

▶ Treatment

Initial treatment for isolated meniscal pathology includes cryotherapy, RoM exercises, NSAIDs, and weight bearing as tolerated. In a young, active individual early surgical referral should be considered. In those middle-aged and older a course of conservative treatment including physical therapy, corticosteroid injection, and bracing can be initially prescribed. Indications for surgical referral include failure to respond to nonsurgical treatment or recurrent episodes of catching, locking, or giving way. When radiographs show substantial degenerative change, menical tears should be treated as arthritis.

Neogi DS et al. Role of nonoperative treatment in managing degenerative tears of the medial meniscus posterior root. *J Orthopaed Traumatol.* 2013.

Salata M, Gibbs AE, Sekiya JK. A systematic review of clinical outcomes in patients undergoing menisectomy. *Am J Sports Med.* 2010; 38:1907.

Taylor SA, Rodeo SA. Augmentation techniques for isolated meniscal tears. *Curr Rev Musculoskel Med.* 2013; 6(2):95–101.

Osteoarthritis of the Knee

ESSENTIALS OF DIAGNOSIS

▶ Insidious onset of joint pain and decreased range of motion.

▶ Pain and stiffness is worst after prolonged immobilization and activity.

▶ Joint line pain, grinding, effusion, and muscle weakness are common on physical exam.

▶ General Considerations

Osteoarthritis (OA) is a degenerative condition that affects >20 million people in the United States. It is often progressive, and risk factors include increasing age, gender, genetics, ethnicity, nutrition, obesity, previous joint injury/trauma, malalignment, and excessive exercise. OA involves the articular surfaces of bones. Typically, over time with normal wear and tear, the cartilage degrades and results in focal loss and joint space narrowing. This causes pain and stiffness, especially after prolonged periods of immobilization and activity. It is often seen in the weight-bearing or larger joints such as the knees and hips; however, it can occur along any articular surface.

▶ Clinical Findings

A. Symptoms and Signs

Onset of pain usually occurs over months to years. Patients typically complain of pain and stiffness in the morning or after prolonged immobilization and activity. They may also describe a "grinding" sensation and complain of intermittent joint swelling. Pain is often diffused and described in many ways, such as aching, burning, sharp, or dull. It is not unusual for the pain to radiate proximally or distally.

Physical examination of the knee may reveal a decreased range of motion and effusion. Pain may be palpated along the length of the joint line, usually medially more than laterally. There is likely associated muscle weakness in the supporting musculature. Crepitus can usually be palpated with joint motion.

B. Imaging Studies

Standard radiographs of the knee are obtained with close attention to views of the weight-bearing joints. Joint space narrowing, osteophytes, subchondral sclerosis, and cyst formation are the most common findings.

C. Lab Studies

If other rheumatologic disorders are suspected, a laboratory analysis should be obtained. A CBC, CMP, urinalysis, ESR, C-reactive protein, RF, anti-CCP, and ANA should be considered. The inflammatory markers, ESR and CRP, may be slightly elevated during the symptomatic phase; all others should be normal.

▶ Differential Diagnosis

Differential diagnosis includes rheumatoid arthritis, menical tears, gout, pseudogout, bursitis, psoriatic arthritis, avascular necrosis, and insufficiency fracture.

▶ Treatment

Treatment of osteoarthritis is aimed at conservative therapy. Topical NSAIDs or other topical analgesics should be first line and may be beneficial in the early stages. Acetaminophen, aspirin, and NSAIDs are commonly used medications for pain relief in OA. A nonimpact exercise program is important to maintain range of motion and strength. In cases of increased BMI, weight reduction alone can aid in pain relief and decrease further risk of advancing arthritis. Hydrotherapy is a great way to get active without significant joint stress. With aerobic exercise on land, bracing can be used for overall support. Certain braces are able to offload the medial or lateral joint, and other braces facilitate patellar tracking. Glucosamine and chondroitin sulfate are beneficial for some people in reducing osteoarthritis pain, but their true benefit/efficacy is still being determined.

If a significant effusion is present, an aspiration and an intraarticular corticosteroid injection can aid in temporary pain relief. Risk/benefit of corticosteroid in uncontrolled diabetics must be considered, given the temporary increase in glucose that occurs. Viscosupplementation with intraarticular hyaluronic acid provides prolonged benefit in some patients and can be repeated every 6 months if effective. Clinicians are still investigating the use and benefits of platelet-rich plasma intraarticular injections for osteoarthritis of the knee. When conservative therapy is exhausted and daily activities are limited secondary to pain and decreased mobility, then partial or full joint replacement should be considered and referral to an orthopedic surgeon should be initiated.

Bhatia D, Bejarano T, Novo M. Current interventions in the management of knee osteoarthritis. *J Pharm Bioallied Sci.* 2013;5(1):30–38.

Fakhari A, Berland C. Applications and emerging trends of hyaluronic acid in tissue engineering, as a dermal filler and in osteoarthritis treatment. *Acta Biomaterialia* 2013; 9(7):7081–92 (journal homepage: www.elsevier.com/locate/actabiomat).

Filardo G, et al. Platelet-rich plasma intra-articula knee injections for the treatment of degenerative cartilage lesions and osteoarthritis. *Knee Surg Sports Traumatol Arthrosc.* 2011;19:528–535.

ANKLE SPRAINS

ESSENTIALS OF DIAGNOSIS

▶ Mechanism of injury is forced inversion and plantar flexion (lateral sprain) or forced eversion and dorsiflexion (medial and/or high ankle sprain).

▶ Pain with palpation over the affected ligaments.

▶ Pain worse with ambulation, swelling, and ecchymosis over the lateral or medial ankle with instability of the ankle joint are common physical findings.

▶ General Considerations

Ankle ligament sprains are the most common ankle injuries and the majority (80%) involves the lateral ankle ligaments: anterior talofibular ligament (ATFL), the calcaneofibular ligament (CFL), and the posterior talofibular ligament. They occur after the ankle is placed under extreme inversion and plantar flexion. Syndesmotic or "high ankle sprains" occur when the ankle is dorsiflexed and everted. The recovery from a syndesmotic sprain can be prolonged and is important to identify. Medial ankle sprains are less common and involve the deltoid ligament complex.

▶ Clinical Findings

A. Symptoms and Signs

Patients present with pain over the injured ligaments after "rolling" their ankle and sometimes hearing a "pop." Swelling, ecchymosis, and difficulty with weight bearing are the typical presentation but can be variable.

On physical examination it is important to observe the patient's gait. Often pain can be palpated over the injured ligaments. Range of motion is often decreased. A complete exam should include palpating the proximal fibula and foot for concurrent injury.

B. Imaging Studies

The Ottawa ankle rules provide high-yield criteria for ordering radiographs (level of evidence).. Indications for radiographs include bony tenderness at the distal (6 cm), posterior portions of the lateral or medial malleoli, inability to bear weight immediately and during the examination, and pain with palpation of the navicular or base of the 5th metatarsal. Routine radiographs include anterior, lateral, and weight-bearing mortise views to assess for fracture, widening of the mortise (indicates instability of the joint), OCD injury. MRI is considered to evaluate the ligaments in patients with chronic instability, and CT scan is utilized if occult fracture is suspected.

C. Special Tests

Anterior drawer: Stabilize the distal tibia with one hand, then grasp the calcaneus in the palm of the other hand, and apply an anterior force. Excessive anterior motion or a "clunk" suggests disruption of the ATFL.

Talar tilt: Stabilize the tibia with one hand, then grasp the calcaneus in the palm of the opposite hand, and invert the hind foot. Significant laxity with inversion suggests disruption of the ATFL and CFL. A reverse talar tilt assesses for laxity of the deltoid ligament.

▶ Differential Diagnosis

Differential diagnosis includes tibia or fibula fracture, talus or calcaneus fracture, osteochondral defect in the talus, or anterior or posterior ankle impingement.

▶ Treatment

Initial treatment of isolated, acute lateral ankle sprains consists of RICE: rest, ice, compression or support, and elevation. Occasionally, crutches, a posterior splint, cast, or walking boot are required if there is concern for fracture. Once fracture has been ruled out, early motion and weight bearing have been shown to facilitate return to activity. This includes a timely physical therapy referral for rehabilitation focusing on restoring motion, strength, and flexibility. Return to play is allowed after full, pain-free strength and range of motion are achieved and there are no limitations with sport-specific activities. Often athletes will benefit from taping or a lace-up ankle support once functional.

Syndesmotic sprains require early diagnosis and a more conservative treatment course. If weight-bearing mortise view shows clear space widening, immediate surgical referral is indicated. If the joint is stable, there is some variability in treatment protocols. This will immobilize in a tall walking boot for 1–2 weeks prior to initiating an aggressive rehab program. It is important to inform your patient that this injury will take longer to recover than a typical ankle sprain.

Fong DT, Chan YY, Mok KM, et al. Understanding acute ankle ligamentous sprain injury in sports. *Sports Med Arthrosc Rehab Ther Technol.* 2009;1:14. [PMID: 19640309]
Kamper SJ, Sanneke JM. Surgical versus conservative treatment for acute ankle sprains. *Br J Sports Med.* 2012;46:77–78.

MEDIAL TIBIAL STRESS SYNDROME

ESSENTIALS OF DIAGNOSIS

► Distal, posteromedial tibia pain worse at the beginning and after activity, and resolves with rest.
► If untreated, pain can advance and occur during activity.
► Pain is diffuse as opposed to localized.

▶ General Considerations

Medial tibial stress syndrome (MTSS) is a common overuse injury that causes activity-related pain over the posteromedial aspect of the distal two-thirds of the tibia. Runners are most commonly affected, but MTSS is also quite prevalent in athletes who participate in jumping sports such as basketball, tennis, volleyball, and gymnastics. Risk factors may be pes planus, leg length discrepancy, tight Achilles tendons, higher BMI, female sex, excess hind foot valgus, and recent change in footwear or running surface.

▶ Clinical Findings

A. Symptoms and Signs

Initially, patients may present with pain at the beginning of workout or physical activity that may be relieved with continued activity or rest. However, as the injury progresses, pain may last throughout the duration of activity and continue during rest. The pain is referred to as a dull ache over the distal one-third of the posteromedial tibia.

Physical examination reveals diffuse tenderness along the posteromedial border of the distal tibia. In some cases, swelling may be present. Pain is reproduced with passive dorsiflexion and plantar flexion, standing toe raises, and one- or two-legged hop.

B. Imaging Studies

Radiographs of the tibia (AP and lateral) are typically negative, but should be obtained to evaluate for stress fracture or tumor. If conservative therapy fails, an MRI or three-phase bone scan should be obtained for further assessment. An MRI is considered the gold standard as it shows greater anatomic detail.

▶ Differential Diagnosis

Differential diagnosis of exertional leg pain includes MTSS, deep venous thrombosis, fascial herniations, muscle strains, posterior tibial tendinitis, nerve or artery entrapment, chronic exertional compartment syndrome, stress fracture, and neoplasm.

▶ Treatment

Initial treatment of MTSS consists of activity modification and avoidance of aggravating factors using pain as a guide. Cross-training activities such as swimming, biking, and jumping are encouraged to maintain cardiovascular fitness during the recovery phase. Impact activities can be increased gradually thereafter, advancing only if asymptomatic at each stage. Ice massage, NSAIDs, shock absorbent inserts, heel cord stretching, and correction of malalignment can aid in treatment and pain relief. Physical therapy with massage, electrical stimulation, ultrasound, and iontophoresis should be considered. Surgical referral for posteromedial fasciotomy is reserved for patients with extraordinarily resistant and painful symptoms. A clinician must have a high index of suspicion for stress fracture and consider early imaging if any doubt exists.

Brewer RB, Gregory AJM. Chronic lower leg pain in athletes: a guide for the differential diagnosis, evaluation, and treatment. *Sports Health.* 2012; 4(2):121–127.
Edwards P Jr., et al. Practical approach for the differential diagnosis of chronic leg pain in the athlete. *Am J Sports Med.* 2005; 33(8):1241–1249.

PLANTAR FASCIITIS

ESSENTIALS OF DIAGNOSIS

► Heel pain at the medial, plantar aspect of the calcaneus.
► Heel pain and tightness with first steps of morning.

General Considerations

The plantar fascia is the fibrous aponeurosis that provides static support and dynamic shock absorption for the longitudinal arch of the foot. After a recent change in distance, intensity. or duration of activity, the plantar fascia can develop microtears and eventually chronic degenerative changes as a result of overuse. This is referred to as *plantar fasciitis*, a common cause of heel pain. Risk factors include pes cavus or pes planus, prolonged standing, excessive training, decreased flexibility of the Achilles tendon and intrinsic foot muscles, obesity, and sedentary lifestyle. Diagnosis is based primarily on history and physical examination. Typically patients have heel pain in their first steps in the morning and with palpation of the medial aspect of the calcaneus.

Clinical Findings

A. Symptoms and Signs

Classically, patients present with insidious onset of pain on the plantar surface of the heel that is worse with the first steps in the morning or when standing after a prolonged period of rest. Pain usually diminishes with rest but may reccur at the end of the day. Athletes report that running, hill climbing, and sprinting exacerbate the pain.

Physical examination generally demonstrates tenderness along the anteromedial aspect of the calcaneus that intensifies with stretching of the plantar fascia by passive dorsiflexion of the toes. Limited ankle dorsiflexion associated with a tight heel cord may also be noted.

B. Imaging Studies

Radiographs are rarely indicated for the initial diagnosis and treatment of plantar fasciitis. Heel spurs on the anterior calcaneus can be misleading; these are present in 15–25% of the general population without symptoms, and many symptomatic patients do not have spurs. For chronic, recalcitrant cases, radiographs of the foot (AP, lateral, oblique views) can guide further treatment plans.

Differential Diagnosis

The differential diagnosis of heel pain includes calcaneal stress fracture, plantar fascia rupture, fat pad atrophy, retrocalcaneal bursitis, nerve entrapment syndromes, arthropathies, Achilles tendinopathy, posterior tibial tendinitis, heel contusion, calcaneal apophysitis, or even tumor.

Treatment

Plantar fasciitis is a self-limiting condition, and regardless of therapy, most will resolve within a year and 90% of patients will improve with conservative treatment. This includes activity modification, NSAIDs, heel cushions or arch supports, and an aggressive Achilles and plantar fascia stretching

program. Deep myofascial massage and iontophoresis have been used by physical therapists with positive benefit in many cases. Corticosteroid injections may provide short-term benefit, but can cause fat pad atrophy or plantar fascia rupture. Custom orthotics in combination with night splints may be beneficial in patients with recalcitrant symptoms. After 6 months of conservative therapy, extracorporeal shockwave therapy is a promising option but seldom covered by medical insurance. After a prolonged period of conservative treatment with continued pain, surgical release or fasciotomy can also be considered.

Goff J, Crawford R Diagnosis and treatment of plantar fasciitis. *Am Fam Physician.* 2011;84(6).

Greater Trochanteric Bursitis

ESSENTIALS OF DIAGNOSIS

▶ Pain over lateral aspect of hip.
▶ Symptoms worsened with pressure on lateral hip such as rolling on side at night.

General Considerations

The greater trochanteric bursa is located on the lateral aspect of the hip and can be a source of pain for individuals of all ages. Inflammation can be either the result of direct trauma or insidious. Historically this pathology has been described as a single source of pain, the bursae. However, more recent evidence suggests broader inflammation and involvement of the iliotibial band and gluteus medius muscle.

Clinical Findings

A. Signs and Symptoms

Patients will complain primarily of lateral hip pain with tenderness to palpation at the greater trochanteric bursae. The patient typically has full hip range of motion and full strength; however, both extremes of motion and manual muscle testing may bring on symptoms.

B. Imaging Studies

Plain radiographs of the hip and pelvis help rule out other pathology such as osteoarthritis or bony hip deformities.

Treatment

Initial treatment includes physical therapy with a focus on iliotibial band stretching and hip strengthening. Often, adding the modality of a foam roller can be helpful in treating this entitiy. Pain should be controlled with ice and NSAIDs.

For most patients a single corticosteroid injection provides improvement of symptoms. A cure rate with conservative interventions can be expected to exceed 90%. However, recurrence is common, and for those with ongoing pain after an extended course of conservative care, surgery may be considered.

Ilizaliturri VM, Camacho-Galindo J, Ramirex ANE, et al. Soft tissue pathology around the hip. *Clin Sports Med.* 2011; 30:391–415.

Lustenberger DP, Ng VY, Best TM, Ellis TJ. Efficacy of treatment of trochanteric bursitis: a systemic review. *Clin J Sports Med.* 2011; 21(5):447–453.

Hip Impingement/Labral Tear

ESSENTIALS OF DIAGNOSIS

▶ Deep anterior groin pain.

▶ Reproduced with flexion and internal rotation of the hip.

▶ General Considerations

Femoroacetabular hip impingement (FAI) and labral tears are modern orthopedic concepts with a constantly expanding body of literature. The two pathologies are intimately related in that a large majority of patients with impingement are found to have labral tears.

Hip impingement is described as an osseous abnormality of femoral head-neck offset (cam) or excessive coverage of the acetabular rim (pincer) resulting in early chondrolabral damage, osteoarthritis, and hip pain. The cause of the bony abnormalities remains unclear at this time.

A labral tear has been found to frequently coexist with hip impingement. The labrum of the hip is a triangular fibrocartilaginous structure located circumferentially around the bony acetabulum that plays a crucial role in hip mechanics. The etiology of tears falls into four categories: traumatic, degenerative, idiopathic, and congenital.

▶ Clinical Findings

A. Symptoms and Signs

The majority of patients with both impingement and labral tears will present with anterior groin pain. The majority will be insidious (50–65%), but some will follow a traumatic event. Patients will occasionally complain of mechanical symptoms such as clicking, catching, locking, or giving way. Most will have decreased hip motion and weakness on exam. Symptoms typically worsen with activity. Nearly all patients will have a positive anterior impingement [flexion, adduction, and internal rotation (FADIR)] test, which is described below.

B. Imaging Studies

Plain radiographs will demonstrate the abnormal morphology of impingement. Anteroposterior (AP) weight-bearing pelvis and cross-table lateral views should be ordered. The cross-table lateral view will show a classic "pistol-grip deformity" in cam impingement. The "crossover sign" suggests acetabular overcoverage as is seen in pincer impingement.

An MRI arthrogram of the hip is necessary to visualize labral pathology and is considered the gold standard diagnostic study.

C. Special Tests

The anterior impingement test is a provocative test that is commonly used and is nearly always positive in patients with FAI and labral tears. However, it must be interpreted with caution as it is also positive in many other situations such as hip osteoarthritis. The patient is positioned supine and the hip is passively flexed to 90° followed by forced adduction and internal rotation (FADIR). The presence of anterior groin pain during this maneuver is considered a positive test.

▶ Treatment

Initial treatment should be conservative, combining physical therapy focusing on hip strengthening, NSAIDs, and activity modification. An intraarticular injection of a long-acting anesthetic combined with a corticosteroid can be both therapeutic and diagnostic for this pathology. If the injection relieves symptoms, even for a brief period, the pain generator is presumed to be intraarticular. A patient who continues to have symptoms after 6–8 weeks of conservative treatment should be referred to an orthopedic surgeon who is experienced in hip arthroscopy for further evaluation.

Ejnisman L, Philippon MJ, Lertwanich P. Acetabular labral tears: diagnosis, repair and a method for labral reconstruction. *Clin Sports Med.* 2011; 30:317–329.

Ejnisman L, Philippon MJ, Lertwanich P. Femoroacetabular impingement: the femoral side. *Clin Sports Med.* 2011; 30:369–377.

Freehill MT, Safran MR. The labrum of the hip: diagnosis and rationale for surgical correction. *Clin Sports Med.* 2011; 30:293–315.

Samora JB, Ng VY, Ellis TJ. Femoroacetabular Impingement: a common cause of hip pain in young adults. *Clin J Sports Med.* 2011; 21(1):51–56.

PEDIATRIC AND ADOLESCENT MUSCULOSKELETAL DISORDERS

SPONDYLOLYSIS

ESSENTIALS OF DIAGNOSIS

▶ Lumbar pain that worsens with extension.

General Considerations

Spondylolysis is one of the most common causes of back pain in active young children and adolescents. It is defined as a defect, or *stress fracture*, in the pars interarticularis of the posterior neural arch of the vertebrae. It occurs at the L5 level in ≤95% of cases and is bilateral in approximately 80% of cases. The etiology is typically repetitive hyperextension of the lumbar spine as is seen in sports such as gymnastics, football, diving, and pole vaulting.

Clinical Findings

A. Symptoms and Signs

Spondylolysis is usually characterized by the insidious onset of low back pain that increases with activity and lumbar extension. Pain may be severe at times, but neurologic symptoms and radiculopathy are rare. Physical examination may be relatively normal, or the patient may have localized lumbosacral tenderness or reproducible pain with gentle extension.

B. Imaging Studies

The initial imaging for suspected spondylolysis includes anterioposterior (AP), lateral, and right and left oblique radiographs of the lumbar spine. The most common radiographic finding is a fracture through the collar of the "Scotty dog" on oblique radiographs. If clinical suspicion remains high despite normal radiographs, more advanced imaging is warranted. Several other modalities have proved useful in detecting pars defects, including bone scan, single-photon emission CT (SPECT), conventional CT, and MRI.

C. Special Tests

The "stork test" is performed by standing on one leg while hyperextending the spine. Reproduction of pain indicates a positive test.

Differential Diagnosis:

The differential diagnosis of acute low back pain in the pediatric population includes spondylolisthesis, scoliosis, lumbrosacral strain, and discogenic pain. Inflammatory arthropathies should be considered in the context of chronic pain. Night pain, fever, or other systemic symptoms should prompt an evaluation for infection or neoplasm.

Treatment

Treatment of symptomatic spondylolysis generally involves a combination of activity modification, bracing, and rehabilitation. Antilordotic bracing will often reduce pain. Rehab protocols should focus on core strengthening and hamstring stretching. Finally, a gradual return to play will result in 95%

of patients returning to their preinjury activity level. Surgical management is indicated if pain persists despite conservative treatment.

Gurd DP. Back pain in the young athlete. *Sports Med Arthrosc Rev.* 2011;19(1):7–16.

LEGG-CALVE-PERTHES DISEASE & SLIPPED CAPITAL FEMORAL EPIPHYSIS

ESSENTIALS OF DIAGNOSIS

▶ Adolescent, often overweight male, presents with limp and diffuse hip pain.

General Considerations

Legg-Calves-Perthes disease (LCPD) is defined as idiopathic osteonecrosis and collapse of the femoral head. Most cases occur between 4 and 8 years of age. Boys are more commonly affected. *Slipped capital femoral epiphysis* (SCFE) is defined as the posterior and inferior slippage of the proximal femoral epiphysis on the metaphysis (femoral neck), which occurs through the epiphyseal plate (growth plate). The peak incidence occurs in early adolescence at 12–13 years of age. There is predominance in overweight males. The etiology of SCFE is assumed to be multifactorial and may include obesity, growth surges, and less commonly, endocrine disorders. Both conditions may be found bilaterally in the same individual.

Clinical Findings

A. Signs and Symptoms

The presentations of both LCPD and SCFE are characterized by diffuse aching pain in the groin, medial thigh, or knee. Pain is often accompanied by an altered gait or limp, and it is usually worsened by activity. SCFE may present as knee pain in ≤23% of cases, and it cannot be overstated that the investigation of knee pain in children should include a history and physical examination that addresses the hips as well.

Physical examination may produce pain at the extremes of motion, particularly in hip abduction and internal rotation. Both disorders will present with loss of normal motion, particularly in internal rotation.

B. Imaging Studies

Anteroposterior (AP) and frogleg lateral and/or cross-table lateral radiographs of both hips should be obtained. Plain radiographs nearly always confirm the diagnosis of SCFE by demonstrating displacement of the femoral head. The LCPD radiographic findings present a continuum of changes as the disease progresses. In the early stages of LCPD, plain radiographs may be normal. However, over time there can be widening of the joint space, sclerosis of the femoral head, cystic changes, and *coxa magna*, which is defined as flattening and widening of the femoral head.

Differential Diagnosis

The differential diagnosis includes developmental dysplasia of the hip, septic arthritis, transient synovitis, labral pathology, and benign or malignant neoplasms. Inflammatory causes (juvenile rheumatoid arthritis, spondyloarthropathies, Lyme disease arthritis) are possible as well.

Treatment

Legg-Calves-Perthes disease is a self-limiting condition, but symptoms may persist for ≤4 years. The primary goal of treatment for LCPD is pain reduction, and this sometimes requires bracing/casting and protected weight bearing. Operative intervention may be indicated in older patients or those with advanced disease. Surgery is the preferred treatment for SCFE and typically involves emergent stabilization of the femoral head with metallic fixation devices. Delays in treatment may lead to further displacement and osteonecrosis, ultimately compromising postoperative outcomes.

Peck D. Slipped capital femoral epiphysis: diagnosis and management. *Am Fam Physician*. 2010; 82(3):258–262.

Wheeless CR, ed. Legg Calve Perthes disease. In: *Wheeless' Textbook of Orthopaedics* (available at http://www.wheelessonline.com/ortho/legg_calve_perthes_disease; published Jan. 3, 2013; accessed March 26, 2013).

OSTEOCHONDRITIS DESSICANS

ESSENTIALS OF DIAGNOSIS

▶ Active adolescent with poorly localized joint pain.

General Considerations

Osteochondritis dissecans (OCD) is described as an idiopathic lesion of the cartilage and subchondral bone in the skeletally immature patient. The "classic" location for this lesion is the lateral aspect of the medial femoral condyle; however, it can also be seen in the other knee compartments, ankle, and elbow. The pathology is not entirely understood, but the etiology is believed to be repetitive trauma. There is a male predominance.

Clinical Findings

A. Symptoms and Signs

The clinical presentation is poorly localized knee pain that is worsened by activity. There may be a mild limp. In more advanced disease the patient may report mechanical symptoms, such as locking or catching. An effusion is present in only <20% of patients and thus should not be used to rule in or out this pathology. Wilson's test has been described for this lesion; however, evidence shows it to be positive in only 16% of knees with proven OCD lesions and thus should not be considered a dependable test.

B. Imaging Studies

Most OCD lesions can be diagnosed on plain radiographs. Lesions can be difficult to visualize on standard views, so four views of the knee should be ordered: anteroposterior, lateral, tunnel, and Merchant views. There should be a low threshold for imaging the contralateral knee for comparison and the possibility of bilateral lesions. MRI is recommended to assess the size, location, and character of the OCD lesion.

Treatment

To classify treatment, two points need to be determined: (1) whether the patient is skeletally mature and (2) whether the lesion is stable. If the lesion is stable and the patient is skeletally immature, then nonsurgical treatment should be first-line. There is no exact timetable, but most clinicians agree on a period of restricting sports participation (perhaps with casting) for 6 weeks. As the lesion heals radiographically, gradual return to activity is allowed. This is a very subjective process that is open for broad interpretation. Those lesions that are unstable or do not respond to conservative care should be treated surgically.

Polousky JD. Juvenile osteochondritis dissecans. *Sports Med Arthrosc Rev*. 2011; 19(1):56–63.

APOPHYSEAL INJURIES

ESSENTIALS OF DIAGNOSIS

▶ Insidious pain over growth plate in skeletally immature individual.
▶ Overuse injury.

General Considerations

An *apophysis* is a growing bony prominence at which secondary ossification occurs in the skeletally immature individual.

Apohysitis is a painful, inflammatory condition at the tendinous insertion onto these bony prominences. This condition is unique to active youth and, by definition, not existent in skeletally mature individuals. Repetitive stress and traction on the apophysis ("overuse") are the offending causes. There seems to be a period of risk surrounding growth spurts. The most common sites of apophysitis are the tibial tuberosity (Osgood-Schlatter disease), inferior patella (Sinding-Larsen-Johansson syndrome), posterior calcaneus (Sever disease), medial epicondyle of elbow ("Little League elbow"), and humeral head ("Little League shoulder"). It is important to note that tendinopathies are unusual in children since the apophysis is intrinsically weaker and more susceptible to injury than the tendon.

Clinical Findings

A. Symptoms and Signs

These conditions are diagnosed clinically by history and physical examination. Patients generally describe an insidious onset of well-localized pain at the site of injury or inflammation. Pain is uniformly present during or shortly after activity. Tenderness is easily elicited by palpation. The presence of mechanical symptoms (locking, catching, or loss of motion), particularly in the elbow, should prompt consideration of an alternate diagnosis.

B. Imaging Studies

While plain radiographs may serve to exclude other causes of pain, they are not routinely necessary in establishing the diagnosis.

Treatment

Apophysitis is generally self-limited and resolves once skeletal maturity is reached and the apophysis fuses. In the meantime, treatment is accomplished by activity modification, ice, NSAIDs, and rehab focused on stretching and strengthening. In most cases a candid discussion with the athlete and her/his family will reveal training patterns that can be altered to prevent further injury. In the case of baseball pitchers, proper throwing mechanics and adhering to pitch count recommendations will be helpful.

Franklin CC, Weiss JM. Stopping sports injuries in kids: an overview of the last year in publications. *Curr Opin Pediatr.* 2012; 24:64–67.

39

Common Upper & Lower Extremity Fractures

W. Scott Black, MD
Robert G. Hosey, MD
Joshua R. Johnson, MD
Kelly Lee Evans-Rankin, MD
Wade M. Rankin, DO

▼ UPPER EXTREMITY FRACTURES

CLAVICLE FRACTURES

▶ Clinical Findings

A. Symptoms and Signs

Clavicle fractures (**Figure 39-1**) are relatively common, accounting for 2–5% of all fractures in adults. The typical mechanism of injury is a fall on an outstretched arm or a direct blow to the shoulder or clavicle. The patient will complain of pain involving the affected shoulder and will typically hold the arm in adduction and internal rotation, avoiding any motion. There may be swelling, discoloration, and deformity at the fracture site. Displaced fractures may cause visible tenting of the skin.

B. Imaging Studies

Clavicle fractures are best seen on an AP view. An AP view with the beam directed 30°–45° cephalad is sometimes necessary to lessen rib interference. A computed tomography (CT) scan can better visualize poorly seen medial or lateral one-third fractures. Additional x-rays of the ipsilateral shoulder may be necessary to evaluate for associated injuries. All x-rays need to be carefully examined for the presence of a concomitant scapular fracture resulting in a floating shoulder.

▶ Complications

Complications may include injuries to the subclavian blood vessels or brachial plexus. Associated pneumothorax is also a rare complication. Fractures displaced ≥100% appear to be at increased risk for nonunion. Excessive callus formation can lead to cosmetic deformity or more rarely, compromise of neurovascular structures. It may require years for a large callus to remodel. Intraarticular fractures on either the medial or lateral end can lead to degenerative arthritis.

▶ Treatment

Nonsurgical management is the treatment of choice for most clavicle fractures and involves a sling for comfort, analgesics, and avoidance of overhead activity. This includes minimally displaced midshaft fractures as well as the vast majority of lateral and medial one-third fractures. Indications for operative management include open fractures, fractures that compromise the airway or neurovascular structures, the presence of significant displacement and/or tenting of the skin, or a floating shoulder. Radiographs should be obtained at 2-week follow-up to assess for displacement and angulation. Visible callus typically forms between 4 and 6 weeks, coinciding with significant clinical improvement. Once the fracture is clinically and radiographically healed, radiographs can be discontinued. The patient may return to normal activity when the clavicle is painless, the fracture is healed on radiograph, and the shoulder has a full range of motion and near-normal strength. Noncontact sports may often be resumed at 6 weeks, but return to contact sports may require ≤4 months.

Pecci M, Kreher JB. Clavicle fractures. *Am Fam Physician*. 2008;77(1):65–70.
Van der Meijden OA, Gaskill TR, Millet PJ. Treatment of clavicle fractures: current concepts review. *J Shoulder Elbow Surg*. 2012; 21:423–429.

COLLE FRACTURES (DISTAL RADIUS FRACTURES)

▶ Clinical Findings

A. Symptoms and Signs

A fall-on-outstretched-hand (FOOSH) injury can lead to a fracture of the distal radius, commonly called a *Colle fracture* (**Figure 39-2**). Patients typically present with pain, swelling,

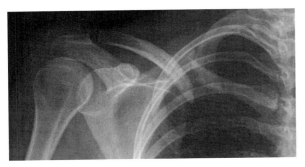

▲ **Figure 39-1.** Clavicle midshaft fracture. (Reproduced with permission of Justin Montgomery, MD; University of Kentucky Radiology.)

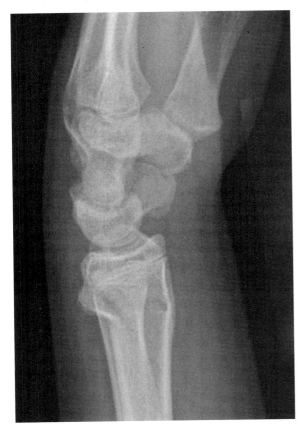

▲ **Figure 39-2.** Colles fracture with dinner fork deformity. (Reproduced with permission of Justin Montgomery, MD; University of Kentucky Radiology.)

and tenderness at the distal forearm. On examination a "dinner fork" deformity (dorsal displacement of the distal fragment and volar angulation of the distal intact radius with radial shortening) may be identified.

B. Imaging Studies

Imaging requires at least AP and lateral radiographs. Additional oblique views are often required to fully assess the extent of the fracture. Intraarticular fractures, concomitant carpal injuries, injuries involving the distal radioulnar joint, or additional upper extremity fractures warrant orthopedic referral. The fracture is at greatest risk of displacement during the first 3 weeks of treatment; therefore it is important to reassess at weekly intervals with x-rays during that timespan.

▶ Complications

Initial complications can include median nerve compression, tendon damage, ulnar nerve contusion or compression, or acute compartment syndrome. Later, patients may develop stiffness of the wrist or hand, cosmetic changes of the wrist, malunion, nonunion, and/or chronic pain of the radioulnar joint during supination.

▶ Treatment

Distal radius fractures are often associated with more long-term disability than commonly realized. Newer surgical techniques may provide better functional outcomes; therefore primary care physicians should carefully consider early surgical referral for any of these fractures.

An impacted or minimally displaced fracture with no extension into the joint space can be managed by the primary care provider. Initially, immobilization may require a volar or sugar-tong splint if significant swelling is present.

Definitive treatment following splinting depends on patient and fracture characteristics. Patients with good bone density and a nondisplaced fracture can often be treated with a functional brace, while patients with minimally displaced fractures or osteopenia should be placed in a cast. Any cast or splint should not obstruct motion of the elbow, metacarpophalangeal (MCP) joints, or fingers.

Fractures that require reduction are often unstable and might be better treated with internal fixation; therefore these fractures are best managed by an orthopedic surgeon.

Reevaluation including x-rays should be performed at weekly intervals for the first 3 weeks. Evidence of displacement warrants orthopedic referral. At 6–8 weeks bridging callus should be visualized and a cast can usually be converted to a functional brace. At the 8–12-week follow-up, additional callus should be seen. The brace can be discontinued at that time. Finger motion exercises should be encouraged as long as the wrist is immobilized.

Black WS, Becker JA. Common forearm fractures in adults. *Am Fam Physician.* 2009; 80(10):1096–1102.

SCAPHOID FRACTURES

▶ Clinical Findings

A. Symptoms and Signs

Scaphoid fractures are caused by a forceful hyperextension of the wrist. This is typically due to a FOOSH with the wrist dorsiflexed and radially deviated. Fracture locations are the distal pole, waist, proximal pole, and tubercle. Another important factor is stability of the fracture. A scaphoid fracture is stable unless there is (1) displacement >1 mm, (2) scapholunate angulation >60°, or (3) radiolunate angulation >15°. Associated injuries to look for include perilunate dislocation, lunate dislocation, trapezium fractures, triquetrum fractures, radial styloid fractures, distal radius fractures (Colle fractures), fractures of metacarpals 1 and 2, and capitate fractures. Patients present with a painful wrist and may report swelling or paresthesias of the affected hand. On examination, there is maximal tenderness in the anatomic snuffbox, pain with radial deviation of the wrist, and pain with axial compression of the thumb.

Bone healing occurs at different rates depending on the location of the fracture. A tuberosity fracture usually heals in 4–6 weeks, and a scaphoid waist fracture in 10–12 weeks. A proximal pole fracture can require 16–20 weeks for healing.

B. Imaging Studies

Traditional PA and lateral radiographs of the wrist obtained at the time of initial injury may not reveal a scaphoid fracture. Oblique radiographic views (45° in pronation and supination) and PA view with the wrist in ulnar deviation (scaphoid view) are often necessary to visualize the fracture. If the initial radiographs are normal and the patient notes persistent pain after 2–3 weeks of immobilization, repeat radiographs should be obtained. If still normal, an MRI should be considered.

▶ Complications

A delay in the diagnosis of a scaphoid fracture can lead to several complications, including delayed union (no healing at 3 months), avascular necrosis (radiographs show sclerosis and cyst development), compartment syndrome (rare), compressive neuropathy (rare), and nonunion (no healing at 4–6 months). Malunion or nonunion resulting in a humpback deformity can lead to carpal instability, loss of wrist extension, weak grip, carpal collapse, and degenerative changes in the wrist. Scaphoid injuries can be associated with additional wrist ligamentous injury, resulting in perilunar instability and need for urgent surgical referral.

▶ Treatment

Nondisplaced or minimally displaced (<1 mm) scaphoid fractures **(Figure 39-3)** are placed in a thumb spica cast. A short arm cast is used for tuberosity fractures and long arm casts for all other nondisplaced or minimally displaced scaphoid fractures. Some studies advocate the use of long arm cast for an initial 4–6 weeks to eliminate scaphoid motion due to forearm rotation followed by a short arm cast for another 4–6 weeks. Although patient expectations of rapid return to work and athletic activities have accelerated the decision of some physicians to recommend early percutaneous screw fixation for nondisplaced or minimally displaced scaphoid fractures, long-term outcomes do not appear to differ between conservative and surgical options. Surgery may allow for earlier clinical evidence of union as well as a quicker return to functional activities, but this decision should be made after a discussion between physician and patient regarding the associated risks accompanying surgical intervention.

When treating nonsurgically, follow-up should occur at 2 weeks with AP, lateral, and oblique radiographic views, checking for stepoffs, angulation, and displacement.

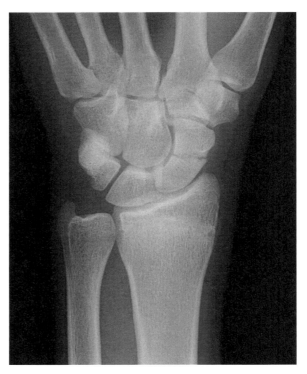

▲ **Figure 39-3.** Scaphoid waist fracture. (Reproduced with permission of Justin Montgomery, MD; University of Kentucky Radiology.)

Trabecular bone may be visible across the fracture line at 4–6 weeks. At 8–12 weeks the fracture line begins to disappear. The normal trabecular bone pattern returns in 12–16 weeks. Rehabilitation takes 3–6 months. Union rates vary; for a nondisplaced fracture the rate is close to 100%. Angulated fracture union rates are 65%, and displaced rates are 45%. The proximal one-third fracture union rate range is 60–70% with immobilization.

Consultation is required for open reduction and internal fixation for displaced fractures, delayed union, and non-union scaphoid fractures. Referral is also appropriate for a patient initially presenting at >3 weeks after the injury.

Alshryda S, et. al. Acute fracture of the scaphoid bone: systemic review and meta-analysis. *Surgeon.* 2012;10(4):218–219.

Kawamura K, Chung KC. Treatment of scaphoid fractures and nonunions. *J Hand Surg Am.* 2008;33(6):988–997.

METACARPAL FRACTURES

▶ Clinical Findings

A. Symptoms and Signs

Metacarpal fractures encompass up to two-thirds of all hand fractures. Most are due to trauma from either a direct blow to the hand or a fall. Patients present with local tenderness and swelling, decreased grip strength, and decreased range of motion. The majority of these fractures are nondisplaced and extraarticular. Often, these fractures are stable and may be managed conservatively. Complications arise from unstable comminuted, displaced, spiral, and oblique fractures resulting in metacarpal shortening and angulation. Such fractures affect functional outcomes and often require surgical consultation and subsequent intervention.

B. Imaging Studies

At a minimum, AP and lateral radiographs are recommended and comparison views are sometimes helpful. In addition, it is recommended that initial radiographs of fractures of the fourth and fifth metacarpals include oblique pronated views. A CT scan may be helpful for fractures of the metacarpal head and base and intraarticular fractures.

▶ Complications

Common complications associated with metacarpal fractures include decreased grip strength and range of motion, painful grip, prolonged dorsal swelling, and intrinsic muscle contraction. Psuedoarthrosis, malunions, nonunion, dorsal radial and ulnar sensory nerve irritation, and arthritis are all described in the literature as possible complications as well.

▶ Treatment

Most metacarpal fractures are inherently stable and do not require fixation. Immobilization via casting is appropriate for 3–4 weeks with range-of-motion (RoM) activities beginning thereafter. If there is no tenderness, no motion at the fracture site, and adequate callus formation, a protective splint can be considered for an additional 2 weeks; otherwise casting should continue until symptomatic resolution and clinical healing have occurred. At 2 weeks postcasting a radiograph should be checked for loss of correction. Bridging callus should be seen at 4–6 weeks. Spiral or oblique fractures, multiple metacarpal shaft fractures, open fractures, fractures with significant shortening, and intraarticular base fractures require further surgical consultation and intervention.

Specific considerations for metacarpal fracture treatment depend on the metacarpal involved, location, ability of the fracture to be reduced, and ultimate stability once reduction is obtained. Fractures are typically described in four distinct locations: base, shaft, neck, and head.

A fracture at the base of the first metacarpal resulting in two dislocated bony segments is known as a *Bennett fracture*. These fractures require either closed reduction and percutaneous fixation or open reduction with internal fixation. For the remainder of extraarticular, minimally displaced metacarpal base fractures, closed reduction with casting for 4–6 weeks until bony healing is usually appropriate. Displaced or intraarticular fractures often require surgical intervention to restore bony congruity and ensure proper return of range of motion and strength.

Shaft and neck (eg, boxer's fracture) fractures usually display apex dorsal angulation due to interosseous muscle pull. For shaft fractures closed reduction is required for angulation >10° in second and third metacarpals, 20° in fourth metacarpal, and 30° in fifth metacarpal fractures (**Figure 39-4**). Accepted angulation for neck fractures is <15° for index and middle metacarpal fractures, and <30° for ring and little-finger metacarpal injuries. If reduction alone is unable to maintain these cited angulations, surgical management must be considered.

Metacarpal head fractures are, by definition, intraarticular injuries and can involve avulsion of the collateral ligaments. Nondisplaced fractures may be treated with splinting, and displaced fragments or fractures involving >20% of the articular surface often require surgical fixation.

Hardy MA. Principles of metacarpal and phalangeal fracture management: a review of rehabilitation concepts. *J Orthop Phys Ther.* 2004;34(12):781–799.

Jones NF, Jupiter JB, Lalonde DH. Common fractures and dislocations of the hand. *Plast Reconst Surg.* 2012;130(5):722e–736e.

RADIAL HEAD FRACTURES

▶ Clinical Findings

A. Symptoms and Signs

Radial head fractures account for up to one-third of all elbow fractures. The typical mechanism of injury is a FOOSH

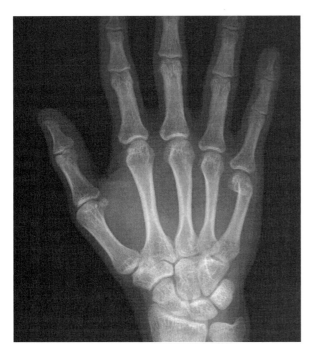

▲ **Figure 39-4.** Boxer's fracture of the fifth metacarpal. (Reproduced with permission of Justin Montgomery, MD; University of Kentucky Radiology.)

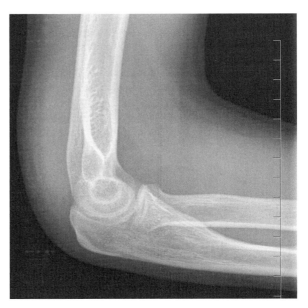

▲ **Figure 39-5.** Fat pad sign with a proximal radial head fracture. (Reproduced with permission of Justin Montgomery, MD; University of Kentucky Radiology.)

with a pronated forearm or with the elbow in slight flexion. Alternatively, a direct blow to the lateral elbow can also produce these fractures. Patients present with elbow pain, swelling, and pain on movement of the forearm. The elbow will be tender to palpation over the radial head, just distal to the lateral epicondyle.

B. Imaging Studies

Anteroposterior and lateral x-rays of the elbow are generally adequate to detect a fracture, although an oblique or radio-capitellar view may be necessary for visualization of subtle fractures or to better evaluate displacement. Sometimes, an elbow joint effusion (sail sign and/or visualization of the posterior fat pad) is the only x-ray evidence of a fracture **(Figure 39-5)**. Follow-up radiographs should be obtained at 2 weeks to assess for displacement. Bone healing is visible between 6 and 8 weeks.

▶ Complications

Loss of elbow motion is the most common complication. For this reason, elbow movement is encouraged as early as possible according to the type of fracture (see Mason classification below) and the patient's symptoms. Additional complications can include posttraumatic arthritis, heterotopic ossification, complex regional pain syndrome, and wrist pain from an associated distal radioulnar joint (DRUJ) injury.

The Mason classification system is as follows:

Type I: nondisplaced fracture; no mechanical obstruction to movement

Type II: displacement >2 mm or angulation >30°

Type III: comminuted fractures

Type IV: fracture with associated elbow dislocation

▶ Treatment

Mason type I fractures can be managed without orthopedic referral. The elbow can be placed in a posterior splint or sling for ≤7 days as needed to control pain. Early movement should be encouraged. If symptoms allow, these fractures can also be treated without immobilization with patients allowed movement of the elbow as tolerated. Repeat x-rays in 1–2 weeks to ensure alignment has been maintained. Resolution of pain and return of normal elbow function are usually obtained by 2–3 months.

Orthopedic referral is generally indicated for Mason type II–IV fractures.

Black WS, Becker JA. Common forearm fractures in adults. *Am Fam Physician.* 2009; 80(10):1096–1102.

STRESS FRACTURES

▶ General Considerations

Management of traumatic fractures of the lower extremity long bones is relatively straightforward if a few simple rules are recognized. Orthopedic referral is required for any traumatic fracture that is displaced or involves a joint line. The goal of this section is to guide the primary care physician through a basic understanding of concepts surrounding bone stress pathogenesis, including epidemiology, clinical signs and symptoms, physical examination, radiographic diagnostic aids, and treatment of four difficult-to-treat areas of stress reaction in the lower extremities. The population most at risk for stress reaction is athletes. This population presents therapeutic challenges secondary to their increased activity, predilection to overuse injury, and desire to return to competition as quickly as possible, which may lead them to compete before the stress injury fully resolves.

Stress fractures are estimated to make up 10% of all athletic injuries. Ninety-five percent of stress injuries occur in the lower extremities secondary to the extreme repetitive weight-bearing loads placed on these bones. The peak incidence occurs in people aged 18–25 years. There is a decreased incidence of stress fracture in men secondary to greater lean body mass and overall bone structure. It has been estimated that female military recruits have a relative risk of stress fracture that is 1.2–10 times greater than men while engaging in the same level of training. In athletic populations a gender difference is not as evident, possibly because athletic women are more fit and better conditioned. Incidence is estimated to be comparable for all races.

Stress fracture is most common after changes in an athlete's training regimen. Injury is especially prevalent in unconditioned runners who increase their training regimen. Training error, which can include increased quantity or intensity of training, introduction of a new activity, poor equipment, and change in environment (ie, surface), is the most important risk factor for stress injury. Low bone density, dietary deficiency, low BMI, menstrual irregularities, hormonal imbalance, sleep deprivation, and biomechanical abnormalities also place athletes at risk. Keeping this in mind and recognizing the increasing incidence of female athletic triad (amenorrhea, disordered eating and osteoporosis), it is easy to understand why women can have an increased risk for stress injury.

▶ Clinical Findings

A. Symptoms and Signs

Stress fractures are related to a maladaptive process between bone injury and bone remodeling. Bone reacts to stress by early osteoclastic activity (old-bone resorption) followed by strengthening osteoblastic activity (new-bone formation). With continued stress, bone resorption outpaces new-bone formation and a self-perpetuating cycle occurs, with continued activity allowing weakened bone to be more susceptible to continued microfracture and ultimately progressing to frank fracture. The initiation of stress reaction is unclear. It has been postulated that excessive forces are transmitted to bone when surrounding muscles fatigue. The highly concentrated muscle forces act across localized area of bone, causing mechanical insults above the stress-bearing capacity of bone.

Athletic stress fracture follows a crescendo process. Symptoms start insidiously with dull, gnawing pain at the end of physical activity. Pain increases over days to the point where the activity cannot be continued. At first pain decreases with rest, then shorter and shorter duration of activity causes pain. More time is then needed for pain to dissipate until it is present with minimal activity and at night. After a few days of rest, pain resolves, only to return once again with resumption of activity. More specific historical and physical examination findings are discussed below in conjunction with specific anatomic regions.

B. Imaging Studies

The diagnosis of stress fracture is primarily clinical and is based on history and physical examination. It is prudent to start with plain radiographs, which have poor sensitivity but high specificity, as the initial study. The presence of stress reaction is confirmed by the presence of periosteal reaction, intramedullary sclerosis, callus, or obvious fracture line. Plain films typically fail to reveal a bony abnormality unless symptoms have been present for at least 2–3 weeks.

The technetium triple-phase bone scan is often employed to improve diagnostic power. Stress reactions can often be visualized within 48–72 hours from symptom onset. Triple-phase bone scan can differentiate soft-tissue and bone injuries. All three phases can be positive in an acute fracture. In soft-tissue injuries, with no bony involvement, the first two phases are often positive, whereas the delayed image shows minimal or no increased uptake. In conditions such as medial tibial stress syndrome (MTSS), in which there is early bony stress reaction, the first two phases are negative and the delayed image is positive. Nuclear medicine bone scans should not be used to monitor fracture healing because the fracture line is not clearly visualized and delayed images continue to demonstrate increased uptake for ≥12 months after initial studies.

Computed tomographic scans can identify conditions that mimic stress fracture on bone scan, confirm fracture suspected on bone scan, or help to make treatment decisions as with navicular stress fractures.

Magnetic resonance imaging offers the advantage of visualizing soft-tissue changes in anatomic regions in which the soft-tissue structures often cloud the differential diagnosis. Clinically the high sensitivity of bone scan and MRI is necessary only when the diagnosis of stress fracture is in question or the exact location or extent of injury must be known in order to determine treatment. MRI is currently the gold standard for stress fracture imaging.

Kaeding CC, Najarian RG. Stress fractures: classification and management. *Phys Sportsmed* 2010;38(3):45–54.
Knapp TP, Garrett WE. Stress fractures: general concepts. *Clin Sports Med*. 1997; 16:339. [PMID: 9238314]

Femoral Stress Fractures

▶ General Considerations

Stress fractures involving the femur can occur in a variety of locations, most commonly the femoral shaft and neck. One study that looked at 320 athletes with bone scan–positive stress fractures revealed the femur to be the fourth most frequent site of injury.

▶ Differential Diagnosis

The symptom most commonly encountered with stress fractures of the femur is pain at the anterior aspect of the hip. Differentiating the diagnosis can be difficult secondary to the multiple number of structures in the hip that have the potential to produce similar pain syndromes and the deep nonpalpable structures of the anatomic region. Diagnosis can be made complex by the multitude of structures in this region from which pain may emanate; thus, the physician must be attuned to the history to narrow the differential down to a list in which stress fracture is prominent. This is important in order to avoid severe complications associated with fractures of the femoral neck.

▶ Femoral Shaft Fractures

Femoral shaft stress fractures are more common than expected, with an incidence of 3.7% among athletes. Onset of pain can be gradual over a period of days to weeks. Average time from symptom onset to diagnosis is approximately 2 weeks. The fulcrum test is well suited to act as a guide for ordering radiologic tests and thereby decreasing time to diagnosis. It is also a useful clinical test to assess healing. For this test, the athlete is seated on the examination table with legs dangling as the examiner's arm is used as a fulcrum under the thigh. The examiner's arm is moved from the distal to proximal thigh as gentle pressure is applied to the dorsum of the knee with the opposite hand. A positive test is elicited by sharp pain or apprehension at the site of the fracture. Plain films are rarely sensitive in detecting stress fractures within the first 2–3 weeks of symptoms. Bone scan or MRI may be useful in this time period to aid in diagnosis.

The most common site of injury in athletes is the midmedial or posteromedial cortex of the proximal femur.

Once diagnosis is confirmed, treatment depends on the underlying causes responsible for the injury. If the fracture is consistent with a compression-sided fracture (**Figure 39-6**), treatment consists of rest with gradual resumption of activity. This usually is adequate for healing of nondisplaced fractures. Treatment protocols are based on empiric data gathered from clinical observation. An example of a treatment protocol may consist of rest for a period of 1–4 weeks of toe-touch weight bearing progressing to full weight bearing. This would be followed by a phase of low-impact activity (ie, biking, swimming). Once patients are able to perform low-impact activity for a prolonged time without pain, they may gradually advance to high impact. Resumption of full activity averages between 8 and 16 weeks. Surgical treatment should be considered if there is displacement of the fracture, delayed union, or nonunion following conservative therapy.

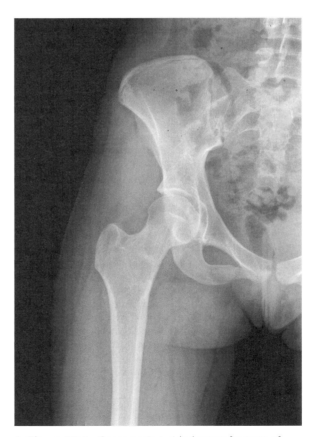

▲ **Figure 39-6.** Compression-sided stress fracture of the right femoral neck. Note sclerotic line perpendicular to medial cortex. (Reproduced with permission of Justin Montgomery, MD; University of Kentucky Radiology.)

Femoral Neck Fractures

Stress fractures of the femoral neck are uncommon but carry a high complication rate if the diagnosis is missed or the fracture is improperly treated. The primary presenting symptom is pain at the site of the groin, anterior thigh, or knee. Pain is exacerbated by weight bearing or physical activity. The athlete may have an antalgic gait or painful, limited hip range of motion in internal rotation or external rotation. MRI is the diagnostic modality of choice for evaluating femoral neck stress fractures.

Stress fractures of the femoral neck are divided into two categories: compression (occurring along the inferior or medial border of the neck) and tension (along the superior or lateral neck) type. Compression fractures are more common in younger patients. The fracture line, if seen on the radiograph, can propagate across the femoral neck. A nondisplaced, incomplete compression fracture is treated with rest until the patient is pain free with full motion. Non-weight-bearing ambulation with the patient on crutches follows until radiographic healing as shown on plain films is complete. Frequent radiographs may need to be obtained to monitor propagation of the fracture. If the compression fracture becomes complete, or fails to heal with rest, then internal fixation may be necessary. Patients treated nonsurgically may not achieve full activity for several months. Tension (distraction)-sided femoral neck fractures are an emergency because of the potential for complications (ie, nonunion or avascular necrosis). The patient is immediately rendered non-weight-bearing and will acutely need internal fixation. If the fracture is displaced, the patient will need open reduction and internal fixation urgently.

McCormick F, Nwachukwu BU, Provencher MT. Stress fractures in runners. *Clin Sports Med* 2012; 31:291–306.

Tibial Stress Fracture

General Considerations

Tibial stress fractures account for half of all stress fractures diagnosed. Most tibial stress fractures in athletes are secondary to running. Two sites located within the tibia are most commonly associated with stress fractures. The first of these is located between the middle and distal third of the tibia along the posteromedial border. This type of injury is most often associated with running. The second site is along the middle third of the anterior cortex. This injury is most commonly associated with activities involving a great deal of jumping (eg, dancing, basketball, gymnastics).

Clinical Findings

A. Symptoms and Signs

On history the patient commonly describes pain occurring in the region of the fracture with activity (eg, running or jumping) and resolving with rest. The pain eventually progresses and lasts longer after the activity until the patient is symptomatic at rest. Physical examination often reveals localized pain to palpation. Sometimes persistent thickening, secondary to periosteal reaction, can be appreciated by palpation along the tibia.

B. Imaging Studies

Diagnosis by radiographic plain film may be possible if symptoms have been present for at least 4–6 weeks. Triple-phase bone scan is very sensitive and may allow diagnosis within 48–72 hours of symptom onset. Tibial stress fractures can be seen clearly on MRI with sensitivity comparable to that of triple-phase bone scan. Both bone scan and MRI allow differentiation of medial tibial stress syndrome and stress fracture.

Differential Diagnosis

Medial tibial stress syndrome (MTSS) is the most commonly confused diagnosis in the classification of tibial stress injuries with stress fracture. MTSS usually occurs diffusely along the middle and distal third of the posteromedial tibia and is commonly seen in runners. This condition, however, can also be seen with activities involving persistent jumping. The symptom spectrum commonly progresses, as does that of stress fractures, with continued activity. MTSS represents a stress reaction within bone whereby the usual remodeling process becomes maladaptive. This injury responds well to rest in a shorter time period as compared with stress fracture and is easily differentiated from stress fracture on triple-phase bone scan.

Treatment

Once the diagnosis of tibial stress fracture has been made, a distinction between a compression versus tension-sided injury must be made. Fractures along the posteromedial border are considered compression stress injuries and respond well to conservative therapy (**Figure 39–7**). The average recovery time for this injury is approximately 12 weeks when the patient is treated with rest alone. Most guidelines for treatment of this injury involve relative or absolute rest. These stress fractures can be effectively treated in a pneumatic leg brace. Athletes treated in the pneumatic brace (long leg air cast) showed decreased time to pain-free symptoms (14 ± 6 days) and time to competitive participation (21 ± 2 days) versus traditional mode non-weight-bearing treatment (77 ± 7 days). Athletes in the brace may continue exercising, but modifications of the training routine must be made to maintain pain-free activities. Patients are treated on the basis of a functional activity progression as outlined by Swenson and colleagues.

Tibial stress fractures of the midanterior cortex, also known as "the dreaded black line," radiographically (**Figure 39–8**), are

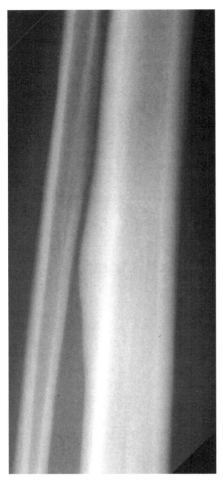

▲ **Figure 39-7.** Periosteal stress reaction at the posterior medial aspect of the tibia.

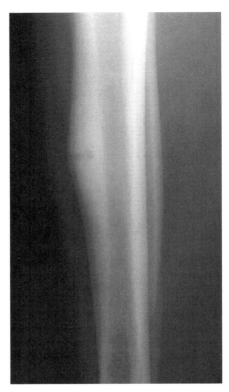

▲ **Figure 39-8.** Dreaded black line at the anterior medial aspect of the tibia.

Shindle MK, Endo Y, Warren RF, et al. Stress fractures about the tibia, foot, and ankle. *J Am Acad Orthop Surg* 2012; 20(3):167–176.

Tarsal Navicular Stress Fracture

▷ General Considerations

Tarsal navicular stress fractures are an underdiagnosed source of prolonged, disabling foot pain predominantly seen in active athletes involved in sprinting and jumping. One study, involving 111 competitive track and field athletes, found that navicular stress fractures are the second most common lower extremity stress fracture.

▷ Clinical Findings

A. Symptoms and Signs

These fractures are prone to misdiagnosis secondary to the vague nature of the pain. The pain may radiate along the medial arch and not directly over the talonavicular joint. Sometimes pain radiates distally, causing the physician to suspect a Morton neuroma or metatarsalgia. The pain often

very difficult to manage conservatively. This fracture occurs at the tension side of the tibial cortex, most commonly in athletes who jump. Delayed union and complete fracture are two significant complications associated with this area. The average time to symptom-free return to activity from symptom onset is >12 months with conservative care. Conservative treatment revolves around rest, or immobilization, or both. Patients who do not respond to conservative treatment or are involved in activities (career or competitive athletics) would benefit from surgical treatment with tibial intramedullary nailing. Patients with these fractures should be referred to a sports medicine specialist.

McCormick F, Nwachukwu BU, Provencher MT. Stress fractures in runners. *Clin Sports Med.* 2012; 31:291–306.

disappears with a few days of rest, often tricking the athlete into not believing the potential seriousness of the diffuse foot pain. The diagnosis is also clouded because the fractures are rarely seen on plain film.

Symptoms suggesting a clinical diagnosis consists of (1) insidious onset of vague pain over the dorsum of the medial midfoot or over the medial aspect of the longitudinal arch; (2) ill-defined pain, soreness, or cramping aggravated by activity and relieved by rest; (3) well-localized tenderness to palpation over the navicular bone or medial arch; and (4) little swelling or discoloration. Certain foot abnormalities, including short first metatarsal and metatarsus adductor and limited dorsiflexion of the ankle, may concentrate stress on the tarsal navicular region, predisposing to stress.

B. Imaging Studies

Initial imaging for tarsal navicular stress fractures includes plain radiographs. Plain radiographs should be obtained in AP, lateral, and oblique standing positions. Unfortunately, sensitivity is low because a majority of these fractures are incomplete and therefore difficult to see on plain radiographs. Also, bony resorption requires 10 days to 3 weeks to allow visualization. Most fractures are located in the central third of bone along the proximal articular surface, which is a relatively avascular region.

The next recommended diagnostic procedure is a triple-phase bone scan. These are positive at an early stage and almost 100% sensitive. CT scanning is the gold stardard for optimal evaluation once bone scan has demonstrated increased uptake in the navicular bone. The best images are obtained with ≤1.5-mm slices. As imaging devices and technique have improved, MRI has been used with increased frequency and is almost as sensitive as bone scan in the detection of these fractures. MRI carries the additional advantage of no radiation exposure and evaluation of surrounding structures.

Treatment

Data indicate that 6–8 weeks of non-weight-bearing cast immobilization compares favorably with surgical treatment for failed weight-bearing treatment. Surgery is recommended for a displaced, complete fracture with a small transverse fragment (ossicle), or failure of conservative management. Surgical treatment often consists of either bone graft or screw fixation followed by non-weight-bearing cast immobilization for 6 weeks.

After 6 weeks of non-weight-bearing cast immobilization, fracture healing is followed clinically by palpation of the fracture site along the dorsal proximal region of the navicular bone. Persistent tenderness over this "N" spot requires an additional 2 weeks of non–weight-bearing immobilization before reassessment. If the fracture site is not tender after casting, the patient may begin weight bearing.

Imaging may remain positive up to 6 months following the injury. For this reason the recommendation is not to repeat imaging, but instead to rely on clinical examination (palpation of the N spot).

Fowler JR, Gaughan JP, Boden BP, Pavolov H, Torg JS. The non-surgical and surgical treatment of tarsal navicular stress fractures. *Sports Med.* 2011; 41(8):613–619.

Khan KM, et al. Outcome of conservative and surgical management of navicular stress fracture in athletes: eighty-six cases proven with computerized tomography. *Am J Sports Med.* 1992;20:657.

Metatarsal Stress Fractures

General Considerations

Metatarsal stress fractures in athletes are very common. Depending on the study referenced, they are either third or fourth in incidence. These fractures are also known as "march fractures" because of the large numbers of military recruits who obtained these fractures after sudden increases in their level of activity. The second metatarsal is the most common location, followed by the third and fourth metatarsals. The second metatarsal is subjected to 3–4 times body weight during loading and pushoff phases of gait.

Clinical Findings

A. Symptoms and Signs

Clinical suspicion for this injury is raised when the athlete complains of forefoot or midfoot pain of insidious onset. On examination these injuries present as areas of point tenderness overlying the metatarsal shaft.

B. Imaging Studies

Radiographs are usually sufficient to document stress fracture, which is visualized as a frank fracture or periosteal reaction at the affected site. As with most stress fractures, the patient may be symptomatic 2–4 weeks prior to visualizing the fracture on radiograph. If the diagnosis is in question, bone scan and MRI have significantly higher sensitivity and specificity for detecting these injuries at an earlier timeframe.

C. Treatment

Treatment is easily managed by the primary care physician. The injury is treated symptomatically, allowing the athlete to participate in activities that are not painful. Immobilization in the form of a steel shank insole or stiff, wooden-soled shoe may be necessary for a limited time, until the pain disappears. At times the patient may benefit from a short leg walking cast or removable walking boot for severe pain. Four weeks of rest is usually sufficient for healing. During these

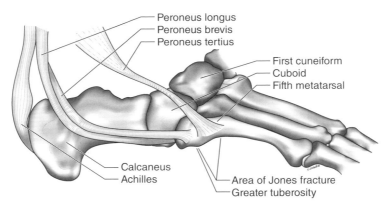

Peroneus longus
Peroneus brevis
Peroneus tertius

First cuneiform
Cuboid
Fifth metatarsal

Calcaneus
Achilles

Area of Jones fracture
Greater tuberosity

▲ **Figure 39-9.** Anatomy of the proximal fifth metatarsal. (Reproduced with permission of Ellsworth C. Seeley, MD.)

4 weeks, the athlete may continue modified conditioning with non-weight-bearing exercises (eg, swimming and pool running), followed by cycling and stair climbing.

Although most of these fractures heal well with conservative management, fractures of the proximal fifth metatarsal have a high incidence of delayed union and nonunion. A thorough understanding of the classification and anatomy of fractures in this location is required for proper identification to determine conservative versus surgical treatment.

FRACTURES OF THE PROXIMAL FIFTH METATARSAL

The fifth metatarsal consists of a base tuberosity, shaft (diaphysis), neck, and head. (**Figure 39-9**). Fractures of the proximal fifth metatarsal include tuberosity avulsion fractures, acute Jones fractures, and diaphyseal stress fractures.

Tuberosity Avulsion Fractures

Tuberosity fractures are typically known as "dancer fractures" because they are usually associated with an ankle inversion plantar flexion injury. This injury is likely secondary to the plantar aponeurosis pulling from the base of the fifth metatarsal. Nondisplaced fracture carries an excellent prognosis, almost always healing in 4–6 weeks with conservative therapy. The athlete's treatment consists of limited weight bearing to pain with modified activity such as that used with second, third, and fourth metatarsal injuries. If needed, the athlete can be immobilized in a walking cast, wooden (or steel shank)-soled shoe, or walking boot. The immobilization can usually be removed by 3 weeks (average 3–6 weeks) in favor of modified footwear if pain has diminished. The patient then may gradually return to vigorous activity; most athletes return to full sports activity in 6–8 weeks. Bony union usually takes place by 8 weeks. Orthopedic referral is needed for displaced fractures or

comminuted fractures involving >30% of the cubometatarsal articular surface or stepoff of >2 mm. Sometimes small displaced fractures at this site may require surgical removal if bony union does not occur secondary to chronic irritation.

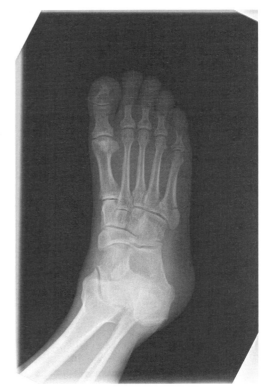

▲ **Figure 39-10.** The Jones fracture. (Reproduced with permission of Justin Montgomery, MD; University of Kentucky Radiology.)

Jones Fractures

Jones fractures consist of a transverse fracture at the junction of the diaphysis and metaphysis (**Figure 39-10**). The Jones fracture is believed to occur when the ankle is in plantar flexion and a large adduction force is applied to the forefoot. It is important to realize that this is a midfoot injury with no prodromal symptoms. Therefore, the injury is classified as acute.

Torg and colleagues showed that this fracture, in nonathletes, could heal in 6–8 weeks with strict non-weight-bearing immobilization. However, secondary to low vascularization and high stresses at the site of the Jones fracture, the injury is associated with a poor outcome; it is plagued by delayed union and nonunion if treated conservatively in athletic patients. Those who undergo conservative treatment are placed on a non-weight-bearing immobilization protocol and in a plaster cast for 6–8 weeks. If there is lack of clinical healing by 6–8 weeks, therapy is individualized. If clinical healing is present by 6–8 weeks, immobilization is continued in a fracture brace with range of motion and gradual weight bearing. If there are no signs of clinical healing, treatment must be individualized either with continued cast immobilization or surgical intervention. Surgical intervention for Jones fracture consists of either intramedullary screw fixation or bone grafting.

Diaphyseal Fractures

Stress fractures distal to the site of Jones fractures and acute-on-chronic fractures occurring in the same position as Jones fractures are commonly seen in athletes who run.

Pain is usually over the lateral aspect of the foot, over the fifth metatarsal base. Usually no significant trauma has been associated with these fractures. Prodromal symptoms occurring weeks to months in advance of an acute injury can often be elicited in the history.

Treatment of choice for acute nondisplaced diaphyseal stress fracture is non-weight-bearing immobilization. More extensive fractures require individualized treatment. Conservative treatment may take ≤20 weeks and result in nonunion. Complications of prolonged immobilization include recurrence of fracture and significant dysfunction from muscle atrophy and loss of range of motion. For athletes, surgical options are recommended. Casting and prolonged immobilization of acute or chronic fractures frequently fail, giving rise to delayed or nonunion fractures. Surgery is often needed and is the recommended procedure of choice.

The difference between screw fixation and bone grafting is recovery time. It takes up to 12 weeks to return to pre-fracture activity with grafting versus 6–8 weeks with screw fixation. Grafting carries a higher failure rate. Screw fixation is now recommended first and bone grafting if fixation fails.

Kerkhoffs GM, Versteegh VE, Sierevelt IN, Kloen P, van Dijk CN. Treatment of proximal metatarsal V fractures in athetes and non-athletes. *Br J Sports Med*. 2012; 46:644–648.

Polzer H, Polzer S, Mutschler W, Prall W. Acute fractures to the proximal fifth metatarsal bone: development of classification and treatment recommendations based on the current evidence. *Injury*. 2012; 43:1626–1632.

Shindle MK, Endo Y, Warren RF, et al. Stress fractures about the tibia, foot, and ankle. *J Am Acad Orthop Surg*. 2012; 20(3):167–176.

Healthy Aging & Geriatric Assessment

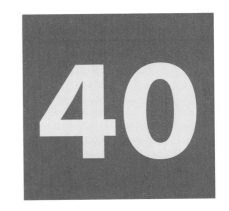

Lora Cox-Vance, MD

CHARACTERISITICS OF AGING

The population of the United States, similar to that of other industrialized nations, is aging. The US population of adults aged ≥65 years increased at a faster rate (15.1%) between 2000 and 2010 than did the total US population (9.7%). Between the years 2010 and 2050, the number of Americans aged ≥65 years is projected to have doubled. In the rapidly changing arena of healthcare financing and delivery, services that promote or improve functional abilities, prevent or delay disease progression, and improve the overall health status of this aging population are essential. This chapter defines successful and healthy aging, highlights recommendations for health promotion and disease prevention, and describes key elements in geriatric assessment.

Aging is a physiologic process, and the term *healthy aging* does not imply an absence of limitations, but rather an adaptation to the changes associated with the aging process that is acceptable to the individual. Successful or healthy aging appears to include three factors: (1) low probability of disease and disability, (2) higher cognitive and physical functioning, and (3) an active engagement with life (**Table 40-1**). Healthcare providers can promote healthy aging by assisting the older adult in developing competence in directing and managing future roles, thereby maintaining autonomy and a sense of self-worth.

While there are common physiologic changes associated with aging, the geriatric population is a highly heterogeneous group with varying degrees of chronic disease, and physical and cognitive disability within individuals. A number of chronic conditions commonly affect this population (**Table 40-2**). The overall health status and well-being of older adults is highly complex and results from many interacting processes, including risk factor exposure (tobacco, alcohol, drugs, diet, sedentary lifestyle), biological age-related changes, and the development and consequences of functional impairments. Many of the conditions previously considered "normal aging" are now known to be modifiable or even preventable with appropriate disease prevention and health promotion strategies.

Bryant LL, et al. In their own words: a model of healthy aging. *Soc Sci Med*. 2001; 53:927. [PMID: 11522138]

Fried LP: Epidemiology of aging. *Epidemiol Rev*. 2000; 22:95. [PMID: 10939013]

Kyle L. A concept analysis of healthy aging. *Nurs Forum*. 2005; 40:45.

Peel N, et al. Behavioral determinants of healthy ging. *Am J Prevent Med*. 2005; 28:298.

United States Census Bureau. *2010 Census Briefs; The Older Population: 201*; issued 2011 (available at http://www.census .gov/prod/cen2010/briefs/c2010br-09.pdf; accessed March 22, 2013).

United States Census Bureau. *The Next Four Decades. The Older Population in the United States: 2010 to 2050*; issued May 2010 (available at http://www.aoa.gov/AoARoot/Aging Statistics/ future_growth/DOCS/p25-1138.pdf; accessed March 22, 2013).

PREVENTION & HEALTH PROMOTION

Prevention in geriatrics attempts to delay morbidity and disability and should be a primary goal of any medical practice caring for older individuals. The primary strategy for prevention lies in the alteration of lifestyle and environmental factors that contribute to the development or progression of chronic disease. A prospective cohort study of older adults with an average baseline age of 68 years found that participants with fewer lifestyle risk factors experienced lower disability and mortality with the benefits persisting through the ninth decade of life.

Frailty is a complex geriatric syndrome associated with several chronic conditions, many of which may be preventable (**Table 40-3**). Important evidence of frailty includes slow walking speed, low physical activity, weight loss, and cognitive impairment. Preventive services for older adults should be implemented with a goal of preventing frailty, preserving function, and optimizing quality of life.

Table 40-1. Factors associated with healthy aging.

"Going and doing" is worthwhile and desirable to the individual
Social activities
Reading
Travel
Housework
Fishing
Creative outlets: eg, music, arts, dance, needlework
Sufficient abilities to accomplish valued activities
Mobility
Vision
Cognitive functioning
Coping
Independence
Having appropriate resources to support the activity
Valued relationships: friends and family
Healthcare and health information
Optimistic attitude
Self-esteem, self-efficacy, self-confidence

Data from Bryant LL, et al. In their own words: a model of healthy aging. *Soc Sci Med.* 2001; 53:927. [PMID: 11522138]

Health promotion is a broad term that encompasses the objective of improving or enhancing the individual's current health status. The purpose of health promotion, especially as applied to the elderly, is the prevention of avoidable decline, frailty, and dependence, thereby promoting healthy aging.

For health promotion to be effective with older adults, it must be individualized, factoring in age, functional status, comorbid conditions, life expectancy, patient goals and preferences, and culture. Culture is important in understanding the older adult's health belief system. Without this

Table 40-2. Most common conditions associated with aging.

Arthritis
Hypertension
Heart disease
Hearing loss
Influenza
Injuries
Orthopedic impairments
Cataracts
Chronic sinusitis
Depression
Cancer
Diabetes mellitus
Visual impairments
Urinary incontinence
Varicose veins

Table 40-3. Conditions associated with frailty.

Advanced age, usually ≥85 years
Functional decline
Falls and associated injuries (hip fracture)
Polypharmacy
Chronic disease
Dementia and depression
Social dependence
Institutionalization or hospitalization
Nutritional impairment

Data from Hammerman D. Toward an understanding of frailty. *Ann Intern Med.* 1999; 130:945.

understanding, a healthcare provider may be unable to negotiate a health promotion and prevention strategy that is acceptable to the patient and the provider.

Ahmed N, et al. Frailty: an emerging geriatric syndrome. *Am J Med.* 2007;120:748-753. [PMID: 17765039]

Chakravarty EF, et al. Lifestyle risk factors predict disability and death in healthy aging adults. *Am J Med.* 2012; 125(2):190-197. [PMID: 22269623]

Rothman MD, et al: Prognostic significance of potential frailty criteria. *J Am Geriatr Soc.* 2008; 56:2211-2216. [PMID: 19093920]

HEALTH PROMOTION & SCREENING

Many of the leading causes of death in the geriatric population (**Table 40-4**) are amenable to both primary and secondary preventive strategies, especially if targeted early in life. The major targets of prevention should therefore be focused at the major causes of death—including coronary heart

Table 40-4. Leading causes of death age ≥65 years, United States, 2010

Cause of Death	Number
Cardiovascular disease	477,338
Cancer	396,670
Lung disease	160,877
Stroke	109,990
Alzheimer's disease	82,616
Diabetes mellitus	49,191
Nephritis	41,994
Unintentional injury	41,300

Data from National Center for Health Statistics. *Leading Causes of Death Reports* (available at http://webappa.cdc.gov/sasweb/ncipc/leadcaus10_us.html; accessed March 29, 2013).

disease, cancer, lung disease, and stroke—with the goals of reducing premature mortality caused by acute and chronic illness, maintaining function, enhancing quality of life, and extending active life expectancy. A priority in screening should be given to preventive services that are both easy to deliver and associated with beneficial outcomes.

Primary, secondary and tertiary preventive efforts should be considered in older adults as enthusiastically as they are employed in younger adults. In developing screening and preventive strategies for individual patients, a number of factors must be considered, including major causes of death and related risk factors, the burden of comorbidity, functional ability, cognitive status, life expectancy, and patients' goal and preferences. These considerations should guide the patient-provider discussion and decision making.

A review of the literature reveals controversy and variation in some specific recommendations across sponsoring medical specialties. This is largely related to a lack of randomized clinical trials in patients aged >75 years. As the number of quality clinical trials including older adults, these recommendations will further evolve.

The US Preventive Services Task Force (USPSTF) has set the standard for providing recommendations for clinical practice on preventive interventions, including screening tests, counseling interventions, immunizations, and chemo-prophylactic regimens. These standards are established by a review of the scientific evidence for the clinical effectiveness of each preventive service. A detailed discussion of health promotion and preventive screening strategies relevant to the geriatric population, including recommendations from the USPSTF, can be found in Chapter 15, on health maintenance for adults. The Agency for Healthcare Research and Quality provides an electronic resource, the Electronic Preventive Services Selector, to assist providers in identifying age-appropriate preventive and screening measures. (This tool is available online at http://epss.ahrq.gov/PDA/index.jsp or for download on most smartphones.)

Albert RH, Clark MM. Cancer screening in the older patient. *Am Fam Physician.* 2008; 78:1369.

PHYSICAL ACTIVITY & EXERCISE IN OLDER ADULTS

Exercise and physical activity as a form of primary prevention have many benefits, even for sedentary older adults. Even leisure activities can serve as a form of primary prevention and have many benefits in older adults. The Leisure World Cohort Study of activities and mortality in the elderly suggests that as little as 15 minutes of leisure physical activity per day decreases mortality risk, with the greatest reduction noted at 45 minutes of physical activity per day. A specific aim of the US Government Healthy People 2020 Initiative is to increase the proportion of older adults with reduced physical or cognitive function who engage in leisure-time physical activities by 10%.

A meta-analysis of physical activity and well-being in advanced age concluded that the maximum benefit of physical activity was in the area of self-efficacy, and that improvements in cardiovascular status, strength, and functional capacity also improved well-being. Engaging in leisurely physical activities has been shown to increase levels of exercise in sedentary populations.

The American Heart Association (AHA) and American College of Sports Medicine (ACSM) recommend the following exercise goals for older adults: (1) moderate aerobic activity for 30 minutes on 5 days per week, (2) 10 repetitions of 8–10 strength training exercises at least 2 days per week, and (3) balance exercises for community-dwelling adults at risk for falls. When engaging in moderate aerobic exercise, the older adult should be advised to work hard enough to sweat but below the point at which increased breathing efforts make conversation difficult.

The AHA recommends a pre-participation history and physical exam (**Table 40-5**) for sedentary older adults planning to begin an exercise program. The ACSM recommends exercise stress testing for older adults before engaging in a vigorous exercise program such as strenuous cycling or running (**Table 40-6**). Conditions that are absolute and relative contraindications to exercise stress testing or embarking on an exercise program should be evaluated (**Table 40-7**).

Recommendations for exercise should be provided to older patients in writing and include the frequency, intensity, type, and duration of exercise. It is important for older adults to gradually increase their physical activity levels over

Table 40-5. Contents of a physical activity preparticipation evaluation for older adults.

History, to include
Patient's lifelong pattern of activities and interests
Activity level in past 2–3 months to determine a current baseline
Concerns and perceived barriers regarding exercise and physical activity:
Lack of time
Unsafe environment
Cardiovascular risks
Limitations of existing chronic diseases
Level of interest and motivation for exercise
Social preferences regarding exercise.
Physical examination, with emphasis on
Cardiopulmonary systems
Musculoskeletal, and sensory impairments

Reproduced with permission from Fletcher GF, et al. AHA scientific statement: exercise standards for testing and training; a statement for healthcare professionals from the American Heart Association. *Circulation.* 2001; 104:1694.

Table 40-6. Graded exercise test (GXT) recommendations according to coronary heart disease (CHD) risk factors[a] and exercise stratification.

Risk	Moderate Intensity Exercise	Vigorous Intensity Exercise
	Walking at 3–4 mph Cycling for pleasure <10 mph Moderate effort swimming Racket sports; pulling or carrying golf clubs	Walking briskly uphill or with a load Cycling fast or racing >10 mph Swimming, fast tread or crawl Singles tennis or racquetball
Low Men aged <45 years and women aged <55 years with ≤1 CHD risk factor and asymptomatic	GXT not necessary GXT not necessary	GXT not necessary GXT recommended
Moderate Men aged ≥54 and women ≥55 years or those with ≥2 CHD risk factors	GXT not necessary	GXT recommended
High Individuals with symptoms of disease or known metabolic, cardiovascular, or pulmonary disease	GXT recommended	GXT recommended

[a]CHD risk factors: family history, cigarette smoking, hypertension, dyslipidemia, impaired fasting glucose tolerance, obesity, sedentary lifestyle. Data from American College of Sports Medicine. *ACSM's Guidelines for Exercise Testing and Prescription*, 6th ed. Lippincott Williams & Wilkins; 2000.

time and for providers to set realistic and obtainable goals as part of each exercise prescription. Older adults should be advised to increases their exercises every 1–2 weeks and have follow-up arranged every 4–6 weeks when initiating an exercise program.

Promotion of an active lifestyle is important at all ages, and the benefits to older adults are numerous. Providers should help older adults understand that exercise need not be strenuous or prolonged to be beneficial. Just encouraging patients to get up out of their chairs and start moving

Table 40-7. Absolute and relative contraindications to exercise stress testing or starting an exercise program.

Absolute Contraindications	Relative Contraindications
Acute myocardial infarction within 2 days	Left main coronary stenosis
Critical or severe aortic stenosis	Moderate stenotic valvular heart disease
Active endocarditis	Tachyarrhythmias or bradyarrhythmias
Decompensated heart failure	Atrial fibrillation with uncontrolled ventricular rate
High-risk unstable angina	Hypertrophic cardiomyopathy
Active myocarditis or pericarditis	Electrolyte abnormalities
Acute pulmonary embolism or infarction	Mental impairment leading to an inability to cooperate
Serious cardiac arrhythmias causing hemodynamic compromise; acute noncardiac condition that may affect exercise performance or may exacerbate the condition (infection, renal failure, thyrotoxicosis)	High-degree atrioventricular block
Physical disability that precludes safe and adequate test performance Inability to obtain consent	

Reproduced with permission from Fletcher GF, et al. Exercise standards for testing and training: a statement for healthcare professions from the American Heart Association. *Circulation*. 2001; 104:1649.

will improve not only the quality but also the quantity of disability-free years.

American College of Sports Medicine. Exercise and physical activity for older adults. *Med Sci Sports Exerc.* 2009; 41:1510-1530. [PMID: 19516148]

DiPietro L. Physical activity in aging: changes in patterns and their relationship to health and function. *J Gerontol A Biol Sci Med Sci.* 2001; 56 (special issue 2):13. [PMID: 11730234]

Metkus TS Jr. Exercise prescription and primary prevention of cardiovascular disease *Circulation.* 2010; 121(23):2601-2604. [PMID: 20547940]

Nelson M, et al. Physical activity and public health in older adults: recommendation from the American College of Sports Medicine and the American Heart Association. *Med Sci Sports Exerc.* 2007; 39(8):1435-1445. [PMID: 17762378]

Netz Y, et al. Physical activity and psychological well-being in advanced age: a meta-analysis of intervention studies. *Psychol Aging* 2005; 20:272. [PMID: 16029091]

Paganini-Hill A, et al. Activities and mortality in the elderly: the World Leisure Cohort Study. *J Gerontol A Biol Med Sci.* 2011;66A(5):559-567. [PMID: 21350247]

Pescatello LS. Exercising for health: the merits of lifestyle physical activity. *West J Med.* 2001; 174:114. [PMID: 11156922]

US Department of Health and Human Services. *Healthy People 2020* (available at https:www.healthypeople2020.gov/topicsobjectives2020; accessed March 20, 2013).

NUTRITION IN OLDER ADULTS

Achieving healthy nutrition and weight status in older adults is a priority, according to *Healthy People 2020*. As individuals age, chronic diseases, functional impairments, polypharmacy, and age-related physiologic and socioeconomic changes may all act in concert to place an older adult at risk for malnutrition and undernutrition. *Malnutrition* is defined as a state in which a deficiency, excess, or imbalance of energy or other nutrients causes adverse physiologic effects. Malnutrition is a major factor associated with mortality in older persons. A multitude of interrelated factors can place an older adult at nutritional risk (**Tables 40-8 and 40-9**). Poor nutritional status may be the result of insufficient dietary intake, leading to undernutrition; excess dietary content for actual expenditure, leading to obesity; and inappropriate dietary intake, exacerbating such conditions as diabetes, hypertension, and renal insufficiency.

Weight tends to increase with aging until the seventh decade, when it stabilizes or begins to decline. Obesity tends to be a problem for patients aged <75 years, whereas undernutrition is commonly encountered in those aged >85 years. Energy requirements decrease in the elderly. The recommended daily allowance (RDA) of 2300 kcal for a 77-kg man and 1900 kcal for a 65-kg woman should be reduced by 10%, based on basal energy expenditure between ages 51 and 75 years, with an additional 10–15% reduction after age 75. Although animal studies have indicated increased longevity with lower body weight and caloric restriction without

malnutrition, studies on the relative risk of obesity to mortality in older adults are inconsistent, ranging from a protective effect for hip fractures to increased functional disability.

Weight loss should be considered clinically significant when the change in baseline weight is >5% in 3 months or >10% in 6 months. An older adult with a basal metabolic index (BMI) of <17 kg/m² also warrants further evaluation. Because anorexia, weight loss, and undernutrition in older persons have such deleterious effects, factors that can be treated or reversed are of major importance. Often, a review of the status of underlying medical conditions, medications, functional limitations, and socioeconomic circumstances will reveal reversible factors contributing to weight loss. Use of oral supplements has been shown to produce small but consistent increases in weight in older adults. Use of appetite-stimulating agents such as megestrol, dronabinol, and oral steroids to promote weight gain is controversial, given the known side effects of these drugs and the absence of quality studies to support their use in most elderly patients. These medications are not recommended as part of a routine strategy to address weight loss in older adults.

The significance of mild to moderate obesity in the elderly is unclear. Height/weight charts for ideal body weight based on life insurance tables are probably less accurate in older adults, and BMI calculations may underestimate body fat, especially in those with reduced muscle mass. Older adults with rapid weight gain should be assessed for underlying congestive heart failure, renal disease, and other such illness. For those with chronic obesity, recommending weight loss should be done with caution and consideration of patient-specific factors. For patients aged <70 years who are 20% above ideal body weight, a weight loss strategy including dietary modification and increased physical activity should be recommended. For patients aged >70 years, weight loss should be recommended if a medical condition such as hypertension, diabetes, or degenerative joint disease exists and is likely to be significantly improved. A nutritionist can further assist the primary care physician in formulating a weight loss program for older patients, with a goal of 0.5–1 lb of weight loss per week.

Promotion of a balanced, healthy diet for all older adults, including recognition and remediation of macronutrient deficiencies, should be incorporated into the health promotion strategies of all primary care physicians caring for older adults. To be most beneficial, nutritional assessments and body weight measurements of older adults should be performed on a periodic basis. Levels of sodium, protein, fiber, fluid, and micronutrient intake are all important factors in providing nutritional counseling to older adults with recommendations tailored to individuals. The United States Department of Agriculture (USDA) *2010 Dietary Guidelines for America* and the USDA MyPlate (ChooseMyPlate.gov) methods offer specific food guidelines useful for both patients and providers.

Table 40-8. Nutrient requirements in older adults, with signs of excess and deficiency.

Nutrient	Requirement	Signs of Deficiency	Signs of Excess
Vitamin A	Requirements decrease with advancing age; 3333 IU for men, 2667 IU for women	Loss of bright, moist appearance; dry conjunctiva; gingivitis	Toxic effects include headache, lassitude, anorexia, reduced white blood cell count, impaired hepatic function, and bone pain with hypercalcemia; hip fracture
Vitamin B₁ (thiamine)	1.1–1.2 mg/d	Common in alcoholic elderly and institutionalized elderly; disordered cognition (delirium), neuropathies, and cardiomegaly	Liver damage and exacerbation of peptic ulcer disease, especially with those using megadoses
Vitamin B₂ (riboflavin)	1.1–1.3 mg/d	Cheilosis, angular stomatitis, gingivitis; changes to tongue papillae	
Vitamin B₆ (pyroxidine)	1.5–1.7 mg/d	Glossitis, peripheral neuropathy, and dementia especially related to alcohol abuse	Liver damage and nervous system dysfunction, especially with those using megadoses
Vitamin B₁₂	2.4 µg/d	Pallor, optic neuritis, hyporeflexia, ataxia, anorexia; loss of proprioception, vibratory sense, and memory loss; megaloblastic anemia	
Vitamin C		Gingival hypertrophy, bleeding gums, petechiae, and ecchymoses	Megadose use can cause diarrhea, oxalate kidney, and bladder stones; result in simpaired absorption of vitamin B₁₂; interfere with serum and urine glucose testing; produce false-negative hemoccult testing
Vitamin D	10–15 µg/d (400–600 IU/d)	Osteomalacia; severe bone pain and osteoporosis; muscular hypotonia; pulmonary macrophage dysfunction	Nausea, headache, anorexia, weakness, and fatigue; interferes with vitamin K absorption
Vitamin K	Widely distributed in food and provided by synthesis of intestinal bacteria; supplements advised for fat malabsorption syndromes and long-term antibiotic therapy	Hemorrhages in skin or gastrointestinal tract; unexplained prolongation of prothrombin time	Unknown
Folic acid	400 µg/d	Pallor, stomatitis, glossitis, memory impairment, depression	
Vitamin E	400 IU/d	Deficiency is rare; abundant in diet	Interferes with vitamin K metabolism; thrombophlebitis; gastrointestinal (GI) distress; possible reduction in wound healing
Niacin	14–16 mg/d	Fissured tongue; dry, thickened, scaling, hyperpigmented skin; diarrhea; dementia	Histamine flush; liver toxicity
Calcium	1200–1500 mg/d	Osteoporosis	
Iron		Rare secondary to increased iron stores; usually secondary to pathologic blood loss	Constipation; excess iron usually given when anemia of chronic disease is misdiagnosed as iron deficiency anemia; some association between neoplasia and coronary artery disease
Zinc		Impaired wound healing; diarrhea; decreased vision, olfaction, insulin, and immune function; anorexia; impotence	GI disturbance; sideroblastic anemia from impaired copper absorption; adverse effect on cellular immunity; interfere with other vitamin absorption

Data from Johnson L. Vitamins and aging. In Morley JE, et al., eds. *The Science of Geriatrics*, Vol. 2. Springer Publishing, 2000: 379; and Dywer JT et al. Assessing nutritional status in elderly patients. *Am Fam Physician.* 1993; 47:613.

Table 40-9. Factors associated with undernutrition in the elderly.

Depression
Dementia
Anorexia
Poor dental health
Medications
Pain
Fatigue
Sensory alterations
Impaired function
Dietary restrictions (more common in women)
Social isolation
Impecuniousness, alcoholism
Swallowing dysfunction
Dieting (low fat, low cholesterol)

Data from Stechmiller JK. Early nutritional screen of older adults. *J Infusion Nurs.* 2003; 26:170; Morley JE: Anorexia and weight loss in older persons. *J Gerontol Med Sci.* 2003; 58A:131.

Alibhai SM, et al. An approach to the management of unintentional weight loss in elderly people. *Can Med Assoc J.* 2005; 172:773. [PMID: 15767612]

American Dietetic Association. Position of the American Dietetic Association: nutrition, aging and the continuum of care. *J Am Diet Assoc.* 2000; 100:580. [PMID: 10812387]

De Castro JM. Age-related changes in the social, psychological, and temporal influences on food intake in free-living, healthy, adult humans. *J Gerontol A Biol Sci Med Sci.* 2002; 57:M368. [PMID: 12023266]

Kennedy RL, et al. Obesity in the elderly: who should we be treating, and why, and how? *Curr Opin Clin Nutr Metab Care.* 2004; 7:3. [PMID: 1509896]

Loreck E, et al. Nutritional assessment of the geriatric patient: a comprehensive approach toward evaluating and managing nutrition. *Clin Geriatr.* 2012; 20(4):20-26.

Lui L, et al. Undernutrition and risk of mortality in elderly patients within 1 year of hospital discharge. *J Gerontol A Biol Sci Med Sci.* 2002; 57:M741. [PMID: 12403803]

US Department of Health and Human Services. *Healthy People 2020* (available at https:www.healthypeople2020.gov/topicsobjectives2020; accessed March 20, 2013).

Vollmer W, et al. Effects of diet and sodium intake on blood pressure: subgroup analysis of the DASH-sodium trial. *Ann Intern Med.* 2001; 135(12):1019-1028. [PMID:11747380]

GERIATRIC ASSESSMENT

The geriatrtic assessment is a multidimensional assessment designed to evaluate an older adult's physical and mental health, functional abilities, cognitive status, and social circumstances (**Table 40-10**). Older adults may be affected by several chronic conditions and syndromes (**Table 40-11**) that place them at higher risk for impairment. Healthcare providers

Table 40-10. Goals of geriatric assessment.

To define the functional capabilities and disabilities of older patients
To appropriately manage acute and chronic diseases of frail elders
To promote prevention and health
To establish preferences for care in various situations (advanced care planning)
To understand financial resources available for care
To understand social networks and family support systems for care
To evaluate an older patient's mental and emotional strengths and weakness

can diagnose severe functional impairments by clinical observation alone but have difficulty identifying moderate impairments. Geriatric assessment helps to identify older adults at risk for increasing frailty and provides an opportunity to intervene in a manner that may enhance general health, function, and quality of life. Social assessment is important in the development of an effective care plan.

Not all older adults will require a comprehensive geriatric assessment. Rather, this tool should be employed in older adults with chronic conditions and syndromes that place them at risk to screen for impairments. A validated self-administered screening tool, the Vulnerable Elders Survey-13 (VES-13), assesses functional and health status and can be used as a case finding tool before implementing more extensive screening. (The VES-13 can be accessed online at http://www.rand.org/health/projects/acove/survey.html.) Another screening tool that can be used by nonphysician office staff to screen ambulatory older patients can be found in **Table 40-12**.

Table 40-11. Common chronic syndromes among the vulnerable elderly.

Dementia
Depression
Diabetes mellitus
Falls and mobility disorders
Hearing impairment
Heart failure
Hypertension
Ischemic heart disease
Malnutrition
Osteoarthritis
Osteoporosis
Pneumonia and influenza
Pressure ulcers
Stroke and atrial fibrillation
Urinary incontinence
Vision impairment

Data from Wegner NS, et al. Quality indicators for assessing care of vulnerable elders. *Ann Intern Med.* 2001; 135[Suppl (8; Pt 2)]:653 (available at http://www.acponline.org).

Table 40-12. A geriatric screening for impaired ambulatory elderly.

1. Medications
   Did the patient bring in all bottles or a list of medications?
   List all medications.
   Remember to ask about over-the-counter medications.
   Remember to ask about supplements and herbs.
2. Nutrition
   Weigh patient and record.
   Have you lost more than 10 lb in the last 6 months?
   Positive screen: 10 lb weight loss or < 100 lb.
   Intervention: Further evaluation with the Mini-Nutritional Assessment.
3. Hearing
   Use handheld audioscope at 40 dB and screen both ears at 1000 and 2000 Hz.
   Positive screen: Patient unable to hear 1000 or 2000 Hz frequency in both ears or unable to hear the 1000 and 2000 Hz frequency in *one* ear.
   Intervention: Evaluate for cerumen impaction; refer to audiology.
4. Vision
   Ask: "Do you have any problems driving, watching TV, reading, or doing any of your activities because of your eyesight?" If yes
   Do Snellen eye chart
   Positive screen: 20/40 or greater
   Intervention: Refer to optometry or ophthalmology
5. Mental status
   Ask to remember three objects: "ball, car, and flag" (have them repeat objects after you)
   Positive screen: Unable to remember all three items after 1 min
   Intervention: Administer more formal mental status testing such as the 7-Minute Neurocognitive Screening Battery or MMSE; assess for causes of cognitive impairment including delirium, depression, and medications
6. Depression
   Ask: "Are you depressed?" or "Do you often feel sad or depressed?"
   Positive screen: Yes.
   Intervention: Perform a more thorough depression screen (Geriatric Depression Scale); evaluate medications; consider pharmacological treatment, and/or refer to psychiatry.
7. Urinary incontinence
   Ask: In the last year have you ever lost urine or gotten wet? If *yes*,
   Ask: Have you lost urine in at least 6 separate days?
   Positive screen: Yes to both
   Intervention: Initiate workup for incontinence; consider urology referral.
8. Physical disability
   Ask: Are you able to do strenuous activities like fast walking or biking? Heavy work around the house like washing windows, floors, and walls? Go shopping for groceries or clothes? Get to places out of walking distance? Bathe, either sponge bath, tub bath, or shower? Dress, like putting on a shirt, buttoning and zipping, and putting on your shoes?
   Positive screen: Unable to do any of the above independently or able to do only with assistance from another.
   Intervention: Corroborate responses if accuracy uncertain with caregivers; determine reason for inability to perform task; institute appropriate medical, social, and environmental interventions; patient may benefit from physical and/or occupational therapy and a home visit.
9. Mobility
   Ask: Do you fall or feel unbalanced when walking or standing?
   Positive screen: Yes.
   Intervention: "Get up and go" test: Get up from the chair, walk 20 feet, turn, walk back to the chair, and sit down (walk at normal, comfortable pace).
   Positive screen: Unable to complete the task in 15 s
   Intervention: Refer to physical therapy for gait evaluation and assistance with use of appropriate adaptive devices; home safety evaluation; patient may need to be instructed in strengthening of both upper and lower extremities.
10. Home environment
    Ask: Do you have trouble with stairs either inside or outside of your house? Do you feel safe at home?
    Positive Screen: Yes.
    Intervention: Supply the older patient or caregiver with a home safety self-assessment checklist; consider making a home visit or use a visiting nurse or other community resource to evaluate the home; make appropriate referrals to help remediate safety issues.
11. Social support
    Ask: Who would be able to help you in case of an illness or emergency?
    Record identified person(s) in medical record with contact information.
    Intervention: Become familiar with available resources for the elderly within your community or know who can provide you with that assistance.

Data from Lachs MS, et al. A simple procedure for general screening for functional disability in elderly patients. *Ann Intern Med.* 1990; 112:699; Moore AA, Siu AL. Screening for common problems in ambulatory elderly: a clinical confirmation of a screening instrument. *Am J Med.* 1996; 100:438.

Table 40-13. Components of geriatric assessment.

A. Functional assessment
  1. Basic activities of daily living (BADLs): fundamental to self-care:
    Bathing
    Dressing
    Toileting
    Transfers
    Continence
    Feeding
  2. Instrumental activities of daily living (IADLs): complex daily activities fundamental to independent community living and interactions);[a]
    Housework: Can you do your own housework?
    Traveling: Can you get places outside of walking distance?
    Shopping: Can you go shopping for food and clothing?
    Money: Can you handle your own money?
    Meal preparation: Can you prepare your own meals?
  3. Advanced activities of daily living (AADLs) : "functional signature"
    Gait-mobility and balance
    Upper extremity evaluation
B. Cognitive and affective assessment
  Dementia
  Depression
  Suicide
  Alcohol misuse
  Sensory impairments
  Nutrition
  Incontinence
C. Social assessment (caregivers, environment, finances)
  Driving
  Sexuality
  Advance care planning

[a]In order of most difficult to least difficult—knowing a person can perform one item indicates they can perform item below it.
Data from Gallo JJ, et al. *Handbook of Geriatric Assessment*, 4th ed. Jones & Bartlett; 2005; Katz S, et al. Studies of illness in the aged: the index of ADL: a standardized measure of biological and psychosocial function. *JAMA.* 1963;185:914; Fillenbaum G. Screening the elderly: a brief instrumental activities of daily living measure. *J Am Geriatr Soc.* 1985;33:683.

Family physicians who care for older adults should strive to incorporate the geriatric assessment tool into their clinical practice. If impairments are identified as part of the geriatric assessment, a comprehensive, interdisciplinary approach should be employed to address those impairments, optimize function, and improve quality of life. **Table 40-13** outlines several components of the geriatric assessment, and a more detailed discussion of several of these components follows in the remainder of this chapter.

Elsawy B, et al. The geriatric assessment. *Am Fam Physician.* 2011; 83(1):48-56.
Ensberg M, Gerstenlauer C. Incremental geriatric assessment. *Prim Care Clin Office Practice.* 2005; 32:619. [PMID: 16140119]

Saliba D, et al. The Vulnerable Elders Survey: a tool for identifying vulnerable older people in the community. *J Am Geriatr Soc.* 2001; 49:1691. [PMID: 11844005]

► Functional Assessment

A. Predictors of Functional Decline

The ability to function independently in the community is an important public health and quality-of-life issue for all older adults. A recent trend toward declining disability has been noted among older persons, especially those with higher levels of education. For example, older adults who walk a mile at least once a week show decreasing decline in functional limitations and disability than their sedentary counterparts. However, these trends are not indicative of the total population. Non-Hispanic Afro American and Mexican American older adults generally report more functional limitations and disability and represent a vulnerable subpopulation within the United States.

Several predictors of functional decline and mortality have been reported. Health status belief and decreased abilities in activities of daily living (ADLs) appear to be important predictors of mortality. Older adults with depression have increased risk of ADL disability, as it appears that depressive symptoms undermine efforts to maintain physical functioning.

Kivela SL, Pahkala K. Depressive disorder as a predictor of physical disability in old age. *J Am Geriatr Soc.* 2001; 49:290. [PMID: 11300240]
Ostchega Y et al: The prevalence of functional limitations and disability in older persons in the US: data from the National Health and Nutrition Examination Survey III. *J Am Geriatr Soc.* 2000; 48:1132. [PMID: 10983915]

B. Evaluation of Functional Status

The capacity to perform functional tasks necessary for daily living can be used as a surrogate measure of independence or a predictor of decline and institutionalization. Functional status needs to be assessed objectively and independently of medical, laboratory, and cognitive evaluation because specific functional loss is not disease-specific and cognitive impairment does not necessarily imply inability to function independently in a familiar environment. Limitations noted on functional assessment should prompt the search for contributing and modifiable conditions, including musculoskeletal dysfunction, cognitive impairment, depression, substance abuse, adverse medication reactions, or sensory impairment.

Knowledge of how older adults spend their time can give physicians a reference point for potential functional decline at subsequent visits. Functional assessment can be considered as a hierarchy ranging from advanced, independent, and basic activities of daily living. An older adult may be fully independent, require assistance, or be fully dependent in any or all of these activities. Individuals may move across levels of assistance or dependence, especially during and after an acute illness. Assessment of these activities allows providers to match services to needs.

The advanced activities of daily living (AADLs) include very-high-level tasks that may be considered the "functional signature" of a well community-dwelling older individual. These tasks include voluntary social, occupational, or recreational activities. An older person who does not successfully participate in such activities may not be impaired, but the presence of significant involuntary loss AADLs may be an important risk factor for further functional losses.

The instrumental activities of daily living (IADLs) are intermediate-level activities (**Table 40-13**) and are required for independent living Older adults living in the community who cannot perform IADLs may have difficulty functioning at home and may be appropriate for assisted living or personal care home settings.

The basic activities of daily living (BADLs) include self-care activities (**Table 40-13**) that are at the most basic level of functioning. Loss of BADLs tends to progress from those involving lower extremity strength to those activities that rely on upper extremity strength such that mobility and toileting are lost before dressing and feeding. Dependence for toileting has been shown to be an indicator of overall poor performance that should alert the provider to the need for increased care. Older adults requiring assistance for BADLs may be appropriate for a nursing home setting. (Online reference tools for completing a detailed functional assessment can be found at http://www.healthcare.uiowa.edu/igec/tools/categoryMenu.asp?categoryID=5.)

De Vriendt P, et al. The process of decline in advanced activities of daily living: a qualitative explorative study in mild cognitive impairment. *Int Psychogeriatr.* 2012; 24(6):974-986.

Katz S, et al. Studies of illness in the aged: the index of ADL. *JAMA.* 1963; 185:914-919.

Lawton MP, et al. Assessment of older people: self-maintaining and instrumental activities of daily living. *Gerontologist.* 1969; 9(3):179-186.

Sherman FT. Functional assessment: easy-to-use screening tools to speed initial office work-up. *Geriatrics.* 2001; 56:36. [PMID: 11505859]

C. Other Geriatric Assessment Elements

Issues relating to mobility and balance (Chapter 40), incontinence (Chapter 41), depression (Chapter 52), and sensory impairments (Chapter 44) are covered in this book, and the reader is referred to those chapters for more detailed information. The remainder of this chapter focuses on issues that need to be addressed in the evaluation of older adults.

Table 40-14. Social support screening.

How many relatives do you see or hear from in the course of a month?
Tell me about the relative with whom you have the most contact.
How many relatives do you feel close to—such as to discuss private matters?
How many friends do you see or hear from in the course of a month?
Tell me about the friend with whom you have the most contact.
When you have an important decision to make, do you have someone you can talk to about it?
Do you rely on anybody to assist you with shopping, cooking, doing repairs, cleaning house, etc?
Do you help others with shopping, cooking, transportation, childcare, etc?
Do you live alone?
With whom do you live?

Data from Gallo JJ, et al. *Handbook of Geriatric Assessment,* 4th ed. Jones & Bartlett; 2005.

1. Social support—Social networks consist of informal supports such as family and close longtime friends, formal supports including social services and healthcare delivery agencies, and semiformal supports such as church groups and neighborhood organizations. Relationships with family and friends may be complex and can have important implications for the vulnerable elder. The availability of assistance from family or friends frequently influences whether a functionally dependent older adult remains at home or is institutionalized. **Table 40-14** contains questions that may be incorporated into social support screening.

2. Caregiver burden—Adults providing care for a frail or cognitively impaired person can face overwhelming demands. Older adults may be either the provider or recipient of such caregiving. Caregiver burden describes the strain or load borne by these providers. A caregiver's perceived burden is closely linked to the caregiver's ability to cope and handle stress. Caregivers are at higher risk for mortality if there is increased mental or emotional strain. Physicians should be vigilant for signs of possible caregiver burnout in any caregiver. These signs include multiple somatic complaints, anxiety or depression, social isolation, and weight loss. Formal assessment tools include the Caregiver Strain Index and the Zarit Burden Interview.

Bedard M, et al. The Zarit Burden Interview: a short version and screening version. *Gerontologist.* 2001; 41:652. [PMID: 11574710]

Kasuya RT, et al. Caregiver burden and burnout: a guide for primary care physicians. *Postgrad Med.* 2000; 108:119. [PMID: 1126138]

Schulz R, Beach SR. Caregiving as a risk factor for mortality: the Caregiver Health Effects Study. *JAMA.* 1999; 282:2215. [PMID: 10605972]

3. Economic factors—Economic factors have important consequences with respect to an older adult's health, nutrition, and living environment. Economic factors may influence an older adult's access to food, medications, assistive technology, and various healthcare services. The physician can inquire as to whether older individuals have sufficient financial resources to meet their needs and whether proposed treatments or interventions will cause the patient an economic burden. The primary care provider should have a working knowledge of Medicare and be familiar with state and local resources.

4. Physical environment—An older adult's physical environment, including their home, neighborhood, and transportation system, is critical to maintaining independence. Environmental hazards within the home are common and can place an older adult at increased risk for falls and injury. Common, modifiable, home hazards include loose throw rugs, obstructed pathways, poor lighting, absence of stair handrails, absence of bathroom grab bars, and low or loose toilet seats. The physician should inquire about the safety of the neighborhood and if older adults have access to transportation or transportation services. This is especially important for elders who are dependent on caregivers for instrumental activities of daily living (IADLs) and are still living within the community.

Environmental hazards are not easily detected during an office visit. A home visit either by the physician or a community agency provider can reveal problems in the living situation, such as wandering, household hazards, social isolation and loneliness, family stress, nutrition problems, financial concerns, and even alcohol abuse. (An environmental checklist that the older person or family member can use for a self-assessment can be found at http://assets.aarp.org/external_sites/caregiving/checklists/checklist_homeSafety.html.)

Kao H, et al. The past, present, and future of house calls. *Clin Geriatr Med.* 2009; 25:19-34.

5. Driving competence—Evaluating the driving competence of an older adult is challenging. The ability to drive allows the older adult to maintain important links within the community, and is closely linked to independence and self-esteem. Older adults who are unable to drive or who stop driving risk social isolation, depression, and functional decline. Many older drivers voluntarily modify their driving habits by driving shorter distances; driving only during daylight; and avoiding rush hour, major highways, and inclement weather.

Older drivers should be counseled on the importance of safety restraints, obeying speed limits, use of a helmet if riding a motorcycle or bicycle, taking a driving refresher course, and avoidance of alcohol and use of mobile phones while driving. Adults aged ≥65 years account for 16% of all traffic fatalities. Driving accidents with older adults are less likely to involve high speeds or alcohol, but more likely to involve visual-spatial difficulties and cognitive and motor skills. Heart disease and hearing impairment are also commonly associated with adverse driving events.

Driving involves a set of complex tasks that require not only physical but also mental integrity. Chronic illness, functional status, or even cognitive status cannot consistently predict adverse driving events. Assessment of the older driver should include a review of the driving record, medications, alcohol use, and functional measures including vision, hearing, attention, visual-spatial skills, muscle strength, and joint flexibility. Providers can consider use of the 4Cs screening tool (crash history, family concerns, clinical condition, and cognitive functions) to identify at at-risk drivers. It is important for primary care physicians to (know the laws of their state with regard to driving and reportable medical conditions. The American Medical Association's physician guide to assessing and talking to older drivers can be accessed online at http://www.ama-assn.org/ama/pub/physician-resources/public-health.)

Carr DB, et al. Older drivers with cognitive impairment. *Am Fam Physician.* 2006; 73:1029-1034, 1035-1036.

Hogan DB. Which older patients are competent to drive? Approaches to office-based assessment. *Can Fam Physician.* 2005; 51:362-368.

Molnar FJ, et al. In-office evaluation of medical fitness to drive: practical approaches for assessing older people. *Can Fam Physician.* 2005; 51:372-379.

National Highway Traffic Safety Administration. *Traffic Safety Facts: Older Population*; 2009 (DOT HS 811 391).

O'Connor M, et al. The 4Cs (crash history, family concerns, clinical condition, and cognitive rfunctions): a screening tool for the evaluation of the at-Risk driver. *J Am Geriatr Soc.* 2010. 58:1104–1108.

6. Alcohol misuse—Alcohol consumption and alcoholism are commonplace among the elderly, with 10.5% of men and 3.9% of women in one primary care practice reporting problematic alcohol use. Alcohol misuse places an older adult at increased risk for falls, injury, hypertension, and cognitive impairment. The National Institute on Alcohol Abuse and Alcoholism recommends that people aged >65 years have no more than seven drinks a week and no more than three drinks on any one day. Preventive care should include screening all elders at least once to detect problems or hazardous drinking by taking a history of alcohol use and using a standard screening questionnaire, such as the four-item CAGE or the 10-item AUDIT. (Information for older adults about alcohol misuse can be found at: http://www.nia.nih.gov/health/publication/alcohol-use-older-people.)

Blow F, et al. Alcohol and substance misuse in older adults. *Curr Psychiatr Rep.* 2012;14:310-319.

Table 40-15. Five steps to successful advanced care planning.

Steps	Process
1. Introduce the topic	During a wellness visit or some other time when the individual is in a good state of health, explain the purpose and nature of the discussion Inquire into how familiar the individual is with advanced care planning and define terms as necessary Be aware of the comfort level of the patient—give information and be supportive Suggest that family members, friends, or even members of the community explore how to manage potential burdens Discuss the identification of a proxy decision maker Encourage the patient to bring the proxy decision maker to the next visit
2. Engage in structured discussions	Convey commitment to patients to follow their wishes and protect patients from unwanted treatment or undertreatment Involve the potential proxy decision maker in discussions and planning Allow the patient to specify the role he/she would like the proxy to assume if the patient is incapacitated—follow patient's explicit wishes, or allow the proxy to decide according to the patient's best interests Elicit the patient's values and goals Use a validated advisory document available at http://www.medicaldirective.org
3. Document patient preferences	Review advanced directives with patient and proxy for inconsistencies and misunderstandings Enter the advanced directives into the medical record Recommend statutory documents be completed by the patient that comply with state statutes Distribute directives to hospital, patient, proxy decision maker, family members, and all healthcare providers Include advanced directives in the care plan
4. Review and update the directive regularly	
5. Apply directives to actual circumstances	Most advanced directives go into affect when the patient can no longer direct her/his own medical care Assess the patient's decision-making capacity Never assume advanced directive content without reading it thoroughly Advanced directives should be interpreted in view of the clinical facts of the case Physician and proxy decision maker will need to work together to resolve ambiguous or uncertain situations If disagreements between physician and proxy cannot be resolved, seek the assistance of an ethics consultant or committee

Data from Emanuel LL, et al. Advance care planning. *Arch Fam Med.* 2000; 9:1181.

National Institute on Alcohol Abuse and Alcoholism. *Older Adults* (available at http://www.niaaa.nih.gov/alcohol-health/special-populations-co-occurring-disorders/older-adults; accessed March 29, 2013).

Ringler SK. Alcoholism in the elderly. *Am Fam Physician.* 2000; 61:1710-1716.

7. Sexual health—Sexual health remains an important consideration in older adults. Older adults may not initiate discussions about sexual health on their own; thus the provider should routinely include discussion of sexual health in their assessment. Using open-ended questions allows the individual to give as much or as little information as is comfortable. The physician needs to have an understanding of the older adult's previous and present normal sexual patterns and interests and whether any changes that have occurred affect sexual functioning and intimacy. These may include medical conditions, medications, physical disabilities, mood disturbance, or cognitive impairment. A sexual assessment may include questions about quality of erection and orgasm for men, and lubrication and orgasm for women. If a problem is uncovered, a more thorough assessment and evaluation should be undertaken.

The physician should inquire into the nature of the older adult's sexual quality of life by asking how affection is displayed and how physical intimacy is expressed. Because not all older persons are in committed heterosexual relationships, it is important that the physician express openness to answers conveyed. Sexually active older adults engaging in high-risk sex practices should be counseled on safer sex practices. (Patient education related to sexual health and aging can be accessed at: http://www.healthinaging.org/aging-and-health-a-to-z/topic:sexual-health/)

Gingold H. The graying of sex. *NYS Psychologist.* 2007; 9(4): 8-23.

Gott M, et al. Barriers to seeking treatment for sexual problems in primary care: a qualitative study with older people. *Fam Practice.* 2003; 20:690-695.

Taylor A, et al. Sexuality in older age: essential considerations for healthcare professionals. *Age Ageing.* 2011; 40:538-543.

8. Spirituality—Information about an older adult's spirituality can provide insight into factors affecting their care decisions and help providers understand the patient's resources to cope with illness and other stressors. The spiritual assessment may include questions about their concept of God or deity, afterlife, value and meaning in life, and any specific religious practices. Older adults can suffer from spiritual distress that may be expressed as depression; crying; fear of abandonment; or hopelessness, anxiety, and despair. This distress may occur in the setting of illness, after the loss of a significant other, following a family or personal disaster, or when there is a disruption in the usual religious activities. Inquiring into the spirituality of patients requires empathy on the part of the physician, strong interpersonal skills, and a closely established physician-patient relationship.

Sulmasy DP. Spirituality, religion and clinical care. *Chest*. 2009; 135:1634-1642.

9. Advanced care planning—Advanced care planning is the process of planning for the medical future in which the patient's preferences will guide the nature and intensity of future medical care, particularly if the patient is unable to make independent decisions. It is important for the physician to learn about the patient's personal values, goals, and preferences for care (**Table 40-15**).

Older adults should indicate the type or level of care that they would and would not want to receive in various situations. Advanced care planning is designed to ensure that the patient's wishes are known and respected. Older adults should be encouraged to share their wishes with family members, and the provider can assist in facilitating this discussion. Advanced care planning is further outlined in Chapter 63.

Fried TR, et al. Understanding advance care planning as a process of health behavior change. *J Am Geriatr Soc*. 2009;9:1547-1555.
Kahana B, et al. The personal and social context of planning end-of-life care. *J Am Geriatr Soc*. 2004;52:1163. [PMID: 15209656]

Websites

Administration on Aging: http://www.aoa.gov
AGS Foundation for Health in Aging: http://www.healthinaging
American Association of Retired Persons: http://www.aarp.org
American Geriatrics Society: http://www.americangeriatrics.org
American Medical Directors Association: http://www.amda.com
American Society of Consultant Pharmacists: http://www.ascp.com
Assisted Living Federation of America: http://www.alfa.org
Children of Aging Parents: http://www.caps4caregivers.org
CDC National Prevention Information Network: http://www.cdcnpin.org
Family Caregiver Alliance: http://www.caregiver.org
Medicare Hotline: http://www.medicare.gov
National Adult Day Services Association: http://www.nadsa.org
National Council on the Aging: http://www.ncoa.org
National Institute on Aging: http://www.nia.nih.gov

Common Geriatric Problems

Daphne P. Bicket, MD, MLS

The syndromes of failure to thrive, pressure ulcers, and falls share features that make them particularly challenging. Their etiologies are multifactorial; they require an interdisciplinary approach to maximize care; and they often herald disability, institutionalization, and death. Interventions in multiple domains can improve outcomes. However, in patients with low functional reserve the physician should be prepared to transition from cure to palliative care. Open and frank communication is vital and should employ the skills needed to address life-changing diagnoses while continuing to supply hope and support. Eliciting patient's goals, what they want and what they want to avoid, is fundamental to crafting an end-of-life framework that is consistent with their values and preferences. The physician can and should maintain a therapeutic relationship with the patient and the family beyond the time when medical therapies are effective. Home visits enhance this relationship and often reveal opportunity for interventions and support.

FAILURE TO THRIVE

 ESSENTIALS OF DIAGNOSIS

▶ Weight loss of more than 5%.
▶ Functional decline.
▶ Depression.
▶ Cognitive impairment.

▶ General Considerations

The National Institute on Aging defined *failure to thrive* (FTT) as "a syndrome of weight loss, decreased appetite and poor nutrition, and inactivity, often accompanied by dehydration, depressive symptoms, impaired immune function,

and low cholesterol." The concepts, cachexia and sarcopenia, have enhanced our understanding of the pathophysiology of FTT and should be considered in the approach to the patient. *Cachexia* is the catabolic state seen in illnesses such as cancer, end-stage renal disease, lung disease, and heart failure. It is progressive and characterized by weight loss, anorexia, inflammation, and insulin resistance; nutrition therapy does not alter the course. *Sarcopenia* is loss of muscle mass that occurs with aging. It is associated with functional decline, disability, and falls; it is mitigated by exercise.

▶ Clinical Findings

A. Symptoms and Signs

Weight loss is an essential feature. Functional decline contributes to falls, poor grooming, depression, and cognitive decline. As in infants, FTT can occur from organic and nonorganic causes, necessitating an approach that includes medical, psychological, functional, and social domains.

B. History and Physical Examination

The history provided by the patient and caregiver can help identify common acute triggers: change in medication, infection, constipation, pain, loss, or grief. Undiagnosed chronic diseases, such as endocrine disorders, tuberculosis, dementia, depression, substance abuse, and rarely, hypoactive delirium, may trigger FTT.

Assess, do not assume, medication compliance; have the patient demonstrate how he/she is taking all prescription and over-the-counter (OTC) medications. Drug effects and interactions should not be underestimated. Alendronate, antiarrhythmics, antihistamines (eg, H_2-blockers, α-antagonists, benzodiazepines, β-blockers, calcium antagonists, colchicine, and digoxin, even within therapeutic range), diuretics, iron or zinc, metformin, metronidazole, neuroleptics, nonsteroid anti-inflammatory drugs (NSAIDs), narcotics,

Table 41-1. Targeted physical examination.

Physical examination details and considerations
Vital signs: BMI <21 or percentage of weight loss since last visit, BP and HR in 2 positions, pulse for 60 seconds; abnormal if >88/min or irregular, respiratory rate/effort
Ears: hearing defects or tinnitus lead to social isolation
Eyes: cataracts or other vision disturbance lead to depression and isolation
Oral health: tooth or gum disease impair eating
Swallowing: aspiration and cough (ACE inhibitor) can negatively impact eating; have patient swallow liquid in your presence if any question of aspiration
JVD: a sensitive marker for CHF exacerbation
Breast mass: will often go unnoticed or unreported
Abdomen: masses, constipation, urinary bladder distention
Skin: sacrum and feet, axillae, panniculus, and groin for breakdown/candida/impetigo
Feet: any condition causing gait or balance disturbance
Motor: gait: bradykinesia, consider Parkinson disease; shoulder/hip weakness, consider polymyalgia rheumatica
Mental status: test for variance from baseline and screen for depression

steroids, SSRIs, tricyclic antidepressants, and xanthines have been associated with FTT. Levels are nonspecific; normal therapeutic levels can have adverse effects. Be aware of genetic and racial variation in drug metabolism.

A comprehensive physical examination should focus on the appropriate items noted in **Table 41-1.** Laboratory evaluations should include complete blood count (CBC), comprehensive metabolic panel (CMP), thyroid-stimulating hormone (TSH), erythrocyte sedimentation rate (ESR), total 25-OH vitamin D, and vitamin B_{12} (if within 200–400 pmol/L, check a methylmalonic level or empirically replace). Additional workup could include fecal occult blood, purified protein derivative, and urinalysis.

Treatment

A. Assessment and Plan

Address modifiable medical conditions. Discuss risk/benefit of watchful waiting for conditions whose interventions carry high morbidity and mortality. Appetite stimulants are neither approved nor recommended and carry significant side effects. As medical interventions become more limited, palliative or hospice services should be initiated.

B. Team Approach

Simplify medications with help of a PharmD. Enlist the help of the Area Agency on Aging (AAA) [www.aoa.dhhs.gov or (800) 677–1116, "Elder Care Locater"]. Concerns about neglect or abuse should be discussed openly and nonjudgmentally; and should be reported. Home Health can supply

short-term nursing, social worker, dietician, physical and occupational therapy, and aide services.

Agarwal K. Failure to thrive in elderly adults. *UpToDate*; Nov. 28, 2012.

PRESSURE ULCERS

ESSENTIALS OF DIAGNOSIS

▶ A skin ulcer caused by ischemia due to prolonged pressure or pressure in combination with shear and/or friction.

▶ Occur on weight bearing or bony prominences (eg, sacrum, hip, heel).

▶ Differentiate from ulcers caused by venous or arterial insufficiency.

Pathogenesis

Extrinsic and intrinsic factors cause pressure ulcers. Extrinsic factors are prolonged pressure, moisture, friction, and shear. Intrinsic causes are the susceptibility of aged skin (less thickness and elasticity), loss of sensation, circulatory compromise, immobility, weight loss, dehydration, malnutrition, and cognitive impairment including sedation.

Prevention

When admitting a patient to acute or long-term care, document the condition of the occiput, spinous processes, scapulae, elbows, sacrum, ischia, greater trochanters, malleoli, and heels. Extra vigilance is needed in cognitively or sensorially impaired elders who wear support stockings, casts, or other orthopedic devices. These should be removed for inspection when possible. The admitting nurse will also do a complete skin assessment; the physician should review, verify, and document concurrence with the findings. **Table 41-2** summarizes the AHRQ (Agency for Healthcare Research and Quality) guidelines for pressure ulcer prevention. Screening scales such as Braden and Norton help quantify risk and tailor treatment plans. The downside to these scales is the misconception that low- and moderate-risk patients are not as vulnerable; it takes them 2 hours to develop a stage I ulcer, the same as the high-risk patient. Although never studied, patient repositioning every 2 hours remains a mainstay in clinical practice.

Differential Diagnosis

Among the differential diagnoses for pressure ulcers are vascular ulcers, diabetic ulcers, and cellulitis. Venous ulcers are the result of prolonged venous hypertension and are

Table 41-2. AHRQ guidelines for pressure ulcer prevention.

Assess risk and institute care plan within 8 hours of admission
Inspect high-risk patients daily (all vulnerable sites)
Keep skin clean with mild soap and water
Keep *clean skin* dry with moisture barrier
Minimize friction and shear with lift sheet, bed trapeze, or both
Post a turning schedule near patient
Relieve heel pressure with inflatable heel elevators
Avoid doughnut cushions
Leave head of bed flat when possible
Use pressure-relieving chair cushion; reposition frequently
Maintain and promote mobility; avoid bed rest
Address nutrition in patients who are hypoalbuminemic or anemic, or in whom BMI is abnormal
Educate patient and family about prevention

Modified from the Agency for Healthcare Research and Quality. *Pressure Ulcer Treatment, Quick Reference Guide for Clinicians.* AHRQ; 1994.

usually located over the medial malleolus. Arterial ulcers are predominantly caused by atherosclerotic vessels, and may be located between toes, over phalangeal heads, or around the lateral malleolus. Diabetic ulcers are produced by a variety of factors: micro- and macrovascular injury, peripheral neuropathy, and mechanical changes in the bony architecture of the foot. These are usually located on the plantar aspect of the foot, metatarsal heads, or under the heel. Cellulitis is an acute inflammation of the dermis and subcutaneous tissue and thus blanches with palpation.

▶ **The National Pressure Ulcer Advisory Panel (NPUAP) Classification**

A. Stage I

Stage I ulcers are characterized by intact skin with non-blanchable redness of a localized area usually over a bony prominence. Darkly pigmented skin may not have visible blanching; its color may differ from the surrounding area. The area may be painful, firm, soft, warmer, or cooler as compared to adjacent tissue. Stage I may be difficult to detect in individuals with dark skin tones and may indicate "at risk" persons (a heralding sign of risk).

Preventive efforts should be intensified. Transparent films like Op-site or Tegaderm can be used; they provide barrier, prevent contamination, and reduce friction. The wound should be pressure-free. Donut cushions and bunny boots worsen ulcers. Use foam or gel overlay for beds or chairs, and inflatable heel elevators to protect feet. Compared with standard hospital mattresses, these devices decrease the incidence of ulcers. For a stage I, use group 1 support surfaces. (A good description of support surfaces

can be found at www.wocn.org/pdfs/WOCN_Library/Fact_Sheets/medicare_part_b.pdf.)

B. Stage II

Stage II is characterized by partial thickness loss of dermis presenting as a shallow open ulcer with a red pink wound bed, without slough. It may also present as an intact or open/ruptured serum-filled blister, or as a shiny or dry shallow ulcer without slough or bruising. (Bruising indicates suspected deep-tissue injury.) This stage should not be used to describe skin tears, tape burns, perineal dermatitis, maceration, or excoriation.

1. Management—Cleansing around the wound with cleanser rather than normal saline has been shown to promote healing in stage II–IV ulcers, with stage II gaining the greatest benefit in healing time. Normal saline is fine if cleanser is not available. Do not use old favorites such as hydrogen peroxide, povidone-iodine (Betadine), liquid detergent, acetic acid, or hypochlorite solutions. Even when diluted, they are potentially toxic to both fibroblasts and white blood cells. Occlusive or semipermeable dressing that will maintain a moist wound environment should be used after cleansing. Hydrogel alone (Intrasite, Solosite) or hydrogel sheets (eg, NuGel) or hydrogel-impregnated gauze (eg, Normlgel) are appropriate. Wet/dry dressing should be avoided, as these ulcers need little debridement. If the wound is exudating, then use a dressing that will absorb the exudate such as alginate (Sorbsan or Aquacel) or NaCl-impregnated gauze (Mesalt.). If multiple stage II ulcers develop while patient is on a group 1 surface for ≥1 month, consider a group II device. Seventy-five percent of stage II ulcers will heal in 8 weeks.

C. Stage III

Stage III is characterized by full-thickness tissue loss. Subcutaneous fat may be visible, but bone, tendon, or muscle are not exposed. Slough may be present but does not obscure the depth of tissue loss. This stage may include undermining and tunneling. The depth of a stage III pressure ulcer varies by anatomical location. The bridge of the nose, ear, occiput, and malleolus do not have subcutaneous tissue, and stage III ulcers can be shallow. In contrast, areas of significant adiposity can develop extremely deep stage III pressure ulcers. Bone/tendon is not visible or directly palpable.

1. Management—Use a sterile Q-tip while examining in order to document tunneling. Do not use this to culture the wound; it will not yield reliable results, as it is not a sterile culture. If necrotic tissue or slough is present, sharp debridement is the best management. Exceptions are heel ulcers, thrombocytopenia, or patient refusal. Other methods of debridement are pulse lavage, whirlpool, wet to dry dressings (NaCl-impregnated gauze several times daily), chemical debridement (Santyl), or autolytic debridement via an occlusive dressing (Duoderm). Occlusive dressings are good for eschar attached to intact skin; once separated, it is more easily debrided mechanically or chemically. Combinations are also effective: Santyl with pulse lavage is an example.

D. Stage IV

Full-thickness tissue loss with exposed bone, tendon, or muscle. Slough or eschar may be present on some parts of the wound bed. This stage often includes undermining and tunneling.

As in stage III, the depth of a stage IV pressure ulcer varies by anatomical location. Stage IV ulcers can extend into muscle and/or supporting structures (eg, fascia, tendon, or joint capsule), which could result in osteomyelitis. Exposed bone/tendon is visible or directly palpable.

These are bad wounds; only 62% ever heal, and only 52% heal within 1 year. They should be managed as in stage III. If after 14 days there is no sign of healing, consider infection; see appropriate management under the section on treatment, later.

Two other stages are grouped with stage IV because of their similar severity levels.

E. Unstageable

Ulcers characterized by full-thickness tissue loss, in which the base of the ulcer is covered by slough (yellow, tan, gray, green, or brown) and/or eschar (tan, brown, or black) in the wound bed, cannot be staged.

Until enough slough and/or eschar is removed to expose the base of the wound, the true depth, and therefore stage, cannot be determined. Stable (dry, adherent, intact without erythema or fluctuance) eschar on the heels serves as "the body's natural (biological) cover" and should not be removed.

F. Suspected Deep-Tissue Injury

A purple or maroon localized area of discolored intact skin or a blood-filled blister may indicate damage of underlying soft tissue from pressure and/or shear. The area may be preceded by tissue that is painful, firm, mushy, boggy, warmer, or cooler as compared to adjacent tissue. Deep-tissue injury may be difficult to detect in individuals with dark skin tones. Evolution may include a thin blister over a dark wound bed. The wound may further evolve and become covered by thin eschar. Evolution may be rapid, exposing additional layers of tissue even with optimal treatment.

► Complications

The most common complications are cellulitis, osteomyelitis, and sepsis. If local erythema of ≥1 cm occurs around the wound, topical antibiotics such as mupirocin should be used. If the erythema is rapidly expanding, with heat, edema, or induration, the patient should be treated for cellulitis with systemic antibiotics. Use local susceptibility patterns to guide therapy. If the patient exhibits systemic symptoms, such as fever, rigors, delirium, or leukocytosis, draw blood cultures and obtain a sterile wound culture by needle aspiration or punch biopsy. We recommend consulting infectious disease specialists if any infection is suspected. Update tetanus immunity.

Osteomyelitis is another complication and should be suspected in painful and nonhealing ulcers and whenever bone is visible. The ^{99m}Tc bone scan and magnetic resonance imaging (MRI) have equal sensitivity. CT has good specificity, poor sensitivity. Needle biopsy of bone is the most useful single test, with a sensitivity of 73% and a specificity of 96%.

Sepsis is a serious consequence of infected pressure ulcers and a frequent cause of death, with mortality rates as high as 48%.

► Treatment

A. Management

We recommend a team approach once a stage 1 ulcer is identified. The wound should be checked daily and documentation of healing performed weekly. A tool to document healing has been developed by the NPUAP. The pressure ulcer status for healing (PUSH) tool measures three components—size, exudate amount, and tissue type. This tool has been validated, has good inter-rater reliability, and is sensitive to change over time.

Enlist the care of a wound team. A physical therapist will mobilize the patient. Unless contraindicated, no elder should be on bed rest. An occupational therapist can assist with positioning for safety and recommend devices to minimize pressure. A wound nurse will document and often photograph the wound, and will recommend appropriate dressings and support surfaces.

Nutrition is essential to healing. A dietician will assist with protein, calorie, and water recommendations as well as nutritional deficiencies. A BMI of <19, with >5% weight loss in 30 days or >10% loss in 180 days, and a serum albumin of <3.5 g/dL suggest malnutrition. Daily administration of 30–40 kcal/kg body weight, 1.2–1.5 g protein/kg body weight, and minimum fluid intake of 30 mL/kg body weight is recommended for at-risk patients. Those with ulcers are in a catabolic state and will require a more intensive and tailored approach by a clinical dietician. While supplements of vitamin C and zinc are commonly recommended, there is no evidence that they enhance wound healing unless the patient is deficient. Zinc at 100 mg daily can cause nausea and vomiting. A speech therapist and oral surgeon/dentist should be involved as needed.

Urinary and fecal incontinence must be managed on a case-by-case basis. The risk of Foley catheter urinary tract infection must be weighed against the projected benefit of a dry wound site. Fecal incontinence can cause skin breakdown and impair healing. Toilet ambulatory patients frequently, manage diarrhea, and use containment devices when necessary.

Attend to pain management: both physical and psychic. Patient dignity should be valued and respected. While use of sedation is associated with significantly increased risk of ulcers, pain from them must be addressed. This is especially important before dressing changes. Topical narcotics may be effective and have the added advantage of minimal systemic absorption, sedation, and constipation.

▶ B. Alternative Therapies

As of 2013 no benefits have been established for a number of therapies in the frail elderly, including platelet-derived growth factors, therapeutic ultrasound, electromagnetic therapy, nutritional supplements, hyperbaric oxygen, infrared, UV, low energy, laser irradiation, and most recently, honey.

C. Cultural Considerations

Some studies have shown higher incidence and severity of pressure ulcers in the African American and Native American populations. Postulated contributing factors are dark skin color and economic factors.

D. Patient Education

Caring for a patient with pressure ulcers is demanding. It is likely that the patient who develops a pressure ulcer has significant comorbidities that necessitate palliative treatment and, in fact, may indicate imminent end of life. Direct caregivers to resources such as AAA, Home Health, and support groups.

For chronically or terminally ill patients with longstanding or recurrent ulceration, aggressive treatment may not be beneficial. Under these circumstances, maintaining patient comfort should be the primary goal rather than instituting major invasive procedures.

Berlowitz D. Prevention and treatment of pressure ulcers. *UpToDate* (available at www.uptodate.com; accessed April 14, 2010; last updated Feb.2013).

Websites

www.ahrq.gov
www.bradenscale.com/images/bradenscale.pdf
www.npuap.org/PDF/push3.pdf

FALLS

ESSENTIALS OF DIAGNOSIS

▶ A sudden, unintentional change in position causing an individual to land at a lower level.

▶ Not caused by paralysis, seizure, or trauma.

▶ Responsible for increased morbidity and mortality in the elderly population.

▶ Often multifactorial.

▶ General Considerations

More than one-third of community-dwelling elders will fall each year. Overall, 20–30% will suffer moderate to severe injuries such as hip fractures and head trauma that reduce mobility and independence. Falls have psychological and social consequences such as fear of falling, anxiety, social isolation, and loss of self-confidence.

▶ Pathogenesis

Understanding the following construct will guide your exam and interventions. Most falls in older people result from the interaction of multiple intrinsic (age-related physiologic changes, medications, gait or balance disturbance, risk taking) and extrinsic factors (environmental hazards, lighting, footwear). Assessment of an acute fall event or of patients at risk for falls warrants a multidimensional approach incorporating (1) postural stability, (2) medical comorbidities, (3) overall function, and (4) environment.

Postural stability is maintained in three phases: input, processing, and output. Input includes vision, vestibular apparatus, and proprioception. Processing requires an intact nervous system: both central processing and competent efferent command. Output requires a motor system characterized by strength, flexibility, absence of pain, and cardiovascular endurance. Impairment of any one phase increases the risk for falls, and the risk is cumulative. Conversely, interventions to modify any of these impairments will decrease the risk for falls.

Chronic diseases, and the medications that we use to treat them, constitute the second key area of assessment. Conditions and drugs that affect the components of postural stability are suspect, and there are usually more than one. Conditions to consider are autonomic dysfunction; arrhythmia; seizure; movement disorder; and central nervous system (CNS) pathology, including dementia, vertigo, or vision impairment. Any medication or combination can contribute to falls; the following are particularly notorious: psychotropics, narcotics, benzodiazepines, antihistamines, antiarrhythmics, the cumulative effect of antihypertensives, combination of more than any four drugs, and alcohol.

Finally, the concept of functional thresholds places the data into a framework that identifies the point at which a particular patient exceeds his/her compensatory abilities. A detailed history and focused physical and performance examination will provide key information on function. For those frail elders, who most commonly fall at home, a home assessment completes the evaluation.

▶ Prevention

A systematic review of scientific studies has identified several strategies, targeting both intrinsic and environmental risk factors that are likely to be beneficial in preventing falls. The only evidence-based strategies shown to reduce fall risk are exercise programs targeting at least two areas: strength, balance, flexibility, and endurance; individually prescribed exercise programs at home; a 15-week tai chi group exercise program of other group exercise; home hazard modification for at-risk patients; withdrawl of psychotropic or sedating medications and decreasing number of medications; cardiac pacing for fallers with cardioinhibitory cardotid sinus hypersensitivity; cataract surgery; and vitamin D supplementation in deficient patients.

Risk reduction should also include advice on appropriate footwear (hard-soled, flat, closed-toed shoes); adequate lighting for all activities, and caution with any activity that requires balance. Seniors should not climb stairs without a hand on the railing, stairways should be well illuminated, and the stairs should be in good repair. Climbing ladders should be discouraged. Robust elders should be cautioned about activities that increase their risk for falls (skiing, skating, etc) and that would hence place them at higher risk for fractures. Patients identified as having balance difficulty or with a history of multiple falls will benefit from muscle strengthening and balance retraining. Assistive devices may prevent falls when used correctly within a targeted intervention. Hip protectors may be necessary to prevent serious injuries such as hip fractures. Environmental modification is of known benefit as part of an overall targeted intervention in the subgroup of older patients who are at known risk for falls.

▶ Clinical Findings

A. Signs and Symptoms

The history should elicit the exact details and circumstances surrounding the fall as precisely as possible. The clinician should ask questions regarding when the fall or near-fall occurred (what time of the day, postprandial), where the patient was (indoors, outdoors), what the patient was doing (getting up from seated position, climbing stairs, turning, reaching, stooping, micturating), how the patient fell (tripped or stumbled, lost balance, lost consciousness), whether there was pain (severe arthritis) or other symptoms

(chest pain, shortness of breath, dizziness/lightheadedness, vertigo, diaphoresis, numbness and weakness of extremities, loss of consciousness), what medications were taken (prescription or OTC), and whether the patient had ingested alcohol.

Pinpointing the patient's subjective complaints is very helpful. Lightheadedness or a near-faint is consistent with cerebral ischemia and would suggest orthostasis, arrhythmias, and other cardiovascular conditions. Muscular weakness, the sense that their legs cannot hold them up, would be more consistent with deconditioning, or neuromuscular disease. Dysequilibrium or the sensation of failed coordination between the legs and the walking surface is suggestive of vestibulospinal tract, proprioception, somatosensory, and cerebellar lesions. Finally, the sensation of movement within the patient or of the room spinning is true vertigo. Clinical examination in itself can provide some useful information about the events surrounding a fall; for example, wrist fractures by a fall on an outstretched hand suggest that consciousness was preserved while falling, or bilaterally damaged patellas suggest drop attacks.

B. Physical Examination

Integrate both pathogenesis and the history to guide a targeted physical exam. Refer to **Table 41-3** for details.

C. Performance Assessment

Gait speed is currently the best predictor of mobility problems and correlates with future disability and life expectancy. The timed "get up and go" test is a simple, well-validated office tool for assessing gait and balance disturbance in frail elders. The patient sits in a straight-backed chair, then rises and walks 10 feet, turns, walks back, and sits on the chair. The patient may use whatever assistive device she/he normally uses and should be allowed one trial before being timed. Completion of the test in <10 seconds represents no risk and can be expected from nonfrail elders. A score of 10–19 seconds represents minimal risk; 20–29 seconds, moderate risk; and >30 seconds, a definite risk for falling. Referral to physical therapy is warranted for patients scoring ≥20 seconds.

D. Laboratory Findings

While lacking evidence, the following are reasonable: complete blood count and serum electrolytes, including calcium, blood urea nitrogen, vitamin B_{12}, vitamin D, and thyroid function tests. Neuroimaging can be useful for a person with a head injury or a new neurologic deficit. Electroencephalography is rarely helpful but may be indicated if there is high suspicion of seizure. Persons with unexplained falls may benefit from ambulatory electrocardiography (Holter monitor), although this has been associated with high false positives and false negatives.

Table 41-3. Focused physical examination.

Vital signs: orthostatic blood pressure and heart rate, sitting and standing pulse for 1 minute
Height: loss of height and kyphosis indicate osteoporosis; intervention may reduce fracture risk
Body mass index: if <21, patient is at risk of malnutrition and/or depression; decreased padding leads to increased injury risk
Vision: visual acuity, field testing, pupillary size, depth perception; visual field loss and depth perception have a much greater impact on mobility and vision function than acuity; dark adaptation time increases with age and is contingent on pupil size, lens opacification, and duration and brightness of light aggravate the problem further; an annual ophthalmologic examination is recommended for all elders; alert the ophthalmologist to your concerns
Vestibular function: have patient march in place with eyes closed; abnormal response is moving more than a few degrees or moving more than a foot in any direction
Cardiovascular: assess for dysrhythmia, valvular disease, congestive heart failure
Neuromuscular
  Proximal muscle weakness suggests polymyalgia rheumatica, polymyositis, adrenal, thyroid, or parathyroid disease
  Distal muscle weakness more suggestive of peripheral neuropathy.
Peripheral neuropathy: ≥20% of elders will have peripheral neuropathy—common causes are diabetes, alcohol, chronic lung disease, monoclonal gammopathy, neoplasm, medication (dilantin, lithium, isoniazid, vincristine), renal disease, thyroid disease, and vitamin B_{12} deficiency; neuropathy occurs before weakness or ataxia; further testing includes vibratory sense—patients should be able to feel a 128-Hz tuning fork at malleolus for 10 seconds; absence of position sense and Achilles reflex help confirm the diagnosis
Generalized muscle weakness: consider toxic myopathy from alcohol, glucocorticoids, HMG coenzyme A reductase inhibitors, and colchicine; atrophy suggests deconditioning; overall weakness suggests electrolyte imbalance
Muscle tone and postural reflexes should be assessed to rule out Parkinson disease or movement disorders
Range of motion: joint, neck, spine and hip, knee, and ankle should be assessed; restriction impairs reflex time and precision; cervical spondylosis is a significant cause of falls
Feet: in addition to peripheral neuropathy, check for deformities such as bunions, callouses, ulcers, hammertoes, and nail pathology; Achilles reflex suggests peripheral neuropathy but is absent in ≤70% of normal elderly individuals; note footwear—thick, soft-soled shoes increase fall risk
Cognitive ability: this can be screened by clock draw test, Mini-Cog or Montreal Cognitive Assessment (MoCA)

E. Environmental Assessment

A home assessment is warranted for frail elders and for anyone who has fallen at home. This may be done by the physician or occupational therapist and should include the environment itself as well as a replay of the circumstances of the fall. (See **Table 41-4.**)

Table 41-4. Environmental checklist.

Approach—outside: uneven sidewalk or walkway, exterior lighting, steps, ease of opening screen/storm/front door, proximity of steps to front door, ease of unlocking door
Interior lighting: especially on stairs and thresholds, loose electrical cords, accessibility of light switches
Carpets: scatter rugs, frayed or worn or high pile carpets
Floors: slippery, polished, unkempt (water, oil, clutter)
Bathroom: toilet height and ease of use, grab bars or bilateral grab bars if needed, bathing site including ease of entry, lighting, surface features, visibility of shower threshold; for overall safety ask about water temperature at this time, should be ≤120°F
Kitchen: location of most commonly used items, reaching and stooping, unstable stools, chair, or pedestal or glass table; smoke alarm
Stairs: lighting, handrail, condition of steps ease of use, nonskid surface
Furnishings: sharp edges, location in trafficked areas, height of bed and chairs
Assistive devices: in good repair, appropriate height for patient, stored out of the way when not in use
Presence of pets such as dogs and cats

▶ Conclusion

In conclusion, falls, like other syndromes of the elderly, are multifactorial and require a multidisciplinary approach. Assessment that identifies intrinsic and extrinsic causes helps focus targeted interventions. A team approach that incorporates the patient, specialists (physiatrist, ophthalmologist, optometrist, podiatrist, orthopedist), and occupational and physical therapists will maximize outcomes.

Gillespie LD, et al. Interventions for preventing falls in elderly people. *Cochrane Database Syst Rev.* 2012; 9:CD007146.
Studenski S. Gait speed and survival in older adults. *JAMA.* 2011; 305(1):50–58. [PMID: 21205966]

Websites (for Patient Education)

National Center for Injury Prevention and Control: http://www.cd.gov/ncipc/falls
National Institute on Aging http://www.niapublications.org/engagepages/falls.asp
Nice information on how to get up after a fall: http://www.stritch.luc.edu/depts/injprev/Falls/adult.htm

Urinary Incontinence

Robert J. Carr, MD

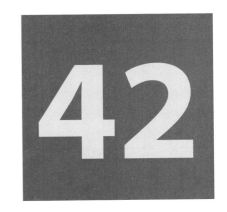

PHYSIOLOGY OF NORMAL URINATION

Urinary incontinence is the involuntary loss of urine that is so severe as to have social or hygienic consequences. A basic understanding of the normal physiology of urination is important to understand the potential causes of incontinence, and the various strategies for effective treatment.

The lower urinary tract consists primarily of the bladder (detrusor muscle) and the urethra. The urethra contains two sphincters: the internal urethral sphincter (IUS), composed predominantly of smooth muscle, and the external urethral sphincter (EUS), which is primarily voluntary muscle. The detrusor muscle of the bladder is innervated predominantly by cholinergic (muscarinic) neurons from the parasympathetic nervous system, the stimulation of which leads to bladder contraction. The sympathetic nervous system innervates both the bladder and the IUS. Sympathetic innervation in the bladder is primarily β-adrenergic and leads to bladder relaxation, whereas α-adrenergic receptors predominate in the IUS, leading to sphincter contraction. Thus, in general, sympathetic stimulation promotes bladder filling (relaxation of the detrusor with contraction of the sphincter), whereas parasympathetic stimulation leads to bladder emptying (detrusor contraction and sphincter relaxation).

The EUS, on the other hand, is striated muscle and under primarily voluntary (somatic) control. This allows for some ability to voluntarily postpone urination by tightening the sphincter and inhibiting the flow of urine. Additional voluntary control is provided by the central nervous system (CNS) through the pontine micturition center. This allows for central inhibition of the autonomic processes described earlier, and for further voluntary postponement of the need to urinate until the circumstances are more socially appropriate or until necessary facilities are available.

The physiologic factors influencing normal urination, summarized in **Table 42-1**, are important considerations when discussing urinary disorders and treatment.

AGE-RELATED CHANGES

Contrary to common perception, urinary incontinence is not inevitable with aging. Most elderly patients remain continent throughout their lifetimes, and a complaint of incontinence at any age should receive a thorough evaluation and not be dismissed as "normal for age." Nonetheless, many common age-related changes predispose elderly patients to incontinence and increase the likelihood of its development with advancing age.

The frequency of involuntary bladder contractions (detrusor hyperactivity) increases in both men and women with aging. In addition, total bladder capacity decreases, causing the voiding urge to occur at lower volumes. Bladder contractility decreases, leading to increased postvoid residuals and increased sensation of urgency or fullness. Elderly patients excrete a larger percentage of their fluid volume later in the day than younger persons. This, in addition to the other changes listed, often leads to an increase in the incidence of nocturia with aging, and more frequent nighttime awakenings.

In women, menopausal estrogen decline leads to urogenital atrophy and a decrease in the sensitivity of α-receptors in the IUS. In men, prostatic hypertrophy can lead to increased urethral resistance, and varying degrees of urethral obstruction.

It is important to remember that these age-related changes are found in many healthy, continent persons as well as those who develop incontinence. It is not completely understood why the predisposition to urinary problems is stronger in some patients than in others, which emphasizes the multifactorial basis of incontinence.

Table 42-1. Physiologic factors influencing normal urination.

Bladder filling	Sympathetic nervous system	β-Adrenergic	Detrusor relaxation
		α-Adrenergic	IUS contraction
Bladder emptying	Parasympathetic nervous system	Cholinergic	Detrusor contraction
Voluntary control	Somatic nervous system	Striated muscle	EUS contraction
	Central nervous system	Pontine micturition center	Central inhibition of urinary reflex

EUS, external urethral sphincter; IUS, internal urethral sphincter.

▶ Clinical Findings

A. Symptoms and Signs

1. Incontinence outside the urinary tract—Incontinence is often classified according to whether it is related to specific urogenital pathology or to factors outside the urinary tract. Terms such as *transient versus established, acute versus persistent,* and *primary versus secondary* have been used to highlight this distinction. The mnemonic DIAPPERS is helpful in remembering the many causes of incontinence that occur outside the urinary tract (**Table 42-2**). These "extraurinary" causes are very common in the elderly, and it is important to identify or rule them out before proceeding to a more invasive search for primary urogenital etiologies.

Delirium, depression, and disorders of excessive urinary output generally require medical or behavioral management of the primary cause rather than strategies relating to the bladder. Once the primary causes are corrected, the incontinence often resolves. Urinary tract infections, although easily treated if discovered, are a relatively infrequent cause of urinary incontinence in the absence of other classic symptoms (dysuria, urgency, frequency, etc). Asymptomatic bacteriuria, which is common even in well elderly, does not cause incontinence.

Pharmaceuticals are a particularly important and very common cause of incontinence. Because of the many neural receptors involved in urination (see Table 42-1), it is easy to understand why so many medications used to treat other common problems can readily affect continence. Medications frequently associated with incontinence are listed in **Table 42-3**. Many of these medications are available over the counter and in combination (**Table 42-4**). In addition, commonly used substances such as caffeine and alcohol can contribute to incontinence by virtue of their diuretic effects or their effects on mental status. For this reason, some medications and substances associated with a patient's incontinence may not be considered important or readily volunteered during a medication history unless the physician specifically asks about them.

Restricted mobility or the inability to physically get to the bathroom in time to avoid incontinence is also referred to as "functional" incontinence. The incontinence may be temporary or chronic, depending on the nature of the physical or cognitive disability involved. Physical therapy or strength and flexibility training may be helpful, as well as simple measures such as a bedside commode or urinal.

Stool impaction is very common in the elderly and may cause incontinence either through its local mass effect or by stimulation of opioid receptors in the bowel. It has been reported to be a causative factor in ≤10% of patients referred to incontinence clinics for evaluation. Continence can often be restored by a simple disimpaction.

2. Urologic causes of incontinence—Once secondary or transient causes have been investigated and ruled out, further evaluation should focus on specific urologic pathology that may be causing incontinence.

The urinary tract has two basic functions: the emptying of urine during voiding and the storage of urine between voiding. A defect in either of these basic functions can cause

Table 42-2. Causes of urinary incontinence without specific urogenital pathology.[a]

D	Delirium/confusional state
I	Infection (symptomatic)
A	Atrophic urethritis/vaginitis
P	Pharmaceuticals
P	Psychiatric causes (especially depression)
E	Excessive urinary output (hyperglycemia, hypercalcemia, congestive heart failure)
R	Restricted mobility
S	Stool impaction

[a]Also known as *transient, acute,* or *secondary incontinence.*

Table 42-3. Pharmaceuticals contributing to incontinence.

Pharmaceutical	Mechanism	Effect
α-Adrenergic agonists	IUS contraction	Urinary retention
α-Adrenergic blockers	IUS relaxation	Urinary leakage
Anticholinergic agents	Inhibit bladder contraction, sedation, immobility	Urinary retention and/or functional incontinence
Antidepressants		
Antihistamines		
Antipsychotics		
Sedatives		
β-Adrenergic agonists	Inhibits bladder contraction	Urinary retention
β-Adrenergic blockers	Inhibits bladder relaxation	Urinary leakage, urgency
Calcium channel blockers	Relaxes bladder	Urinary retention
Diuretics	Increases urinary frequency, urgency	Polyuria
Narcotic analgesics	Relaxes bladder, fecal impaction, sedation	Urinary retention and/or functional incontinence

IUS, internal urethral sphincter.

incontinence, and it is useful to initially classify incontinence according to whether it is primarily a defect of storage or of emptying. An *inability to store* urine occurs when the bladder contracts too often (or at inappropriate times), or when the sphincter(s) cannot contract sufficiently to allow the bladder to store urine and keep it from leaking. Thus the bladder rarely, if ever, fills to capacity and the patient's symptoms are generally characterized by frequent incontinent episodes of relatively small volume. An *inability to empty* urine occurs when the bladder is unable to contract appropriately, or when the outlet or sphincter(s) is (are) partially obstructed (either physically or physiologically). Thus, the bladder continues to fill beyond its normal capacity and eventually overflows, causing the patient to experience abdominal distention and continual or frequent leakage.

Whether the primary problem is the inability to store or the inability to empty can often be determined easily during the history and physical examination according to the patient's incontinence pattern (intermittent or continuous) and whether abdominal (bladder) distention is present.

Table 42-4. Nonprescription agents contributing to incontinence.

Agent	Mechanism	Effect	Common Examples
Alcohol	Diuretic effect, sedation, immobility	Polyuria and/or functional incontinence	Beer, wine, liquor, some liquid cold medicines
α-Agonists	IUS contraction	Urinary retention	Decongestants, diet pills
Antihistamines	Inhibit bladder contraction, sedation	Urinary retention and/or functional incontinence	Allergy tablets, sleeping pills, antinausea medications
α-Agonist/antihistamine combinations	IUS contraction and inhibition of bladder contraction	Marked urinary retention	Multisymptom cold tablets
Caffeine	Diuretic effects	Polyuria	Coffee, soft drinks, analgesics

IUS, internal urethral sphincter.

Determination of postvoid residual is also helpful in making this distinction (see section on history and physical findings, later). This initial classification is important in narrowing down the specific etiology of the incontinence, and in ultimately deciding on the appropriate management strategy.

3. Symptomatic classification—Once it is determined whether the primary problem is with storage or with emptying, incontinence can be further classified according to the type of symptoms that it causes in the patient. The most common categories are discussed below. The first two types, urge incontinence and stress incontinence, result from an inability to store urine. The third type, overflow incontinence, results from an inability to empty urine. Because the term "overflow" has been widely deemed confusing and imprecise, the terms *incomplete bladder emptying* and *urinary retention* are now often used instead. A patient may have a single type of incontinence or a combination of more than one type (mixed incontinence). **Table 42-5** summarizes the major categories of incontinence, the underlying urodynamic findings, and the most common etiologies for each.

A. Urge incontinence—Urge incontinence is the most common type of incontinence in the elderly. Patients complain of a strong, and often immediate, urge to void followed by an involuntary loss of urine. It is rarely possible to reach the bathroom in time to avoid incontinence once the urge occurs, and patients often lose urine while rushing toward a bathroom or trying to locate one. Urge incontinence is most frequently caused by involuntary contractions of the bladder, often referred to as *detrusor instability*. These involuntary contractions increase in frequency with age, as does the ability to voluntarily inhibit them. Although the symptoms of urgency are a hallmark feature of this type of incontinence, detrusor instability can sometimes result in incontinence without these symptoms. Although most patients with detrusor instability are neurologically normal, uninhibited contractions can also occur as the result of neurologic disorders such as stroke,

dementia, or spinal cord injury. In these cases it is often referred to as *detrusor hyperreflexia*. Detrusor instability and urgency can also be caused by local irritation of the bladder as with infection, bladder stones, or tumors. The term *overactive bladder syndrome* (OABS) is now commonly used to describe the symptoms of urgency caused by detrusor instability and to emphasize that they can occur either with or *without* incontinence. OABS is described by the International Continence Society as voiding ≥8 times during a 24-hour period, and awakening ≥2 times during the night. Treatment of OABS is similar regardless of whether incontinence is present.

B. Stress incontinence—Stress incontinence is much more common among women than men and is defined as a loss of urine associated with increases in intraabdominal pressure (Valsalva maneuver). Patients complain of leakage of urine (usually small amounts) during coughing, laughing, sneezing, or exercising. In women, stress incontinence is most often caused by urethral hypermobility resulting from weakness of the pelvic floor musculature, but it can also be caused by intrinsic weakness of the urethral sphincter(s), most commonly following trauma, radiation, or surgery. Stress incontinence is rare in men, unless they have suffered damage to the sphincter through surgery or trauma. In diagnosing stress incontinence, it is important to ascertain that the leakage occurs exactly *coincident* with the stress maneuver. If the leakage occurs several seconds after the maneuver, it is more likely caused by an uninhibited bladder contraction that has been triggered by the stress maneuver, and is urodynamically more similar to urge incontinence. This is sometimes known as *stress-induced detrusor instability*.

C. Incomplete bladder emptying (overflow incontinence)—This is a loss of urine associated with overdistention of the bladder. Patients complain of frequent or constant leakage or dribbling, or they may lose large amounts of urine without warning. Incomplete emptying may result either from a defect in the bladder's ability to contract

Table 42-5. Types and classification of urinary incontinence.

Underlying Defect	Symptomatic Classification	Most Common Urodynamics	Possible Etiologies
Inability to store urine	Urge (U)	Detrusor hyperactivity	Uninhibited contractions; local irritation (cystitis, stone, tumor); central nervous system causes
	Stress (S)	Sphincter incompetence	Urethral hypermobility; sphincter damage (trauma, radiation, surgery)
Inability to empty urine	Overflow (O) (incomplete emptying)	Outlet obstruction	Physical (benign prostatic hyperplasia, tumor, stricture); neurologic lesions, medications
		Detrusor hypoactivity	Neurogenic bladder (diabetes, alcoholism, disc disease)
	Functional (F)	Normal	Immobility problems; cognitive deficits
	Mixed	U + S, U + F	

(*detrusor hypoactivity*) or from obstruction of the bladder outlet or urethra. Detrusor hypoactivity is most commonly the result of a *neurogenic bladder* secondary to diabetes mellitus, chronic alcoholism, or disk disease. It can also be caused by medications, primarily muscle relaxants and β-adrenergic blockers. Outlet obstruction can be physical (prostatic enlargement, tumor, stricture), neurologic (spinal cord lesions, pelvic surgery), or pharmacologic (α-adrenergic agonists). Because neurogenic bladder is relatively rare in the geriatric population, it is important to rule out possible causes of obstruction whenever the diagnosis of overflow incontinence is made.

D. FUNCTIONAL INCONTINENCE—The term *functional incontinence* is used to describe physical or cognitive impairments that interfere with continence even in patients with normal urinary tracts (see section on incontinence outside the urinary tract, Table 42-2, and the DIAPPERS mnemonic, earlier).

E. MIXED INCONTINENCE—*Mixed incontinence* describes various combinations of the preceding four types. When present, it can make the diagnosis and management of incontinence more difficult. The term is most frequently used to describe patients who present with a combination of stress and urge incontinence, although other combinations are also possible. Functional incontinence, for example, can coexist with stress, urge, or overflow incontinence, further complicating the treatment of these patients. Side effects of medications being used to treat other comorbidities can also cause a mixed picture when combined with underlying incontinence of any type. Mixed stress and urge incontinence is particularly common among elderly women. When present, it is helpful to focus on the symptom that is most bothersome to the patient, and to direct the initial therapeutic interventions in that direction.

B. Screening

Screening for incontinence in all women is recommended because of its high prevalence and low degree of self-reporting by patients. Elderly women and those with neurologic diseases or diabetes are at the highest risk. Screening women aged ≥65 years for urinary incontinence is one of the *quality reporting measures* adopted by the Centers for Medicare and Medicaid Services in their 2013 Physician Quality Reporting System (PQRS) initiative, as is characterizing the type of incontinence and developing a plan of care.

C. History and Physical Findings

The history and physical examination of a patient presenting with incontinence should have the following goals:

1. To evaluate for and rule out causes of incontinence outside the urinary tract (DIAPPERS)

2. To determine whether the primary defect is an inability to store urine or an inability to empty urine

3. To determine the type of incontinence according to the patient's symptoms and likely etiologies

4. To determine the pattern of incontinence episodes and its effect on the patient's functional ability and quality of life

1. History—A thorough medical history should include a special focus on the neurologic and genitourinary history of the patient as well as any other medical problems that may be contributing factors (see Table 42-2). Information on any previous evaluation(s) for incontinence, as well as their degree of success or failure, can be helpful in guiding the current evaluation and in determining patient expectations. A careful medication history is very important, focusing on the categories of medications listed in Table 42-3 and remembering to include nonprescription substances (see Table 42-4). Finally, the pattern of incontinence is important in helping to classify its type and in planning appropriate therapy. While many urinary symptoms (eg, dribbling, frequency, hesitancy, nocturia) may lack diagnostic specificity, symptoms of urgency (the sudden urge to void with leakage before reaching the toilet) are very sensitive and specific for the diagnosis of urge incontinence. Urine leakage with coughing or other stress maneuvers is a sensitive indicator of stress incontinence, but is less specific than urge because of overlap with other conditions. A voiding diary or bladder record can be a very useful tool in obtaining additional diagnostic information. The patient or caregiver is given a set of forms and is asked to keep a written record of each incontinent episode for several days. A sample form is shown in **Table 42-6**. Incontinent episodes are recorded in terms of time, estimated volume (small or large), and precipitating factors. Fluid intake, as well as any episodes of urination in the toilet, is also recorded. When completed accurately, the bladder record can often elucidate the most likely type of incontinence and provide a clue to possible precipitating factors. Continuous leakage, for example, may be more consistent with overflow incontinence, whereas multiple, large-volume episodes may be more consistent with urge. Smaller-volume episodes associated with coughing or exercise may be more consistent with stress incontinence, whereas incontinence occurring only at specific times each day may suggest an association with a medication or other non–urinary tract cause. Although other information from the physical and laboratory evaluations will obviously be needed, the physician can often make significant progress toward determining the type of incontinence and possible precipitating factors from the history and voiding record alone.

2. Physical examination—In addition to a thorough search for nonurologic causes of incontinence, the physical examination should focus on the cardiovascular, abdominal, genital, and rectal areas. Cardiovascular examination should focus on signs of fluid overload. Evidence

Table 42-6. Sample voiding record.

Bladder Record

Name: _____

Date: _____

Instructions: Place a check in the appropriate column next to the time you urinated in the toilet or when an incontinence episode occurred. Note the reason for the incontinence and describe your liquid intake (for example, coffee, water) and estimate the amount (for example, one cup).

Time Interval	Urinated in Toilet	Had a Small Incontinent Episode	Had a Large Incontinent Episode	Reason for Incontinent Episode	Type/Amount of Liquid Intake
6–8 a.m.					
8–10 a.m.					
10–noon					
Noon–2 p.m.					
2–4 p.m.					
4–6 p.m.					
6–8 p.m.					
8–10 p.m.					
10–midnight					
Overnight					

Number of pads used today: _____

Number of episodes: _____

Comments: _____

of bladder distention on abdominal examination should raise suspicion for overflow incontinence. Genital examination should include a pelvic examination in women to assess for evidence of atrophy or mass, as well as any signs of uterine prolapse, cystocele, or rectocele. A rectal examination is helpful in ruling out stool impaction or mass, as well as in evaluating sphincter tone and perineal sensation for evidence of a neurologic deficit. A prostate examination is usually included, but several studies have demonstrated a poor correlation between prostate size and urinary obstruction. A neurologic examination focusing on the lumbosacral area is helpful in ruling out a spinal cord lesion or other neurologic deficits.

3. Special tests—Two additional tests, specific to the diagnosis of incontinence, should be added to the general physical examination.

A. PROVOCATIVE STRESS TESTING—This test attempts to reproduce the symptoms of incontinence under the direct visualization of the physician and is useful in differentiating stress from urge incontinence. The patient should have a full bladder and preferably be in a standing position (although a lithotomy position is also acceptable for patients unable to stand). The patient should be told to relax, and then to cough vigorously while the physician observes for urine loss. If leakage occurs simultaneously with the cough, a diagnosis of stress incontinence is likely. A delay between the cough and the leakage is more likely caused by a reflex bladder contraction and is more consistent with urge incontinence.

B. POSTVOID RESIDUAL (PVR)—This measurement should be obtained for incontinent patients suspected of urinary retention and potential obstruction. This includes men with severe urinary symptoms, women with prior gynecological or pelvic surgery, persons with neurological disorders or diabetes, and those who have failed initial empiric therapy. PVR measurement is traditionally done by urinary catheterization; however, portable ultrasound scanners for this purpose are now available that also provide very accurate readings. These ultrasound devices minimize the risks of instrumentation and infection that are inherent in catheterization, especially in male patients. Prior to measurement, the patient should be asked to empty the bladder as completely as possible. Residual urine in the bladder should be measured within a few minutes after emptying using either in-and-out catheterization or ultrasound. A PVR of <50 mL is normal; >200 mL indicates inadequate bladder emptying and is consistent with overflow incontinence. PVRs between 50 and 199 mL can sometimes be normal but may also exist with overflow incontinence, and results should be interpreted in light of the clinical picture. Patients with elevated PVRs should generally be referred for further evaluation and to rule out obstruction prior to treatment of the incontinence symptoms.

C. OTHER DIAGNOSTIC MANEUVERS—Other maneuvers, or "bedside urodynamics," have often been recommended to help in the diagnosis of incontinence. The best known of these are the Q-tip test to diagnose pelvic laxity and the Bonney (Marshall) test to determine whether surgical intervention will be helpful. Although these tests may be useful in some settings, recent studies have cast doubt on their predictive value, and in the family practice setting they are unlikely to add clinically useful information that would help in sorting out the small percentage of patients whose diagnosis remains unclear after a thorough history and physical examination.

C. Laboratory and Imaging Evaluation

Like the history and physical examination, the laboratory evaluation should be focused on ruling out the nonurologic causes of incontinence. A urinalysis is very helpful in screening for infection as well as in evaluating for hematuria, proteinuria, or glucosuria. It must be remembered, however, that asymptomatic bacteriuria is very common in the elderly and is not a cause of incontinence. Antibiotic treatment of asymptomatic bacteriuria has not been shown to reduce morbidity or to improve incontinence in either the institutionalized elderly or ambulatory women. Thus, antibiotic treatment in the face of incontinence and bacteriuria should be reserved for patients whose incontinence is of recent onset, has recently worsened, or is accompanied by other signs of infection. Hematuria, in the absence of infection, should be referred for further evaluation to rule out carcinoma.

Additional laboratory studies that are recommended and may be helpful include measurement of renal function [blood urea nitrogen (BUN) and creatinine] and evaluation for metabolic causes of polyuria (hypercalcemia, hyperglycemia). Radiologic studies are not routinely recommended in the initial evaluation of most patients with incontinence; however, a renal ultrasound study is useful in patients with obstruction to evaluate for hydronephrosis.

Abrams P, et al. eds. *Incontinence*, 3rd ed. Health Publications; 2005.

Abrutyn E, et al. Does asymptomatic bacteriuria predict mortality and does antimicrobial treatment reduce mortality in elderly ambulatory women? *Ann Intern Med*. 1994; 121:827. [PMID: 7818631]

Centers for Medicare and Medicaid Services. *2013 Physician Quality Reporting System* (PQRS) *Measures List* (downloaded from http://www.cms.gov/Medicare/Quality-Initiatives-Patient-Assessment-Instruments/PQRS/MeasuresCodes.html).

Fantl JA, et al. *Urinary Incontinence in Adults: Acute and Chronic Management*. Clinical Practice Guideline 2, 1996 update. US Department of Health and Human Services. Public Health Service, Agency for Health Care Policy and Research. AHCPR Publication 96-0682; 1996.

Holroyd-Leduc JM, et al. What type of urinary incontinence does this woman have? *JAMA*. 2008; 299:1446.

Ouslander JG. Management of overactive bladder. *N Engl J Med*. 2004; 350:786. [PMID: 14973214]

Resnick NM. Urinary incontinence. *Lancet*. 1995; 346:94. [PMID: 7603221]

▶ Treatment

If nonurologic or functional causes are found as major contributors to the patient's incontinence, treatment should be targeted at the underlying illnesses and improving any functional disability. In addition to medical management of the underlying disorder(s), physical therapy and the use of assistive devices may be helpful in improving the patient's level of function and ability to reach the bathroom prior to having an incontinent episode. For the ambulatory patient, a home visit is often useful in assessing for any environmental hazards that may be contributing to functional incontinence.

Simple lifestyle modifications may be helpful in mild cases of urinary incontinence. Fluid restriction and avoidance of caffeine and alcohol, especially in the evening, can be recommended as an initial step. Weight loss can be recommended if the patient is obese, and the use of a bedside commode or urinal can also be helpful. For patients with more severe incontinence, however, including most patients with urologic causes, further treatment measures usually are necessary.

Treatment for urinary incontinence is divided into three categories: behavioral and nonpharmacologic therapies, pharmacotherapy, and surgical intervention.

A. Behavioral and Nonpharmacologic Therapies

Lifestyle measures and behavioral therapies should be the first-line treatments in most patients with urge or stress incontinence, as they have the advantages of being effective in a large percentage of patients with few, if any, side effects. Lifestyle measures include limiting excessive fluid intake, avoiding caffeinated and alcoholic beverages, and attaining a healthy weight. Weight loss in overweight and obese women has been shown to be effective in reducing episodes of stress incontinence, but urge incontinence was not decreased. Behavioral therapies range from those designed to treat the underlying problem and restore continence (eg, bladder training, pelvic muscle exercises) to those designed simply to promote dryness through increased attention from a caregiver (eg, timed voiding, prompted voiding). The former category requires a motivated patient who is cognitively intact, whereas the latter category can be used even in patients with significant cognitive impairment.

1. Bladder training—This technique is designed to help patients control their voiding reflex by teaching them to void at scheduled times. The patient is asked to keep a voiding record for approximately 1 week to determine the pattern of incontinence and the interval between incontinent episodes. A voiding schedule is then developed with a scheduled voiding interval significantly shorter than the patient's usual incontinence interval. (For example, if the usual time between incontinent episodes is 1–2 hours, the patient should be scheduled to void every 30–60 minutes.) The patient is asked to empty the bladder as completely as possible at each scheduled void regardless of whether an urge is felt. Patients who have the urge to void at unscheduled times should try to stop the urge through relaxation or distraction techniques until the urge passes, and then void at the next scheduled time. If the urge between scheduled voids becomes too uncomfortable, the patient should go ahead and void, but should still void again as completely as possible at the next scheduled time. As the number of incontinent episodes decreases, the scheduled voiding intervals should be gradually extended each week, until a comfortable voiding interval is reached.

Fantl and colleagues, in a well-publicized albeit relatively small trial of bladder retraining (Fantl et al. 1991), demonstrated significant improvement in both the number of incontinent episodes and the amount of fluid lost in incontinent elderly women. Although the benefit was greatest in women with urge incontinence, women with stress incontinence also demonstrated improvement. In a later study, their group also demonstrated a significant improvement in quality of life following institution of bladder training. Studies in a family practice setting, in a home nursing program, and in a health maintenance organization also demonstrated significant benefit from a program of bladder training. The latter, a randomized controlled trial published in 2002, included patients with stress, urge, and mixed incontinence. Overall, patients had a 40% decrease in their incontinent episodes with 31% being 100% improved, 41% at least 75% improved, and 52% at least 50% improved.

2. Pelvic muscle exercises—These exercises, also known as *Kegel exercises*, are designed to strengthen the periurethral and perivaginal muscles. They are most useful in the treatment of stress incontinence but may also be effective in urge and mixed incontinence. Patients are initially taught to recognize the muscles to contract by being asked to squeeze the muscles in the genital area as if they were trying to stop the flow of urine from the urethra. While doing this, they should ensure that only the muscles in the front of the pelvis are being contracted, with minimal or no contraction of the abdominal, pelvic, or thigh muscles. Once the correct muscles are identified, patients should be taught to hold the contraction for at least 10 seconds followed by 10 seconds of relaxation. The exercises should be repeated between 30 and 80 times per day. Patients are then taught to contract their pelvic muscles before and during situations in which urinary leakage may occur to prevent their incontinent episodes from occurring.

A recent systematic review of 43 published clinical trials concluded that pelvic muscle exercises are effective for both stress and mixed incontinence, but that their effectiveness for urge incontinence remains unclear. Biofeedback has been used effectively to improve patients' recognition and contraction of pelvic floor muscles, but the required equipment and expertise can make this impractical in a primary care setting. Weighted vaginal cones and electrical stimulation have also been used to enhance pelvic muscle exercises. These modalities are provided by many physical therapy or geriatric departments and can be considered as additional options for women who are unsuccessful with pelvic muscle exercises or who have obtained only partial improvement. The Cochrane group concluded that weighted vaginal cones, electrostimulation, and pelvic muscle exercises are probably similar in effectiveness. There was insufficient evidence to conclude that the addition of cones or biofeedback is more effective than pelvic muscle exercises alone. The effectiveness of pelvic muscle exercises has not been well studied in men, but pelvic muscle exercises have been shown to improve incontinence following prostatectomy.

3. Timed voiding—Timed voiding is a passive toileting assistance program that is caregiver-dependent and can be used for patients who are either unable or unmotivated to participate in more active therapies. Its goal is to prevent incontinent episodes rather than to restore bladder function. The caregiver provides scheduled toileting for the patient on a fixed schedule (usually every 2–4 hours), including at night. There is no attempt to motivate the patient to delay voiding or resist the urge to void as there is in bladder training. The technique can be used for patients who can toilet independently as well as those who require assistance. It has been used with success in both male and female patients and has achieved improvements of ≤85%. Timed voiding has also been used effectively in postprostatectomy patients as well as in patients with neurogenic bladder.

A variation of timed voiding, known as *habit training*, uses a voiding schedule that is modified according to the patient's usual voiding pattern rather than an arbitrarily fixed interval. The goal of habit training is to preempt incontinent episodes by scheduling the patient's toileting interval to be shorter than the usual voiding interval. Both timed voiding and habit training are most commonly used in nursing homes but may also be used in the home if a motivated caregiver is available.

4. Prompted voiding—Prompted voiding is a technique that can be used for patients with or without cognitive impairment; it has been studied most frequently in the nursing home setting. Its goal is to teach patients to initiate their own toileting through requests for help and positive reinforcement from caregivers. Approximately every 2 hours, caregivers prompt the patients by asking whether they are wet or dry and suggesting that they attempt to void. Patients are then assisted to the toilet if necessary and praised for trying to use the toilet and for staying dry. A recent systemic analysis of controlled trials of prompted voiding concluded that the evidence was suggestive, although inconclusive, that prompted voiding provided at least short-term benefit to incontinent patients. The addition of oxybutynin to a prompted voiding program may provide additional benefit for some patients. A recent nursing home trial demonstrated that prompted voiding is most effective for reducing daytime incontinence, and that routine nighttime toileting was not effective in reducing incontinent episodes during the night.

B. Pharmacotherapy

Medications may be used alone or in conjunction with behavioral therapy when degree of improvement has been insufficient. There are very few studies comparing drug therapy with behavioral therapy, but both have been found more effective than placebo. An accurate diagnosis of the type of incontinence is necessary in order to choose appropriate pharmacotherapy for each patient.

1. Urge incontinence—Anticholinergic medications are the drugs of choice for urge incontinence, and six medications in a total of 12 formulations are now available. Oxybutynin, the earliest of these medications, is now available in a transdermal patch (Oxytrol) that can be dosed twice weekly, as well as a long-acting formulation (Ditropan XL) and a gel (Gelnique) that can both be dosed once daily. It is also available in a generic formulation that is significantly less expensive, but requires dosing (2.5–5 mg) 2–4 times a day.

Tolterodine is also available in both short-acting (Detrol) and long-acting (Detrol LA) formulations that can be dosed either once or twice daily. No direct trial has yet been published comparing the long-acting forms of the two drugs. A study of long-acting oxybutynin versus short-acting tolterodine found oxybutynin was modestly more effective with a similar side effect profile and cost. A meta-analysis of four comparative trials (studying mainly the short-acting formulations) concluded that oxybutynin is superior in efficacy, but that tolterodine is better tolerated with fewer dropouts because of medication side effects. The most common side effects of anticholinergic medications include dry mouth, blurred vision, constipation, dizziness, and headache. Urinary retention and delirium can also occur. These effects are less common with tolterodine, and dry mouth seems less common with the transdermal and gel formulations of oxybutynin, due to a lower production of metabolite.

Four newer anticholinergic medications have been released to compete with oxybutynin and tolterodine. Trospium (Sanctura), released in 2004, offers the advantage of fewer drug-drug interactions because it is not metabolized by the cytochrome P450 system and is cleared by the kidney. It now has an extended-release formulation available that allows once-daily dosing. Solifenacin (Vesicare) and darifenacin (Enablex), both released in 2005, are more selective for the M3 muscarinic receptors in the bladder than the more traditional agents. Both are dosed once daily. M3 receptors are found preferentially in smooth muscle, the salivary glands, and the eyes. This selectivity may lead to a lower incidence of drowsiness and dizziness in some patients; the most common side effects are dry mouth and constipation. The industry-sponsored STAR trial found solifenacin to be somewhat more effective than tolterodine in reducing urgency and frequency, but dry mouth and constipation were more frequent with solifenacin. Fesoterodine (Toviaz), released in 2009, is similar to Detrol LA and has the same active metabolite. It is supplied in a higher-dose formulation (8 mg) than Detrol, which may increase its efficacy but likely also its side effects.

Mirabegron (Myrbetriq), released in 2012, is the first β_3-agonist, and is marketed for use in overactive bladder syndrome and urge incontinence. Stimulation of β_3-receptors helps to relax the bladder and increase storage capacity, and this drug can be used as an alternative to anticholinergics for patients who don't tolerate or respond adequately to them. Mirabegron has been shown to slightly increase heart rate and blood pressure, so these parameters should be monitored in patients on this drug. In addition, mirabegron can lead to increased drug levels of digoxin, metoprolol, desipramine, and other medications metabolized by the cytochrome P450-2D6 system. There is no current evidence for the safety of efficacy of combination therapy with mirabegron and any of the anticholinergic medications.

The tricyclic antidepressant imipramine has traditionally been widely used to treat urge incontinence, but its use has now largely been supplanted by these newer agents with more favorable side effect profiles and better documented efficacy.

2. Stress incontinence—Medical treatment is most effective for patients with mild to moderate stress incontinence and without a major anatomic abnormality. The α-agonist pseudoephedrine, at a dosage range of 15–60 mg 3 times a day, is the drug of choice for patients without contraindications. Side effects include nausea, dry mouth, insomnia, and restlessness. Studies using phenylpropanolamine (now removed from the market) demonstrated improvement in 19–60% of women and cure in 9–14%. One study indicated that a significant number of patients referred for surgical intervention could avoid surgery with α-agonist therapy.

Traditionally, estrogen therapy has been used in conjunction with α-agonists to increase α-adrenergic responsiveness and improve urethral mucosa and smooth-muscle tone. However, the recent Heart and Estrogen/Progestin Replacement Study (HERS) demonstrated estrogen therapy to be less effective than placebo for symptoms of urinary incontinence, with only 20.9% of the treatment group reporting improvement and 38.8% reporting worsening of their incontinence (compared with 26% improvement and 27% worsening in the placebo group). Data from the Women's Health Initiative study, indicating that patients on an estrogen-progestin combination demonstrated increased risk for heart disease, stroke, breast cancer, and pulmonary embolism, also cast significant doubt on the advisability of long-term estrogen use for this indication. Although the risks and benefits of topical estrogen are not completely known, prescription of oral estrogen for the treatment of incontinence is not currently recommended.

3. Overflow incontinence—Overflow incontinence associated with outlet obstruction is seldom treated with medications because the primary therapy is removal of the obstruction. In men, outlet obstruction is most commonly caused by prostatic enlargement secondary to infection (prostatitis), benign prostatic hyperplasia, or prostate cancer. Prostatitis can be treated with a 2–4-week course of a fluoroquinolone or trimethoprim-sulfamethoxazole. Once prostate cancer has been ruled out, benign prostatic hyperplasia may be treated with α-blockers, finasteride, surgery, or transurethral microwave thermotherapy. α-Blockers have been shown to be ineffective in "prostatismlike" symptoms in elderly women.

Medical treatment of overflow incontinence caused by bladder contractility problems is rarely highly efficacious. The cholinergic agonist bethanechol may be useful subcutaneously for temporary contractility problems following an overdistention injury but is generally ineffective when given orally or when used on a long-term basis.

C. Surgical Intervention

Surgical therapy may be indicated for patients with incontinence resulting from anatomic abnormalities (eg, cystocele, prolapse), with outlet obstruction resulting in urinary retention, or for patients in whom more conservative methods of treatment have not provided sufficient relief. Beyond the correction of anatomic abnormalities or obstruction, surgical therapy is most effective for stress incontinence or for mixed incontinence in which stress incontinence is a primary component. Numerous surgical options are available for the management of stress incontinence, including injection of periurethral bulking agents, transvaginal suspensions, retropubic suspensions, slings, and sphincter prostheses. Choice of procedure is based on the relative contributions of urethral hypermobility versus intrinsic sphincter deficiency, urodynamic findings, the need for other concomitant surgery, the patient's medical condition and lifestyle, and the experience of the surgeon.

D. Electrical Stimulation

These devices are sometimes used to treat incontinence that has been refractory to other methods. The goals are to stimulate contractions of the pelvic floor muscles and/or inhibit overactive bladder contractions. Noninvasive stimulation electrodes can be placed in either the vagina or the anus. Current evidence does not support the efficacy of these methods as being better than behavioral training alone. Electrodes can also be implanted in the sacral nerve roots, the bladder, or the peripheral tibial nerve. These appear to be more effective than noninvasive stimulation, but are reserved for carefully selected patients who have been refractory to less invasive measures.

E. Pads, Garments, Catheterization, and Pessaries

The use of absorbent pads and undergarments is extremely common among the elderly. Although they are not recommended as primary therapy before other measures have been tried, they may be useful in patients whose incontinence is infrequent and predictable, who cannot tolerate the side effects of medications, or who are not good candidates for surgical therapy. The main purpose of these pads and garments is to contain urine loss and prevent skin breakdown. However, very few studies have compared the numerous absorbent products available and their degree of success or failure in meeting these objectives. A recent Cochrane review concluded that disposable products may be more effective than nondisposable products in decreasing the incidence of skin problems, and that superabsorbent products may perform better than fluff pulp products. More comparative studies are needed in this area to assist patients and caregivers in making better-informed decisions.

Although urethral catheterization should be avoided as a general rule, it is sometimes indicated in cases of overflow incontinence or in patients for whom no other measures have been effective. External collection devices (eg, Texas catheters) are preferable to indwelling catheters, but acceptable external devices are not widely available for women, and adverse reactions such as skin abrasion, necrosis, and urinary tract infection may occur. When internal catheterization is needed, intermittent or suprapubic catheterization has been shown to be preferable to indwelling catheterization in reducing the incidence of bacteriuria and its consequent complications. Indwelling urethral catheterization should be limited to very few circumstances, including comfort measures for the terminally ill, for prevention of contamination of pressure ulcers, and for patients with inoperable outflow obstruction.

Pessaries are intravaginal devices used to maintain or restore the position of the pelvic organs in patients with genitourethral prolapse. Although there are few comparative data on their use in incontinence, they can sometimes be useful in patients with intractable stress incontinence who are poor candidates for, or who do not desire, surgery.

F. Primary Care Treatment versus Referral

Once the information from the history, physical examination, voiding record, provocative stress testing, PVR measurement, and laboratory data is available, a presumptive diagnosis can be made in the large majority of patients. If the patient has uncomplicated urge or stress incontinence, or a mixture of urge and stress, primary treatment can be initiated by the family physician. If the patient has overflow incontinence, manifested by an elevated PVR, referral is indicated to rule out obstruction prior to attempting medical or behavioral management. In the minority of patients in whom the type or cause of incontinence remains unclear, referral for urodynamic testing is indicated if a specific diagnosis will be helpful in guiding therapy. Urodynamic testing in the routine evaluation of incontinence is not indicated as studies have not shown an improvement in clinical outcome between patients diagnosed by urodynamics and patients whose treatment was based on history and physical examination.

Other indications for referral include incontinence associated with recurrent symptomatic urinary tract infections, hematuria without infection, history of prior pelvic surgery or irradiation, marked pelvic prolapse, suspicion of prostate cancer, lack of correlation between symptoms and physical findings, and failure to respond to therapeutic interventions as would be expected from the presumptive diagnosis.

Appell RA, et al. Overactive Bladder: judging Effective Control and Treatment Study Group: prospective randomized controlled trial of extended-release oxybutynin chloride and tolterodine tartrate in the treatment of overactive bladder: results of the OBJECT study. *Mayo Clin Proc.* 2001; 76:358. [PMID: 11322350]

Benson JT. New therapeutic options for urge incontinence. *Curr Womens Health Rep.* 2001; 1:61. [PMID: 12112953]

Eustice S, et al. Prompted voiding for the management of urinary incontinence in adults. *Cochrane Database Syst Rev.* 2000; (2):CD002113. [PMID: 10795861]

Fantl JA, et al. Efficacy of bladder training in older women with urinary incontinence. *JAMA.* 1991; 265:609. [PMID: 1987410]

Fink HA, et al. Treatment interventions in nursing home residents with urinary incontinence: a systemic review of randomized trials. *Mayo Clin Proc.* 2008; 83:1332.

Glazener CM, Lapitan MC. Urodynamic investigations for management of urinary incontinence in adults. *Cochrane Database Syst Rev.* 2002; (3):CD003195. [PMID: 12137680]

Godec CJ. "Timed voiding"—a useful tool in the treatment of urinary incontinence. *Urology.* 1994; 23:97. [PMID: 6691214]

Grady D, et al. Postmenopausal hormones and incontinence: the Heart and Estrogen/Progestin Replacement Study. *Obstet Gynecol.* 2001; 97:116. [PMID: 11152919]

Harvey MA, et al. Tolterodine versus oxybutynin in the treatment of urge urinary incontinence: a meta-analysis. *Am J Obstet Gynecol.* 2001; 185:56. [PMID: 11483904]

Hay-Smith EJ, et al: Pelvic floor muscle training for urinary incontinence in women. Cochrane Database Syst Rev 2001; (1): CD001407. [PMID: 11279716]

MacDonald R, et al. Pelvic floor muscle training to improve urinary incontinence after radical prostatectomy; a systematic review of effectiveness. *BJU Int.* (*British Journal of Urology International*) 2007;100(1):76–81 (review). [PMID: 17433028].

Madersbacher H, et al. Conservative management in the neuropathic patient. In: Abrams, P et al. eds. *Incontinence: first International Consultation on Incontinence. Recommendations of the International Scientific Committee: The Evaluation and Treatment of Urinary Incontinence.* Health Publication Ltd.; 1999.

PL Detail-Document. *Medications for Overactive Bladder.* Pharmacist's Letter/Prescriber's Letter; Oct. 2012.

Rossouw JE, et al. Writing Group for the Women's Health Initiative Investigators: Risks and benefits of estrogen plus progestin in healthy postmenopausal women: principal results from the Women's Health Initiative randomized controlled trial. *JAMA.* 2002; 288:321. [PMID: 12117397]

Shamliyan T, Wyman JF, Ramakrishnan R, Sainfort F, Kane RL. Benefits and harms of pharmacologic treatment for urinary incontinence in women: a systematic review. *Ann Intern Med.* 2012;156:861–874.

Shirran E, Brazzelli M. Absorbent products for the containment of urinary and/or faecal incontinence in adults. *Cochrane Database Syst Rev.* 2000;(2):CD001406. [PMID: 10796783]

Subak LL, et al. Weight loss to treat urinary incontinence in overweight and obese women. *N Engl J Med.* 2009; 360:481.

Subak LL, et al. The effect of behavioral therapy on urinary incontinence: a randomized controlled trial. *Obstet Gynecol.* 2002; 100:72. [PMID: 12100806]

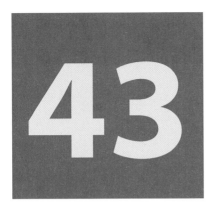

Elder Abuse

David Yuan, MD, MS

Jeannette E. South-Paul, MD, FAAFP

► General Considerations

As hidden as the other forms of family violence may be, domestic elder abuse is even more concealed within our society. As the baby boomers age, the number of elders in the United States will continue to increase. The societal cost for the identification and treatment of elder abuse is also projected to rise as the baby boomers enter the elder years. Elder abuse is now recognized as a pervasive and growing problem. Vastly underreported, for every case of elder abuse and neglect that is reported to authorities, as many as five cases are not reported.

Many physicians feel ill-equipped to address this important social and medical problem. The most common reporters of abuse are family members (17%) and social services agency staff (11%). Physicians reported only 1.4% of the cases. Healthcare professionals consistently underestimate the prevalence of elder abuse. Concerns for patient safety and retaliation by the caregiver, violation of the physician-patient relationship, patient autonomy, confidentiality, and trust issues are quoted as reasons for low reporting. Studies have shown that healthcare professionals attest to viewing cases of suspected elder abuse but yet fail to report them. One study revealed that physicians report only 2% of all suspected cases.

Older victims who suffer from neglect or physical abuse are likely to seek care from their primary care physician or gain entry into the medical care system through an emergency department. Except for the older person's caregivers, physicians may be the only ones to see an abused elderly patient.

Cooper C, Selwood A, Livingston G. Knowledge detection and reporting of abuse by health and social care professionals: a systematic review. *Am J Geriatr Psychiatry.* 2009; 17(10): 826–838. [PMID: 19916205]

Lachs MS, Pillemer K. Elder abuse. *Lancet.* 2004; 364:1263. [PMID: 15464188]

Schmeidel AN, et al. Health care professionals' perspectives on barriers to elder abuse detection and reporting in primary care settings. *J Elder Abuse Negl.* 2012; 24(1):17–36. [PMID: 22206510]

A. Definition and Types of Abuse

Elder abuse encompasses all types of mistreatment and abusive behaviors toward older adults. The mistreatment can be either acts of commission (abuse) or acts of omission (neglect). The National Center on Elder Abuse (NCEA) describes seven different types of elder abuse: physical abuse, sexual abuse, emotional abuse, financial exploitation, neglect, abandonment, and self-neglect (**Table 43-1**). *Self-neglect* is defined as the behavior of an elderly person that threatens her/his own health and safety. Labeling a behavior as abusive, neglectful, or exploitative is difficult and can depend on the frequency, duration, intensity, severity, consequences, and cultural context. Currently, state laws define elder abuse and definitions vary considerably from one jurisdiction to another.

Wood EF. *The Availability and Utility of Interdisciplinary Data on Elder Abuse: A White Paper for the National Center on Elder Abuse.* American Bar Association Commission on Law and Aging for the National Center on Elder Abuse. National Center on Elder Abuse at American Public Human Services Association; 2006.

B. Prevalence

It is estimated that 4% of adults aged > 65 years are subjected to mistreatment in the United States. In almost 90% of cases the perpetrator of the abuse is known, and in two-thirds of cases the perpetrators are spouses or adult children. Because of underreporting, poor detection, and differing definitions, the true estimate of elder abuse may be far greater. In a nationally representative survey of almost 6000 subjects, the prevalence of elder abuse was 0.6% for sexual abuse, 1.6% for

Table 43-1. Elder abuse: definitions.

Physical abuse	Use of physical force that may result in bodily injury, physical pain, or impairment
Sexual abuse	Nonconsensual sexual contact of any kind with an elderly person
Emotional abuse	Infliction of anguish, pain, or distress through verbal or nonverbal acts
Financial/material exploitation	Illegal or improper use of an elder's funds, property, or assets
Neglect	Refusal, or failure, to fulfill any part of a person's obligations or duties to an elderly person
Abandonment	Desertion of an elderly person by an individual who has physical custody of the elder or who has assumed responsibility for providing care to the elder
Self-neglect	Behaviors of an elderly person that threaten the elder's health or safety

Data from National Center on Elder Abuse. *Major Types of Elder Abuse* (available at www.ncea.aoa.gov; accessed 2012).

Table 43-2. Risk factors for elder abuse.

Cognitive impairment
Aggressive behaviors
Psychological distress
Lower levels of social network and social support
Lower household income
Need for ADL assistance

Data from Mosqueda L, et al. Elder abuse and self-neglect. JAMA 2011;b306(5):532-40.

than for unimpaired adults. In a recent systematic review, caregiver burden/stress was a significant risk factor. Care setting also seems to influence risk of elder abuse. Most elder abuse and neglect occur in the home. Paid home care has a relatively high rate of verbal abuse, and assisted-living settings have an unexpectedly high rate of neglect. Moving from paid home care to nursing homes has been shown to more than triple the odds of the elder experiencing neglect. In one study >70% of nursing home staff reported that they had behaved at least once in an abusive or neglectful way toward residents over a one-year period. Risk factors commonly cited for elder mistreatment are listed in **Table 43-2**.

Characteristics of perpetrators of elder abuse can be seen in **Table 43-3**.

A typology of abusers has also been suggested to better delineate who may perpetrate abuse. Five types of offenders have been postulated:

1. *Overwhelmed offenders* are well intentioned and enter caregiving expecting to provide adequate care; however, when the amount of care expected exceeds their comfort level, they lash out verbally or physically.

physical abuse, 4.6% for emotional abuse, 5.1% for neglect, and 5.2% for financial abuse by a family. Psychological abuse is more prevalent than physical abuse. Neglect—the failure of a designated caregiver to meet the needs of a dependent elderly person—is the more common form of elder maltreatment. The prevalence of elder financial abuse is difficult to gauge. One researcher estimates that for every known case of financial exploitation, 24 go unreported. Elder self-neglect is an important public health concern that is the most common form of elder abuse and neglect reported to social services.

Acierno R, et al. Prevalence and correlates of emotional, physical, sexual, and financial abuse and potential neglect in the United States: the National Elder Mistreatment Study. *Am J Public Health*. 2010; 100(2):292–297. [PMID: 20019303]

Gibson SC, et al. Assessing knowledge of elder financial abuse: a first step in enhancing prosecutions. *J Elder Abuse Negl*. 2013; 25(2):162–182. [PMID: 23473298]

Mosqueda L, et al. Elder abuse and self-neglect. *JAMA*. 2011; 306(5):532–540. [PMID: 21813431]

C. Risk Factors

Several explanations have been proposed to explain the origins of elder mistreatment. These explanations have focused on overburdened or mentally disturbed caregivers, dependent elders, a history of childhood abuse and neglect, and the marginalization of elders in society. Abuse among older adults with cognitive impairment is markedly higher

Table 43-3. Characteristics of perpetrators of elder abuse.

Relationship	Percentage (%)
Family member	89.7
Adult child	47.3
Spouse	19.3
Other relatives	8.8
Friend	6.2
Home service provider	2.8
Out-of-home service provider	1.4

Data from US Department of Health and Human Services Administration on Aging and the Administration for Children and Families. *The National Elder Abuse Incidence Study*. Washington, DC: National Center for Elder Abuse; 1998

2. *Impaired offenders* are well intentioned, but have problems that render them unqualified to provide adequate care. The caregiver may be of advanced age, have physical or mental illness, or have developmental disabilities.

3. *Narcissistic offenders* are motivated by anticipated personal gain and not the desire to help others. These individuals tend to be socially sophisticated and gain a position of trust over the vulnerable elder. Maltreatment is usually in the form of neglect and financial exploitation.

4. *Domineering or bullying offenders* are motivated by power and control and are prone to outbursts of rage. This abuse may be chronic and multifaceted, including physical, psychological, and even forced sexual coercion.

5. *Sadistic offenders* derive feelings of power and importance by humiliating, terrifying, and harming others. Signs of this type of abuse include bite, burn, and restraint marks and other signs of physical and sexual assault.

Johannesen M, et al. Elder abuse: a systematic review of risk factors in community-dwelling elders. *Age Ageing*. 2013; 42(3): 292–298. [PMID: 23343837]

McDonald L, et al. Institutional abuse of older adults: what we know, what we need to know. *J Elder Abuse Negl*. 2012; 24(2):138–160. [PMID: 22471513]

Page C, et al. The effect of care setting on elder abuse: results from a Michigan survey. *J Elder Abuse Negl*. 2009; 21(3):239–252. [PMID: 19827327].

Ramsey Klawsnik H. Elder-abuse offenders: a typology. *Generations*. 2000; 24:17.

▶ Clinical Findings

Several medical and social factors make the detection of elder abuse more difficult than other forms of family violence. The elderly dependent patient may fear retaliation from the abuser and may be reluctant to come forward with information. Given the higher prevalence of chronic diseases in older adults, signs and symptoms of mistreatment may be misattributed to chronic disease, leading to "false negatives," such as fractures that are ascribed to osteoporosis instead of physical assault. Alternatively, sequelae of many chronic diseases may be misattributed to elder mistreatment, creating "false positives," such as weight loss because of cancer erroneously ascribed to intentional withholding of food.

A. Screening

The US Preventive Services Task Force (USPSTF) found insufficient evidence to recommend for or against routine screening of older adults or their caregivers for elder abuse. The American Medical Association recommends that older

Table 43-4. American Medical Association screening questions for abuse.

1. Has anyone ever touched you without your consent?
2. Has anyone ever made you do things you didn't want to do?
3. Has anyone taken anything that was yours without asking?
4. Has anyone ever hurt you?
5. Has anyone ever scolded or threatened you?
6. Have you ever signed any documents you didn't understand?
7. Are you of afraid of anyone at home?
8. Are you alone a lot?
9. Has anyone ever failed to help you take care of yourself when you needed help?

Reproduced with permission from Geroff AJ, Olshaker JS. Elder abuse. *Emerg Med Clini North Am*. 2006;24:491-505.

patients be asked about family violence even when evidence of such abuse does not appear to exist. A careful history is crucial to determining whether suspected abuse or neglect exists. The physician should interview the patient and caregiver separately, and if the caregiver does not allow this, abuse potential should be considered. A physician's suspicions should be heightened if the caregiver dominates the medical interview. General questions about feeling safe at home and who prepares meals and handles finances can open the door to more specific questions. Ask if the caregiver is yelling or hitting, making the elder wait for meals and medications, confining the elder to a room, or threatening institutionalization. It is also important to inquire about the possibility of sexual abuse (unwanted touching) or financial abuse (stolen money, being coerced to sign legal documents without understanding the consequences). Self-neglect may be present if the patient begins to miss appointments, gets lost on the way to appointments, or is unable to take medications correctly. **Table 43-4** lists important questions to ask when screening for suspected abuse.

Avoid confrontation and blame when interviewing the caregiver. Ask about caregiver burden. Be alert if a caregiver has poor knowledge of a patient's medical problems. If a caregiver has excessive concerns about costs or is financially dependent on the elder, be alert for financial abuse. A study of 2800 older adults found that elder mistreatment was associated with an increased risk for nursing home placement and all-cause mortality. Self-neglect is associated with increased rates of hospitalization and mortality as well.

Dong X et al. Elder self neglect and abuse and mortality risk in a community-dwelling population. *JAMA*. 2009; 302(5):517–526. [PMID: 19654386]

US Preventive Services Task Force. *Screening for Intimate Partner Violence and Abuse of Elderly and Vulnerable Adults* (recommendation statement; available at http://www.uspreventiveservicestaskforce.org; accessed 2013).

Table 43-5. Findings suggestive of physical abuse.

Finding	Bruising	Burns
Size	>5 cm	
Shape	Resembling implement used, eg, hand, shoe, belt, or cane	Resembling implement used, eg, cigarette, clothing iron
Location	Face, side of right arm, or back of torso	Immersion burns may appear in stocking/glove distribution
Miscellaneous	Color not indicative of age of bruise	Characteristic similar to burns seen in children

Adapted with permission from Palmer M et al. Elder abuse: dermatologic clues and critical solutions. *J Am Acad Dermatol.* 2013; 62(2):e37-e42.

Table 43-6. Factors affecting the reporting and recognition of elder abuse and neglect.

Medical care providers might not report abuse for the following reasons:
Might not recognize the abuse/neglect and therefore attribute the patient's medical condition to another cause
Might feel constrained by time
Might be concerned about offending the patient and family or in denial that a family member is abusing, especially if the potential abuser is also a patient of the physician
Is unfamiliar with mandatory reporting laws
Is unfamiliar with available resources
Is concerned about personal safety and is afraid of involvement
Is unfamiliar with screening tools
Misinterprets the patient's signs as indicative of another disease process

Data from Abbey L. Elder abuse and neglect: when home is not safe. *Clin Geriatr Med.* 2009; 25:47-60.

B. Physical Examination

There are no pathognomonic signs of elder abuse, and physical abuse is not the most common type of elder abuse. Yet a thorough physical examination is critical as the elder victim may not be forthcoming about the abuse. Particular attention to the functional and cognitive status of the elder is important to understanding the degree of dependence that the elder may have. Neglect or self-neglect should be suspected when a patient appears disheveled or has evidence of poor hygiene. **Table 43-5** lists findings suggestive of physical abuse.

Detailed documentation of the physical examination is important as it may be used as evidence in a criminal trial. Documentation must be complete and legible, with accurate descriptions and annotations on sketches or, when possible, with the use of photographic documentation.

Palmer M, et al. Elder abuse: dermatologic clues and critical solutions. *J Am Acad Dermatol.* 2013; 62(2):e37–e42. [PMID: 23058875]
US Administration on Aging. *National Center on Elder Abuse Administration on Aging* (available at http://www.ncea.aoa.gov).

▶ Intervention & Reporting

Barriers to reporting elder abuse are listed in **Table 43-6**. Forty-four US states have mandatory reporting laws that require healthcare professionals to report a reasonable suspicion of abuse or self-neglect. Most states have anonymous reporting and Good Samaritan laws that can offer an alternative to a direct physician report if there are significant concerns for maintaining the physician-patient relationship. By emphasizing the treatment of the health consequences of the abuse, the elderly patient and caregiver may feel less threatened. Reporting should be done in a caring and compassionate manner in order to protect the autonomy and self-worth of the elder while ensuring his/her continued safety.

The victim should be told that a referral will be made to Adult Protective Services (APS). Involving the caregiver in the discussion must be carefully considered with regard to potential retaliation on the victim. The law enforcement implications of APS should be downplayed, and the social support and services offered by APS should be offered as part of the medical management of the victim. Victims may deny the possibility of abuse or fail to recognize its threat to their personal safety. In financial abuse the victim, the offender, or both may not acknowledge the abuse. If the victim refuses the APS referral, the clinician may explain that s/he is bound to adhere to state regulations and that the regulations were developed to help older persons who were not receiving the care they needed.

The safety of the patient is the most important consideration in any case of suspected abuse. If the abuse is felt to be escalating, as may occur with physical abuse, law enforcement as well as APS should be contacted. Hospitalization of the elder may be a temporary solution to removing the victim from the abuser.

If elders have decision-making capacity, their wishes to either accept interventions for suspected abuse or refuse those interventions must be respected. If an abused elder refuses to leave an abusive environment, the primary care physician can still help. This may include helping the older victim to develop a safety plan, such as when to call 911, or installing a lifeline emergency alert system. Close follow-up should be offered.

If older victims no longer retain decision-making capacity, the courts may need to appoint a guardian or conservator to make decisions about living arrangements, finances, and care. This is typically coordinated through APS. The physician's role is to provide documentation of impaired decision-making capacity and of the findings of abuse.

Intervention can be complicated when self-neglect is suspected. Patients may be capable of understanding their actions even if their choices disagree with recommendations of family or professionals. Assessment of cognition and decision-making capacity are critical and may be challenging if individuals refuse assessment. Behavioral health professionals, ethics committees, the guardianship process, and court system are invaluable in assisting families and physicians.

Because of confidentiality guidelines it may be difficult to enlist clergy and other community organizations for help.

As the size of the elderly population continues to grow, physicians need to be vigilant in identifying patients at risk for elder abuse. The physician's role is to recognize elder abuse and self-neglect, treat any associated medical problems, and provide a safe disposition for the patient.

Bond MC, et al. Elder abuse and neglect: definitions, epidemiology, and approaches to emergency department screening. *Clin Geriatr Med.* 2013; 29(1):257–273. [PMID: 23177610]

Movement Disorders

Yaqin Xia, MD, MHPE

Movement disorders (MDs) are a broad spectrum of motor and nonmotor disturbances arising from the dysfunction of subcortical motor control circuitry, including basal ganglia and thalamus, as well as other parts of the nervous system, involving the cortex, cerebellum, central, and peripheral autonomic nervous system. Patients suffering from MDs have normal muscle strength and sensation, but their normal voluntary motor activities are influenced or impaired by involuntary movement, alteration in muscle tone or posture, and loss of coordination or regulation—either facilitation or inhibition—of pyramidal motor activities as a result of malfunction. MDs can be classified into the following categories on the basis of their clinical manifestations: tremor, chorea and choreoathetosis, dystonia, myoclonus, tics, and ataxia. MDs include less movement (hypokinesia or akinesia), or excessive movement (hyperkinesias), or both (**Table 44-1**).

PARKINSON'S DISEASE

ESSENTIALS OF DIAGNOSIS

- ▶ Cardinal motor features
  - ▶ Bradykinesia
  - ▶ At least one of the following: 4–6-Hz resting tremor, muscular rigidity, postural instability (late presentation).
- ▶ Absence of a secondary cause.
- ▶ At least three supportive criteria: unilateral onset, progressive, resting tremor, persistent asymmetry affecting side of onset most, excellent reponse (70–100%) to levodopa, severe levodopa-induced chorea, levodopa response for ≥5 years, or clinical course of ≥10 years.

▶ General Considerations

Parkinson's disease (PD) is the second most common progressive neurodegenerative disorder after Alzheimer's disease but remains the only neurodegenerative disease for which symptoms can be effectively controlled medically. It affects 1% of the global population aged 65 years and may double in 2030 with aging of the population. Numerous hypotheses have been explored to explain the process of the neurodegeneration, such as the effects of environment, genetics, or inflammatory processes, or defects in mitochondrial function, or oxidative stress, but without a definitive conclusion. Aging is the greatest risk factor associated with PD. Approximately 95% of PD cases are idiopathic/sporadic and occur in people aged >50 years. The incidence of PD is 1.5–2 times higher in males. Other risk factors include head trauma and exposure to pesticides or herbicides in association with rural living or exposure to well water. Five genes, including the best studied leucine-rich repeat kinase 2 (LRRK2, autosomal-dominant) and parkin (autosomal-recessive), may be the cause of 2–3% of PD. New genetic foci have been identified or investigated. An individual may have a doubled risk if there is a family history in a first-degree relative.

▶ Pathogenesis

More recent studies of functional brain imaging in PD and other MDs have identified, circuit disorders in PD, including increased metabolic activity in the putamen/globus pallidus, thalamus, pons, cerebellum, and sensorimotor cortex, with relatively reduced premotor and parietal association cortex activity. PD results from the loss of dopaminergic projection neurons and axons in the substantia nigra (SN) and striatum. It is a progressive and degenerative process. Patients will become symptomatic when ~30% of DAergic SN neurons or 50–60% of their axon terminals are impaired or dead

Table 44-1. Classification of movement disorders.

Hypokinetic Disorders	Hyperkinetic Disorders
Parkinson's disease (idiopathic)	Tremor
Secondary parkinsonism:	Tics (Tourette's syndrome)
Drug-induced parkinsonism	Chorea (Huntington's disease)
Vascular parkinsonism	Myoclonus
Normal pressure hydrocephalus	Dystonia/athetosis
(NPH)	Ataxia
Other: infections, toxins,	Akathisia (almost always affects
metabolic disorders	the legs)
Parkinson-plus syndromes	Hemiballismus
DLB	Stereotype
PSP	Restless legs syndrome
MSA (Shy-Drager, OPCA, SND)	Dyskinesia
CBGD	Gait disorders

CBGD, corticobasal ganglionic degeneration; DLB, dementia with Lewy bodies; MSA, multisystem atrophy; OPCA, olivopontocerebellar atrophy; PSP, progressive supranuclear palsy; SND, striatonigral degeneration.

and there is a 20–50% dopamine decrease in the striatum. One side of the SN is usually more severely affected than the other, which results in more prominent symptoms on one side of the body. The treatment of PD aims at supplementation of levodopa (L-dopa), or decreased metabolism/degradation of dopamine. Neuroprotection of the dopaminergic neurons in SN is still under investigation.

Lewy bodies, typical α-synuclein (αSyn) immunoreactive intracytoplasmic eosinophilic inclusions in neurons, are a neuropathologic hallmark of PD. PD may also involve other CNS, peripheral, and enteric nervous systems, with Lewy bodies located in the olfactory nucleus, amygdala, brainstem, neocortex, vagal nerve nucleus, and the sympathetic nervous system. αSyn is also found in the intramural enteric nervous system, skin, retina, submandibular gland, cardiac nervous system, and other visceral organ nervous systems. Lewy bodies are also associated with Alzheimer's disease, Down syndrome, and other neurologic diseases.

▶ **Clinical Findings**

A. Symptoms and Signs

The diagnosis of PD is based on its characteristic cardinal motor manifestations, not by infections or primary visual, vestibular, cerebellar, proprioceptive, or other neurodegenerative disorders. The patients' excellent and sustained response to dopaminergic treatment supports the diagnosis. The most common initial finding is an asymmetric resting tremor in an upper extremity. The cardinal signs may eventually become bilateral after several years but will remain more prominent on one side of the body. Early referral to PD

specialists is crucial when a patient has atypical or secondary parkinsonism.

1. Cardinal motor signs—Resting tremors are the presenting symptoms in 50–70% of patients, with hands, fingers, forearms, and feet most frequently affected. The tremors are a characteristic oscillating or pill-rolling movement of one hand at a regular rhythm (4–6 Hz). They diminish during sleep and voluntary movement. Other parts of the body such as the jaw or face may also be affected. *Bradykinesia* refers to slow movement, the initiation of movement, or the sudden stopping of movement. Patients may make short, shuffling steps with a decreased arm swing or manifest an expressionless masklike face, freezing gait, or difficulty turning in bed. They cannot perform rapid repetitive movements, such as tapping the fingers or heels repeatedly. Rigidity or increased muscle tone in the affected limb manifests as a "lead pipe" with continuous resistance or "cogwheel type" movement with passive flexion or extension of the elbow. Patients with PD may experience impaired balance and postural reflexes when standing, known as *postural instability*, which will increase the risk of falls. Other clinical presentations include hypophonia, difficulty swallowing, muscle spasm, and micrographia.

2. Nonmotor symptoms—PD is no longer considered a pure motor disorder. The nonmotor symptoms may begin subtly, long before the motor signs start. They affect patients' emotional, cognitive, behavioral, and general health. Recognizing these premotor symptoms may aid in the early diagnosis of PD, so preventive measures and treatment can be started early to achieve more favorable results. The major nonmotor/premotor features are listed in **Table 44-2**. The significance of these nonmotor features in early diagnosis of PD requires further investigation.

Olfactory impairment precedes motor features of PD by many years in most patients with PD. Olfactory testing should be considered in order to differentiate PD from progressive supranuclear palsy and corticobasal degeneration. It is not currently recommended for diagnosing PD. It is not specific, but may be used to identify people either at risk for developing PD or in a presymptomatic stage of PD.

3. Cognitive and psychiatric symptoms—Dementia may affect a third of patients in late PD. Lewy body deposition is associated with dementia in PD. It can be a result of medications with anticholinergic property, or other medical conditions that can affect patients' mental status, such as infection, dehydration, or intracranial bleeding. Once detected, it should be treated with rivastigmine or donepezil because of their small but significant effect on the improvement in cognitive scales and activities of daily living. Polypharmacy should be assessed and avoided. A withdrawal of anticholinergic medications, including amantadine, dopamine

Table 44-2. Nonmotor/premotor symptoms of Parkinson disease.

Clinical Areas Involved	Clinical Features and Potential Complications
Hyposmia	Impairment of odor detection, identification, and discrimination (90% of cases)
Dysautonomia	Orthostatic hypotension, hyperhidrosis GU: neurogenetic bladder urgency, frequency and nocturia, erectile dysfunction and anorgasmia GI: gastroparesis, constipation (60–80%), diarrhea
Cognitive symptoms	Frontal executive dysfunction Dementia
Sleep	Insomnia Reduced REM sleep Excessive daytime sleepiness RLS/PLMS (30–80%)
Neurologic symptoms	Impaired color discrimination, pain (50%), paresthesias (40%) Fatigue Speech and voice disorders (89%) Nocturnal akinesia
Psychiatric disorders	Stress from the illness Anxiety Depression (50%) Psychosis (20–40%) Hallucinations

PLMS, periodic limb movement disorder; RLS, restless leg syndrome.

agonists, and MAO-B inhibitors, may be needed. Major depression is seen in ~17% and milder depression in another ~35% of PD patients. The somatic and cognitive symptoms in PD, such as psychomotor retardation, or anhedonia resulting from inability to perform usual activities, overlap with that of depression, which makes it difficult to diagnose. The Hamilton Depression Rating Scale (Ham-D) or the Montgomery-Asberg Depression Rating Scale (MADRS) should be used in conjunction with a structured patient interview in all circumstances to eliminate DSM exclusion criterion.

Psychosis occurs late (10 years after the diagnosis) in the disease process. These symptoms are often the side effects of antiparkinsonian medications. Both dopaminergic and dopamine receptor agonists pose a higher risk for psychosis, which is independent of dosage and treatment duration. Other underlying disease processes, for example, dementia, advanced age, depression, insomnia, and preexisting psychiatric conditions (which usually occur early in PD), are also risk factors for psychosis. Visual hallucinations are the most common clinical manifestation. Auditory hallucinations are less frequent and typically occur concomitantly with visual hallucinations. Vivid dreaming, illusions, or delusions may also occur. Quetiapine and clozapine are effective in treating psychotic symptoms in PD.

B. Laboratory Findings

Genetic tests should be considered in patients with a family history or early onset of PD before age 40 years.

C. Imaging Studies

Researchers have been trying to identify changes in brain structural and functional imaging studies to assist PD diagnosis, especially in the premotor stage. Early diagnosis is critical in redefining the importance of neuroprotective treatment. Routine use of imaging studies is currently not recommended for PD diagnosis.

The dopamine transporter ligand ioflupane with single-photon emission computed tomography scanning, (123) I-FP-CIT SPECT, was approved by the FDA in 2011 for use in differentiating PD from essential tremor and for evaluating parkinsonian syndromes. It cannot differentiate PD from secondary etiologies of parkinsonism.

Both CT and MRI can be ordered for atypical clinical presentations to rule out other intracranial pathologic processes; examples are midbrain atrophy in possible progressive supranuclear palsy, cerebellar/brainstem atrophy/gliosis in possible multisystem atrophy (MSA), normal-pressure hydrocephalus (NPH), and vascular or other causes of parkinsonism. MRI measurement of iron deposition transcranial sonography (TCS) can differentiate PD from progressive supranuclear palsy and MSA by detecting hyperechogenicity of the substantia nigra.

▶ **Differential Diagnosis**

It is important to differentiate PD from other parkinsonian syndromes (see Table 44-1) in order to produce a favorable response to antiparkinsonian treatment. An imaging study of the brain is usually required to rule out other parkinsonian syndromes if a patient has an atypical presentation, such as being unresponsive to levodopa, early falls in the disease course, symmetric signs without tremor, rapid disease process, and early dysautonomia. Patients with secondary parkinsonism may have a positive medication or medical history. Parkinson-plus syndromes related to underlying neurodegenerative conditions are relatively uncommon and have characteristic clinical presentations and different neurologic imaging findings. Progressive supranuclear palsy is the most common Parkinson-plus syndrome. It is characterized by a downward-gaze palsy, minimal tremor, and severe postural instability with frequent falls starting during the first year of the disease process. Corticobasal ganglionic degeneration (CBGD) demonstrates asymmetric symptoms but also severe limb apraxia and dystonia.

▶ Complications

Both motor and nonmotor clinical features of PD cause progressive disability that interferes with daily activities in all age groups and at all stages of the illness. The frequent reasons for hospitalization include motor disturbances, reduced mobility, lack of adherence to treatment, inappropriate use, falls, fractures, and pneumonia. Other potential complications of PD include weight loss, malnutrition and risk of aspiration, cognitive deterioration and depression, problem with speech, worsening of vision, and loss of smell. The risk of osteoporosis may double in PD. Table 44-2 lists common nonmotor symptoms and complications.

Motor complications, dyskinesias, and motor fluctuations usually start 4–6 years after initiation of treatment. They are assumed to be induced by pulsatile plasma levodopa levels. Dyskinesias are involuntary movements that can present as choreiform movements, dystonia, and myoclonus. Patients with motor fluctuations may experience a sudden loss of levodopa effects and switch from an "on" symptom-controlled period to an "off" symptomatic period, an end-dose "wearing-off" effect, and "freezing" during "on" periods.

▶ Treatment

Treatment of PD is aimed at cardinal symptom control, disease process modification, nonmotor manifestation treatment, and management of motor and nonmotor complications in late stages of PD. Although no treatment has been shown conclusively to slow down progression of the disease, several pharmacologic and surgical therapies are available to control patients' symptoms.

The goals of treatment vary depending on the disease stage. In early PD, treatment goals are to modify the disease process, delay and control motor symptoms, and maintain patients' independent functions; in more advanced PD, the goals are to maximize medication effectiveness, manage motor complications from levodopa, and control complications due to PD progression. Nonmotor symptom treatment should be started early and monitored throughout the disease process.

A. Pharmacotherapy

When to start PD therapy is a collaborative decision relying on effective communication between the physician, patient, and family. A variety of factors will be considered, such as the degree of impairment and its effect on the patient's daily life and employment, the patient's understanding of PD, and the patient's attitude toward medications. The traditional wait and watch approach, to start treatment when the patient begins to experience functional impairment, has been challenged.

1. Motor symptom therapy—Levodopa with a dopa decarboxylase inhibitor (DDI) is the most effective medication for PD symptom control and has a more favorable safety profile compared with other regimens, especially in older patients. However, the motor complications, such as dyskinesia, motor fluctuation, or hypertonia, appearing several years after initiation of levodopa, can compromise its effects and limit its long-term use.

Strategies to extend levodopa treatment and minimize motor complications have been explored, such as continuous administration of intravenous levodopa or administration via duodenal infusion (effective but not clinically applicable). Sustained-release levodopa has not been shown to decrease motor complications. Adding a catechol-O-methyltransferase (COMT) inhibitor to levodopa reduces "off" periods by limiting dopamine metabolism and prolonging levodopa half-life. Domperidone can be used for nausea and vomiting, which are common side effects of levodopa. There is no sufficient evidence to support the concerns of neurotoxicity from chronic use of L-dopa *in vivo* and postmortem studies. The fear of the side effects and motor complications may delay the use of levodopa and result in undertreatment of PD, but alternative medications may be used as first-line treatment to reduce dyskinesias.

Dopamine agonists (DAs) are used by many physicians as the first monotherapy to control PD motor symptoms, especially in younger patients. DAs have shown significant improvement in the Unified Parkinson Disease Rating Scale (UPDRS) in early PD with fewer motor side effects, but their other side effects (**Tables 44-3–44-5**) have limited its use especially in those aged > 65 years or those with alcohol, OCD, or mood disorders. Together with levodopa, they increase dopamine levels in the brain and reduce motor fluctuation. Compared with bromocriptine, levodopa has a demonstrated advantage in motor function, disability scores, and physical dysfunction, but may have no significant difference in mortality, dyskinesias, motor fluctuations, and dementia. Ergoline DAs, including bromocriptine, pergolide, lisuride, and cabergoline, are almost never used now because they are associated with moderate to severe cardiac valvulopathy, and pleural, pericardial, and retroperitoneal serosal fibrosis.

Early use of the irreversible monoamine oxidase (MAO-B) inhibitors has shown effectiveness in some clinical trials in controlling motor symptoms, and providing disease-modifying, levodopa-sparing relief when used simultaneously with a dopamine agonist, and less functional decline. MAO-B inhibitors, alone or together with a dopamine agonist, are preferred by some physicians to initiate PD treatment, but they have demonstrated conflicting effectiveness on motor fluctuation. Table 44-5 lists the common antiparkinsonian medications.

Pergolide was withdrawn from the market in 2007 because of its potential serious side effect of heart valve damage. The rotigotine patch was recalled in the United States

Table 44-3. Medications based on PD stages

PD Stages	Medications	Evidence[a]
Early PD with motor symptoms		
	Levodopa with a dopa decarboxylase inhibitor	A
	Oral/transdermal dopamine agonists	A
	Monoamine Oxidase B inhibitors	A
Advanced PD motor complications		
	Dopamine agonists, preferably nonergot	A
	MOBI	A
Medications may be considered to decrease "off" time		
	COMTI COMT inhibitors	A
	Apomorphine, intermittent, subcutaneous	A
Drugs should not be used as first line treatment		
	Anticholinergics	B
	Ergot-derived dopamine agonists	B

[a]Level of evidence: **A**—at least one high-quality meta-analysis, systematic review of RCTs, or RCT with a very low risk of bias and directly applicable to the target population; **B**—high-quality systematic reviews of case-control or cohort studies, and high-quality case-control or cohort studies with a very low risk of confounding or bias and a high probability that the relation is causal and that the reviews are directly applicable to the target population and with overall consistency of results; **C**—well-conducted case-control or cohort studies with a low risk of confounding or bias and a moderate probability that the relation is causal and that the studies are directly applicable to the target population and with overall consistency of results; **D**—nonanalytic studies: case reports, case series, or expert analysis.

in April 2008 secondary to the formation of rotigotine crystals, which decrease the delivery and thus the efficacy of the medication.

2. Neuroprotective/disease-modifying therapy—Neuroprotective treatment should be the final goal of PD treatment. Ideally, it should be started as soon as the diagnosis of

Table 44-4 Management of motor complications.

Levodopa treatment-associated motor complications	Strategies in general: 1. Dosage adjustment 2. More invasive treatments: apomorphine infusion and intraduodenal levodopa 3. Neurosurgery: DBS 4. Withdrawal of drugs
End of dose wearing off	Add COMT inhibitors
Dyskinesias	Amantadine
Motor fluctuations on/off	1. Add MAO-B inhibitors: "on" and "off" 2. DAs: reduce "off" time; nonergot preferred 3. COMT inhibitors: reduce "off" time

PD has been made or even before the nonmotor or premotor symptoms are identified. The insidious onset and wide variety of possible etiologies renders PD difficult to identify and prevent. There is insufficient evidence to support the neuroprotective or modifying effects of the MAO-B inhibitors selegiline and rasagiline. There is little or no evidence to substantiate the disease-modifying effects of vitamins, anti-inflammatory medications, nutritional supplements, or CoQ10. How to identify at-risk patients and diagnose PD early to start preventive or protective treatment, which is under investigation, also needs to be addressed.

3. Nonmotor symptom therapy—Medications and other management methods are chosen based on each specific symptom or problem, such as SSRI antidepressants for depression and baclofen for pain and spasm control. For patients with cognitive impairment, antiparkinsonian medications such as anticholinergics, dopamine agonists, amantadine, and selegiline may need to be decreased or discontinued. Cholinesterase inhibitors may be considered for dementia and fludrocortisone or midodrine for orthostatic hypotension. Sleep disturbance may improve with adjusting levodopa dosage, discontinuing nighttime use of antiparkinsonian drugs, discontinuing dopamine agonists, or starting clonazepam. Methylphenidate may help improve gait and decrease the risk of falls.

The first step in controlling psychosis is to decrease the dosage of antiparkinsonian medication or gradually remove some medications in the order of anticholinergics, selegiline, amantadine, dopamine receptor agonists, COMT, and finally, levodopa (switch to short-acting). Antipsychotic agents are considered if the patient still has symptoms. The atypical antipsychotic agents clozapine and quetiapine have fewer extrapyramidal and prolactin-elevating adverse effects. Other second-generation antipsychotic medications, such as ziprasidone, risperidone, and olanzapine, and the third-generation antipsychotic aripiprazole are not recommended because they may be not as effective or may have worse extrapyramidal adverse effects. Cholinesterase inhibitors (except rivastigmine), such as donepezil, galantamine, and tacrine, have shown inconsistent results and may worsen PD or have other side effects. Electroconvulsive therapy (ECT) should be used as a last resort for psychiatric disorders or depression when medications are not effective. By stimulating the D_3 dopamine receptors in the mesolimbic pathways, ropinirole has been shown to control motor symptoms and mood fluctuation, including depression and anxiety in patients with motor fluctuations.

B. Surgical Intervention

Surgery is an effective treatment option in more advanced PD. Subthalamic nucleus (STN) deep-brain stimulation (DBS) is effective in improving motor function and alleviating motor complications. It is reserved for motor complications from levodopa treatment. Potential neurorestoration

Table 44-5. Pharmacotherapy for Parkinson disease.

Class/Drug	Usual Daily Dosage	Clinical Use and Side Effects
Dopaminergic drugs Precursor amino acid: Levodopa		Nausea and vomiting, dyskinesia, motor fluctuations, somnolence, ICDs and DDS, psychosis, hypotension, peripheral edema, melanoma, weight loss
Carbidopa/levodopa (Sinemet)	10/100, 25/100, 25/250, 200/2000 mg/d TID	Increase by one tablet every day or every other day to a maximum of eight tablets per day
Controlled release (Sinemet CR)	25/100, 50/200, 200–1400 mg/d BID	Increase by one tablet every 3 days to a maximum of eight tablets per day
Carbidopa/levodopa/entacapone (Stalevo)	12.5/50/200 mg BID	Used when other medications become less effective; increase slowly to a maximum of eight tablets per day
Dopamine agonists		Excessive somnolence (caution with driving), ICDs, hallucinations, orthostatic hypotension, edema, vomiting, dizziness, confusion; higher risk in older patients
Bromocriptine	Initially, 1.25 mg BID 100 mg/d maximum	Adjust every 2–4 weeks; ergot dopamine agonist (see text for detailed side effects).
Pramipexole	0.125 mg TID	Adjust every week ≤1.5 mg TID
Ropinirole	Initially, 0.25 mg TID or once daily 3–24 mg/d	Adjust every week as needed
Apomorphine	2–6 mg/d SC approved in the United States	For rescue therapy for "off" episodes; nausea (requires trimethobenzamide initially), hypotension
Rotigotine	1–8 mg/24 hours transdermal	
Monamine oxidase B (MAO–B) Inhibitor		Sleep disturbance, lightheadedness, nausea, abdominal pain, confusion, hallucinations; avoid tyramine–containing food, such as aged cheese, sausages, salamis, or soy sauce (cause uncontrolled hypertension); be aware of drug interactions; no dose titration required; possibly neuroprotective
Selegiline	1.25–2.5 mg daily (PO or rapidly dissolving in mouth)	
Rasagiline	0.5–1 mg/d	
N–Methyl–D–aspartate (NMDA) receptor inhibitor Amantadine	100–300 mg/d	Hallucinations, dry mouth, livedo reticularis, ankle swelling, myoclonic encephalopathy in setting of renal failure; avoid in cognitive impairment Insufficient evidence in treatment of early PD
Catechol–O–methyl transferase (COMT) inhibitors		Effective only with levodopa; worsening of levodopa–induced dyskinesias, diarrhea, nausea, vivid dreams, visual hallucinations, sleep disturbances, daytime drowsiness, headache
Tolcapone	100 or 200 mg TID	Hepatotoxicity; strict licensing criteria; blood level monitoring needed
Entacapone	200 mg, 2–8 times per day with each dose of carbidopa/levodopa	No hepatotoxicity.
Anticholinergics Trihexyphenidyl Biperidine	2–15 mg/d 1–8 mg/d	Limited use for significant neuropsychiatric and cognitive adverse effects Confusion, sleepiness, blurred vision, constipatio. May worsen motor symptoms on discontinuation; tapering needed

BID, twice daily; DDS, dopamine dysregulation syndrome; ICD, impulse control disorder; TID, 3 times daily.

with dopaminergic or stem cell replacement may also bring hope in controlling dopamine deficiency–related disabilities. Other options such as thalamotomy and pallidotomy are effective in controlling motor complications but can cause destructive lesions.

C. Ancillary Treatment and Supportive Measures

Psychological counseling and therapy, such as cognitive-behavioral therapy, supportive therapy, and coping skill development, may help patients with psychiatric manifestations.

Supportive treatment is important in terms of maintaining function and general health. It includes allied health interventions; occupational therapy; physical therapy; and speech, swallowing, and voice therapy. Physical exercise is a very important component in PD treatment. It can improve PD patients' motor performance as well as their learning, memory, and mental health. It may repair or reverse the neurochemical damage through facilitating synaptogenesis and neurotrophy. To provide support to the family and caregivers is also crucial. Information regarding PD and other resources should be provided to caregivers. Patients and their families can be referred to various support groups, including the American Parkinson Disease Association (http://www.apdaparkinson.com), the National Parkinson Foundation (http://www.parkinson.org), and the Michael J. Fox Foundation for Parkinson Research (http://www.michaeljfox.com). Other websites providing PD information include the Worldwide Education and Awareness for Movement Disorder (http://www.wemove.org/) and the Movement Disorder Society (http://www.movementdisorders.org/).

Prevention

The role of hormones (ie, estrogen, testosterone, or growth hormone) in neuroprotection has been under investigation with uncertain clinical value. Haaxma et al. (2007) reported that estrogen may play a role in the lower prevalence of PD, delayed and milder symptoms, and slower progression of PD in females. Some potential protective factor have been identified in some studies, such as caffeine and smoking. Smoking, however, is not an option, for obvious reasons. Nonsteroidal anti-inflammatory drugs (NSAIDs) may have a potential role in preventing the neuroinflammatory destruction of dopaminergic neurons and decreasing the risk of PD development.

Prognosis and Disease Process Monitoring

Parkinson disease is a chronic and progressive disease with a mean survival of >10 years. Older age at onset and the presence of rigidity or hypokinesia as initial symptoms predict a more rapid rate of motor progression, as do other associated morbidities such as stroke, auditory deficits, visual impairments, gait disturbances, and male sex.

Caring for PD patients involves a long-term assessment of disease progress and monitoring for the effects and adverse effects of treatment in order to modify the management plan as needed. Clinical rating scales can be used to evaluate the patients' function, satisfaction, and severity of motor and non-motor symptoms. The Unified Parkinson Disease Rating Scale (UPDRS) is widely used and contains six sections to assess mood and cognition; activities of daily living in both "on" and "off" states; motor abilities; complications of therapy; disease severity; and global function, including level of disability, mood, and both disease- and treatment-related manifestations of PD. Other monitoring/evaluating instruments include the Parkinson Psychosis Rating Scale (PPRS), Mini-Mental State Examination (MMSE), and the Parkinson Disease Quality of Life questionnaire (PDQL), to name only a few.

Dorsey ER, et al. Projected number of people with Parkinson disease in the most populous nations, 2005 through 2030. *Neurology*. 2007;68:384–386. [PMID: 17082464]

Haaxma CA, et al. Gender differences in Parkinson's disease. *J Neurol Neurosurg Psychiatr*. 2007;78:819–824. [PMID: 17098842]

Hughes AJ, Daniel SE, Kilford L, Lees AJ. Accuracy of clinical diagnosis of idiopathic Parkinson's disease. A clinicopathological study of 100 cases. *J Neurol Neurosurg Psychiatr*. 1992;55:181–184.

Jankovic J, et al. Therapies in Parkinson's disease. *Curr Opin Neurol*. 2012; 25:433–447.

Jellinger KA. Neuropathology of sporadic Parkinson's disease. *Movement Dis*. 2012; 27(1).

Malaty IA, et al. Neuroendocrinologic considerations in Parkinson disease and other movement disorders. *Neuroendocrinology* 2009; 15(2; Continuum issue):125–147.

Scottish Intercollegiate Guidelines Network. *Diagnosis and Pharmacological Management of Parkinson'sDdisease* (a national clinical guideline; available at www.sign.ac.uk; published Jan.2010).

Shtilbans A, et al. Biomarkers in Parkinson's disease: an update. *Curr Opin Neurol*. 2012; 25:460–465.

We Move Website (available at http://www.wemove.org/; accessed June 30, 2009).

Whitton PS. Inflammation as a causative factor in the aetiology of Parkinson's disease. *Br J Pharmacol*. 2007;150:963–976. [PMID: 17339843]

TREMOR

Tremor is a rhythmic oscillation of one part of the body from regular contractions of reciprocally innervated antagonistic muscles. It is the most common movement disorder. Tremor can occur at rest, when body parts are held in a fixed posture (postural), or during certain actions (intentional). **Table 44-6** lists different types of tremor due to different physiologic or pathologic etiologies.

ESSENTIAL TREMOR

 ESSENTIALS OF DIAGNOSIS

► Core criteria:
  ►Postural or kinetic tremor of the hands and forearms or at least one arm.
  ►Head tremor with no signs of dystonia.
  ►Absence of other etiologic factors and neurologic signs: medications, alcohol, parkinsonism, dystonia, hyperthyroidism.

► Additional diagnostic criteria (not consistently applied):
  ►Bilateral.
  ►Duration (>1 year to longstanding).
  ►Severity (interferes with activities of daily living, handwriting, vocalization).
  ►Positive family history.
  ►Beneficial effect of alcohol.

Table 44-6. Classification of tremors.

Category	Tremor Characteristics	Medical Conditions
Action tremor		
Postural tremor	Occurs when a body part (limb) is maintaining a posture against the force of gravity (4–12 Hz[a])	(Enhanced) physiologic tremor (most common tremor) Essential tremor (second most common) Orthostatic tremor Writing tremor Musician's tremor Psychogenic tremor Rubral tremor Neuropathic tremor Dystonic tremor
Kinetic: Simple kinetic tremor	Occurs with voluntary but non-target-directed movement of extremities (eg, pronation-supination or flexion-extension wrist movement) (3–10 Hz)	Cerebellar and cerebellar outflow tract disease: eg, MS, trauma, stroke tumor, vascular, Wilson, drugs, toxins, rubral tremor
Intentional tremor Task-specific intention tremor	Occurs with target-directed movement (finger-to-nose) (5 Hz) Involves task-specific, skilled, highly learned motor acts (eg, writing, sewing, playing musical instruments) (5–7 Hz)	Primary writing tremor
Isometric tremor	Occurs with muscle contraction against a stationary object (eg, squeezing examiner's fingers) (4–6 Hz)	Musician's tremor
Resting tremor	Frequency: low to medium (3–6 Hz)	Parkinsonism (third most common) Rubral (midbrain) tremor Wilson disease Severe essential tremor
Miscellaneous		Myoclonus Convulsions Asterixis Fasciculation Clonus Psychogenic

[a]Hz, hertz; the number of tremor cycles per second.

General Considerations

Essential tremor (ET) is the most common movement disorder. It starts at a mean age of 45 years and affects ~4% of those aged > 40 years, and the prevalence increases with age. The prevalence of ET varies widely among studies because of different criteria used in making the diagnosis. It affects both males and females. ET is a chronic and slowly progressive disorder with both upper extremities most commonly affected. It is postural and kinetic in nature and can be disabling and affect the quality of life. Family aggregation is noted in more than half of the patients and seems to follow an autosomal dominant pattern of inheritance. Linkage of genes on chromosomes 3q13 (ETM1) and 2p24.1 (ETM2) to ET and their clinical significance need to be further investigated. Environmental factors such as β-carboline alkaloids, which include harmine and harmane, may also play a role in the development of ET.

Clinical Findings

A. Symptoms and Signs

Essential tremor is diagnosed on the basis of its clinical features compiled through a detailed medical history regarding tremor, family history, social history (alcohol, caffeine, and drug use), and medications (eg, β-agonists, corticosteroids, valproic acid, amphetamines, thyroid hormones, lithium, neuroleptic agents, tricyclic antidepressants), as well as a thorough physical examination. The tremor typically starts from either hands or forearms (~95%) or less commonly from one hand (usually dominant) in 10–15% of cases with upper extremity involvement as the initial presentation.

The tremor can be postural, occurring with outstretched arms, or kinetic, occurring during action such as finger-to-nose movement, pouring and drinking water from a cup, writing, or drawing Archimedean spirals. With more advanced age, the tremor will be slower but have greater amplitude, which can be more disabling. Other parts of the body can be affected in isolation or concomitantly with hand tremor, such as head (34%), legs (30%), voice (12%), chin, tongue, or trunk. The patient may present with head shaking (no-no) or nodding (yes-yes), a shaky or trembling voice, or an unsteady gait (eg, tandem gait disturbance). Ethanol reduces tremor in two-thirds of cases with prompt improvement within 15 minutes. Many tremor scales are available for assessing severity, for example, the tremor rating scale from the Washington Heights–Inwood Genetic Study of Essential Tremor (score 0–5) and the Fahn-Tolosa-Marin tremor rating scale (score 0–40). In **Table 44-7**, the classic phenomena of essential tremor are described and contrasted with features of tremor resulting from other physiologic and pathologic causes.

B. Laboratory and Other Tests

Routine laboratory tests such as thyroid function; liver function; electrolytes, including calcium, magnesium, and phosphorous; and blood glucose level may be ordered. Other lab tests or imaging studies should be ordered according to each clinical scenario. In patients whose tremor started before age 40 years, blood and urine should be checked to rule out Wilson disease. Physiologic studies such as electromyography and accelerometry are available in specialized labs. They are not part of the routine evaluation but can assist with atypical tremor diagnosis and measure tremor severity and its influence on patients by assessing frequency, rhythmicity, and amplitude of the tremor.

▶ Nonmotor Complications

Essential tremor is not as benign as once believed. It can cause substantial physical, cognitive, and psychosocial disability. Patients may lose or have to quit their jobs owing to

Table 44-7. Clinical and differential diagnosis of tremors.

Tremor	Clinical Features	Diagnostic Tests and Management
Essential tremor	An 8–12-Hz tremor is seen in young adults and a 6–8-Hz tremor in elderly people; there are negative neurologic signs with normal muscle tone and coordination, worsening with stress, fatigue, and voluntary movement; improves with alcohol ingestion	Only for differential diagnosis or atypical presentations
Enhanced physiologic tremor	High frequency, 10–12 Hz, lower amplitude; involves hands; occurs under various conditions, eg, stress, fatigue, hypoglycemia, thyroid and adrenal gland disorders, alcohol withdrawal, and medication use; no other neurologic signs; responsive to offending medication or toxin reduction or removal, treatment of endocrine disorders, and stress management	Chemistry profile (glucose, liver function tests); thyroid function tests; review of medications; propranolol prior to stressful events may help
Parkinsonism	Late age onset; asymmetric; slow (4–6 Hz), high amplitude, rest tremor biplanar; pill-rolling; possible action tremor; worse under stress, better with voluntary movement; unaffected by alcohol; onset in hands or legs; additional parkinsonian symptoms	See text
Cerebellar tremor	Intentional tremor on the ipsilateral side of the body; 3–4 Hz; positive ataxia; dysmetria; nystagmus; other cerebellar signs	Appropriate imaging and other tests
Orthostatic tremor	Occurs exclusively while standing (13–18 Hz); late onset; rare family history; tremor limited to legs and paraspinal muscles	Response to gabapentin, pramipexole, and clonazepam
Neuropathic tremor	Associated with peripheral nerve pathology, eg, hereditary neuropathies, Guillain-Barré syndrome, chronic inflammatory demyelinating polyneuropathy; not responsive to propranolol or other therapy	
Psychogenic tremor	Variable tremor; intermittent; somatization in past history; tremor changes with voluntary movement of contralateral limb	Electrophysiologic testing
Wilson disease	Postural or intentional, wing-beating tremor (4–6 Hz); ascites, jaundice, signs of hepatic disease; intracorneal ring-shaped pigmentation; rigidity, muscle spasms; mental symptoms	Liver function tests; serum ceruloplasmin; urine copper; slit-lamp examination for Kayser-Fleischer rings
Task-specific intention tremors	Involves skilled, highly learned motor acts, eg, writing, sewing, playing musical instrument (5–7 Hz)	Treatment: botulinum toxin injection; surgery effective; oral medicine less effective

the uncontrollable tremor and memory and other cognitive impairments. Activities of daily living, as simple as drinking and eating, are significantly affected. The impact of ET on the patient's physical, psychologic, and social health status needs to be assessed from the patient's point of view. The health-related quality-of-life (QoL) evaluation for ADL abilities is also essential to management.

Nonmotor, cognitive-neuropsychological presentations of ET also contribute to the patient's health status and may influence functional disability. Depression, anxiety, low vigor, mild executive dysfunction, possible mild cognitive impairment, and personality changes are some of the nonmotor manifestations of ET. Patients with late onset are more likely to have dementia. A disease-specific questionnaire, for example, the Quality of Life (QoL) in Essential Tremor Questionnaire, will assist in a comprehensive evaluation of ET to improve management and QoL.

▶ Treatment

The goal of ET treatment is to decrease functional disability and improve the patient's health status and QoL. Treatment may be initiated when symptoms are present. Both pharmacologic and surgical approaches are available. The response to medical treatment varies; some patients may not benefit from any medications or have only a partial response. Propranolol and primidone are recommended as initial therapy in ET, either alone or in combination (**Table 44-8**). More recent studies do not report sufficient evidence to support or refute the use of antipsychotics (clozapine and olanzapine), pregabalin, or zonisamide in ET. Levetiracetam and 3,4-diaminopyridine are not recommended for limb tremor in ET, based on 2001 evidence-based guideline update from the American Academy of Neurology. In medically refractory cases, deep-brain stimulation (DBS) of the thalamus and unilateral thalamotomy (level C) have shown moderate to marked improvement of tremor in most patients. DBS of the ventral intermediate (VIM) thalamic nucleus (level C) has fewer adverse events than thalamotomy and the flexibility for adjustment but is more expensive.

Physical or occupational therapy with lightweight training of wrists may help improve hand stability and function.

▶ Prognosis

Essential tremor is a slowly progressive disorder with a potential 7% increase in tremor amplitude each year. More than two-thirds of patients report significant changes in their daily living and socializing, and approximately 15% are seriously disabled, more notably men, in a longitudinal, prospective study. Complications secondary to difficulty in ambulating, falls, pneumonia, and other functional disabilities may have contributed to the increased mortality.

Louis ED. Essential tremor. *Clin Geriatr Med.* 2006; 22:843–857. [PMID: 17000339]

Louis ED, et al. A population-based study of mortality in essential tremor. *Neurology.* 2007; 69:1982–1989. [PMID: 18025392]

Louis ED, et al. Diagnostic criteria for essential tremor: a population perspective. *Arch Neurol.* 1998; 55:823–828. [PMID: 9626774]

Woods SP, et al. Executive dysfunction and neuropsychiatric symptoms predict lower health status in essential tremor. *Cogn Behav Neurol.* 2008; 21:28–33. [PMID: 18327020]

Zesiewicz TA, et al. Practice parameter: therapies for essential tremor: report of the Quality Standards Subcommittee of the American Academy of Neurology. *Neurology.* 2005;64:2008-2020. [PMID: 15972843]

Zesiewicz TA, et al. AAN evidence-based guideline update: treatment of essential tremor: report of the Quality Standards Subcommittee of the American Academy of Neurology, *Neurology.* 2011; 77:1752–1755.

Zesiewicz TA, et al. Practice parameter: therapies for essential tremor: report of the Quality Standards Subcommittee of the American Academy of Neurology. *Neurology.* 2005; 64:2009.

TIC DISORDERS: TOURETTE SYNDROME

 ESSENTIALS OF DIAGNOSIS

▶ Two or more motor tics and one or more vocal tics are present (not necessarily concurrent).

▶ The tics occur many times a day nearly every day over >1 year without a tic-free period of > 3 consecutive months.

▶ Disease onset before age 18 years.

▶ Other causes of tics ruled out (eg, substance uses, stimulants, Huntington disease, CNS infection, stroke).

▶ General Considerations

Tourette syndrome (TS) is a serious, chronic neuropsychiatric disorder. It affects 4–6 per 1000 children. The mean age of onset is ~5 years with males 4–5 times more than females. Both genetic (likely complex inheritance) and environmental factors (eg, stress, postinfection autoimmune disease, intrauterine exposure, fetal or neonatal hypoxia) play a role in the development of TS.

▶ Clinical Findings

A. Symptoms and Signs

Tics are sudden, brief (0.5–1-second), uncontrollable, repetitive, nonrhythmic, stereotyped, and purposeless movements (motor tics) or vocalizations (vocal tics). Tics can be either simple, such as blinking, grimacing, head jerking, shoulder

Table 44-8. Pharmacotherapy for essential tremor.

Class/Drug	Usual Daily Dosage	Clinical Use and Side Effects
β-Adrenergic blockers Propranolol (A[a])	60–800 mg/d (divided TID) Optimal: 160–320 mg/d Long-acting: 80–320 mg/d	50% improvement Well tolerated; titrate every 3–7 d Fatigue, mild to moderate bradycardia and reduced blood pressure, exertional dyspnea, depression
Atenolol (B[a])	50–150 mg/d	25–37% improvement
Sotalol (B[a])	75–200 mg/d	28% improvement
Anticonvulsants (GABA receptor) Primidone(A[a])	50–750 mg/d (divided TID)	50% improvement Tolerance may develop Sedation, fatigue, unsteadiness, vomiting, acute toxic reaction, ataxia, vertigo
Gabapentin(B[a])	1200–1800 mg/d	33–77% improvement Drowsiness, nausea, dizziness, unsteadiness
Topiramate (B[a])	Maximum 400 mg/d	22–37% improvement Dizziness, ataxia, somnolence, depression, nausea, weight loss, paresthesia
Benzodiazepines (GABA receptor)		Sedation and cognitive slowing; potential for abuse
Alprazolam(B[a])	0.125–3 mg/d	25–35% improvement
Clonazepam(C[a])	0.5–6 mg/d	Efficacy varies; 26–71% improvement Withdrawal following abrupt discontinuance
Botulinum toxin injection (C[a])		Produces focal weakness; reduces tremor effectively but may not improve function; postinjection pain
For hand tremor	50–100 units per arm	20–27% improvement
For head tremor	40–400 units	Significant clinical improvement but no statistical significance
For voice tremor	0.6–15 units (uni- or bilateral)	22–30% improvement Difficulty swallowing

[a]*Level of evidence:* A—at least one high-quality meta-analysis, systematic review of RCTs, or RCT with a very low risk of bias and directly applicable to the target population; B—high-quality systematic reviews of case-control or cohort studies, and high-quality case-control or cohort studies with a very low risk of confounding or bias and a high probability that the relation is causal and that the studies are directly applicable to the target population and with overall consistency of results; C—well-conducted case-control or cohort studies with a low risk of confounding or bias and a moderate probability that the relation is causal and that the studies are directly applicable to the target population and with overall consistency of results; D—nonanalytic studies: case reports, case series, or expert analysis.

shrugging, and throat clearing, or other meaningless utterances/noises, or more coordinated and purposeful complex features, such as jumping, kicking, abdomen thrusting, stuttering, echolalia (involuntary repetition of other people's words), echopraxia (imitating others' gestures), and coprolalia (speaking obscenities). Ninety percent of patients with TS have premonitory sensations, or unpleasant somatosensory urges (burning, tingling, itching, or pain) preceding tics. They are relieved by the execution of tics. Tics typically start early, at 3–5 years of age, and peak around 9–12 years; the severity improves at the end of adolescence. Simple and transient tics are common in children, with 6–20% affected.

Tics are the only positive findings on neurologic examination in TS. They usually start in the upper body, especially the eyes or other parts of the face, in the form of simple motor or vocal tics. As TS gradually progresses, the tics can involve other parts of the body such as the extremities and torso, where they will become complex in nature and vary in type and combination, severity, and location. The phenotype of TS involves not only tics but also behavioral components and commonly associated comorbidities (**Table 44-9**). Frustrated or embarrassed by the involuntary and sometimes disabling tics, together with the misconception of family and others that tics can be controlled, patients may develop anxiety, depression, or even social withdrawal, which impairs academic and social performance. Comorbid conditions include obsessions such as repeatedly counting, hand washing, or touching, and the need to scratch out

Table 44-9. Tourette syndrome phenotype and comorbidities.

Tic Component	Simple or Complex Features
Socially inappropriate behaviors	Coprophenomena (coprolalia, mental coprolalia, copropraxia) Echophenomena (echolalia, echopraxia) Paliphenomena (palilalia, palipraxia) spitting, hitting and kicking, self-injury
Compulsive behaviors	Forced touching, repetitive looking at objects, other ritualized behaviors
Comorbidities	ADHD (60%[a]) OCD (50%[a]) Depression Anxiety Learning disability (20%[a]) Problems with executive planning, organization, and social problem solving

[a]Percentage of the comorbidity in patients diagnosed with TS. ADHD, attention deficit hyperactivity behaviour; OCD, obsessive-compulsive disorder.

a word. A comprehensive physiopsychosocial evaluation (eg, Yale Global Tic Severity Scale, Global Assessment of Functioning, Health-Related Quality of Life Scale, Child Behaviour Checklist, or Youth Self-Report) is necessary for children with tics. Comorbid ADHD may impact cognitive performance. A neuropsychological assessment may be considered. Coping strategies for the patient, family, and teachers need to be explored.

B. Laboratory and Other Test Findings

Tourette syndrome is a clinical diagnosis based on a thorough personal and family history, physical examination, and close observation of the disease process. Laboratory tests, EEG, and brain imaging studies (CT, MRI, or PET) may be considered to rule out infections or other neurologic conditions that can either cause tics or mimic tics.

Differential Diagnosis

Other medical conditions that may cause tics or be misdiagnosed as tics need to be ruled out before starting treatment. Tics may be mistaken for other hyperkinetic movement disorders such as chorea, myoclonus, dystonia, tardive dyskinesia, seizure, periodic limb movements of sleep, and restless leg syndrome. Tics can also be caused by other medical conditions such as stroke, infections, dystonia, essential tremor, and dementia.

Treatment

The goal of TS treatment is to control disabling symptoms and comorbidities; improve academic, occupational, or social performance and quality of life; and support patient and family. It is important to prioritize treatment to the most bothersome symptoms and to achieve symptom control to the level at which the patient can function. Patients and families need to realize that complete resolution of symptoms is difficult to achieve. TS with mild symptoms that do not interfere with the patient's daily functioning can be followed clinically without medical treatment.

A. Medical Treatment

α_2-Agonists are the current first-line treatment (see **Table 44-10** for these and other treatment recommendations). They may help reduce tics by ~30% and can improve comorbid ADHD symptoms. They are preferred to antipsychotics because they do not cause tardive dyskinesia or weight gain. Neuroleptics (haloperidol, pimozide, fluphenazine, and risperione) are the most effective in treating TS, but are usually reserved as second-line medications for moderate to severe TS because of their side effects, including weight gain and diabetes. They can reduce the severity of tics by 25–50%. Acute dystonic reactions may occur with initiation of these agents. Anticholinergics can be added to decrease their risk. Tardive dyskinesia may develop during neuroleptic treatment and is not always reversible after treatment is discontinued. Pergolide, tetrabenazine, and topiramate are also effective in decreasing tics. Stimulants or SSRIs may be started for attention deficit hyperactivity behaviour (ADHD), obsessive compulsive disorder (OCD), and other comorbidities.

B. Behavioral Therapy and Counseling

Habit reversal therapy through awareness training and competing response practice is as effective as antipsychotics and supportive therapy. Assertiveness training, cognitive therapy, relaxation therapy, and habit reversal therapy are widely used to improve patients' social functioning and the undesirable behaviors associated with tics. Education should be provided to the family and at school to create a supportive and understanding environment and decrease misconceptions and intolerance.

C. Other Therapies

Botulinum toxin injection and deep-brain stimulation are available for medically refractory tics.

Prognosis

Tics typically wax and wane, with the most severe tics occurring between 8 and 12 years of age. Many patients will experience significant improvement by the end of adolescence.

However, if tics persist into adulthood (20%), TS can cause severe behavioral and social dysfunction.

Bloch M, et al. Recent advances in Tourette syndrome. *Curr Opin Neurol.* 2011;24:119–125.

Cath DC, et al. European clinical guidelines for Tourette syndrome and other tic disorders. Part I: assessment. *Eur Child Adolesc Psychiatr.* 2011;20:155–171.

Kenney C, et al. Tourette's syndrome. *Am Fam Physician.* 2008;77:651–658, 659–660. [PMID: 18350763]

Robertson MM, et al. Principal components analysis of a large cohort with Tourette syndrome. *Br J Psychiatr.* 2008;193:31–36. [PMID: 18700215]

Roessner V, et al. European clinical guidelines for Tourette syndrome and other tic disorders. Part II: pharmacological treatment. *Eur Child Adolesc Psychiatr.* 2011; 20:173–196.

Websites

http://www.wemove.org
hppt://www.tsa-usa.org

RESTLESS LEGS SYNDROME (RLS)

 ESSENTIALS OF DIAGNOSIS

► Core criteria:
  ► An urge to move the legs, usually accompanied by uncomfortable and unpleasant sensations in the legs.
  ► The urge to move or unpleasant sensations beginning or worsening during periods of rest or inactivity such as lying down or sitting.
  ► The urge to move, or unpleasant sensations that are partially or totally relieved by movement, such as walking or stretching, as least as long as the activity continues.
  ► The urge to move or unpleasant sensations are worse or only occur in the evening or at night.
► Supportive features:
  ► Family history of RLS.
  ► Positive response to dopaminergic therapy.
  ► Occurrence of periodic leg movements (PLMs) in sleep (PLMS) or during wakefulness (PLMW).
► Additional diagnostic criteria for children aged 2–12 years:
  ► Children must express leg discomfort in their own words, for example, tickle, bugs, or feeling shaky.
  ► Have two of the following: sleep disturbance, parent with definite RLS, and elevated periodic limb movement index on polysomnography.

General Considerations

Restless leg syndrome (RLS) is a chronic neurologic movement disorder with a prevalence of 5–10% in the adult population; it affects approximately 2% of children aged 8–17 years. It affects 12 million people in the United States, with a 2:1 female predominance, and it is also more severe in females. Primary RLS is idiopathic and occurs sporadically, but it demonstrates a strong genetic component with familial inheritance (60%). Pathogenesis of RLS is related to low brain iron and may involve the subcortical dopaminergic system. Several genes for RLS have been identified. Secondary RLS can be associated with other medical conditions such as anemia, thyroid problems, diabetes, kidney failure, peripheral neuropathy, ADHD, fibromyalgia, rheumatoid arthritis, Sjögren's syndrome, cyanocobalamin deficiency, folic acid deficiency, and pregnancy. Medications that can aggravate RLS symptoms include antinausea drugs (prochlorperazine, metoclopramide), anticonvulsants (phenytoin, droperidol), antipsychotic drugs (haloperidol), tricyclic and SSRI antidepressants, and over-the-counter (OTC) cold and allergy medications.

Clinical Findings

A. Symptoms and Signs

Diagnosis of RLS is based on a detailed history, including symptoms, medications, family history, and a thorough neurologic evaluation. Its typical presentation includes unpleasant sensations due to paresthesias and dysesthesias (burning, itching, tingling, cramping, or aching) deep in the legs (calves), which subside only with voluntary movement of the legs. The sensation may present on only one side of the body and may move to another part of the body. The motor restlessness occurs with the urge to relieve the sensation, and the patient may move voluntarily with repetitive stereotypical movements such as pacing, rocking, and stretching. Patients with RLS usually have sleep disturbances, such as difficulty falling asleep or maintaining sleep, leg movement during sleep, and daytime fatigue. PLMS and PLMW are stereotyped, repetitive movements with dorsiflexion of the ankles or big toes. Abnormal physical findings and positive test results may be due to associated conditions in secondary RLS. Smoking, alcohol consumption, poor sleep hygiene, and fatigue may aggravate symptoms of RLS.

B. Laboratory and Other Test Findings

A complete blood count, ferritin iron level, electrolytes, glucose level, thyroid hormone, and kidney function should be ordered. PLMS can be assessed and monitored by the International Restless Leg Syndrome scale (IRLS). Polysomnography is not routinely ordered. It may be considered when the presentation is not diagnostic for RLS,

Table 44-10. Pharmacotherapy for Tourette syndrome.

Class/Drug	Usual Daily Dosage	Clinical Use and Adverse Effects
α-Agonists		First-line agents
Clonidine (oral, transdermal) (A[a])	0.05 mg at bedtime, increased by 0.05 mg every few days to a maximum of 0.2 mg TID Most patients respond to 1 tablet (0.1 mg) TID	Initial treatment of TS Sedation, orthostatic hypotension and constipation Withdrawal: taper over 7–10 d
Guanfacine	0.5 mg at bedtime; maximum 1 mg TID	Fewer side effects; well tolerated
Antipsychotics (dopamine receptor blockers)		Second-line agents; may be added to α-agonist or mono-therapy First-line agents: for patients with severe tics Acute dystonic reaction
Risperidone (A[a])	0.25 mg at bedtime; maximum 2 mg BID	Sedation and weight gain Less risk of tardive dyskinesia
Olanzapine (B[a])	1.25 mg at bedtime; maximum 5 mg BID	Similar to risperidone
Haloperidol (A[a])	0.25–2 mg/d	Used when atypical antipsychotics listed above are ineffective Tardive dyskinesia
Pimozide (A[a])	0.5 mg at bedtime; maximum 3 mg BID	Prolonged QTc interval, ventricular arrhythmia
Fluphenazine	0.5 mg at bedtime; maximum 3 mg TID	Safer than haloperidol; more controlled studies needed
Other drugs Baclofen Topiramate Lorazepam	5 mg daily; maximum 20 mg TID 25 mg at bedtime; maximum 200 mg daily 0.25 mg at bedtime; maximum 1 mg TID	Alternative to antipsychotics; safe and effective; weight loss

[a]*Level of evidence*: **A**—at least one high-quality meta-analysis, systematic review of RCTs, or RCT with a very low risk of bias and directly applicable to the target population; **B**—high-quality systematic reviews of case-control or cohort studies, and high-quality case-control or cohort studies with a very low risk of confounding or bias and a high probability that the relation is causal and that the studies are directly applicable to the target population and with overall consistency of results; **C**—well-conducted case-control or cohort studies with a low risk of confounding or bias and a moderate probability that the relation is causal and that the studies are directly applicable to the target population and with overall consistency of results; **D**—nonanalytic studies: case reports, case series, or expert analysis.

there is suboptimal response to treatment, or other nocturnal conditions such as sleep apnea are suspected.

Differential Diagnosis

Among the many medical conditions that need to be differentiated from RLS, polyneuropathy is the most commonly encountered. The sensory symptoms of polyneuropathy do not improve with movement, and there will be positive findings from the neurologic examination, nerve biopsy, and neurophysiologic examination. The differential diagnosis includes nocturnal leg cramps, obstructive sleep apnea syndrome, intermittent claudication, pathophysiologic insomnia, Tourette syndrome, and orthostatic tremor.

Treatment

The goal of RLS treatment is to minimize the unpleasant sensations and motor restlessness, reduce sleep disturbance, and improve quality of life.

A. Nonpharmacotherapy

Identify any conditions that may cause or aggravate RLS, such as offensive medications, smoking, and excessive alcohol consumption. Give iron supplementation when ferritin is low and vitamin supplementation. Monitor kidney function. A healthy lifestyle will help alleviate RLS with moderate daily exercise, leg movement and massage, and hot baths. Cognitive behavioral and exercise therapy are under investigation.

B. Pharmacotherapy

Medications should be started when patients are experiencing daily symptoms that are affecting their quality of life. The nonergot dopamine agonists (DAs) ropinirole and pramipexole are the medications of choice for primary RLS (high evidence). DAs are 70–90% effective in relieving symptoms. They can be administered 1–3 hours before the onset of symptoms, and their effect is immediate. Adverse effects include nausea, peripheral edema, daytime somnolence, and impulsivity. Levodopa (high evidence) is fast-acting and can be taken 1–2 hours before symptoms start. However, augmentation, worsening of RLS symptoms from ongoing treatment, may develop with long-term use or high doses (>200 mg) of dopaminergic medications, especially carbidopa/levodopa. It is recommended for treatment of intermittent RLS. Levodopa is less favored as an initial medication than DAs because of its motor side effect as well as the augmentation.

There is ample evidence that gabapentin enacarbil, the prodrug of gabapentin, is effective in RLS treatment. There is insufficient evidence to support the use of gabapentin, pregabalin, opioids, carbamazepine, and clonidine. Oral iron treatment may reduce RLS symptoms in patients with iron deficiency or refractory RLS (minimal evidence). Benzodiazepines are effective in improving sleep quality but not periodic leg movement (PLM).

Aurora RN, et al. The treatment of restless legs syndrome and periodic limb movement disorder in adults—an update for 2012: practice parameters with an evidence-based systematic review and meta-analyses. *SLEEP*. 2012; 35(8):1039–1062.

Ball E, Caivano CK. Internal medicine: guidance to the diagnosis and management of restless legs syndrome. *South Med J*. 2008; 101:631–634. [PMID: 18475241]

Salas RE, et al. Update in restless legs syndrome, *Curr Opin Neurol*. 2010;23:401–406

Wolf DS, Singer HS. Pediatric movement disorders: an update. *Curr Opin Neurol*. 2008; 21:491–496. [PMID: 18607212]

Website

http://www.wemove.org

CHOREA

Chorea is an irregular, rapid, involuntary jerky movement that flows randomly to any part of the body. Multiple etiologies, such as Huntington disease (see next section), vascular disorders, electrolyte imbalance, medications (antiparkinsonian, anticonvulsants, cocaine, neuroleptics), infection (HIV, encephalitis), and autoimmune disorders (SLE, Sydenham chorea), have been identified as causing chorea by affecting the basal ganglia. Chorea usually affects the hands, feet, face (eg, nose wrinkling), and trunk. Laboratory tests may be ordered to differentiate the causes, such as throat culture and streptococcal blood antigen for Sydenham chorea, liver function tests, complement levels, ANA, antiphospholipid antibody titers, TSH, and electrolytes. Brain CT, MRI, and PET scan may also aid in diagnosis.

HUNTINGTON'S DISEASE

Huntington's disease (HD) is an adult-onset (ages 35–50 years), autosomal-dominant progressive neurodegenerative disorder caused by a mutation with CAG repeats in the IT15 gene on chromosome 4. It affects approximately 1 in 10,000 people. Dopamine and glutamate neurotransmitters are thought to be affected. It is characterized by chorea, cognitive decline, and psychiatric impairment. Its clinical features include chorea, gait disturbance, dysarthria and dysphagia, eye movement disorders, and associated cognitive and behavioral disorders (dementia, depression, OCD, suicidal ideation). The Unified Huntington Disease Rating scale (UHDRS) measures the motor, cognitive, behavioral and functional impairment in HD and have been used to evaluate clinical progression in research. Its application in clinical settings needs further investigation. Imaging studies may show abnormalities such as putamen atrophy on MRI, enlarged ventricles on CT, and decreased glucose and oxygen metabolism in caudate nuclei on PET. Genetic confirmatory testing may be offered to patients with clear symptoms of HD and a family history of HD. Testing for fatal HD in individuals without symptoms but with a documented family history can cause enormous stress and emotional concerns. Genetic counseling before and after the test regarding implications of possible results and potential family, social, and ethical issues is important for informed decision making and patient and family support. Individuals who have a positive test result will experience a gradually increasing sense of hopelessness as the onset of the disease approaches. Some will suffer severe depression with suicidal ideation. They will demonstrate increased avoidance behaviors, and close monitoring is warranted.

Treatment is mainly symptomatic to control chorea, behavioral comorbidities (by means of antidepressants), and potential complications (rhabdomyolysis, local trauma from falls, and aspiration pneumonia). Tetrabenazine, a monoamine-depleting agent, is the only FDA-approved drug for HD. It is likely effective in chorea control. Its serious side effects include depression, parkinsonism, prolonged QT interval, and neuroleptic malignant syndrome. Amantadine and nabilone (a synthetic cannabinoid) may be effective in decreasing HD chorea. Riluzole, with antiglutamatergic and antiexcitotoxic effects, is moderately effective at a higher dose, 200 mg/d. Liver function and suicidal thoughts need to be monitored. There is no sufficient date to support the use of clozapine, coenzyme Q10, donepezil, or creatine. Supportive management and a multidisciplinary approach, including speech and physical and occupational therapy, are important in maintaining patients' quality of life. Patients can be referred to several national support groups and organizations, including the Huntington Disease Society of America (http://www.hdsa.org) and the Hereditary Disease Foundation (http://www.hdfoundation.org/home.php).

Armstrong MJ. Evidence-based guideline: pharmacologic treatment of chorea in Huntington disease. Report of the Guideline Development Subcommittee of the American Academy of Neurology. *Neurology*. 2012;79:597–603.

Kalman L, et al. Development of genomic reference materials for Huntington disease genetic testing. *Genet Med.* 2007;9:719–723. [PMID: 18073586]

Satija P, Ondo WG. Restless legs syndrome: pathophysiology, diagnosis and treatment. *CNS Drugs.* 2008;22:497–518. [PMID: 18484792]

Timman R, et al. Adverse effects of predictive testing for Huntington disease underestimated: long-term effects 7-10 years after the test. *Health Psychol.* 2004;23:189–197. [PMID: 15008664]

Websites

http://www.wemove.org
http://www.hdsa.org
http://www.hdfoundation.org/home.php

OTHER MOVEMENT DISORDERS

Dystonia

Dystonia is characterized by sustained, directional, uncoordinated, or simultaneous agonist and antagonist muscle contractions, which result in repetitive twisting movements or abnormal postures with a body part flexed or twisted along its longitudinal axis. The same group of muscles are repeatedly involved. The excessive random movements are worsened with intentional movements and improve at rest. Dystonic movements can be triggered by specific actions such as hand cramps with writing, called *task-specific dystonia*; they can extend beyond the commonly affected body parts, called *overflow dystonia*. Mirror movements may be seen in unaffected extremities when repetitive tasks, such as writing or finger sequences, are performed in the most affected body side; in a more severe form than action dystonia, they can occur at rest, called *rest dystonia*. Finally, the movements become fixed postures or positions, referred to as *permanent contractures*. A sensory trick (*geste antagonistique*) is a phenomenon of dystonic movements. Patients may suppress dystonic movements by touching affected or adjunctive body parts. In primary dystonia, this is the only neurologic abnormal finding and is associated with a genetic cause in autosomal dominant fashion (such as DYT phenotypes). It is considered a neurodevelopmental circuit disorder of the cortical, subcortical, and cerebellar pathways. Early-onset (<26 years) primary dystonia usually affects an extremity. Late-onset (>26 years) primary dystonia affects the neck or cranial muscles and tends to remain focal. Secondary dystonia is associated with an exogenous etiology such as drug use, head trauma, infection, and hypoxia. Other abnormal neurologic examination findings are present, for example, HD, PD, neurodegeneration, Wilson disease, CNS tumor, and stroke. Dopa-responsive dystonia (DRD, Segawa syndrome) is a childhood-onset dystonia plus parkinsonism that responds to levodopa.

The diagnosis of dystonia is based on history, typical clinical presentation, and neurologic examination. Dopamine transporter (DAT) scans are typically normal in primary dystonia. MRI of the brain and appropriate laboratory investigations (eg, serum ceruloplasmin, CSF analysis, ANA, ESR, and metabolic panels) can help assess secondary dystonia. Genetic testing for early-onset dystonia may be considered. Genetic counseling should be provided to patients and family before and after the testing.

Treatment of dystonia is aimed at underlying causes and symptom control. Botulinum toxin injection is the first choice for most focal dystonias. Other symptomatic treatments include oral medication (benzodiazepines, dopamine agonists or dopaminergic agents, anticholinergics, or baclofen); and surgery, such as DBS, epidural premotor stimulation or peripheral denervation. Early-onset dystonia should have a trial of levodopa for possible DRD. Physical therapy such as stretching exercises and sensory tricks may be used to help maintain range of motion or interrupt muscle twisting.

Albanese A. Update on dystonia. *Curr Opin Neurol.* 2012;25: 483–490,

Geyer HL, Bressman SB. The diagnosis of dystonia. *Lancet Neurol.* 2006;5:780–790. [PMID: 16914406]

Kartha N. Dystonia. *Clin Geriatr Med.* 2006;22:899–914. [PMID: 17000342]

Website

http://www.wemove.org

Myoclonus

Myoclonus refers to sudden, quick, jerklike, involuntary spasmodic movements of a muscle or a group of muscles. Positive myoclonus is due to involuntary muscular contractions; negative myoclonus (asterixis) is due to sudden brief loss of muscle tone. It is not preceded by an urge to move and not suppressible. It is not interrupted by a geste antagoniste such as in dystonia. They can be focal, segmental, axial, or generalized; arrhythmic, rhythmic, or oscillatory. Based on etiology, myoclonus can be classified into four categories. *Physiologic myoclonus* is a normal and benign movement that occurs commonly, such as hiccups, hypnic jerks, anxiety-induced or exercise-induced jerks, and benign infantile myoclonus with feeding. The movements are usually self-limited and not disabling. *Essential myoclonus* is a multifocal movement disorder, which can be sporadic or hereditary in an autosomal dominant pattern (associated with dystonia). Even though myoclonic movements are the one abnormal clinical finding on neurologic examination, they occur more frequently at any time, affecting patients' daily lives. *Epileptic myoclonus* occurs with seizure activities and demonstrates EEG and electromyographic changes.

Secondary (symptomatic) myoclonus is the most common type of myoclonus (~70%) and occurs as the result of central or peripheral nervous system insult or damage from a wide variety of medical conditions, which can be metabolic (inborn errors of metabolism, Hashimoto encephalopathy) or neurodegenerative (PD, HD), or due to trauma or infection; medications (eg, anesthetic agents, opiates, and anticonvulsants), or toxin exposure (pesticides, gases). Electrophysiologic studies (EEG-EMG), MRI and transcranial magnetic stimulation (TMS) can be employed for the diagnosis and to evaluate origin of myoclonus at cortical, subcortical, spinal, and peripheral levels. Laboratory investigations and genetic testing should be ordered on the basis of suspected underlying conditions. Treatment of myoclonus is aimed at the secondary causes such as removal medications or correction of metabolic imbalances. Evidence for symptomatic treatment is disappointing. Different medications are used according to the level of the nervous system involved, such as levetiracetam and piracetam, which are first choices for cortical myoclonus; clonazepam is used in subcortical and spinal myoclonus; botulinum toxin injection is used for peripheral myoclonus. Other medications have been used to control myoclonus, such as trihexyphenidyl, rituximab, ACTH, valproic acid, and primidone. DBS may be effective in certain cases of myoclonus.

Borg M. Symptomatic myoclonus. *Neurophysiol Clin.* 2006;36:309–318. [PMID: 17336775]

Chang VC. Myoclonus. *Curr Treat Options Neurol.* 2008;10:222–229.

Dijk JM. Management of patients with myoclonus: available therapies and the need for an evidence-based approach. *Lancet Neurol.* 2010;9:1028–1036.

Website

http://www.wemove.org

Hearing & Vision Impairment in the Elderly

Archana M. Kudrimoti, MD

Saranne E. Perman, MD

Sensory impairment affects up to two-thirds of the geriatric population. Identification, evaluation, and treatment of these conditions (**Table 45-1**) may improve patients' quality and quantity of life. The impact of sensory impairments is significant. The same objective level of sensory function can result in different levels of disability depending on the needs and expectations of patients. Poor hearing is associated with depression as well as decreased quality of life; poor mental health; and decreased physical, social, and cognitive functioning. Vision impairment increases the risk of death and is associated with an elevated risk of falling and hip fracture, depression, medication errors, and problems with driving.

Research has yet to demonstrate that community-based screening of asymptomatic older people results in improvements in vision or hearing. The US Preventive Services Task Force (USPSTF) and the American Academy of Family Physicians (AAFP) recommend screening for hearing difficulties by questioning elderly adults about hearing impairment and counseling them regarding the availability of treatment when appropriate. In a 2009 update, AAFP and USPSTF concluded that there is inadequate direct evidence that screening for impairment of visual acuity by primary care physicians improves functional outcomes in elderly; yet there is adequate evidence that early treatment of refractive error, cataracts, and age-related macular degeneration (AMD) improves or prevents loss of visual acuity.

COMMON CAUSES OF HEARING IMPAIRMENT IN THE ELDERLY

PRESBYCUSIS

ESSENTIALS OF DIAGNOSIS

▶ Age-related high-frequency sensorineural hearing loss.

▶ Difficulty with speech discrimination.

▶ General Considerations

Presbycusis is the most common form of hearing loss in the elderly, although it often goes unrecognized. It occurs more frequently with advancing age and in patients with a positive family history. This multifactorial disorder is due to a combination of structural and neural degeneration and genetic predisposition. Risk factors for presbycusis include noise exposure, smoking, and medications such as aminoglycoside antibiotics, loop diuretics, and cardiovascular risk factors such as hypertension. Presbycusis is a diagnosis of exclusion.

▶ Prevention

Until the exact pathophysiology of presbycusis is understood, attempts at prevention will be limited. Limitation of noise exposure may reduce the hearing loss. Although several studies have evaluated the role of vitamins, antioxidants, smoking cessation, and diet in preventing presbycusis, there have been no conclusive findings in humans.

▶ Clinical Findings

Patients with this disorder may present with a chief complaint of hearing loss and difficulty understanding speech. However, presbycusis is often diagnosed only after complaints are raised by close patient contacts, or hearing loss is noted on routine screening in a patient without hearing-related complaints. The Hearing Handicap Inventory of the Elderly Screening Version (HHIE-S) is a widely accepted subjective screening tool for hearing disability. Abnormalities of the whisper test are found as the level of hearing loss increases. Results of the Weber tuning-fork test remain normal as long as the hearing loss is symmetric. Results of Rinne testing are normal, because presbycusis is a sensorineural hearing loss and not a conductive one.

An audiogram of a patient with presbycusis typically shows bilaterally symmetric high-frequency hearing loss.

Table 45-1. Differential diagnosis of geriatric hearing and vision impairment.[a]

Hearing Impairment	Vision Impairment
Presbycusis	**Presbyopia**
Cerumen impaction	**Age-related macular degeneration**
Noise-induced hearing loss	**Glaucoma**
Central auditory processing disorder	**Senile cataract**
Otosclerosis	**Diabetic retinopathy**
Chronic otitis media	Central retinal artery or vein occlusion
Glomus tumor or vascular anomaly	Posterior vitreous or retinal detachment
Cholesteatoma	Vitreous hemorrhage
Autoimmune hearing loss	Temporal arteritis
Perilymph fistula	Optic neuritis
Ménière disease	Corneal pathology
Acoustic neuroma	Iritis

[a]The most common causes are indicated in bold type.

Treatment

The treatment of presbycusis consists of hearing rehabilitation, which often involves fitting for digital and analog types of hearing aids. Patients are more likely to perceive benefit from hearing aids if they view their hearing loss as a problem. Cochlear implantation is reserved for patients with profound hearing loss that is unresponsive to hearing aids. Additional tools include lip-reading classes; television closed captioning; sound-enhancing devices for concerts, church, or other public gatherings; and telephone amplifiers. A combined approach involving the patient, hearing loss specialist, family physician, and close contacts of the patient is likely to produce the best overall treatment plan.

Suggested topics for patient education include patient self-advocation as well as the proper use of hearing aids and other assistive devices.

Prognosis

The expectation of slow progression of this hearing loss should be communicated to the patient. Complete deafness, however, is not typical of presbycusis.

NOISE-INDUCED HEARING LOSS

 ESSENTIALS OF DIAGNOSIS

▶ History of occupational or recreational noise exposure.

▶ Bilateral notch of sensorineural hearing loss between 3000 and 6000 Hz on audiogram.

▶ Problems with tinnitus, speech discrimination, and hearing in the presence of background noise.

General Considerations

Noise-induced hearing loss is the second most common sensorineural hearing loss (**Table 45-2**) after presbycusis. Up to one-third of patients with hearing loss have some component of their deficit that is noise-induced. The degree of hearing loss is related to the level of noise and the duration of exposure. Excessive shear force from loud sounds or long exposure results in cell damage, cell death, and subsequent hearing loss.

Prevention

Hearing protection programs are prevalent in industrial settings and typically include the use of earplugs, intermittent audiograms, and limiting exposure. Patient commitment to the use of hearing protection is critical for the success of prevention programs.

Clinical Findings

Patients may present with tinnitus, decreased speech discrimination, and difficulty hearing when background noise is present. Patients identified through hearing protection

Table 45-2. Causes of hearing loss.[a]

Conductive Hearing Loss	Sensorineural Hearing Loss
Outer ear	**Inner ear**
Otitis externa	Presbycusis
Trauma	Noise exposure
Cerumen	Ménière's disease
Osteoma	Ototoxic drugs
Exostosis	Meningitis
Squamous cell carcinoma	Viral cochleitis
Middle ear	Barotraumas
Otitis media	Acoustic neuroma
Tympanic membrane perforation	Meningioma
Cholesteatoma	Multiple sclerosis
Otosclerosis	Vascular disease
Glomus tumors	
Temporal bone trauma	
Paget disease	

[a]The most common causes are indicated in bold type.

programs may be asymptomatic. Results of the whisper test or office-based pure-tone audiometry may be normal or abnormal, depending on the degree of hearing loss.

Audiometric evaluation of noise-induced hearing loss reveals a bilateral notch of sensorineural hearing loss between 3000 and 6000 Hz.

Treatment

When prevention fails, treatment involves hearing rehabilitation, as previously outlined in the treatment of presbycusis. Education about the risks of loud noise exposure should begin when patients are young, because hearing loss can occur from significant recreational noise. The importance of adhering to hearing protection programs should also be emphasized.

Prognosis

Nothing can be done to reverse cell death from noise-induced hearing loss; however, some patients exposed to brief episodes of loud noise exhibit only hair cell injury and may recover hearing over time. These patients are more susceptible to noise-induced hearing loss on reexposure.

Cerumen Impaction

ESSENTIALS OF DIAGNOSIS

▶ Mild, reversible conductive hearing loss.

▶ Cerumen buildup in ear canal, limiting sound transmission.

▶ Direct visualization of wax plug confirms diagnosis.

General Considerations

Impaction of wax in the external auditory canal is a common, frequently overlooked problem in the elderly. Removal of cerumen has been shown to significantly improve hearing ability. The incidence of cerumen impactions increases in the elderly population. Chronic skin changes lead to loss of normal migration of skin epithelium leading to exfoliated cell debris accumulation. Cerumen gland atrophy results in drier wax that is more likely to become trapped by the large tragi hairs in the external ear canal. The likelihood of impaction is increased by hearing aid or earplug use.

Prevention

Cerumen impactions may be prevented by the regular use of agents that soften wax. Readily available household agents such as water, mineral oil, cooking oils, hydrogen peroxide, or glycerin may be used. Commercially available

ceruminolytic compounds, such as carbamide peroxide, triethanolamine polypeptide, and docusate sodium liquid, are also efficacious, but not more so than less-expensive options.

Clinical Findings

Patients presenting with cerumen impaction may complain of sudden or gradual hearing loss, tinnitus affecting one or both the ears, and interference with hearing aids. Examination of the external canal reveals partial or complete occlusion of the ear canal with cerumen.

Complications

Various removal methods are associated with ear discomfort and potential for ear canal trauma. Canal trauma can result in bleeding, canal swelling, or infection. Warm water should be used for ear irrigation, because cold water can induce vertigo.

Treatment

The management of impactions may be approached in various ways. When the wax is soft, gentle irrigation of the canal with warm water may be sufficient to remove the offending material. In the case of firmer wax, ceruminolytic agents may be applied, followed by irrigation. Any cerumen remaining after these maneuvers may be removed using a curette in combination with an otoscope for direct visualization. The patient may experience an improvement of symptoms even with partial removal of the impaction. Patients should be instructed about ear cleaning techniques and home use of ceruminolytics.

Prognosis

Cerumen impaction has an excellent prognosis, and hearing can be dramatically improved with relatively simple interventions. However, recurrence of impaction is common.

CENTRAL AUDITORY PROCESSING DISORDER

ESSENTIALS OF DIAGNOSIS

▶ Hearing impairment due to insult to central nervous system.

▶ Reduction in speech discrimination exceeds hearing loss.

General Considerations

Central auditory processing disorder (CAPD) is the general term for hearing impairment that results from central nervous system (CNS) dysfunction. Any insult to the nervous system such as stroke or dementia can cause CAPD. The disorder is characterized by a loss of speech discrimination that is more profound than the associated loss in hearing.

Prevention

It may be postulated that the protection of the CNS provided by aspirin therapy and hypertension control could reduce the incidence of CAPD.

Clinical Findings

Patients with CAPD have difficulty understanding spoken language but may be able to hear sounds well. A patient may have difficulty following verbal instructions but understand written ones. There are no specific physical findings of CAPD, but patients may have other evidence of neurologic abnormalities.

Treatment

Treatment of CAPD is limited. If CNS dysfunction is caused by a reversible entity, then treatment for the underlying cause should be initiated. Identifying and treating other causes of sensory impairment may improve the patient's level of disability; however, CAPD may decrease the effectiveness of auditory rehabilitation. Patient education efforts should focus on educating friends and family about the disorder and options for hearing rehabilitation. The prognosis for patients with CAPD is determined by the underlying disorder.

Gates GA, et al. Presbycusis. *Lancet*. 2005; 366(9491):1111–1120. [PMID: 16182900]

Pacala JT. Hearing deficits in the older patient: "I didn't notice anything." *JAMA*. 2012;307(11):1185–1194. [PMID: 22436959]

Sprinzl GM, et al. Current trends in treating hearing loss in elderly people: a review of the technology and treatment options- a mini-review. *Gerontology*. 2010; 56(3):351–358. [PMID: 20090297]

Websites

National Institute on Deafness and Other Communication Disorders: http://www.nidcd.nih.gov/health/pages/default.aspx

National Institute on Aging: www.nia.nih.gov/health/publication/hearing-loss

COMMON CAUSES OF VISION IMPAIRMENT IN THE ELDERLY

Visual impairment is defined as binocular acuity of 20/40 or worse. Legal blindness is when acuity is worse than 20/200. Older adults with good visual acuity show problems with visual function in real-life situations as testing is usually done in an optimum condition with maximum contrast and illumination with minimal glare. Testing for visual problems with decreased contrast sensitivity, decreased illumination, and increased glare is not practical for primary care providers, and hence it is important that they ask questions routinely to screen for performance under these circumstances. Educating the patient about simple measures to improve the environment may help with their quality of life.

PRESBYOPIA

 ESSENTIALS OF DIAGNOSIS

► Age-related decrease in near vision.
► Distance vision remains unaffected.

General Considerations

Presbyopia is an age-associated progressive loss of the focusing power of the lens. Its incidence increases with age. The cause of this disorder is the ongoing increase in the diameter of the lens as a result of continued growth of the lens fibers with aging. This thickened lens accommodates less responsively to the contraction of muscles in the ciliary body, limiting its ability to focus on near objects.

Clinical Findings

Patients presenting with this disorder frequently complain of eye strain or of blurring of their vision when they quickly change from looking at a nearby object to one that is far away. On examination, the only abnormality noted is a decrease in near vision.

Treatment

Because presbyopia is due to normal age-related changes of the eye, there is no proven prevention. In patients with normal distance vision, treatment for this disorder is as simple as purchasing reading glasses. For patients requiring correction of their distance vision, options include spectacle correction with bifocal or trifocal lenses, monovision contact lenses in which one eye is corrected for distance vision and the other eye for near vision, or contact lens correction of distance vision and simple reading glasses for near vision. Surgical treatment of presbyopia is an evolving science, including procedures on the cornea, lens, and sclera.

Prognosis

All patients should be educated to anticipate a decline in near vision with aging. When left uncorrected, problems may occur with reading, driving, or other activities of daily living.

AGE-RELATED MACULAR DEGENERATION

 ESSENTIALS OF DIAGNOSIS

▶ Slowly progressive central vision loss with intact peripheral vision.

▶ Vision problems in low light intensity and Amsler grid distortion.

▶ Drusen located in the macula of the retina.

General Considerations

Age-related macular degeneration (AMD/ARMD) is the leading cause of severe vision loss in older Americans. It is characterized by atrophy of cells in the central macular region of the retinal pigment epithelium, resulting in the loss of central vision. Peripheral vision generally remains intact. AMD is typically classified as early and intermediate (usually dry type) or advanced/late AMD, which is divided into atrophic or nonneovascular (dry) or exudative or neovascular (wet) forms. The exudative form occurs in only 10% of patients with AMD, but it is responsible for the majority of severe vision loss related to the disease.

Prevention

Multiple risk factors for this disorder have been studied, including genetic factors, white race, obesity, and cardiovascular disease; only increasing age and tobacco abuse have consistently been associated with AMD. Because smoking has been strongly implicated as a risk factor and continued tobacco use is associated with a worse response to laser photocoagulation, tobacco avoidance and smoking cessation should be highly recommended to all patients. Hypertension has also been linked to a worse response to laser therapy; thus, effective blood pressure control is desirable, as well. Finally, antioxidants play a role in tertiary prevention. Patients with intermediate AMD or unilateral advanced AMD had a ~25% reduction of their risk for developing advanced AMD if treated with a high-dose combination of vitamin C, vitamin E, β-carotene, and zinc. Patients with early or no AMD did not have the same benefit.

Clinical Findings

A. Symptoms and Signs

Patients may report onset of blurred central vision that is either gradual or acute with difficulty reading in dim light and night driving. Wavy or distorted central vision, known as *metamorphopsia*; intermittent shimmering lights; and central blind spots, termed *scotoma*, may all occur. Clinical findings include decreased visual acuity, Amsler grid distortion, and characteristic abnormalities on dilated funduscopic examination. In early disease, the most common findings are drusen: yellowish-colored deposits deep in the retina. In late disease of the atrophic type, areas of depigmentation are seen in the macula. In the exudative form, abnormal vessels (subretinal neovascularization) leak fluid and blood beneath the macula.

B. Special Examinations

Fluorescein angiography may be used by a specialist to confirm the diagnosis and to help determine whether a patient has atrophic or exudative AMD.

Treatment

A. Referral

An ophthalmologist will play a critical role in care of the patient with known or suspected AMD. Urgent referral to an eye specialist should occur if a patient with suspected or known AMD presents with *acute* visual changes. Treatment of exudative AMD is a rapidly advancing field with many ongoing clinical trials of surgical and pharmaceutical interventions. Current treatment options include laser photocoagulation, photodynamic therapy (Verteporfin), and intravitreal antiangiogenic therapy [antivascular endothelial growth factor (VEGF)]. No effective treatments exist for patient with dry AMD.

Vision rehabilitation is the cornerstone to helping patients maximize their remaining vision and maintain their level of function for as long as possible. Low-vision professionals along with social workers can be of great assistance in recommending optical aids and devices and accessing local, state, and federal resources for the visually impaired. Direct-illumination devices, magnifiers, high-power reading glasses, telescopes, closed-circuit television, large-print publications, and bold-lined paper are some of the many devices that can be employed.

B. Patient Education

Patient education topics include the importance. (Its use is described at http://www.amd.org.)

Prognosis

Many patients with mild dry AMD will not experience significant worsening of their vision. It is difficult to predict which patients will develop advancing disease and further loss of central vision. This condition is generally progressive but is not completely blinding. Peripheral vision should not be affected by AMD.

Bourla DH, et al. Age-related macular degeneration: a practical approach to a challenging disease. *J Am Geriatr Soc.* 2006; 54 (7):1130–1135. [PMID: 16866687]

Jager RD, et al. Age-related macular degeneration. *N Engl J Med.* 2008; 358(24):2606–2617. [PMID: 18550876]

Lim LS, et al. Age-related macular degeneration. *Lancet.* 2012; 379(9827):1728–1738. [PMID: 22559899]

GLAUCOMA

 ESSENTIALS OF DIAGNOSIS

▶ Optic neuropathy with variably progressive vision loss.

▶ Intraocular pressure (IOP) is often elevated but may be normal.

General Considerations

Glaucoma is the second leading cause of blindness in the United States. Although glaucoma is most often associated with elevated IOP, it is the optic neuropathy that defines the disease. Normal IOP is generally accepted to be between 10 and 21 mmHg. The majority of patients with an IOP of > 21 mmHg will not develop glaucoma, and 30–50% of patients with glaucoma will have an IOP of < 21 mmHg. Despite these facts, it has been clearly shown that as IOP increases, so does the risk of developing glaucoma. Other identified risk factors for glaucoma include family history and advancing age and African-American race. Additional possible risk factors include diabetes mellitus, hypertension, and myopia.

Prevention

The AAFP and the USPTF do not recommend screening for glaucoma, citing insufficient evidence to recommend for or against routine screening by primary care clinicians for elevated IOP or early glaucoma. The American Academy of Ophthalmology recommends screening for glaucoma by an ophthalmologist every 1–2 years after age 65.

Clinical Findings

A. Symptoms and Signs

Patients with acute angle-closure glaucoma typically present with unilateral intense pain and blurred vision. Patients may report seeing halos around light sources and complain of photophobia, headache, nausea, and vomiting. Physical examination shows a middilated pupil, conjunctival injection, and lid edema. Patients generally have markedly elevated IOP, usually between 60 and 80 mmHg.

Primary open-angle glaucoma is a more insidious disease with a long asymptomatic phase. Patients may notice a gradual loss of peripheral vision. Examination may reveal diminished visual fields, elevated IOP, and abnormalities of the optic disk on direct ophthalmoscopy (symmetrically enlarged cup-to-disk ratio, cup-to-disk ratio asymmetry between the two eyes, or a highly asymmetric cup in one eye).

B. Special Tests

Intraocular pressure may be measured using a variety of tools. The most readily available tool is the physician's hand. Palpation of the globe through a lightly closed lid can reveal asymmetric hardness or bilaterally firm eyeballs and provide a very gross measure of IOP. More accurate tools include the Tono-Pen (a handheld applanation tonometer), Goldmann applanation tonometry, and pneumotonometry (puff test).

Treatment

Patients with significant risk factors or physical findings that raise concern for glaucoma should be referred to an ophthalmologist for further evaluation and confirmation of diagnosis.

A. Acute Angle-Closure Glaucoma

Acute angle-closure glaucoma is a medical emergency that requires immediate referral and treatment.

B. Primary Open-Angle Glaucoma

The treatment of primary open-angle glaucoma consists of pharmacologic and surgical interventions aimed at decreasing the IOP. Although elevated IOP is not required for the diagnosis of glaucoma, it has been shown that reduction of IOP in patients with glaucoma slows the progression of disease. Even patients with normal pressures can benefit from reduction in IOP.

1. Pharmacotherapy—Topical eyedrops or oral medications aimed at decreasing aqueous humor production or increasing outflow are used. Topical agents such as β-blockers and prostaglandin analogs are first-line therapy, and α-adrenergic agents and carbonic anhydrase inhibitors are second-line of therapy. Topical miotics and epinephrine compounds are now infrequently used. Oral medications include carbonic anhydrase inhibitors such as acetazolamide. Topical glaucoma agents have varying degrees of systemic absorption and are capable of producing systemic side effects and drug-drug interactions. Patients should be educated on the importance of routine eye care and of taking medications as prescribed.

2. Surgical intervention—When medical management is unsuccessful, surgical intervention is considered. Laser trabeculoplasty and laser or conventional trabeculectomy are the most commonly performed procedures.

Prognosis

Untreated glaucoma can result in blindness. Rapid treatment of acute angle-closure glaucoma may preserve vision.

Treatment of primary open-angle glaucoma can prevent further loss of vision, but typically does not restore lost vision.

Kwon YH, et al. Primary open-angle glaucoma. *N Engl J Med.* 2009;360(11):1113–1124. [PMID: 19279343].

Quigley HA. Glaucoma. *Lancet.* 2011;377(9774):1367–1377. [PMID: 21453963].

CATARACTS

ESSENTIALS OF DIAGNOSIS

▶ Opacity or cloudiness of the crystalline lens.

▶ General Considerations

Any opacification of the lens is termed a *cataract.* Cataract disease is the most common cause of blindness worldwide and the most common eye abnormality in the elderly. Risk factors for cataracts include advancing age, exposure to ultraviolet (UV) B light, glaucoma, smoking, alcohol abuse, diabetes, and chronic steroid use. Diet and vitamins do not play a role in development or progression of the disease. Because cataracts tend to develop slowly, the patient may not be fully aware of the degree of vision impairment.

▶ Prevention

Prevention of cataracts is aimed at the modifiable risk factors. Physicians should use steroids at as low a dose as is therapeutic and discontinue them when possible. Patients should be advised on how to minimize UV light exposure as well as the benefits of smoking cessation and control of chronic diseases.

▶ Clinical Findings

Patients may report blurring of vision, "ghosting" of images, difficulty seeing in oncoming lights (glare) and difficulty with night driving, and monocular diplopia. The patient may also complain of a decrease in color perception and even note "second sight," which is an improvement in near vision with a nuclear cataract. Examination of the eye reveals opacification of the lens. Cataracts may be easier to see with dilation of the eye and a direct ophthalmoscope at +5D (diopters) setting held 6 inches from the patient's eye.

▶ Treatment

The treatment of cataracts is predominantly surgical. Although small cataracts may be treated by an updated eyeglass prescription, most patients with significant symptoms from a cataract benefit from surgical removal and replacement of the lens. Factors influencing the timing of surgery include life expectancy, current level of disability, status of other medical illnesses, family and social situations, and patient expectations.

Family physicians may aid patients in understanding the surgery and assisting with preoperative management. Cataract surgery is a low-risk procedure. Routine use of laboratory testing and electrocardiogram screening has not improved surgical outcome. Individuals should receive a history and physical examination prior to undergoing surgery. Additional testing is recommended only if findings are abnormal. Cataract surgery is often accomplished under local anesthesia with minimally invasive techniques. In this case, there is no need to discontinue anticoagulation for the procedure. Surgeons should be made aware if patients are taking α-blockers as this is associated with a complication called *intraoperative floppy iris syndrome.*

▶ Prognosis

Cataracts do not resolve and may progress without treatment. The prognosis with surgical treatment is excellent, and ≤95% of patients obtain improved vision after surgery.

Asbell PA. Age-related cataract. *Lancet.* 2005;365(9459):599–609. [PMID: 15708105].

Eichenbaum JW. Geriatric vision loss due to cataracts, macular degeneration, and glaucoma. *Mt Sinai J Med.* 2012;79(2):276–294. [PMID: 22499498].

DIABETIC RETINOPATHY

ESSENTIALS OF DIAGNOSIS

▶ Asymptomatic, gradual vision loss or sudden vision loss in a diabetic patient.

▶ Characteristic fundoscopic findings of micro aneurysms, flame hemorrhages, exudates, macular edema, and neovascularization.

▶ General Considerations

Diabetic retinopathy (DR) is the leading cause of blindness in adults in the United States. It is important to consider diabetic retinopathy as a disease of the aging eye because prevalence increases with duration of diabetes mellitus. The risk of blindness attributable to this disorder is greatest after 30 years of illness. DR is divided into two major forms: nonproliferative (NPDR) and proliferative (PDR), named for the absence or presence of abnormal new blood vessels emanating from the retina, respectively. NPDR can be further classified into mild, moderate, severe, and very severe categories depending on the extent of nerve fiber layer infarcts (cotton-wool spots), intraretinal hemorrhages, hard exudates, and microvascular abnormalities. The severity of proliferative retinopathy can be classified as early, high-risk, and severe depending on the severity and extent of neovascularization.

Prevention

Patients with diabetes mellitus type 2 should have a comprehensive eye examination by an ophthalmologist shortly after diagnosis to screen for signs of retinopathy. Meticulous glycemic control decreases the risk of development and progression of retinopathy in all patients with diabetes. In addition, tight control of blood pressure also significantly reduces a patient's risk of developing retinopathy.

Clinical Findings

Many patients presenting with diabetic retinopathy are free of symptoms; even those with the severe proliferative form may have 20/20 visual acuity. Others may report decreased vision that has occurred slowly or suddenly, unilaterally or bilaterally. Scotomata or floaters may also be reported. Funduscopic examination reveals any or all of the following: microaneurysms, dot and blot intraretinal hemorrhages, hard exudates, cotton-wool spots, boat-shaped preretinal hemorrhages, neovascularization, venous beading, and macular edema.

Fluorescein angiography may be performed by an ophthalmologist to further assess the degree of disease.

Treatment

Untreated proliferative retinopathy is relentlessly progressive, leading to significant vision impairment and blindness. In addition to maximizing glucose and blood pressure control, focal and pan-retinal laser photocoagulation surgery or vitrectomy is the mainstay of acute and chronic treatment and may preserve vision in certain patients. There is emerging evidence that intravitreal anti-VEGF treatment can be used in the management of retinopathy. When vision loss has occurred, vision rehabilitation should be initiated, as described earlier in the discussion of AMD. Topics to review with patients include the importance of an annual, comprehensive eye examination, glycemic control, and hypertension management.

Prognosis

Early diagnosis and treatment, as well as tight glycemic and blood pressure control, improve prognosis and prevents blindness.

Antonetti D, et al. Diabetic retinopathy. N Engl J Med. 2012; 366(13):1227–1239. [PMID: 22455417].

Mohamed Q, et al. Management of diabetic retinopathy: a systemic review. JAMA. 2007; 298:902–916. [PMID: 17712074]

Websites

Lighthouse International (health information on vision disorders, treatment, and rehabilitation services): http://www.lighthouse.org

National Institute on Aging (patient education handout on the aging eye and hearing loss): www.nia.nih.gov/health/publication/aging-and-your-eyes

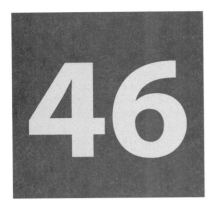

Oral Health

Wanda C. Gonsalves, MD

Although the nation's oral health is believed to be the best it has ever been, oral diseases remain common in the United States. In May 2000, the first report on oral health from the US Surgeon General, *Oral Health in America: A Report of the Surgeon General*, called attention to a largely overlooked epidemic of oral diseases that is disproportionately shared by Americans: This epidemic strikes in particular the poor, young, and elderly. The report stated that although there are safe and effective measures for preventing oral diseases, these measures are underused. The report called for improved education about oral health, for a renewed understanding of the relationship between oral health and overall health, and for an interdisciplinary approach to oral health that would involve primary care providers.

DENTAL ANATOMY & TOOTH ERUPTION PATTERN

In utero, the 20 primary teeth evolve from the expansion and development of ectodermal and mesodermal tissue at approximately 6 weeks of gestation. The ectoderm forms the dental enamel, and the mesoderm forms the pulp and dentin. As the tooth bud evolves, each unit develops a dental lamina that is responsible for the development of the future permanent tooth. The adult dentition is composed of 32 permanent teeth. **Figure 46-1** shows the anatomy of the tooth and supporting structures. **Table 46-1** outlines the eruption pattern of the teeth.

DENTAL CARIES

ESSENTIALS OF DIAGNOSIS

▶ Nonlocalized pain when exposed to heat, cold, or sweats.

▶ Painless white spot (demineralized areas of enamel) near gingival margins (white or brown spots).

▶ As infection proceeds to pulp, pain becomes localized.

▶ Visible pits or holes in the teeth.

▶ Poor oral hygiene and frequent snacking between meals are risk factors.

▶ General Considerations

Dental caries (tooth decay) is the single most common chronic childhood disease, 5 times more common than asthma and 7 times more common than hayfever among children aged 5–7 years. Minority and low-income children are disproportionately affected. According to the Centers for Disease Control and Prevention (CDC), among children aged 2–4 years and 6–8 years, tooth decay is more prevalent in Mexican American, and African American, non-Hispanic communities. Among adults aged 35–44 years in those same communities, untreated tooth decay is 2 times more prevalent than among white non-Hispanics. In addition, one-third of persons of all ages have untreated tooth decay, 8% of adults aged >20 years have lost at least one permanent tooth to dental caries, and many older adults suffer from root caries.

▶ Pathogenesis

Dental caries is a multifactorial, infectious, communicable disease caused by the demineralization of tooth enamel in the presence of a sugar substrate and of acid-forming cariogenic bacteria that are found in the soft gelatinous biofilm plaque (**Figure 46-2**). Thus, the development of caries requires a susceptible host, an appropriate substrate (sucrose), and the cariogenic bacteria found in plaque. *Streptococcus mutans* [also known as *mutans streptococci* (MS)] is considered to be the primary strain causing decay. Additionally, when plaque

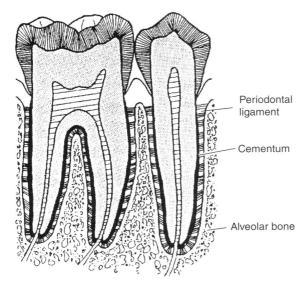

▲ **Figure 46-1.** Anatomy of the tooth and supporting structures.

- Periodontal ligament
- Cementum
- Alveolar bone

Table 46-1. Eruption pattern of teeth.

Teeth	Eruption Date
Primary dentition	
Mandibular central incisor	6 months
Maxillary central incisor	7 months
Mandibular lateral incisor	7 months
Maxillary lateral incisor	9 months
Mandibular first molar	12 months
Maxillary first molar	14 months
Mandibular canine	16 months
Maxillary canine	18 months
Mandibular second molar	20 months
Maxillary second molar	24 months
Permanent dentition	
Mandibular central incisors	6 years
Maxillary first molars	6 years
Mandibular first molars	6 years
Maxillary central incisors	7 years
Mandibular lateral incisors	7 years
Maxillary lateral incisors	8 years
Mandibular canines	9 years
Maxillary first premolars	10 years
Mandibular first premolars	11 years
Maxillary second premolars	11 years
Mandibular second premolars	11 years
Maxillary canines	11 years
Mandibular second molars	12 years
Maxillary second molars	12 years
Mandibular third molars	17–21 years
Maxillary third molars	17–21 years

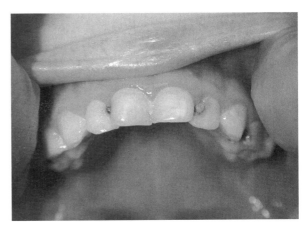

▲ **Figure 46-2.** Dental caries due to plaque.

is not regularly removed, it may calcify to form calculus (tartar) and cause destructive gum disease.

Finally, the development of caries is a dynamic process that involves an imbalance between demineralization and remineralization of enamel. When such an imbalance is caused by environmental factors such as low pH or inadequate formation of saliva, dissolution of enamel occurs and caries result.

▶ Clinical Findings

A. Symptoms and Signs

When enamel is repeatedly exposed to the acid formed by the fermentation of sugars in plaque, demineralized areas develop on the tooth surfaces, between teeth, and on pits and fissures. These areas are painless and appear clinically as opaque or brown spots (**Figures 46-3–46-5**). If infection

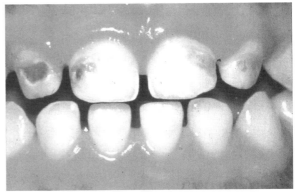

▲ **Figure 46-3.** Brown spots indicating demineralized areas in enamel.

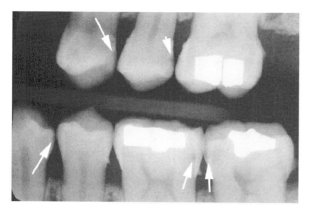

▲ **Figure 46-4.** Opaque areas indicating demineralized areas in enamel.

is allowed to progress, a cavity forms that can spread to and through the dentin (the component of the tooth located below the enamel) and to the pulp (composed of nerves and blood vessels; an infection of the pulp is called *pulpitis*), causing pain, necrosis, and, perhaps, an abscess.

B. Diagnosis

Carious lesions progress at various rates and occur at many different locations on the tooth, including the sites of previous restorations. Demineralized lesions (white or brown spots) generally occur at the margins of the gingiva and can be detected visually; they may not be seen on radiographs. Advanced carious lesions such as those spread through dentin can be detected clinically or, if they occur between the teeth, by radiographs. Root caries, commonly seen in older adults, occur in areas from which the gingiva has receded.

Dental professionals use a dental explorer to detect early caries in the grooves and fissures of posterior teeth. To diagnose secondary caries (caries formed at the site of

restorations), dental professionals use digitally acquired and postprocessed images.

▶ Risk Assessment

Caries can develop at any time after tooth eruption. Early teeth are principally susceptible to caries caused by the transmission of MS from the mouth of the caregiver to the mouth of the infant or toddler. This type of caries is called *early childhood caries* (ECC) or *baby bottle tooth decay* (BBTD). According to the American Academy of Pediatric Dentistry, ECC "is defined as 'the presence of one or more decayed (noncavitated or cavitated lesions), missing (due to caries), or filled tooth surfaces' in any primary tooth in a child 71 months of age or younger." In children aged <3 years, any sign of smooth-surface caries is called *severe early childhood caries* (S-ECC). Children with a history of ECC or S-ECC are at a much higher risk of subsequent caries in primary and permanent teeth. (Guidelines on caries risk assessment and management may be found on the American Academy of Pediatric Denistry website: http://www.aapd.org/media/Policies_Guidelines/G_CariesRiskAssessment.pdf).

Early childhood caries contribute to other health problems, including chronic pain, poor nutritional practices, and low self-esteem, which may lead to lack of self-esteem among older children and a great reduction in their ability to succeed in life.

The risk factors for adult caries are similar to those for childhood caries.

▶ Differential Diagnosis

Developmental defects or pits in the tooth surface or visible groove is the differential diagnosis.

▶ Prevention & Treatment

Fluoride, the ionic form of the element fluorine, is widely accepted as a safe and effective practice for the primary prevention of dental caries. Fluoride slows or reverses the progression of existing tooth decay by (1) being incorporated into the enamel before tooth eruption, (2) inhibiting demineralization, (3) enhancing remineralization, and (4) inhibiting bacterial activity in plaque. Unfortunately, only 73.9% of the US population has access to community water fluoridation, according to the CDC census in 2010. Systemic fluoride supplements (tablets, drops, lozenges) are recommended for children aged <6 months who are at high risk of the development of caries; for infants with ECC; for children aged 6 months to 16 years who live in nonfluoridated water areas; and for adults whose water is not fluoridated or who have diseases that produce a decrease in salivary flow, receding gums, or mental or physical disabilities. A supplemental fluoride dosage schedule is shown in **Table 46-2**. Topical fluoride supplements such as gels and varnishes are

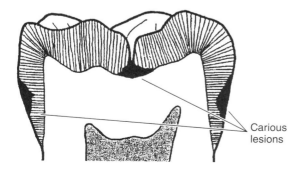

Carious lesions

▲ **Figure 46-5.** Dental caries.

Table 46-2. Supplemental fluoride dosage schedule.

Age	Fluoride Ion Level in Drinking Water (ppm)[a]		
	<0.3 ppm	0.3-0.6 ppm	>0.6 ppm
Birth–6 mo	None	None	None
6 mo–3 yr	0.25 mg/d[b]	None	None
3–6 yr	0.50 mg/d	0.25 mg/d	None
6–16 yr	1.0 mg/d	0.50 mg/d	None

[a]1 ppm = 1 mg/L.
[b]2.2 mg sodium fluoride contains 1 mg fluoride ion.
mo, months; yr, years.
Data from http://www.cdc.gov/FLUORIDATION/other/spplmnt_schdl.htm.

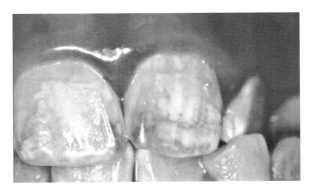

▲ **Figure 46-6.** Fluorosis.

highly concentrated fluoride products that are professionally applied by a dental health provider or a parent (for gels). Varnishes, which are less toxic than gels and more effective than mouth rinses, are applied 3 times a week, once a year by disposable brushes, cotton-tipped applicators, or cotton pellets. (To learn more about fluoride varnish application visit the Smiles for Life website, www.smilesforlifeoralhealth.org).

Before prescribing supplemental fluoride, the primary care provider must determine the fluoride concentration in the child's primary source of drinking water. Other sources of fluoride include well water exposed to fluorite minerals, certain fruits and vegetables grown in soil irrigated with fluoridated water, beverages, and foods such as meats or poultry that may contain 6–7% of total dietary fluoride. Although fluoride supplementation is not recommended for persons who live in communities whose water is optimally fluoridated (0.7–1.2 ppm or >0.6 mg/L), the bottled water used by many families may contain low levels of fluoride. Parents and caregivers should be educated about the benefits of fluoride and the possible side effects of too much fluoride, a condition called *fluorosis*. Fluorosis results when too much fluoride is obtained from any source when the permanent tooth is forming (**Figure 46-6**). Overall, 22% of children and adolescents aged 6–19 years have very mild or greater fluorosis. The benefits and side effects of fluoride use should be weighed against the risk of tooth decay among children at high risk of caries.

A second method of preventing dental caries is proper oral hygiene. Before the teeth erupt, a parent may use a washcloth or cotton gauze to clean an infant's mouth and to transition the child to toothbrushing. Parents should supervise brushing and should discourage children aged <6 years from using fluoridated dentifrices because of the risk that toothpaste may be swallowed during brushing. A pea-sized amount of toothpaste is recommended for brushing.

Generally speaking, children aged <2 years should avoid fluoride toothpaste.

Dental sealants, first introduced in the 1960s, are plastic films that coat the chewing surfaces of primary or permanent teeth. Sealants prevent decay from developing in the pits and fissures of teeth. Dental professionals often use sealants in combination with topical fluorides (**Figure 46-7**).

Older children and adults should avoid frequent consumption of drinks and snack foods containing sugars. Chewing sugar-free gum or cheese after meals has a saliva buffer effect that may counter plaque acids. Xylitol has been proposed as preventing caries, however, its recommendation lacks consistent evidence.

American Academy of Pediatric Dentistry. Policy on use of xylitol in caries prevention. *Pediatr Dent.* 2010; 32(special issue):36–38 (see also the AAPD website: http://www.aapd.org).

Fontana M, Gonzalez-Cabezasc C. Are we ready for definitive clinical guidelines on xylitol/polyol use? *Adv Dent Res.* 2012; 24(2):123–128.

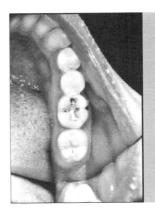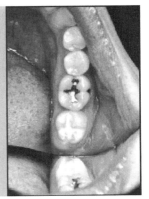

▲ **Figure 46-7.** Dental sealants.

National Institutes of Health. *Diagnosis and Management of Dental Caries throughout Life* (NIH Consensus Statement Online, March 26–28, 2001; 18:1; available at http://consensus.nih.gov/cons/115/115_statement.htm).

PERIODONTAL DISEASE

 ### ESSENTIALS OF DIAGNOSIS

▶ Swelling of the intradental papillae followed by swelling of the gingiva.

▶ Mild gingivitis is painless and may bleed when brushing or eating hard foods.

▶ Shifting or loose teeth with associated alveolar bone loss.

▶ General Considerations

Periodontal disease is the most common oral disease in adults affecting one of every two adults aged >30 years, according to the CDC. Three forms exist: gingivitis, chronic periodontitis, and aggressive periodontitis. It is uncommon among young children, affecting <1%; however in some studies, ≤25% of Hispanic children aged 12–17 years were affected. Like dental caries, periodontal diseases are caused by bacteria in dental plaque that create an inflammatory response in gingival tissues (gingivitis) or in the soft tissue and bone supporting the teeth (periodontitis). Risk factors that contribute to the development of periodontal disease include poor oral hygiene, environmental factors such as crowded teeth and mouth breathing, steroid hormones, smoking, comorbid conditions such as weakened immune status or diabetes, and low income.

Severe gum disease is defined as a 6-mm loss of attachment of the tooth to the adjacent gum tissue. Severe gum disease affects approximately 14% of adults aged 45–54 years and 23% of those aged 65–74 years. Approximately 25% of adults aged ≥65 years no longer have any natural teeth. The severity of periodontal disease does not increase with age. Rather, the disease is believed to occur in random bursts after periods of quiescence.

▶ Pathogenesis

A. Gingivitis

Gingivitis is caused by a reversible inflammatory process that occurs as the result of prolonged exposure of the gingival tissues to plaque. Gingivitis may develop as a result of steroid hormones, which encourage the growth of certain bacteria in plaque during puberty and pregnancy and in women taking oral contraceptive pills.

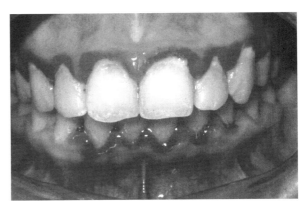

▲ **Figure 46-8.** Gingivitis.

No special tests are needed to diagnose gingivitis; rather, the disease is diagnosed by clinical assessment. Simple or marginal gingivitis may be painless and is treated by good oral hygiene practices such as toothbrushing and flossing. This type of gingivitis occurs in 50% of the population aged ≥4 years. The inflammation worsens as mineralized plaque forms calculus (tartar) at and below the gum surface (sulcus). Gingivitis may persist for months or years without progressing to periodontitis; this fact suggests that host susceptibility plays an important role in the development of periodontitis. Additionally, gingivitis (**Figure 46-8**) can be either acute or chronic. A severe form, acute necrotizing ulcerative gingivitis (ANUG), also known as *Vincent disease* or "trench mouth," is associated with anaerobic fusiform bacteria and spirochetes. ANUG (**Figure 46-9**) is painful, ulcerative, and edematous and produces halitosis and bleeding gingival tissue. Predisposing factors include conditions that contribute to a weakened immune status, such as HIV infection,

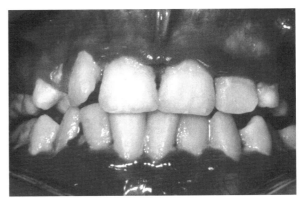

▲ **Figure 46-9.** Acute necrotizing ulcerative gingivitis (ANUG).

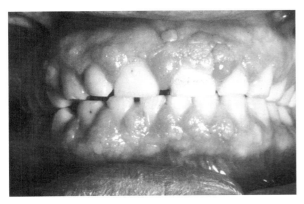

▲ **Figure 46-10.** Gingival enlargement due to drugs.

smoking, malnutrition, viral infections, and, possibly, stress. Chronic gingivitis affects >90% of the population and results in gingival enlargement or hyperplasia that resolves when adequate plaque control is instituted. Generalized gingival enlargement or swelling (gingiva hyperplasia) may be caused by drugs such as calcium channel blockers, phenytoin, and cyclosporin (**Figure 46-10**); by pregnancy; or by systemic diseases such as leukemia, sarcoidosis, and Crohn's disease.

B. Periodontitis

Chronic periodontitis (CP) is caused by chronic inflammation of gingival soft tissue and supporting structures by plaque microorganisms, specifically gram-negative bacteria that affect gingival soft tissues and supporting structures, with resultant loss of periodontal attachment and bony destruction. CP is common in adults, affecting >50% of the population. Adult-onset periodontitis begins in adolescence and is reversible if treated in its early stages, when minimal pockets (gaps) have formed between the tooth and the periodontal attachment. Severe periodontitis is characterized by a 6-mm loss of tooth attachment as detected by the dental health professional by means of dental probes.

If periodontitis is found in children or young adults or if it progresses rapidly, the primary care provider should be alert to the possibility of a systemic cause such as diabetes mellitus, Down syndrome, hypophosphatasia, neutropenia, leukemia, leukocyte adhesion deficiency, or histiocytosis. A less common, rapidly progressing form of adult periodontitis begins in the third or fourth decade of life and is associated with severe gingivitis and rapid bone loss. Several systemic diseases, including diabetes, HIV infection, Down syndrome, and Papillon-Lefèvre syndrome, have been associated with this rare form of periodontitis. Localized juvenile periodontitis (LJP) and localized prepubertal periodontitis (LPP) are forms of early onset periodontitis seen in young children and teenagers, respectively, without the evidence of systemic disease. LJP is more common among African American children. It affects the first molars and incisors, with rapid destruction of bone. Although there is some evidence for autosomal transmission, it is likely heterogenous. Both LJP and LPP are believed to be the result of a bacterial infection (specifically implicated is *Actinobacillus actinomycetemcomitans*) and, possibly, host immunologic deficits.

Clinical Findings

A. Symptoms and Signs

Clinical signs of gingivitis and periodontitis include interdental papillae edema, erythema, and bleeding on contact during tooth brushing or dental probing (**Figure 46-11**). The amount of gingival inflammation and bleeding and the probing depth of gingival pockets determine the severity of periodontal disease. Tartar, gum recession, and loose teeth are characteristics of severe periodontal disease. For children aged <4 years, loss of primary teeth may be the first clinical sign of periodontal disease and the systemic manifestation of hypophosphatasia. Dental probing by the dental health professional will detect sulcus depth.

B. Imaging Studies

Bone loss can be detected by radiographs and bone density scans.

Periodontal Health & Systemic Disease

Emerging evidence, particularly from the dental literature, suggests that periodontal disease may be a risk factor for systemic conditions such as cardiovascular disease, diabetes mellitus, and adverse pregnancy outcomes of preterm labor and low birth weight. Current evidence supports a bidirectional relationship between diabetes and periodontal disease. Periodontal disease is a risk factor for poor glycemic control

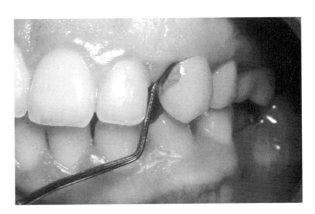

▲ **Figure 46-11.** Gingival inflammation and bleeding.

among diabetic patients, and diabetes is associated with increased severity of periodontal disease. Studies showing the relationship between periodontal disease and cardiovascular disease have proposed that patients with chronic bacterial infection or periodontitis may have (1) a bacteria-induced platelet aggregation defect that contributes to acute thrombolic events, (2) injury to vascular tissue by bacterial toxins, or (3) vascular injury resulting from a host inflammatory response that predisposes the patient to a systemic disorder such as atherosclerosis. Additionally, the link between periodontal disease and preterm labor has several proposed biological mechanisms, one of which is the infection that is mediated by prostaglandins and cytokines among patients with severe periodontitis. This infection causes decreased fetal growth and premature labor.

▶ Differential Diagnosis

Other causes of gingivitis include hormonal changes associated with pregnancy, and systemic disease such as diabetes, Addison disease, HIV, and mechanical injury such as popcorn kernels that might become wedged under the gums.

Gingiva hyperplasia caused by medications such as calcium channel blockers, phenytoin, and cyclosporine cause overgrowth of the gingiva that may occur with or without gingivitis.

▶ Prevention & Treatment

Good oral hygiene is essential for the prevention and control of periodontal diseases. Gingivitis, the mildest form of periodontal disease, is reversible with regular toothbrushing and flossing. Nonsurgical and surgical treatments are available for periodontitis. An added benefit is provided by over-the-counter (OTC) and prescription antimicrobial mouth rinses, such as a 0.1–0.2% chlorhexidine gluconate aqueous mouthwash used twice a day. Caution is advised when chlorhexidine is used because it causes superficial staining of the teeth of patient who drink tea, coffee, or red wine. The treatment of periodontitis includes professional care to remove tartar and may require periodontal surgery.

Because tobacco use is an important risk factor for the development and progression of periodontal disease, patients should be counseled about tobacco cessation. Systemic diseases such as diabetes that may contribute to periodontal disease should be well controlled.

American Academy of Periodontology: http//www.perio.org

Gonsalves W, Chi A. Common oral lesions: part 1. Superficial mucosal lesions. *Am Fam Physician*. 2007; 75:501–507.

Salvi GE, et al. Influences of risk factors on the pathogenesis of periodontitis. *Periodontal*. 2000; 14:173. [PMID: 9567971]

Teng YT, et al. Periodontal health and systemic disorders. *J Can Dent Assoc*. 2002; 68:188. [PMID: 11911816]

Zeeman GG, et al. Focus on primary care: periodontal disease: implications for women's health. *Obstet Gynecol Surv*. 2001; 56:43. [PMID: 11140863]

ORAL & OROPHARYNGEAL CANCERS

ESSENTIALS OF DIAGNOSIS

▶ White or red patch that may progress to ulcer of mucosal surface, endophytic or exophytic growth.

▶ Lesions presenting for >2 weeks need biopsy.

▶ Common distribution of lesions in order of frequency are the tongue, floor of mouth, and lower lip vermilion,

▶ Risk factors include smoking and alcohol use, HPV, lichen planus, and Plummer-Vinson syndrome.

▶ General Considerations

In the United States, cancers of the oral cavity and oropharynx constitute approximately 3% of all cancers among men (the ninth most common cancer among men) and 2% of all cancers among women. The prevalence of these cancers increases with age. Since the 1970s, the incidence of these cancers and the death rates associated with them have been slowly decreasing, except among African American men, for whom the incidence and 5-year mortality estimates are nearly twice as high as for white men.

The overall survival rate for patients with oral and oropharyngeal cancers is only ~51% and has not changed substantially since the early 1990s. However, the 5-year survival estimate for patients with lip carcinoma is >90%; this high survival rate is due in part to early detection. Most oral and oropharyngeal cancers are squamous cell carcinomas that arise from the lining of the oral mucosa. These cancers occur most commonly (in order of frequency) on the tongue, the lips, and the floor of the mouth. Approximately 60% of oral cancers are advanced by the time they are detected, and ~15% of patients have another cancer in a nearby area such as the larynx, esophagus, or lungs. Early diagnosis, which has been shown to increase survival rates, depends on the discerning clinician who recognizes risk factors and suspicious symptoms and can identify a lesion at an early stage.

Table 46-3 shows the risk factors associated with oral and oropharyngeal cancers. Tobacco use and heavy alcohol consumption are the two principal risk factors responsible for 75% of oral cancers. The incidence of oral cancer is higher among persons who smoke or drink heavily than among those who do not.

▶ Prevention

All forms of tobacco, including cigarette, pipe, chewing, and smokeless, have been shown to be carcinogenic in the susceptible host. Alcohol has been identified as another important risk factor for oral cancer, both independently

Table 46-3. Risk factors associated with oral and oropharyngeal cancer.

Tobacco use (smoking or using smokeless tobacco or snuff)
Excessive consumption of alcohol
Viral infections (HSV, HIV, EBV)
Chronic actinic exposure
Betel quid use
Lichen planus
Plummer–Vinson or Paterson–Kelly syndrome
Immunosuppression
Dietary factors (low intake of fruits and vegetables)

EBV, Epstein-Barr virus; HIV, human immunodeficiency virus; HSV, herpes simplex virus.

Table 46-4. Components of an oral cancer examination.[a]

Extraoral examination
Inspect head and neck
Bimanually palpate lymph nodes and salivary glands
Lips
Inspect and palpate outer surfaces of lip and vermilion border
Inspect and palpate inner labial mucosa
Buccal mucosa
Inspect and palpate inner cheek lining
Gingiva/alveolar ridge
Inspect maxillary/mandibular gingiva and alveolar ridges on both the buccal and lingual aspects
Tongue
Have patient protrude tongue and inspect dorsal surface
Have patient lift tongue and inspect ventral surface
Grasping tongue with a piece of gauze and pulling it out to each side, inspect lateral borders of tongue from its tip back to lingual tonsil region
Palpate tongue
Floor of mouth
Inspect and palpate floor of mouth
Hard palate
Inspect hard palate
Soft palate and oropharynx
Gently depressing the patient's tongue with a mouth mirror or tongue blade, inspect soft palate and oropharynx

[a]A good oral examination requires an adequate light source, protective gloves, 2 × 2 gauze squares, and a mouth mirror or tongue blade.

and synergistically when heavy consumers of alcohol also smoke. Therefore, primary prevention in the form of reducing or eliminating the use of tobacco and alcohol has been strongly recommended. The US Preventive Services Task Force (USPSTF) has not endorsed annual screening (secondary prevention) for asymptomatic patients, stating that "there is insufficient evidence to recommend for or against routine screening" and "clinicians may wish to include an examination for cancerous and precancerous lesions of the oral cavity in the periodic health examination of persons who chew or smoke tobacco (or did so previously), older persons who drink regularly, and anyone with suspicious symptoms or lesions detected through self-examination." However, the American Cancer Society and the National Cancer Institute's Dental and Craniofacial Research Group support efforts that promote early detection of oral cancers. The American Cancer Society recommends annual oral cancer examinations for persons aged ≥40 years.

Because primary care providers are more likely than dentists to see patients at high risk of oral and oropharyngeal cancers, providers need to be able to counsel patients about their behaviors and be knowledgeable about performing oral cancer examinations. The primary screening test for oral cancer is the oral cancer examination, which includes inspection and palpation of extraoral and intraoral tissues (**Table 46-4**).

▶ Clinical Findings

A. Symptoms and Signs

Early oral cancer and the more common precancerous lesions (leukoplakia) are subtle and asymptomatic. They begin as a white or red patch, progress to a superficial ulceration of the mucosal surface, and later become an endophytic or exophytic growth. Some lesions are solitary lumps. Larger, advanced cancers may be painful and may erode underlying tissue.

According to the definition of the World Health Organization, leukoplakia is "a white patch or plaque that cannot be characterized clinically or pathologically as any other disease." The lesions may be white, red, or a combination of red and white (called *speckled leukoplakia* or *erythroleukoplakia*). Multiple studies have shown that these lesions undergo malignant transformation. Biopsies have shown that erythroplakia and speckled leukoplakia are more likely than other types of leukoplakia to undergo malignant transformation with more severe epithelial dysplasia. **Figures 46-12** and **46-13** show leukoplakia.

Oropharyngeal carcinomas can be found in the intraoral cavity, the oral cavity proper, and the oropharyngeal sites. The most common intraoral site is the tongue; lesions frequently develop on its posterior lateral border. Lesions also occur on the floor of the mouth and, less commonly, on the gingiva, buccal mucosa, labial mucosa, or hard palate.

A common cancer of the oral cavity proper is lower lip vermilion carcinoma. These lesions arise from a precancerous lesion called *actinic cheilosis*, which is similar to an actinic keratosis of the skin. Dry, scaly changes appear first and later progress to form a healing ulcer, which is sometimes mistaken for a cold sore or fever blister. **Figure 46-14** shows actinic cheilosis.

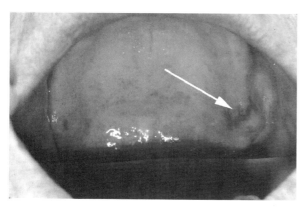

▲ **Figure 46-12.** Leukoplakia.

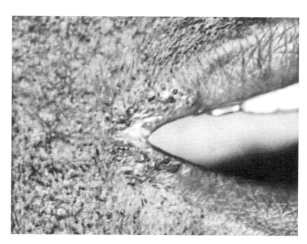

▲ **Figure 46-14.** Actinic cheilosis.

Oropharyngeal carcinomas commonly arise on the lateral soft palate and the base of the tongue. Presenting symptoms may include dysphagia, painful swallowing (odynophagia), and referred pain to the ear (otalgia). These tumors are often advanced at the time of diagnosis. Oral cancer metastasizes regionally to the contralateral or bilateral cervical and submental lymph nodes. Distant metastases are commonly found in the lungs, but oral cancer may metastasize to any other organ.

B. Diagnosis

All patients whose behaviors put them at risk of oral cancer should undergo a thorough oral examination that involves visual and tactile examination of the mouth; full protrusion of the tongue with the aid of a gauze wipe; and palpation of the tongue, the floor of the mouth, and the lymph nodes in the neck. Because oral cancer and precancerous lesions are asymptomatic, primary care providers need to

carefully examine patients who are at risk of oral or oropharyngeal carcinomas. Using a scalpel or small biopsy forceps, the primary care physician should perform a biopsy of any nonhealing white or red lesion that persists for >2 weeks. Alternatively, the patient may be referred to a dentist, an oral surgeon, or a head and neck specialist, who can perform the biopsy. Patients with large lesions or advanced disease should undergo a complete head and neck examination, because 15% of these patients will have a second primary cancer at the time of diagnosis. Neck nodules with no identifiable primary tumor may be evaluated by fine-needle aspiration.

C. Imaging Studies

Imaging studies such as computed tomography with contrast and magnetic resonance imaging of the head and neck are used to determine the extent of disease and involvement of the cervical lymph nodes for the purposes of staging.

▶ Differential Diagnosis

Precancerous white lesions may be confused with frictional keratosis: lesions that result from chronic chewing of the cheek and nicotine stomatitis, a condition with hyerkeratotic epithelial changes on the hard palate as a result of cigarette smoking.

Other white lesions include hairy leukoplakia, geographic tongue, and candidiasis, which should be included in the differential of precancerous lesions.

▶ Treatment

Treatment for oral and lip cancers includes chemotherapy, surgery, radiation, or some combination of these therapies, depending on the extent of the disease. These treatments

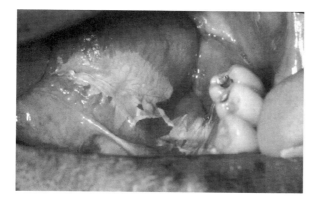

▲ **Figure 46-13.** Leukoplakia.

can cause severe stomatitis (inflammation of the mouth), xerostomia (dry mouth), disfigurement, altered speech and mastication, loss of appetite, and increased susceptibility to oral infection. The management of these complications requires a multidisciplinary team approach by the clinician, oral surgeon, oncologist, and speech therapist. Early diagnosis allows better treatment, cosmetic appearance, and functional outcome and increases the probability of survival. Patients should be encouraged to visit their dental health provider before beginning cancer therapy so that existing health problems can be treated and some complications can be prevented.

Mashberg A, Samit A. Early diagnosis of asymptomatic oral and oropharyngeal squamous cancers. *CA Cancer J Clin*. 1995; 45:328. [PMID: 7583906]

Neville BW, Day TA. Oral cancer and precancerous lesions. *CA Cancer J Clin*. 2002; 52:195. [PMID: 12139232]

Silverman S Jr. Demographics and occurrence of oral and pharyngeal cancers. The outcomes, the trends, the challenge. *J Am Dent Assoc*. 2001; 132; 7S. [PMID: 11803655]

Weinberg MA, Estefan DJ. Assessing oral malignancies. *Am Fam Physician*. 2002; 65:1379. [PMID: 11996421]

▶ Oral Effects of Medications

Medications used to treat certain systemic conditions may have oral manifestations. Most commonly these include xerostomia (dry mouth), gingival hyperplasia, dental caries and erosions, and osteonecrosis of the jaw.

Xerostomia, commonly seen in the elderly, is caused by hypofunction of the salivary gland, but has also been caused by antihypertensives, antidepressants, protease inhibitors, antihistamines, and diuretics. Xerostomia increases the risk of denture sores and caries, since saliva is a lubricant with antimicrobial properties. Symptoms include a sensation of dry mouth. Treatment is avoidance of medications known to cause xerostomia and careogenic foods, good oral hygiene, and salivary substitutes or stimulants.

Gingiva hyperplasia has been associated with calcium channel blockers, methotrexate, cyclosporine, and phenytoin. Dental caries may be caused by syrups such as cough medicines, and dental erosions may follow use of β-blockers, calcium channel blockers, nitrates, and progesterone. Treatment is avoidance of medications associated with gingiva hyperplasia.

Avascular osteonecrosis of the mandible and maxilla have been associated with bisphosphonates. Symptoms include swelling and pain, difficulty eating, bleeding, lower lip paresthesia, and loose and mobile teeth. Since radiographs are nonspecific, lesions should be biopsied for definitive diagnosis. Risk factors include IV bisphosphonates, cancer, invasive dental procedures, smoking, steroid use, radiation therapy, and poor dental hygiene. Patients should be advised to avoid dental procedures while taking these medications.

Gonsalves W, Wrightson AS, Henry R. Common oral problems in older patients. *Am Fam Physician*. 2008; 78(7):845–852.

Ghezzi E, Ship J. Systemic diseases and their treatments in the elderly: impact on oral health. *J Public Health Dent*. 2000; 60(4):289–296.

Turner M, Ship J. Dry mouth and its effects on the oral health of elderly people. *J Am Dent Assoc*. 2007; 138 (suppl):15S–20S.

Global References for Oral Health

Beltram-Aguilar ED, et al. Centers for Disease Control and Prevention: surveillance for dental caries, dental sealants, tooth retention, edentulism and enamel fluorosis—United States, 1988–1994 and 1999–2002. *MMWR Surveill Summ*. 2005; 54:1. [PMID: 16121123]

Office of Disease Prevention and Health Promotion, US Department of Health and Human Services. *Healthy People 2010* (available at http://www.healthypeople.gov/document/html/objectives/21-08.htm; accessed Aug. 23, 2010).

US Department of Health and Human Services. *Oral Health in America: A Report of the Surgeon General—Executive Summary*. DHHS, National Institute of Dental and Craniofacial Research, National Institutes of Health; 2000 (available at http://www.nidr.nih.gov/sgr/execsumm.htm).

Websites

Academy of General Dentistry: http://www.agd.org

American Association of Public Health Dentistry: http://www.aaphd.org

American Dental Association: http://www.ada.org

Centers for Disease Control and Prevention: http://www.cdc.gov/oralhealth

Children's Dental Health Project: http://www.childent.org

Health Resources and Services Administration (HRSA) Oral Health Initiative: http://www.hrsa.gov/oralhealth

National Maternal and Child Oral Health Resource Center: http://www.mchoralhealth.org

Smiles for Life: http://www.smilesfororalhealth.org

US Surgeon General's Report on Children's Oral Health: http://www.nidcr.nih.gov/sgr/sgr.htm

Pharmacotherapy Principles for the Family Physician

Jennie Broders Jarrett, PharmD, BCPS
Elizabeth Cassidy, PharmD, BCPS
Lauren M. Sacha, PharmD

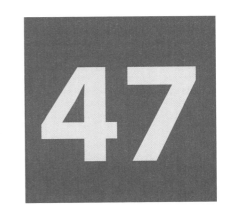

Medication therapy is an integral element of healthcare interventions. In 2011, >4 billion prescriptions were dispensed in the United States. Medication use is often supported by "hard science" and evidence; clinical practice often shifts to the "soft science" of medicine, trying to understand patients, their histories, personalities, medication adherence, and a way to provide the best possible care.

Of the billions of prescriptions filled, it is estimated that half are taken improperly. Achieving a balance between "hard" and "soft" sciences—by providing evidence-based medication therapy that patients will adhere to—becomes paramount. This chapter explores patient adherence; provider's considerations such as evidence, pharmacokinetics/pharmacodynamics, and safety; and healthcare system factors such as formulary systems/resources.

Editorial: the soft science of medicine. *Lancet.* 2004; 363:1247.
Lindsley CW. The top prescription drugs of 2011 in the United States: antipsychotics and antidepressants once again lead CNS therapeutics. *ACS Chem. Neurosci.* 2012; 3(8):630–631.

TAKING A MEDICATION HISTORY

Discrepancies among documented medication therapy records and actual patient use of medications are common and occur with all classes of medications. Therefore, the first step for the provider in determining optimal medication therapy is to understand what medications patients are actually taking and how they are taking them. The physician must also inquire in a nonjudgmental manner whether patients are taking any over-the-counter (OTC) medications, herbal, or vitamin products. Over 17% of the population takes herbal supplements on a yearly basis, but only 45% of these patients report this to their physician. **Table 47-1** lists five concise steps to a medication review. To obtain an accurate medication history, the physician should start by asking open-ended questions; for example, "What medications are you taking?" This approach avoids the common mistake of assuming the patient is taking all their medications as prescribed. Although conducting an open-ended medication history may take more time up front, it may ultimately prevent over- or underprescribing and may also improve patient relationships. *Polypharmacy* is defined as the concurrent use of multiple medications or the prescribing of more medications than are clinically indicated. Polypharmacy can be minimized by a thorough medication regimen review.

Rambhade S, Chakarborty A, Shrivastava A, Patil UK, Rambhade A. A survey on polypharmacy and use of inappropriate medications. *Toxicol Int.* 2012; 19(1):68–73.
Steinke DT, et al. The doctor patient relationship and prescribing patterns: a view from primary care. *Pharmacoeconomics.* 1999;16:599–603.
Tam VC, et al. Frequency, type and clinical importance of medication history errors at admission to hospital: a systematic review. *Can Med Assoc J.* 2005; 173(5):510–515.
Wu CH, Wang CC, Kennedy J. Changes in herb and dietary supplement use in the U.S. adult population: a comparison of the 2002 and 2007 National Health Interview Surveys. *Clin Ther.* 2011; 33(11):1749–1758.

▶ Evaluation & Change

A thorough medication history and safety assessment begins to clarify many aspects of a patient's medication regimen and, paired with evidence, can help the clinician make a solid patient-specific decision about a regimen. *Evidence-based medicine* (EBM) is 'a model for incorporating the tools of clinical epidemiology into clinical practice.' This model entails obtaining the best external evidence to support clinical decisions and is, therefore, not restricted solely to randomized trials and meta-analysis.

Kennedy HL. The importance of randomized clinical trails and evidence-based medicine: a clinician's perspective. *Clin Cardiol.* 1999; 22:6–12.

Table 47-1. Reviewing a medication regimen.

1. Match the medication with the diagnosis
2. Review the regimen for duplication of therapy
3. Elicit from the patient if s/he is taking the medicine
4. Review laboratory results and patient history for efficacy/toxicity of the regimen
5. Strive to remove any unnecessary agents from the regimen

Tilburt JC. Evidence-based medicine beyond the bedside: keeping an eye on context. *J Eval Clin Practice*. 2008; 14(5):721–725.

It is critical to appreciate that EBM does not depend solely on the skills and aptitude of literature evaluation and application of data, but must also incorporate clinical experience. The most commonly reported barrier to practicing EBM is a lack of time. However, the goal of EBM is to provide appropriate allocation of effective and efficient care to all patients. It is estimated that >6 million references have been published in >4000 journals in the National Library of Medicines database, MEDLINE. Slawson and Shaughnessy (2001) propose that the practitioner should approach this "information jungle" with a basic equation:

$$\text{Usefulness} = \frac{\text{Relevance} + \text{Validity}}{\text{Work}}$$

Relevance is directly proportional to its applicability to the physician's practice. Validity relates to the intrinsic methodology, study design, and conclusions. Thus, by maximizing the principles of the usefulness equation, one may locate the best source of information. The mnemonic **p**atient-**o**riented **e**vidence that **m**atters (POEMs) is an easy way for practitioners to focus in on information that can directly affect practice. **Table 47-2** lists EBM-related websites.

Duncan B, et al. Do drug treatment POEMs report data in clinically useful ways? *J Fam Practice*. 2013; 62(2):E1–E5.
Shaughnessy AF, et al. Clinical jazz: harmonizing clinical experience and evidence-based medicine. *J Fam Practice*. 1998; 47:425–428.
Slawson DC, Shaughnessy AF. Becoming an information master. Using "medical poetry" to remove the inequities in health care delivery. *J Fam Practice*. 2001; 50:51–56.
Zwolsman S, et al. Barriers to GPs' use of evidence-based medicine: a systematic review. *Br J Gen Practice*. 2012; 62(600): e511–e521.

EXPLORING THE EVIDENCE: USE OF GUIDELINES & FORMULARIES

Clinical practice guidelines are defined by the Institute of Medicine as "statements that include recommendations intended to optimize patient care which is informed by a

Table 47-2. EBM sources.

Clinical Information Internet Sources
Agency for HealthCare Research and Quality:
 http://www.ahrq.gov
Bandolier:
 http://www.jr2.ox.ac.uk/Bandolier/index.html
Centre for EBM:
 http://www.cebm.net/
The Cochrane Library:
 http://www.cochrane.org
Essential Evidence Plus:
 http://www.essentialevidenceplus.com
Journal of Family Practice POEMS:
 http://www.jfponline.com or http://www.medicalinforetriever.com

Evidence-Based Guideline Websites
Agency for HealthCare Research and Quality:
 http://www.ahrq.gov/clinic
Clinical Evidence, BMJ Publishing Group:
 http://www.clinicalevidence.org
Health Web:
 http://www.health.gov
Institute for Clinical Systems Improvement:
 http://www.ICSI.org
Medical Matrix:
 http://medmatrix.org
National Guideline Clearinghouse:
 http://www.guideline.gov
Primary Care Clinical Practice Guidelines:
 http://medicine.ucsf.edu/resources/guidelines

systematic review of evidence and an assessment of the benefits and harms of alternative care options." Clinical practice guidelines are intended to support clinicians' decision making by providing a comprehensive summary and critique of the available evidence. Several types of evidence-based guidelines exist and the strength of evidence of each is variable. *Evidence-based clinical practice guidelines* incorporate recent literature regarding the effectiveness of therapy and clinical experience. *Expert consensus guidelines* may be the simplest type of guideline; however, limitations to this approach are inherent author bias and limited evidence-based sources. *Outcomes-based guidelines* incorporate measures of effectiveness to validate a positive impact on patient care.

The Cochrane Collaboration produces systematic reviews, maintains a registry of trials, and is a leading provider of evidence-based guidelines. Cochrane reviews may be located in the Cochrane Library, Cochrane Collaboration, or *Cochrane Reviews' Handbook* at the following site: http://www.cochrane.org. In addition to the Cochrane Collaboration, many medical/professional societies, health maintenance organizations, and the Agency for Health Care Policy and Research provide practice guidelines and Internet links to the guidelines.

Coleman CI, et al. A clinician's perspective on rating the strength of evidence of a systematic review. *Pharmacotherapy.* 2009; 29:1017–1029.

Institute of Medicine. *Clinical Practice Guidelines We Can Trust* (available at http://www.iom.edu/Reports/2011/Clinical-Practice-Guidelines-We-Can-Trust.aspx; accessed March 21, 2013).

Formulary systems are fundamental tools of hospitals, health systems, and managed care organizations to designate preferred products and provide rational, cost-effective prescribing decisions. A drug formulary may be defined as "a continuously revised list of medications that are readily available for use within an institution and reflect the current clinical judgment of the medical staff."

Drug formulary policies are based on comparative efficacy, safety, drug interactions, dosing, pharmacology, pharmacokinetics, and cost. Decisions are made by consensus of a pharmacy and therapeutics (P&T) committee made up of healthcare professionals of all major disciplines of practice who serve to represent the medical staff. A P&T committee has been described as "an advisory committee that is responsible for developing, managing, updating, and administering a formulary system." The goal of this body is to guide the appropriate, safe, and cost-effective use of medications.

Boucher BA. Formulary decisions: then and now. *Pharmacotherapy.* 2010; 30:35–41.

Schiff GD, et al. A prescription for improving drug formulary decision making. *PLoS Med.* 2012; 9:1–7.

Taylor LS, et al. ASHP statement on the pharmacy and therapeutics committee and the formulary system. *Am J Health Syst Pharm.* 2008; 65:2384–2386.

BALANCING THE EVIDENCE WITH THE PATIENT

▶ Medication Adherence

"Drugs don't work in patients who don't take them" – C. Everett Coop, MD, former US Surgeon General.

Medication adherence, or the degree to which a patient's medication-taking behaviors comply with a prescribed regimen, represents a serious and insidious barrier to optimal patient care. Many factors may affect adherence to a regimen, including perceived acuity of the disease being treated, regimen complexity, sequelae of the patient's underlying illness, and provider-patient relationships. Regardless of the reasons for nonadherence, it is clear that patients may not receive the full benefit of a medication regimen as a consequence of not taking the medication. In the United States, an estimated 33–69% of medication-related hospitalizations result from poor medication adherence.

While many studies report percentages of "adherence" and "nonadherence" as dichotomous and mutually exclusive variables, the true nature of medication adherence more likely resembles a continuum. Recognizing medication nonadherence and acting to improve patient self-efficacy present opportunities to improve both patient care and provider-patient relationships.

Blaschke TF, et al. Adherence to medications: insights arising from studies on the unreliable link between prescribed and actual drug dosing histories. *Annu Rev Pharmacol Toxicol.* 2012; 52:275–301.

Osterberg L, Blaschke T. Drug therapy: adherence to medication. *N Engl J Med.* 2005; 53:487–497.

Because it is difficult to predict patient adherence behavior, it is critical to identify barriers to adherence that may be controlled or modified. Many techniques may be used to assess compliance, including directly observed therapy, pill counts, review of prescription refill records, and patient interviews. Directly questioning the patient, while efficient and easy to do in an office visit, may create a bias towards perceived compliance that is not actually true. Morisky and colleagues developed a validated four-question assessment to gauge patient adherence behaviors. Patients are asked these questions:

1. Do you ever forget to take your medications?

2. Are you careless at times about taking your medications?

3. When you are feeling better, do you sometimes stop taking your medications?

4. Sometimes if you feel worse, do you stop taking your medications?

Techniques from motivational interviewing may be useful in eliciting useful responses. In particular, empathizing with the patient about their medication regimen may be helpful. For example, a physician might ask about medication adherence while providing support, as in the following example: "I know it is difficult to take all of your medications—how often do you miss taking them?" This approach makes a patient comfortable and allows the physician to gain useful and truthful information.

If nonadherence to a medication regimen is identified, consider assisting the patient by helping them to create a medication list or calendar, provide refill reminders, use a pill organizer, develop a medication reminder chart, or consider electronic devices and compliance services. Additionally, consider referring the patient to their pharmacist for support.

Morisky DE, et al. Current and predictive validity of a self-reported measure of medication adherence. *Med Care.* 1986; 241:67–74.

Clear communication with patients when prescribing new medications is imperative. Improved medication adherence has been associated with patients who receive better general communication, more medication information, and better explanations about how to take medications. Despite the importance of conveying this information, prescribers often fall short. Tarn and colleagues (2006a, b) studied physician communication for new medications and found that physicians failed to describe the medication's name 26% of the time, potential side effects 65% of the time, and cost 88% of the time.

The measurement tool used by Tarn and colleagues, known as the *medication communication index* (MCI), was developed from national guidelines for communication about new medications. This simple five-category index can be used as a guide for the five points to discuss with patients each time a new medication is started: (1) name of the medication, (2) purpose or justification for use, (3) duration of intake, (4) directions for use, and (5) potential adverse effects.

Kripalani S, et al. Development and evaluation of a medication counseling workshop for physicians: can we improve on 'take two pills and call me in the morning?' *Med Educ Online.* 2011; 16:7133.

Tarn DM, et al. Physician communication when prescribing new medications. *Arch Intern Med.* 2006a; 166:1855–1862.

Tarn DM, et al. Physician communication about the cost and acquisition of newly prescribed medications. *Am J Managed Care.* 2006; 12:657–664.

▶ Managing Medication Cost

In 2011, spending on prescription drugs in the United States amounted to $263 billion, or 9.7% of national health expenditures. These costs continue to rise from year to year; between 2001 and 2011, prescription drug spending increased by almost 90%. For patients who have trouble affording their prescriptions, there are several ways to combat the high costs of drug therapy.

If the patient has prescription insurance coverage, prescribing within the payer's formulary will aid in reducing out of pocket costs. Many third-party payers now post their formularies online where patients and providers may easily reference them. Prescribing of generic or lowest-tier drugs is encouraged whenever possible. Some retail pharmacy chains provide generic drug pricing plans that can decrease patients' medication costs even further. Overall medication burden may also cause financial strain for patients. In this case, a thorough medication regimen review may identify drugs that can be discontinued, if medically appropriate.

Centers for Medicare and Medicaid Services. *National Health Expenditure Data.* (available at https://www.cms.gov/Research-Statistics-Data-and-Systems/Statistics-Trends-and-Reports/NationalHealthExpendData/downloads/tables.pdf; accessed March 21, 2013).

National Council on Patient Information and Education. *Enhancing Prescription Medicine Adherence: A National Action Plan* (available at http://www.talkaboutrx.org/documents/enhancing_prescription_medicine_adherence.pdf; accessed March 21, 2013).

For patients who do not have insurance, a few options can be pursued to help them obtain medications at a reduced cost:

1. *A patient aged ≥65 years can apply for drug coverage through Medicare Part D.* To determine which plans the patient is eligible for, and associated costs, visit www.medicare.gov.

2. *Determine whether your patient qualifies for any federal, state, or military-operated program.* Income restrictions apply.

3. *Have contact information available for state Medicaid programs.*

4. *Consider applying for medication assistance programs sponsored by pharmaceutical manufacturers.* Pharmaceutical manufacturers supplied free or low-cost medications to >5 million people in the United States. Several Internet sites are available to aid in obtaining information on how to use these programs, including www.needymeds.com, www.rxhope.com, and www.themedicineprogram.com.

Felder TM, et al. What is the evidence for pharmaceutical patient assistance programs? A systematic review. *J Health Care Poor Underserved* 2011; 22:24–49.

Partnership for prescription assistance: http://www.pparx.org/en/prescription_assistance_programs (accessed March 21, 2013).

ENSURING MEDICATION SAFETY

Patient harm as a consequence of a medical error or drug effect is a common, costly, and largely preventable problem. Fatalities related to adverse drug reactions (ADRs) have been estimated to rank between the fourth and sixth leading cause of death in the United States.

During premarketing trials, if ≥1500 patients are exposed to a drug, the most common ADRs will be detected. However, >30,000 patients must be exposed to the drug in the postmarketing period to detect an ADR in one patient with a power of 0.95 to discover an incidence of 1 in 10,000. For both new and older medications alike, primary care providers play an important role in detecting and reporting unexpected or previously unreported reactions to medications. Physicians can anonymously report ADRs simply by (1) logging onto www.fda.gov/MEDWATCH or calling 800-FDA-1088, or (2) if in a hospital or nursing home setting, contacting the pharmacy or local drug information center. Adverse reactions to vaccines should be reported to the, Vaccine Adverse Event Reporting (VAERS) program, which is cosponsored by the CDC and FDA.

Bates DW, et al. Incidence of adverse drug events and potential adverse drug events: implications for prevention. *JAMA.* 1995;274:29–34.

The Federal Food and Drug Administration (FDA). *Safety Information and Adverse Drug Reporting Program* (available at http://www.fda.gov/Safety/MedWatch/default.htm; accessed March 22, 2013).

Pirmohamed M, et al. Fortnightly review: adverse drug reactions. *Br Med J.* 1998; 316:1295–1298.

Vaccine Adverse Event Reporting System: http://vaers.hhs.gov/esub/index (accessed March 22, 2013).

von Lau NC, et al. The epidemiology of preventable adverse drug events: review of the literature. *Wien Klin Wochenschr.* 2003; 115(12):407–415.

MATCH THE PATIENT & THE DRUG: PHARMACOKINETIC & PHARMACODYNAMIC PRINCIPLES

Although a subset of ADRs is unpredictable, those that are preventable include drug-drug interactions. A grasp of basic pharmacokinetic/pharmacodynamic principles is needed to prevent interactions. Pharmacokinetics characterizes the rate and extent of absorption, distribution, metabolism, and elimination of a drug. Pharmacodynamics is the study of the relationship between the drug concentration at the site of action and the patient response. In reviewing the patient history, consider the following characteristics in relation to drug pharmacokinetics:

- **Age**: Most drugs are studied in adult patients and recommended dosages may vary in different age groups.

- **Gender**: Although data are limited, male and female patients can metabolize and eliminate drugs differently, so the optimal drug dosages may differ.

- **Weight**: For patients who are obese or cachectic, changes in drug absorption, clearance, or volume of distribution may necessitate dosage adjustments or selection of a different drug or dosage form.

- **Disease conditions**: Three conditions that must be approached with special caution when prescribing any drug are heart failure (HF), renal disease, and hepatic failure. As HF progresses, bodily organ blood flow declines; the ensuing drug clearance decline necessitates lower dosages for many agents. As kidney or liver function declines, the renal and hepatic elimination of drugs decreases, leading to lower dosage requirements for renally and hepatically cleared agents, respectively. Additionally, fluid retention that is commonly seen with these diseases may affect drug dosing.

- **Genetics**: Pharmacogenomics is the study of the relationship of genetics in drug metabolism and response. In a systematic review by Phillips and colleagues, of 27 drugs known to frequently cause ADRs, 59% were known to be influenced by individual patient genetic characteristics.

El Desoky ES. Pharmacokinetic-pharmacodynamic crisis in the elderly. *Am J Ther.* 2007; 14(5):488–498.

Kirchheiner J, Seeringer A. Clinical implications of pharmacogenetics of cytochrome p450 drug metabolizing enzymes. *Biochim Biophys Acta.* 2007; 1770(3):489–494.

Pai MP. Drug dosing based on body surface area: mathematical assumptions and limitations in obese patients. *Pharmacotherapy.* 2012; 32:856–868.

Schwartz JB. The current state of knowledge on age, sex, and their interactions on clinical pharmacology. *Clin Pharmacol Ther.* 2007; 82(1):87–96.

DRUG-DRUG INTERACTIONS: UTILIZING PHARMACOKINETIC & PHARMACODYNAMIC PRINCIPLES

Once the patient-specific characteristics noted in the preceding section have been established, the physician can begin to examine the drug-specific characteristics. The main enzymatic system responsible for drug metabolism is the cytochrome P450 (CYP) system. Metabolism through the CYP system occurs mainly in the liver, but CYP isozymes are also found in the intestines and other organs. Identifying different CYP isozymes is an area of ongoing research. There are six isozymes for which there is a reasonable amount of knowledge: CYP 1A2, 2C9, 2C19, 2D6, 2E1, and 3A4. Understanding this system allows prediction of drug-drug interactions among many patients. To do this, it is necessary to identify which drugs are metabolized by the CYP 450 system, and how they interact with the enzyme system. There are three ways in which a drug can interact with the isozymes:

- **Substrate**: Drug is metabolized by an isozyme that is specific for an individual CYP receptor.

- **Inducer**: Drug activates the isozyme system, allowing a greater metabolism capacity.

- **Inhibitor**: Drug competes with another drug(s) for a specific isozyme-binding site, rendering the isozyme inactive.

A review of the patient's medication list may reveal drugs that compete or use the same enzyme system. A change in drug selection may prevent a drug interaction. Physicians may check on whether a drug is a CYP substrate, inducer, or inhibitor in the "interactions" section of drug information resources.

Cupp MJ, Tracy TS. Cytochrome P450: new nomenclature and clinical implications. *Am Fam Physician.* 1998; 57:107–116.

Gex-Fabry, M et al. Therapeutic drug monitoring databases for postmarketing surveillance of drug-drug interactions. *Drug Safety*. 2001; 24:947–959.

KEEPING UP WITH THE LITERATURE

Subscribing to survey services is one way to stay current with the pertinent literature, while decreasing the amount of work and time required. Survey services provide an efficient means of reviewing a host of medical journals and articles. However, one should do this cautiously because of the potential for bias toward positive conclusions or embellishment of study results. The conclusions and recommendations presented by such services should be critically evaluated before applying the information in practice.

Castillo DL, Abraham NS. Knowledge management: how to keep up with the literature. *Clin Gastroenterol Hepatol*. 2008; 6:1294–1300.

Three basic categories of survey services exist: (1) abstracting services, (2) review services, and (3) traditional newsletters. Abstracting services for family medicine practitioners include, but are not limited to, the *ACP Journal Club*, the *Journal of Family Practice*, and *Journal Watch Online*. All have a goal of providing relevant information in a timely manner. *ACP Journal Club* (http://acpjc.acponline.org/) is published by the American College of Physicians–American Society of Internal Medicine. This service provides brief, high-level summaries of current original articles and systematic reviews in a structured abstract format. The *ACP Journal Club* reviews over 100 journals and uses prestated criteria to select and evaluate data. Pertinent information summaries are provided to subscribers on a bimonthly basis. The *Journal of Family Practice* (http://www.jfponline.com) provides family practice physicians with timely, reliable information supplemented with expert commentary on clinically applicable topics. *Journal Watch Online* (http://www.jwatch.org) is supported by the publishers of the *New England Journal of Medicine*. This service, similar to the others, provides current summaries of the most important primary literature. An editorial board, composed of physicians from many specialty areas reviews, analyzes, and summarizes 55–60 critically important articles. The summaries are published on a bimonthly basis. In addition, this service features *Clinical Practice Guidelines Watch* and editorials of the year's top medical stories.

ACP Journal Club: http://acpjc.acponline.org (accessed March 21, 2013).
Journal Watch Online: http://www.jwatch.org (accessed March 21, 2013).
The Journal of Family Practice: http://www.jfponline.com (accessed March 21, 2013).

Review Services provide a succint summary of a specific topic, rather than a survey of the literature. One example of a review service is *The Medical Letter* (http://www.medletter. com). *The Medical Letter* is published by an independent nonprofit organization and provides critical appraisals of new medications or uses for medications in a clinical context, comparing and contrasting the new medications to similar established agents. This concise publication is printed bimonthly. Another example of a review service is *Primary Care Reports* (http://www.ahcpub.com/ahc_root_html/products/newsletters/pcr.html). This service is printed bimonthly and is intended to provide review articles on critical issues in primary care; treatment recommendations are provided with each review.

Primary Care Reports: http://www.ahcpub.com (accessed March 21, 2013).
The Medical Letter: http://www.medletter.com (accessed March 21, 2013).

Traditional newsletters provide brief reviews of current literature with topics from news media and other sources. Examples of this type of newsletter include The *Drug and Therapeutics Bulletin* and *Therapeutics Letter*. The *Drug and Therapeutics Bulletin* (http://www.dtb.bmj.com) is a concise monthly bulletin that provides evaluations of medications and summarizes randomized, controlled, clinical trials, and consensus statements. This service provides informed and unbiased assessments of medications and their overall place in therapy. The *Therapeutics Letter* (http://www.ti.ubc.ca/ TherapeuticsLetter) is a bimonthly newsletter that targets problematic therapeutic issues and provides evidence-based reviews written and edited by a team of specialists and working groups of the International Society of Drug Bulletins.

Drug and Therapeutics Bulletin: http://dtb.bmj.com (accessed March 21. 2013).
Therapeutics Initiative Evidence-Based Drug Therapy: http://www.ti.ubc.ca/TherapeuticsLetter (accessed March 21, 2013).

It is recommended that physicians use these services as a filtering tool to determine which primary literature articles are critical to read in-depth. Survey services provide condensed forms of information, but it is the clinician's responsibility to analyze, interpret, and apply this information effectively in patient care decisions.

DRUG INFORMATION/PHARMACOTHERAPY IN THE DIGITAL ERA

Traditionally, textbooks have been the cornerstone reference for physicians for drug information such as the *Physician's Desk Reference* (PDR), *American Hospital Formulary Services* (AHFS), *Drug Facts and Comparisons* (*Facts & Comparisons*), and the *Drug Information Handbook*. However, as we move into this digital era where instantaneous, accurate information is expected, physicians and residents alike are turning toward their computers and handheld devices for drug information resources.

> Cohen JS. Dose discrepancies between the physician's desk reference and the medical literature, and their possible role in the high incidence of dose-related adverse drug events. *Arch Intern Med.* 2001; 16:957–964.

There are numerous drug information resources available to address general or specific pharmaceutical categories (eg, ADRs, drug interactions, therapeutic use, dosing) that are well referenced with the prescribing information from drug manufacturers, counseling tips and FDA warnings. *MICROMEDEX* is a computerized drug information resource that contains facts from the DRUGDEX Information System. This is a well-referenced, easily searchable, expansive drug information reference, housing information on prescription, nonprescription, and herbal products. *Facts & Comparisons* contains information on prescription and nonprescription medications. This reference provides tables and comparative drug class data along with patient counseling information. *Clinical Pharmacology* is another digital resource available to address drug questions including interaction information and a wide array of printouts available for patient-friendly information. Finally, *Lexicomp* is a thorough drug information resource to search for drug information questions. With a user friendly mobile application, *Lexicomp* is a widely utilized resource.

With increases of natural products, *The Natural Medicines Comprehensive Database* and the National Library of Medicine are two electronic references that consistently provide valid natural production information. *ePocrates Rx* has been advocated by insurance companies and government agencies to enhance clinical management and decrease medication errors.

> *Clinical Pharmacology*: http://www.clinicalpharmacology.com/ (accessed March 30, 2013).
> *ePocrates Rx.* http://www.epocrates.com (accessed March 30, 2013).
> *Facts and Comparisons*: http://www.factsandcomparisons.com/ (accessed March 30, 2013).
> *Lexicomp*: http://www.lexi.com/ (accessed March 30, 2013).
> *MICROMEDEX 2.0*: http://www.micromedex.com/ (accessed March 30, 2013).
> *Natural Medicines Comprehensive Database*: http://www.naturaldatabase.com (accessed March 30, 2013).
> Sweet BV, et al. Usefulness of herbal and dietary supplement references. *Ann Pharmacother.* 2003; 37:494–499.

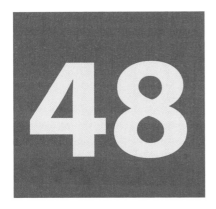

48

Genetics for Family Physicians

W. Allen Hogge, MD

A common misconception in the medical community is that genetic disorders consist of a collection of extremely rare conditions that are seldom relevant to day-to-day clinical practice. In fact, essentially every medical condition affecting humankind has at least some genetic component to its etiology. The study of how mutations in single genes cause rare disease (genetics) is gradually being eclipsed by research on how mutations in multiple genes interact with each other and the environment to result in health and disease (genomics). Knowledge derived from genomic discoveries is reshaping the underpinnings of much of medical practice, and will continue to do so for decades to come. At a practical level, recent advances have taught us a tremendous amount about the basis of common conditions such as diabetes, heart disease, and cancer. This new knowledge is being rapidly translated into approaches for disease risk assessment, prevention, and treatment. Likewise, the study of how genes affect drug metabolism (pharmacogenetics) is being increasingly used to inform drug prescribing (see Chapter 49). Importantly, primary care physicians should not lose sight of the fact that so-called rare single-gene disorders collectively represent a significant proportion of pediatric and adult illnesses.

Primary care physicians are in a unique position to diagnose genetic disorders because they are often the first contact for patients and also provide care for multiple family members. Recognition of, and subsequent attention to, the presence of genetic risk factors for disease in an individual can be lifesaving for individuals and their relatives. Further, as pharmacogenetics becomes increasingly important to drug therapy, primary care providers will need to be aware of and comfortable with ordering and interpreting this type of testing prior to prescribing a variety of medications.

Feero W, et al. Genomic medicine—an updated primer. *N Engl J Med.* 2010; 362:2001–2011. [PMID: 18349096]

GENETIC EVALUATION

▶ Family History

Most common diseases result from a combination of exposure to environmental factors and the effects of variations in multiple genes. Inherited variations confer individual risks that can be distinguishable from the population-based average, and hundreds of such variations have been discovered over the last several years for conditions ranging from schizophrenia to Parkinson disease to coronary artery disease. However, for most conditions the genetic variations discovered to date explain only a small fraction of the heritable component of disease risk in any given individual—for example, in type 2 diabetes well over a dozen genetic variations have been discovered, yet collectively they explain only 5–10% of heritable disease risk.

Obtaining a medical family history provides the most effective current method to rapidly determine whether an individual is at genetic risk of developing common disorders. Additionally, for most individuals family history captures at least some of the environmental and cultural contributors to disease risk. For many common diseases, patient-reported family history of disease in first-degree relatives is highly sensitive and specific. Importantly, common disorders often have modifiable risk factors that can be addressed or for which screening interventions can be instituted (**Table 48-1**). Family history evaluation can also be useful in identifying rare conditions that may not otherwise be considered in a differential diagnosis. For example, a child with developmental delay may have other family members who have had developmental delays or more severe congenital abnormalities. The Office of the US Surgeon General provides an excellent free patient-focused, web-based tool for family history collection called *My Family Health Portrait*.

Sometimes specific questions will suffice when screening for a particular disease. However, recording family

Table 48-1. Disorders for which a positive family history may change screening practices or disease management.

Anemia
Breast cancer
Cardiomyopathy
Colon cancer
Coronary artery disease
Developmental delay
Diabetes mellitus
Dyslipidemia
Emphysema
Gastric cancer
Hearing impairment
Heart failure
Hip dysplasia
Hypertension
Kidney cancer
Liver cancer
Osteoporosis
Pancreatitis
Prostate cancer
Syncope
Thromboembolism
Thyroid cancer
Thyroid disease
Urticaria
Visual impairment

Data from National Human Genome Research Institute, National Institutes of Health, Bethesda, MD.

medical history in the form of a pedigree (**Figure 48-1**) can provide a concise visual tool for recording and interpreting medical information. When obtaining or updating a pedigree, the following general information may be recorded: patient name; date recorded or updated; consanguinity (note relationship); ethnic background of each grandparent, if known; and name and credentials of the person who recorded the pedigree. It is often helpful to include a key that explains symbols used in the pedigree (see Figure 48-1). Specific information such as age, relevant health information, age at diagnosis, age at death (with year, if known), cause of death, infertility (if known), and information about pregnancies (including miscarriages, stillbirths, and pregnancy terminations, along with gestational ages) is then obtained for each listed family member.

The American College of Medical Genetics recommends the followings five questions as good starting points for obtaining information on key genetic issues:

1. Are there any health problems that are known to run in your family, or that close relatives have been told are genetic?

2. Has anyone in your family had cancer, heart disease, or other adult-onset medical conditions at an early age (between 20 and 50 years old)?

3. Does/did anyone in the family have intellectual disabilities, have learning problems, or have to go to a special school?

4. Have there been early deaths in the family, including stillbirths, infant deaths, multiple miscarriages, or childhood deaths?

5. Has any relative had extreme or unexpected reactions to medications or anesthesia?

As a family medicine physician, you should ask an important sixth question:

6. Have there been any problems with pregnancy, issues with infertility, or birth defects in your family?

It is essential to use terminology that is understandable to the family. Although, the medically correct term is *intellectual disability*, the patient may regard the uncle as having "mental retardation" or as being "slow." Likewise, all bleeding disorders may be described as "hemophilia," even in women. When the pedigree suggests a potential risk to the patient or her offspring, obtaining medical records is essential to providing adequate genetic counseling.

▶ **Inheritance Patterns**

A pedigree can help to identify a pattern of inheritance for a particular disorder, which can be useful in establishing a diagnosis. For example, if mental retardation is present in more than one generation in a family and only male family members are affected, an X-linked disorder should be considered. **Table 48-2** reviews clues to determine patterns of inheritance. Unfortunately, limited collection of family history data, small family size, nonpaternity, delayed age of onset of symptoms, mild expression of disease symptoms, and sex-limited expression of disease symptoms (eg, a woman with a healthy father whose sisters have breast and ovarian cancer) can complicate the identification of patterns of inheritance.

▶ **Ethnic and Racial Background Implications**

As part of the pedigree, the racial and ethnic origins of the patient and her spouse should be noted. Certain geographic, ethnic, and racial groups are at relatively high risk for otherwise rare genetic disorders. The high frequency reflects both evolutionary forces, and geographic/cultural isolation. For example, sickle cell carriers of African ancestry seem to carry some protection from malaria. On the other hand, individuals of Ashkenazi Jewish ancestry are at risk for certain disorders, such as Tay-Sachs disease, because of a combination of geographic and cultural issues that are part of their heritage. **Table 48-3** outlines diseases prevalent in certain racial/ethnic groups.

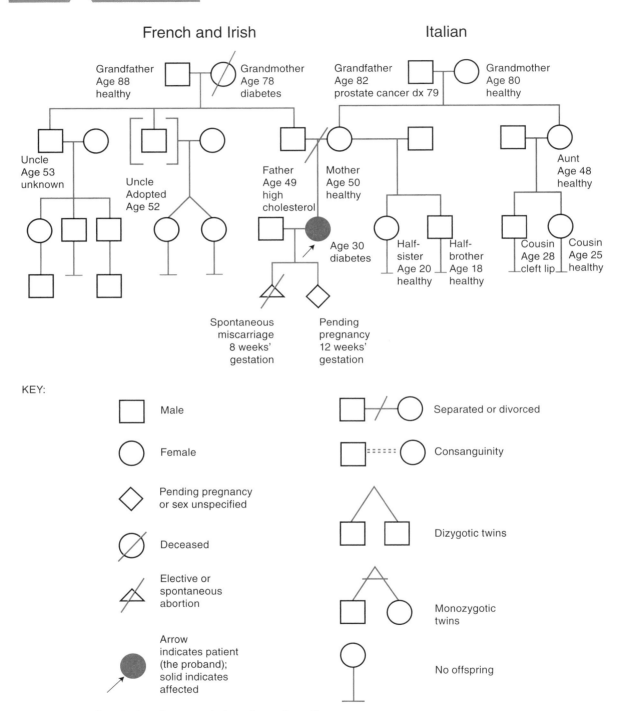

▲ Figure 48-1. Standard pedigree symbols and sample pedigree.

Table 48-2. Clues to determine patterns of inheritance.

Pattern[a]	Diagnostic Clues
Autosomal-dominant	Males and females equally affected Transmission passes from one generation to another (vertical inheritance) 50% risk for each offspring to be affected Variable expressivity: affected individuals in the same family may demonstrate varying degrees of phenotypic expression (severity) Reduced penetrance: some individuals who have inherited a genetic mutation may not express the phenotype ("skipped generations" may be seen)
Autosomal-recessive	Males and females equally affected Multiple affected offspring and unaffected parents (horizontal inheritance) 25% risk for each offspring to parents with an affected child
X-linked-recessive	Affects more males than females Heterozygous females are usually normal or have mild manifestations Inheritance is through maternal side of the family (diagonal inheritance) Female carriers have a 50% risk for each daughter to be a carrier and a 50% risk for each son to be affected All daughters of an affected male are carriers, and none of his sons are affected
Multifactorial or complex	Risk highest for closest relatives to affected individuals Multiple genes and environmental factors may contribute to risk No well-defined pattern of inheritance in pedigree; "runs in the family"

[a]For more complex patterns of inheritance, see Korf B. Basic genetics. *Prim Care Clin Office Practice.* 2004; 31:461.

▶ Medical History "Red Flags"

In addition to family history, there are certain clinical clues derived from the patient that should alert a clinician to consider a genetic cause for a medical condition (**Table 48-4**). Important issues to consider in all age groups are multiple congenital anomalies, earlier than usual onset of common conditions, extreme pathology (eg, rare tumors or multiple primary cancers), developmental delay or degeneration, and extreme laboratory values (eg, extremely high cholesterol level).

Whelan A, et al. Genetic red flags: clues to thinking genetically in primary care practice. *Prim Care Clin Office Practice.* 2004; 31:497. [PMID: 15331244]

Websites

The American Medical Association has a pamphlet available online entitled *Family Medical History in Disease Prevention*: http://www.ama-assn.org/ama1/pub/upload/mm/464/family_history02.pdf.

The US Department of Health and Human Services, through the Surgeon General's Family Health History Initiative, makes available *My Family Health Portrait Tool*, which can be used by families to create a family history (https://familyhistory.hhs.gov).

The National Society of Genetic Counselors has available a guide for constructing a family history that is family-friendly: http://www.nsgc.org/Publications/ShopNSGC/tabid/55/pid/33/default.aspx.

CLINICAL GENETICS

▶ Genetic Counseling

Although there have been many attempts to define what it means to provide genetic counseling, the provision of genetic counseling is a process that needs to vary depending on the specific clinical circumstances. In the case of a patient seeking genetic counseling because of a cousin with cystic fibrosis, the components of the session likely will include a discussion of the natural history of cystic fibrosis, an explanation of autosomal-recessive inheritance and the risk that the patient and her partner are carriers of the gene, and finally a summary of available testing to determine their exact carrier status. Prior to providing this in-depth information a complete medical, family, and social history would be obtained to identify any other factors that could impact a future pregnancy.

Counseling in their circumstance should be nondirective; that is, the counselor provides the information necessary for the individual or couple to make informed decisions. This type of counseling is important, especially in a circumstance where both members of the couple are subsequently found to be carriers of the cystic fibrosis gene. The reproductive options available to them should be explained fully, and without bias. These options will range from not having children to preimplantation genetic diagnosis. The role of the counselor (either a trained genetic professional or a primary care physician) is to provide an explanation of each option,

Table 48-3. Examples of genetic disorders seen in specific ethnic and racial groups

Racial or Ethnic Group	Genetic Disorder	Inheritance
African American	Sickle cell disease	AR
	Glucose-6-phosphate dehydrogenase deficiency	XLR
Amish/Mennonite	Maple syrup urine disease	AR
	Chondroectodermal dysplasia (Ellis–van Crevald syndrome)	AR
	Cartilage-hair hypoplasia	AR
	McKusick-Kaufman syndrome	AR
	Limb girdle muscular dystrophy	AR
	Glutaric aciduria type I	AR
Ashkenazi Jewish	Tay-Sachs disease	AR
	Canavan disease	AR
	Gaucher disease type 1	AR
	Hereditary breast/ovarian cancer	AD
	Sensorineural deafness	AR
	Familial dysautonomia	AR
	Mucolipidosis type IV	AR
	Niemann-Pick disease type A	AR
Finnish	Hereditary nephrosis	AR
	Cartilage-hair hypoplasia	AR
	Infantile neuronal ceroid lipofuscinosis	AR
French Canadian	Leigh syndrome, French Canadian type	AR
	Hereditary multiple intestinal atresia	AR
	Tyrosinemia type I	AR
	Tay-Sachs disease	AR
	Cystinosis	AR
	Pseudo–vitamin D deficiency rickets	AR
Mediterranean (Italian, Greek, North African)	β-Thalassemia	AR
	Glucose-6-phosphatate dehydrogenase deficiency	XLR
Middle Eastern	β-Thalassemia	AR
	Familial Mediterranean fever	AR
Portuguese	Machado-Joseph disease	AR
Puerto Rican	Hermansky-Pudlak syndrome	AR
Southeast Asians	α-Thalassemia	AR
	β-Thalassemia	AR

AD, autosomal-dominant; AR, autosomal-recessive; XLR, X-linked-recessive.

including the risks and benefits of each approach. There is no place for the provision of "recommendation."

On the other hand, providing genetic counseling to a 35-year-old woman who has just been found to be carrying a **BRCA1** mutation is likely to include precise information on current recommendation regarding prophylactic mastectomy and oophorectomy. The role of the counselor is to recognize when there are clear evidence-based guidelines, and present the options available to ensure that the patient's decisions will be based on balanced and complete information.

The current standard of care dictates that genetic counseling should be provided to patients prior to initiating DNA-based, clinically driven genetic testing. However, this model is impractical for certain commonly ordered tests in primary care (eg, thrombophilia testing), and will be increasingly problematic as more single-platform tests for predisposition for multiple common conditions become available. Depending on the primary care provider's level of comfort with the disorder to be tested for and the testing modality being offered, counseling might best be delivered by that provider or by a genetic specialist. Appropriate counseling, regardless of who provides the service, has several key elements. Pretest counseling should involve discussion of the mode of inheritance and risk of the condition for the patient

Table 48-4. Genetic "red flags."

Preconceptual/Prenatal	Pediatric	Adult
Personal or family history of known or suspected genetic disorder or congenital abnormality Two or more pregnancy losses Unexplained infertility Ethnic predisposition to genetic disorder Mother ≥aged 35 years at time of delivery (increased risk of chromosome abnormalities) Abnormal maternal serum screening Abnormal fetal ultrasound Exposure to teratogen Maternal condition that affects fetal development Parents with close biological relationship	One or more major malformations or dysmorphic features Abnormal newborn screening Abnormal development Congenital hearing loss Congenital blindness or cataracts Constellation of features suggestive of genetic disorder or chromosome abnormality Family history of known or suspected genetic disorder Personal or family history of hereditary cancers Development of degenerative neurologic disorder or unexplained seizures	Family history of known or suspected genetic disorder Diagnosis of common disorder with earlier age of onset than typical, especially if multiple family members are affected (eg, cancer, heart disease, stroke, diabetes mellitus, hearing or vision loss, degenerative neurologic disorder), unusual manifestation of disease (eg, male breast cancer, multiple primary cancers) Pediatric indications that have not yet been evaluated

and family members; the natural history of the condition; prognosis; presentation of appropriate testing options and interventions, including their risks, benefits, and limitations; discussion of the voluntary nature of genetic testing; and exploration of the social and familial implications of testing. These issues constitute the basis for informed consent, which should be documented before initiating DNA testing.

Posttest counseling involves the proper interpretation of results to the patient, including implications for further testing, management, and risks for other family members. It also may involve continued emotional support and referral to mental health professionals or disease-specific support groups, even for those who have tested negative for a particular disorder that may run in their family, due to feelings of guilt or sadness.

Family medical history or clinical clues may lead a clinician to consider genetic testing. Many primary care providers may be unfamiliar with a particular genetic disorder or the availability of genetic testing for a disorder. GeneTests (http://www.genetests.org) is a web-based resource that contains concise reviews and information on genetic testing availability for many genetic disorders. This website also provides information regarding access to genetic specialists, including medical geneticists (physicians who have residency training in genetics), genetic counselors (individuals with master's degree–level training in genetics), and PhD-qualified individuals with formal clinical genetics training.

Overview of Genetics

Human genetic information is contained in DNA and is present in nearly every cell in the human body. DNA consists of two long, paired strands of chemical bases called *nucleotides*. When cells divide, the DNA is compacted into complex structures composed of DNA and proteins called *chromosomes*; somatic cells have 46 chromosomes that are arranged in 23 pairs. The first 22 pairs, called *autosomes*, contain the genetic information for both men and women. The chromosomes that determine sex (X and Y) are paired as XX for females and XY for males. One chromosome from each pair is inherited from the mother and the other from the father. The germ cells or gametes (sperm and egg cells) contain only 23 chromosomes.

Chromosomes contain the thousands of genes that are the basis of inheritance. It is estimated that the human genome consists of ~20,000 protein coding genes. Genes consist of short segments of DNA along each chromosome that encode the blueprint for a protein or RNA molecule along with sequences of DNA that are likely involved in the control of gene expression. Each gene comes in a pair; one copy of each gene is inherited from an individual's father and the other from his/her mother. The coding region of each gene specifies the instructions for a particular protein or RNA molecule according to the order in which the nucleotides are arranged. Proteins are responsible for the development and functioning of our bodies. RNA molecules play important roles. During cell replication and division, errors can occur in the DNA sequence (*mutations*), resulting in a protein that does not function properly or is present in insufficient amounts. Occasionally errors such as large deletions or rearrangements of chromosome structure occur that affect the function of multiple genes.

Methods of Genetic Testing

It is difficult to define what constitutes a "genetic" test. A test involving DNA or chromosome studies may be considered a genetic test but may not provide information about a person's inherited genetic identity. An example of this type of "genetic" testing is the use of chromosome studies in the subclassification of leukemia. Conversely, tests that are considered routine, and not necessarily "genetic," such as a cholesterol panel, have the potential to reveal genetic information about individuals and their family members.

The test method used to detect a genetic disorder depends on what the genetic change associated with a particular condition primarily affects [eg, in the chromosomes, genes, or proteins (gene products)]. The primary laboratory methods used are cytogenetic analysis, DNA testing, and biochemical tests.

The type of genetic test used for testing has moved increasingly toward some form of DNA-based methodology. Classic cytogenetic analysis to identify abnormalities in the number or structure of chromosomes is still used in certain circumstances when a change in number of chromosomes (eg, Down syndrome) is expected. However, in most diagnostic circumstances, molecular cytogenetics, using techniques such as fluorescence *in situ* hybridization (FISH) and array comparative genomic hybridization (microarrays), is used to detect small genetic changes that are below the resolution of traditional cytogenetic methods.

Several methods are used to detect single-gene mutations. These include Southern blot analysis, multiplex polymerase chain reaction analysis, allele-specific oligonucleotide hybridization, microarrays, and direct gene sequencing. Direct gene testing may be indicated for patients affected by or predisposed to a condition for which the gene change(s) that cause the condition have been identified (eg, cystic fibrosis, thrombophilia, hereditary breast and ovarian cancer syndrome). It may also be indicated in the setting of prescribing certain medications in order to avoid side effects [eg, abacavir hypersensitivity in human immunodeficiency virus (HIV) therapy] or to select appropriate therapies for patients (eg, *KRAS* mutation testing prior to using cetuximab in colorectal cancer).

Biochemical techniques such as metabolite testing, organic acid analysis, amino acid analysis, and assays of specific enzymes or proteins are used to identify or quantify absent or accumulated metabolites or measure the activity of a specific enzyme. These tests are commonly used to help diagnose and monitor disorders such as hemochromatosis, familial hyperlipidemia, and the thrombophilias. Classically, biochemical tests are used to confirm the diagnosis of an inborn error of metabolism (eg, phenylketonuria, Tay-Sachs disease, Hurler syndrome).

What a Genetic Test Can Reveal

Before ordering testing for heritable disorders, clinicians should carefully consider the relevance and the implications of the testing for their patient. Genetic testing is typically considered to fall into several major categories, which help to determine how the test can be used for clinical decision making for a patient or her/his family members. *Diagnostic testing* is used to confirm or identify a known or suspected genetic disorder in a symptomatic individual. This type of testing may also include assays that help to inform prognosis and treatment decisions in someone with an established disease diagnosis. *Predictive testing* is offered to an asymptomatic individual with or without a family history of a genetic disorder to better define their risk of developing a given condition. Patients are further defined as *presymptomatic* if eventual development of symptoms is certain (eg, Huntington disease) or *predispositional* if eventual development of symptoms is likely but not certain (ie, colon cancer). *Carrier testing* is offered to appropriate individuals who have a family member with an autosomal-recessive or X-linked condition (eg, the sister of a boy with Duchenne muscular dystrophy) or individuals in an ethnic group known to have a high carrier rate for a particular disorder (eg, sickle cell anemia in the African American population). *Pharmacogenetic* testing is used to help guide selection and dosing of medications for drug therapy. *Prenatal testing* is performed during a pregnancy and is offered when there is an increased risk of having a child with a genetic condition. *Preimplantation testing* is performed on early embryos during *in vitro* fertilization and offered to couples who are at increased risk of having a child with a genetic condition. *Newborn screening* is performed during the newborn period and identifies children who may have an increased risk of a specific genetic disorder so that further evaluation and treatment can be initiated as soon as possible.

Table 48-5 summarizes points to consider with each type of genetic testing.

Ethical, Legal, & Social Issues

Many issues can arise when individuals are faced with the diagnosis of or susceptibility to a genetic disorder. Critical issues to consider include, but certainly are not limited to

- Privacy (the rights of individuals to control access to information about themselves).

- Informed consent (giving permission to do genetic testing with the knowledge of the risks, benefits, effectiveness, and alternatives to testing).

- Confidentiality (acknowledgment that genetic information is sensitive, and that access should be limited to those authorized to receive it).

- Insurance and employment discrimination. In 2008 the Genetic Information Nondiscrimination Act (GINA) became law, providing baseline national protections in the United States that prohibit the use of genetic test results (including family history) to discriminate for employment or health insurance purposes in asymptomatic individuals. It does not prevent the use of such

Table 48-5. Considerations in the use of genetic testing.

Type of Test	Considerations
Diagnostic	Confirming a diagnosis may alter medical management Genetic testing may yield diagnostic information at a lower cost and with less risk than other procedures May have reproductive or psychosocial implications for patient and other family members Negative result requires further testing or follow-up May be used to provide prognosis
Predictive	Indicated if early diagnosis allows interventions that reduce morbidity or mortality When possible and appropriate, identification of the specific genetic mutation should be established in an affected relative first Likelihood of showing disease symptoms is increased but is frequently considerably <100% Can have psychosocial implications and can influence life Testing of asymptomatic children at risk for adult-onset disorders is strongly discouraged when no medical intervention is available
Pharmacogenetic	Testing for metabolism of one drug may have implications for other drugs Relatively unlikely to have psychosocial implications
Carrier	Identification of the specific genetic mutation in an affected family member may be required May have reproductive or psychosocial implications Can improve risk assessment for members of ethnic groups that are more likely to be carriers for certain genetic disorders
Prenatal	Invasive prenatal diagnostic procedures (eg, amniocentesis, chorionic villus sampling) have an associated risk to fetus In most cases, a specific genetic mutation must be known in an affected relative (eg, mother with myotonic dystrophy) Prenatal testing for adult-onset disorders is controversial, and parents should receive a complete discussion of the issue
Preimplantation	Only performed at a few centers and available for a limited number of disorders Because of possible errors in preimplantation procedures and DNA analysis, traditional prenatal diagnostic procedures (amniocentesis, chorionic villus sampling) are recommended Cost is very high and may not be covered by insurance
Newborn screening	Usually legally mandated and varies by state Not designed to be diagnostic Further clinical evaluation and patient education is necessary with positive screening results Parents may not realize that testing was done

information in life, long-term care, or disability insurance underwriting. Several states have enacted laws to protect individuals from genetic discrimination by insurance companies or in the workplace. The Health Insurance Portability and Accountability Act (HIPAA) also provides some protection from discrimination.

- Nonpaternity or unknown adoption. This information can be unexpectedly revealed through genetic testing.

- Duty to warn (the obligation to disclose information to at-risk relatives if they are in clear and imminent danger). On rare occasions, this duty may require a healthcare professional to consider breaching patient confidentiality.

- Patient autonomy (the obligation to respect the decision-making capacities of patients who have been fully informed with accurate and unbiased information).

- Professional limitations (the duty of clinicians to realize the extent of their knowledge, skills, attitude, or behavior as they pertain to their practice and the laws, rules, regulations, and standards of care).

Clayton E. Ethical, legal, and social implications of genomic medicine. *N Engl J Med.* 2003; 349:562. [PMID: 12904522]

Hudson K, et al. Keeping pace with the times—the Genetic Information Nondiscrimination Act of 2008. *N Engl J Med.* 2008; 358:2661. [PMID: 18565857]

Website

National Human Genome Research Institute: http://www.genome.gov/PolicyEthics/.

EXAMPLES IN PRACTICE

▶ Case 1

A 25-year-old patient presents to you for an annual examination. Evaluation of her family history reveals that her paternal grandmother and a paternal aunt died of breast cancer in their early 40s.

Screening for familial cancer is an important part of the initial evaluation of a patient, and should be a regular part of each subsequent visit to assess any changes in the family history. Primary care physicians have an important role in identifying those patients with a potentially hereditary cancer syndrome. Although practicing physicians are not expected to be familiar with all the hereditary cancer syndromes, they should be able to recognize the key features in a family history that suggest that the patient may be at risk, and make an appropriate referral for evaluation and counseling.

Hereditary Cancer Syndromes

1. Hereditary breast and ovarian cancer—This is a dominantly inherited syndrome most commonly caused by germline mutations in the genes *BRCA1* and *BRCA2*. In the general population the mutated gene is found in approximately one in every 500 persons, but in those of Ashkenazi Jewish ancestry the cancer frequency is 1 in every 40 individuals. However, the majority of breast and ovarian cancers are sporadic, as only 5–10% of them are caused by a *BRCA1* or *BRCA2* (*BRCA1/2*) mutation.

Key features strongly suggestive of a *BRCA1/2* mutation would be early onset of breast or ovarian cancer in a patient, a family history with multiple affected members, or the presence in the family history of both breast and ovarian cancer. It is important to recognize that males who carry one of these mutations may be asymptomatic, but also are at risk for breast, prostate, and pancreatic cancer. Even in women with the mutation, the gene is not completely penetrant. For a female with the mutation there is 40–66% lifetime risk of breast cancer, and ≤46% risk of ovarian cancer. These risks are significantly higher than the US general population risk of 12% for breast cancer and 1.5% for ovarian cancer. In addition, many of these cancers will occur before age 50. Equally of concern is the risk of breast cancer in the contralateral breast, which is between 40% and 65% over a lifetime, and ≤30% 10 years postdiagnosis.

Patients with early-onset breast or ovarian cancer, or those with family histories similar to that seen in the case study, should be referred to individuals trained in cancer genetic counseling for evaluation and genetic testing. If the patient is found to carry a pathogenic mutation, an appropriate management plan needs to be developed to include both screening options and prophylactic surgical options.

The absence of a known pathogenic mutation does not exclude the possibility that the family has a hereditary form of breast and/or ovarian cancer. In addition to the other known syndromes outlined below, there are likely many other cancer-causing gene mutations that have yet to be discovered. In the presence of a strong family history, but negative gene testing, it is essential that a comprehensive screening plan be developed for the potentially at-risk patient.

2. Hereditary nonpolyposis colon cancer (Lynch syndrome)—A family history of early-onset colon cancer, and other cancers, such as ovarian or endometrial, should raise suspicion of Lynch syndrome, and prompt a referral for genetic counseling and gene testing for the DNA mismatch genes that are commonly mutated in this disorder. In addition to the associated gynecologic cancers, a wide variety of other cancers may be found in these families, including gastric, small intestine, biliary, brain, skin, and pancreatic. In the patient identified with the Lynch syndrome, a comprehensive screening plan including both a gastroenterologist and a gynecologist is essential, as the risk for ovarian cancer and endometrial cancer may be ≤12% and ≤60%, respectively.

3. Li-Fraumeni syndrome—This condition is highly penetrant with a 90% risk of cancer by age 60. Most cases are due to germline mutations in the tumor suppression genes, *p53* and *CHEK2*. Soft-tissue sarcomas, often expressed in children or young adults, are the most common cancers. However, breast cancer is a commonly associated cancer, as are bone, brain, and adrenal cancers. Unlike most of the other cancer-predisposing genes, the frequency of *de novo* mutations is quite high (7–20%). In certain circumstances gene testing may be offered in the absence of a positive family history.

▶ General Considerations

Patients with family history or a personal history of early-onset cancers, bilateral cancers in paired organs, male breast cancer, or cancer affecting multiple generations should be referred for genetic counseling (see **Table 48-6**). Current guidelines suggest that even in the absence of any family history of breast or ovarian cancer that patients with ovarian, primary peritoneal, and fallopian tube cancers should be referred for genetic counseling and possible *BRCA1/2* mutation testing. In patients of Ashkenazi Jewish descent, a personal history of breast cancer at any age may be considered an indication for genetic testing. Assessing both the

Table 48-6. Indicators of hereditary cancer susceptibility in a family.

Cancer in two or more first-degree relatives
Multiple cancers in multiple generations
Early age of onset (ie, <50 years for adult-onset cancers)
Multiple cancers in a single individual
Bilateral cancer in a paired organ such as breasts, kidneys, or ovaries
Presence of rare cancers in family (eg, male breast cancer)
Recognition of a known association between etiologically related cancers in the family, such as breast and ovarian cancer (hereditary breast ovarian cancer) or adrenocortical carcinoma and breast cancer (Li-Fraumeni syndrome)
Presence of congenital anomalies associated with an increased cancer risk
Presence of precursor lesions known to be associated with cancers (atypical nevi and risk of malignant melanoma)
Recognizable pattern of inheritance

maternal and paternal family history is important because the gene mutation, although inherited in an autosomal dominant fashion, may not manifest in a male. Genetic counseling provides the patient a detailed risk assessment, options for genetic testing, and appropriate interpretation of the results of testing, if done. Patients found to be at risk for a hereditary cancer syndrome should be managed by a multidisciplinary team with expertise in cancer genetics.

Overview of Genetic Testing for Hereditary Cancer

When a decision is made to proceed with genetic testing, the testing should first be offered to the person affected by the cancer in question. If that person is positive for one of the known gene mutations, then precise testing should be available for other, potentially at-risk, but unaffected, relatives; such testing is equally important for the person affected, as any information of a positive test for a relative places the person at risk for a second primary cancer, and an appropriate surveillance plan must be put in place.

If a mutation is identified in the family, a negative test in other relatives removes them from the high-risk category. On the other hand, they remain at risk for sporadic cancers, and should have screening that is appropriate for the general population. A positive test for a *BRCA1/2* mutation requires a multidisciplinary approach to management. **Table 48-7** outlines a sample management plan, but these guidelines can change rapidly, and consultation with a cancer genetics professional should always precede implementation of any management plan.

Table 48-7. Management of a Patient with BRCA 1/2 Mutation

Screening for breast cancer
Monthly breast self-exam beginning at age 18
Physician breast exams every 6–12 months beginning at age 25
Mammography beginning at age 25; frequency should be at least annually; more often, and to include breast MRI, if clinically indicated

Screening for ovarian cancer
Bimanual pelvic exam every 6–12 months from age 25
Serum CA-125 at least annually beginning at age 30
Transvaginal ultrasound with Doppler assessment, beginning at age 35

Risk reduction options
Consider tamoxifin after age 35
Consider oral contraceptives for both contraception and ovarian cancer risk reduction
Consider prophylactic mastectomy
Oophorectomy is strongly recommended by age 40, or when childbearing is complete

Data from Peshkin BN, Isaacs C. Evaluation and management of women with BRCA1/2 mutations. *Oncology.* 2005; 19:1451-1459.

In addition to the development of a management plan, cancer geneticists can address only psychological effects of a positive diagnosis, and provide information to the patient on implications for other family members who may be at risk.

There are two problematic areas in genetic testing. The first is that of the *indeterminate negative*. In these families the family history is strongly suggestive of autosomal-dominant inheritance, but no causative mutation is found in the family. These patients should be cautioned against interpreting the failure to find a mutation as a negative result. These patients should be treated as high-risk patients with increased surveillance, despite the absence of a common genetic mutation.

The second area of confusion for patients is the **indeterminate positive** result. Full sequencing of *BRCA1/2*, as well as other cancer susceptibility genes, may detect variants of uncertain clinical significance (VUS). These variants, often a single nucleotide change, have an unknown impact on protein function. Population studies will, in some cases, identify the variant as either benign or deleterious, but most will not have been categorized. In general the finding of a VUS should not be used to modify the care of a patient or her family.

Aarnio M, Sankila R, Pukkala E, et al. Cancer risk in mutation carriers of DNA-mismatch-repair genes. *Int J Cancer.* 1999; 81(2):214–218. [PMID: 10188721]

Chen S, Parmigiani G. Meta-analysis of *BRCA1* and *BRCA2* penetrance. *J Clin Oncol.* 2007; 25(11):1329–1333. [PMID: 17416853] [PMCID: PMC2267287]

Daly MB, Axilbund JE, Buys S, et al. Genetic/familial high-risk assessment: breast and ovarian. *J Natl Compr Canc Netw.* 2010; 8(5):562–594. [PMID: 20495085]

Gonzalez KD, Buzin CH, Noltner KA, et al. High frequency of de novo mutations in Li-Fraumeni syndrome. *J Med Genet.* 2009; 46(10):689–693. [PMID: 19556618]

Kurian AW. *BRCA1* and *BRCA2* mutations across race and ethnicity: distribution and clinical implications. *Curr Opin Obstet Gynecol.* 2010; 22(1):72–78. [PMID: 19841585]

Peshkin BN, Isaacs C. Evaluation and management of women with BRCA1/2 mutations. *Oncology.* 2005; 19:1451–1459. [PMID: 16370446]

Case 2

Mr. Jones, a 45-year-old man, presented with a 1-year history of gradually worsening fatigue and diffuse arthralgias. His friends frequently compliment him on his healthy tan. Laboratory testing showed mildly elevated liver transaminases, despite his lack of recreational sun exposure. Testing for viral hepatitis was negative, but his ferritin level was elevated. Further testing revealed a markedly elevated fasting transferrin iron saturation. Genetic testing confirmed hereditary hemochromatosis.

Hemochromatosis is a disorder of iron metabolism in which toxic iron overload occurs. It can be inherited or acquired. The most common genetic form has a prevalence of ~1 in 300 in Caucasian populations and is inherited in an autosomal-recessive manner. The disorder becomes symptomatic in the fourth or fifth decades of life in men and about a decade later in women. Typical symptoms and signs include arthralgias, fatigue, abdominal pain, and bronzing of the skin. The classic triad of symptoms includes bronze skin, diabetes, and cirrhosis, but this is probably an uncommon presentation. Untreated, the disease can progress to liver cirrhosis or cardiomyopathy, either of which can be fatal. Diagnosis can be made without gene testing by measuring serum transferrin and iron saturation levels, with confirmatory liver biopsy showing elevated iron stores. Early, repeated phlebotomy to decrease body iron stores is very effective in treating the disease.

Since 2003 or so, a handful of specific mutations in the *HFE* gene have been shown to cause a majority of the genetic cases of hemochromatosis. Most individuals are either homozygous for the *C282Y* mutation (85%) or compound heterozygotes for the mutations *C282Y* and *H63D* (<10%) in the *HFE* gene. This gene encodes a protein that regulates cellular iron uptake. Although genetic testing is available for this disorder, population screening in asymptomatic individuals is not currently recommended. Less common forms caused by gene mutations at other loci exist, including a rather severe juvenile form.

Beutler E, et al. Penetrance of 845G–> A (C282Y) HFE hereditary haemochromatosis mutation in the USA. *Lancet.* 2002; 359:211. [PMID: 11812557]

Pietrangelo A. Hereditary hemochromatosis—a new look at an old disease. *N Engl J Med.* 2004; 350:2383. [PMID: 15175440]

Website

US Preventive Services Task Force, Screening for Hemochromatosis: http://www.ahrq.gov/CLINIC/USPSTF/uspshemoch.htm.

FUTURE DIRECTIONS & CURRENT CHALLENGES

Knowledge of human genetics has improved considerably since the early 1990s, and many new mutations causal of single-gene disorders have been identified. Completion of the International HapMap Project, an extension of the Human Genome Project, has facilitated a large number of "genomewide association studies" that have yielded a wealth of new data on the genetic underpinnings of many common disorders. Current studies are explaining an ever-increasing amount of the inherited component of disease risk for these conditions. This information will lead to the development of new diagnostic and screening tests, novel therapies, and strategies for the prevention of diseases. Pharmacogenetics and the use of genetic tests to guide screening, prevention, and treatment of cancers are already changing day-to-day clinical practice. The next wave of genomic discovery will be driven by the advent of extremely low-cost whole-genome sequencing. The consequences of this will be myriad for clinical medicine.

Genomics is a rapidly moving field. This presents a challenge to efficiently conducting clinical trials that inform clinical guideline development for genomic applications. Therefore, it is incumbent on healthcare providers to increase their individual knowledge base regarding genomics. Primary care physicians face major challenges in the realm of clinical applications of genomics: (1) they must decide which portion of this new, complex healthcare delivery process they feel comfortable managing, and identify specialty resources to assist them with patient-care questions or patient referral; (2) they must become familiar with the standard components of the genetic testing process, including pretest counseling, informed consent, proper interpretation of test results, posttest discussion of the implications of test results for their patient and family members, and implementation of appropriate risk reduction and surveillance recommendations; and (3) they must keep pace with the new genomic discoveries that are made every year and the most current versions of rapidly evolving disorder-specific evaluation and management recommendations.

Given the complexity and fast pace of genomic advances, a collaborative, multidisciplinary approach to patient care in the primary care setting will likely afford maximum benefits for the individual and their family.

Websites

Centers for Disease Control and Prevention: http://www.cdc.gov/node.do/id/0900f3ec8000e2b5.

Medline Plus/National Institutes of Health: http://www.nlm.nih.gov/medlineplus/geneticdisorders.html.

National Cancer Institute/National Institutes of Health: http://www.nci.nih.gov/cancertopics/pdq/genetics.

National Coalition of Health Professional Education in Genetics: http://www.nchpeg.org.

Acknowledgment

The author would like to acknowledge the work of Christine M. Mueller, DO, and W. Gregory Feero, MD, PhD as authors of earlier editions of this chapter.

Pharmacogenomics

Matthew D. Krasowski, MD, PhD

OVERVIEW OF PHARMACOGENOMICS

Pharmacogenomics (also known as *pharmacogenetics*) is a component of individualized ("personalized") medicine that addresses how genetic factors impact drug therapy, with the goal of optimizing drug therapy and ensuring maximal efficacy with minimal side effects. The effect of drugs is traditionally divided into pharmacokinetics (how drugs are absorbed, distributed, metabolized, and eliminated) and pharmacodynamics (the molecular target or targets underlying the therapeutic effect). In principle, genetic variation can influence pharmacokinetics, pharmacodynamics, or both. Currently, most clinical applications of pharmacogenomics involve drug metabolism, but over time more attention will likely shift to pharmacodynamics. Many of the current pharmacogenomic clinical applications focus on the cytochrome P450 (CYP) enzymes. The sequencing of the human genome and intensive research into how genetic variation affects drug response holds the promise of altering the paradigms for medication therapy. However, current clinical applications utilizing pharmacogenomics are still rather limited. The coming years should see steady growth in this field that will allow primary care providers and other health professionals to better manage drug therapy.

Genetic Variability

The most common type of genetic variation is single-nucleotide polymorphism (SNP), a situation in which some individuals have one nucleotide at a given position while other individuals have another nucleotide (eg, cytosine vs adenosine, C/A). If this occurs in the coding region of a gene (ie, within coding exons), it may result in a change in the amino acid sequence that results when DNA is transcribed into RNA and the RNA is then translated into protein. Other less common types of genetic variation include insertions or deletions (sometimes referred to collectively as *indels*),

partial or total gene deletion, alteration of mRNA splicing (ie, the process of removing introns from genomic DNA sequences that contain exons and introns), variation in gene promoters, and gene duplication or multiplication.

Genetic variants are named in a historical but often confusing system to those new to the field. By definition, the normal allele (individual copy of a gene on a chromosome) is defined as *1 (eg, CYP2D6*1). In order of historical discovery, variant alleles were designated *2, *3, *4, and so on added later on. Unfortunately, this nomenclature does not give any clue to the nature of the genetic variation. For instance, *4 and *6 could represent fairly benign genetic variants whereas *5 could signify a variant that results in complete absence of enzyme activity. However, this nomenclature is what is commonly used.

Pharmacogenomics Involving Drug Metabolism

Although numerous nongenetic factors influence the effects of medications—including disease, organ function, concomitant medications, herbal therapy, age, and gender—there are now many examples in which interindividual differences in medication response are due to variants in genes encoding drug targets, drug-metabolizing enzymes, and drug transporters. Currently, most well-established applications of pharmacogenomics involve drug metabolism. Several organs can metabolize (biotransform) drug molecules, with the liver being the dominant organ for this purpose in humans. The proteins that have been studied in greatest depth are the CYP enzymes, a complicated group of enzymes expressed in liver, intestines, kidneys, lungs, and some other organs. Several CYP enzymes account for the majority of drug metabolism in humans: CYP3A4/5, CYP2D6, CYP2C9, and CYP2C19. CYP3A4, in particular, has been shown to play a role in the metabolism of >50% of the prescribed drugs in the United States.

Genetic variation of CYP2D6 was one of the first classic examples of pharmacogenomics. In the 1970s, the experimental (and now obsolete) antihypertensive drug debrisoquine was being tested. For the majority of individuals, this drug provided safe control of hypertension. However, some individuals developed prolonged hypotension after receiving the drug, with the hypotension lasting for days in some people. Debrisoquine was later found to be metabolized mainly by CYP2D6, an enzyme found in the liver that is now known to metabolize ~25% of all drugs currently prescribed in the United States. Of the CYP enzymes, CYP2D6 shows the greatest range of genetic variation, with common genetic variants that include total gene deletion (CYP2D6*5) and gene duplication, with rare individuals documented that have over four functional copies of the CYP2D6 gene. Genetic variation of CYP2D6, as will be discussed below, has clinical importance for psychiatric, cardiac, and opiate medications. Individuals with low CYP2D6 activity may experience severe adverse effects to standard doses of certain drugs, whereas those with higher-than-average activity may degrade a drug so quickly that therapeutic concentrations are not achieved with standard doses.

The CYP enzymes also underlie a number of clinically important drug-drug or drug-food interactions. For example, erythromycin is a powerful inhibitor of multiple CYP enzymes, including CYP3A4. Erythromycin thus has potentially dangerous interactions with drugs metabolized by CYP3A4 such as the immunosuppressive drug cyclosporine, if appropriate dose reductions are not made. On the contrary, several compounds markedly increase (induce) the expression of CYP enzymes, including rifampin, phenytoin, carbamazepine, phenobarbital, and the herbal antidepressant St. John's wort. By increasing the expression of CYP enzymes and other proteins involved in drug metabolism and elimination, inducers such as rifampin can cause increased metabolism not only of other drugs but also of endogenous compounds such as steroid hormones and vitamin D. This is the mechanism underlying unintended pregnancy that can result in women using estrogen-containing oral contraceptives who also receive a CYP inducer such as St. John's wort. CYP inducers greatly increase the metabolism of the estrogen component of combined oral contraceptives, resulting in therapeutic failure. CYP inducers are also known to cause osteomalacia by accelerating the metabolism and clearance of the active form of vitamin D (1α, 25-dihydroxyvitamin D$_3$).

There is some nomenclature related to pharmacogenomics of drug-metabolizing enzymes that can be confusing to those new to the field. *Poor metabolizers* represent individuals with little or no enzymatic activity, due either to lack of expression of the enzyme or mutations that reduce enzymatic activity (eg, a mutation that alters the active catalytic site). *Extensive metabolizers* are considered the "normal" situation and generally represent individuals with two normal copies of the enzyme gene on each chromosome.

Intermediate metabolizers have enzymatic activity roughly half that of extensive metabolizers. The most common genetic reason underlying intermediate activity is one copy of the normal gene and one variant copy associated with low activity (ie, heterozygous for the mutation). *Ultrarapid metabolizers* have enzymatic activity significantly greater than that of the average population. This often results when an individual has more than the normal two copies of a gene. Gene duplication or multiplication is not seen with many genes but can occur with CYP2D6. For example, an individual may have three or more functional copies of the CYP2D6 gene instead of the normal two copies.

Two common drugs, clopidogrel and codeine, are *prodrugs* that are inactive until converted to active metabolites by CYP enzymes. Clopidogrel is activated by CYP2C19, and codeine is converted to morphine by CYP2D6. For these prodrugs, poor metabolizers of the respective CYP enzyme will be more likely to show lack of efficacy.

For many other drugs, CYP enzymes inactivate the drug and thus play an important role in clearance. Poor metabolizers may thus experience drug toxicity with standard doses due to slower drug clearance. Ultrarapid metabolizers may see little clinical effect with standard drug doses due to rapid clearance of the drug.

Pharmacogenomics Involving Pharmacodynamics

Understanding the genetic variation involving pharmacodynamics has developed more slowly than that of pharmacokinetics. In part, this is because the molecular targets of certain drugs are incompletely understood. An example of pharmacodynamic genetic variation is for the β_2-adrenergic receptor, the target of β-agonists used in asthma therapy such as albuterol and salmeterol. Genetic variation of the receptor influences how well β-agonist therapy works. However, genetic testing of the β_2-adrenergic receptor has not had much impact clinically. The other example of pharmacogenomics involving pharmacodynamics is the molecular target of warfarin, the vitamin K epoxide reductase complex subunit 1 (VKORC1) protein, which will be discussed below. The importance of understanding pharmacodynamic variation is that it holds the potential of predicting therapeutic efficacy (or lack thereof). This could be especially valuable for disorders such as depression where weeks or even months may be required to determine effectiveness of a drug.

O'Donnell PH, Ratain MJ. Germline pharmacogenomics in oncology: decoding the patient for targeting therapy. *Mol Oncol.* 2012; 6:251–259. [PMID: 22321460]

Swen JJ, Guchelaar HJ. Just how feasible is pharmacogenetic testing in the primary healthcare setting? *Pharmacogenomics.* 2012; 13:507–509. [PMID: 22462740]

Wilke RA, Dolan ME. Genetics and variable drug response. *JAMA.* 2011; 306:306–307. [PMID: 21771992]

Table 49-1. Possible indications for pharmacogenomic testing.

Provide guidance for drug and dose selection
Predict drug toxicity
Evaluate cause of adverse drug reaction
Investigate reason for therapeutic failure
Familial testing if other family member known to have pharmacogenomic variant

Clinical Applications

Pharmacogenomics may be useful for a number of clinical indications (**Table 49-1**). Although pharmacogenomics is far from fulfilling its promise of developing a patient-specific pharmacologic profile, there are areas in which genetic testing is being applied clinically. **Table 49-2** lists pharmagenomic associations mentioned in package inserts for approved medications.

Clopidogrel & CYP2C19

Clopidogrel (Plavix) is a commonly used antiplatelet drug administered to reduce risk of myocardial infarction, stroke, and peripheral vascular events. Clopidogrel is converted to an active thiol metabolite mainly by CYP2C19. Patients who are CYP2C19 poor metabolizers (most commonly the *2 and *3 alleles) may show "Plavix resistance" and pose higher risk for therapeutic failure and cardiovascular events while on clopidogrel. The TRITON-TIMI 38 trial demonstrated that patients with CYP2C19 loss-of-function mutations had a relative 53% increased risk of death from cardiovascular causes (myocardial infaction, stroke) and a threefold increased rate of stent thrombosis compared to patients with normal CYP2C19 genotype. The FDA issued a label warning update in March 2010 for CYP2C19 poor metabolizers.

CYP2C19 genotyping for patients who are candidates for clopidogrel therapy has not been widely adopted. One important point is that the CYP2C19 function is only one factor of many that can influence clopidogrel response, with drug-drug interactions also of importance. A task force of three societies in 2011 did not recommend routine screening for clopidogrel resistance, by either CYP2C19 genotyping or platelet function testing. However, CYPC19 genotyping may be clinically useful for high-risk patients, especially those receiving coronary stents. Large-scale randomized, prospective clinical trials are planned. The related drug prasugrel is an alternative antiplatelet agent for patients with poor clinical response to clopidogrel.

Table 49-2. Selected pharmacogenomic biomarkers and drugs with package insert data on pharmacogenomics.

Biomarker	Drug Categories Affected	Specific Drugs
CYP2C9	Analgesics	Celecoxib
CYP2C9, VKORC1	Anticoagulant	Warfarin
CYP2C19	Cardiovascular Neurologic and psychiatric Gastrointestinal	Clopidogrel Carisoprodol, citalopram, clobazam, diazepam Proton pump inhibitors: dexlansoprazole, esomeprazole, lansoprazole, omeprazole, pantoprazole, rabeprazole
CYP2D6	Analgesics Cardiovascular Neurologic and psychiatric	Codeine Carvedilol, metoprolol, propranolol *Antidepressants* (SSRIs/SNRIs): citalopram, fluoxetine, fluvoxamine, nefazodone, paroxetine, venlafaxine *Antidepressants* (tricyclics): amitriptyline, clomipramine, desipramine, doxepin, imipramine, nortriptyline, protriptyline *Antipsychotics*: aripiprazole, clozapine, iloperidone, perphenazine, risperidone *Other*: atomoxetine, chlordiazepoxide, modafinil
HLA-B*1502	Neurologic	Carbamazepine, phenytoin
HLA-B*5701	Antivirals	Abacavir
TPMT	Oncologic/rheumatologic	Azathioprine, 6-mercaptopurine
UGT1A1	Oncologic	Irinotecan

Data from US Food and Drug Administration: http://www.fda.gov/Drugs/ScienceResearch/ResearchAreas/Pharmacogenetics/ucm083378.htm.

Other Drugs Metabolized by CYP2C19

Several other categories of drugs are inactivated by CYP2C19 metabolism. These include carisoprodol (muscle relaxant), citalopram, clobazam, diazepam, and most of the "proton pump inhibitors" used to treat gastroesophageal reflux (eg, lansoprazole, omeprazole). CYP2C19-poor metabolizers may experience drug toxicity at standard doses. The frequencies of CYP2C19 inactivating genetic variants are highest in Asians (~15–25%) and Polynesians (up to ~75%) and lower in African-American (4%) and Caucasian (2–5%) populations. Genotyping of CYP2C19 has been much more widely applied in Japan than in the United States because of the prevalence of CYP2C19-poor metabolism in the Japanese population. CYP2C19 genotyping may be helpful in patients with poor clinical response or unusual toxicity to drugs metabolized by CYP2C19.

Levine GN, et al. 2011 ACCF/AHA/SCAI Guideline for Percutaneous Coronary Intervention. A report of the American College of Cardiology Foundation/American Heart Association Task Force on Practice Guidelines and the Society for Cardiovascular Angiography and Interventions. *J Am Coll Cardiol*. 2011; 58:e44–e122. [PMID: 22070834]

Ma JD, et al. Clinical application of pharmacogenomics. *J Pharm Practice*. 2012; 25:417–427. [PMID: 22689709]

Mega JL, et al. Dosing clopidogrel based on CYP2C19 genotype and the effect on platelet reactivity in patients with stable cardiovascular disease. *JAMA*. 2011; 306:2221–2228. [PMID: 22088980]

Warfarin

Warfarin remains the most commonly prescribed oral anticoagulant, although the recent introduction of other oral anticoagulants (eg, direct thrombin and factor X inhibitors) has reduced warfarin usage. Warfarin-related bleeding complications occur in ~3% of patients in the first 3 months of therapy, with the highest risk also in the first 3 months of therapy. During maintenance therapy there is a risk of bleeding complications of 7.6–16.5 per 100 patient-years. Thus, there is a need to accurately predict both the initial and maintenance doses of warfarin.

Two major genes are involved in warfarin pharmacogenomics: CYP2C9 and VKORC1. CYP2C9 metabolizes warfarin to an inactive metabolite. VKORC1 is the molecular target inhibited by warfarin, thus reducing the production of vitamin K–dependent clotting factors. CYP2C9-poor metabolizers are at risk for warfarin toxicity at standard doses because of reduced clearance of the drug. The two most common mutations are CYP2C9*2 and *3. VKORC1 has several genetic variants that influence warfarin sensitivity or resistance. Collectively, genetic variation in CYP2C9 and VKORC1 account for approximately one-third of the observed variation in warfarin dosage that leads to stable anticoagulation.

Various algorithms are available to predict optimal warfarin dosage. The most widely used (www.warfarindosage.org) is open-access and allows the clinician to input various factors that influence warfarin response (eg, age, gender, concomitant medications such as statins and trimethoprim/sulfamethoxazole, cigarette smoking, weight, CYP2C9 genotype, VKORC1 genotype). The algorithm does not require genetic information if unavailable. The output of the algorithm is an estimated maintenance dose of warfarin. A 2010 case-control study reported that genotyping-guided warfarin dosing can lower hospitalizations and thromboembolic complications. However, large-scale randomized prospective clinical trials have not yet demonstrated long-term efficacy and cost-effectiveness of warfarin genotyping.

Anderson JL, et al. A randomized and clinical effectiveness trial comparing two pharmacogenetic algorithms and standard care for individualizing warfarin dosing (CoumaGen-II). *Circulation*. 2012; 125:1997–2005. [PMID: 22431865]

Klein TE, et al. Estimation of the warfarin dose with clinical and pharmacogenetic data. *N Engl J Med*. 2009; 360:753–764. [PMID: 19228618]

Verhoef TI, et al. A systematic review of cost-effectiveness analyses of pharmacogenetic-guided dosing in treatment with coumarin derivatives. *Pharmacogenomics*. 2010; 11:989–1002. [PMID: 20602617]

Codeine & CYP2D6

Codeine is a prodrug that needs to be converted by CYP2D6 to morphine for therapeutic effect. CYP2D6 poor metabolizers are likely to get poor therapeutic effect from codeine due to lack of morphine conversion. Such patients more often benefit from other opiates such as hydrocodone, oxycodone, or morphine itself. However, as mentioned above, there are also individuals who are CYP2D6 ultrarapid metabolizers. Such patients convert codeine to morphine rapidly and may even experience morphine toxicity. Life-threatening codeine toxicity due to rapid CYP2D6 metabolism has been especially seen in the pediatric population, with some fatalities. Codeine toxicity may occur in CYP2D6 ultrarapid metabolizing children administered codeine (eg, for pain relief for dental surgery) or in breastfeeding infants whose mothers are CYP2D6 ultrarapid metabolizers prescribed codeine. In either case, the excess of morphine can cause respiratory depression and other symptoms of opiate overdose. FDA issued separate warnings on use of codeine in breastfeeding mothers and for postsurgical pain management for children in 2007 and 2012, respectively.

Other Drugs Metabolized by CYP2D6

Numerous other drugs are metabolized by CYP2D6. In contrast to the activation of codeine by CYP2D6, many drugs are inactivated by CYP2D6-mediated metabolism, often representing the major route of elimination for these drugs. The major categories of CYP2D6 substrates include β-adrenergic receptor antagonists (carvedilol, metopropol, propranolol), antidepressants (including some selective serotonin reuptake inhibitors, serotonin-norepinephrine reuptake inhibitors, and tricyclic antidepressants), and antipsychotics (both typical and atypical agents) (see Table 49-2). For drugs inactivated by CYP2D6, poor metabolizers are at risk for drug toxicity at standard doses, due to slow clearance of the drug. Poor metabolizers may require reduced dosage or use of an alternative drug. Ultrarapid metabolizers may show lack of efficacy at standard dosages and need higher doses to compensate for more rapid metabolism.

Madadi P, et al. Genetic transmission of cytochrome P450 2D6 (CYP2D6) ultrarapid metabolism: implications for breastfeeding women taking codeine. *Curr Drug Safety.* 2011; 6:36–9. [PMID: 21241245]

Seeringer A, Kirchheiner J. Pharmacogenetics-guided dose modifications of antidepressants. *Clin Lab Med.* 2008; 28:619–626. [PMID: 19059066]

Willmann S, et al. Risk to the breast-fed neonate from codeine treatment to the mother: a quantitative mechanistic modeling study. *Clin Pharmacol Ther.* 2009; 86:634–643. [PMID: 19710640]

Cancer Pharmacogenomics

There are increasing pharmacogenomic applications involving cancer therapy. Some examples are related to drug metabolism, while others involve the mechanism of action.

Azathioprine and 6-mercaptopurine (6MP) are agents used in the treatment of cancers (eg, acute lymphoblastic leukemia) and autoimmune disorders such as rheumatoid arthritis and inflammatory bowel disease. Azathioprine is the prodrug of 6MP. One route for inactivation and clearance of 6MP is by the enzyme thiopurine methyltransferase (TPMT). Although azathioprine and 6MP both have the potential for bone marrow suppression if used in high doses, approximately 1 in 300 Caucasians (less in most other populations) experiences very profound bone marrow toxicity following standard doses of azathioprine and 6MP.

Many of the patients experiencing severe toxicity in response to azathioprine or 6MP therapy have very low TPMT enzymatic activity (they are "PMT-poor metabolizers"). Several clinical laboratory tests can predict up front whether individuals will have difficulty metabolizing 6MP and azathioprine. In 2004–2005, the package inserts for azathioprine and 6MP were revised to include warnings on toxicity related to genetic variation of TPMT. TPMT-poor metabolizers can still receive 6MP or azathioprine but need markedly reduced doses.

A second oncology application involves the drug irinotecan, a chemotherapeutic agent used in the treatment of colorectal cancer. Irinotecan has complicated metabolism but is inactivated by glucuronidation mediated by UDP-glucuronosyltransferase 1A1 (UGT1A1), an enzyme that also carries out conjugation of bilirubin. A variety of rare, severe mutations in UGT1A1 can result in the Crigler-Najjar syndrome, a devastating disease that can be fatal in childhood unless liver transplantation is performed. A milder mutation, designated UGT1A1*28, is the most common cause of a mostly benign condition called *Gilbert syndrome*, a condition often diagnosed incidently in the primary care setting following detection of (usually mild) unconjugated hyperbilirubinemia. These individuals are, however, at high risk for severe toxicity following irinotecan therapy. With standard doses, such individuals may develop life-threatening neutropenia or diarrhea poorly responsive to therapy. A genetic test for UGT1A1*28 became FDA-approved and, similar to 6MP and azathioprine, the package insert for irinotecan now includes specific information on UGT1A1 genetic variation. However, genetic screening for UGT1A1 has not been adopted universally.

Pharmacogenomics also finds application in oncology in targeted therapies for certain cancers. One of the best examples is the use of trastuzumab (Herceptin) for breast cancers overexpressing the HER2 protein. In the pathology workup of breast cancer, determination of HER2 expression status determines whether trastuzumab is a therapeutic option.

A recent trend in oncology is the emergence of *paired diagnostics*, where a drug and its companion diagnostic test are approved simultaneously. An example is vemurafenib (Zelboraf), a drug that targets metastatic melanoma with a specific mutation in *BRAF*. Vemurafenib and the companion test to determine *BRAF* mutation status were approved simultaneously by the FDA. Health insurance coverage for vemurafenib generally will occur only if used for cancers with the specific *BRAF* mutation. The future will likely see many more similar type strategies of cancer treatment.

Duffy MJ, et al. Use of molecular markers for predicting therapy response in cancer patients. *Cancer Treat Rev.* 2011; 37: 151–159. [PMID: 20685042]

Wang L, et al. Genomics and drug response. *N Engl J Med.* 2012; 364:1144–1153. [PMID: 21428770]

Abacavir & Carbamazepine Hypersensitivity

Drug hypersensitivity is a relatively common problem and may manifest on a spectrum from mild symptoms to more severe presentations such as Stevens-Johnson syndrome and toxic epidermal necrolysis. Genetic variation in the human leukocyte antigen (HLA)-B gene has now been strongly linked to severe hypersensitivity to abacavir (antiviral used to treat human immunodeficiency virus, HIV) and carbamazepine (anticonvulsant).

Approximately 5–8% of HIV patients develop hypersensitivity to abacavir. Presence of the HLA-B*5701 allele carries a high risk of hypersensitivity. If the HLA-B*5701 is absent, the risk of hypersensitivity is very low. Label warning to abacavir was issued in July 2008.

For carbamazepine, the HLA-B∗1502 allele is positively correlated to hypersensitivity. This allele occurs mainly in individuals of southeast Asian descent and is uncommon in other populations. Label warning for carbamazepine was issued in December 2007. The HLA-B∗1502 is also linked to hypersensitivity to phenytoin and its prodrug fosphenytoin.

Mallal S, et al. HLA-B∗5701 screening for hypersensitivity to abacavir. *N Engl J Med.* 2008; 358:568–579. [PMID: 18256392]

Yip VL, et al. HLA genotype and carbamazepine-induced cutaneous adverse drug reactions: a systematic review. *Clin Pharmacol Ther.* 2012; 92:757–765. [PMID: 23132554]

DISCUSSION & FUTURE DIRECTIONS

The clinical application of pharmacogenomics has developed slowly, with so far only mild impacts on primary care. So far, few studies have clearly demonstrated clinical efficacy and cost-effectiveness of genetic testing to guide pharmacotherapy. Consequently, pharmacogenomic therapy is often used retrospectively to try to determine why a particular patient has experienced toxicity or unexplained lack of efficacy to a drug. Clinicians also need to realize that genetics may account for only a minor portion of variability in response to a drug. Other factors such as concomitant medications or organ failure may be more important in some circumstances. Clinical experience and ongoing research trials should better define useful applications of pharmacogenomics so that testing will become more common in the primary care setting.

Complementary & Alternative Medicine

Wayne B. Jonas, MD

Mary P. Guerrera, MD

Background

According to the World Health Organization, between 65% and 80% of the world's health care services are classified as traditional medicine. These practices become relabeled as complementary, alternative, or unconventional medicine when they are used in Western countries. In April 1995, a panel of experts, convened at the National Institutes of Health (NIH), defined *complementary and alternative medicine* (CAM) as "a broad domain of healing resources that encompasses all health systems, modalities, practices and their accompanying theories and beliefs, other than those intrinsic to the politically dominant health system of a particular society or culture in a given historical period." Similar definitions have been used since then by other organizations. Surveys of CAM use by the public and health professionals have defined it as those practices used for the prevention and treatment of disease that are not an integral part of conventional care, and are neither taught widely in medical schools nor generally available in hospitals. **Table 50-1** lists the major types and domains of complementary and alternative medicine, while recognizing that there can be some overlap, adapted from the National Center for Complementary and Alternative Medicine (NCCAM) at NIH.

A. Use of Complementary and Alternative Medicine

Practices that lie outside the mainstream of "official" or current conventional medicine have always been an important part of the public's management of their personal health. Complementary, alternative, and unconventional medicine has become increasingly popular in the United States. Two identical surveys of unconventional medicine use in the United States, done in 1990 and 1996, showed a 45% increase in use of CAM by the public. Visits to CAM practitioners increased from 400 million to >600 million per year. The amount spent on these practices rose from $14 billion to

$27 billion—most of it not reimbursed. Recent data from the National Health Interview Survey (NHIS) have increased this estimate to $33.9 billion. Professional organizations are now beginning the "integration" of these practices into mainstream medicine. In 2007, the number of those using CAM was similar between 1997 and 2002, and rose in 2007 (36.5%, 36.0% and 38.3%; respectively $P = .21$). The greatest relative increase in single CAM use was seen for deep breathing (12.1%, 11.6%, and 12.7 respectively) and meditation (3.7%, 7.6%, and 9.4% respectively).

The public uses these practices for both minor and major problems. Multiple surveys have now been conducted on populations with cancer, human immunodeficiency virus (HIV), children, minorities, and women on CAM use. Rates of use are significant in all these populations. For example, >50% of women surveyed have been found to explore and use CAM both for themselves and as healthcare decision makers for their family. A recent national survey showed that 12% of children use CAM regularly. More than 68% of patients with cancer or HIV will use unconventional practices at some point during the course of their illness. Immigrant populations often use traditional medicines that they experienced in their country of origin and not commonly used in the West.

As the public's use of CAM has grown, so, too, has the call to action of our research institutions and training centers. Will CAM treatments offer hope as we grapple with the growing burden of chronic illness and rising costs currently stressing our health systems? Are new educational and research training paradigms needed? Such efforts have emerged and are evolving. For example, the budget of the Office of Alternative Medicine at the US National Institutes of Health rose from $5 million to the present $123.1 million in 10 years and changed from a coordination office to a large government agency: the National Center for Complementary and Alternative Medicine (NCCAM). The NCCAM

Table 50-1. Complementary and alternative medicine (CAM) systems of healthcare, therapies, or products.

Major Domains of CAM	Examples under Each Domain
Whole medical systems	Ayurvedic medicine Homeopathic medicine Native American medicine (eg, sweat lodge, medicine wheel) Naturopathic medicine Traditional Chinese medicine (eg, acupuncture, Chinese herbal medicine) Tibetan medicine
Mind-body medicine	Meditation/mindfulness Hypnosis Yoga and tai chi Guided imagery Dance therapy Music therapy Art therapy Prayer and mental healing Biofeedback
Biology-based therapies	Herbal therapies Dietary supplements Biologics
Manipulative and body-based practices	Massage Chiropractic Osteopathy
Energy therapies	Qigong Reiki Therapeutic touch
Bioelectromagnetic therapies	Magnet therapy Electromagnetic devices

Adapted from the major domains of CAM and examples of each developed by the National Center for Complementary and Alternative Medicine, National Institutes of Health.

2012–enacted Congressional budget was $128,299,000. The 2013 Congressional budget request is $127,930,000, a reduction of <1% from fiscal year 2012. During fiscal year 2012, 248 research grants and 5 research centers were funded by the NCCAM. Since the early 1990s, more than 2500 research projects have been funded by NCCAM.

Our current medical and health professions students are the future. How are they learning about the potential healing power and possible pitfalls of CAM? Currently >95 of the nation's 125 medical schools require their medical students to enroll in either required or elective CAM coursework. A significant development in residency training, lead by family medicine educators, is the Integrative Medicine in Residency (IMR) national curriculum project. Launched in 2008 via eight pilot sites, the IMR was the first time that integrative medicine education became a required component of graduate medical education. IMR has been successfully disseminated to 42 residencies, including family medicine, internal medicine, and pediatrics (http://integrativemedicine.arizona.edu/education/imr.html). An increasing percentage of hospitals have developed complementary and integrative medicine programs offering both in- and outpatient services. Some health management organizations have "expanded" benefits packages that include specific alternative practitioners and services with a reimbursement option. A recent survey of CAM use in the US hospitals showed that 37% of hospitals offer CAM services. The majority of all services are offered on an outpatient basis, with massage therapy (54%), acupuncture (35%), and relaxation training (27%) among the most popular. On an inpatient basis, the top modalities offered are pet therapy (46%), massage therapy (40%), and music/art therapy (30%).

As the interface of CAM and conventional medicine grew, there emerged the concept of *integrative medicine* as a way to bridge the best of both worlds. The Consortium of Academic Health Centers for Integrative Medicine has defined *integrative medicine* (IM) as the practice of medicine that reaffirms the importance of the relationship between practitioner and patient; focuses on the whole person; is informed by evidence; and makes use of all appropriate approaches, healthcare professionals, and disciplines to achieve optimal health and healing. The application of integrative medicine can be defined as the purposeful, coordinative application of appropriate preventive and treatment modalities that support and stimulate the patient's inherent healing and self-recovery capacities. As such, these treatments are derived from various practices and healthcare systems from around the world. Thus, the term *integrative medicine* encompasses concepts from various healing philosophies, such as person-centered care, humanistic medicine, holistic healthcare, and the medical home.

Complementary and alternative medicine, and more specifically integrative medicine, is finding an important and growing place in American medical practice. Indeed, its significance is demonstrated by the newly formed American Board of Integrative Medicine® (ABOIM) under the auspices of the American Board of Physician Specialties (ABPS) (http://www.abpsus.org/integrative-medicine). Undoubtedly, these philosophies and practices will continue to be debated informally among medical staff and physicians and formally in peer-reviewed publicaitons, as well as medical societies, academies, and organizations. More importantly, the individual Western-trained medical physician will continue to be the primary arbitrator and counselor for the patient through the time-honored fundamentals of the therapeutic alliance; that is, compassion coupled with trust, integrity, and empathy; concern coupled with caring and active listening; competence coupled with skill, intellect, and common sense; and communication coupled with availability, continuity, and follow-through.

B. Conventional Physician Use of CAM in Practice

Family physicians are frequently faced with questions about CAM. Some also refer patients for CAM treatment and, to a lesser extent, provide CAM services. A review of 25 surveys of conventional physician referral and use of CAM found that 43% of physicians had referred patients for acupuncture, 40% for chiropractic services, and 21% for massage. The majority believed in the efficacy of these three practices. Rates of use of CAM practices ranged from 9% (homeopathy) to 19% (chiropractic and massage). National surveys have confirmed that many physicians refer for and fewer incorporate CAM practices into their professional practice. However, as CAM and IM physician training and fellowships programs (eg, AzCIM's IMF: http://integrativemedicine.arizona.edu/education/fellowship/index.html and the ABOIM's listing of current IM fellowships: http://www.abpsus.org/integrative-medicine-fellowships) continue to grow, so will the direct incorporation of CAM and IM into clinical care.

C. Risks of CAM

The amount of research on CAM systems and practices is relatively small compared with that on conventional medicine. There are >1000 times more citations on conventional cancer treatments in the National Library of Medicine's bibliographic database, MEDLINE, than on alternative cancer treatments. With increasing public use of CAM, inadequate communication between patients and physicians about it, and few studies on the safety and efficacy of most CAM treatments, risks are increased for misuse and harm. In response to inadequate communication about CAM use, NIH launched the "time to talk" campaign to increase awareness (http://nccam.nih.gov/timetotalk/forpatients.htm?nav=gsa). Many practices, such as acupuncture, homeopathy, and meditation, are low-risk but require practitioner competence to avoid inappropriate use. Botanical preparations can be toxic and produce herb-drug interactions. Contamination and poor quality control also exist with these products, especially those harvested, produced, and shipped from Asia and India.

D. Potential Benefits of CAM

Both CAM and IM practices have value for the way we manage health and disease. In botanical medicine, for example, there is research showing the benefit of herbal products such as *ginkgo biloba* for improving conditions due to *circulation* problems (although not Alzheimer disease), *Butterbur* for migraine prophylaxis and other herbal preparations, and the prevention of heart disease with garlic. A number of placebo-controlled trials have been performed showing that *Hypericum* (St. John's wort) is effective in the treatment of mild to moderate depression. Additional studies report that *Hypericum* is as effective as some conventional antidepressants but produces fewer side effects and costs less. However, the quality of too many of these trials does not reach the standards set for drug research in this country. Thus, physicians need to have and apply basic skills in the evaluation of clinical literature.

Ananth S. CAM: an increasing presence in US hospitals (published in *Hosp Health Netw* Jan.2009; available at http://www.hhnmag.com/hhnmag_app/jsp/articledisplay.jsp?dcrpath=HHNMAG/Article/data/01JAN2009/090120HHN_Online_Ananth&domain=HHNMAG).

Astin JA. Why patients use alternative medicine: results of a national study. *JAMA.* 1998; 279(19):1548.

DeKosky ST, et al. Ginkgo Evaluation of Memory (GEM) Study Investigators. *Ginkgo biloba* for prevention of dementia: a randomized controlled trial. *JAMA.* 2008; 300(19):2253–2262.

Federation of State Medical Boards. *Report on Health Care Fraud from the Special Committee on Health Care Fraud.* Federation of State Medical Boards of the United States, Inc.; 1997.

Le Bars PL, et al. A placebo-controlled, double-blind, randomized trial of an extract of ginkgo biloba for dementia. *JAMA.* 1997; 278(8):1327–1332. [PMID: 9343463]

Marwick C. Alterations are ahead at the OAM. *JAMA.* 1998; 280:1553–1554. [PMID: 9820244]

NCCAM. *Fiscal Year 2013 Budget Request* (available at http://nccam.nih.gov/about/budget/congressional/2013#Org; accessed May 2, 2013).

NCCAM. *Congressional Justification*; 2013 (available at http://nccam.nih.gov/about/budget/congressional/2013?nav=gsa#Bud; accessed May 2, 2013).

NCCAM. *Exploring the Science of Complementary and Alternative Medicine*, Third Strategic Plan 2011–2015, National Center for Complementary and Alternative Medicine, US Dept of Health and Human Services, National Institutes of Health Publication 11-7643/D458; Feb. 2011; p. 47.

Panel on Definition and Description. Defining and describing complementary and alternative medicine. *Altern Ther Health Med.* 1997; 3(2):49–57. [PMID: 9061989]

Saper RB, et al. Lead, mercury and arsenic in US and Indian-manufactured Ayurvedic medicines sold via the Internet. *JAMA.* 2008; 300(8):915–923. [PMID: 18728265]

Tindle HA, et al. Trends in use of complementary and alternative medicine by US adults: 1997–2002. *Altern Ther Health Med.* 2005; 11(1):42–49. [PMID: 15712765]

Wahner-Roedler DL, et al. Physicians' attitudes toward complementary and alternative medicine and their knowledge of specific therapies: a survey at an academic medical center. *Evid Based Complement Alternat Med.* 2006; 3(4):495–501. [PMID: 17173114]

White House Commission on Complementary and Alternative Medicine. *Policy Final Report*; 2002 (available at http://www.whccamp.hhs.gov/).

Websites

http://nccam.nih.gov/news/camstats/2002/graphics2002.htm.

http://nccam.nih.gov/sites/nccam.nih.gov/files/news/camstats/2007/72_dpi_CHARTS/chart4.htm.

http://nccam.nih.gov/news/camstats/NHIS.htm (accessed May 13, 2013).

http://www.aha.org/presscenter/pressrel/2008/080915-pr-cam.shtml (accessed May 2, 2013).

National Center for Complementary and Alternative Medicine (NCCAM) at the National Institutes of Health: http://nccam.nih.gov/about/offices/od/directortestimony/0607.htm.

Role of the Family Physician

What is the role of the family physician in the management of CAM? The goal is to help patients make informed choices about CAM as they do in conventional medicine. Specifically, physicians must continue to apply the ethical principle of beneficence and autonomy and play the role of patient advocate—a professional should protect, permit, promote, and partner with patients about CAM practices as appropriate.

A. Protecting Patients from Risks of CAM

Many practices, such as acupuncture, biofeedback, homeopathy, and meditation, are low- risk if delivered by competent practitioners. However, if used in place of more effective treatments, CAM may result in harm. The practitioners who apply these modalities should be qualified to help patients avoid inappropriate use. Many herbal preparations contain powerful pharmacologic substances with direct toxicity and herb-drug interactions. Contamination and poor quality control occur more often than with conventional drugs, especially if preparations are obtained from overseas. The family physician can help distinguish between CAM practices with little or no risk of direct toxicity (eg, homeopathy, acupuncture) and those with greater risk of toxicity (eg, megavitamins and herbal supplements). Physicians should be especially cautious about those products that can produce toxicity, work with patients to ensure that they do not abandon proven care, and alert patients to signs of possible fraud or abuse. "Secret" formulas, cures for multiple conditions, slick advertising for mail order products, pyramid marketing schemes, and any recommendation to abandon conventional medicine are "red flags" and should be suspect.

B. Permitting Use of Nonspecific Therapies

Spontaneous healing and placebo effects account for the improvement seen in many illnesses. The medical literature does contain essays and polemics that attempt to separate and often denigrate these factors from those that are considered identifiable, tangible, specific aspects of a therapy. The clinician, however, is interested in how to combine both specific and nonspecific factors for maximum benefit. Many CAM systems emphasize high-touch, personalized approaches for the management of chronic disease and the crises associated with acute illness. The physician can permit the integration of selected CAM approaches that are not harmful or expensive, that may enhance these nonspecific factors.

C. Promoting CAM Use

Proven therapies that are safe and effective should be available to the public. As research continues, more CAM practices will be found to be effective. Gradually, physicians and patients will have more options for management of disease. In arthritis, for example, there are studies suggesting improvements with homeopathy, acupuncture, vitamin and nutritional supplements, botanical products, diet therapies, mind-body approaches, and manipulation. A similar collection of studies exists for other conditions such as heart disease, depression, asthma, and addictions. The Cochrane Collaboration conducts systematic reviews (SRs) of randomized controlled trials (RCTs) on both conventional and complementary medicine and is an excellent source for evidence-based evaluation of such studies. Other groups such as RAND, AHRQ, EPIC, and Samueli Institute also conduct such reviews. Samueli Institute has developed a streamlined but effective way to do these reviews called the *rapid evidence assessment of the literature*. As research accumulates, rational therapeutic options can be developed in these areas.

As CAM information is presented in peer-reviewed professional journals, the challenge will be to implement its coordinated application via integrative medicine strategies within clinical teams into holistic care models in hospitals, offices, clinics, and other care venues. The availability of pluralistic care delivery with onsite, certified, and licensed CAM practitioners will require the training of physicians who will guide the appropriate selection of modalities using indication and evaluation methods related to safety and efficacy. In fact, an increasing number of team-based care and group visits will be required to accomplish this. Although the physician may be the cornerstone of this team, optimal care will require collaboration among all members with honest communication, generous listening, a shared commitment to treating the whole person, integrated care plans, and appropriate referral when necessary.

D. Partnering with Patients about CAM Use

Over 60% of patients who use CAM practices do not reveal this information to their conventional physicians. Thus, there is a major communication gap between physicians and the public about CAM. Patients use alternative practices for various reasons: their culture or social network, dissatisfaction with the results of their conventional care, or an attraction to CAM philosophies and health beliefs. The overwhelming majority of patients use CAM practices as an *adjunct* to conventional medicine. Fewer than 5% use CAM *exclusively*. Patients who use alternative medicine do not foster antiscience or anti–conventional medicine sentiments or represent a disproportionate number of the uneducated, poor, seriously ill, or neurotic. Patients often do not understand the role of science in medicine and will accept anecdotal evidence or slick marketing as sufficient justification for use. The family physician can play a role in examining the research base of these medical claims and partner with patients to incorporate more evidence into their healthcare decisions. Quality research on CAM practices provide this evidence, and the physician can help bridge this gap with patients.

Other social factors have also influenced the emergence of CAM. These include rising rates of chronic disease, increasing access to health information, growing "computerization" of medical decision making, declining faith that science will benefit personal health, and increasing interest in spirituality. In addition, both the public and health professionals are increasingly concerned about side effects, errors, and the escalating costs of conventional care. Physicians and scientists who ignore CAM only broaden the communication gap between the public and the profession that serves them. Thus, as patient advocates, physicians will best meet their patients' needs by learning about these practices and openly engaging in dialogue.

Chez RA, Jonas WB. The challenge of complementary and alternative medicine. *Am J Obstet Gynecol.* 1997; 177(5):1156–1161. [PMID: 9396912].

Eisenberg DM, et al. Perceptions about complementary therapies relative to conventional therapies among adults who use both: Results from a national survey. *Ann Intern Med.* 2001; 135: 344–351. [PMID: 11529698].

Eisenberg DM, et al. Trends in alternative medicine use in the United States 1990–1997: results of a follow-up national survey. *JAMA.* 1998; 280:1569–1575. [PMID: 9820257]].

Lewith G, et al. *Clinical Research in Complementary Therapies: Principles, Problems and Solutions.* London: Churchill Livingstone; 2010.

Websites

Cochrane Collaboration: www.cochrane.org
Samueli Institute: www.SamueliInstitute.org

▶ **Evidence Hierarchy or Evidence House?**

We all need good evidence to make medical decisions. Evidence comes in a variety of forms, and what may be good for one purpose may not be good for another. The term *evidence-based medicine* (EBM) has become a synonym for "good" medicine recently, and is often used to support and deny the value of complementary medicine. EBM uses the "hierarchy of evidence" (**Figure 50-1**). In this hierarchy, SRs are seen as the "best" evidence, then individual RCTs, then nonrandomized trials, then observational studies, and finally case series. All efforts are focused on approximating evidence at the top of the pyramid, and lower levels are considered inferior. Clinical experiments on causal links between an intervention and outcomes become the gold standard when this model is used.

All family physicians have seen patients who recover from disease because of complex factors, many of which are not additive and cannot be isolated in controlled experiments. Under these circumstances, observational data from clinical practice may provide the best evidence rather than controlled trials. Patients' illnesses are the human experience of the disease—the manifestation of the patient's beliefs, fears, and expectations. As such, they are complex, and holistic phenomena cannot be reduced to single, objective measures. Often highly subjective judgments about life quality may be the best information with which to make a decision. Such experiences may be captured only with qualitative research, not with scans or blood tests. Often the meaning that patients infer regarding their illness and recovery is the "best" evidence for medical decisions.

Sometimes the "best" evidence comes from laboratory tests. For example, the most crucial evidence for management

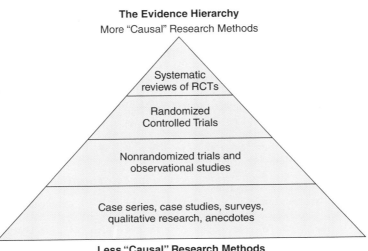

The Evidence Hierarchy

More "Causal" Research Methods

Systematic reviews of RCTs

Randomized Controlled Trials

Nonrandomized trials and observational studies

Case series, case studies, surveys, qualitative research, anecdotes

Less "Causal" Research Methods

▲ **Figure 50-1.** The evidence hierarchy.

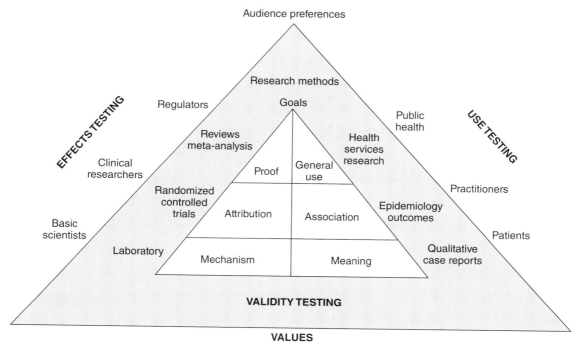

▲ Figure 50-2. The evidence house.

of St. John's wort in patients on immunosuppressive medications originates from a laboratory finding that it accelerates drug metabolism via cytochrome P450. Arranging evidence in a hierarchy obscures the fact that the "best" evidence may be neither related to cause and effect, nor objective, nor clinical.

We suggest that family physicians not use an evidence hierarchy but rather build an evidence "house" (**Figure 50-2**). On the left side of this house is evidence for causal attributions, for mechanisms of action, and for "proof." If physicians confine themselves to the left side of the house, they will never know about the relevance of a treatment for patients or what happens in the real world of clinical practice. They will also not know whether proven treatments can be generalized to populations such as the ones they see or the healthcare delivery system in which they practice. The "rooms" on the right side of the house provide evidence about patient relevance and usefulness, in practices both proven and unproven.

How evidence is approached has ethical implications. Different groups prefer different types of evidence. Regulatory authorities are most interested in RCTs or SRs (left side), which may never be done because of the logistics of time, cost, and access. Healthcare practitioners usually want to know the likelihood of benefit or harm from a treatment (right side). Patients are intensely interested in stories and descriptions of cures (right side). Rationalists want to

know how things work and so need laboratory evidence (left side). If one type of evidence is selected to the exclusion of others, science will not allow for full public input into clinical decisions. A livable house needs both a kitchen and a bathroom and places to sleep and play. Each type of evidence has different functions and value, and all types need to be of high quality.

Jonas WB. Evidence, ethics and evaluation of global medicine. In: Callahan D, ed. *Ethical Issues in Complementary and Alternative Medicine.* Hastings Center Report; 2001.

Lewith G, Walach H, Jonas W. *Clinical Research in Complementary Medicine,* 2nd ed. New York: Elsevier; 2012.

Linde K, Jonas WB. Evaluating complementary and alternative medicine: the balance of rigor and relevance. In: Jonas WB, Levin J, eds. *Essentials of Complementary and Alternative Medicine.* Philadelphia: Lippincott Williams & Wilkins; 1999.

▶ An Evidence-Based Approach

Fortunately, most treatment decisions need information only on whether a practice has a specific effect and on the magnitude of that effect in practice. This is evidence from randomized controlled trials and outcomes research, respectively. An evidence-based practice would then involve clinical expertise, informed patient communication, and quality research. This presumes that the physician has good clinical and communication skills. Medical training and experience address these, but evaluation of the CAM research evidence may not be something that physicians feel fully prepared to undertake. Obtaining research, selecting appropriate research for clinical situations, and then evaluating the quality of that research in CAM are essential for a fully evidence-based practice that addresses these topics.

A. Finding and Selecting Good Information

Where can the family physician obtain research on CAM? A number of groups have collated and produced CAM-specific databases (Cochrane Collaboration, Evidence Based Medicine Reviews, Samueli Institute, and Natural Standard). **Table 50-2** lists some good sources of clinical information on CAM and what they provide. When searching these databases, look for the following key terms: (1) meta-analyses, (2) RCTs, and (3) observational or prospective outcomes data. Although there are many other types of studies, it is necessary to be cautious about using these for problem-oriented decision making in practice. If no research information is found from the databases listed, it is likely that there is little relevant evidence for the practice on that clinical condition. A search for this information need not take up a lot of time. A trained research

Table 50-2. Sources of CAM information for healthcare practitioners.

Source of CAM Information	Description	Where to Go
Cochrane Library	Database of Systematic Reviews: systematic reviews of RCTs of CAM and conventional therapies Controlled Trials Register: extensive bibliographic listing of controlled trials and conference proceedings	http://www.cochrane.org http://gateway.ovid.com
Natural Medicines Comprehensive Database	Comprehensive listing and cross-listing of natural and herbal therapies, separate "all known uses" and "effectiveness" sections, safety ratings, mechanisms of action, side effects, herb-drug interactions, and review of available evidence	http://www.naturaldatabase.com

National Library of Medicine	Powerful search engine that allows searches of PubMed and all government guidelines combined
	Includes "synonym and related terms" option
		Search engine: hstat.nlm.nih.gov
		Individual guidelines at:
		  http://www.guideline.gov
		  http://www.cdc.gov/publications

Focus on Alternative and Complementary Therapies (FACT)	Quarterly review journal of CAM therapies Contains evidence-based reviews, focus articles, short reports, news of recent developments, and book reviews on complementary medicine	http://www.exeter.ac.uk/FACT
PubMed Clinical Queries Search Engine	The old standby has a clinical queries filter to limit your search results Click on "Clinical Queries" on the left blue banner to access the filter For the most comprehensive search, use the keywords "complementary medicine"	http://www.pubmed.org
National Center for Complementary and Alternative Medicine (NCCAM)	Clinical Trials Section: listing of clinical trials indexed by treatment or by condition Crosslinked to http://www.clinicaltrials.gov and PubMed	http://www.nccam.nih.gov
Agency for Healthcare Research and Quality (AHRQ)	For information on the quality, safety, efficiency, and effectiveness of healthcare for all Americans	http://www.ahrq.gov
Clinical Evidence	Promotes informed decision making by summarizing what is known, and not known, about >200 medical conditions and >2000 treatments	http://www.clinicalevidence.com/ceweb/condition/index.jsp
TRIP	Allows health professionals to easily find the highest-quality material available on the Internet	http://www.tripdatabase.com
Family Physicians Inquiry Network	Provides clinicians with answers to 80% of their clinical questions in 60 seconds	http://www.fpin.orgs/

CAM, complementary and alternative medicine; RCT, randomized controlled trial.
Adapted with permission from Beutler AI, Jonas WB. Complementary and alternative medicine for the sports medicine physician. In: Birrer RB, O'Connor FG, eds. *Sports Medicine for the Primary Care Physician*. Boca Raton, FL: CRC Press, 2004: 315.

assistant or librarian can often do the search, streamlining time spent on this process. Many librarians, especially those at health centers and hospitals, are now receiving training in literature searching methodology and growing awareness and expertise in CAM databases. After a literature search, the physician can be confident in knowing the quantity of evidence on the therapy (Figure 50-3). Patients are usually grateful for this effort as they will come to their physician in the hopes of obtaining science-based information they can trust.

B. Risks and Types of Evidence for Practice

If there are studies on a specific type of CAM practice, then the risk of toxicity and the cost of the therapy indicate which types of data are needed. Low-risk practices include OTC homeopathic medications, acupuncture and gentle massage or manipulation, meditation, relaxation and biofeedback,

other mind-body methods, and vitamin and mineral supplementation below toxic doses. Low-cost therapies involving self-care are also often low-risk. High-risk practices include herbal therapies, high-dosage vitamins and minerals, colonics, and intravenous administration of substances. Some otherwise harmless therapies can produce considerable cost if they require major lifestyle changes. Herbal therapies can produce serious adverse effects secondary to their impact on cell function, including enzymatic reactions or contamination with toxic materials. Because patients frequently take herbal products along with calculated dose prescription medications, physicians should specifically inquire about their use. High-risk or high-cost practices and products require RCT data.

Under some circumstances, observational (outcomes) data are more important, and in other circumstances RCT data are more important. Outcomes research provides the probability of

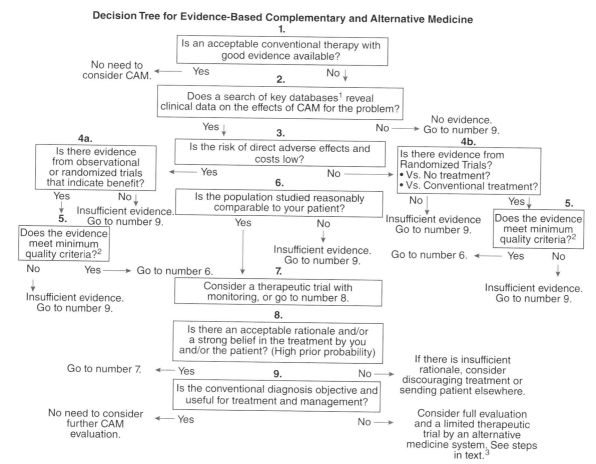

▲ **Figure 50-3.** Decision tree for evidence-based complementary and alternative medicine.

an effect and the absolute magnitude of effects in the context of normal clinical care. It is more similar to clinical practice and usually involves a wide variety of patients and variations of care to fit the patient's circumstances. It does not provide information on whether a treatment is specific or better than another treatment.

With low-risk practices, the physician wants to know the probability of benefit from the therapy. Quality observational data from practices are preferable to RCT data if the data are collected from actual practice populations similar to those of the practitioner. This may be sufficient evidence for making clinical decisions. Often, it will be the only useful information available for chronic conditions. For example, if quality outcome studies report a 75% probability of improving allergic rhinitis using a nontoxic, low-cost, homeopathic remedy, this information can assist in deciding on its use.

For high-risk, high-cost interventions, the physician should use randomized controlled trials (or meta-analyses of those trials). RCTs address the relative benefit of one therapy over another (or no therapy). RCTs can determine whether the treatment is the cause of improvement and how much the treatment adds to either no treatment or placebo treatment. RCTs provide relative (not absolute) information effects between a CAM and control practice. They are difficult to do properly for more than short periods and difficult if the therapy being tested is complex and individualized or if there are marked patient preferences. In addition, RCTs remove any choice about therapy and, if blinded, blunt expectations—both of which affect outcomes. Placebo-controlled RCT differences are dependent largely on the control group, which requires careful selection and management. Strong patient preferences for CAM, differing cultural groups, and informed consent may also alter RCT results. RCTs are more important if we need to know more about specific benefit-harm comparisons, such as with high-risk, high-cost interventions. Recently *comparative effectiveness research* (CER) has emerged as an important goal and set of methods. CER may be a valuable addition to CAM research, allowing whole systems of care to be compared to other different systems.

The more a CAM practice addresses chronic disease and depends on self-care (eg, meditation, yoga, biofeedback), or involves a complex system (eg, classical homeopathy, traditional Chinese medicine, Unani-Tibb), the more local, observational data are important. The more a CAM practice involves high-risk or high-cost interventions, the more essential RCT data become.

C. Evaluating Study Quality

Once data are found and the preferred type of study is selected, the practitioner should apply some minimum quality criteria to these studies. Three items can be quickly checked: (1) blind and random allocation of subjects to comparison groups (in RCTs) or blind outcome assessments (in observational research), (2) the clinical relevance and reliability of the outcome measures, and (3) the number of subjects that could be fully analyzed at the end of the study compared to the number entered. These same minimum quality criteria apply to RCTs or observational studies, except that blinded, random allocation to treatment and comparison groups does not apply in the latter. However, evaluation of effects before/after treatment can be blinded to the treatment given in any study. Detailed descriptions of patients, interventions, and dropouts are hallmarks of a quality outcomes trial.

Finally, one can ask if the probability of benefits reported in the outcomes study is worth the inconvenience, risk of side effects, and costs of the treatment and, in addition, whether confidence intervals were reported. *Confidence intervals* are the range of minimum to maximum effects expected in 95% of similar studies. If confidence intervals are narrow, the physician can be confident that similar results will occur with other patients. If confidence intervals are broad, the chance of obtaining those effects from treatment in other patients will be less predictable.

If the quality screening questions reveal marked quality flaws in the studies retrieved, the evidence in the study is insufficient and should not be used as a basis for clinical decisions.

D. The Population Studied

Even if good evidence is found for a practice, physicians should determine whether the population in the studies is similar to the patient being seen. Although this matching is largely subjective, the physician can compare five areas. Specifically, determine whether the study was done (1) in a primary, secondary, or tertiary referral center; (2) in a Western, Eastern, developing, or industrialized country; and (3) with diagnostic criteria similar to the patient (eg, the same criteria were used to diagnose osteoarthritis or congestive heart failure). Also, determine whether the age (4) and gender(s) (5) of the study population were similar. If the study population is not similar to the patient being seen, then the data, even though valid, cannot be applied to the situation. The study country may be especially important for some CAM practices. For example, data on use of acupuncture to treat chronic pain may come from China. Pain perception and reporting is different in China from that in the United States. Results from a study done in one country may not be applicable in another. If the study and clinic population match, an appropriate body of evidence for moving forward with a therapeutic trial exists.

E. Balancing Beliefs

Belief in the treatment by the physician and the patient needs to be explicitly considered in CAM. In conventional medicine, both patient and physician accept the plausibility of treatment. Belief has long been known to affect outcome. Strong belief enhances positive outcomes, and weak belief interferes with them. A physician may feel that a CAM practice has incredibly low plausibility although the patient may have a strong belief in the therapy. This "prior probability" (or belief) by the physician and patient should be considered in the decision to allow or not allow the patient to use a treatment. If physician and patient have similar beliefs, then a decision is easily made. Sometimes, however, the patient has a strong belief in the therapy, but the physician finds it unbelievable. In such situations, the physician should work with the patient to decide the best action—including referral elsewhere as an option.

F. Alternative Diagnoses

Some diagnoses are not very useful for management of a patient's illness. If the family physician's conventional diagnosis is not helping a patient, the clinician may want to consider an evaluation by an alternative system. Chinese medicine uses energy diagnosis, for example, and homeopathy has a remedy classification system. Sometimes, obtaining an assessment from a practitioner experienced in a CAM system may prove useful. For example, a 51-year-old woman with several years of idiopathic urticaria had obtained no relief from several conventional physicians. A homeopathic assessment showed that she might benefit from the remedy Mercurius 200C (mercurius virax). She was given several small doses and the urticaria cleared.

The physician should also be alert to practitioners who pursue CAM diagnoses that are not useful. A complicated CAM evaluation and treatment with little effect might be managed simply and effectively by conventional medicine. For example, a 57-year-old man with cardiovascular disease and recurrent bouts of angina was treated by a CAM practitioner for 3 years with special diets and nutritional supplements without help. Consultation with a conventional practitioner shows that he had myxedema. A thyroid supplement cleared his angina rapidly. In cases in which the diagnostic approach of the medical system fails, a professional consultation may be needed. In situations in which the alternative system's diagnostic and treatment approach is clear, a limited therapeutic trial with specific treatment goals and follow-up can be attempted. Of course, quality products and qualified practitioners must be located. In situations of serious disease, such as cancer, desperate patients may seek out CAM treatments. Under these circumstances, good training and clinical experience and protection of patients from harm (even from themselves) should prevail.

Evidence-based medicine can be applied to complementary and alternative medicine. **Table 50-3** summarizes questions for CAM management. Although evidence-based CAM may initially seem like a large task, appropriate data-driven clinical decisions can be made with CAM as with all medical care.

Table 50-3. Questions for evidence-based CAMT management.

A patient is using a complementary and alternative medicine therapy (CAMT) or an alternative treatment is sought. The following questions should be answered.
1. Has the patient received proper conventional medical care?
2. Is the CAMT likely to produce direct toxic or adverse effects or is it expensive?
3. Are there clinical data from randomized trials or outcomes research on the CAMT?
4. Do the studies meet minimum quality criteria?
5. Is the study population similar to the patient using or seeking the CAMT?
6. Is the plausibility of the therapy acceptable to both patient and physician?
7. Can a quality product or a qualified practitioner be accessed?
8. Can the patient be monitored while undergoing the CAMT?
9. Is a full diagnostic assessment by a conventional or CAM system in order?

Summary

American medicine continues to evolve in its focus, capabilities, technology, and demands. Our population is aging, and with that comes more chronic disease. By definition, chronic disease cannot be cured—patients may suffer with disability, diminished function, emotional challenges, economic burden, and overall challenges to quality of life. Conventional medicine is failing to provide the necessary and required care that these patients deserve. Although cure is not always the physician's primary goal, the provision of individualized, person-centered care suffused with empathy and compassion remains the foundation of all medical practice. The knowledgeable use of integrative medicine, combining the best of CAM and conventional therapies, will empower patients to participate in a process of healing with their physician by engaging in their inherent healing capacities, expectation, hope, understanding, and belief that well-being can and will manifest.

Eisenberg DM. Advising patients who seek alternative medical therapies. *Ann Intern Med.* 1997; 127:61–69. [PMID: 9214254]

Gatchel RJ, Maddrey AM. Clinical outcome research in complementary and alternative medicine: an overview of experimental design and analysis. *Alt Ther Health Med.* 1998; 4(5):36–42. [PMID: 9737030]

Jonas WB. Clinical trials for chronic disease: randomized, controlled clinical trials are essential. *J NIH Res.* 1997; 9:33.

Jonas WB, et al. How to practice evidence-based complementary and alternative medicine. In: Jonas WB, Levin JS, eds. *Essentials of Complementary and Alternative Medicine.* Philadelphia: Lippincott Williams & Wilkins, 1999.

Kirsch I. *How Expectancies Shape Experience.* American Psychological Association; 1999.

Websites

Clinical Pearls News. Current Research on Nutrition and Preventive Medicine: www.clinicalpearls.com.

National Center for Complementary and Alternative Medicine (NCCAM): www.altmed.od.nih.gov/NCCAM.

Acknowledgment

Special thanks to Cindy Crawford and Viviane Enslein in helping collecting background information and preparing the manuscript.

51

Chronic Pain Management

Ronald M. Glick, MD

Dawn A. Marcus, MD

General Considerations

Pain is defined by the International Association for the Study of Pain as "an unpleasant sensory or emotional experience associated with actual or potential tissue damage or described in terms of such damage." This definition emphasizes that the pain experience is multidimensional and may include sensory, cognitive, and emotional components. Additionally, the latter part of the definition allows for the possibility, as in chronic pain states, that the overt tissue damage may no longer be present. Pain persisting for >3–6 months is defined as chronic pain. Pain persisting for 3 months, however, is unlikely to resolve spontaneously and may continue to be reported by patients after 12 months. In addition, many of the secondary problems associated with chronic pain, such as deconditioning, depression, sleep disturbance, and disability, begin within the first few months of the onset of symptoms of pain. Studies indicate that early patient identification and treatment are essential to reduce pain chronicity and prevent further disability.

Chronic pain is one of the most common complaints seen in primary care. A survey of 89 general practices in Italy showed pain as a complaint for 3 of every 10 patients seen. Among these patients, pain was chronic for over half (53%). According to a recent Center for Disease Control and Prevention (CDC) survey, women are twice as likely as men to have chronic pain conditions such as migraines. A monograph from the Institute of Medicine, *Relieving Pain in America,* notes that 100 million Americans experience chronic pain with estimated annual medical and indirect costs of approximately $600 billion. Low back pain is most common, followed closely by migraines, neck pain, and other arthritic joint pain complaints.

Committee on Advancing Pain Research Care, and Education– Board on Health Sciences Policy. *Relieving Pain in America: A Blueprint for Transforming Prevention, Care, Education and Research.* Institute of Medicine; June 29, 2011.

Koleva D, et al. Pain in primary care: an Italian survey. *Eur J Public Health.* 2005; 15:475. [PMID: 16150816]

Schiller JS, Lucas JW, Peregoy JA. Summary health statistics for U.S. adults: National Health Interview Survey, 2011. National Center for Health Statistics. *Vital Health Stat.* 2012; 10(256). 2012.

Pathogenesis

Acute pain occurs following some form of tissue injury (eg, ankle sprain) and is treated with RICE (rest, immobilization, compression, and elevation) and pain-soothing treatments, such as heat, ice, and massage. During the acute period of tissue injury and healing, patients appropriately limit activity to reduce risks of further injury (eg, development of a Charcot joint in a patient with neuropathy who risks aggravation of the injury because of impaired sensation). Studies show that patients improve best after acute injury when they reduce activities to what can be tolerated and allow healing to occur, in contrast to patients treated with either bed rest or acute physical therapy.

Chronic pain occurs after the acute healing period has been completed or in the context of chronic conditions (eg, neuropathy or arthritis). Restriction of activity in patients with chronic pain leads to deconditioning, with muscle and bone loss that increases pain and the risk for reinjury, and also promotes psychological sluggishness, if not depression. Consequently, the RICE approach will actually aggravate the symptoms of chronic pain. The natural response of restricting activities when experiencing pain is appropriate for acute injury pain but aggravates chronic pain. Patients with chronic pain require an active, progressive exercise program. They must learn appropriate strategies for treating pain, avoid a tendency to restrict activity excessively, and resume more normal activity levels through a stepwise, progressive activity program.

► Clinical Findings

The most common chronic pain conditions in young and middle adulthood are low back pain, neck pain, and headaches. Musculoskeletal diseases rank fifth in generating hospital expenses and first in generating expenses related to work absenteeism and disability. The most common cause of chronic pain in older adults is degenerative joint and disk diseases, with arthritis causing chronic pain in >80% of elderly patients with pain. Other causes of chronic pain that occur more frequently with increasing age are pain related to cancer, vascular disease, and neuropathy (eg, postherpetic neuralgia). Throughout the lifecycle, pain can be associated with various general medical conditions, such as Crohn's disease or sickle cell anemia.

The overall pain experience includes primary pain-generating signals, along with common secondary problems that may develop regardless of pain etiology and that complicate pain management (**Figure 51-1**). Both physical (eg, joint restrictions and deconditioning) and psychological (eg, depression and anxiety) changes frequently accompany chronic pain. Psychological distress is common. In a survey of 500 patients with chronic low back, hip, or knee pain, depression or anxiety accompanied pain complaints for 46% of patients. Both depression and anxiety were identified in 23%, with depression alone in 20% and anxiety alone in 3%. Patients with pain plus the combination of depression and anxiety experienced significantly greater pain severity and disability (*P*<.0001 for each). Psychosocial stress may result from difficulties related to school or work, family relationships, social isolation, and legal and financial areas. Although the possibility of secondary gain (eg, litigation) may increase pain complaints, true malingering and factitious disorders are uncommon, occurring in only 1–10% of patients. The *Diagnostic and Statistical Manual of Mental Disorders,* 5th edition (*DSM*-5) recognizes that regardless of the etiology, many individuals may experience persistent thoughts and a high level of anxiety may be related to the pain problem. The diagnosis of *somatic symptom disorder with predominant pain* reflects an understanding that for such individuals psychological factors may greatly compound the level of distress and dysfunction. The family physician is in a unique position to identify and treat the physical and psychosocial factors influencing complaints of pain.

American Psychiatric Association, *Desk Reference to the Diagnostic Criteria from DSM-5.* Arlington, VA: American Psychiatric Association; 2013.

Bair MJ, et al. Association of depression and anxiety alone and in combination with chronic musculoskeletal pain in primary care patients. *Psychosom Med.* 2008; 70:890. [PMID: 18799425]

► Treatment

Chronic pain management focuses on reduction in symptoms and improvement of function rather than on disease cure. Both medication and nonpharmacologic modalities effectively decrease primary and secondary symptoms of chronic pain, with a range of treatments often provided through a treatment team (**Table 51-1**). However, physicians and patients must accept the fact that complete resolution of pain complaints may not be possible. Thus they need to work toward rehabilitative goals of reducing symptoms and

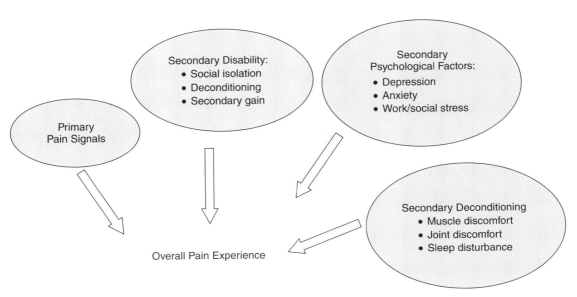

▲ **Figure 51-1.** Primary and secondary features of chronic pain.

Table 51-1. Comprehensive treatment of chronic pain.

Specialist	Treatment Modalities
Physician	Analgesics, adjunctive medications, nerve blocks, medical counseling to foster self-management
Physical/occupational therapist	Musculoskeletal dysfunction, deconditioning, work simplification
Psychology/psychiatry	Address locus of control, depression therapy, anxiety therapy
Complementary/alternative therapist	Acupuncture, yoga/tai chi, meditation, chiropractic therapy

minimizing disability. Although modern medicine and rehabilitation techniques can be beneficial, the patient's mindset must shift from searching for a medical cure to engaging in collaborative rehabilitation, geared toward decreasing pain and optimizing function. Goals of chronic pain rehabilitation are improvement in both pain and secondary symptoms, including deconditioning, depression, and disability (**Table 51-2**). Early identification and treatment should reduce the severity of secondary symptoms.

A. Psychological Approaches

Cognitive behavioral therapy (CBT) is an effective psychological treatment technique that challenges dysfunctional precepts or perception of pain ("My pain must be cured. I can't do anything if I have pain.") and replaces it with one that is more conducive to change ("Pain limits me from

Table 51-2. Appropriate treatment goals.

General Goal	Specific Treatment Target
Decreased pain	Pain reduction to moderate levels; reduced frequency and duration of flares
Improved function	Return to school or work; increased number of household chores; increased participation in leisure activities
Improved sleep	Reduced number of wake-ups; improved overall sleep to 5 hours per night
Improved mood	Increased participation in social activities; reduced time in bed/being inactive; improved nutrition intake
Reduced use of medical resources	Reduced emergency department visits; reduced use of excessive analgesics; decreased repeat consultations or studies

lifting 25 pounds, but I can still carry a bag of groceries."). Cognitive behavioral therapy helps change patients' perceptions or locus of control from external (believing that pain is not controllable by the patient) to internal (believing that the patient can positively influence symptoms). When patients endorse an external locus of control, they see themselves as victims of pain and as powerless to improve their situation. This results in the expectation that only fate or the physician can help when pain becomes severe. When expectations are not met, these patients seek alternative evaluations and treatments (eg, another physician, a different diagnostic test, or surgical procedures) that may not be in their best interest. The clinician must help patients to move into a pain self-management–internal locus of control belief system, in which patients perceive themselves as the agent for change. Greater perceived self-control of pain decreases both pain and secondary symptoms. Although CBT is typically the purview of psychologists, the family physician can reinforce these concepts through interactions with the patient. Mindbody approaches can be very helpful and are often integrated with CBT in a self-management program (see section on complementary and alternative therapies).

Additionally, counseling should be directed toward issues concerning mood, sleep, and other psychosocial factors. Severe symptoms of depression or anxiety or significant psychosocial stressors may necessitate a psychiatric referral.

Jensen MP, et al. Changes after multidisciplinary pain treatment in patient pain beliefs and coping are associated with concurrent changes in patient functioning. *Pain.* 2007; 131:38. [PMID: 17250963]

B. Physical and Occupational Therapy

Identification and treatment of musculoskeletal dysfunctions and decisions concerning limitations on activity often require consultation with physical or occupational therapists. Reconditioning, active stretching and strengthening exercises, and graded activity programs are effective for managing chronic pain. Physical therapists should instruct patients in a daily exercise routine as well as flare management techniques (eg, trigger point massage, oscillatory movements, and use of heat and ice). Furthermore, exercise therapy effectively reduces pain in elderly patients with osteoarthritis. Obesity is associated with increased inflammatory cytokines, weakness (particularly of the quadriceps), and increased disability associated with osteoarthritis of the knees. Conversely, exercise reduces weight and inflammatory markers, improves strength, and reduces pain and associated disability.

Occupational therapists will address work simplification, body mechanics, and pacing skills. Occupational therapists can facilitate returning to a more normal activity schedule (eg, returning to work or school), even on a modified basis. Prolonged absence from normal activities increases the difficulty of reducing disability. Return to normal activity as soon as possible, however, should be the primary goal of pain management, and the physician should work to expedite that return, with modifications if needed. Conflicts with an employer, fear of losing a job and benefits, or other intervening factors need to be identified and addressed to facilitate a successful return to work.

Jan MH, et al. Effects of weight-bearing versus nonweight-bearing exercise on function, walking speed, and position sense in participants with knee osteoarthritis: a randomized controlled trial. *Arch Phys Med Rehab.* 2009; 90:897. [PMID: 19480863]

Jessep SA, et al. Long-term clinical benefits and costs of an integrated rehabilitation programme compared with outpatient physiotherapy for chronic knee pain. *Physiotherapy.* 2009; 95:94. [PMID: 19627690]

Messier SP. Diet and exercise for obese adults with knee osteoarthritis. *Clin Geriatr Med.* 2010; 26(3):461–477. [PMID: 20699166]

C. Pharmacotherapy

Medications are prescribed to treat an underlying medical condition (eg, disease-modifying medications in rheumatoid arthritis), relieve symptoms of pain and secondary symptoms (eg, depression, anxiety, or sleep disturbance). Most medications used to treat chronic pain address the latter two factors (**Table 51-3**).

1. Pain relievers—Analgesics rarely eliminate pain entirely and may result in either significant adverse effects or habituation. Treatment should begin with simple analgesics, such as acetaminophen or nonsteroidal anti-inflammatory drugs (NSAIDs). There is debate over the appropriate maximum dosage of acetaminophen, historically 4 g per day, but recently reduced by McNeil PPC Inc to 3 g given concerns of toxicity. Acetaminophen should be restricted in patients with significant alcohol intake or liver disease. A variety of available NSAIDs share similar efficacy and tolerability.

Tramadol is a novel analgesic that has weak serotonergic and noradrenergic properties as well as weak μ-opioid activation. Despite the opioid agonist effect, in the absence of a history of opioid dependence, tramadol does not pose the same level of concern regarding abuse potential, physical tolerance, and psychological dependence as the true opioids. It thus offers an option falling between first-tier of agents (ie, acetaminophen and NSAIDs) and the stronger opioid medications. Common side effects include sedation, dizziness, and nausea. Although the full dosage is 100 mg 4 times daily, a lower dosage (eg, 50 mg times daily) is commonly prescribed, with extra dosing on an as-needed basis. The 400-mg maximum dose should be strictly adhered to given the potential for seizures at higher doses. For older adults or those taking other centrally acting agents, a maximum of 200–300 mg/d is a more reasonable maximum. As noted later, there is great concern regarding risk for falls and impaired cognition with these medications in older adults. Finally, the potential exists for inducing a serotonin syndrome when tramadol is used in combination with antidepressants or other serotonergic agents [eg, selective serotonin reuptake inhibitors (SSRIs) such as paroxetine or escitalopram, tricyclic antidepressants (TCAs) such as amitriptyline or nortriptyline, or novel agents such as trazodone or mirtazapine]. This syndrome can be seen as a paradoxical excitation associated with excessive activation of central nervous system (CNS) serotonin, with psychological effects that include hyperarousal, irritability, and agitation; neuromotor effects that include tremor, jitteriness, rigidity, and (at an

Table 51-3. Medication management of chronic pain.

Symptom Treated	Medication Class	Examples
Pain	Analgesics	Acetaminophen NSAIDs Tramadol
	Long-acting opioids	Sustained-release morphine, oxycodone, or transdermal fentanyl
Neuropathic pain	Antidepressants Anticonvulsants	Duloxetine, 30–60 mg BID Gabapentin, 300–1200 mg TID Pregabalin, 75–200 mg TID
Muscle spasm	Muscle relaxants	Tizanidine, 2–8 mg at bedtime to TID
Sleep disturbance	Antidepressants	Nortriptyline, 25–75 mg at bedtime Trazodone 50–150 mg at bedtime
Depression	Antidepressants	Bupropion, extended release, 150–300 mg daily Citalopram 20–40 mg daily

BID, twice daily; NSAIDs, nonsteroidal anti-inflammatory drugs; TID, 3 times daily.

extreme) seizures; and cardiac effects that include tachycardia and hypertension.

Including opioids in the management of chronic pain is controversial. Although isolated treatment with opioids is not effective for managing chronic pain, opioids can provide a safe, cost-effective adjunctive pain therapy because of reduced morbidity and cost associated with organ toxicity from analgesics. Chronic opioid use has been shown to reduce both pain and disability. Opioids may be considered in patients with severe, disabling chronic pain that is unrelieved with simple analgesics and is associated with significant impairment in daily functioning and quality of life. Opioids are most appropriately used when they are included as part of a more comprehensive rehabilitation program rather than as monotherapy. Relative contraindications include a history of substance abuse, serious psychopathology, and lack of motivation to engage in an appropriate therapy program or to improve functioning. Patients with no history of substance abuse are at low risk for abuse with prescribed medications. Patients with current addiction problems should be referred to a drug rehabilitation facility before pain management is initiated. Patients with recent substance abuse or addiction problems should be managed by a pain specialist, ideally in conjunction with a counselor specializing in treating patients with these types of problems. Misusing or abusing opioids occurs in about one in three chronic pain patients prescribed opioids. Guidelines from the American Pain Society and the American Academy of Pain Medicine can help identify patients who may be more appropriate candidates for opioid therapy and offer document recommendations to reduce liability. The Screener and Opioid Assessment for Patients with Pain (SOAPP; available at https://www.painedu.org/soapp.asp) and Opioid Risk Tool (ORT; available at http://www.opioidrisk.com/ node/884) are brief screening tools to help identify patients at higher risk for opioid misuse or abuse. The Current Opioid Misuse Measure (COMM; available at https://www.painedu.org/soapp.asp) helps determine whether patients prescribed long-acting opioids may be misusing their medications. Implementation of Risk Evaluation and Mitigation Strategy (REMS) programs designed to educate prescribers and patients about abuse risks is intended to help minimize opioid misuse and abuse.

Patients who have severe chronic pain that is constantly present are best managed with long-acting medication rather than frequent dosing with immediate-release agents. Short-acting medications are best used infrequently for intermittent, short-lived pain flares. Long-acting opioids include sustained-release morphine sulfate, sustained-release oxycodone, oxymorphone, transdermal fentanyl, and methadone. Methadone is least expensive (about 10% the cost of brand-name opioids); however, titration is difficult because of individual variability in metabolism. Opioid equivalence charts may be helpful when converting patients from one medication to another (**Table 51-4**). For example, the amount of opioid administered from a 100-μg/h fentanyl patch is roughly equivalent to an oral dose of 240 mg morphine sulfate daily. In general, musculoskeletal pain is more responsive to opioids than neuropathic pain, chronic headache, or fibromyalgia. Opioids may be a useful adjunctive treatment to other neuropathic medications in patients with neuropathic pain and, because of the high cost of gastrointestinal and renal effects of chronic analgesic therapy, can provide a cost-effective alternative for patients with chronic pain when properly monitored. Meperidine should be avoided, given the potential for adverse effects related to accumulation of metabolite normeperidine and a somewhat greater addictive potential.

Table 51-4. Opioid conversion chart.[a]

Drug	Oral Dose (mg)	Transdermal Dose (μg/h)	Intravenous Dose (mg)	Brand Names
Morphine sulfate	15		5	MS Contin, Kadian, Oramorph
Hydromorphone	4		0.8	Dilaudid
Oxycodone	10			Percocet, Roxicet, OxyContin
Hydrocodone	15			Vicodin, Lorcet, Norco
Oxymorphone	5			Opana
Meperidine[b]	150		35	Demerol
Fentanyl		6.25		Duragesic

[a]Dose conversions are approximate, with variation based on both individual patients and drug preparations.
[b]Should be avoided (see text).

Cepeda MS, et al. Tramadol for osteoarthritis. *Cochrane Database Syst Rev.* 2006; (3):CD005522. [PMID: 16856101]

Chou R, et al. Clinical guidelines for the use of chronic opioid therapy in chronic noncancer pain. *J Pain.* 2009; 10:113–130. [PMID: 19187889]

Khan MI, et al. Opioid and adjuvant analgesics: compared and contrasted. *Am J Hosp Palliat Care.* 2011; 28:378–383. [PMID: 21622486]

Krenzelok EP, Royal M. A. Confusion: acetaminophen dosing changes based on NO evidence in adults. *Drugs R&D.* 2012; 12(2):45–48. [PMID: 22530736]

Stillman M. Clinical approach to patients with neuropathic pain. *Cleve Clin J Med.* 2006; 73:726. [PMID: 16913197]

2. Adjunctive medications—Adjunctive medications supplement the benefits from analgesics, treat neuropathic or central pain, and treat secondary complaints. In addition, effective use of adjunctive agents often reduces the need for analgesic medications. Adjunctive agents interact with the mechanism of neuropathic or central pain and chronic headache by reducing *nervous system windup*, the process by which the nervous system amplifies and eventually perpetuates pain signals in the absence of ongoing nociceptive input from the periphery.

The two primary categories of adjunctive analgesics are antidepressants and anticonvulsants. Among the antidepressants, the greatest analgesia is achieved by dual serotonin- and norepinephrine-activating agents, with efficacy demonstrated for fibromyalgia, chronic headaches, and neuropathic pain. TCAs, venlafaxine, and duloxetine have good evidence supporting pain relief for fibromyalgia, neuropathic pain, and chronic headaches. Nortriptyline is often better tolerated, especially in older patients, than amitriptyline with comparable efficacy.

Comorbid depression, anxiety symptoms, sleep disturbance, and loss of energy are commonly seen in individuals with chronic pain. Many patients do not tolerate antidepressant medications or experience adverse effects (eg, sexual dysfunction with SSRIs). For such individuals, it may be preferable to find a tolerated agent that will help with mood and associated symptoms. For example, an anergic overweight woman with fibromyalgia may benefit from treatment with bupropion; alternatives to TCAs for a patient with depression and a sleep disturbance would include mirtazapine or trazodone.

Anticonvulsants, particularly gabapentin, have become a mainstay in the treatment of neuropathic pain. They are also beneficial for treating chronic headaches and may be beneficial for treating fibromyalgia. Valproate has also demonstrated efficacy for reducing neuropathic pain. Topiramate may also be beneficial. Some have multiple mechanisms of action, including membrane stabilization involving sodium and calcium channels, N-methyl-D-aspartate blockade, and GABAergic (γ-aminobutyric) effects. Pregabalin and gabapentin are related anticonvulsants with indications for pain associated with diabetic peripheral neuropathy and postherpetic neuralgia. Pregabalin is approved for fibromyalgia as well.

Most muscle relaxants (eg, carisoprodol and cyclobenzaprine) used to treat acute musculoskeletal pain are associated with significant sedation, reducing their usefulness as a treatment for chronic pain, for which the primary focus is on reducing disability and time spent in bed. Tizanidine, a unique muscle relaxant with both antispasticity and α-adrenergic effects, results in reduced spasticity and reduced pain perception with both acute and chronic use. In addition to reducing spasticity related to neurologic conditions (eg, multiple sclerosis, stroke, or spinal cord injury), tizanidine can also reduce symptoms associated with myofascial pain, fibromyalgia, and headaches, with some evidence of benefit for neuropathic pain. Tizanidine is often used in low doses (2–8 mg daily) given at bedtime or divided into three daily doses. Tizanidine is mildly sedating, which can assist with associated sleep disturbance.

Regarding dosing, medical mythology suggested that low doses of adjunctive agents were analgesic. The older agent, gabapentin, has nonlinear pharmacokinetics, complicating optimal dosage selection. Dose-response studies with both duloxetine and pregabalin have demonstrated a fairly linear response, indicating that efficacy may be found at higher doses among patients with a limited initial response to a low dose. The clinical applicability of this linear response with duloxetine and pregabalin has been confirmed in controlled clinical trials.

Bril V et al. Evidence-based guideline: treatment of painful diabetic neuropathy: report of the American Academy of Neurology, the American Association of Neuromuscular and Electrodiagnostic Medicine, and the American Academy of Physical Medicine and Rehabilitation. *Neurology.* 2011; 76:1758–1765. [PMID: 21482920]

Häuser W et al. The role of antidepressants in the management of fibromyalgia syndrome: a systematic review and meta-analysis. *CNS Drugs.* 2012; 26:297–307. [PMID: 22452526]

Silberstein SD, Holland S, Freitag F, et al. Evidence-based guideline update: pharmacologic treatment for episodic migraine prevention in adults: report of the Quality Standards Subcommittee of the American Academy of Neurology and the American Headache Society. *Neurology.* 2012; 78:1337–1345. [PMID: 22529202]

Thakur R, Philip AG. Chronic pain perspectives: treating herpes zoster and poster herpetic neuralgia: an evidence-based aproach. *J Fam Practice.* 2012; 61(9Suppl):S9–S15. [PMID: 230006700]

Verdu B et al. Antidepressants for the treatment of chronic pain. *Drugs.* 2008; 68(18):2611–2632. [PMID: 19093703]

3. Adverse events with chronic pain medications—Gastric ulcers occur in 15–30% of chronic NSAID users. Frequent use of NSAIDs or acetaminophen has also been linked with increased risk for developing hypertension and renal insufficiency. NSAIDs must be used with particular caution in the elderly, as their use reduces the effectiveness of diuretics and doubles the risk for hospitalization from congestive heart failure. Cyclooxygenase-2 (COX2) inhibitors were initially widely used in patients with chronic pain to minimize costs from gastric toxicity; however, postmarketing identification of increased risk for myocardial infarction and stroke has restricted use, especially in older patients.

Opioids are not associated with organ toxicity. Practitioners must monitor for evidence of the development of tolerance (reduced effectiveness of the medication over time) or abuse (failure to identify prescribed opioids on random urine testing or repeated, lost, or overused medications). The most common side effects experienced with opioids are constipation, fatigue, nausea, sleep disturbances, and poor appetite. Depression and sexual dysfunction may also occur. Patients who are prescribed daily opioids need an appropriate bowel regimen, including increased fluid and fiber intake and stool softeners/laxatives.

Newer anticonvulsants used to treat neuropathic pain do not require the frequent laboratory monitoring that is common with older anticonvulsants (eg, carbamazepine and sodium valproate). Gabapentin is cleared by the kidneys, requiring dose adjustment or reduced frequency of administration in patients with renal insufficiency. Dialysis patients receive gabapentin dosing after each treatment with hemodialysis.

Tricyclic antidepressants (TCAs), typically prescribed in low to moderate doses to treat neuropathic pain, are still associated with a small risk for cardiac arrhythmia. All prepubertal children treated with TCAs should receive a baseline electrocardiogram (ECG), followed by regular assessments of heart rate and blood pressure, periodic testing of antidepressant drug levels, and repeat ECGs. Similarly, older adults or individuals with a history of cardiac disease should also be monitored with blood tests and ECGs when TCA doses approach the low therapeutic range. For historical reference, we note that QTc prolongation led the FDA to pull propoxyphene from the market in the United States. This reminds us that the combination of agents such as citalopram and methadone may share this risk.

Selective serotonin reuptake inhibitors (SSRIs) and bupropion have been associated with seizures in higher doses and should be used with caution in individuals with tendencies to seizure. Venlafaxine and milnacipran can have a cardiac stimulatory effect at higher doses, and blood pressure should be monitored. Antidepressants, particularly those with a prominent serotoninergic effect, have been associated with the potential for suicidality and should be monitored closely in patients at risk and in children or adolescents. Combining serotonergic agents have the potential to create a serotonin syndrome, characterized by tremors, irritability, and cardiac excitation. One should exert caution with combining agents such as a classical antidepressant, trazodone for sleep, and tramadol for pain.

Tizanidine, duloxetine, and milnacipran have been associated with hepatotoxicity and should be avoided in individuals with a history of liver problems. Periodic liver enzyme screening should be obtained in patients taking these agents chronically.

Gooch K, et al. NSAID use and progression of chronic kidney disease. *Am J Med.* 2007; 120:280.e1–e7. [PMID: 17349452]
Stanos S. Evolution of opioid risk management and review of the classwide REMS for extended-release/long-acting opioids. *Phys Sportsmed.* 2012;40:12–20. [PMID: 23306411]
Vonkeman HE, van de Laar MA. Nonsteroidal anti-inflammatory drugs: adverse effects and their prevention. *Semin Arthritis Rheum.* 2010; 39:294–312. [PMID: 18823646]

4. Medication management in pediatric patients and in older patients—Chronically administered opioids are generally avoided in pediatric patients, although there are certainly exceptions with chronic disease states such as hemophilia and sickle cell disease. Acetaminophen and NSAIDs should be considered first-line therapy for pediatric patients with pain. TCAs and gabapentin have been extensively utilized for neuropathic pain in pediatric patients, and pediatric dosing guidelines are available. As noted, caution must be taken regarding the potential for cardiac conduction disturbance with the use of TCAs in prepubertal children.

When selecting medication for older adults, physicians need to strongly consider the side effect profiles, particularly for agents that have central nervous system (CNS) effects—including opioids, antidepressants, and anticonvulsants. As opposed to the mild sedation or dizziness experienced by younger individuals, geriatric patients may experience more profound drowsiness, confusion, delirium, and increased risk for falls. Medical comorbidities and medications for these conditions increase the risk for adverse events in geriatric patients. The potential for activation or inhibition of cytochrome P450 pathways is problematic in patients taking multiple medications, particularly agents with a narrow therapeutic index, such as digoxin and warfarin. With the exception of gabapentin, the dosing of adjunctive analgesics typically is lower for older adults.

Low to modest doses of opioids may be a very useful part of the treatment regimen for geriatric patients with pain, particularly because of good tolerability at low doses. As the degree of degenerative disease progresses, benefits from NSAIDs may be limited, necessitating stronger analgesia. When used judiciously, opioids typically are well tolerated and can allow individuals to retain a level of functioning sufficient to maintain their independence.

D. Interventional Pain Management

Interventional techniques are considered for patients failing conservative therapy or when specific nervous system pathology has been identified. Lumbar epidural steroid injections are effective for treating herniated disks or spinal stenosis. Sympathetic blocks reduce the burning pain of complex regional pain syndrome or reflex sympathetic dystrophy that may develop after acute extremity injury or surgery. Trigger point injections are useful for localized muscle pain. The benefit from injections is often transient, so these techniques are generally used in conjunction with physical therapy and medication management. Radiofrequency treatment (including ablative therapy and pulsed treatment) may be considered for patients with recalcitrant musculoskeletal or nerve pain. Conventional radiofrequency ablation is used for lumbar zygapophyseal joint pain, while pulsed treatment is more effective for cervical radicular pain and shoulder joint pain. Pulsed treatment may also have a role for treating discogenic pain, chronic inguinal herniorrhaphy pain, and chronic testicular pain.

Implantable devices, including intrathecal pumps and dorsal column stimulators, can be used to treat individuals with cancer-related pain or severe incapacitating pain resulting from nonmalignant conditions. Intrathecal medications are considered for patients requiring high medication doses when side effects from oral medications become intolerable. Dorsal column stimulators are most commonly used for treating patients with persistent severe back pain after surgery (failed back syndrome) and complex regional pain syndrome. For the treatment of pain resulting from nonmalignant conditions, it is essential to obtain psychological consultation prior to the surgery.

Nerve blocks may be particularly beneficial for postherpetic neuralgia, which can be quite difficult to treat. Nerve blocks, particularly thoracic epidural local anesthetics or intercostal blocks, can be used in the acute or chronic stage. Early use of nerve blocks, especially within the first 2 months of onset of symptoms, greatly decreases the incidence and severity of postherpetic neuralgia.

Chua NH, et al. Pulsed radiofrequency treatment in interventional pain management mechanisms and potential indications—a review. *Acta Neurochir.* 2011;153:763–771. [PMID: 21116663]

Manchikanti L, et al. Comprehensive evidence-based guidelines for interventional techniques in the management of chronic spinal pain. *Pain Physician.* 2009;12:699. [PMID: 19644537]

Patel VB, et al. Systematic review of intrathecal infusion systems for long-term management of chronic non-cancer pain. *Pain Physician.* 2009; 12:345. [PMID: 19305484]

Rainov NG, et al. Long-term intrathecal infusion of drug combinations for chronic back and leg pain. *J Pain Symptom Manage.* 2001; 22:862. [PMID: 11576803]

Yampolsky C, et al. Dorsal column stimulator applications. *Surg Neurol Int.* 2012; 3(Suppl4):S275–S289. [PMID: 23230533]

E. Complementary and Alternative Therapies

Complementary and alternative treatments are used by 40% of chronic pain sufferers. As in the discussion of psychological approaches, one tries to place the greatest emphasis on active strategies that can enhance an individual's self-management skills. Mind-body approaches such as mindfulness meditation and movement approaches such as yoga and tai chi fall within this model and have shown efficacy for a number of pain conditions. A recent meta-analysis revealed benefit of acupuncture for chronic conditions, including back and neck pain, osteoarthritis, headache, and shoulder pain. They noted a significant contribution from nonspecific factors as well. Chiropractic treatment is recommended for acute spinal pain, but there is no clear consensus on the effectiveness of chiropractic manipulation for chronic pain, and controlled studies are needed to provide efficacy data. Among biologically based treatments, glucosamine sulfate and chondroitin sulfate have had mixed success in studies, but they may provide an alternative to chronic nonsteroidal treatment for some patients, particularly with knee osteoarthritis. Another agent that merits further study for possible analgesic and anti-inflammatory effects is fish oil, in a dose of 1–2 g/d.

Clegg DO, et al. Glucosamine, chondroitin sulfate, and the two in combination for painful knee osteoarthritis. *N Engl J Med.* 2006; 354(8):795–808. [PMID: 16495392]

Posadzki P, Ernst E, Terry R, Lee MS. Is yoga effective for pain? A systematic review of randomized clinical trials. *Complement Ther Med.* 2011; 19(5):281–287. [PMID: 21944658]

Santilli V, et al. Chiropractic manipulation in the treatment of acute back pain and sciatica with disc protrusion: a randomized double-blind clinical trial of active and simulated spinal manipulations. *Spine J.* 2006; 6:131. [PMID: 16517383]

Vickers AJ, Cronin AM, Maschino AC, et al. Acupuncture for chronic pain: individual patient data meta-analysis. *Arch Intern Med.* 2012; 172(19):1444–1453. [PMID: 22965186]

Walker BF, French SD, Grant W, Green S. A Cochrane review of combined chiropractic interventions for low-back pain. *Spine.* 2011; 36(3):230–242. [PMID: 20393942]

Wang C, Schmid CH, Rones R, et al. A randomized trial of tai chi for fibromyalgia. *N Engl J Med.* 2010;363(8):743–754. [PMID: 20818876]

Weiner DK, et al. Complementary and alternative approaches to the treatment of persistent musculoskeletal pain. *Clin J Pain.* 2004; 20(4):244–255. [PMID: 15218409]

Wong SY, Chan FW, Wong RL, et al. Comparing the effectiveness of mindfulness-based stress reduction and multidisciplinary intervention programs for chronic pain: a randomized comparative trial. *Clin J Pain.* 2011; 27(8):724–734. [PMID: 21753729]

In Memoriam

We mourn the loss of Dawn A. Marcus, MD (1961–2013). Dr. Marcus was a respected neurologist, researcher, medical writer, and educator, as well as an Animal Friends volunteer.

Travel Medicine

Deepa Burman, MD, D.ABSM

William Markle, MD, FAAFP, DTM&H

In 2012 the United Nations World Tourism Organization reported that the international arrivals across boundaries surpassed the 1 billion mark for the first time in history, up from 996 million in 2011. This represents over a 71% increase in 15 years growing at a rate of 3–4% every year. There were 59 million international departures from the United States in 2011. Travelers may be business travelers to large cities where there are special dangers related to urban travel, but increasingly travelers are seeking out exotic locations as tourist destinations. Pretravel advice is often an afterthought for these travelers. Unfortunately, travel can also lead to health problems that range from unpleasant to life-threatening illnesses.

It is estimated that fewer than half of travelers seek any kind of pretravel advice. Many people ask their family physicians for recommendations, and at times the advice that they receive is either uninformed or outdated. Individuals returning to their country of origin are even less likely to consult a physician before travel, and preventable systemic illness is seen more commonly in this group than other tourists. It is important for all primary care physicians to be prepared to give accurate advice to travelers about both pretravel preparation and how to deal with illnesses contracted abroad. Sometimes there is not enough time to obtain the required immunizations, and priorities must be established. The goal of this chapter is to enable the family physician to provide guidance to patients wishing to be prepared for illnesses and emergencies related to travel.

Hudson TW, Fortuna J. Overview of selected infectious disease risks for the corporate traveler. *J Occup Environ Med.* 2008; 50:924–934. [PMID: 18695451]

Jong EC, Sanford C. *The Travel and Tropical Medicine Manual*, 4th ed. Philadelphia: Saunders Elsevier; 2008.

Leder K, et al. Illness in travelers visiting friends and relatives: a review of the GeoSentinel Surveillance Network. *Clin Infect Dis.* 2006; 43:1185. [PMID: 17029140]

World Tourism Organization. *Tourism Highlights*. Madrid: UNWTO; 2012 (available at http://mkt.unwto.org/sites/all/files/docpdf/unwtohighlights12enlr_1.pdf; accessed 3/10/13).

PRETRAVEL PREPARATION & CONCERNS

 Case 1

A 28-year-old man in good health is planning a 2-month trip to Kenya. He will be working in Nairobi but also plans to visit game parks and participate in outdoor activities.

- What history must be obtained?
- What specific advice should the patient be given, especially regarding hygiene, safety, and food preparation?
- What immunizations are needed?
- What malaria prophylaxis is recommended?
- Where can the physician find the answers to these questions?

The first step is to obtain a thorough history—including any preexisting medical conditions and use of medications that may have side effects or may interact with other drugs that will be prescribed—and to perform a thorough physical examination. What is the patient's exact itinerary, what countries will he visit en route, and in what order? What accommodations will he have? Will he remain in urban areas or visit some rural regions? What is his immunization history? This information will help determine necessary immunizations and prophylaxis. The physician can also help the traveler ensure that he has potentially essential items, such as insect repellent. If the patient has a chronic illness, he should be given pertinent portions of his medical record and a list of medications and allergies to take along in case he must seek medical care abroad.

Several websites provide helpful information about travel and health requirements (see listing at the end of this chapter). After reviewing these requirements, the physician would find that this patient faces several risks that should be discussed:

- Malaria, especially at lower elevations such as in game parks.
- Diarrhea, caused by parasites or bacteria such as *Escherichia coli* or *Shigella*.
- Typhoid fever and other salmonelloses.
- Hepatitis A, B, C, and E.
- Schistosomiasis, especially if swimming or wading in local bodies of water.
- Violence and petty thievery, especially in urban areas such as Nairobi.
- HIV/AIDS and other sexually transmitted diseases.
- Poor infrastructure for dealing with serious emergencies, such as motor vehicle accidents, especially outside of urban areas.

In the United States, as 78 million baby boomers approach retirement age, increasing numbers of older adults will plan for international travel. They will require the same steps pretravel, but since they are more likely to have chronic conditions and special needs, they may need some additional preparation.

Schlaudecker JD, Moushey EN, Schlaudecker EP. Keeping older patients healthy and safe as they travel. *J Fam Practice*. 2013; 62(1):16–23. [PMID: 23326818]

▶ Travelers' Medical Kit

Every traveler should carry a medical kit that addresses basic care for common illnesses and injuries. The essential components of such a kit are listed in **Table 52-1**, but they must be adjusted, depending on individual needs. If a patient uses a medication that is taken regularly, s/he should be advised to carry along enough to last for the entire trip and probably 1 or 2 weeks' extra. This will allow for unexpected changes in travel plans. A small supply should be kept in the carry-on bags, in case luggage is lost or delayed. All applicable airline regulations regarding carry-on baggage must be observed to ensure that the medication is not confiscated. Travelers should carry a letter from their physician if they plan to take along any controlled substance. This letter will help answer questions from immigration officials and other authorities in case questions are raised. Travelers should not forget to bring spare eyeglasses or contact lenses, contact lens solution, and their ophthalmologic prescription, in case of loss or breakage.

If the traveler is planning a long stay, the physician may be asked to supply prescribed medications on a regular basis from the United States, particularly if the drug in question is not available at the international destination. Increasingly, however, medications prescribed in the United States are available abroad (often much more cheaply) and can be

Table 52-1. Medical kit for travelers.

Contact card with important addresses and phone numbers of healthcare providers at home, medical insurance information, travel insurance, area hospitals or clinics, and US embassy
Insect repellent with ≤30% DEET, picaridin, or oil of lemon eucalyptus
Permethrin spray for clothing and mosquito nets, if traveling to the tropics
Sunscreen (minimum SPF15)
Syringes and needles (3–5-mL syringes, 21–25-gauge needles), if traveling in less developed countries where instrument sterilization may be uncertain
Extra pair of contact lenses or prescription glasses if applicable

Basic First Aid Items
Dressings, gauze pads, adhesive tape, adhesive bandages, small bottle of disinfectant, elastic bandage (eg, ACE), scissors, tweezers, cotton swab
Thermometer
Moleskin, if extensive hiking is planned
Hand wipes, liquid soap, hand sanitizer, facial tissues
First aid quick reference guide

Medications
Aspirin, acetaminophen, or other analgesic drug
Antidiarrheal (eg, diphenoxylate, loperamide, bismuth subsalicylate)
Antacid (eg, calcium carbonate), H_2-blocker (eg, cimetidine)
Eyedrops (for allergy and infection)
Eardrops (if risk of external otitis)
Dimenhydrinate or scopolamine, if motion sickness is a problem with air or water travel
Throat lozenges and cough drops
Sleep aid
Laxative
Condoms and contraceptives
Antihistamines (preferably a nonsedating agent such as loratadine, but diphenhydramine may be useful as a sleep aid in addition to its antihistamine activity)
Cold and cough medications
Asthma medications and inhalers if needed
Prednisone or other steroid
Topical antibiotics, antifungals, steroids, and vaginal antifungal drugs
Antibiotics (eg, ciprofloxacin, sulfamethoxazole-trimethoprim, amoxicillin, amoxicillin-clavulanate, azithromycin, doxycycline)[a]
Malaria prophylaxis (see text)
Water purification kit or filter (see text)
Acetazolamide, if travel is contemplated to elevations >8000 ft (>2500 m) above sea level
Injectable epinephrine if traveler has a history of anaphylactic reactions to foods or insect bites

[a]Inclusion of antibiotics depends on familiarity of the traveler with these medications and the likelihood they will be needed, based on the itinerary.
DEET, N,N-diethyl-meta-toluamide; SPF, sun protection factor.

obtained without difficulty by a knowledgeable traveler. Travelers should be cautioned to carefully examine any medications bought overseas, because ingredients may differ from those used in the US products, and some ingredients may not be considered safe by the US standards.

Jong EC, Sanford C. *The Travel and Tropical Medicine Manual*, 4th ed. Philadelphia: Saunders Elsevier; 2008.

Insurance

Travelers should check their health insurance policies to determine whether they include coverage for medical expenses incurred abroad. If coverage is provided, they should bring a blank insurance form in case it is needed or it becomes necessary to contact the insurance company. Term travel health insurance policies are also available. Evacuation insurance is essential in the event of a serious accident or medical problem. Some policies will return travelers to their home cities; others will evacuate them to the nearest location where they can receive medical care comparable to that available in their home country. Among the better-known companies offering evacuation insurance and emergency travel insurance are CSA Travel Protection (http://www.csatravelprotection.com), International SOS (http://www.internationalsos.com), MEDEX Insurance (http://www.medexassist.com), MedjetAssist (http://www.medjetassistance.com), and Multi-National—HCC Medical Insurance Services, LLC (http://www.hccmis.com/legal/). Policies can also be obtained through travel agencies. Finally, the traveler may wish to purchase trip insurance. This type of insurance ensures reimbursement in case a trip must be canceled for medical or other reasons beyond the traveler's control. (It should be noted that most trip insurance policies do not cover cancellation for personal reasons, such as a change in plans.) This insurance is especially attractive for older travelers, who are more likely to have a medical emergency that prevents them from traveling. The US Department of State answers questions about medical coverage on their website (http://travel.state.gov/travel/cis_pa_tw/cis/cis_1470.html; accessed 3/10/13).

Air Travel Concerns

Some medical conditions require special attention during air travel. These conditions include many severe, common illnesses, including anemia, clotting disorders, disfiguring dermatoses, dyspnea at rest, incontinence, otitis media, pulmonary or acute upper respiratory infections, and sickle cell hemoglobinopathies. Medical contraindications to air travel are listed in **Table 52-2**. Any traveler with an acute infectious disease should be cleared by a physician before traveling. If there is any question about the diagnosis, the individual should not travel until the risk is known. Exposure to tuberculosis and other serious infections can occur during flight, and an individual with a serious infectious disease should not travel on a commercial flight. Ill or handicapped travelers must notify the airline 72 hours before departure to ensure that the plane is properly equipped. Services such as a wheelchair, oxygen, stretcher, and other necessary equipment can usually be provided with advance notice.

Table 52-2. Contraindications to air travel.

Unstable angina
Myocardial Infarction in past 2 weeks (or 6 weeks if complicated)
Active bronchospasm
Neurosurgery or skull fracture in the past 2 weeks
Uncontrolled cardiac disease (congestive heart failure or arrhythmia)
Percutaneous coronary intervention in past 5 days (or 2 weeks if complicated)
Cerebral infarction in past 2 weeks
Pneumothorax in past 2–3 weeks
Colonoscopy with polypectomy in past 24 hours
Late pregnancy after 36 weeks gestation (long flights)
Highly contagious diseases, including active tuberculosis
Major uncontrolled psychiatric disorders
Cyanosis
Pulmonary hypertension
Recent middle ear surgery
Scuba diving in past 24 hours
Hemoglobin <7.5 g/dL
Heart, lung, or gastrointestinal surgery in past 3 weeks
Noncommunicating lung cysts

A. Use of Respiratory Assistive Devices on Aircraft

Patients with sleep apnea or requiring oxygen should carry their portable machines with them especially during long travels. In May 2009, the US Department of Transportation (DOT) issued a final ruling that all air carriers conducting passenger service (on aircraft originally designed for a passenger capacity of ≥19 seats) must permit someone with a disability to use a ventilator, respirator, continuous positive airway pressure (CPAP) machine, or an FAA-approved portable oxygen concentrator (POC), unless the device fails to meet applicable FAA requirements for medical portable electronic devices (M-PEDs) and does not display a manufacturer's label indicating that the device meets those FAA requirements. Currently, all FAA-approved POCs meet FAA requirements for M-PEDs.

US DOT. *Info for Operators*. Washington DC: FAA, 2009 (available at http://www.faa.gov/other_visit/aviation_industry/airline_operators/airline_safety/info/all_infos/media/2009/info09006.pdf; accessed 3/10/13).

Travel Health at Sea or on Cruise Ships

The sea has drawn adventurers, explorers, and settlers, as well as recreational travelers, to its shores and beyond for centuries. In 2008, the North American cruise industry, which makes up most of the global cruise market, comprised 161 ships carrying more than 13 million passengers to destinations worldwide. Nearly 9 million cruise passengers departed from US ports.

Exposure to dry, recirculated air, unfamiliar viral and bacterial pathogens, and new environmental allergens make respiratory illness the most common diagnosis in a ship's infirmary. Most cases are self-limited and should be treated symptomatically. Isolated cases of gastrointestinal illness aboard cruise ships are common, representing 5—10% of sickbay visits. Many of these cases are precipitated by changes in diet, overindulgence, and food and water ingested off the ship in developing countries. Fortunately, outbreaks of food- and waterborne illness are rare. As with shore-side outbreaks, more than half are due to the Norwalk (or related) viruses or undetermined agents. The rest are due to various bacterial agents, most notably enterotoxigenic *Escherichia coli*, salmonella, shigella, *Staphylococcus aureus*, *Clostridium perfringens*, and campylobacter. The Vessel Sanitation Program (VSP), developed and administered by the CDC, has been instrumental in the steady decline of gastrointestinal outbreaks aboard cruise ships.

Slaten DD, Mitruka K. *Cruise Ship Travel*. Atlanta: CDC; 2011 (available at http://wwwnc.cdc.gov/travel/yellowbook/2012/chapter-6-conveyance-and-transportation-issues/cruise-ship-travel.htm; accessed 3/10/13).

Zuckerman JN, ed. *Principles and Practice of Travel Medicine* (electronic resource published online). Hoboken, NJ: Wiley; 2002.

▶ Food and Water Sanitation

Many infectious diseases can be prevented by attention to food and water sanitation and good hygiene. These diseases include intestinal viral, bacterial, and parasitic infections. Travelers should be advised to avoid eating food that has not been cooked adequately or peeled by them. Cooking must be thorough, not just warming, and a clean knife must be used for peeling. If fish are eaten, they should be fresh, not dried or old-looking. Cans should be inspected for bulging or gas formation. Only dairy products that have been pasteurized should be consumed, and products that have been ultrapasteurized by the ultraheat treatment (UHT) method are preferred. Avoid raw vegetables and unpeeled fruits. Fruits and vegetables should be peeled by the traveler before consumption. Hands must be kept clean and fingernails trimmed. Clean silverware and plates should be used; these can be rinsed in boiling water or bleach rinse to sterilize them.

Travelers should be advised that bottled or canned drinks are safe as long as the seal is intact. Iced and lukewarm drinks should not be trusted, but hot drinks such as coffee or tea are generally safe if prepared recently and still hot when served. Tap water can be purified by either boiling it, treating it with iodine or chlorine, or filtering it with a reliable ultrafilter water purification system, as described below:

- Bring water to a rolling boil for 1 minute. Although the actual temperature reached will be slightly lower at higher elevation, this does not seem to have clinical relevance.

- Treat the water with iodine (10 drops of tincture per liter) and let stand for 30 minutes, or treat it with chlorine (1–2 drops of 5% chlorine bleach per liter of water) and let stand for 30 minutes. Although chlorine may not kill all parasitic cysts or viruses, water treated with chlorine has a better taste than iodized water; furthermore, chlorine does not affect thyroid function over long periods of use.

- Reliable water filtration systems are available through various sources [eg, Campmor (http://www.campmor.com) includes information on several systems]. A pore size of 0.2 μm is needed to filter out all enteric bacteria and parasites. If the water is cloudy or especially dirty-looking, some gross filtration or sedimentation must be done first before using a small-pore filter. Adding iodine resins to the filter will kill viruses if contact is sufficient.

Backer HD. Field water disinfection. In: Auerbach PS, ed. *Wilderness Medicine*, 6th ed. Philadelphia: Mosby; 2011: 1324–1359.

▶ Injury Prevention & Personal Security

The leading cause of mortality in travelers is motor vehicle accidents. Drivers should be aware of local motor vehicle laws and never mix alcohol with driving or any activity that requires mental alertness. Other common accidents that occur during travel include drowning, carbon monoxide poisoning, electric shock, and drug reactions. Travelers should be aware that jet lag and other causes of drowsiness while traveling (eg, medications to alleviate motion sickness) may heighten the risk of injury. If a traumatic injury occurs, travelers should be cautioned not to agree to blood transfusions unless absolutely necessary.

Although the risks to personal security in many parts of the world may be similar to those encountered in many urban areas of the United States, travelers may be at greater risk in areas where they are obviously foreigners or tourists. Most commonly, the risks to personal security are related to theft of personal belongings and the occasional violent methods used, especially in the urban areas of Africa and Latin America.

Another rarely discussed but important area of personal security is that of sexual activity while traveling. The freedom from a daily schedule and uniqueness of the situation may cause travelers to let down their normal guard. The incidence of sexually transmitted diseases, especially HIV, is quite high in many popular tourist destinations, including much of Africa, the Caribbean, Thailand, and some parts of Latin America. Travelers should be cautioned to use good judgment (especially in situations involving alcohol use), barrier protection such as condoms, and caution with oral-genital contact.

Sanford C. Urban medicine: threats to health of travelers to developing world cities. *J Travel Med*. 2004;11:313–327. [PMID: 15544716]

▶ Obtaining Medical Care Abroad

Obtaining reliable medical care abroad can be difficult. Frequent travelers may wish to become members of the International Association for Medical Assistance to Travelers (IAMAT), which provides up-to-date advice on where to seek competent medical care for virtually any area of the world. [Contact information: 1623 Military Rd., No. 279, Niagara Falls, NY 14304-1745; (716) 754-4883; www.iamat .org.] The International Society of Travel Medicine (www .istm.org) and the American Society of Tropical Medicine and Hygiene (www.astmh.org) are also excellent resources for those seeking to find travel clinics anywhere in the world.

▶ Immunizations

No vaccines are currently *required* for travel, with the exception of yellow fever vaccine if travel is planned through an endemic area. However, travelers from the United States should be up-to-date on all routine immunizations, including diphtheria, pertussis, tetanus, measles, mumps, varicella-zoster, rubella, influenza, pneumonia, and for children *Haemophilus influenzae* type b (see Chapter 7). For previously immunized adults, a single dose of polio vaccine is recommended for travel to an area with a risk of polio. Europe, Australia and the Western Pacific, and the Western Hemisphere have been certified polio-free.

Yellow fever vaccine is recommended for travelers to certain areas of Africa and Latin America. If there is a definite risk, the vaccine is recommended for all travelers at least 9 months of age. In some areas it is not generally recommended unless the person is at high risk (prolonged travel, heavy exposure to mosquitoes or inability to avoid mosquito bites). In areas without transmission, the vaccine is not recommended.

Typhoid and hepatitis A vaccines are recommended for travelers to most areas of the world. Two typhoid vaccines are currently available in the United States: Ty21a and Vi. Efficacy of both vaccines is 50–80%. Ty21a is a live oral vaccine that conveys protection for 5 years. It is taken as a series of four tablets, one every other day. The tablets must be refrigerated until ingested. Vi is a parenteral vaccine that provides protection for 2 years. Persons receiving this vaccine have a higher incidence of systemic reactions such as fever or malaise for the first 2–3 days after administration than those who receive the oral vaccine, and they may also develop injection site soreness.

Meningococcal vaccine is indicated for travelers to areas of sub-Saharan Africa and any area where meningococcal disease is endemic or epidemic. Saudi Arabia now requires that Hajj and Umrah visitors be vaccinated with a tetravalent vaccine before entering the country. Meningococcal conjugate vaccine group 4 (MCV4) is preferred among persons aged 11–55 years, and meningococcal polysaccharide vaccine group 4 (MPSV4) is the recommended vaccine among children aged 2–10 years and adults >55 years. Duration of immunity lasts at least 5 years, and adverse reactions are generally mild. Japanese encephalitis (JE) vaccine is recommended for travelers to endemic areas of rural Asia during periods of transmission, especially if the traveler plans to live there or stay for >30 days.

Cholera vaccine is no longer available in the United States; however, an oral vaccine, *Vibrio cholerae* whole-cell/B subunit vaccine (Dukoral), is available abroad. This vaccine also provides limited protection against infection with enterotoxic *E. coli.* No country now requires cholera vaccination; however, some local authorities may ask for this documentation. A single dose of the oral vaccine is sufficient; or a medical waiver written on physician letterhead will satisfy this request.

Rabies vaccine is recommended for travelers to high-risk developing countries and countries where rabies immune globulin is not available. Long-term travelers or those who may have extensive outdoor or nighttime exposure and those whose occupations place them at risk should consider this vaccine. Postexposure vaccination is still required.

Hepatitis B vaccine is recommended for travelers to high-risk areas, especially long-term travelers, and those engaging in high-risk sexual behaviors. Medical workers must be vaccinated, as should the future adoptive parents of children from a developing country.

All travelers are at a risk of pertussis, and all adults aged >19 years who have not received a prior Tdap or are in close contact with infants should receive a single dose of Tdap even if a Td booster has been administered recently.

Table 52-3 summarizes information for these and other vaccines. Up-to-date immunization information can be obtained from the Centers for Disease Control and Prevention (CDC; www.cdc.gov/travel).

Brunette GW, ed. *CDC Health Information for International Travel 2008.* US Dept of Health and Human Services, Public Health Service, Centers for Disease Control and Prevention. New York: Oxford University Press 2012.

TREATMENT & PREVENTION OF TRAVEL-RELATED ILLNESSES

Travelers' Diarrhea

 ESSENTIALS OF DIAGNOSIS

▶ Twofold increase in the frequency of unformed bowel movements, usually more than four or five stools per day.

▶ Abrupt onset while traveling or soon after returning home.

▶ Usually associated with abdominal cramps, rectal urgency, bloating, and malaise.

▶ Generally is self-limiting after 3–4 days.

Table 52-3. Vaccines that may be administered to travelers.

Vaccine	Efficacy (%)	Partial Protection Begins	Duration of Protection
Live vaccines			
MMR	>95	28 days after first dose	Lifelong
Tuberculosis (BCG)	Variable	6–8 weeks	Variable
Typhoid Ty21a (oral)	50–80	After 3rd dose	5 years
Varicella	>99	After 4–6 weeks	≥10 years
Yellow fever	>99	After 10–14 days	≥10 years
Inactive vaccines			
Cholera (oral)	80–85	After 7 days	≥6 months
Diphtheria	95–97	After 2nd dose	5–10 years
Hepatitis A	95–100	2 weeks after 1st dose	Lifelong after series completed
Hepatitis B	90–95	4 weeks after 2nd dose	Lifelong after series completed
Influenza (inj)	86–87	1–2 weeks	6 months–1 year
Japanese encephalitis	80–91	10 days after 2nd dose	2–4 years
Meningococcal	75–100	After 14 days	≥5 years depending on vaccine
Pertussis	80–86	After 2nd dose	≥2 years
Pneumococcal PCV7	>90	After 2nd dose for invasive disease	Unknown
Pneumococcal 23	56–81	Variable	5–10 years
Polio (inj)	>95	After 3rd dose	Probably lifelong
Rabies	>99	7 days after 2nd dose	2 years
Tetanus	>99	After 2nd dose	10 years
Tickborne Encephalitis	95–100	2 weeks after 2nd dose	3 years
Typhoid Vi (inj)	50–80	After 10 days	2 years

BCG, bacillus Calmette-Guérin; inj, injectable; MMR, measles, mumps, rubella.

▶ General Considerations

Travelers' diarrhea occurs in a significant number of people who travel to foreign countries, and approximately 30–50% of travelers to high-risk areas (Mexico, Latin America, Africa, Asia, and the Middle East) will develop diarrhea during a 1–2 week stay. It is caused by fecal-oral contamination of food or water by bacteria, parasites, and viruses. The condition is more common in young adults, and the best chance for prevention involves strict attention to hygiene, sanitation, and food preparation, as outlined earlier. Food from restaurants and street vendors are common sites for exposure, and thus eating in a private home may be safer. It is extremely difficult to avoid all dangers in food and drink, and multiple studies have shown no correlation between personal hygiene measures and travelers' diarrhea. Nevertheless, it is prudent to follow basic hygiene measures while abroad.

In contrast to the developed world, where viruses are the most common cause of diarrhea, enterotoxigenic *E. coli* and other bacteria such as *Shigella, Salmonella, Vibrio,* and *Campylobacter* species, are the most common causes of diarrhea in most parts of the developing world. There are significant regional differences.

Clinical Findings

Travelers' diarrhea is characterized by the abrupt onset of at least a twofold increase in loose stools, usually four to five stools per day. Most episodes begin 4–14 days after arrival but can occur sooner if the concentration of bacteria ingested is sufficiently high. Common signs and symptoms include loose or watery stool, abdominal cramping, bloating, urgency, malaise, and nausea. Vomiting occurs in ≤15% of those affected. Symptoms usually resolve in 3–4 days if not treated but can last longer. Depending on the cause, fever, bloody stool, and painful defecation may occur, but these symptoms are not common. Physical findings include a benign abdomen with diffuse tenderness but no rigidity and increased bowel sounds. Patients may appear dehydrated depending on the severity of the diarrhea. Although travelers' diarrhea rarely is life-threatening, it can result in significant morbidity; one in five travelers with diarrhea is bedridden for a day, and >33.3% have to alter their activities. Stool examination and culture may yield a causative agent, but in 40–70% of cases no pathogen is identified. It is very difficult to differentiate enterotoxic and nonpathogenic *E. coli*. Examination for *C. parvum,C. microsporidium*, or other less common organisms should be initiated only when diarrhea has persisted for >10–14 days.

Treatment

Treatment for travelers' diarrhea includes fluid replacement and usually includes fluoroquinolone antibiotics (or in children, azithromycin) (**Table 52-4**). Trimethoprim-sulfamethoxazole and doxycycline are no longer generally recommended because of the development of widespread resistance. Rifaximin can also be used to treat noninvasive *E. coli*–induced travelers' diarrhea. It is very useful in Latin America and Mexico, but is less useful when *Campylobacter* is the causative pathogen. In some countries, particularly Thailand and Nepal, *Campylobacter* infections may be resistant to fluoroquinolones; thus azithromycin or other antibiotics may be needed. Although a 3–5-day course on antibiotics is usually recommended, there is evidence that 1–2 days of treatment may be sufficient.

Bismuth subsalicylate can be used by chewing two tablets (or taking 1 oz of liquid) every 30 minutes in up to eight doses. The potential for salicylate toxicity should be considered in patients taking aspirin, pregnant women, or children. Loperamide or diphenoxylate may be used for adults but never in the presence of high fever or bloody stool. Generally, it is best to combine these agents with antibiotics, especially if diarrhea is moderate or severe.

Fluid replacement using World Health Organization ORS salts are available in most countries. In the United States the salts can be obtained through Cera Products (www.ceraproductsinc.com). A simple rehydration solution can be prepared at home using ½ teaspoon of table salt, ½ teaspoon of baking soda, and 4 tablespoons of sugar in 1 L of water; orange juice can be added to provide potassium. Adults should drink 8 oz after every diarrheal stool. Children aged <2 years should be given 2–4 oz and those aged 2–10 years, 4–7 oz. Acetorphan (Racecadotril), available in Europe but not in the United States, may be an effective adjunct to oral rehydration solutions. Women who are breastfeeding an infant with diarrhea should continue to do so. Patients can also be instructed to eat boiled rice, which often leads to faster resolution of the diarrhea.

Prevention

Although, as mentioned earlier, the effectiveness of dietary precautions have not been conclusively proven to prevent travelers' diarrhea, it is important for travelers to observe good hygiene and sanitation and pay strict attention to food preparation and avoid high-risk food and adventuresome eating behavior.

The CDC does not recommend antibiotic prophylaxis for most travelers; however, it may be indicated in patients with active inflammatory bowel disease, brittle diabetes mellitus type 1, AIDS and other immunosuppressive disorders, unstable heart disease, and those on proton pump inhibitors. Travelers planning an exceptionally critical short trip, where even 1 day of illness could impact the purpose of the trip, may wish to use a prophylactic medication.

Fluoroquinolones have been found to provide ~90% protection. Ciprofloxacin 500 mg daily, levofloxacin 500 mg daily, norfloxacin 400 mg daily, or ofloxacin 300 mg daily, have all been used. Rifaximin has also been found to be safe

Table 52-4. Antibiotics used for the treatment of travelers' diarrhea.

Antibiotic	Dosage	Comments
Ciprofloxacin (Cipro)	500 mg BID for 1–3 days	Other quinolones (eg, ofloxacin, norfloxacin, and levofloxacin are presumed to be effective as well)
Rifaximin (Xifaxan)	200 mg TID for 3 days	Not effective in persons with dysentery
Azithromycin (Zithromax)	In adults, 500 mg daily for 3 days or 1000 mg in single dose; in children, 10 mg/kg daily for 3 days	Antibiotic of choice in children and pregnant women, and for quinolone-resistant *Campylobacter*

and effective and provides 72% protection against travelers' diarrhea. Bismuth subsalicylate (Pepto-Bismol two tablets 4 times a day) provides ~ 60% protection against travelers' diarrhea. Probiotics have also been studied, but results are not conclusive. They seem to reduce the risk of travelers' diarrhea by ~8%. There is no antibiotic with proven efficacy for prophylaxis against *Campylobacter* species, which are a more common cause of travelers' diarrhea in South and Southeast Asia

Brunette GW, ed. *CDC Health Information for International Travel 2008.* US Dept of Health and Human Services, Public Health Service, Centers for Disease Control and Prevention. New York: Oxford University Press, 2012.

Drugs for travelers' diarrhea. *Med Lett.* 2008; 28:50(1291):58–59.

Dupont HL, et al. A randomized, double-blind, placebo-controlled trial of rifaximin to prevent travelers' diarrhea. *Ann Intern Med.* 2005; 142:805. [PMID: 15897530]

Hill DR, Ericsson CD, Pearson RD, Keystone JS, Freedman DO, Kozarsky PE, et al. The practice of travel medicine: guidelines by the Infectious Diseases Society of America. *Clin Infect Dis.* 2006; 43(12):1499–1539..

Shah N, et al. Global etiology of travelers' diarrhea: systematic review from 1973 to the present. *Am J Trop Med Hyg.* 2009; 80(4):609–614. [PMID: 19346386]

Malaria

ESSENTIALS OF DIAGNOSIS

▶ Abrupt onset of fever, headache, chills, myalgias, and malaise during or after returning from an area in which malaria is endemic.

▶ Recurrence of symptoms every 1–2 days (highly variable).

▶ Thick and thin Giemsa-stained blood smears showing *Plasmodium* (diagnostic gold standard), or confirmation by rapid diagnostic testing for malaria.

▶ General Considerations

Malaria is a major international public health problem, responsible for considerable morbidity and mortality around the world each year. At least 40% of the world's population live in areas in which malaria is endemic, and ~5% are infected at any one time. It causes an estimated 1 million deaths per year. Although 90% of cases occur in sub-Saharan Africa, the disease is found throughout the tropics. In most countries the distribution is spotty. Few Americans know much about the disease because it was eradicated in the United States in the 1940s. In the United States about 1500 cases of malaria acquired abroad are reported annually to the CDC.

Malaria is caused by infection with *Plasmodium falciparum*, *P. vivax*, *P. malariae*, *P. ovale* (two subspecies:

Table 52-5. *Plasmodium* species causing human malaria.

Species[a]	Average Incubation Period (days)	Duration of Untreated Infection (years; max)	Duration of Attack (hours)	Periodicity
P. falciparum	7–14	2	>16	Daily or none
P. vivax	13	4	8-12	48 h
P. malariae	13–28	≥40	8-10	72 h
P. ovale	14–17	4	8-12	48 h
P. knowlesi	10–12	Unknown	>16	24 h

[a]*Plasmodium* genus.

P. ovale curtisi and *P. ovale wallikeri*) or *P. knowlesi*. The first two species account for the majority of infections, and most cases of severe infection and death are due to *P. falciparum*. The vector for transmission to humans is the female *Anopheles* mosquito. With the exception of Central America and parts of the Middle East, most *P. falciparum* infections are resistant to chloroquine, and some strains of *P. vivax* are also resistant. Travelers to the tropics should receive prophylaxis based on the latest CDC recommendations.

Incubation periods differ among the *Plasmodium* species (**Table 52-5**), and at times they may be much longer than those usually reported. *P. falciparum*, *P. malariae* and *P. knowlesi* do not form hypnozoites and do not produce chronic liver infection. Thus, infected patients should not relapse if treatment is adequate. This is not the case with *P. vivax* and *P. ovale*. Reactivation of dormant hypnozoites in the liver can occur with these species leading to relapse—sometimes decades after the original infection.

▶ Clinical Findings and Diagnosis

A. Symptoms and Signs

Classical symptoms of malaria in a nonimmune person are fever, chills and sweats, headache, and muscle and joint pains. Nausea, vomiting, abdominal pain, and diarrhea can also occur. Symptoms usually begin 10 days to 4 weeks after infection; however, malaria symptoms might start as early as 7 days or as late as 1 year, depending on the species, after the traveler returns from a malarial area. Physical findings include fever, tachycardia, and flushed skin; mental confusion and jaundice may be present. The spleen and liver are often palpable, especially in persons who have had repeated infections. Symptoms may be much milder in a semi-immune person and may be only a headache or general body aches.

Severe malarial infection, usually due to *P. falciparum*, causes a multitude of complications, including cerebral malaria (with seizures, coma, or death), renal failure, hemo-globinuria (also called "black water fever"), hemolytic anemia, acute respiratory failure, shock, and hypoglycemia. Long-term complications include hypersplenism, nephrotic syndrome, and a seizure disorder.

B. Laboratory Findings

The gold standard for diagnosis remains detection of parasites by Giemsa-stained thick and thin blood smears. Thick films are more sensitive for picking up infections and for measuring parasite density, and thin films are more accurate for identification of species. The films must be fixed and stained properly, and experience is required to interpret the findings. Reputable laboratories can be difficult to identify by a traveler abroad. Also, where malaria is no longer endemic (ie, the United States), healthcare providers may not be familiar with the disease. Clinicians seeing a febrile patient may not consider malaria among the potential diagnoses and thus would not order the needed diagnostic tests. Laboratory workers may lack experience with malaria and fail to detect parasites when examining blood smears.

Data have now emerged to support routine use of rapid diagnostic tests (RDT) for diagnosis of malaria in endemic areas as the standard of care. Thus far only one RDT has been approved by the US FDA: the BinaxNOW malaria test kit. It tests for the histidine-rich protein II (HRP2) antigen specific for *P. falciparum* plus a panmalarial antigen specific for all human plasmodia. Sensitivity and specificity to *P. falciparum* is 95% and 94%, respectively. *P. vivax* sensitivity and specificity are 69% and 100%, respectively.

Limitations of the BinaxNOW® malaria test kit include: samples containing *P. falciparum* are needed as a positive control, negative results require confirmation by thick and thin smears, and both viable and nonviable organisms are detected, including gametocytes are sequestered *P. falciparum* parasites. Therefore, this test may not be used for monitoring response to therapy since antigen persists after elimination of the parasite. HRP2-based techniques may also be limited by mutations of the HRP2 gene or antibody interference at high levels of HRP2.

Some representative websites with information on rapid diagnostic tests for malaria include http://www.alere.com/us/en.html, http://www.rapidtest.com, and http://www.premiermedcorp.com. Complete information about these diagnostic tests is also available from the WHO web site at http://www.wpro.who.int/malaria/sites/rdt/.

Hendriksen IC, Mtove G, Pedro AJ, Gomes E, Silamut K, Lee SJ, et al. Evaluation of a PfHRP2 and a pLDH-based rapid diagnostic test for the diagnosis of severe malaria in 2 populations of African children. *Clin Infect Dis.* 2011; 52(9): 1100.

Masanja MI, McMorrow M, Kahigwa E, et al. Health workers' use of malaria rapid diagnostic tests (RDTs) to guide clinical decision making in rural dispensaries, Tanzania. *Am J Trop Med Hyg.* 2010; 83(6):1238.

McCutchan TF, Piper RC, Makler MT. Use of malaria rapid diagnostic test to identify *Plasmodium knowlesi* infection. *Emerg Infect Dis.* 2008; 14(11):1750.

C. Differential Diagnosis

The differential diagnosis of malaria includes most febrile tropical illnesses prevalent in the area that the traveler has visited (see the section on fever in a returning traveler, later in this chapter). The illnesses most often confused with malaria include influenza and viral infections, dengue fever, babesiosis, relapsing fever, yellow fever, hepatitis, typhoid fever, kala-azar, urinary tract infections, tuberculosis, endocarditis, and meningitis (especially in patients with cerebral symptoms).

▶ Treatment

The medications used for the treatment of malaria vary and are frequently used in combinations. Ideally, determination of the correct treatment involves identification of the species of malaria, knowledge of where the traveler has been, and the medical history of the patient. No one drug acts on all stages of the disease, and different species of parasites show different responses. Full discussion of the treatment of malaria is beyond the scope of this chapter and may be found at www.cdc.gov/malaria/diagnosis_treatment/treatment.html.

A traveler who plans to visit a remote area without adequate medical facilities may wish to take along a reliable supply of medication for a full course of presumptive treatment if symptoms of malaria develop. Presumptive self-treatment should never take the place of being evaluated at a medical facility; however, it could be lifesaving if there is no nearby help. **Table 52-6** includes two suggestions for presumptive self treatment: atovaquone-proguanil (Malarone) or artemether-lumefantrine (Coartem). Malarone should not be used if the patient is taking this as prophylaxis, and Coartem should not be used in patients taking mefloquine prophylaxis.

Artemisinin derivatives such as artemether and artesunate are well tolerated and are given in combination with another drug such as amodiaquine, sulfadoxine-pyrimethamine, mefloquine, or lumefantrine. Artemether-lumefantrine is the only artemisinin-based combination therapy (ACT) currently available in the United States, but others are available abroad. There have been a few reports of resistance to artemisinin. Combination therapy has the advantages of slowing the development of resistance, reducing the length of the required treatment course, and more effectiveness.

For more information about malaria in general, visit the Roll Back Malaria website at http://www.rbm.who.int. CDC clinicians are also on-call 24 hours to provide advice to clinicians on the diagnosis and treatment of malaria and can be reached through the Malaria Hotline 770-488-7788 (or toll-free at 855-856-4713).

Table 52-6. Prophylaxis and presumptive treatment dosages for malaria.

Drug	Adult Dosage	Dosage in Children
Malaria Presumptive Treatment Atovaquone-proguanil[a,b] Adult tabs = 250 mg atovaquone + 100 mg proguanil Pediatric tabs = 62.5 mg atovaquone + 25 mg proguanil	4 adult tabs once daily for 3 days	5–8 kg: 2 pediatric tabs/d for 3 days 9–10 kg: 3 pediatric tabs/d for 3 days 11–20 kg: 1 adult tab/d for 3 days 21–30 kg: 2 adult tabs/d for 3 days 31–40 kg: 3 adult tabs/d for 3 days >40 kg: use adult dose
Artemether-lumefantrine[b,c] 20 mg artemether + 120 mg lumefantrine per tablet	Adult and pediatric doses based on weight 5–14 kg 1 tablet per dose 15–24 kg 2 tablets per dose 25–34 kg 3 tablets per dose ≥35 kg 4 tablets per dose 2nd dose given 8 hours after 1st dose, then a dose is given BID for next 2 days for a total of 6 doses over 3 days	Pediatric doses based on weight as in adult dose
Malaria Prophylaxis Chloroquine phosphate	300 mg base (500 mg salt) per week; start 1–2 weeks before travel and continue for 4 weeks after last exposure	5 mg base/kg per week (8.3 mg salt/kg) to maximum of adult dose
Hydroxychloroquine sulfate	310 mg base (400 mg salt) per week; start 1–2 weeks before travel and continue for 4 weeks after last exposure	5 mg base/kg per week (6.5 mg salt/kg) to maximum of adult dose
Mefloquine[d]	228 mg base (250 mg salt) per week Start 2–3 weeks before travel and continue for 4 weeks after last exposure	4.6 mg base/kg per week (5 mg salt/kg) per week: 9–19 kg: ¼ adult tablet per week 20–30 kg: ½ adult tablet per week 31–45 kg: ¾ adult tablet per week > 45 kg: 1 adult tablet per week
Atovaquone-proguanil[a,b]	1 adult tablet (250 mg atovaquone + 100 mg proguanil) per day; start 1–2 days before travel and continue for 7 days after last exposure	Pediatric tabs contain 62.5 mg atovaquone + 25 mg proguanil; dosages based on child's weight: 5–8 kg: ½ pediatric tab daily 9–10 kg: ¾ pediatric tab daily 11–20 kg: 1 pediatric tab daily 21–30 kg: 2 pediatric tabs daily 31–40 kg: 3 pediatric tabs daily > 40 kg: 1 adult tab daily
Doxycycline[e]	100 mg/d Start 1–2 days before travel and continue for 4 weeks after last exposure	Children ≥8 years: 2.2 mg/kg daily up to max of adult dose
Primaquine[f,g] For short duration exposure in areas with primarily *P. vivax*	30 mg base (52.6 mg salt) daily Start 1–2 days before travel and continue for 7 days after return	0.5 mg base/kg (0.8 mg/kg salt) up to adult dose daily
For terminal prophylaxis in people with prolonged exposure to or infection with *P. vivax* and/or *P. ovale*	30 mg base (52.6 mg salt) daily for 14 days after leaving area	0.5 mg base/kg (0.8 mg/kg salt) daily up to adult dose for 14 days after leaving area

[a]Contraindicated with severe renal impairment.
[b]Not for use in children <5 kg, pregnancy or lactating women breastfeeding an infant <5 kg.
[c]Do not use if taking mefloquine prophylaxis.
[d]Cautious use in pregnancy
[e]Contraindicated in pregnant or lactating women and in children younger than 8 years
[f]Contraindicated with G6PD deficiency and in pregnancy and lactation unless the infant has a documented normal G6PD level
[g]All patients should have a documented normal G6PD level before taking primaquine.
Tab, tablet.

▶ Prevention

A common approach to malaria prevention is to follow the "A, B, C, D" rule. (**a**wareness of risk, **b**ite avoidance, compliance with chemoprohylaxis, and prompt **d**iagnosis in case of fever).

A. General Measures

Travelers to endemic areas should be advised about basic measures to prevent mosquito bites, including wearing long sleeves, long pants, and light-colored clothing at dusk; avoiding perfumes that might attract mosquitoes; and treating bed nets with permethrin. A mosquito repellent containing 30–50% DEET (*N,N*-diethyl-meta-toluamide) is recommended. In Europe, 20% of picaridin and 35% of DEET have shown comparable efficacy for protection against malaria vectors for ≤8 hours after application.

Advice for Travelers. Treatment guidelines, *Med Lett*. 2006; 4: 25.

B. Malaria Prophylaxis

Chemoprophylaxis is a strategy that uses medications before, during, and after the exposure period to prevent the disease caused by malaria parasites. The aim of prophylaxis is to prevent or suppress symptoms caused by blood-stage parasites. In addition, presumptive antirelapse therapy (also known as *terminal prophylaxis*) uses a medication (primaquine) toward the end of the exposure period (or immediately thereafter) to prevent relapses or delayed-onset clinical presentations of malaria caused by dormant liver stages of *P. vivax* or *P. ovale*.

In choosing an appropriate chemoprophylactic regimen, the traveler and the healthcare provider should consider several factors. The travel itinerary should be reviewed in detail to determine whether the traveler is actually at risk for acquiring malaria. The next step is to determine whether significant antimalarial drug resistance has been reported in that location. Resistance to antimalarial drugs has developed in many regions of the world. Healthcare providers should consult the latest information on resistance patterns before prescribing prophylaxis for their patients.

Five medications are currently available and approved in the United States for malaria prophylaxis: chloroquine (or hydroxychloroquine), mefloquine, doxycycline, atovaquone/proguanil and primaquine. See Table 52-6 for prophylactic dosages in adults and children.

1. Chloroquine (or hydroxychloroquine)—This drug is still effective for prophylaxis in Central America above the Panama Canal and in some areas of the Middle East. It should not be used for prophylaxis in other areas. Most strains of *P/ falciparum* and some strains of *P. vivax* have developed resistance to chloroquine. Some of its side effects are pruritus, headache, blurred vision, myalgia, alopecia, and spotty depigmentation. It can cause exacerbations of psoriasis, eczema, and dermatitis, and caution should be used if it is prescribed to people with these disorders. Retinal injury may occur with lifetime doses of >100 g. Chloroquine is safe in pregnancy and breastfeeding. Prophylaxis should begin 1–2 weeks before the traveler's planned arrival in a malaria-endemic area and should continue for 4 weeks after return.

2. Mefloquine—This agent is effective for prophylaxis in most of the world except the border areas between Thailand, Myanmar, Cambodia, and Vietnam. *P. falciparum* shows a patchy, but increasing, resistance to the drug in some areas. It is considered safe to use in pregnancy and breastfeeding, although small amounts of drug are passed in breast milk. The most serious side effects are neuropsychiatric, such as bad dreams, paresthesias, hallucinations, and even psychotic reactions. Other side effects include vertigo, seizures, hepatotoxicity, headache, confusion, gastrointestinal upset, pruritus, and depression. It is contraindicated with serious psychiatric disorders or seizures. Caution is advised in patients with cardiac conduction abnormalities. Prophylaxis should begin at least 2 weeks before arrival in a malaria-endemic area and continue for 4 weeks after return.

3. Atovaquone/proguanil—This drug is effective and safe for children, but there is insufficient evidence to recommend it for use in pregnant women, children weighing <5 kg, or women breastfeeding infants weighing <5 kg. It is contraindicated in patients with severe renal impairment (creatinine clearance <30 mL/min). Side effects are generally mild and include abdominal pain, vomiting, and headache. Prophylaxis should begin 1–2 days before arrival in a malaria-endemic area and continue for 7 days after return.

4. Doxycycline—This agent is efficacious, safe, and the least expensive choice for prophylaxis. Its use is contraindicated in pregnancy, breastfeeding, and in children aged <8 years. Side effects include gastrointestinal upset, esophagitis, vaginal yeast infection, phototoxicity, hepatic toxicity, pseudomembranous colitis, and increased intracranial pressure. Prophylaxis should begin 1 day before arrival in a malaria-endemic area and continue for 4 weeks after return.

5. Primaquine—Primaquine may be used as primary prophylaxis in areas with primarily *P. vivax*. It is taken 1–2 days before travel to a malarial area and daily for 7 days after return. Terminal prophylaxis is not needed if primaquine is used as primary prophylaxis. When used as terminal prophylaxis, it is taken daily for 14 days after leaving the malarial area. Adverse effects include gastrointestinal upset. In patients with glucose-6-phosphate dehydrogenase (G6PD) deficiency, it can cause hemolysis, which can be severe and even fatal. It should be used only in those with documented evidence of a normal (G6PD) level.

Alto WA. *The Little Black Book of International Medicine.* Sudbury, MA: Jones and Bartlett; 2009.

Brunette GW, ed. *CDC Health Information for International Travel 2008*. US Deparmentt of Health and Human Services, Public Health Service, Centers for Disease Control and Prevention. New York: Oxford University Press; 2012.

Freedman DO. Malaria prevention in short-term travelers. *N Engl J Med*, 2008;359(6): 603–612. [PMID: 18687641]

TREATMENT OF THE RETURNING TRAVELER

Despite the best preparations, many travelers become sick while abroad or are ill on their return home. Of the 50 million travelers to the developing world each year, >50% will have a travel-related health impairment and 10–20% will consult a physician, either while abroad or after returning home, due to a travel related illness. This section describes three common problems faced by the family physician—fever, diarrhea, and eosinophilia—with the goal of assisting the physician make a final diagnosis and provide appropriate treatment to the returning traveler. The differential diagnosis depends on the traveler's itinerary and other factors, and all possibilities cannot be covered here. Fever and eosinophilia, in particular, may occur as symptoms in a wide range of infectious and inflammatory conditions.

Fever in a Returning Traveler

Fever in a returning traveler requires a thorough history (including immunizations and any use of prophylactic medications, illness in companions, sexual activities, and any nonprescribed drug use) and physical examination. Often localized symptoms or signs (eg, respiratory symptoms, jaundice) help narrow the diagnosis. See **Table 52-7** for the physical findings in various disorders. If the diagnosis is not immediately obvious, diseases that are endemic in the area(s) visited should be considered. Stable patients may be safely observed for a few days, and most fevers will resolve spontaneously. No definite cause is found in ≥25% of returning travelers with a fever; however, in a 2007 report from the GeoSentinel Network, 21% of patients were found to have malaria, 6% to have dengue fever, and 17% to have a disease preventable by a vaccine or chemoprophylaxis. Fever usually has an infectious cause, but occult malignancies and rheumatologic conditions should be considered in the differential diagnosis.

If illness persists or the patient is unstable or seriously ill, laboratory investigation becomes the key to the diagnosis. Laboratory studies that may be appropriate include a complete blood count; malaria smear, and smears for *Borrelia, Babesia,* and *Filaria*; typhoid culture or antigen test, including urine for *Salmonella* and *Legionella* antigens; urinalysis; liver function tests; cultures of blood, urine, and possibly cerebrospinal fluid; stool examination; biopsy of skin lesions, lymph nodes, or other masses, bone marrow aspirate; hepatitis serology; and other serologies depending on the patient's possible exposures. Acute and convalescent sera can be helpful in making a final diagnosis.

Table 52-7. Possible diagnoses with certain physical findings in febrile travelers.

Finding	Possible Associated Diseases
Rash	Dengue, typhoid, rickettsial infections, syphilis, gonorrhea, brucellosis, hemorrhagic fever viruses, Chikungunya and other viral illnesses including arboviruses, acute HIV infection, measles
Jaundice	Hepatitis, malaria, yellow fever, leptospirosis, relapsing fever
Lymphadenopathy	Mononucleosis and other viruses, rickettsial infections, brucellosis. dengue, acute HIV, visceral leishmaniasis, Lassa fever, toxoplasmosis
Hepatomegaly	Amebiasis, malaria, hepatitis, leptospirosis
Splenomegaly	Malaria, relapsing fever, trypanosomiasis, typhoid, brucellosis, visceral leishmaniasis, typhus, and dengue
Eschar	Rickettsial infections (especially Tsutsugamushi disease), *Borrelia*, Crimean-Congo hemorrhagic fever
Hemorrhage	Dengue, meningococcemia, leptospirosis, Lassa fever, Marburg and Ebola fever, Crimean-Congo fever, Rift Valley fever, yellow fever, rickettsial infections (Rocky Mountain spotted fever, louseborne typhus).

Data from Leggat PA. Assessment of febrile illness in the returned traveller. *Austral Fam Phys.* 2007; 36(6):328–333 and Wilson ME. Fever in Returning Travelers. Atlanta: CDC, 2011 (available at http://wwwnc.cdc.gov/travel/yellowbook/2012/chapter-5-post-travel-evaluation/fever-in-returned-travelers.htm#1954; accessed 3/10/13).

A chest radiograph should generally be done in febrile patients, especially if tuberculosis is suspected, and purified protein derivative (PPD) testing for tuberculosis should be performed. Seriously ill patients must be hospitalized, and any patient suspected of having a highly contagious condition must be isolated. This is especially true of travelers returning from Africa with hemorrhagic fever. Any case of suspected viral hemorrhagic fever must be reported to the local health department and to the CDC.

It is important to remember that "the common is still common," and, in fact, the most common causes of fever in returned travelers are routine illnesses such as upper and lower respiratory tract infections, sinusitis, urinary tract infections, and influenza. A more extensive differential diagnosis of fever is listed in **Table 52-8**, but these diseases should be considered only if a more common cause is not readily apparent.

Malaria is one of the more common and worrisome causes of fever in a returning traveler. Most cases of serious

Table 52-8. Selected causes of fever in a traveler returning from the tropics (not in order of frequency).

Short Incubation (<28 days)	Long Incubation (>28 d)
Arboviruses such as Chikungunya	Brucellosis (some cases)
Babesiosis	Filariasis
Bacterial diarrhea	Fungal diseases
Bartonellosis	Hepatitis B, C, E, and A (some cases)
Borreliosis	Leishmaniasis
Brucellosis (some cases)	HIV infection
Cytomegalovirus and other viruses	Liver abscess (amoebic)
Dengue fever, yellow fever, and hemorrhagic fever viruses	Malaria (some cases)
Endocarditis	Melioidosis
Hepatitis A (some cases)	Schistosomiasis
Histoplasmosis and other fungal diseases	Syphilis
Influenza and other acute respiratory infections	Trypanosomiasis (American and African)
Leptospirosis	Tuberculosis
Listeriosis	
Malaria (some cases)	
Meningococcemia	
Plague	
Rickettsial diseases	
Sepsis	
Toxoplasmosis	
Typhoid or paratyphoid fever and enteric fever	

fever requiring hospitalization in travelers are due to malaria. Infections, particularly with *P. falciparum*, frequently occur within 2 weeks of the mosquito bite, but may occur up to 5 years after exposure, especially if caused by *P. vivax* or *P. ovale*. In a seriously ill febrile traveler to a malarial area, for whom no cause can be found, it may be wise to include empiric treatment for malaria, even if the results of the blood smears are initially negative.

Leggat PA. Assessment of febrile illness in the returned traveller. *Austral Fam Phys.* 2007; 36(6):328–333.

Speil C, et al. Fever of unknown origin in the returning traveler. *Infect Dis Clin North Am.* 2007; 21:1091–1113.

Wilson ME, et al. Fever in returned travelers: results from the GeoSentinel Surveillance Network. *Clin Infect Dis.* 2007; 44:1560.

Diarrhea in a Returning Traveler

As discussed earlier, travelers' diarrhea is an acute condition that usually resolves within 2 weeks. Most acute bacterial infections can be treated successfully with ciprofloxacin or other antibiotics. Some travelers, however, develop persistent diarrhea or other gastrointestinal (GI) symptoms that can be difficult to diagnose and treat. In fact, a recent study showed diarrhea and other GI symptoms constitute 35% of

Table 52-9. Selected causes of persistent diarrhea in a returning traveler.

Parasites, especially *Giardia, Entamoeba histolytica, Cyclospora, Cryptosporidium*, microsporidia (especially if immunocompromised)

Bacteria, eg, *Campylobacter, E. coli* spp (enteropathogenic or toxin-producing stains), *Shigella, Salmonella, Aeromonas, Vibrio cholerae* and noncholera vibrios, *Yersinia, Clostridium difficile*

Lactase deficiency and other disaccharidase deficiencies

Bacterial overgrowth and tropical sprue

Irritable bowel syndrome

Inflammatory bowel disease

Idiopathic (Brainerd diarrhea)

all problems in travelers presenting to their family physicians. Some travelers develop a transient lactase deficiency after any bacterial, viral, or parasitic infection. This problem usually responds to lactose restriction for 7–10 days. Some travelers, especially those not careful with their diet, may develop a small bowel bacterial overgrowth, which may require antibiotic treatment. In some travelers, just a change from their usual diet or the consumption of treated or boiled water or unpasteurized milk can cause a lingering diarrhea termed *Brainerd diarrhea*.

Some causes of persistent diarrhea in a returning traveler are listed in **Table 52-9**. If a patient's response to antibiotic treatment is inadequate or the diarrhea persists for >7 days, a stool examination should be performed. Preferably three stools should be examined. In addition to checking for ova and parasites, an evaluation for *Giardia* antigen and bacterial cultures should also be performed. If symptoms of rectal disease are present, anoscopic and sigmoidoscopic examination should be done with biopsies as needed. If the results of these tests are negative, the physician should consider an empiric trial of metronidazole for the treatment of a possible *Giardia* or other protozoan infection. Irritable bowel syndrome (IBS) and, less commonly, inflammatory bowel disease may develop after travel in those who experience a bout of bacterial or viral diarrhea. In fact, one study showed that 63% of a group of 97 healthy student travelers to Mexico, who returned a questionnaire, developed diarrhea compatible with travelers' diarrhea. Six months later, 18% still reported loose stools, 18% reported abdominal pain, and 9% had fecal urgency. Of the 60 patients who had acquired diarrhea in Mexico, 7 (11.7%) met the criteria for IBS 6 months later. Finally, sometimes underlying GI pathology, such as celiac sprue and other malabsorption disorders and even gastrointestinal malignancy, can be unmasked after a bout of diarrhea in a traveler.

Caumes E, et al. Health problems in returning travelers consulting general practitioners. *J Trav Med.* 2008; 15(6):457–459.

Okhuysen PC, et al. Post-diarrhea chronic intestinal symptoms and irritable bowel syndrome in North American travelers to Mexico. *Am J Gastroenterol.* 2004; 99:1774–1778.

Rosenblatt JE. Approach to diarrhea in returned travelers. In: Jong EC, Sanford C, eds. *The Travel and Tropical Medicine Manual,* 4th ed. Philadelphia: Saunders Elsevier; 2008.

Eosinophilia in a Returned Traveler

A high level of eosinophilia (>450 eosinophils/μL), which almost always indicates a parasitic infection, is characteristically found in helminthic infections, especially for those helminthes that have an extraintestinal migration phase and produce tissue infection. Strongyloides and lymphatic and tissue filariasis cause some of the highest levels, and infection in humans can persist for many years if not treated. Protozoans, such as *Giardia* and *Plasmodium* species, rarely cause eosinophilia, with the exceptions noted in **Table 52-10**. Schistosomiasis has become a serious problem for people swimming or rafting in freshwater in Africa. Allergic disorders, such as allergic rhinitis or asthma, can also cause eosinophilia. In one study from Israel, 82 of 995 travelers (8.2%) were found to have significant eosinophilia. Of these, 44 (53.7%) were found to have schistosomiasis mostly acquired in sub-Saharan Africa. Of the remaining 38 cases, a definitive parasitological diagnosis could be made in only 9 (23.7%) travelers. This is compatible with other studies. A therapeutic trial of albendazole was given to most of the cases without a specific diagnosis, and ~90% reported a favorable response with resolution of symptoms and a significant decrease in the eosinophil count after 2 months.

The workup for a traveler with eosinophilia must include multiple stool examinations, including stool concentration if schistosomiasis is suspected. Biopsy specimens of skin lesions (onchocerciasis) or swollen lymph nodes (filariasis) can be examined for definitive diagnosis. Several serologic tests are available from the CDC and other specialized laboratories. These include tests for toxocariasis, strongyloidiasis, filariasis, trichinosis, schistosomiasis, cysticercosis, and paragonimiasis. A therapeutic trial of albendazole is probably warranted as above if no diagnosis is found.

Meltzer E, et al. Eosinophilia among returning travelers: a practical approach. *Am J Trop Med Hyg.* 2008; 78(5):702–709.

Table 52-10. Selected causes of eosinophilia in a returned traveler.

Infectious Causes

Helminthic: angiostrongyliasis, ascariasis, capillariasis, clonorchiasis, cutaneous larva migrans, echinococcosis, enterobiasis, fasciolopsiasis, filariasis, gnathostomiasis, hookworm, loiasis, onchocerciasis, paragonimiasis, schistosomiasis, strongyloidiasis, toxocariasis, trichinosis

Protozoal: *Blastocystis hominis, Dientamoeba fragilis, Isospora belli*

Fungal: bronchopulmonary aspergillosis

Viral: hepatitis B, HIV

Ectoparasitic: scabies

Other: tropical pulmonary eosinophilia (related to tissue filarial infections)

Noninfectious Causes

Allergic disorders: atopic eczema, urticaria, asthma, allergic rhinitis, drug reaction

Inflammatory bowel disease

Malignancy

Vasculitis

HIV, human immunodeficiency virus.

Websites

http://www.cdc.gov/travel (This site has advice regarding special needs, children, and pets. There is information about vaccines, and the site also has safety information about cruise ships. Finally, there is also information about recent disease outbreaks.)

http://www.paho.org (The Pan-American Health Organization web site has information on countries in the western hemisphere.)

http://www.promedmail.org (ProMED is a listserv that monitors for emerging diseases worldwide.)

https://www.travmed.com (This website has general information on travel medicine with links to many other sites.)

http://www.who.int (The World Health Organization web site has much useful information, including worldwide disease surveillance.)

Tickborne Disease

Niladri Das, MD, UPMC

ESSENTIALS OF DIAGNOSIS

▶ Tick bites are typically painless, and <50% of patients with tickborne disease present with a known bite.

▶ Consider tickborne diseases (TBDs) in the summer months for patients who present with fever, myalgias, and headaches but without GI or upper respiratory symptoms who live in tick-endemic regions of the United States.

▶ Diagnosis can be difficult because of nonspecific symptoms and difficulty in timely confirmatory testing.

▶ Treatment with doxycycline should be initiated when Rocky Mountain Spotted Fever, human granulocytic anaplasmosis, and/or ehrlichiosis is included in the differential diagnosis.

General Considerations

Tickborne diseases are on the rise in the United States. Several factors contribute to this surge, including suburban development, climate change, a rise in human outdoor activities, and an increase in vector hosts such as White-Tailed deer. Lyme disease is the most widely known tickborne illness to the public, as well as the most common. During 2000–2010 there were 250,000 reported cases of Lyme disease in the United States, although there has not been an incremental increase in the number of cases reported each year. However, the incidence of reported cases of anaplasmosis, babesiosis, ehrlichiosis, and Rocky Mountain Spotted Fever have all increased over that period of time and are the next most common TBDs after Lyme. The tickborne illnesses mentioned above will be discussed in detail in this chapter. Numerous other diseases are associated with ticks as vectors, many of which are emerging. (For more information regarding these

illnesses, visit the following CDC webpage: http://www.cdc.gov/ticks/).

One factor that is essential to the diagnosis and treatment of TBD is the geographic distribution of the particular disease (**Figure 53-1**). Lyme disease, Rocky Mountain Spotted Fever (RMSF), ehrlichiosis, human granulocytic anaplasmosis (HGA), and babesiosis are all associated with particular species of ticks. **Table 53-1** lists the six tick species of significance for this chapter, including their distribution and primary hosts. However, the patient rarely presents with the actual tick attached, and therefore visual identification of species is typically unnecessary.

Decker CF. Tick-borne illnesses: an overview *Dis Mon.* 2012; 58(6):327–329 [PMID: 22608118]

Centers for Disease Control and Prevention. *Tickborne Diseases of the United States: A Reference Manual for Health Care Providers*; 2013 (available at http://www.cdc.gov/lyme/resources/TickborneDiseases.pdf).

Pathogenesis

As is the case in any vector borne disease, ticks require hosts to survive and to transmit pathogens. Their lifecycle consists of egg, larval, nymph, and adult stages. Only ticks in the nymph and adult stages are able to attach to humans. These stages are most active during the summer months hence the seasonality of most TBDs. Humans are incidental, not primary, hosts. Primary hosts (mice, deer, dogs) serve as reservoirs for the diseases. Ticks attach to any host from outdoor contact with grasses, shrubs, and foliage, but vector-to-vector attachment can occur. Ticks feed on blood. In order to do so, they extend a mouthpiece to the host, secreting saliva with anesthetic properties. This saliva is where TBD pathogens are contained. In cases where saliva and blood contact is made, transmission can occur.

The pathogens themselves complicate the diagnosis of TBD. In the United States the causative organism of

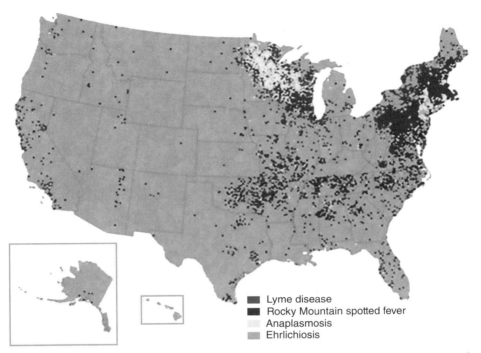

▲ **Figure 53-1.** Distribution of key tickborne diseases 2010 (babesiosis not included). (Data from Centers for Disease Control and Prevention, March 30, 2013.)

- ■ Lyme disease
- ■ Rocky Mountain spotted fever
- ▢ Anaplasmosis
- ▨ Ehrlichiosis

Lyme disease (*Borrelia burgdorferi*) is a spirochete, RSMF (*Rickettsia rickettsii*) is a gram-negative intracellular bacillus, ehrlichiosis (*Ehrlichia chaffeensis/ewingii*) and HGA (*Anaplasma phagocytophilum*) are intracellular gram-negative coccobacilli, and babesiosis (*Babesia microti*) is an intraerythrocyte protozoa. The atypical nature of these organisms makes for complicated pathophysiology in disease, but also complicates diagnosis and treatment.

CDC. *Tick Life Cyle and Host-Ticks*; March 2013 (available at /Ticks/). Salinas LJ, et al. Tickborne Infections in the southern United States. *Am J Med Sci.* 2010; 340(3):194–201 [PMID: 20697259]

▶ **Prevention**

Primary prevention of tickborne disease is achieved through a reduction of bites. Wearing light-colored clothing to facilitate

Table 53-1.

Tick (Common Name/Species Name)	Primary Range	Transmits	Additional Facts
Black-legged tick/deer tick (*Ixodes scapularis*)	Northeastern USA, Great Lakes region	Lyme, HGA, babesiosis	Can remain active in warmer winters
Western black-legged tick (*Ixodes pacificus*)	Pacific Coast, particularly northern CA	Lyme, HGA	Rates of infection are low
American dog tick (*Dermacentor variabilis*)	East of Rockies	RMSF	Also known as wood tick
Rocky Mountain wood tick (*Dermacentor andersoni*)	Rocky Mountain states	RMSF	Live in elevations 4000–10,500 feet
Lone Star tick (*Amblyomma americanum*)	Southeast USA, but can be Texas to Maine	Ehrlichiosis	Bites can be particularly irritating
Brown dog tick (*Rhipicephalus sanguineus*)	Throughout USA	RMSF	Primary host–dogs

HGA, human granulocytic anaplasmosis; RMSF, Rocky Mountain Spotted Fever.

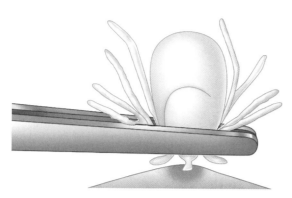

▲ **Figure 53-2.** (1) Use fine-tipped tweezers to grasp the tick as close to the skin's surface as possible; (2) pull upward with steady, even pressure—don't twist or jerk the tick, as this can cause the mouthparts to break off and remain in the skin (if this happens, remove the mouthparts with tweezers; if you are unable to remove the mouthparts easily with clean tweezers, leave it alone and let the skin heal); (3) after removing the tick, thoroughly clean the bite area and your hands with rubbing alcohol, an iodine scrub, or soap and water. (Data from Centers for Disease Control and Prevention, CDC-Tick Removal /ticks/, March 30, 2013.

tick visualization, as well as decreasing exposed skin area, has been demonstrated to be effective. Skin examination and showering within 2 hours after spending extended periods outdoors is recommended in tick-endemic areas. If a tick is discovered, forceps (**Figure 53-2**) or a commercial tick removal device should be utilized to mechanically remove the arthropod. No chemical means of removal are recommended.

Environmental alterations such as cutting tall grass and reducing brush and leaf piles will reduce outdoor areas where people would likely be affected by ticks. These measures also prevent attracting native hosts such as deer and mice. An environmental pesticide can also be extremely useful in endemic areas for total tick population reduction. At the present there are no TBD vaccines available on the market for humans. A previously available Lyme disease vaccine has been off the market for many years. Those who were inoculated using this product should no longer consider themselves immunized against Lyme disease. Of the personal repellents, products with *N,N*-diethyl-3-metylbenzamide (DEET) are the most effective. DEET product concentration ranges from 5% to 100%. The American Academy of Pediatrics advises against using any concentration that is >30%, although the CDC specifically recommends concentrations >20% for tick bite prevention. Children aged >2 months can use DEET. Its efficacy in patients of all ages

lasts between 1 to 5 hours depending on the concentration and extended periods outdoors merits reapplication to skin and clothing. The same rule applies for picaridin, which is effective for ≤3 hours and can been applied to the skin as well as clothing. No other repellents can be safely applied to the skin, but clothing immersed in permethrin solutions have been shown to be effective tick repellents.

Lyme disease is the only TBD for which antibiotic prophylaxis is recommended. If a patient presents with the history of tick attachment for >36 hours, antibiotic prophylaxis may be given within 72 hours after the removal. Doxycycline is the only antibiotic indicated for this: 200 mg by mouth (PO) once or ≤200 mg per 8 mg/kg for children aged >8 years. Prophylaxis with doxycycline is recommended only in the Lyme-endemic areas, which include locations with a tick infection rate of >20%. These areas are the Northeast from Maryland to Maine, Minnesota and Wisconsin, but not the West Coast when prevalence rates are low.

CDC. *CDC Features-DEET, Showers, and Tick Checks Can Stop Ticks* (available at /stopticks/; Jan.21, 2014).

Clark RP, Hu LT. Prevention of Lyme disease and other tick-borne infections. *Infect Dis Clin North Am.* 2008; 22(3):381–396. [PMID: 18755380]

LYME DISEASE

▶ **General Considerations**

A. Symptoms & Signs

Overall, 94% of Lyme cases are reported from Connecticut, Delaware, Maine, Maryland, Massachusetts, Minnesota, New Jersey, New Hampshire, New York, Pennsylvania, Virginia, and Wisconsin. Although Lyme disease is the most common vectorborne disease in the United States, the diagnosis is complicated by two potential stages of illness with variable presentations involving dermatologic, musculoskeletal, neurologic, and cardiac findings.

The localized stage of Lyme disease is most likely to present in the summer months 3–30 days after a tick bite. The hallmark of localized Lyme disease is erythema migrans (EM) (**Figure 5-3**). EM is typically at the site of prior tick attachment, often presenting for 7 days after the initial bite. It is characterized by an erythematous, ring or target macular lesion, typically measuring ≥5 cm. Rashes at the site of tick bites in the first 48 hours after a bite are typically local reactions and not indicative of TBD. EM is diagnostic of Lyme disease, and its presence is the only instance in which confirmatory testing is not necessary. This Lyme rash can present alternatively as a nontargetoid bluish lesion, as a rash with central crusting and no clearing, or as multiple red lesions with dusky centers known collectively as *disseminated erythema migrans*, which is indicative of disease spread. 70-80% of patients with Lyme disease present with EM, which typically resolves within 3–4 weeks without treatment. Along with

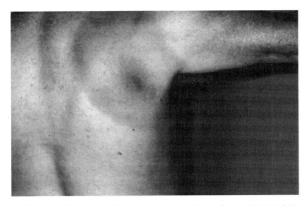

▲ **Figure 53-3.** Erythema migrans. (Data from CDC Public Health Image Library: http://phil.cdc.gov/; Jan. 2014.)

EM, the most common presenting symptoms of Lyme are fever, headache, myalagias, malaise, and fatigue, which are mostly consistent with a flulike illness but lack upper respiratory or gastrointestinal symptoms (**Table 53-2**).

The disseminated stage of Lyme disease typically occurs weeks after the initial infection. This can be manifested as disseminated EM as well as the persistence of flulike symptoms. Disseminated Lyme should be suspected in patients presenting in late summer/fall with aseptic meningitis,

cranial nerve palsies (particularly Bell palsy), atrioventricular block, myocarditis/pericarditis, migratory joint pain, and large joint monoarthritis or oligoathritis. Late-stage Lyme can manifest with one or more of these symptoms, and in endemic areas it is important to include TBD in the differential for any of these symptoms so that proper laboratory workup can be performed (Table 53-2).

B. Laboratory Findings

Laboratory evaluation in localized Lyme is often nonspecific. An elevated erythrocyte sedimentation rate, elevated liver enzymes, and hematuria or proteinuria can be seen. If a patient is suspected to have aseptic meningitis presenting with fever and headache, the cerebrospinal fluid (CSF) can demonstrate elevated lymphocytes/lymphocytic predominance, mild increase in protein, and normal glucose. The CDC has two accepted diagnosis methodologies for Lyme disease: EM and the presence of at least one sequela of late-stage disease and confirmatory testing. Serologic antibody testing is the laboratory diagnosis of choice. However, antibody testing is not helpful for early disease, as IgM does not develop until 2–4 weeks after initial disease and IgG typically takes longer than 4 weeks to develop. When ELISA testing is ordered, positive or indeterminate tests are typically followed by Western blot confirmation as false positives are common. Lyme disease–specific antibodies from CSF may be helpful in diagnosing cases of meningitis (Table 53-2).

Table 53-2. Diagnosis of tickborne diseases.

Disease	Incubation	Signs and Symptoms	General Labs	Confirmatory Labs
Localized Lyme disease	3–30 days	Erythema migrans (EM), flulike illness	Elevated ESR (typically <80), mild LFT elevation	Not typically applicable; see below; EM diagnostic
Disseminated Lyme disease	Month(s) after bite	Disseminated EM, large-joint arthritis, CN palsies, meningitis	CSF lymphocytic pleocytosis, elevated ESR/CRP	IgG/IgM; if +antibodies, then Western blot confirmation
RMSF	2–14 days	Fever, maculopapular rash 2–5 days after fever, petechiae after day 6, severe headache, AMS, meningismus	Thrombocytopenia, mild LFT elevation, hyponatremia	IgG + 7–10 days after onset of illness, fourfold increase after 2–4 weeks IgM false + common, early disease seronegative
Ehrlichiosis	7–14 days	Fever, headache, malaise, rash in 60% of children	Mild anemia, thrombocytopenia, leukopenia, elevated LFTs	Ehrlichia IgG + 1 week after onset of illness, fourfold increase after 2–4 weeks +PCR before abx
HGA	7–14 days	Fever, headache, myalgias	Mild anemia, thrombocytopenia, leukopenia, elevated LFTs	IgG + 1 week after onset of illness, fourfold increase after 2–4 weeks +PCR before abx
Babesiosis	7 days–2+ months	Fever, malaise, dark urine, nausea	Hemolytic anemia, thrombocytopenia, elevated BUN/Cr	Blood smear ID of protozoa, +PCR, antibody testing

abx, antibiotics; AMS, altered mental status; BUN/Cr, blood urea nitrogen/creatinine; CN, cranial nerve; CSF, cerebrospinal fluid; EM, erythema migrans; LFT, liver function test(s); PCR, polymerase chain reaction.

C. Other Considerations

Imaging studies may be useful in ruling out other etiologies when considering Lyme disease. The differential diagnosis should include other tickborne diseases, especially HGA, babesiosis, and Southern Tick-Associated Rash Illness (STARI). STARI is an emerging tick-borne disease with unknown etiology, but very similar presentation to early Lyme. At present the CDC recommends using the same antibiotics to treat STARI that are used to treat Lyme (**Table 53-3**). Non-tick related differentials for EM include local tick bite reaction, cellulitis, erythema multiforme, nummular eczema, granuloma annulare, contact dermatitis, and alternative arthropod bites. For late stage Lyme the differential includes juvenile idiopathic arthritis, rheumatoid arthritis, septic arthritis, gout, pseudogout, viral meningitis, multiple sclerosis, other etiologies of Bell palsy, and lymphoma.

► Treatment

The treatment of Lyme disease is complicated by the local and disseminated stages. Treatment options for those presenting with erythema migrans are doxycycline, cefuroxime, and amoxicillin for a ≥14-day course. There is some evidence supporting doxycycline use for only 10 days. Intravenous dosing with cetriaxone, cefotaxime, and penicillin G is indicated in patients with central nervous system (CNS) and cardiac manifestations. Arthritis manifestations without CNS manifestations can be treated with the aforementioned oral medications for 28 days (Table 53-3).

► Prognosis

Prognosis for Lyme is good, especially with early treatment. Even if disease progresses to disseminated stage, disability is

Table 53-3. Treatment of tickborne diseases.

Disease	First-Line Antibiotics (Adults)	First-Line Antibiotics (Children)	Duration	Alternative Regimens/Comments
Localized Lyme Disease[a]	Doxycycline 100 mg PO BID, amoxicillin 500 mg PO TID Cefuroxime 500 mg POD BID	Doxycycline 4 mg/kg divided doses BID, amoxicillin 50 mg/kg divided doses TID, cefuroxime 30 mg/kg divided doses BID	14 days, although can be extended to 21 days depending on case presentation	Macrolides can be used for patients who are intolerant of antibiotics listed They are less effective; doxycycline 200 mg can be given as single-dose prophylaxis
Disseminated Lyme disease	CNS/carditis: Ceftriaxone 2 g IV once daily Cefotaxime 2 g IV every 8 hours Penicillin G 18–24 million units/day in 6 divided doses Arthritis without CNS: treat with antibiotics for localized disease	CNS/carditis: ceftriaxone 50–75 mg/kg IV Arthritis without CNS: treat with antibiotics for localized disease	CNS/carditis: 14–28 days Arthritis without CNS: 28 days	Doxycycline 200–400 mg/day orally in 2 divided doses if unable to tolerate β-lactam antibiotics Carditis patients should preferentially be treated with ceftriaxone
RMSF	Doxycycline 100 mg PO or IV BID	Doxycycline 2.2 mg/kg per dose PO or IV BID	At minimum 3 days after resolution of fever; minimum 5–7 days	Use doxycycline if RMSF suspected in all cases, including children; other antibiotics increase likelihood of mortality
Ehrlichiosis/ HGA	Doxycycline 100 mg PO or IV BID		At minimum 3 days after resolution of fever; minimum 5–7 days	Rifampin is an alternative in special circumstances
Babesiosis	(1) Atovaquone 750 mg PO q12h + azithromycin 500–1000 mg PO on day 1 and 250 mg once daily thereafter (2) Clindamycin 300–600 mg IV q6h or 600 mg PO q8h + quinine 650 mg PO q6–8h	(1) Atovaquone 20 mg/kg PO q12h + azithromycin 10 mg/kg PO on day 1 and 5 mg/kg once daily thereafter (2) Clindamycin 7–10 mg/kg IV or PO q6–8h + quinine 8 mg/kg PO q8h	Treat for at least 7–10 days	Clindamycin plus quinine is the standard for severe babesiosis, but not as well tolerated Treatment not recommended for asymptomatic patients

[a]The treatment recommendations for STARI at present are to use the same antibiotics indicated for localized Lyme disease.
CNS, central nervous system.

uncommon. Treatment at any stage portends a high likelihood of symptom resolution, but lasting symptoms typically consist of arthralgias and/or sensory deficits (CN VII). Chronic Lyme disease is a separate entity with symptoms typically consisting of musculoskeletal pain and fatigue. Chronic or posttreatment Lyme continues to be an area of controversy. Studies are ongoing as to potential etiologies, but continued antibiotic treatment after resolution of active disease is not indicated.

Centers for Disease Control and Prevention. *Tickborne Diseases of the United States: A Reference Manual for Health Care Providers*; 2013 (available at http://www.cdc.gov/lyme/resources/TickborneDiseases.pdf).

Graham J, et al. Tick-borne illness: a CME update. *Pediatr Emerg Care*. 2011; 27(2):141–147. [PMID: 21293226]

Wormser GP, et al. The clinical assessment, treatment and prevention of Lyme disease, human granulocytic anaplasmosis, and babesiosis: clinical practice guidelines by the Infectious Diseases Society of America. *Clin Infect Dis*. 2006; 43:1089–1134. [PMID: 17029130]

ROCKY MOUNTAIN SPOTTED FEVER (RSMF)

▶ General Considerations

A. Symptoms & Signs

Rocky Mountain Spotted Fever cases have been reported in most US states. It is a medical misnomer as 60% of cases occur in North Carolina, Oklahoma, Arkansas, Tennessee, and Missouri. RMSF is considered to be the most severe tickborne illness in the United States as it causes a systemic, small vessel vasculitis and has a mortality rate of ≥25% without treatment. The classic presentation of RMSF is fever, rash, and headache 2–14 days after a tick bite. However, myalgias, nausea, and changes in mental status are common on acute presentation. The hallmark rash of RMSF is maculopapular and occurs in ≤90% of patients, typically 2–5 days after the fever presents. The rash classically first appears as discrete, blanchable lesions on the wrists, ankles, and forearms that spreads to the trunk, palms, and soles (**Figure 53-4**). However, diagnosis should not be based on the appearance of a rash, as this can delay treatment (Table 53-2).

Because of the vasculitic nature of the disease, petechiae can occur after 6 days of symptoms. Development of petechiae often occurs in untreated disease and is a poor prognostic sign. Another poor prognostic sign is CNS involvement with meningismus and altered mental status. Clinical diagnosis is imperative to initiating proper treatment, which significantly reduces morbidity.

B. Laboratory Findings

Early disease is associated with thrombocytopenia (most common), a mild elevation in liver enzymes, anemia, and

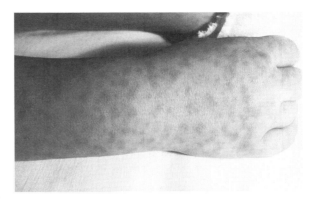

▲ **Figure 53-4.** Maculopapular rash of Rocky Mountain Spotted Fever. (Data from CDC Public Health Image Library: http://phil.cdc.gov/; Jan.2014.)

hyponatremia. Again, RMSF is a clinical diagnosis as antibodies are detectable only 7–10 days after illness onset. In the event of a positive IgG antibody test, repeat testing 2–4 weeks following the initial testing is recommended. If the follow-up IgG testing demonstrates a fourfold titer increase, RMSF is confirmed. For those patients presenting with CNS symptoms, cerebrospinal fluid analysis is typically unremarkable (Table 53-2).

C. Other Considerations

Twenty percent of RSMF cases are in children, making the diagnosis even more difficult given initial symptom overlap with other viral illnesses as well as other TBDs. It is important to bear in mind that 90% of cases are reported between April and September. In those patients who are acutely ill, it is important to obtain infectious disease consultation early in the course of the evaluation and treatment.

▶ Treatment

The key treatment decision when RMSF is considered in the differential is to select doxycycline as the antibiotic of choice. Clinical suspicion merits treatment. Doxycycline is first-line therapy for patients of all ages, including children. There is no evidence to show permanent teeth discoloration with limited dosing, and unfortunately the use of other antibiotics has been shown to increase mortality (Table 53-3).

▶ Prognosis

In patients who receive early antibiotics, the mortality rate with RMSF is approximately 2–3%. A delay in antibiotic treatment to >5 days increases that rate to >20%. Although most patients who are treated with antibiotics recover without long-term complications, some patients have persistent neurologic symptoms such as gait abnormalities, speech difficulty, dysphagia, and/or encephalopathy. These symptoms may resolve over time, but reinforce the critical nature of early treatment with doxycycline.

Centers for Disease Control and Prevention. *Tickborne Diseases of the United States: A Reference Manual for Health Care Providers*; 2013 (available at http://www.cdc.gov/lyme/resources/TickborneDiseases.pdf).

Decker CF. When to suspect tick-borne illness. *Dis Mon*. 2012; 58(6):330–334. [PMID: 22608119]

Salinas LJ, et al. Tickborne infections in the southern United States. *Am J Med Sci*. 2010; 340(3):194–201. [PMID: 20697259]

Woods CR. Rocky Mountain spotted fever in children. *Pediatr Clin North Am*. 2013; 60(2):455–470. [PMID: 23481111]

HUMAN GRANULOCYTIC ANAPLASMOSIS (HGA) AND EHRLICHIOSIS

► General Considerations

A. Symptoms & Signs

Ehrlichiosis and HGA have similar clinical manifestations, but are associated with two different species of ticks. HGA, commonly known as *anaplasmosis*, is associated with the *Ixodes* species and is also the tick that carries Lyme disease. Therefore coinfection is possible as HGA is found in the same primary range of the Great Lakes and northeastern United States. Ehrlichiosis is reported most frequently in the southeastern United States. Both diseases present with fever, headache, malaise, and myalgias 1–2 weeks after tick bite. These nonspecific symptoms make the diagnosis difficult, and occasionally nausea, vomiting, and a maculopapular rash (particularly in children) complicate the diagnostic picture, due to a clinical presentation similarity to RSMF or Lyme.

► Laboratory Findings

Nonspecific findings for both HGA and ehrlichiosis include mild anemia, thrombocytopenia, leucopenia, and liver enzyme elevation. During the early phase of illness morulae, or HGA/Ehrlichial inclusion bodies, may be visualized in leukocytes and are highly indicative of acute infection. However, the absence of morulae on peripheral smears does not exclude either diagnosis.Similar to RMSF, antibody testing is the gold standard for confirmation of disease. Initial IgG antibody titers positive for HGA or ehrlichiosis occur 7–10 days after symptoms start. Confirmation of disease is made by repeating IgG testing in 2–4 weeks and noting a fourfold increase in titers. Unlike RMSF, early polymerase chain reaction (PCR) testing is available, but most sensitive in the first week of illness, particularly before the administration of antibiotics.

► Treatment

Despite the complexity in diagnosis plus overlapping range and symptoms with other TBDs, ehrlichiosis, HGA, Lyme, and RMSF can all be treated with doxycycline (Table 53-3). The rule of thumb should be if a serious TBD is considered in the differential, use doxycycline for treatment. It can easily be discontinued or treatment refined if an alternative diagnosis is made. However, as with RMSF, doxycycline is the only antibiotic that is highly effective against HGA and ehrlichiosis. As in the case with all TBDs and pregnancy, consider an infectious disease consultation.

► Prognosis

Mortality rates with HGA and ehrlichiosis are between 1% and 3% of those with known infections. Although 35–50% of patients will require hospitalization, a majority of those will recover completely with no long-term affects. The elderly and immunocompromised patients are at higher risk.

Centers for Disease Control and Prevention. *Tickborne Diseases of the United States: A Reference Manual for Health Care Providers*; 2013 (available at http://www.cdc.gov/lyme/resources/TickborneDiseases.pdf).

Qasba N. A case report of human granulocytic anaplasmosis (ehrlichiosis) in pregnancy and a literature review of tick-borne diseases in the United States during pregnancy. *Obstet Gynecol Surv*. 2011; 66(12):788–796.

Salinas LJ, et al. Tickborne infections in the southern United States. *Am J Med Sci*. 2010; 340(3):194–201. [PMID: 20697259] Wormser GP et al. The clinical assessment, treatment and prevention of Lyme disease, human granulocytic anaplasmosis, and babesiosis: clinical practice guidelines by the Infectious Diseases Society of America. *Clin Infect Dis*. 2006;43:1089–1134. [PMID: 17029130]

BABESIOSIS

► General Considerations

A. Symptoms & Signs

Unlike the TBDs described above, babesiosis is a protozoan-induced infection. It is reported in the northeastern United States and Great Lakes region, but sporadic cases have been noted across the country, and its incubation period ranges from 1 week to >2 months. The geographic variability and delayed presentation also confirm that babesiosis can be contracted via blood transfusion, which is unique among TBDs. There are approximately 10 such case reports a year.

Babesiosis can be asymptomatic, with only 60% of children and 80% of adults presenting with signs of infection. Typical symptoms include fever, chills, malaise, arthralgias, anorexia, nausea, and dark urine. The physical exam may demonstrate hepatosplenomegaly and jaundice secondary to hemolysis. Patients with hemolysis can have fulminant disease.

B. Laboratory Findings

Anemia secondary to this hemolysis is often noted in babesiosis, as is elevated blood urea nitrogen (BUN) and serum creatinine. Acutely, elevated liver enzymes and thrombobo-cytopenia may also be noted. Microscopic identification of *Babesia* in the erythrocytes by peripheral blood smear is diagnostic, but the sensitivity is low. PCR analysis positive for *Babesia* is confirmatory, and IgG testing can be supportive, but does not distinguish between acute and past infection.

Treatment

Similar to malaria, babesiosis requires the use of antiprotozoals. Two combination therapies are recommended: atovaquone plus azithromycin or quinine plus clindamycin. The latter combination is recommended in cases of serious infection. Treatment duration of 7–10 days is usually adequate.

Prognosis

Symptoms of fatigue may persist weeks to months after successful treatment, but complete resolution is common without persisting disability. Recurrence of infection, particularly in the elderly, immunocompromised and asplenic requires extended treatment.

Cable RG, Leiby D. Risk and prevention of transfusion-transmitted babesiosis and other tick-borne diseases. *Curr Opin Hematol.* 2003;10(6):405–411. [PMID: 14564169]

Vannier E, Krause PJ. Human babesiosis. *N Engl J Med.* 2012; 366(25):2397–2407 [PMID: 22716978]

Wormser GP, et al. The clinical assessment, treatment and prevention of Lyme disease, human granulocytic anaplasmosis, and babesiosis: clinical practice guidelines by the Infectious Diseases Society of America. *Clin Infect Dis.* 2006;43:1089–1134. [PMID: 17029130]

Tuberculosis

N. Randall Kolb, MD

Tuberculosis remains an important infectious disease for primary care physicians. Significant problems exist in recognizing and diagnosing active tuberculosis and in using correct treatment to prevent the development of multidrug-resistant tuberculosis. Recognizing and treating tuberculosis in patients with AIDS is a major challenge. The impaired immune response leads to a lack of common signs and symptoms and more difficulty in providing effective treatment.

▶ Definitions

Tuberculosis infection is caused by *Mycobacterium tuberculosis*, generally affecting the lungs but can occur at many locations in the body [*Treatment of Tuberculosis Guidelines* 4th ed.; 2009 (available at WHO/HTM/TB/2009.420)]. *Multidrug-resistant tuberculosis* is defined as *M. tuberculosis* resistant to isoniazid and rifampin. *Extensively drug-resistant* (XDR) *tuberculosis* is defined [*MMWR* 2006; 55(43):1176] as *M. tuberculosis* isolates resistant to isoniazid, rifampin, any fluroquinolone, and at least one of three injectable second-line drugs (amikacin, kanamycin, or capreomycin). *Latent tuberculosis* is exposure to *M. tuberculosis* without active disease. *Primary tuberculosis infection* is active disease due to *M. tuberculosis*. Secondary tuberculosis infection in patients previously sensitized to M. tuberculosis usually occurs as reactivation TB, but may occur with reinfection with a new strain of M. tuberculosis. Extrapulmonary tuberculosis refers to localized infection at a site other than the lungs, such as lymph nodes, pleura, kidney, genitalia, bones or joints, heart, nervous system (particularly meninges), any intraabdominal organ (particularly at terminal ileum and cecum), peritoneum, and pericardium.

▶ General Considerations

A. Global Overview

Tuberculosis (TB) (see *WHO Fact Sheet* 104; reviewed Feb. 2013) is second only to HIV/AIDS as the greatest killer worldwide, due to a single infectious agent even though the TB death rate dropped by 41% between 1990 and 2011. In 2011, 8.7 million people contracted TB and 1.4 million died from it. Most TB deaths (>95%) occur in low- and middle-income countries, and it is among the top three causes of death for women aged 15–44. In 2010, approximately 10 million children were orphaned as a result of TB deaths among parents. TB is a leading killer of people living with HIV, causing 25% of all deaths in this group of people.

Tuberculosis occurs in every part of the world. In 2011, the largest number of new TB cases occurred in Asia, accounting for 60% of new cases globally. However, sub-Saharan Africa carried the greatest proportion of new cases per population with over 260 cases per 100,000 people. Multidrug-resistant TB (MDR-TB) is present in virtually all countries surveyed.

In 2012, a total of 9951 new TB cases were reported in the United States, with an incidence of 3.2 cases per 100,000 population. However, the rate of TB increased in certain minority populations in United States. For instance, in 2012 the rate of TB among non-Hispanic Asians was 25 times greater than that among non-Hispanic whites, 7.3 times greater among non-Hispanic Afro Americans, and 6.6 times greater among Hispanics.

In the United State, the most commonly affected groups are foreign-born, HIV-positive, and homeless persons, as well as individuals who are incarcerated, report excessive alcohol use, and are international adoptees who have a TB infection rate of 12% [*Pediatrics* 2004;120(3):e610].

B. Multidrug-Resistant Tuberculosis

In 2011, a total of 127 cases of multidrug-resistant TB (MDR-TB) were reported in the United States. In 2012, one case of extensively drug-resistant TB was reported in the United States [*MMWR* 2013;62:101]. Worldwide, 3.7% of new cases and 20% of previously treated cases were estimated to have MDR-TB. India, China, the Russian

Federation, and South Africa have almost 60% of the world's cases of MDR-TB. The highest proportions of TB patients with MDR-TB are in eastern Europe and central Asia (*WHO Global Tuberculosis Report 2012*).

▶ Prevention

Adults with active tuberculosis are the most common source of tuberculosis, so prevention depends on timely diagnosis of active TB. Active TB can be prevented by treating latent TB infection (LTBI) in persons likely to develop active TB. Public health programs with intensive screening, treatment, and preventive therapy for household contacts of active TB cases may modestly decrease TB incidence rates by effectively preventing new cases of active TB. Tuberculin skin testing is the primary screening method in the United States.

Administration of the tuberculin skin test (TST) [previously referred to as the *purified protein derivative* (PPD) test] is as follows:

- Inject 0.1 mL PPD intradermally.
- This should produce a wheal of 6–10 mm.
- Read 48–72 hours after placement—do not let healthcare workers (HCWs) read their own results.
- Find and measure induration—do not measure redness.
- Employ the Sokal ballpoint pen method as follows:
  - Place tip of ballpoint pen 1–2 cm away from margin of skin test reaction.
  - Move pen slowly toward center of reaction while applying moderate pressure.
  - Maintain skin tension if necessary by applying slight traction on skin behind pen in direction opposite pen movement.
  - When ballpoint reaches margin of induration and definite resistance to further movement is noted, lift pen.
  - Repeat procedure from opposite side of reaction.
  - Measure distance between margins of induration and record result.

If the TST reaction is read as ≥15 mm up to 7 days after placement, the result can be considered positive. Pregnant patients require no modification in testing or interpretation of results.

Interpretation of tuberculin skin test in adults is as follows [*MMWR Recomm Rep*. 2000; 49(RR-6):1]:

- Induration ≥15 mm considered positive in persons with no risk factors for tuberculosis (TB)
- Induration ≥10 mm considered positive in
  - Injection drug users
  - Persons with high-risk clinical conditions

- Silicosis
- Diabetes mellitus
- Chronic renal failure
- Some hematologic disorders (eg, leukemias and lymphomas)
- Other specific malignancies (eg, head, neck, or lung carcinoma)
- Weight loss ≥10% of ideal body weight
- Gastrectomy
- Jejunoileal bypass
- Recent immigrants (within previous 5 years) from high-TB-prevalence countries
- Persons from medically underserved, low-income populations
- Residents and employees of high-risk congregate settings (prisons, nursing homes and other long-term care facilities, residential facilities for patients with AIDS, homeless shelters); ≥15 mm induration considered positive for employees who are otherwise at low risk and are tested at start of employment
- Mycobacteriology laboratory personnel
- Induration ≥5 mm considered positive in patients with
  - HIV infection or risk factors for HIV infection with unknown status
  - Recent contact with individual with active TB (household, social, or unprotected occupational exposure similar in duration and intensity to household contact)
  - Fibrotic chest x-ray (consistent with healed TB)
  - Organ transplants or receiving immunosuppressive therapy (equivalent of prednisone ≥15 mg/day for > 1 month)

Interpretation of tuberculin skin test in children and adolescents is as follows [*Pediatrics* 2004; 114(Suppl 4):1175]:

- Induration ≥15 mm considered positive in children ≥4 years old with no known risk factors
- Induration ≥10 mm considered positive in
  - Children or adolescents at increased risk of disseminated disease
  - Children < 4 years old
  - Those with concomitant medical conditions (eg, Hodgkin disease, lymphoma, diabetes mellitus, chronic renal failure, or malnutrition)
  - Children or adolescents with increased risk of exposure to cases of TB disease
    - Those born in or travel to a country with high prevalence of TB cases
    - Those with parents born in a country with high prevalence of TB cases

- Those frequently exposed to adults with risk factors for TB disease (eg, adults with HIV infection, homeless adults, users of illicit drugs, those who are incarcerated, or migrant farm workers)

- Induration ≥5 mm considered positive in

  - Children or adolescents in close contact with a known or suspected case of infectious TB

  - Children or adolescents with suspected TB disease–finding on chest radiograph consistent with active or previously active TB or clinical evidence of TB disease

  - Children or adolescents who are immunosuppressed (eg, receiving immunosuppressive therapy or immunosuppressive conditions)–specific dose, frequency, and length of treatment with corticosteroids that increase risk for false negative not known

Interpretation of positive test based on the criteria listed above should not be affected by patient history of bacille Calmette-Guérin (BCG) vaccination.

Priorities for screening populations are identified [*MMWR Recomm Rep.* 2005;54(RR-12):1] by employing a tiered approach, determined by the relative likelihood of TB infection in a population and the ease of implementing a screening program. Screening includes identification of risk factors, assessment for signs of active TB, and placement of a tuberculin skin test:

- Tier 1 (high risk, easily accessible, with good likelihood of completing therapy)

  - Workers and patients in clinics serving persons with HIV infection

  - Prisoners

  - Legal immigrants and refugees with TB notification status

  - Recently arrived refugees

  - Well-defined groups in congregate living facilities

  - Patients in substance abuse treatment programs

- Tier 2 (high risk, easily accessible, with lower likelihood of completing therapy due to transient status)

  - Jail detainees

  - Residents or staff of homeless shelters

  - Immigrants reporting for adjustment of status

- Tier 3 (high prevalence of latent TB but risk for TB disease not increased, not easily accessible group)

  - Foreign-born high-risk persons immigrating within 5 years from a country with high incidence of TB

Screening children in the United States consists in identifying children at increased risk and then screening them using a tuberculin skin test. The New York City Department of Health questionnaire is a useful tool for identifying at-risk children. The questionnaire with at least one positive response has a 5.6% positive predictive value (PPV) and 99.8% negative predictive value (NPV) for a positive tuberculin skin test [*JAMA* 2001;285(4):451]. The questionnaire asks about contact with a TB case, birth in or travel to endemic areas, regular contact with high-risk adults, and HIV infection.

Tuberculin skin testing is recommended before treatment with tumor necrosis factor α inhibitors: infliximab (Remicade), etanercept (Enbrel), and adalimumab (Humira).

Tuberculin skin test (TST) boosting is an issue in populations who will have repeated TST over time. Boosting occurs when a person with LTBI has a negative TST reaction when tested many years after the initial infection. The initial TST may stimulate (boost) T cell ability to react, and then any positive reactions to subsequent TSTs could be misinterpreted as a recent converter indicating recent infection. This problem is avoided by using the two-step testing for the initial TST. Testing with a blood assay for *Mycobacterium. tuberculosis* (BAMT) such as QFT-Gold, which does not boost, and involves a single-baseline test, is adequate.

Tuberculin skin text (TST) two-step testing is employed for initial baseline *M. tuberculosis* testing for those who will be given TST periodically (eg, HCWs or staff in homeless shelters):

- No previous TST: perform two-step test.

- First test positive: consider TB-infected.

- First test negative: retest in 1–3 weeks (after first TST result was read).

- Second test positive: consider TB-infected.

- Second test negative: consider not infected.

When serial testing identifies a staff member who converts to a positive TST (ie, ≥10 mm increase in TST) or new positive BAMT, perform a problem evaluation with contact investigation. This includes determining the likelihood and extent to which *M. tuberculosis* transmission occurred; identifying persons exposed and, if possible, the source of potential transmission; identifying factors that could have contributed to transmission such as failure of isolation procedures; and ensuring that exposure to *M. tuberculosis* has been terminated and conditions leading to exposure have been eliminated.

Treatment of latent tuberculosis (also called *prophylaxis*) is indicated for

- Household members and other close contacts of potentially infectious persons

- Newly infected persons [positive tuberculin skin test (TST) within 2 years]

- Positive TST and age <35 years

- Patients with past tuberculosis (TB) or significant TST reaction and abnormal chest x-ray in whom current active TB has been excluded

- Positive TST with silicosis, diabetes mellitus, long-term steroids, immunosuppression, AIDS, HIV, reticuloendothelial cancer, end-stage renal disease, rapid weight loss, or chronic undernutrition (postgastrectomy, chronic malabsorption, chronic peptic ulcer disease)

Drug treatment of latent TB infection consists in administration of the following agents:

- Isoniazid 300 mg once daily (or 10-15 mg/kg up to 900 mg twice weekly) for 9 months is drug of choice.
- Rifampin 600 mg daily for 4 months is alternative regimen in patients intolerant to isoniazid or exposed to patients with isoniazid-resistant TB.
- Pyrazinamide plus ethambutol or quinolone if exposed to TB resistant to both isoniazid and rifampin.
- Rifampin plus pyrazinamide for 2 months *not recommended* because of hepatotoxicity (earlier protocol).

To prevent TB in adults and adolescents with HIV infection, the Centers for Disease Control and Prevention (CDC) recommends the following. Advise patients with HIV infection that time spent in congregate settings identified as possible sites of TB transmission (such as correctional facilities, homeless shelters, nursing homes) might increase their likelihood of TB infection. In healthcare facilities, physically separate all patients with known or presumed infectious TB from other patients, especially from patients with HIV infection. Patients with infectious TB should not return to congregate settings or any setting in which susceptible persons might be exposed until they have completed adequate treatment for >2 weeks, have three consecutive negative acid-fast bacilli (AFB) smear results from good-quality sputum samples >8 hours apart (including 1 during early morning), and show clinical improvement. Treat patients with HIV infection presumptively for latent TB infection, if they have substantial history of TB exposure regardless of diagnostic testing results.

The diagnosis of latent TB infection in patients with HIV infection includes testing for latent TB infection (LTBI) at the time of HIV diagnosis regardless of TB risk category. Retest persons with initial negative diagnostic tests for LTBI, who have CD4 count of <200 cells/µL and without indications for starting empiric LTBI treatment once they start antiretroviral therapy and attain CD4 count of ≥200 cells/µL. Annual testing for LTBI is recommended for high-risk persons, including those who are or have been incarcerated, live in congregate settings, are active drug users, or have other sociodemographic risk factors for TB.

In patients with HIV infection, antiretroviral treatment (ART) may reduce overall mortality and incidence of TB, and isoniazid prophylaxis may reduce risk of TB. Isoniazid prophylaxis in children with HIV infection not receiving ART reduces mortality and incidence of TB. Screening by chest x-ray does not appear to be helpful in asymptomatic patients with HIV infection seeking prophylaxis.

Drug treatment of latent TB in patients with HIV infection is indicated for patients with a history of tuberculin skin test (TST) ≥5 mm or recent close contact with patient with active TB. The preferred regimen is INH 300 mg orally once daily and pyridoxine 50 mg orally once daily for 9 months. Alternative regimens include rifampin 600 mg orally once daily for 4 months (10–20 mg/kg daily for 6 months in children) or isoniazid 15 mg/kg (maximum 900 mg) plus rifapentine 900 mg (reduced dose if <50 kg) once weekly under direct observation for 12 weeks if not taking antiretroviral medications. Isoniazid plus rifampin for 3 months might be as effective as INH for 12 months.

For BCG vaccination, per CDC guidelines [*MMWR Recomm Rep.* 1996;45(RR-4):1], consider vaccination for an infant or child who has negative TST result if there is continual exposure to either (1) an untreated or ineffectively treated patient with infectious pulmonary TB, and if the child cannot be separated from the infectious patient or given long-term primary preventive therapy; or (2) a patient with infectious pulmonary TB caused by *M. tuberculosis* strains resistant to isoniazid and rifampin, and if the child cannot be separated from the infectious patient.

The CDC recommends BCG vaccination among healthcare workers in high-risk settings. These include settings where a high percentage of TB patients are infected with *M. tuberculosis* strains resistant to both isoniazid and rifampin, or if transmission of drug-resistant *M. tuberculosis* strains to healthcare workers is likely, and in settings where comprehensive TB infection control precautions have been implemented and have not been successful. Healthcare workers considered for BCG vaccination should be counseled regarding the risks and benefits associated with both BCG vaccination and TB preventive therapy, including variable data regarding the efficacy of BCG vaccination, and possible interference with diagnosing a newly acquired *M. tuberculosis* infection by TST in a BCG-vaccinated person. The risk of possible serious complications of BCG vaccine in immunocompromised persons, especially those infected with HIV; the lack of data regarding efficacy of preventive therapy for *M. tuberculosis* infections caused by strains resistant to isoniazid and rifampin; and the risks for drug toxicity associated with multidrug preventive therapy regimens should be considered. BCG vaccination is not recommended for children with HIV infection or adults in United States

Isolation and quarantine are components of preventing the spread of tuberculosis. Federal air travel restrictions allow health officers to notify CDC and place a person with active TB on the "Do not board" list, which prevents boarding of commercial aircraft in the United States. Patients with active TB are considered noninfectious and can board aircraft if they are on adequate drug therapy, show clinical response, and have two consecutive negative smears. Patients with MDR-TB represent a greater public health risk, and two consecutive negative cultures are recommended before removal from the "Do not board" list (http://www.who.int/tb/publiations/2008/WHO_HTM_TB_2008:399_eng.pdf).

While they are hospitalized patients with confirmed or suspected active TB should be placed in respiratory isolation using the following standards:

- Place in an airborne infection isolation (AII) room. In existing healthcare settings, AII rooms should have airflow of ≥6 air changes per hour (ACH); 12 ACH recommended in new or renovated rooms.

- Healthcare workers should wear N95 disposable filtering facepiece respirators; they must be fitted properly.

- The N95 respirator is designed to filter out droplet nuclei, and is *not* to be worn by the patient.

- Patients should be in single room with separate bathroom.

- Infectious patients should wear a surgical mask to stop droplet nuclei from being exhaled; surgical masks are *not* to be worn by healthcare workers or visitors.

Patients can be removed from respiratory isolation when (1) infectious TB is unlikely and another diagnosis is made that explains the syndrome; or (2) the patient has three consecutive negative AFB sputum smear results obtained at least 8 hours apart, has received standard antituberculosis treatment (minimum of 2 weeks), and has demonstrated clinical improvement. For patients with MDR-TB, maintain isolation until they have a negative culture. Hospitalization for respiratory isolation is *not* required for newly diagnosed patients who can be treated as outpatients when DOT treatment has been arranged and the patient is willing to remain inside until noninfectious. In situations where household contacts are at high risk of contracting TB (immunocompromised person or aged <4 years), strongly consider alternate housing until the index patient is noninfectious.

▶ **Clinical Findings of Active Tuberculosis**

A. History

- Pulmonary tuberculosis (TB):
  - Cough may be productive or nonproductive but is seldom present in AIDS patients.
  - Unexplained productive cough of > 2 weeks' duration is common.
  - Hemoptysis is possible (but is a sign of advanced infection).

- Pulmonary and extrapulmonary TB symptoms:
  - Fever
  - Loss of appetite
  - Weight loss
  - Weakness
  - Night sweats
  - Malaise

- Symptoms in extrapulmonary TB are often slight or absent until the disease is advanced and depend on the system/organ involved, but may include the following:
  - Lymphadenopathy
  - Painful urination, blood in urine, or frequent urination in genitourinary infection
  - Pelvic pain, menstrual irregularities (genitourinary TB in women)
  - Painless scrotal mass (genitourinary TB in men)
  - Pain in bones or joints
  - Headache, neck stiffness, decreased level of consciousness (TB meningitis)
  - Abdominal pain (gastrointestinal TB)
  - Chest pain (pericardial TB)

- Common symptoms in children [WHO. *Guidance for National Tuberculosis Programmes on the Management of Tuberculosis in Children* (available at WHO/HTM/TB/2006.371]:
  - Cough >21 days
  - Fever >38°C (100.4°F) for 14 days
  - Weight loss
  - Pain is the usual presenting symptom in skeletal tuberculosis, additional findings can include the following:
    - Joint swelling
    - Limited range of motion
    - Bone tenderness
    - Limping

Symptom combination may be used to predict pulmonary TB in children in resource-poor settings [*Pediatrics* 2006; 118(5):e1350]. The combination of persistent cough for >2 weeks, documented failure to thrive (weight loss or deviation from growth percentiles) in prior 3 months, and fatigue yielded 82% sensitivity, 90% specificity, and 82% positive predictive value (PPV) in HIV-negative children aged ≥3 years. In HIV-negative children aged <3 years, the combination yielded 52% sensitivity, 92.5% specificity, and 90% PPV.

B. Physical Exam Findings

General:

- Fever.
- Weight loss.
- Children may show poor weight gain or fall off growth curve.

HEENT:

- Choroidal tubercle (granuloma in choroid of retina) strongly suggestive of disseminated tuberculosis.

Neck:

- Lymphadenopathy.
- Extrapulmonary tuberculosis in children is associated with nontender cervical lymphadenopathy accompanied by fistula formation.

Chest:

- Physical findings generally not helpful in diagnosis of pulmonary tuberculosis.
- Assess for rales, wheezes, or decreased breath sounds.
- Assess for tachycardia or friction rub.

Abdomen:

- With disseminated or abdominal tuberculosis:
  - Hepatomegaly
  - Splenomegaly
  - Abdominal tenderness
  - Palpable mass
- Flank pain may be seen with genitourinary involvement.

Back:

- Extrapulmonary tuberculosis in children associated with gibbus (sharply angled kyphosis), especially of recent onset.

▶ Laboratory Testing Overview

When pulmonary tuberculosis is suspected, proceed with the following tests: (1) chest x-ray (may be omitted in resource poor situations); (2) collect an initial sputum specimen and two subsequent morning samples to be tested for *Mycobacterium tuberculosis* identification using microscopy, including acid-fast bacillus (AFB) smear (often negative in persons with HIV and active TB) or nucleic acid amplification testing (NAAT), which helps identify nontuberculous mycobacterium in AFB-positive patients; and (3) send a culture that is the gold standard for diagnosing TB (Table 54-1). The Xpert MTB/RIF test provides a rapid nucleic acid amplification test (NAAT) for diagnosis and detection of rifampin resistance. Sputum collection may require additional approaches in children who cannot produce a specimen. Gastric lavage may have higher yield than bronchoscopy, although nasopharyngeal aspiration may be preferable to gastric aspiration in children.

The NAAT can identify TB in smear-negative cases weeks earlier than culture and identify nontuberculous mycobacterium in smear-positive cases, which helps accurately target contact investigations. CDC recommendations on use of smear and NAAT to direct therapy are as follows:

- If the NAA result is positive and the AFB smear result is positive, presume that the patient has TB and begin anti-TB treatment while awaiting culture results.
- If the NAA result is positive and the AFB smear result is negative, use clinical judgment on whether to begin anti-TB treatment while awaiting culture results and determine whether additional diagnostic testing is needed. Consider testing an additional specimen using NAA to confirm the NAA result. A patient can be presumed to have TB, pending culture results, if two or more specimens are NAA positive.
- If the NAA result is negative and the AFB smear result is positive, a test for inhibitors should be performed and an additional specimen should be tested with NAA. Sputum specimens (3–7%) might contain inhibitors that prevent or reduce amplification and cause false-negative NAA results.
  - If inhibitors are detected, the NAA test is of no diagnostic help for this specimen. Use clinical judgment to determine whether to begin anti-TB treatment while awaiting results of culture and additional diagnostic testing.
  - If inhibitors are not detected, use clinical judgment to determine whether to begin anti-TB treatment while awaiting culture results and determine if additional diagnostic testing is needed. A patient can be presumed to have an infection with nontuberculous mycobacteria if a second specimen is smear positive and NAA negative and has no inhibitors detected.

If the NAA result is negative and the AFB smear result is negative, use clinical judgment to determine whether to begin anti-TB treatment while awaiting results of culture and additional diagnostic tests. Currently available NAA tests are not sufficiently sensitive (detecting 50–80% of AFB smear-negative, culture-positive pulmonary TB cases) to exclude the diagnosis of TB in AFB smear-negative patients suspected to have TB.

Bronchoscopy is useful if active TB is suspected and smear is negative.

When extrapulmonary TB is suspected, collect fluid or tissue to test for *M. tuberculosis* identification. Urinalysis should be sent for lab analysis if genitourinary infection is suspected (ie, showing pyuria or hematuria). Biopsy, needle aspiration, or imaging may be done as appropriate to site of suspected infection. Tests for protein, glucose, cell count, and differential are done on pleural, peritoneal, cerebrospinal, or pericardial fluids of suspected infection site. For HIV-positive patients with no obvious localized infection but with fever, obtain blood or bone marrow culture for *M. tuberculosis*. Tuberculin skin testing (TST) is seldom useful in the diagnosis of active TB but may be helpful in children and can support diagnosis in culture-negative cases. Interferon-γ release assay (IGRA) does not appear accurate for diagnosing or ruling out active pulmonary or extrapulmonary TB, although it may help in diagnosis of pleural TB.

When TB is diagnosed, obtain baseline testing for management, including complete blood count, electrolytes, liver enzyme assay, creatinine, HIV test, and visual acuity and red-green color discrimination if ethambutol is used. The differential diagnosis of tuberculosis is presented in **Table 54-2**.

Table 54-1. Diagnostic tests for tuberculosis.

Test	Sensitivity (%)	Specificity (%)	Notes
Chest radiograph			Primary infection may be normal. Reactivation classic appearance is lesions in the apical-posterior segments of upper lung and superior segments of lower lobe. Cavitary lesions are associated with infectivity. In children most common finding is opacification in the lung together with enlarged hilar or subcarinal lymph glands. HIV-positive patients have atypical radiographic changes more often than the classical findings.
Tuberculin skin test	59–100	44–100	Sensitivity and specificity vary with risk factors and size of induration. Generally positive 2–3 weeks after infection but can be as late as 12 weeks after exposure. Skin test is negative in ~25% of active TB patients. Most useful in diagnosing LTBI.
Interferon-γ (IFNγ) release assays (IGRAs) QuntiFERON-TB Gold®	78	99	For diagnosis of LTBI.
AFB smear	20–80		Early-morning sputum or gastric aspirate (especially useful in children). Sensitivity increases to >90% with multiple specimens. False positive with nontuberculous mycobacteria. Specificity highest in endemic countries, sensitivity varies widely by laboratory. Sensitivity lower in HIV coinfection cohorts, so negative smear has low ability to rule out TB.
Solid media culture (Lowenstein-Jensen media)	67–82	99–100	Gold standard for diagnosis.
Liquid culture media (7H-12 BACTEC™)	93–97	98	Can be used on specimen from any site. Can be positive in 2 weeks.
Nucleic acid amplification (NAAT)	96 66	85 98	Smear-positive sample PPV>95%. Smear-negative sample.
Xpert MTB/RIF automated molecular test identification TB	90 82	98 98	HIV coinfection cohort.
Xpert MTB/RIF automated molecular test for rifampin resistance	89 80	99 97	HIV-negative. HIV-positive.

▶ Treatment

Centers for Disease Control and Prevention (CDC)-recommended treatment regimens for adults and children include an initial phase treatment with isoniazid, rifampin, pyrazinamide, and ethambutol, and then continuation-phase treatment based on chest x-ray and sputum culture results (**Table 54-3**). In children whose visual acuity cannot be monitored, ethambutol is rarely recommended unless there is an increased likelihood of disease caused by isoniazid-resistant organisms or when the child has "adult-type" (upper lobe infiltration, cavity formation) TB. Extrapulmonary TB requires 6 months of therapy, except bone and joint disease requires 6–9 months, and neurotuberculosis requires 9–12 months. Corticosteroids are generally *not* recommended but are strongly recommended in cases of TB pericarditis and neurotuberculosis.

- Initial empiric therapy usually includes four drugs daily for 2 months:
  - Isoniazid orally (PO), intravenously (IV), or intramuscularly (IM) 5 mg/kg daily (maximum 300 mg/day), 10–15 mg/kg daily in children (max 300); weekly adult dose 15 mg/kg (max 900 mg), twice weekly adult dose 15 mg/kg (max 900), children 20–30 mg/kg (max 900).
  - Rifampin PO or IV, adult 10 mg/kg daily (maximum 600 mg/day, children 10–20 mg/kg per day (max 600).
  - Pyrazinamide orally 25 mg/kg per day (maximum 2 g/day), 15–30 mg/kg daily in children.

Table 54-2. Differential diagnosis of TB.

Disease	Characteristics
Nontuberculous mycobacterium	Signs and symptoms may be the same as for *M. tuberculosis*. Typically has less fever and weight loss.
Sarcoidosis	Dyspnea and cough. Chest x-ray: diffuse infiltrative lung disease with bilateral hilar adenopathy. Noncaseating granulomas on biopsy.
Aspiration pneumonia	May have indolent course. Radiologic infiltrates are more common in dependent areas. Look for risk factors such as loss of gag reflex, loss of consciousness.
Lung abscess	Frequently in posterior upper segment of upper lobes. May be acute or indolent. Patient usually has very foul-smelling sputum. Obtain specimen for culture.
Pulmonary fungal infections, such as histoplasmosis or coccididomycosis	Patient may have fever, cough, night sweats. These diseases are usually geographically specific. Chest x-rays may be miliary or can be cavitary. Obtain specimen for fungal stain and culture.
Granulomatosis with polyangiitis (Wegener's)	Patients have fever and cough. Necrotizing granulomas in the lung and necrotizing glomerulonephritis. Chest x-ray often shows a cavitary lesion
Actinomycosis	Cough, hemoptysis, and eventually draining sinuses with sulfur granules seen on stain are characteristic. Indolent course is common.
Neoplasm	Patients may have weight loss and cough similar to TB findings. Primary lung cancer, lymphoma, metastasis. Obtain specimen for cytology or biopsy.

- Ethambutol orally 15 mg/kg per day (maximum 1.6 g/day), 20 mg/kg per day in children.
- Streptomycin 15 mg/kg per day may be an additional drug or substituted for ethambutol in some patients.
- Regardless of initial regimen, continuation phase typically is 4 months with isoniazid and rifampin.

The CDC-recommended number of doses to complete therapy is defined by completion of the recommended total number of doses, not necessarily the expected duration of therapy. If the specified number of doses cannot be administered in the expected timeframe, the initial phase can be extended to 3 months and doses for an 18-week continuation phase can be extended for 6 months If the longer timeframe is not feasible, consider as interrupted therapy. A 5-day/wk treatment with directly observed therapy (DOT) is considered equivalent to a 7-day/wk.

The WHO recommendations for dosing frequency in treatment of pulmonary TB in adults (http://whqlib.doc.who.int/publications/2010/9789241547833_eng.pdf) include DOT as the preferred initial management, and all patients receiving drugs <7 days a week must receive DOT. New patients with pulmonary TB may receive a daily intensive phase followed by 3 times weekly continuation phase if each dose is directly observed. New patients with pulmonary TB may receive 3 times weekly dosing throughout therapy, provided that every dose is directly observed therapy and the patient is *not* HIV-positive or living in an HIV-prevalent setting.

The standard regimen for new patients with TB is isoniazid, rifampin, pyrazinamide, and ethambutol orally daily for 2 months, followed by isoniazid and rifampin for 4 months. In countries with high levels of isoniazid resistance, in new patients, and where isoniazid drug susceptibility testing results are unavailable before the continuation phase begins, add ethambutol to 4-month isoniazid, rifampin continuation phase (recommendation based on expert opinion not evidence).

The WHO recommendations for treatment of TB in children (note higher dose of pyrazinamide compared to CDC) are as follows:

- Recommended doses of anti-TB medications:
  - Isoniazid: 10 mg/kg (range 10–15 mg/kg); maximum dose 300 mg/day
  - Rifampicin: 15 mg/kg (range 10–20 mg/kg); maximum dose 600 mg/day
  - Pyrazinamide: 35 mg/kg (30–40 mg/kg)
  - Ethambutol: 20 mg/kg (15–25 mg/kg)

▶ A. Treatment of Active TB in Patients with HIV

Initiation of antiretroviral therapy (ART) during antituberculosis therapy is associated with not only increased survival but also an increase in the risk of immune reconstitution inflammatory syndrome (IRIS). This paradoxical response as the patient is responding to the antiretroviral treatment

Table 54-3. Treatment regimens for patients with culture-positive pulmonary tuberculosis caused by drug-susceptible organisms (CDC guidelines).

Initiation Phase		Continuation Phase			
Agents	Dosage and Minimal Duration	Agents	Dosage and Minimal Duration	Length of Therapy (Total Doses)	Notes
Isoniazid (INH), rifampin (RIF), pyrazinamide, ethambutol	Once daily for 8 weeks (56 doses) *or* 5 times per week for 8 weeks (40 doses DOT)	Isoniazid and rifampin	Once daily for 18 weeks (126 doses) *or* 5 times per week for 18 weeks (90 doses DOT)	26 weeks (130–182)	Preferred regimen. Directly observed therapy (DOT) required for <7 times a week dosing. Daily regimen is required if HIV- positive. When susceptibility testing shows sensitivity to INH and RIF, then ethambutol may be discontinued. If sputum is smear-positive at 2 months, repeat smear at 3 months.
		Isoniazid and rifampin	Twice weekly for 18 weeks (36 doses DOT)	26 weeks (76–92)	Intermittent dosing not recommended for HIV- positive patients.
		Isoniazid and rifampin	Once weekly for 18 weeks (18 doses DOT)	26 weeks (58–74)	Only for HIV-negative patients with no cavity on CXR and negatove sputum at 2 months.
		Isoniazid and rifampin	Daily for 31 weeks (217 doses, 155 DOT)	39 weeks (195–273)	If cavity on CXR and sputum positive at 2 months, maintain continuation phase for 31 weeks.
		Isoniazid and rifampin	Twice weekly for 31 weeks (62 doses DOT)	39 weeks (102–118)	
Isoniazid, rifampin, pyrazinamide, ethambutol	Once daily for 2 weeks, then twice weekly for 6 weeks (26 doses DOT) *or* 5 times per week for 2 weeks, then twice weekly for 6 weeks (22 doses DOT)	Isoniazid and rifampin	Twice weekly for 18 weeks (36 doses DOT)	26 weeks (58–62)	Intermittent dosing not recommended for HIV-positive patients
		Isoniazid and rifapentine	Once weekly for 18 weeks (18 doses DOT)	26 weeks (40–44)	Only for HIV-negative patients with no cavity on CXR and negative sputum at 2 months.
Isoniazid, rifampin, pyrazinamide, ethambutol	3 times per week for 8 weeks (24 doses DOT)	Isoniazid and rifampin	3 times per week for 18 weeks (54 doses DOT)	26 weeks (78)	
Isoniazid, rifampin, ethambutol	Once daily for 8 weeks (56 doses) *or* 5 times per week for 8 weeks (40 doses DOT)	Isoniazid and rifampin	Once daily for 31 weeks (217 doses) *or* 5 times per week for 31 weeks (155 doses DOT)	39 weeks (195–273)	May withhold pyrazinamide if pregnant, severe liver disease, or gout with extended continuation phase.
		Isoniazid and rifampin	Twice weekly for 31 weeks (62 doses DOT)	39 weeks (102–118)	

is attributed to the stronger immune response to TB and includes fever, worsening pulmonary infiltrates, and lymphadenopathy and rarely, death.

The United States Department of Health and Human Services (DHHS) recommendations for timing of ART in patients with HIV and *Mycobacterium tuberculosis* (TB) coinfection [*DHHS Guidelines on Use of Antiretroviral Agents in Adolescents and Adults with HIV-1 Infection* (available at AIDSinfo2013Feb12PDF)] are as follows:

- Start TB treatment immediately in patients with HIV infection and active TB.

- All patients with HIV infection and active TB should be given ART:

  - For patients with CD4 counts <50 cells/µL, start ART within 2 weeks of starting TB treatment to improve survival.

  - In patients with CD4 counts ≥50 cells/µL and no severe clinical disease, there is less evidence that early ART improves survival with treatment of active TB. ART can be delayed to 8–12 weeks to reduce the risk of IRIS.

  - In pregnant women, start ART as early as possible, for maternal health and prevention of mother-to-child transmission.

  - In patients with documented multidrug-resistant and extensively drug-resistant TB, start ART within 2–4 weeks of confirmation of TB drug resistance and initiation of second-line TB therapy.

Recommended initial treatment is four drugs for 2 months, consisting of INH plus rifampicin (or rifampin) plus pyrazinamide plus ethambutol; rifabutin is substituted for rifampin in patients taking protease inhibitors or maraviroc. The preferred continuation therapy is INH plus rifampicin for 4 months, given once daily or 2–3 times weekly (but not twice weekly if CD4 counts <100 cells/µL). Duration of therapy is 6 months, except 9 months for patients with cavitary lung disease, delayed response to therapy, or extrapulmonary TB. Extending treatment from 6 months to 12 months in HIV-positive patients with pulmonary TB may reduce relapse rates. Long-term isoniazid plus sulfadoxine-pyrimethamine may reduce recurrence and sick days after recovery from pulmonary TB in patients with HIV infection.

Trimethoprim-sulfamethoxazole (cotrimoxazole) reduces mortality in HIV-positive patients treated for pulmonary TB. Add corticosteroids when treating central nervous system (CNS) and pericardial disease. Adjunctive prednisolone therapy may reduce mortality in patients with tuberculous pericarditis. Recommended daily doses are dexamethasone 0.3–0.4 mg/kg tapered over 6–8 weeks or prednisone 1 mg/kg for 3 weeks and then tapered for 3–5 weeks.

The World Health Organization (WHO) proposes the following approach that is useful in limited resource environments for the diagnosis and treatment of TB in HIV prevalent settings. For ambulatory patients with cough for 2–3 weeks and no danger signs [ie, respiratory rate >30/minute, fever >39°C (102.2°F), pulse rate > 120/minute, inability to walk unaided], obtain an acid-fast bacilli (AFB) and an HIV test at the first visit. Treat patients who are HIV-positive or whose status remains unknown as follows:

- If AFB-positive–treat for TB, cotrimoxazole, HIV assessment.

- If AFB-negative–chest x-ray, sputum AFB and culture, clinical assessment (all at same time wherever possible to decrease visits and time to diagnosis).

  - If TB likely–treat for TB, cotrimoxazole, HIV assessment

  - If TB unlikely–HIV assessment and one of following: (1) treat for bacterial infection plus cotrimoxazole; (2) treat for *Pneumocystis carinii* pneumonia, especially if hypoxic; (3) if there is a response, advise to return if symptoms recur; (4) if there is no or only partial response, reassess for TB.

The WHO recommendations for dosing regimens in HIV-positive and HIV-negative children are as follows:

- Four-drug regimen of isoniazid, rifampin, pyrazinamide, and ethambutol for 4 months followed by isoniazid and rifampin regimen for 4 months should be given in any of following cases:

  - Children with extensive pulmonary disease.

  - Children living in places with high isoniazid resistance or high HIV prevalence (≥ 1% in adult pregnant women or ≥ 5% in patients with TB) who have suspected/confirmed either

    - Pulmonary TB

    - Tuberculous peripheral lymphadenitis

- Three-drug regimen (isoniazid, rifampin, pyrazinamide) for 2 months followed by a two-drug regimen of isoniazid and rifampin for 4 months can be given to children without HIV infection living in places with low HIV prevalence and isoniazid who have suspected/confirmed either

  - Pulmonary TB

  - TB peripheral lymphadenitis

- Avoid intermittent (2 times weekly or 3 times weekly) dosing regimens in children with HIV infection or in any children living in high-HIV-prevalence areas with suspected/confirmed pulmonary TB or tuberculous peripheral lymphadenitis.

- During continuation phase, consider 3 times weekly regimens for HIV-negative children in settings with well-established DOT.

- Treat children with suspected or confirmed tuberculous meningitis or osteoarticular TB with standard four-drug regimen of isoniazid, rifampin, pyrazinamide, and ethambutol for 2 months, followed by standard two-drug regimen of isoniazid and rifampin for 10 months, for a total duration of treatment of 12 months.

The WHO recommendations for dosing frequency in HIV-positive patients are as follows:

- TB patients with known positive HIV status and all TB patients living in HIV-prevalent settings should receive daily TB treatment at least during the intensive phase.

- Optimal dosing frequency during continuation phase is also daily for these patients.

- If a daily continuation phase is not possible for these patients, 3 times weekly dosing during the continuation phase is an acceptable alternative.

▶ B. Treatment of Multidrug-Resistant Tuberculosis (MDR-TB)

1. CDC recommendations–Never add only one new drug to an ineffective regimen. When starting or changing treatment, use at least three previously unused drugs that have demonstrated in vitro susceptibility and include one injectable agent in the regimen (two simultaneous injectable agents not recommended). Use more than three agents if other previously unused drugs likely to be active are available. In patients with multidrug-resistant TB resistant to isoniazid, rifampin, and other first-line agent regimens, consider regimens with four to six medications and institute hospital-based or home-based DOT for oral medications; intermittent therapy for injectable agents after 2–4 months of daily therapy is also an option.

Drug resistance patterns are as follows:

- Rifampin resistance usually associated with cross-resistance to rifabutin and rifapentine; avoid rifabutin unless *in vitro* susceptibility is demonstrated.

- No cross-resistance between streptomycin and other injectable agents amikacin, kanamycin, and capreomycin.

- Cross-resistance between amikacin and kanamycin is universal.

- If mono-resistance to pyrazinamide is demonstrated without resistance to other first-line drugs, evaluate for infection with *Mycobacterium bovis*.

For INH-resistant *M. tuberculosis*, use rifampin, pyrazinamide, and ethambutol for 6 months and add a fluoroquinolone as a fourth agent in extensive disease.

For RIF-resistant *M. tuberculosis*, use isoniazid, pyrazinamide, ethambutol either daily or 3 times weekly for 12 months. If extensive disease, consider adding a fluoroquinolone. If there is extensive disease, or to shorten duration of treatment, consider adding an injectable agent (streptomycin, amikacin, kanamycin, or capreomycin) during initial 2 months of therapy. Isoniazid, pyrazinamide, and streptomycin for 9 months has demonstrated efficacy, although an injectable agent for 9 months may not be feasible.

For INH- and RIF-resistant *M. tuberculosis*, use fluoroquinolone, pyrazinamide, ethambutol and injectable streptomycin, amikacin, kanamycin, or capreomycin for 18–24 months. If there is extensive disease, consider adding one of following for 18–24 months: ethionamide, cycloserine, *p*-aminosalicylic acid, clarithromycin, amoxicillin/clavulanate, or linezolid. Resectional surgery may be appropriate.

For INH and RIF plus either ethambutol- or pyrazinamide-resistant *M. tuberculosis*, use fluoroquinolone (either ethambutol or pyrazinamide if susceptibility demonstrated on testing), and an injectable agent (streptomycin, amikacin, kanamycin, or capreomycin) for 24 months. If there is extensive disease, consider adding two of the following for 24 months: ethionamide, cycloserine, *p*-aminosalicylic acid, clarithromycin, amoxicillin/clavulanate, or linezolid. Surgery may be appropriate since drug treatment may be very difficult.

2. WHO principles of treatment—WHO (WHO 2007 PDF, National Guideline Clearinghouse 2010 March 1: 13595) recommends using at least four drugs known to be effective. It recommends against using drugs that may have cross-resistance or are not safe, and recommends including drugs from groups 1 to 5 in a hierarchical order based on potency:

- Group 1: first-line oral agents–use any or all of the following drugs if clinical or laboratory suggest susceptibility:

  - Pyrazinamide

  - Ethambutol

  - Rifabutin

- Group 2: injectable agents– use one of the following in the drug regimen if laboratory susceptibility is documented or suspected:

  - Kanamycin

  - Amikacin

  - Capreomycin

  - Streptomycin

- Group 3: fluoroquinolones–use one of the following if laboratory susceptibility is documented or is deemed efficacious:

  - Levofloxacin

  - Moxifloxacin

  - Ofloxacin (if levofloxacin or moxifloxacin unavailable)

- Group 4: oral bacteriostatic second-line agents–use two or three of the following to obtain a regimen of at least four drugs:

  - *p*-Aminosalicylic acid

  - Cycloserine

  - Terizidone

  - Ethionamide

  - Protionamide

- Group 5: agents with unclear role in treatment of drug-resistant TB–use any two of the following in the drug regimen if unable to complete a four-drug regimen from selections in groups 1 to 4:
  - Clofazimine
  - Linezolid
  - Amoxicillin/clavulanate
  - Thioacetazone
  - Imipenem/cilastatin
  - High-dose isoniazid (16–20 mg/kg per day)
  - Clarithromycin

Children with proven or suspected multidrug-resistant pulmonary TB or tuberculous meningitis can be treated with a fluoroquinolone in the context of a well-functioning multidrug-resistant TB control program and within an appropriate multidrug-resistant TB regimen.

In populations with known or suspected high levels of isoniazid resistance, WHO recommends that new TB patients receive isoniazid, rifampin, and ethambutol as therapy in continuation phase as an acceptable alternative to isoniazid and rifampin. Daily dosing during initial intensive phase may also prevent acquired drug resistance in patients with suspected isoniazid resistance.

▶ C. Options for Drug Intolerance

The CDC recommendations for drug intolerance are as follows:

- For patients intolerant of isoniazid [*Am J Respir Crit Care Med.* 2003;167(4):603]:
  - Use rifampin, pyrazinamide, and ethambutol for 6 months.
  - Alternatively, consider using rifampin, pyrazinamide, and ethambutol for 2 months, followed by continuation of rifampin and ethambutol for an additional 10 months.
- For patients intolerant of rifampin:
  - Use isoniazid, pyrazinamide, and ethambutol for ≥2 months, followed by continuation of isoniazid and ethambutol to complete 12–18 months' treatment.
  - Fluoroquinolones may be useful, but optimal length of therapy has not been defined.
  - Rifabutin has been substituted for rifampin in standard regimens if necessary to avoid drug interactions, generally with antiretroviral drugs.
- For patients intolerant of pyrazinamide in initial therapy, use 7 months of isoniazid and rifampin for continuation therapy.

HIV Primary Care

Ramakrishna Prasad, MD, MPH, AAHIVS

ESSENTIALS OF DIAGNOSIS

- Diagnosis of *HIV infection* is made by HIV antibody testing by ELISA, confirmed by Western blot or multispot ELISA.

- Absolute CD4 lymphocyte count is widely used for staging HIV disease. *Acquired immune deficiency syndrome* (AIDS) is defined as a CD4 <200 cells/μL. AIDS represents advanced HIV disease that is associated with opportunistic infections or malignancy in the absence of treatment.

- HIV RNA level (viral load) is used to monitor response to antiretroviral therapy.

General Considerations

As the fourth decade of the HIV/AIDS epidemic unfolds, major shifts in the epidemiology and prognosis of HIV disease have occurred. Significant advances in treatment of HIV infection have transformed this fatal disease into a chronic multisystem disease characterized by multiple comorbidities, with noninfectious complications. The Centers for Disease Control and Prevention (CDC) estimated that there are 1.2 million adults and adolescents currently living with HIV infection in the United States.

Another important shift has been the aging of the HIV-infected population in several countries.

It is estimated that in the USA, by 2017, more than half of all HIV-infected individuals will be over 50 years old. As patients are living longer with HIV, the number of patients with chronic infection has increased steadily.

While older studies indicate an association between optimal clinical outcomes and greater provider expertise in managing HIV infection, in several countries, including the United States, it is projected that there is a strong need

to develop the HIV care provider workforce. In the United States, many of the clinicians involved in HIV care entered this field at the beginning of the epidemic and are nearing retirement; additionally, fewer infectious diseases physicians are choosing to become HIV primary care providers. New CDC recommendations for universal screening will further increase the demand for care, as patients previously unaware of their HIV status are diagnosed. On account of expanded screening, increasing prevalence of HIV infection, the syndemic of HIV and aging related comorbidities, and a looming shortage of HIV primary care providers, primary care providers (PCPs) have a critical role to play in providing care to HIV-infected individuals and populations.

By virtue of their training, family physicians and other primary care providers, including physician assistants and nurse practitioners, are particularly well suited to provide this type of comprehensive, longitudinal care with an emphasis on addressing multiple medical co-morbidities, and preventive care (UN AIDS 2012 Global Report). It is well documented that the quality of HIV care provided by generalists with HIV experience is comparable to that of infectious disease (ID) specialists. Studies have also shown that general practitioners, when compared with ID physicians, are significantly more comfortable with the management of several comorbidities such as depression, diabetes, hypertension, and hyperlipidemia. These conditions are commonly encountered in HIV-infected individuals.

It is well established that effective HIV care leads to effective suppression of viral replication, improved immune status, near-normal life expectancy, enhanced quality of life, and prevention of HIV transmission (Currier and Havlir 2009; Palella, et al. 20006). However, in the United States, for every 100 individuals living with HIV, only 28 are able to adhere to their treatment and sustain undetectable viral loads. The overall cascade of HIV care is shown in **Figure 55-1**. These missed opportunities in detection, delayed entry into care, and cycling in and out of care result in poor clinical outcomes, selection of drug-resistant strains of the virus,

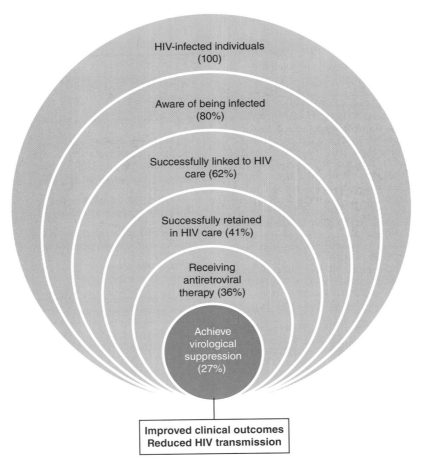

HIV-infected individuals
(100)

Aware of being infected
(80%)

Successfully linked to HIV
care (62%)

Successfully retained
in HIV care (41%)

Receiving
antiretroviral
therapy (36%)

Achieve
virological
suppression
(27%)

Improved clinical outcomes
Reduced HIV transmission

▲ **Figure 55-1.** Spectrum of HIV care toward improving clinical outcomes and reducing HIV transmission to others. In the United States, for every 100 individuals living with HIV, it is estimated that only 80 are aware of their HIV status, 62 have been successfully referred to HIV treatment services (*linkage*), <41 stay in HIV care (*retention*), 36 receive antiretroviral therapy (ART), and finally only 27 are able to adhere to their treatment and sustain undetectable viral loads. (Data from Gardner et al.)

and transmission of HIV to others. Primary care physicians can play a major role in improving the overall cascade of HIV care, including detection, linkage, retention and engagement, and improved outcomes of treatment.

Currier JS, Havlir DV. Complications of HIV disease and antiretroviral therapy. *Top HIV Med*. 2009; 17(2):57–67.
Palella FJ Jr, Baker RK, Moorman AC, et al. HIV Outpatient Study Investigators. Mortality in the highly active antiretroviral therapy era: changing causes of death and disease in the HIV outpatient study. *J Acquir Immune Defic Syndr*. 2006; 43(1):27–34.

This chapter is intended primarily for primary care providers, including family physicians, internists, nurse practitioners, and physician assistants. While the US-based, Department of Health and Human Services (DHHS) guidelines are primarily referred to, most aspects of HIV care discussed here are applicable to other primary care settings worldwide. (Please see http://hivinsite.ucsf.edu/global?page=cr-00-04#SmzguidelineX for country-specific guidelines.)

The aspects of HIV care discussed in this chapter are as follows:

- Screening and diagnosis of HIV-infection
- Natural history and staging of HIV disease
- Initial evaluation and management of an HIV-infected individual, including medical history and physical examination, laboratory assessments, and diagnostic testing
- Principles of treatment of HIV infection, including prevention of opportunistic infections

- Overview of comorbidities, complications, and end-organ dysfunction associated with chronic HIV infection
- Health maintenance and preventive care
- Unique aspects of HIV care in special populations.

Carmichael D, Feinberg, et al. *Averting a Crisis in HIV Care: A Joint Statement of the American Academy of HIV Medicine (AAHIVM) and the HIV Medicine Association (HIVMA) on the HIV Medical Workforce* (available at https://www.hivma.org/WorkArea/DownloadAsset.aspx? id=14752; accessed Sept. 28, 2012).

CDC 2012. *New Estimates of US HIV Prevalence* (available at http://www.cdc.gov/hiv/topics/surveillance/resources/fact-sheets/pdf/prevalence.pdf; accessed Sept.24, 2012).

Chu C, Selwyn PA. An epidemic in evolution: the need for new models of HIV care in the chronic disease era. *J Urban Health.* 2011; 88(3):556–566.

Fultz SL, Goulet JL, Weissman S, et al. Differences between infectious diseases-certified physicians and general medicine-certified physicians in the level of comfort with providing primary care to patients. *Clin Infect Dis.* 2005; 41:738–743.

Gallant, JE, Adimora, AA, Carmichael, JK, et al. Essential components of effective HIV care: a policy paper of the HIV Medicine Association of the Infectious Diseases Society of America and the Ryan White Medical Providers Coalition. *Clin Infect Dis.* 2011;53(11):1043–1050.

Gardner EM, McLees MP, Steiner JF, et al. The spectrum of engagement in HIV care and its relevance to test-and-treat strategies for prevention of HIV infection. *Clin Infect Dis.* 2011;52(6): 793–800.

▶ Epidemiology

The immunodeficiency virus (HIV) is a retrovirus transmitted by (1) unprotected sexual contact, (2) exposure to infected blood through sharing of injection drug use paraphernalia or receipt of contaminated blood products, and (3) perinatal transmission. Studies have yielded estimates of the probability of HIV transmission by various routes in adults and adolescents (**Table 55-1**). Factors such as plasma HIV RNA levels in the source patient; presence of sexually transmitted diseases (STDs), including syphilis, gonorrhea, herpes simplex, chlamydial infection, and human papillomavirus infection; and the quantity of infectious blood transferred influence per exposure probabilities of transmission.

▶ Distribution

A. Global

As of 2011, approximately 34 million individuals were living with HIV infection worldwide. Approximately 2.5 million people, including 390 000 children, became newly infected with HIV in 2011. An estimated 1.7 million people died from AIDS-related causes worldwide. Tuberculosis (TB) is the leading cause of death among HIV-infected individuals. Sub-Saharan Africa is the most affected region, with nearly 1 in every 20 adults living with HIV. Globally, the major routes of transmission are heterosexual (>75%) and from mother to child (5–10%). Access to lifesaving antiretroviral therapy has

Table 55-1. Per exposure probabilities of HIV transmission by route.

Manner of HIV Exposure	Per Exposure HIV Acquisition Risk
Blood transfusion	90–95 in 100
Mother-to-child transmission (without ART)	15 – 40 in 100
Injection drug use (needle sharing)	6.7 in 1000
Percutaneous needlestick (healthcare setting, known HIV-infected blood)	3 in 1000
Needlestick in community setting	Not reported to date
Unprotected receptive anal intercourse	5–32 in 1000
Unprotected insertive anal intercourse	6.5 in 10,000
Unprotected receptive vaginal intercourse	1–3 in 1000
Unprotected insertive vaginal intercourse	3–9 in 10,000
Receptive oral intercourse	1 in 10,000
Insertive oral intercourse	5 in 100,000
Mucous membrane exposure (healthcare setting, known HIV-infected blood)	9 in 10,000

Modified, with permission, from Tolle MA, Schwarzwald HL. Postexposure prophylaxis against human immunodeficiency virus. *Am Fam Physician.* 2010; 82(2):161-166.

been a major game changer in the global fight against HIV/AIDS. However, <50% of infected individuals are currently aware of their HIV status. Consequently, despite dramatic scaleup in terms of access to antiretroviral therapy (ART), out of an estimated 14 million individuals eligible for treatment with ART, only 8 million were currently receiving them.

Smith DK, et al. Antiretroviral postexposure prophylaxis after sexual, injection-drug use, or other nonoccupational exposure to HIV in the United States: recommendations from the U.S. Department of Health and Human Services. *MMWR Recomm Rep.* 2005;54(RR-2):1–20.

B. Distribution in the United States

HIV/AIDS remains a major threat in the United States. The Centers for Disease Control and Prevention (CDC) estimates that there are ~1.2 million adults and adolescents living with HIV infection in the United States. The annual incidence rate is 50,000–60,000 cases per year. Men who have sex with men (MSM) and racial/ethnic minorities disproportionately bear the burden of HIV/AIDS.

The MSM group represents 2% of the US population, but 63% of all HIV diagnoses are attributed to male-to-male sexual contact. African Americans represent 12% of US population but 47% of diagnoses of HIV infection. Male-to-male sexual contact is the most frequently identified risk factor for HIV exposure among adult and adolescent males, accounting for two-thirds of reported HIV/AIDS cases in men. Among men, high-risk heterosexual contact and injection drug use account for 16% and 12% of cases, respectively. Approximately 25% of new cases occur in women. High-risk heterosexual contact accounts for 80% of cases, while injection drug use accounts for ~19% of cases.

Centers for Disease Control and Prevention. *HIV Surveillance Report*; 2011; vol. 23 (availaable at http://www.cdc.gov/hiv/topics/surveillance/resources/reports/; published Feb. 2013; accessed, March 7, 2013).

▶ Screening

The CDC has recommended universal screening for HIV infection since 2006. In 2012, the United States Preventive Services Task Force (USPSTF) also updated its recommendations and now endorses screening all individuals aged 15–65 years for HIV infection, irrespective of risk factors. Thereafter, screening should be repeated upon risk assessment. All pregnant women should also be screened for HIV. Testing should be performed on an "opt-out" basis, meaning that unless patients decline, they should be tested.

Detection of HIV infection represents the first step in HIV treatment. Unless detected, infected individuals have no opportunity to avail themselves of treatment. Furthermore, infected individuals who are unaware of their diagnosis are the main drivers of the HIV epidemic. Risk factor–based HIV testing has not been successful. Approximately 20–25% of individuals living with HIV infection are unaware of their HIV status. This group is thought to account for 50–70% of new infections. Furthermore, at the time of diagnosis, ~33.3% of all individuals diagnosed with HIV infection either already have AIDS or develop it within a year of diagnosis–indicating both advanced disease and delayed diagnosis. Individuals diagnosed at this late stage in their HIV infection typically report at least four encounters with the healthcare system in the year preceding diagnosis at which opportunities to detect HIV infection were missed.

USPSTF 2013. *US Preventive Services Task Force Issues Draft Recommendation on Screening for Human Immunodeficiency Virus (HIV)* (available at http://www.uspreventiveservicestaskforce.org/bulletins/hivbulletin.pdf; accessed 3/9/13).

▶ Diagnosis and Progression of HIV Infection

Diagnosis of HIV infection is based on results of serologic tests that demonstrate the presence of antibodies to HIV. A rapid HIV test or a conventional enzyme-linked immunosorbent assay (ELISA) is used as the initial test. A positive or reactive result is then confirmed by a second confirmatory test such as Western blot, indirect immunofluorescence assay, or multispot ELISA. Both the standard and rapid HIV antibody tests are highly accurate in diagnosing HIV infection (>99% sensitive and specific). Rapid HIV testing may use either blood or oral fluid specimens, and provides results in ~5–40 minutes.

A. Natural History of HIV/AIDS

The progression of HIV disease is well established. On infection, and in the absence of treatment, viral replication progressively depletes the immune system and results in immunodeficiency, which renders the infected individual susceptible to a multitude of opportunistic infections and malignancies (see **Figure 55-2**). The stages of HIV infection are shown in **Table 55-2**. **Table 55-3** lists opportunistic infections by CD4 counts. The rate of progression is variable and in a small number of individuals disease progression may be significantly slower.

Kassutto S, Rosenberg ES. Primary HIV type 1 infection. *Clin Infect Dis.* 2004; 38(10):1447–1453.

B. Comorbidities and Complications of Chronic HIV Infection

Patients with human immunodeficiency virus (HIV) infection often develop multiple complications and comorbidities. A limited account is provided here. Comorbidities and complications could be directly related to HIV infection. However, they could also be completely unrelated to HIV infection and finally arise as a result of HIV drug therapy. Hence, it is important for the clinician providing care to HIV-infected individuals to consider a relatively broad differential diagnosis. **Table 55-4** provides a listing of comorbidities, opportunistic infections, and antiretroviral related adverse effects by organ system.

Chu C, Selwyn PA. Complications of HIV infection: a systems-based approach. *Am Fam Physician*. 2011;83(4):395–406.

C. Initial Evaluation of HIV-Infected Individuals in the Office Setting

The initial evaluation of an HIV-infected individual represents one of the most significant encounters between the patient and the healthcare provider. The diagnosis of HIV infection is often a profound life-altering experience for patients. Often several visits may be needed to achieve these goals. The initial evaluation is discussed in detail in the HIV primary care guidelines from the HIV Medicine Association (HIVMA) and the Infectious Diseases Association of America (IDSA). **Table 55-5** lists the various elements of the initial evaluation.

The main goals of this visit are to (1) lay the foundation for fostering a strong and empathic physician-patient relationship; (2) develop and document a comprehensive understanding of the patient's history, stage of disease, and physical findings; and (3) address psychosocial elements that play a major role in treatment success, including stigma, coping mechanisms, social support, social work needs, and housing.

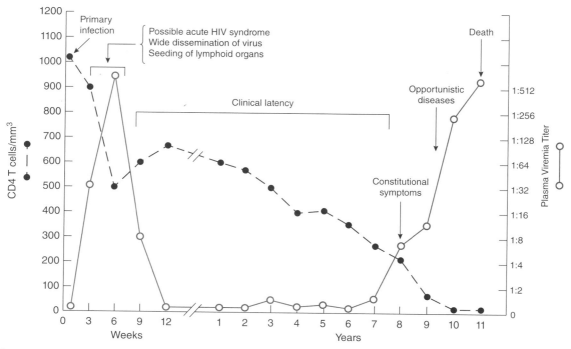

▲ **Figure 55-2.** Progression of HIV disease. (Reproduced with permission from Pantaleo G, Graziosi C, Fauci AS. New concepts in the immunopathogenesis of human immunodeficiency virus infection. *N Engl J Med*. 1993;328:327-335.)

Aberg JA, Gallant JE, Ghanem K.G., et al. HIV Medicine Association of the Infectious Diseases Society of America. Primary care guidelines for the management of persons infected with human immunodeficiency virus: 2009 update by the HIV Medicine Association of the Infectious Diseases Society of America. *Clin Infect Dis*. 2009; 49(5):651–681.

D. History and Physical Examination

Individuals presenting for evaluation with HIV infection may be at any stage of the infection. This can range from asymptomatic individuals to those presenting with full-blown AIDS involving virtually every organ system. In order

Table 55-2. Clinical stages of HIV/AIDS.

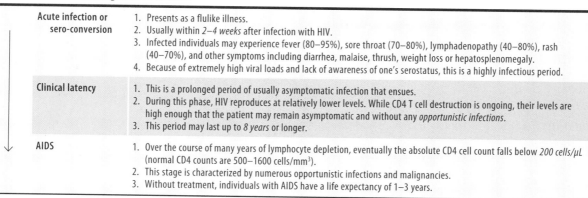

Acute infection or sero-conversion	1. Presents as a flulike illness. 2. Usually within *2–4 weeks* after infection with HIV. 3. Infected individuals may experience fever (80–95%), sore throat (70–80%), lymphadenopathy (40–80%), rash (40–70%), and other symptoms including diarrhea, malaise, thrush, weight loss or hepatosplenomegaly. 4. Because of extremely high viral loads and lack of awareness of one's serostatus, this is a highly infectious period.
Clinical latency	1. This is a prolonged period of usually asymptomatic infection that ensues. 2. During this phase, HIV reproduces at relatively lower levels. While CD4 T cell destruction is ongoing, their levels are high enough that the patient may remain asymptomatic and without any *opportunistic infections*. 3. This period may last up to *8 years* or longer.
AIDS	1. Over the course of many years of lymphocyte depletion, eventually the absolute CD4 cell count falls below *200 cells/μL* (normal CD4 counts are 500–1600 cells/mm³). 2. This stage is characterized by numerous opportunistic infections and malignances. 3. Without treatment, individuals with AIDS have a life expectancy of 1–3 years.

Table 55-3. Common opportunistic infections by CD4 count.

Absolute CD4 Count	Opportunistic Infection/ Malignancy	Specific OI Prophylaxis Recommended
Above 300	Vaginal candidiasis Tuberculosis Skin disease Fatigue Bacterial pneumonia Herpes zoster	No specific opportunistic infection prophylaxis
Below 300	Oral hairy leukoplakia Thrush, Fever, diarrhea, weight loss	
Below 200	Kaposi's sarcoma Non-Hodgkin's lymphoma *Pneumocystis carinii* pneumonia CNS lymphoma	Pneumocystis prophylaxis with Bactrim (1 tablet daily)
Below 100	Toxoplasmosis, Esophageal candidiasis Cryptococcosis	Toxoplasma prophylaxis with Bactrim DS (1 tablet daily)
Below 50	Cytomegalovirus (CMV) *Mycobacterium avium* complex (MAC) CNS lymphoma	MAC prophylaxis with Azithromycin (1200 mg weekly)

to establish a timeline for infection in the individual, the initial evaluation should include inquiries about any previous HIV testing, prior negative test results, occurrence of symptoms, and timing of high-risk activities. In patients who have an established diagnosis, the lowest CD4 cell count and highest HIV load should be ascertained, if possible. Patients should be asked about any prior HIV-associated complications and comorbidities, including opportunistic infections, malignancies, and cardiovascular disease history and risk. Efforts should be made to obtain previous medical records.

1. Past medical history—Information about chronic medical conditions, such as peripheral neuropathy, gastrointestinal disease, chronic viral hepatitis, hyperlipidemia, diabetes mellitus, or renal insufficiency may affect the choice of therapy or response to therapy and hence should be collected. Other medical conditions of significance in HIV-infected patients include a history of chickenpox or shingles, tuberculosis or tuberculosis exposure, STDs, and gynecologic or perianal problems.

2. Medications—It is also critical to obtain a thorough medication history. This is particularly important for patients who have already received antiretroviral therapy. Details including drug combinations taken, response to each regimen, CD4 cell count and viral load, duration of treatment, reasons for treatment changes, any drug toxicities, adherence,

and prior drug resistance test results, should be sought. Patients should be asked about any medications they take, including prescription and over-the-counter (OTC) drugs, methadone, and dietary or herbal supplements, some of which have been shown to interact with antiretroviral drugs. A discussion of allergies should include questions about hypersensitivity reactions to prior therapies, especially sulfa drugs and any antiretroviral agents.

3. Travel and immunizations—It is important to ask patients about travel and where they have lived. For example, patients living in areas endemic for histoplasmosis (eg, Ohio and Mississippi River valleys in the United States) may be at risk for reactivation disease, even after moving to areas in which these infections are not endemic. The status of immunizations, including tetanus toxoid, pneumococcal vaccine, and hepatitis A and B vaccines, should be elicited. A full birth history and review of maternal history and risk factors should be obtained for all children.

4. Social history—The social history should include a discussion of the use of tobacco, alcohol, heroin, and recreational drugs, including marijuana, cocaine, 3,4-methylenedioxy-methamphetamine (ie, "ecstasy"), ketamine, methamphetamine, and bath salts. Active injection drug users should be asked about their drug use practices, the source of their needles, and whether they share needles. It is of paramount importance to obtain sexual history in an open, nonjudgmental manner. Patients should be asked about their partners, sexual practices (including condom and contraceptive use), and whether their partner(s) have been informed of their HIV status. Patients may also be asked if they are aware if any of their sexual contacts is on antiretroviral therapy. Laws vary from state to state regarding the obligation of healthcare providers to notify sex partners, and clinicians should be aware of laws in their own jurisdiction.

5. Social support—Patients should also be specifically asked whom they have informed of their HIV status, how they have been coping with the diagnosis of HIV infection, and what kinds of support they have been receiving. It is important to know about the patient's family, living situation, and work environment and how the patient has been affected by the diagnosis of HIV infection. Other pertinent information includes housing issues, employment, and plans for having children.

6. Family history—As HIV-infected individuals live longer and age, family history may help in assessing their risk of developing certain malignancies, neurologic diseases, and atherosclerotic disease.

7. Review of systems—The review of systems should be comprehensive. Fever, night sweats, weight loss, headaches, visual changes, oral thrush or ulceration, swallowing difficulties, respiratory symptoms, diarrhea, skin rashes or lesions, and changes in neurological function or mental status may be

Table 55-4. Comorbidities and complications by organ system in patients with HIV/AIDS.

	Complications in Patients with HIV/AIDS		
System	Comorbidities and Complications	Important Opportunistic Infections/Malignancies	Antiretroviral Treatment--Related Adverse Effects
Neuropsychiatric	1. HIV-associated neurocognitive disorders 2. neuropathy, radiculopathy, myelopathy 3. Chronic psychiatric disorders	a. Cryptococcal meningitis b. Cerebral toxoplasmosis c. Cytomegalovirus (CMV) encephalitis d. JC virus–related progressive multifocal leukoencephalopathy (PML) e. Primary CNS lymphoma	1. Efavirenz (Sustiva): vivid dreams, sedation 2. NRTIs: peripheral neuropathy
Head and neck	1. HIV-associated retinopathy 2. Gingivitis, dental and salivary gland disease	a. CMV and toxoplasma retinitis b. Acute retinal necrosis and progressive outer retinal necrosis due to varicella zoster virus c. Otitis, sinusitis due to invasive fungi	
Cardiovascular	1. HIV-associated cardiomyopathy 2. Atherosclerosis	a. Pericarditis/myocarditis due to CMV, invasive fungi, *Mycobacterium* species, *Toxoplasma gondii*	1. Abacavir-related cardiotoxicity 2. Protease inhibitor–associated dyslipidemia
Pulmonary	1. HIV-associated pulmonary hypertension 2. Chronic obstructive pulmonary disease 3. Lung cancer	a. Pulmonary tuberculosis: *Mycobacterium tuberculosis* b. Kaposi sarcoma c. Lymphoma d. Pneumonia/pneumonitis due to CMV, invasive fungi, *Pneumocystis jiroveci* (formerly *Pneumocystis carinii*)	
Gastrointestinal	1. HIV-induced enteropathy 2. Viral hepatitis (especially hepatitis B and C) 3. Nonalcoholic fatty liver disease 4. HPV-related malignancies	a. Chronic diarrhea due to *Cryptosporidium, Isosopra, Microsporidium, Cyclospora,* and *Giardia* b. Lymphoma, Kaposi sarcoma c. Oral/esophageal candidiasis d. *Esophagitis due to* CMV and HSV	1. NRTI-associated pancreatitis 2. Protease inhibitor– associated diarrhea, fatty liver
Renal/genitourinary	1. HIV-associated nephropathy 2. Chronic kidney disease not caused by HIV- associated nephropathy 3. Sexually transmitted infections		1. Protease inhibitor–related nephrolithiasis 2. Tenofovir-associated nephrotoxicity
Endocrine	1. Impaired lipid and glucose metabolism 2. HIV-associated wasting 3. Hypogonadism	a. Adrenal gland infiltration by CMV, invasive fungi, and *Mycobacterium* species	1. Protease inhibitor– associated lipid or glucose disorders and lipodystrophy
Musculoskeletal	1. Myopathy/myositis 2. Osteopenia, osteoporosis, 3. Avascular necrosis		1. NRTI or NNRTIs associated with osteomalacia 2. Protease inhibitors with statins increase risk of myopathy
Hematologic or oncologic	1. Anemia of chronic disease 2. Coagulation disorders 3. Multiple myeloma	a. Lymphoma b. Parvovirus B19–related pure red cell aplasia (PRCA) c. Bone marrow infiltration (leading to pancytopenia) by CMV, invasive fungi, and *Mycobacterium* species	1. Zidovudine and trimethoprim/sulfamethoxazole-related anemia
Dermatologic	1. Eosinophilic folliculitis 2. Papulosquamous disorders (eg, eczema, seborrheic dermatitis, psoriasis) 3. Molluscum contagiosum	a. Kaposi sarcoma b. Fungal dermatoses, varicella zoster virus	

Adapted with permission from Chu C, Selwyn PA. Complications of HIV infection: a systems-based approach. *Am Fam Physician.* 2011; 83(4):395-406.

Table 55-5. Elements of the initial evaluation.

Initial Evaluation and Preventive Care	
Psychosocial assessment	Emotional response to illness Support networks Durable power of attorney for healthcare, advance directives.
History	Illnesses High-risk behaviors Travel Drug allergies Medications Cigarette, alcohol, recreational drug use Review of systems
Physical examinations	Complete physical examination Cervical Pap smear for women Consider anal Pap screening for dysplasia
Skin testing and treatment of latent TB infection (LTBI)	PPD and baseline CXR If (+) PPD (>5 mm) and no evidence of old infection on CXR, LTBI should be treated
Vaccines	Pneumococcal vaccine (conjugate and polysaccharide) Hepatitis A vaccine if HepA IgG negative Hepatitis B vaccine if seronegative Flu vaccine if at risk for exposure Tetanus, MMR, HPV, inactivated polio if indicated per usual guidelines
Laboratory data	CD4 count HIV viral load by PCR Complete blood count Electrolytes, creatinine AST, alkaline phosphatase Hepatitis A, B, and C serologies RPR/VDRL, treponemal antibody *Taxoplasma.gondii* IgG G6PD before dapsone Baseline CXR
Counseling	Safer sex and birth control Smoking cessation Alcohol and drug use Nutrition and exercise
Referrals	Registered dietician with HIV expertise Ophthalmologist if CD4 < 50 Dentist Psychotherapist/ drug treatment

AST, aspartate transaminase; CXR, chest radiograph; G6PD, glucose-6-phosphate dehydrogenase; IgG, immunoglobulin G; INH, isoniazid; MMR, measles-mumps-rubella; PPD, purified protein derivative; RPR, rapid plasma reagin; VDRL, Venereal Disease Research Laboratory.

noted in patients with advanced or uncontrolled HIV infection. For women, a menstrual history should be obtained.

8. Depression screening—Depression is common among HIV-infected patients, and the review of systems should include questions focusing on changes in mood, libido, sleeping patterns, appetite, concentration, and memory. As part of the initial evaluation and at periodic intervals thereafter, providers should assess the presence of depression and domestic violence by means of direct questions or validated screening tools such as PHQ-2 or PHQ-9. Women with HIV infection have high rates of adult sexual and physical abuse and of childhood sexual abuse. The prevalence of depression among those with HIV infection is particularly high in the setting of violence or victimization.

9. Physical examination—A complete physical examination should be performed at the initial encounter. Vital signs should be obtained. The height and weight for all patients should be measured. For children aged <3 years, head circumference should also be measured and plotted against standard growth curves. Abnormal measurements should be followed up.

The overall body habitus may reveal cachexia (especially seen in AIDS) or lipodystrophy (especially in patients with a history of receiving older antiretroviral medications). Lipodystrophy may present either as lipoatrophy (eg, loss of subcutaneous fat in the face, extremities, or buttocks) or lipohypertrophy (eg, increased dorsocervical fat pad, gynecomastia, or abdominal protuberance from visceral fat). Please see **Table 55-6** for a listing of common physical findings organized by organ system.

E. Baseline Laboratory Evaluation

A number of initial laboratory studies are indicated for patients presenting with HIV infection (**Tables 55-5** and **55-7**). The tests are used for determining HIV disease status, assessing baseline organ function, and screening for coinfections and comorbidities. From an HIV-disease-specific perspective, the three most important initial laboratory studies are the plasma HIV RNA level (viral load), CD4 cell count, and genotypic resistance test.

The CD4 cell count measures the degree of HIV-associated immunodeficiency. It is the most important criterion for initiation of ART and opportunistic infection (OI) prophylaxis. The viral load measures the amount of viral activity and replication. It is correlated with the risk of transmission and progression of disease and is the most important indicator of the success of ART. Untreated patients with undetectable viral loads should be retested for HIV with a standard EIA and WB to rule out a false-positive result. A genotypic resistance test is used to determine whether the patient was infected with drug-resistant virus, which could affect the choice of initial therapy. In settings where access to resistance testing exists, it should always be performed at

Table 55-6. Physical examination findings in HIV-infected individuals (by organ system).

System	Findings
Skin	Common findings include folliculitis, seborrheic dermatitis, Kaposi sarcoma, superficial fungal infections, psoriasis, and herpes zoster.
Eye	A dilated fundoscopic examination should be performed by an ophthalmologist in patients with advanced HIV disease (CD4 cell count <50 cells/mm^3). Patients with advanced disease or ocular symptoms may have evidence of cytomegalovirus (CMV) retinitis and other ocular manifestations of HIV infection.
Oral cavity	The oropharynx should be carefully examined for evidence of candidiasis, aphthous ulceration, oral hairy leukoplakia, mucosal Kaposi sarcoma, and periodontal disease.
Lymph nodes	Persistent generalized lymphadenopathy is common among HIV-infected patients. However, it does not correlate with prognosis or disease progression. Localized lymphadenopathy, or hepatomegaly or splenomegaly may be a sign of infection or malignancy and should be evaluated further.
Cardiopulmonary	Examination may reveal evidence of pneumonia (including pneumocystis jerovicii pneumonia), COPD, tuberculosis, and peripheral vascular disease.
Anogenital	It is important to perform a careful examination for evidence of rectal lesions (including cancer) and STDs, including condylomata and herpes simplex infection. HIV-infected women should have a pelvic examination. The pelvic examination should include visual inspection of the vulva and perineum for evidence of genital ulcers, warts, or other lesions. Speculum examination is used to assess the presence of abnormal vaginal discharge or vaginal or cervical lesions.
Neurologic	The neurological examination should include a general assessment of cognitive function, as well as motor and sensory testing. Patients with suspected cognitive dysfunction may need formal neuropsychological testing. Developmental assessment is important in infants and children.

baseline, regardless of the need for ART. Resistance testing is also used at the time of virologic failure to choose the subsequent antiretroviral regimen.

Other baseline studies and interventions that are indicated in HIV-infected patients are listed in **Table 55-7**.

Gallant, JE. What does the generalist need to know about HIV infection? *Adv Chronic Kidney Dis.* 2010; 17:5–18.

> **Principles of Antiretroviral Therapy: When to Start & What to Start**

The primary goals for initiating antiretroviral therapy (ART) are to reduce HIV-associated morbidity and prolong the duration and quality of survival, restore and preserve immunologic function, durably suppress plasma HIV viral load to below the detection limit, and to prevent HIV transmission. In recent years, ART has become simpler for patients with respect to pill burden, dosing frequency, and tolerability. In order to prescribe ART safely and effectively, clinicians require an understanding of preferred regimens, drug resistance, drug-drug interactions, medication-associated toxicities, and how comorbidities influence treatment choices. ART recommendations change frequently as new data and drugs become available. The Department of Health and Human Services publishes updated guidelines for reference.

DHHS 2013. Panel on Antiretroviral Guidelines for Adults and Adolescents. *Guidelines for the Use of Antiretroviral Agents in HIV-1-Infected Adults and Adolescents.* Department of Health and Human Services (available at http://aidsinfo.nih.gov/contentfiles/lvguidelines/AdultandAdolescentGL.pdf; section accessed March 9, 2013)

A. When to Start ART

The question of when to start ART has been a moving target. In settings where access to antiretroviral therapy exists, all patients who are motivated and ready to start therapy should start regardless of CD4 count or viral load.

The rationale for this is as follows: HIV infection is now known to cause heightened levels of immune activation and inflammation, which may increase the incidence of myocardial infarction and malignancy independent of CD4 count. There is increasing evidence to support the theory that untreated HIV infection may lead to accelerated aging, with premature loss of bone density and neurocognitive decline. In addition, recent studies such as the HPTN 052 study showed a 96% decrease in HIV transmission validating "treatment as prevention." Successful suppression of viral replication by antiretroviral therapy mitigates these consequences significantly.

Table 55-7. Laboratory studies and other investigations indicated in HIV-infected patients at baseline evaluation.

Investigations/Studies	Common Findings
CBC with differential	May reveal cytopenias such as anemia, neutropenia, and thrombocytopenia that are often associated with HIV disease.
Comprehensive chemistry panel	Allows assessment of transaminases for hepatitis, creatinine for kidney function, and albumin for nutritional status. Kidney function should be further measured by calculation of creatinine clearance.
Urinalysis	May detect proteinuria, a common manifestation of HIV-associated nephropathy (noted particularly in patients of African ancestry or those on tenofovir)
Hepatitis serologies	Hepatitis B surface antigen test and anti–hepatitis C antibody test generally rule out chronic hepatitis B and C, respectively. Seronegative patients with unexplained transaminase elevations may need hepatitis B DNA and/or hepatitis C RNA to rule out seronegative hepatitis, especially for those at high risk or with low CD4 counts. Hepatitis B surface antibody and total hepatitis A antibody are also used to assess the need for vaccination.
Testing for sexually transmitted infections	Serologic testing for syphilis is indicated in all patients at baseline. Assessment for gonorrhea (GC) and *Chlamydia* using urine, vaginal, or rectal swabs cultures (GC and *Chlamydia*) should be done. In patients at risk, throat cultures (GC) may also be useful.
Fasting lipid panel	Helps establish a baseline before starting ART because many antiretroviral agents alter lipid levels.
Screening for latent *Toxoplasma* infection (anti–*Toxoplasma* immunoglobulin G, or IgG)	Determines the need for primary prophylaxis. Those with negative tests should be counseled about the prevention of infection with proper preparation of meat and avoidance of cat feces.
Glucose-6-phosphate dehydrogenase (G6PD) level	If pneumocystis prophylaxis with dapsone is being considered, G6PD level testing helps determine risk of developing hemolytic anemia (this is particularly useful in patients of Mediterranean or African descent).
Tuberculin skin test	Useful to diagnose latent *Mycobacterium tuberculosis* infection (LTBI). The criterion for positivity is 5 mm of induration in HIV-infected patients. LTBI treatment should be offered regardless of age after active tuberculosis has been ruled out.
Pap smears	A cervical Pap smear is recommended at baseline and on a regular basis thereafter in all HIV-infected women. Abnormal results should be followed up with colposcopy. Anal pap smears (with follow-up high-resolution anoscopy as indicated) are increasingly being recommended in HIV-infected men and women, especially those who have had receptive anal intercourse, to screen for human papilloma virus–associated anal dysplasia.

Cohen MS, Chen YQ, McCauley M et al. Prevention of HIV-1 infection with early antiretroviral therapy. *N Engl J Med.* 2011; 365(6):493–505.
http://aidsinfo.nih.gov/guidelines/html/1/adult-and-adolescent-arv-guidelines/2/introduction.

B. What to Start in Terms of ART

The goal of ART is suppression of the viral load to undetectable levels (<50 copies/ mL). Initial antiretroviral regimens typically consist of a "backbone" of two nucleoside analog reverse transcriptase inhibitors (NRTIs) plus a third agent, typically a nonnucleoside reverse transcriptase inhibitor (NNRTI), a protease inhibitor (PI), or an integrase inhibitor. PIs are usually combined with a low dose of ritonavir (RTV), a potent inhibitor of CYP3A4-mediated PI metabolism. RTV "boosting" increases PI drug concentrations, prolongs half-life, simplifies dosing, and helps to prevent the emergence of PI resistance. The preferred first-line regimens and alternatives are listed in **Table 55-8**.

Having a visual chart of available antiretroviral agents is a helpful tool for counseling. One such chart can be found at http://www.positivelyaware.com/2012/12_02/pdfs/2012DrugChart.pdf. This also promotes collaborative decision making between the healthcare provider and the patient. Readers are referred to the DHHS guidelines for updated information and a more detailed discussion of all available antiretrovirals.

C. Monitoring Response to ART

Suppression of viral load should be achieved within 3–6 months, depending on the height of the baseline viral load. Viral suppression is usually accompanied by an increase in the CD4 cell count, with the greatest increase occurring

Table 55-8. Preferred and alternative antiretroviral regimens in treatment of naive individuals.

Preferred Regimens	NNRTI-Based Regimen	Comments
(*Note*: These regimens are deemed optimal because of durable efficacy, favorable tolerability, favorable toxicity profile, and ease of use.)	Efavirenz+tenofovir+emtricitabine (available as single, once-daily pill – Atripla) If Viral load less than 100,000 copies/ml Efavirenz+Abacavir+Lamivudine Rilpivirine+Tenofovir+Emtricitabine (available as a single, once daily pill-Complera) **PI-Based Regimens (same setting)** Ritonavir-boosted atazanavir+ tenofovir+emtricitabine Ritonavir-boosted darunavir+ tenofovir+emtricitabine **INSTI-Based Regimen** Raltegravir+tenofovir+emtricitabine	*Efavirenz* should be used with caution in women who are planning to become pregnant or who are sexually active and not using effective contraception because of teratogenicity concerns. *Tenofovir* should be used with caution in patients with renal insufficiency. *Atazanavir* should not be used in patients who require >20 mg omeprazole equivalent per day. *Abacavir* should only be used if the patient is HLA B5701 negative.

Modified from *Preferred and Alternative Antiretroviral Regimens for Antiretroviral Therapy-Naive Patients* (available at: http://aidsinfo.nih.gov/guidelines; accessed March 9, 2013).

during the first months of therapy, followed by a slower rise that typically continues for several years. Successful ART often leads to weight gain and improvement in overall health, including reversal or resolution of a number of HIV associated conditions.

An increase in viral load to detectable levels after achieving suppression may indicate early treatment failure (often because of nonadherence). However, isolated low viral loads (eg, <200 copies/mL) are common and may be harmless "blips." True virologic failure is defined by persistent viremia. The management of treatment failure is complex and should be directed by an expert. Various forms of resistance testing are usually required, as well as a thorough review of the patient's antiretroviral history in designing salvage therapy. Clinicians may consider consulting an HIV specialist in these situations. Please see **Table 55-9** for laboratory monitoring schedules for patients before and during initiation of antiretroviral therapy.

NIH. Table 3. Laboratory Monitoring Schedule for Patients before and after Initiation of Antiretroviral Therapy (page 1 of 2) (available at http://aidsinfo.nih.gov/contentfiles/lvguidelines/AA_Tables.pdf).

Patient Adherence to HIV Therapy

In the long-term management of HIV-infected individuals, it is critical to realize that suppression of the HIV RNA viral load cannot be fully realized if patients do not adhere to the prescribed regimens. Inadequate adherence to medication regimens remains a major problem worldwide. In the context of HIV management, adherence is of particular concern as patients must consume at least 95% of their medications to avoid problems with viral resistance and therapeutic failure.

Persistent viremia is often due to non-adherence and should be addressed and assessed by the primary care physician before changing medication regimen. Factors that contribute to patient nonadherence to antiretroviral regimens

include poor health literacy, depression, substance abuse, increased pill burden, adverse effects of medications, and poor patient-physician relationships. Currently, some methods used for assessing patient adherence include pill counts, and pharmacy refill data via the electronic medical record. Technologies such as the use of electronic medication event monitoring systems (MEMS) caps, in which a computer chip is embedded in a specially designed pill bottle cap, may be a valuable tool in the future. To facilitate adherence and to assist them in achieving therapeutic goals, physicians should establish open lines of communication with patients to use every visit to stress the value of therapy adherence.

Prevention of Opportunistic Infections (OIs)

The effectiveness of ART has decreased the emphasis on the prevention and management of OIs. However, patients with CD4 cell counts of <200 cells/µL remain at risk for OIs and require primary prophylaxis. Table 55-3 lists the common OIs and the prophylaxis of select infection that are frequently encountered in HIV primary care. Patients who have been treated for OIs often require secondary prophylaxis or maintenance therapy. The diagnosis and management of HIV-related OIs is beyond the scope of this chapter. Details can be found in the OI treatment and prevention guidelines.

Kaplan JE, Benson C, Holmes KH. Guidelines for prevention and treatment of opportunistic infections in HIV-infected adults and adolescents: recommendations from CDC, the National Institutes of Health, and the HIV Medicine Association of the Infectious Diseases Society of America. *MMWR.* 2009; 58 (RR-4):1-207.

Side Effects

Clinicians managing HIV-infected patients should be able to recognize common adverse effects of these agents. These include hepatotoxicity, nephrotoxicity, rash (including

Table 55-9. Monitoring schedule on antiretroviral therapy.

Test	Prior to Initiating Antiretroviral Therapy (Pre-ART Phase)		After Initiating Antiretroviral Therapy (ART Phase)					Treatment failure	Clinically indicated
	Entry into care	Follow-up before ART	ART initiation or modification[a]	2–8 weeks after ART initiation or modification	Every 3–6 months	Every 6 months	Every 12 months		
CD4 count	✓	Every 3–6 months	✓		✓	In clinically stable patients with suppressed viral load, CD4 count can be monitored every 6–12 months		✓	✓
Viral load	✓	Every 3–6 months	✓	✓[b]	✓[c]			✓	✓
Resistance testing	✓		✓[d]					✓	✓
HLA-B*5701 testing			If considering ABC						✓
Tropism testing			✓ if considering a CCR5 antagonist					If considering a CCR5 antagonist or for failure of CCR5 antagonist-based regimen	✓
Hepatitis B serology[e]	✓		✓ May repeat if HBsAg (-) and anti-HBs (-) at baseline						✓
Basic chemistry[f]	✓	Every 6–12 months	✓	✓	✓				✓
ALT, AST, T.bilirubin	✓	Every 6–12 months	✓	✓	✓				✓
CBC with differential	✓	Every 3–6 months	✓	If on ZDV	✓				✓
Fasting lipid profile	✓	If normal, annually	✓	Consider 4–8 weeks after starting new ART		If abnormal at last measurement	If normal at last measurement		✓

(Continued)

Table 55-9. Monitoring schedule on antiretroviral therapy. (*Continued*)

Test	Prior to Initiating Antiretroviral Therapy (Pre-ART Phase)		ART initiation or modification[a]	After Initiating Antiretroviral Therapy (ART Phase)					
	Entry into care	Follow-up before ART		2–8 weeks after ART initiation or modification	Every 3–6 months	Every 6 months	Every 12 months	Treatment failure	Clinically indicated
Fasting glucose	✓	If normal, annually	✓		If abnormal at last measurement	If normal at last measurement			✓
Urinalysis[g]	✓		✓			If on TDF[h]	✓		✓
Pregnancy test			✓ If starting EFV						✓

[a]ARV modification may be done for treatment failure, adverse effects, or simplification.

[b]If HIV RNA is detectable 2–8 weeks, repeat every 4–8 weeks until suppression to <200 copies/mL, then every 3–6 months.

[c]For adherent patients with suppressed viral load and stable clinical and immunologic status for >2–3 years, some experts may extend the interval for HIV RNA monitoring to every 6 months.

[d]For ART-naïve patients, if resistance testing was performed at entry into care, repeat testing is optional; for patients with viral suppression who are switching therapy for toxicity or convenience, resistance testing will not be possible and therefore, not necessary.

[e]If HBsAg is positive at baseline or prior to initiation of ART, TDF+ (FTC or 3TC) should be used as part of ARV regimen to treat both HBV and HIV infections. If HBsAg and anti-HBs are negative at baseline, hepatitis B vaccine series should be administered.

[f]Serum Na, HCO3, Cl, BUN, cretinine, glucose (preferably fasting); some experts suggest monitoring phosphorus while on TDF; determination of renal function should include estimation of creatinine clearance using Cockcroft-Gault equation or estimation of glomerular filtration rate based on MDRD equation.

[g]For patients with renal disease, consult *Guidelines for the Management of Chronic Kidney Disease in HIV-Infected Patients: Recommendations of the HIV Medicine Association of the Infectious Diseases Society of America.*

[h]More frequent monitoring may be indicated for patients with increased risk of renal insufficiency, such as patients with diabetes.

3TC, lamivudine; ABC, abacavir; ALT, alanine aminotransferase; ART, antiretroviral therapy; AST, aspartate aminotransferase; CBC, complete blood count; EFC, efavirenz; FTC, emtricitabine; HBsAg, hepatitis B surface antigen; anti-HBs, hepatitis B surface antibody; HBV, hepatitis B virus; MDD, modification of diet in renal disease (equation); TDF, tenovofir; ZDV, zidovudine.

Adapted from *Laboratory Monitoring Schedule for Patients Before and After Initiation of Antiretroviral Therapy* (page 1 of 2; available at http://aidsinfo.nih.gov/contentfiles/lvguidelines/AA_Tables.pdf.

potentially life-threatening abacavir-related hypersensitivity rash), lipodystrophy, and pancreatitis.

In addition to the potentially serious toxicities, antiretroviral agents can also cause several side effects that can adversely affect adherence or quality of life. These include gastrointestinal side effects such as nausea, diarrhea, and flatulence and central nervous system (CNS) effects such as vivid dreams, dizziness, insomnia, difficulty concentrating, and sometimes mood changes. These side effects may improve with continued dosing, but patients who have severe or persistent side effects may need to switch agents. Readers are referred to the DHHS guidelines for a more detailed discussion of common adverse effects encountered with individual antiretroviral medications.

Drug Interactions

The NNRTIs, PIs, and CCR5 antagonists are especially prone to drug-drug interactions because they are metabolized through the CYP3A4 enzyme system. Before prescribing medications to HIV-infected patients, general practitioners should be aware of common interactions between antiretroviral agents and other medications. Clinicians should be particularly cautious when prescribing warfarin, rifamycins, oral contraceptives, anticonvulsants, statins, clarithromycin, calciumchannel blockers, antiarrhythmics, certain benzodiazepines and opiates, and drugs for erectile dysfunction to patients taking ART regimens that include NNRTIs, PIs, or CCR5 antagonists.

The Liverpool drug interaction charts (http://www.hiv-druginteractions.org/), Johns Hopkins HIV Guide (http://www.hopkins-hivguide.org), and the Clinical Care Options website (http://www. clinicaloptions.com/HIV/Resources/Tool%20 Download.aspx) are well regarded and easy to use resources that can be used at the point of care.

Health Maintenance & Other Primary Care Issues

Many HIV-infected individuals develop multiple complications and comorbidities. Some complications of HIV infection are the direct result of long-term infection, whereas others are the indirect result of aging, antiretroviral therapy, or other patient factors. Primary care providers of HIV-infected individuals should screen patients with routine laboratory monitoring (eg, comprehensive metabolic and lipid panels) and validated tools (eg, the HIV Dementia Scale). Treatment of many chronic complications is similar for patients with HIV infection and those without infection. Many HIV-associated complications, such as dyslipidemia, diabetes, depression, and obesity, are familiar to primary care providers. However, special attention should be given to patients taking antiretroviral drugs because of potential drug interactions. Preventive care, health promotion (eg, safe sex education, smoking cessation, healthy lifestyles), and psychosocial assessments are central to the HIV primary care.

Psychiatric Disorders & Behavioral Risk Reduction Counseling

Studies estimate that ≤50% of patients with HIV infection have concurrent chronic psychiatric and substance use disorders. Depression, anxiety, and substance abuse are highly prevalent among HIV-infected individuals. Psychiatric symptoms may also be manifestations of HIV-related neurocognitive dysfunction. Prompt recognition and treatment of psychiatric comorbidities is central to the effective management of HIV-infected patients.

Behavioral risk reduction counseling is also a cornerstone of HIV primary care. Each visit presents an opportunity to review the patient's sexual and drug use activities. Discussion should focus on risk reduction interventions tailored to the individual's behaviors. Counseling toward limiting the number of sexual partners, engaging in lower-risk sexual activities, and consistent use of latex condoms during sexual intercourse should be provided. Patients should also be strongly encouraged to disclose their serostatus to all sexual partners. The potential for acquiring different and potentially drug-resistant strains of HIV, resulting in treatment failure, should be discussed.

Patients who use injection drugs should be counseled about the risks of continued use, including acquisition of other bloodborne pathogens such as hepatitis B, hepatitis C, and new strains of HIV. In patients who are unable to stop injecting drugs, they should be told not to reuse or share needles. The entry of patients into substance abuse treatment program may need to be facilitated.

Immunizations

Immunizations are an important part of preventive care for HIV-infected patients. The pneumococcal conjugate and polysaccharide vaccine, influenza vaccine, and tetanus toxoid are indicated in all HIV-infected patients. Revaccination with pneumococcal polysaccharide vaccine should be considered 5 years after the initial vaccination or sooner if it was administered when the CD4 count was <200 cells/mm^3 and if the CD4 count has increased to >200 cells/mm^3 on ART. All HIV-infected patients should receive influenza vaccination annually. This is especially important in those who smoke cigarettes or have underlying lung disease. In patients without immunity to hepatitis B or A should be vaccinated against both viruses. This is particularly important if they are coinfected with hepatitis C. All inactivated vaccines are considered safe in this setting, but live-attenuated vaccines should be avoided in patients with advanced HIV disease (CD4 <200). The HPV vaccine is recommended for both males and females below 26 years of age. Point-of-care resources such as the Society of Teachers of Family Medicine (http://immunizationed.org/ShotsOnline.aspx) may be found valuable by clinicians.

Screening for Other Diseases

A. Cervical Cancer Screening

Cervical screening should be performed as part of the initial evaluation in all HIV-infected women. Management in women with abnormal Papanicolaou tests is based on cytologic findings. Please refer to ACOG screening guidelines.

B. Anal Cancer Screening

Human immunodeficiency virus infection is associated with an increased risk for anal cancer in both men and women. In several HIV clinics, anal Pap screening for HPV-associated dysplasia is considered the standard of care among HIV-infected adults. Patients with any abnormality on the anal Pap test should be referred for high-resolution anoscopy and biopsy.

C. Screening for Other Sexually Transmitted Diseases (STDs)

Patients with HIV infection should be screened for other STDs at the initial evaluation. Discussion of sexual practices along with prevention counseling should be incorporated regularly into visits. Periodic screening for STDs should be performed in persons at continued risk. Please refer to the chapter on STDs in this book for a more detailed discussion.

D. Tuberculosis Screening

Prophylaxis against *Mycobacterium tuberculosis* infection is recommended for HIV-infected patients with a positive PPD ($\geq$5 mm induration) or positive interferon-γ test, history of a positive PPD without prior treatment, or contact with a person with active pulmonary TB. A chest x-ray and clinical evaluation should be performed in all patients with a positive TB screening test to exclude active disease prior to the initiation of prophylaxis. Please refer to the CDC guidelines on the treatment of latent TB.

E. Screening for Other Conditions

Age-appropriate screening for breast, colon, and prostate cancer should be performed in HIV-infected patients according to recommendations used for the general population. Please refer to the USPSTF guidelines for more information on these.

Care of Special Populations

A. Gay, Bisexual, and Other Men Who Have Sex with Men (MSM)

The MSM group represents only 2% of the US population. Nonetheless, in 2009, MSM accounted for 61% of new HIV infections in the United Sstates and 79% of infections among all newly infected men. MSM is the only group in the United States in which new HIV infections have been increasing since the early 1990s. Homophobia, stigma, and discrimination put MSM at risk for multiple physical and mental health problems and affect whether MSM seek and are able to obtain high-quality health services. Negative attitudes about homosexuality can lead to rejection by friends and family, discriminatory acts, and bullying and violence. These dynamics make it difficult for some MSM to be open about same-sex behaviors with others, which can increase stress, limit social support, and negatively affect health. Because of these factors, the care of HIV-infected MSM requires particular attention to a sensitive and inclusive approach with an emphasis on risk reduction counseling. Special attention is needed for STDs, anal cancer screening, alcohol and tobacco use, psychological health, domestic violence, and stigma. Physicians should also inquire about "club drugs" such as methamphetamines, whose use has been associated with high-risk sexual behaviors.

B. HIV Infection in Women

Worldwide, almost an equal number of women are infected with HIV compared with men. In some parts of the world (eg, sub-Saharan Africa), they constitute the majority of infected individuals. The burden of HIV in women is significantly complicated by gender inequality and stigma. In the United States, women currently account for >25% of all cases. Primary care of the HIV-infected woman requires special attention to issues such as drug toxicities, contraception, and family planning. A baseline pregnancy test should be performed in women prior to initiation of ART. Certain antiretroviral agents (eg, efavirenz) should be used with caution in women of childbearing age because of teratogenicity-related concerns. Contraceptive methods should be recommended following due consideration of potential interactions between antiretroviral drugs and hormonal contraceptives.

Among HIV-infected pregnant women living in resource-abundant settings, the near elimination of perinatal transmission due to antenatal treatment of HIV infection has been one of the greatest public health success stories in the HIV/AIDS epidemic. In the absence of treatment, the risk of vertical transmission of HIV is as high as 25–30%. With the implementation of HIV testing, counseling, antiretroviral medication, delivery by appropriate use of elective cesarean section, and avoidance of breastfeeding, the mother-to-infant transmission has decreased to <2% in the United States. There are several unique factors to consider in the use of antiretroviral medications in HIV-infected pregnant women, including (1) dosing adjustments relative to physiologic changes associated with pregnancy; (2) potential exacerbation in toxicities of ARV drugs during pregnancy; (3) risk of toxicity to the fetus because of transplacental transfer of drugs; and (4) the potential for preterm birth, teratogenicity, mutagenicity, or carcinogenicity, and other adverse pregnancy outcomes. The US DHHS publishes periodically updated guidelines for the perinatal management of HIV disease.

Perinatal HIV Guidelines Working Group. *Public Health Service Task Force Recommendations for Use of Antiretroviral Drugs in Pregnant HIV-1 Infected Women for Maternal Health and Interventions to Reduce Perinatal HIV-1 Transmission in the United States.* Bethesda, MD: National Institutes of Health (available at http://www.aidsinfo.nih.gov/guidelines/html/3/perinatal-guidelines/0/; accessed March 11, 2013).

C. HIV Infection in Children

While in the developed world, the number of children living with HIV infection is small, worldwide, an estimated 3.4 million children were living with HIV at the end of 2011. More than 90% of these children were in sub-Saharan Africa. Most children acquire HIV from their HIV-infected mothers during pregnancy, birth, or breastfeeding. Pediatric HIV infection may affect normal neurologic and immunologic development at critical phases and present unique management challenges. Some clinical features uniquely seen in HIV-infected children are growth failure/short stature, developmental delay/mental retardation, aspiration and swallowing problems, recurrent ear infections, and delayed puberty. A detailed description of pediatric HIV/AIDS and its management may be found in the *Red Book* published by the American Academy of Pediatrics.

American Academy of Pediatrics. Human inmmunodeficeincy virus infection. In: Pickering LK, ed. *Red Book: 2012 Report of the Committee on Infectious Diseases.* 29th ed. El Grove Village, IL; 2012.

D. HIV Infection in Older Adults

The prevalence and incidence of HIV infection in patients aged >50 is increasing because of the success of potent ART, as well as the occurrence of new primary infections. Treatment of HIV infection in this population is often complicated by comorbidities and an increased potential for drug toxicity and drug-drug interactions. The help of a pharmacist is very valuable in these circumstances. The American Geriatrics Society (AGS) and the American Academy of HIV Medicine (AAHIVM) published a consensus report on the care of older individuals with HIV infection in 2012.

Spivack BS. Caring for older adults with HIV and AIDS. *Clin Geriatr.* 2012;20(1):14–15.

▶ Complementary & Alternative Therapies (CAM) in HIV/AIDS

No alternative and complementary modalities have proven beneficial in HIV treatment or control of infection. However, acupuncture, plant products (eg, herbal supplements), massage, aromatherapy, and meditation are frequently utilized CAM modalities by HIV-infected individuals to improve general health, energy, and overall sense of well-being. They also use these modalities to alleviate ART-related side effects.

Some studies have reported rates of usage to be as high as 74%, particularly among patients with lipodystrophy. Patients seldom disclose their use to their providers. Hence, it is important for providers to ask about the use of herbal supplements. While some CAM therapies, such as meditation, might help to improve the sense of well-being and quality of life, caution should be exercised with the use of herbal supplements. Drug-drug interactions with antiretroviral medications are a significant concern with the use of herbal products. For example, St. John's wort is known to have drug-drug interactions with protease inhibitors and may increase the risk of virologic failure. In order to promote health and diminish the risk of treatment failure, it is extremely important for providers to have an open and ongoing discussion with HIV-infected individuals regarding the use of these therapies.

Cho M, Ye X, Dobs A, et al. Prevalence of complementary and alternative medicine use among HIV patients for perceived lipodystrophy. *J Altern Complement Med.* 2006; 12:475–482.

Littlewood RA, Vanable PA. A global perspective on complementary and alternative medicine use among people living with HIV/AIDS in the era of antiretroviral treatment. *Curr HIV/AIDS Rep.* 2011; 8(4):257–268.

Depression in Diverse Populations & Older Adults

56

Ruth S. Shim, MD, MH
Annelle Primm, MD, MPH

ESSENTIALS OF DIAGNOSIS

Depression is a clinical diagnosis characterized by ≥2 weeks of depressed mood and/or anhedonia (loss of interest or pleasure), and multiple additional symptoms:

- Change in appetite (or weight change)
- Change in sleep pattern
- Change in activity
- Fatigue and/or loss of energy
- Guilt and/or feeling of worthlessness
- Diminished concentration
- Suicidal thoughts

Anxiety symptoms are often common among depressed individuals. Among older adults, cognitive impairment may be associated with depression. Within various cultures, depression can manifest with more somatic symptoms rather than mood symptoms.

General Considerations

Mental health is an essential part of overall health. Unfortunately, some demographic groups are at increased risk for having unmet mental health needs, including children and youth, older adults, and members of medically underserved racial and ethnic groups. Because these groups are most likely to seek treatment for their mental health problems in primary care settings, it is essential that primary care physicians and other allied health practitioners be skilled in providing high-quality mental health services.

Depression is one of the leading causes of disability worldwide. It is a highly prevalent condition, affecting 35% of patients seen in primary care settings, and its prevalence in all age groups has been increasing in recent years. The most common age of onset is between 25 and 35 years of age, and an earlier age of onset of depression is associated with worse prognosis and functional impairment over time. Depression is twice as common among women as men, and African American and Hispanic individuals with a diagnosis of depression are less likely to receive mental health services compared to their white counterparts, as older adults are less likely to receive mental health services compared to younger adults.

Depression is a highly comorbid condition, particularly in later life. Medical illness and disability–more common in the elderly–are risk factors for depression. Depression diminishes quality of life, leads to nonadherence with self-care and treatment recommendations, increases the use of medical services, and is associated with cognitive impairment in adults. Furthermore, depression is often associated with medical and social complexity–patients with depression often have multiple chronic conditions, poor socioeconomic status, and poor social support, which, in turn, increase the risk of developing depression. Major psychosocial risk factors for depression include bereavement, caregiver strain, social isolation, disability, chronic medical illness, and role transitions.

Agency for Healthcare Research and Quality. *2011 National Healthcare Disparities Report*. AHRQ; 2012 (available at http://www.ahrq.gov/research/findings/nhqrdr/nhdr11/index.html; accessed March 20, 2013).

González HM, Vega WA, Williams DR, Tarraf W, West BT, Neighbors HW. Depression care in the United States: too little for too few. *Arch Gen Psychiatr.* 2010; 67(1):37. [PMID: 20048221]

Roca M, Gili M, Garcia-Garcia M, et al. Prevalence and comorbidity of common mental disorders in primary care. *J Affect Disord.* 2009; 119(1–3):52–58. [PMID: 19361865]

World Health Organization. *The Global Burden of Disease: 2004 Update*. WHO; 2008 (available at http://www.who.int/healthinfo/global_burden_disease/GBD_report_2004update_full.pdf; accessed March 21, 2013).

Prevention

Preventive interventions that target individuals at higher risk for depression (or the adverse effects of depression) can allow primary care providers to focus their efforts on promoting whole-person health. Effective primary prevention efforts that decrease the incidence of depression often require a multifactorial, interdisciplinary approach that targets multiple risk factors across various sectors. Interventions may include education about stress-coping techniques; facilitating healthy relationships with friends, family, and support groups; and protecting sleep quality through better sleep hygiene. Secondary prevention strategies include screening tools to enhance detection and treatment of depression. Universal screening in primary care settings, when coupled with effective treatment, can be an important tool in the prevention of depression. Finally, tertiary prevention efforts, which include antidepressant treatment and psychotherapy, have been shown to reduce relapse rates and morbidity associated with depression. Universal, selective, and indicated preventive interventions target the general public or specific individuals at highest risk for developing depression in the future.

O'Connell M, Boat T, Warner K. *Preventing Mental, Emotional, and Behavioral Disorders among Young People: Progress and Possibilities*; 2009 (available at http://www.ncbi.nlm.nih.gov/books/NBK32775/pdf/TOC.pdf; accessed March 15, 2013).

Primm AB, Vasquez MJ, Mays RA, et al. The role of public health in addressing racial and ethnic disparities in mental health and mental illness. *Prev Chronic Dis.* 2010; 7(1). [PMID: 20040235]

van't Veer-Tazelaar PJ, van Marwijk HW, van Oppen P, et al. Stepped-care prevention of anxiety and depression in late life: a randomized controlled trial. *Arch Gen Psychiatr.* 2009; 66(3):297. [PMID: 19255379]

Clinical Findings

The type and level of severity of depression run along a spectrum, ranging from subclinical varieties to major depression. Major depression typically occurs in discrete episodes, each with a clear beginning and end. After an initial episode, >50% of individuals will have additional episodes in their lifetime. Among older adults with depression, approximately 50% had experienced depression earlier in their life, and the other half experienced their first depressive episode after the age of 60.

A. Initial Assessment

Many individuals are reluctant to seek care for mental health problems. In a national sample of people who reported experiencing major depression, >33.3% of individuals did not seek treatment. In addition, many adults are reluctant to report their depressive symptoms to their primary care physicians. Recent data suggest discordance between patients presenting with symptoms of depression and physicians' appraisal of depression symptoms during primary care visits. Even so, primary care physicians prescribe the majority of antidepressant medication in the United States, and have a major responsibility to detect and effectively treat depression in these settings.

Initial assessment should include a focused psychiatric history and examination, and, for older adults, a brief clinical cognitive examination. In addition, a medical history, physical examination, focused neurologic examination, and laboratory studies to rule out physical conditions with similar symptoms are preferred as part of the assessment. It is also important to assess other domains, particularly for older adults, including level of functioning or disability, loss or grief concerns, the physical environment, and psychosocial stressors.

B. Symptoms and Signs

Specific features associated with depressive disorders are described as follows:

- **Depressed mood:** feeling sad, "low," empty, hopeless, gloomy, or "down in the dumps," different from a normal sense of sadness or grief

- **Anhedonia:** inability to enjoy usually pleasurable activities (eg, sex, hobbies, daily routines)

- **Changes in appetite or weight:** a decrease in appetite (most patients) or an increase in appetite associated with craving specific foods

- **Changes in sleep patterns:** insomnia (difficulty falling asleep, staying asleep, or early-morning awakening) in most patients; hypersomnia in some patients

- **Changes in activity:** psychomotor retardation (speech, thinking, movement) or psychomotor agitation (inability to sit still, pacing, hand wringing)

- **Loss of energy:** decreased energy, tiredness, fatigue

- **Cognitive changes:** inability to think, concentrate, or make decisions

- **Sense of worthlessness or guilt:** excessive feelings of low self-esteem, self-blame, and lack of self-worth

- **Suicidal ideation:** thoughts of death or suicide, with and without a plan, or suicide attempts

A total of five of the nine features, including either depressed mood or anhedonia, must be present during the same 2-week period for the patient to be diagnosed with major depressive disorder. Symptoms of depression can present with varying degrees of severity, and may be accompanied by symptoms of anxiety or mania. In addition, symptoms can occur in the context of discrete episodes of depression, or, in cases of more chronic, unremitting symptoms, can be considered a persistent depressive disorder. Among older adults, a key factor is symptom presentation, which may differ considerably from that of younger adults. Older adults are less likely to present with affective symptoms than younger adults. Primary care providers should focus on assessing symptoms of cognitive difficulty, sleep disturbance, psychomotor retardation, and feelings of hopelessness in older adults.

C. Screening Measures

Many validated screening instruments exist for screening depression in diverse populations. Screening for depression in the primary care setting can be initiated using a two-question initial screening test to detect the presence of depressed mood and anhedonia: "Over the past 2 weeks, have you felt down, depressed, or hopeless?" and "Over the past 2 weeks, have you felt little interest or pleasure in doing things?"). This short screening test is often referred to as the *Patient Health Questionnaire-2* (PHQ-2). PHQ-2 scores ≥ 3 are 83% sensitive and 92% specific for diagnosing major depression when used in primary care settings. Patients who screen positive on the PHQ-2 can be further evaluated with the PHQ-9, which has been validated in multiple culturally diverse populations, including African Americans, Africans, Chinese Americans, Hispanics, and others, as well as in older adults. In primary care settings where the quality of depression care is high, patients received universal screening for depression with the PHQ-9.

Among older adults, the Geriatric Depression Scale (GDS) has several versions, including an original 30-item version, as well as 20-, 15-, 12-, 10-, 5-, 4-, and 1-item versions of the scale. The GDS-15 and GDS-5 have been shown to be as effective as the GDS-30 in diagnosing depression in older adults.

The PHQ-9 and GDS-15 has been proven effective in detecting suicidal ideations. Risk factors for attempting suicide include mood disorders and other mental disorders, substance use disorders, history of deliberate self-harm, becoming disabled, and a history of suicide attempts. A majority of individuals who have completed suicide will have seen their primary care physician in the month before their death, which signals an opportunity for primary care providers to provide lifesaving interventions. Once a patient has been deemed to be at higher risk of suicide; immediate referral to specialty mental health services is indicated.

All screening tools should be seen as the initial phase of the assessment, and should be followed by a more detailed assessment to confirm the diagnosis of depression, which includes evaluating for concomitant psychiatric problems (including substance use disorders, manic episodes, or anxiety disorders) and determining the severity of depression. **Table 56-1** lists several screening instruments for depression.

Arroll B, Goodyear-Smith F, Crengle S, et al. Validation of PHQ-2 and PHQ-9 to screen for major depression in the primary care population. *Ann Fam Med.* 2010; 8(4):348–353. [PMID: 20644190]

Table 56-1. Depression and suicide screening instruments.

Patient Health Questionnaire (PHQ-2, PHQ-9)
Geriatric Depression Scale (GDS-15, GDS-30)
Center for Epidemiologic Studies Depression Scale (CES-D)
Beck Depression Inventory (BDI-II)
Zung Self-Rating Depression Scale (SDS)

Bell RA, Franks P, Duberstein PR, et al. Suffering in silence: reasons for not disclosing depression in primary care. *Ann Fam Med.* 2011; 9(5):439–446. [PMID: 21911763]

Fiske A, Wetherell JL, Gatz M. Depression in older adults. *Ann Rev Clin Psychol.* 2009; 5:363. [PMID: 19327033]

Heisel MJ, Duberstein PR, Lyness JM, Feldman MD. Screening for suicide ideation among older primary care patients. *J Am Board Fam Med.* 2010; 23(2):260–269. [PMID: 20207936]

Mark TL, Levit KR, Buck JA. Datapoints: psychotropic drug prescriptions by medical specialty. *Psychiatr Serv.* 2009; 60(9):1167–1167. [PMID: 19723729]

Mitchell AJ, Vaze A, Rao S. Clinical diagnosis of depression in primary care: a meta-analysis. *Lancet.* 2009; 374(9690):609–619. [PMID: 19640579]

Mitchell AJ, Bird V, Rizzo M, Meader N. Diagnostic validity and added value of the Geriatric Depression Scale for depression in primary care: a meta-analysis of GDS30 and GDS15. *J Affect Disord.* 2010; 125(1–3):10–17. [PMID: 19800132]

Mojtabai R. Unmet need for treatment of major depression in the United States. *Psychiatr Serv.* 2009; 60(3):297–305. [PMID: 19252041]

Park M, Unützer J. Geriatric depression in primary care. *Psychiatr Clin North Am.* 2011; 34(2):469. [PMID: 21536169]

▶ Differential Diagnosis

The most critical comorbid health conditions to consider in a person with depression include alcohol and substance use disorders and medications that can cause mood disorders (eg, prednisone). Late-life depression often coexists with cognitive impairment and other illnesses of the central nervous system (CNS), and the concomitance increases the risk of developing symptoms of Alzheimer's disease compared with those with cognitive impairment without depression. Bipolar depression must also be ruled out in patients presenting with depressive symptoms. All patients with depressive symptoms should be screened for a history of manic or hypomanic symptoms. Depending on the clinical presentation, physicians should also assess the patient for a variety of general medical problems that could be contributing to mood symptoms, including cardiac disease, diabetes, and certain types of cancer. Among older adults, accidental misuse of medications and physical, verbal, or emotional abuse by caregivers or relatives should also be evaluated.

Complications

If untreated, depression can lead to multiple complications, including more serious, treatment-resistant forms of the illness, worsening physical condition, and suicide. Individuals with untreated depression are at greater risk for complications from general medical problems, alcohol and substance use disorders, and relationship problems. Impairment in social and occupational functioning can lead to increased disability.

Treatment

Treatment of mental disorders has increased substantially over the past decades, yet a majority of adults with mental disorders do not receive treatment at all, or do not receive treatment in accordance with accepted standards of care. For minority populations, rates of high-quality mental health treatment are even lower.

Selection of an initial treatment modality should be influenced by both clinical factors (eg, severity of symptoms) and patient preference. In general, evidence-based recommendations for treatment of moderate to severe depression in the primary care setting involves a combination of pharmacotherapy and psychotherapy, and for the treatment of mild to moderate depression, psychotherapy or pharmacotherapy alone.

Although the majority of depressed patients are treated in primary care settings, some cases are especially difficult to manage in general medical clinics without specialized services. Specialized psychiatric care is strongly indicated if clinical findings support a diagnosis of psychotic depression, bipolar disorder, active suicidal ideation, depression with comorbid substance abuse, depression with comorbid dementia, treatment-resistant depression, and other needs for a more specialized assessment.

A. Psychotherapeutic Interventions

For patients with mild to moderate major depressive disorder, psychotherapy alone may be appropriate. Cognitive-behavioral therapy (CBT) and interpersonal therapy (IPT) are evidence-based psychotherapeutic approaches used in the treatment of patients with major depressive disorder. Factors to consider when determining how often to see an individual patient include the goals of the psychotherapy, the frequency necessary to create and maintain a therapeutic alliance, the frequency required to ensure treatment adherence, and the frequency necessary to monitor and address suicidality. Often, if a skilled therapist is not available in the primary care setting, referral to a mental health specialist may be indicated (eg, psychiatric nurses, licensed clinical social workers, psychologists, or psychiatrists). Primary care providers should ensure that patients are made aware of psychotherapy as an option and that they are assisted in accessing psychotherapeutic interventions.

B. Pharmacotherapy

Antidepressant medications may be initiated for treatment of patients with mild symptoms of major depressive disorder, and should be initiated for all patients with moderate to severe symptoms. Improvement should be noted within 6–8 weeks of initiating therapy, and the goal of antidepressant therapy is to achieve full remission of depressive symptoms. Studies have shown that maintenance antidepressant therapy is effective in preserving improvements and preventing recurrent depression.

The most commonly used antidepressant mediations are listed in **Table 56-2**. Selective serotonin reuptake inhibitors (SSRIs) are usually first-line therapy, due to greater tolerability and equal efficacy compared to other antidepressants. Other medications likely to be optimal for most patients include nortriptyline, bupropion, venlafaxine, and duloxetine. Because of their potential to cause serious side effects and the need for dietary restrictions, monoamine oxidase inhibitors (MAOIs) are typically reserved for patients with treatment-resistant depression.

Patients prescribed antidepressant medication should be monitored to assess their response to pharmacotherapy as well as side effects and adverse reactions. After dosing antidepressant medication at the recommended starting dose, it is important to increase the medication over time to an efficacious dose. Few patients treated for depression in primary care reach the recommended therapeutic dosage of the medicine. Screening tests can be used to objectively monitor a patient's progress throughout treatment. To maintain consistency with clinical practice guidelines, patients should be seen for follow-up after initiating pharmacological treatment within 2–4 weeks. If no response is seen within the initial 6-8-week period of pharmacological therapy, referral for specialty mental healthcare may be considered.

Stepped-care models have been used in primary care settings to manage diverse conditions such as hypertension, and have been shown to be effective in improving the quality of depression care for patients in primary care settings. Stepped-care models are systematic procedures based on using the most effective, but least intensive, treatment for patients, which includes detailed monitoring and tracking of patients' response to interventions. An example of a stepped-care model for depression treatment is shown in **Table 56-3**.

C. Complementary/Alternative Therapies

Some studies show a beneficial effect of exercise programs in treatment of depression in comparison to antidepressant medication alone. Meditation-based cognitive therapy has been shown to be effective for treatment of and decreasing recurrence of major depressive disorder. A variety of coping and self-management strategies can also be helpful, such as peer support, exercise, good nutrition, progressive muscle

Table 56-2. Medications used in treatment of depression.[a]

Drug Type: Brand (Generic)	Typical Daily[b] Dosage (mg)
Selective Serotonin Reuptake Inhibitors (SSRIs)	
Celexa (citalopram[c])	20–40
Lexapro (escitalopram)	10–20
Paxil (paroxetine[c])	20–50
Paxil CR (paroxetine, controlled-release)	12.5–62.5
Prozac (fluoxetine[c])	20–60
Prozac Weekly (fluoxetine[c])	90
Zoloft (sertraline[c])	50–200
Serotonin and Norepinephrine Reuptake Inhibitors (SNRIs)	
Cymbalta (duloxetine)	60–120
Effexor (venlafaxine[c])	75–375
Effexor XR (venlafaxine, extended-release)	75–225
Pristiq (desvenlafaxine)	50–100
Other	
Remeron (mirtazapine[c])	15–45
(trazodone)	150–400
Wellbutrin, Wellbutrin XL (bupropion[c])	150–450
Wellbutrin SR (bupropion, sustained-release[c])	150–400
Tricyclics	
(amitriptyline)	150–300
Aventyl, Pamelor (nortriptyline[c])	75–150
Norpramin (desipramine[c])	150–300
Sinequan (doxepin[c])	25–300
Tofranil (imipramine[c])	150–200
Monoamine Oxidase Inhibitors (MAOIs)	
Emsam skin patch (selegiline)	6–12
Marplan (isocarboxazid[c])	30–60
Nardil (phenelzine[c])	45–90
Parnate (tranylcypromine[c])	10–60

[a]This list represents the most commonly prescribed antidepressants.
[b]These dosages represent an average range for the treatment of depression. The precise effective dosage varies from patient to patient and depends on many factors. *Starting dosages tend to be lower for older adults.*
[c]Generic version is available at lower cost.
Data from Swartz KL. *The Johns Hopkins White Papers: Depression and Anxiety.* Baltimore, MD: Johns Hopkins Medicine; 2009 (available at www.JohnsHopkinsHealthAlerts.com); Schatzberg AF, Cole JO, DeBattista C. *Manual of Clinical Psychopharmacology,* 7th ed. Washington, DC: American Psychiatric Publishing; 2009 (available from http://psychiatryonline.org/content.aspx?bookid=2&sectionid=1359932).

Table 56-3. Stepped-care model of depression treatment.

Step 1: All known and suspected presentations of depression	Assessment, support, psychoeducation, active monitoring, and referral for further assessment and interventions
Step 2: Persistent subthreshold depressive symptoms, mild to moderate depression	Low-intensity psychological and psychosocial interventions, medication, and referral for further assessment and interventions
Step 3: Persistent subthreshold depressive symptoms or mild to moderate depression with inadequate response to initial interventions; moderate and severe depression	Medication, high-intensity psychological interventions, combined treatment, collaborative care, and referral for further assessment and interventions
Step 4: Severe and complex depression; risk to life; severe self-neglect	Medication, high-intensity psychological interventions, electroconvulsive therapy, crisis service, combined treatments, multiprofessional and inpatient care

Reproduced with permission from National Collaborating Centre for Mental Health. *Depression: Quick Reference Guide.* NICE Clinical Guidelines; 2009 (available from http://www.nice.org.uk/nicemedia/live/12329/45890/45890.pdf).

demonstrated its effectiveness in the treatment of mild to moderate depression. However, St. John's wort has increased medication interactions, particularly in older adults, and is generally not recommended for treatment of depression in most populations. Interactions between St. John's wort and antidepressants are concerning, especially considering that patients are often less likely to share information about herbal supplements that they are taking when discussing their current medications.

Other alternative medication therapies have conflicting reports about efficacy, but include *S*-adenosyl methionine (SAM-e), omega-3 fatty acids, and folic acid supplementation; however, further research is needed to determine their efficacy in the treatment of depression.

D. Combination Therapy

The combination of psychotherapy and medication is recommended for patients with moderate to severe depression. Patients who have a history of only partial response to adequate trials of either treatment modality alone may benefit from combined treatment. Sequential treatment of psychotherapy and pharmacotherapy may also be beneficial. Patients with poor adherence to individual treatments may also benefit from combined treatment of any form.

relaxation, setting aside time for pleasurable activities, and setting small, achievable goals. Furthermore, increasing evidence in the medical literature supports the beneficial role of spirituality in the health of patients.

St. John's wort has been used to treat depression for many years, and multiple randomized clinical trials have

E. Electroconvulsive Therapy

Electroconvulsive therapy (ECT) remains a highly stigmatized treatment modality, but it is an evidence-based, effective therapy for depression, particularly among older adults and patients with psychotic or treatment-resistant depression. Patients often have rapid improvement of symptoms of depression, and usually receive two to three treatments per week for 3–6 weeks. Primary care providers should consider a referral to a mental health specialist for evaluation for ECT in patients who have not responded to multiple trials of medication and psychotherapy.

F. Integrated/Collaborative Care Models

Integrated care and collaborative care models have effectively improved the treatment of depression in primary care settings. An extremely well-studied model of using integrated care to treat depression in older adults is the *Improving Mood-Promoting Access to Collaborative Treatment* (IMPACT) collaborative care management program for late-life depression. The IMPACT model has shown significantly better outcomes for treatment of depression in older adults compared to the usual care. The model embeds a depression care manager (supervised by a psychiatrist and primary care expert) in a primary care setting to provide comprehensive services to older adults with depression.

Integrated care models have shown particular efficacy among older adults, who are more likely to accept treatment for depression in primary care settings rather than in specialty mental health settings. Within diverse populations, integrated care/collaborative care models have also shown efficacy in African American and Hispanic populations, but further research on additional racially/ethnically diverse populations is needed.

G. Addressing Disparities and Cultural Differences in Depression Care

Studies have shown that different racial and ethnic groups, as well as different age and gender groups, experience and communicate symptoms of depression differently and prefer different forms of treatment. If the provider does not speak the patient's native language, a well-trained healthcare interpreter should be used to ensure that accurate information is exchanged. Some minority populations are more receptive to psychotherapy than pharmacotherapy, and patient preferences should be explored in order to practice cultural competence. Because stigma continues to be a pervasive barrier to seeking appropriate mental health treatment, primary care providers should encourage open dialog and help correct any false assumptions about the origins of mental health problems and judgments about individuals with mental health problems.

Patient-provider communication is critical to diagnosis and treatment. The physician should elicit patients'

Table 56-4. Factors affecting cultural competence in assessment, diagnosis, and treatment of depression.

Recognition of language differences
Health literacy barriers
Somatic presentations
Use of cultural idioms of distress
Treatment preferences
Non-Western context of mental illness and treatment
Individually tailored treatment plans

explanatory models (what patients believe is causing their illness) and agendas (what patients seek from treatment), the role of family members in their lives, how those family members will react to the patient being treated, and how patients perceive treatment. For some people, experiences of racism and prejudice may leave people suspicious of diagnoses that do not require radiologic or laboratory examinations. The provider must use excellent communication skills to convey humility, empathy, respect, and compassion, as these are important factors in securing an accurate diagnosis and effective treatment of depression in racially, ethnically, and culturally diverse populations (See **Table 56-4**).

Spirituality is often an important determinant of mental health. The mere presence of a religious affiliation and the saliency of a person's religion have been shown to provide a strong defense against depression and suicide, particularly in older adults with medical illnesses or disability. This is important for providers not only because it may largely influence how patients cope with their illnesses, but also because studies have shown that validating this aspect of a patient's life and incorporating it into treatment plans can positively affect the patient's adherence to treatment and even accelerate rates of remission.

Davidson J. Major depressive disorder treatment guidelines in America and Europe. *J Clin Psychiatr.* 2010; 71:e04. [PMID: 20371031]

Ghods BK, Ford DE, Larson S, Arbelaez JJ, Cooper LA. Patient–physician communication in the primary care visits of African Americans and whites with depression. *J Gen Intern Med.* 2008; 23(5):600–606. [PMID: 18264834]

González HM, Vega WA, Williams DR, Tarraf W, West BT, Neighbors HW. Depression care in the United States: too little for too few. *Arch Gen Psychiatr.* 2010; 67(1):37. [PMID: 20048221]

Ishak WW, Ha K, Kapitanski N, et al. The impact of psychotherapy, pharmacotherapy, and their combination on quality of life in depression. *Harv Rev Psychiatr.* 2011; 19(6):277–289. [PMID: 22098324]

Katon W. Collaborative depression care models. *Am J Prev Med.* 2012;42(5):550–552. [PMID: 22516497]

Nahas R, Sheikh O. Complementary and alternative medicine for the treatment of major depressive disorder. *Can Fam Physician.* 2011; 57(6):659–663. [PMID: 21673208]

National Collaborating Centre for Mental Health. *Depression: Quick Reference Guide.* NICE Clinical Guidelines; 2009 (available at http://www.nice.org.uk/nicemedia/live/12329/45890/45890. pdf; accessed March 20, 2013).

Rasic D, Robinson JA, Bolton J, Bienvenu OJ, Sareen J. Longitudinal relationships of religious worship attendance and spirituality with major depression, anxiety disorders, and suicidal ideation and attempts: findings from the Baltimore epidemiologic catchment area study. *J Ppsychiatr Res.* 2011; 45(6):848–854. [PMID: 21215973]

Richards DA, Borglin G. Implementation of psychological therapies for anxiety and depression in routine practice: two year prospective cohort study. *J Affect Disord.* 2011; 133(1):51–60. [PMID: 21501876]

Rubenstein L, Unutzer J, Miranda J, et al. *Clinician Guide to Depression Assessment and Management in Collaborative Care*; 2009 (available at http://www.communitypartnersincare.org/ depression-care-resources/primary-care/; accessed March 20, 2013).

Shelton RC. St John's wort (Hypericum perforatum) in major depression. *J Clin Psychiat.* 2009; 70:23. [PMID: 19909690]

Unützer J, Park M. Older adults with severe, treatment-resistant depression. *JAMA.* 2012; 308(9):909–918. [PMID: 22948701]

Unützer J, Katon WJ, Fan M-Y, et al. Long-term cost effects of collaborative care for late-life depression. *Am J Manage Care.* 2008; 14:95–100. [PMID: 18269305]

Woltmann E, Grogan-Kaylor A, Perron B, Georges H, Kilbourne AM, Bauer MS. Comparative effectiveness of collaborative chronic care models for mental health conditions across primary, specialty, and behavioral health care settings: systematic review and meta-analysis. *Am J Psychiatr.* 2012; 169(8): 790–804. [PMID: 22772364]

Prognosis

Primary care practitioners are the sole contacts for more than half of patients with mental illness, and therefore are important in ensuring recognition and treatment of depression. The good news is that most patients can be treated to remission, especially if medication and psychotherapy are combined. Depression is generally a chronic, relapsing illness; however, treatment works not only to make patients well but also to keep them well. Treatment provides symptomatic relief, facilitates functional improvements, and prevents relapse and recurrence.

Roca M, Gili M, Garcia-Garcia M, et al. Prevalence and comorbidity of common mental disorders in primary care. *J Affect Disord.* 2009; 119(1-3):52–58. [PMID: 19361865]

57

Anxiety Disorders

Philip J. Michels, PhD
M. Sharm Steadman, PharmD

▶ General Considerations

Anxiety is a diffuse, unpleasant, and often vague subjective feeling of apprehension accompanied by objective symptoms of autonomic nervous system (ANS) arousal. The experience of anxiety is associated with a sense of danger or a lack of control over events. The psychological component varies from individual to individual and is strongly influenced by personality and coping mechanisms.

Many factors contribute to the experience of anxiety by individuals in our society. We live in a rapidly changing culture characterized by continuous technologic advancements, proliferation of increasingly refined information, and a mass media and entertainment industry saturated with violence and sexuality, all of which promote feelings of insecurity. In the workplace, downsizing, restructuring, mergers, and specialization are commonplace; transient work relationships and the elimination of benefits such as health insurance and retirement provisions increase the sense of insecurity.

Anxiety is pathologic when it occurs in situations that do not call for fear or when the degree of anxiety is excessive for the situation. Anxiety may occur as a result of life events, as a symptom of a primary anxiety disorder, as a secondary response to another psychiatric disorder or medical illness, or as a side effect of a medication.

The majority of individuals with mental disorders receive psychiatric care from primary care settings, whereas <20% receive care in specialized mental health settings. Among mental disorders, anxiety disorders have the highest overall lifetime morbidity risk: specific phobia (18.4%), social phobia (13.0%), posttraumatic stress disorder (10.1%), generalized anxiety disorder (9.0%), separation anxiety (8.7%), panic disorder 6.8%), agoraphobia 3.7%), obsessive-compulsive disorder (2.7%), and any anxiety disorder (41.7%), yet only 23–59% of anxious patients receive treatment. The estimated 1-year prevalence rate is 17% with a lifetime prevalence rate at 25%. Patients with anxiety disorders are at increased risk of other medical comorbidities, longer hospital stays, more procedures, higher overall health care costs, failure in school or at work, low-paying jobs, and financial dependence in the form of welfare or other government subsidies.

Kessler RC, Petukhova M, Sampson NA, Zaslavsky AM, Wittchen HU. Twelve-month and lifetime prevalence and lifetime morbid risk of anxiety and mood disorders in the United States. *Int J Methods Psychiatr Res.* 2012; 21(3):169.

Lam RM. Challenges in the treatment of anxiety disorders: beyond guidelines. *Int J Psychiatr Clin Practice.* 2006; 10(Suppl 3):18.

Mendlowicz MV, Stein MB. Quality of life in individuals with anxiety disorders. *Am J Psychiatr.* 2000; 157:669. [PMID: 10784456]

▶ Pathogenesis

A. Biomedical Influences

Because the symptoms of anxiety are so varied and prevalent, several etiologies exist to explain them. A recent meta-analysis revealed a significant genetic component, especially for panic disorder, generalized anxiety, and phobias. Temperament, which has genetic roots, is a broad vulnerability factor for anxiety disorders.

The inhibitory transmitter γ-aminobutyric acid (GABA) occupies ~40% of all synapses and is clearly implicated in the anxiety disorders, as is the endocrine system. Exposure to a stressor activates the release of an endogenous opioid, β-endorphin, which is coreleased with adrenocorticotropic hormone.

B. Psychological and Social Influences

Family dysfunction and parental psychopathology are involved in the development and maintenance of anxiety. Families of anxious children are more involved, controlling, and rejecting, and less intimate than are families who do not manifest anxiety. Parents of anxious children promote cautious and avoidant child behavior.

Behavioral and cognitive explanations define anxiety as a learned response. Anxiety develops in response to neutral or positive stimuli that become associated with a noxious or aversive event. Fearful associations develop from the situational context and the physical sensations present at the time. The patient may generalize (ie, classify objects and events in terms of a common characteristic) and thereby establish new cues to trigger anxiety. Previously neutral situations become feared and avoided. By avoiding anxiety-arousing stimuli, anxiety is diminished.

As panic and avoidance become more chronic, the behaviors involved become more habitual and awareness of one's thoughts in relation to these anxiety states diminishes. Information-processing prejudices such as selectively attending to threatening stimuli become involuntary and unconscious. A person's appraisal of an event, rather than intrinsic characteristics of that event, defines stress, evokes anxiety, and influences the ability to cope. Failure to cope elicits fear and vulnerability.

Kagan J, Snidman N, Early childhood predictors of adult anxiety disorders. *Biol Psychiatr.* 1999; 46:1536. [PMID: 10599481]

▶ Prevention

Training in stress inoculation, relaxation training, and cognitive behavioral therapy can be implemented through an integrated curriculum in public education during the early and middle years. School settings provide furtive environments for group modeling and an opportunity to reach large numbers of people. The work of Dr. Martin Seligman [see Gillham et al. 1995]) demonstrates the sizable advantages of such school-based programs.

Gillham JR, et al. Prevention of depressive symptoms in school-children: two-year follow-up. *Psychol Sci.* 1995; 6:343.

▶ Clinical Findings

A. Symptoms and Signs

Examination of the patient usually yields few clues to assist in establishing the diagnosis of an anxiety disorder. Diagnosis is complicated by the amount of symptoms and their overlap with other disease states; thus anxiety often becomes a diagnosis of exclusion. **Table 57-1** lists various symptoms of anxiety by organ system.

Despite the variety and diffuse nature of many of these symptoms, anxiety disorders can often be identified by exploration of the patient's history, along with a few laboratory values. The symptoms of each anxiety disorder are sufficiently specific to arrive at the diagnosis by taking a thorough history from the patient, including pertinent past, social, and family information. Recognition of anxiety subtypes is often based on history alone.

Table 57-1. Somatic symptoms of anxiety.

System	Symptoms
Musculoskeletal	Muscle tightness, spasms, back pain, headache, weakness, tremors, fatigue, restlessness, exaggerated startle response, jitters
Cardiovascular	Palpitations, rapid heartbeat, hot and cold spells, flushing, pallor
Gastrointestinal	Dry mouth, diarrhea, upset stomach, lump in throat, nausea, vomiting
Bladder	Frequent urination
Central nervous	Dizziness, paresthesias, lightheadedness
Respiratory	Hyperventilation, shortness of breath, constriction in chest
Miscellaneous	Sweating, clammy hands

Data from Sharma R, et al. Anxiety states. In: Flaherty JA, et al, eds: *Psychiatry: Diagnosis and Treatment.* Appleton & Lange; 1993.

B. Diagnostic Criteria

The *Diagnostic and Statistical Manual of Mental Disorders,* 5th edition (*DSM-5*) differentiates several anxiety disorders. Diagnostic criteria for each disorder are presented below.

1. Separation anxiety disorder—This disorder Involves excessive anxiety or fear concerning separation from those whom the individual is attached to.

2. Selective mutism—This disorder involves a consistent failure to speak in specific social situations where there is an expectation to speak despite speaking in other situations.

3. Specific phobias—These phobias involve marked fear or anxiety about a specific object or situation (eg, flying, heights, receiving an injection).

4. Social anxiety disorder—This condition is characterized by marked fear or anxiety about one or more social situations where the individual is exposed to possible scrutiny by others. The individual fears that s/he will act in a certain way or show anxiety that will be negatively evaluated and avoids these social situations or endures them with intense fear or anxiety, out of proportion to the actual threat.

5. Panic disorder—The attack involves an abrupt surge of intense fear or discomfort that reaches a peak within minutes and can be recurrent and unexpected. Symptoms include nausea, dizziness, lightheadedness, tingling sensations, feelings of unreality or being detached from oneself, fear of going crazy, and fear of dying.

6. Agoraphobia—This is a marked fear or anxiety about using public transportation, being in open or enclosed spaces, being in a crowd, or being outside alone.

7. Generalized anxiety disorder (GAD)—At least 6 months of persistent and excessive anxiety and worry occur on most days, with difficulty controlling the worry. Symptoms include restlessness, being on edge, being easily fatigued, difficulty concentrating, irritability, muscle tension, and sleep disturbance. Several validated tools have been developed to screen for GAD, including the two-item and seven-item Generalized Anxiety Disorder scales (GAD2, GAD7). These self-report questionnaires are easy to use and can assist primary care physicians in assessing the severity of GAD as well.

8. Substance/medication-induced anxiety disorder—Anxiety is a direct physiologic consequence of a drug of abuse, medication, or exposure to a toxin.

9. Anxiety disorder due to another medical condition—Panic attacks or anxiety predominate, and there is evidence that the disturbance is the direct pathophysiological consequence of another medical condition.

10. Adjustment disorder with anxious mood—Clinically significant symptoms of anxiety occur in response to an identifiable stressor within 3 months after onset of the stressor and resolve within 6 months after termination of the stressor. However, symptoms may persist longer if they occur in response to a chronic stressor (eg, a disabling chronic medical condition) or to a stressor that has enduring consequences (eg, financial effects of a divorce).

Conner KM, et al. Mini-SPIN: a brief screening assessment for generalized social anxiety disorder. *Depress Anxiety.* 2001;14(2):139.
Spitzer RL, et al. A brief measure for assessing generalized anxiety disorder: the GAD-7. *Arch Intern Med.* 2006;166(10):1092–1097.

C. Laboratory Findings

There are no gold standard laboratory studies on diagnosing anxiety disorders. It is reasonable to perform a limited empiric evaluation to identify the etiology of the symptoms as well as evaluate for comorbid medical problems that may complicate the treatment. This evaluation may include a complete blood count, electrolyte, glucose, creatinine, calcium, liver panel, and thyroid function tests. Further testing should be tailored on an individual basis, depending on the clinical circumstances. Urine drug screening should be considered, because illicit drug use and withdrawal may be a possible differential diagnosis and patients with anxiety may self-medicate with drugs of abuse.

Fricchione G. Clinical practice. Generalized anxiety disorder. *N Engl J Med.* 2004;351:675. [PMID: 15306669]

D. Imaging Studies

Imaging studies are completed only to preclude any laboratory abnormalities or organic disease that may mimic anxiety or panic. Such studies include, but are not limited to, thyroid scan and cardiac diagnostics. Functional magnetic resonance imaging (MRI) is a technique that enables one to map cognitive, affective, and experiential processes onto brain substrates. It is a proxy measure of how complex processes are implemented in different neural systems. Magnetic resonance spectroscopy (MRS) is a noninvasive *in vivo* method used to quantify metabolites that are relevant to a wide range of brain processes. Recent studies have shown that there are significant metabolic differences in various regions of the brain between patients with anxiety disorders and healthy controls.

Paulus MP. The role of neuroimaging for the diagnosis and treatment of anxiety disorders. *Depress Anxiety.* 2008; 25:348. [PMID: 18412061]
Trzesniak C, Araujo D: Magnetic resonance spectroscopy in anxiety disorders. *Acta Neuropsy.* 2008; 20:56.

E. Special Tests

Psychological tests resort to self-report of symptoms and are major assessment tools for anxiety. This is unfortunate as most other medical diagnoses (eg, diabetes mellitus) rely on both symptom self-report and systematic biomedical measurements (eg, the glucose tolerance test).

The State-Trait Anxiety Inventory (STAI) measures the frequency and intensity of transient anxiety processes and anxiety proneness as a character trait, while the Beck Anxiety Inventory-Trait (BAIT) is specific to measuring trait anxiety. Both self-report tests have excellent reliability and validity.

Other validated measures are the Endler Multidimensional Anxiety Scales (EMAS-T), which specifically measures responses to social evaluation, physical danger, and ambiguous and daily routines, while the Three Systems Anxiety Questionnaire (TSAQ) assesses the behavioral, cognitive, and somatic components of anxiety. Comorbidity can comprehensively be assessed by the Minnesota Multiphasic Personality Inventory-II (MMPI-II), a test composed of 567 true/false test items that can be completed in ~2 hours. The Profile of Mood States (POMS) primarily measures mood states in psychiatric outpatients. Its advantage over the MMPI-II is a completion time of ~10 minutes.

Elwood LS, Wolitzky-Taylor K, Olatunji BO. Measurement of anxious traits: a contemporary review and synthesis. *Anxiety Stress Coping J.* 2012;25 (6):647.
Hathaway SR, McKinley C. *Minnesota Multiphasic Personality Inventory-2.* National Computer Systems, University of Minnesota; 1989.
McNair DM, et al. *Profile of Mood States, Revised.* Educational and Industrial Testing Service; 1992.
Spielberger CD. *State-Trait Anxiety Inventory.* Consulting Psychologists Press; 1983.

Differential Diagnosis

Because anxiety is a ubiquitous symptom of numerous conditions, family physicians must be alert to the possibility of alternative medical causes. A thorough evaluation and workup are essential to alleviate patients' concerns that their symptoms are due to other chronic or severe medical conditions.

The first step in planning a diagnostic evaluation is to perform a thorough history and physical examination (H&PE). **Table 57-2** presents the differential diagnosis of other medical conditions that may present with anxietylike symptoms. The clinician must rule out psychiatric disorders and ascertain whether symptoms of anxiety are secondary to a medical illness or to a side effect of a medication. If anxiety did not predate a medical illness, subsequent anxiety may represent an adjustment disorder with anxious mood. The most likely organic cause of anxiety is alcohol and drug use (withdrawal or intoxication). Caffeine toxicity and increased sensitivity to caffeine also commonly mimic symptoms of anxiety.

Symptoms of cardiovascular abnormalities such as chest discomfort, shortness of breath, and palpitations are also cardinal symptoms of anxiety. Many anxious patients function poorly because they believe that they have heart disease. The electrocardiogram can be a useful tool to differentiate anxiety from a significant cardiac abnormality. Further evaluation should be considered according to the patient's symptoms and risk profile.

Table 57-2. Differential diagnosis of anxiety disorders.

Cardiovascular:
  Acute coronary syndrome, congestive heart failure, mitral valve prolapse, dysrhythmia, syncope, hypertension
Drugs:
  β-Agonists, caffeine, digoxin toxicity, levodopa, nicotinic acid, pseudoephedrine, selective serotonin reuptake inhibitors, steroids, stimulants (methylphenidate, dextroamphetamine), theophylline preparations, thyroid preparations
Endocrine disorders:
  Hyper/hypothyroidism, hyperadrenalism
Neoplastic:
  Carcinoid syndrome, pheochromocytoma, insulinoma
Neurologic disorders:
  Parkinsonism, encephalopathy, restless leg syndrome, seizure, vertigo, brain tumor
Pulmonary:
  Asthma (acute), chronic obstructive pulmonary disease, hyperventilation, pneumonia, pneumothorax, pulmonary edema, pulmonary embolus
Psychiatric:
  Affective disorders, drug abuse and dependence/withdrawal syndromes
Other conditions:
  Anaphylaxis, anemia, electrolyte abnormalities, porphyria, menopause

A careful auscultatory examination of the heart may reveal evidence of mitral valve prolapse, the most common valvular abnormality in adults. Long-term studies have shown that complications from mitral valve prolapse are rare, but often these patients present with palpitations and a generalized sense of being unwell that may mimic anxiety.

Musculoskeletal pain syndromes and esophageal disorders, including esophageal motility disorders and gastroesophageal reflux disease (commonly known as "heartburn"), are the most common noncardiac explanations of chest pain. Anxiety exacerbates gastrointestinal conditions such as colitis, ulcers, and irritable bowel syndrome. Treating anxiety often resolves or improves gastrointestinal symptoms and its associated chest pain.

Most patients with chronic unexplained chest pain have concomitant psychiatric diagnoses, especially anxiety. When further cardiac evaluation yields normal results, the anxious patient is more effectively reassured.

The primary care physician must be alert to acute medical conditions that can present with hyperventilation or dyspnea such as pulmonary conditions. The differentiation between these entities can be as simple as checking a pulse oxygen saturation but will often require more advanced diagnostic studies such as chest radiography, computed tomography (CT), or pulmonary angiography. Anxiety, hyperventilation, and dyspnea may accompany recurrent pulmonary emboli with few reliable physical signs. Anxiety has been shown to have a negative impact on quality of life in patients with asthma.

Hyperthyroidism and hypoglycemia may be mistaken for anxiety. Hypoparathyroidism, hyperkalemia, hyperthermia, hyponatremia, hypothyroidism, menopause, porphyria, and carcinoid tumors are less common causes of organic anxiety syndromes.

Depression is the most common psychiatric disorder associated with anxiety. Symptoms that discriminate clinical depression from anxiety include depressed mood, lack of energy, and loss of interest and pleasure.

Ingested substances such as medications or alcohol can elicit anxiety symptoms. Patients with anxiety disorders commonly drink to excess. Alcohol and drug problems involving dependence rather than abuse are most strongly associated with problems involving anxiety. Anxiety disorder and alcohol disorder can each initiate the other, especially in cases of alcohol dependence. Although many alcoholic patients present with anxiety, these symptoms decrease rapidly when the patient stops drinking. Only a small percentage (perhaps 10%) has persistent symptoms of anxiety.

Kushner MG, et al. The relationship between anxiety disorders and alcohol use disorders: a review of major perspectives and findings. *Clin Psychol Rev.* 2000; 20:149. [PMID: 10721495]
Lavoie KL, et al. What is worse for asthma control and quality of life: depressive disorders, anxiety disorders, or both? *Chest.* 2006;130:1039–1047. [PMID: 17035436]

► Treatment

The continuity of care and established physician-patient relationship characteristic of the primary care setting offer treatment advantages for patients with an anxiety disorder. However, physicians often miss signs of psychiatric problems in their patients because of a biomedical orientation. The result is excessive diagnostic testing, increased costs, frustrated patients, and cynical physicians.

Positive patient expectations and trust have a formidable impact on prognosis. By increasing their familiarity with standard cognitive behavioral techniques (CBTs) and psychotropic medications, family physicians can enhance outcomes for patients with anxiety disorders. Several of the CBTs described later can easily be implemented by a busy family physician as supplemental treatment to psychopharmacology. Seeing patients more frequently while maintaining the time constraints of a 15-minute office visit can improve patient functioning without overwhelming the busy family physician. Other interventions can be offered through referral to mental health specialists. If the patient remains unimproved or nonadherent after several 15-minute office visits, referral or consultation is also appropriate.

Other characteristics have also been shown to facilitate the treatment of anxiety disorders. These include female gender, more years of practitioner experience, and social support. Positive characteristics of the organization such as level of expertise, time availability, financial resources, and administrative support are also helpful. A conducive reimbursement system has obvious positive consequences.

A. Pharmacotherapy

Medications provide symptomatic relief but do not cure the underlying anxiety disorder for which they are prescribed. The decision to prescribe medication should be based on the patient's degree of emotional distress, the level of functional disability, and the side effects of the medication. **Table 57-3** provides a summary of the dosage range, indications, and financial costs associated with psychotherapeutic agents commonly used in the treatment of anxiety disorders.

1. Selective serotonin reuptake inhibitors (SSRIs)—SSRIs are now considered the first line of medication treatment for most anxiety disorders, with the exception of situational anxiety. SSRIs are well tolerated, have low potential for overdose, and are not associated with psychological or physical dependence. Relative to benzodiazepines, SSRIs do not impair learning or memory.

Recommendations on dosing have been to start low and titrate slowly upward to therapeutic levels in order to minimize jitteriness and insomnia that may occur with higher initial doses. Exceptions would be the treatment of OCD and PD with or without agoraphobia, which often requires higher-than-usual dosing. When a patient exhibits both depression and anxiety, SSRIs are strongly recommended. Common side effects include nausea, diarrhea, headache, and sexual dysfunction. Interestingly, a recent review of these second-generation antidepressants reveal mild to moderate strength in treating anxiety.

Thaler KJ, Morgan LC, et al. Comparative effectiveness of second-generation antidepressants for accompanying anxiety, insomnia, and pain in depressed patients: a systematic review. *Depress Anxiety.* 2012:29:495.

2. Benzodiazepines—These agents remain the treatment of choice for panic attacks, anticipatory anxiety, phobic avoidance, and transient situational stress reactions. They may be used as short-term therapy of panic disorder until concurrent SSRIs become effective. Use of benzodiazepines should be limited to 2–4 months of continuous therapy to limit the potential for psychological or physical dependence. Common side effects include anterograde amnesia, difficulty in balance, impairment of driving ability, and additive effects with alcohol. Use in elderly patients has been associated with paradoxical excitement and an increased risk of falls and hip fractures, especially with longer-acting agents.

Tolerance to the antianxiety effects is uncommon. The abrupt discontinuation of benzodiazepines, especially those with short half-lives, is associated with withdrawal syndromes of relatively rapid onset. A rebound syndrome, similar to but more transiently intense than the original disorder, may begin over a few days. Abrupt discontinuation of high doses of alprazolam may result in psychotic behaviors or seizures; a slow taper is essential.

Usual treatment initially combines an SSRI and a benzodiazepine. Studies have shown that patients who received combined treatment demonstrated more rapid improvement than those receiving either class of drug alone. There appears to be no additional benefit from taking a benzodiazepine after the first 5 or 6 weeks.

3. Serotonin norepinephrine reuptake inhibitors (SNRIs)— Venlafaxine (Effexor, Effexor XR) and duloxetine (Cymbalta) are both approved for treatment of GAD. Duloxetine is also approved for treatment of peripheral neuropathy and fibromyalgia. Side effects include headache, elevated blood pressure, and increased heart rate. Sexual dysfunction and GI intolerance occur less often than with SSRIs.

4. Buspirone (BuSpar)—Buspirone has an unknown mechanism of action but appears to affect neurotransmitters differently than benzodiazepines. Because of delayed onset of action of ≥2 weeks, it is indicated only in the treatment of GAD. Although studies have found buspirone to be as effective as benzodiazepines for GAD, many patients who previously received benzodiazepines do not perceive it to be as effective because they do not experience the "buzz" they had with benzodiazepines. Buspirone does not impair driving or

Table 57-3. Pharmacotherapy for anxiety disorders.

Drug Name	Usual Dosage Range	FDA-Approved Indications	Comments
Benzodiazepines[a] Alprazolam[b] (Xanax, Xanax XR, Niravam)	0.5–4 mg (3–6, ≤ 10 mg daily for panic) divided into 3 doses	Short-term relief of anxiety Panic disorder	XR dosed once daily Reduce doses for elderly or patients with hepatic disease Physical dependence can occur with relatively short-term use Abrupt discontinuation can result in rebound anxiety or withdrawal symptoms Rapid-dissolve tablet available
Clorazepate[b] (Tranxene)	15–60 mg in divided doses	Short-term relief of anxiety	Reduce doses for elderly or patients with hepatic disease Physical dependence can occur with relatively short-term use
Clonazepam[b] (Klonopin)	0.25–0.5 mg twice daily (max dose 4 mg/d)	Panic disorder	Long duration of effect results in smoother control Rapid-dissolve tablet available
Diazepam[b] (Valium)	2–10 mg 2–4 times daily (max dose 40 mg/d)	Anxiety disorders Short-term relief of anxiety	Reduce doses for elderly or patients with hepatic disease Physical and psychological dependence can occur with continuous use
Lorazepam[b] (Ativan)	2–6 mg in divided doses	Short-term relief of anxiety Anxiety associated with depression	Effective when given orally or by IM/IV injection Preferred in patients with hepatic insufficiency because of no active metabolites
Selective Serotonin Reuptake Inhibitors (SSRIs) Escitalopram (Lexapro)	10 mg once daily	Generalized anxiety disorder	No significant additional benefit if dose increased to 20 mg
Fluoxetine[b] (Prozac)	10–60 mg once daily	GAD Panic disorder OCD PMDD	Doses should be taken in morning Start with low dose and titrate to effective dose
Paroxetine[b] (Paxil, Paxil CR)	10–60 mg (12.5–62.5 mg CR) once daily	Panic disorder Social anxiety disorder GAD PTSD OCD PMDD	Start with low dose and titrate to effective dose Abrupt discontinuation can result in rebound anxiety or withdrawal symptoms CR formulation has lower gastric intolerance
Sertraline (Zoloft)	25–200 mg once daily	Panic disorder Social anxiety disorder OCD PTSD Pediatric OCD	Start with low dose and titrate to effective dose Abrupt discontinuation can result in rebound anxiety or withdrawal symptoms
Miscellaneous Venlafaxine (Effexor, Effexor XR)	75–225 mg in 2–3 divided doses	GAD Social anxiety disorder	Initiate with 37.5 mg daily and titrate up to effective dose XR formulation dosed once daily Taper dose on discontinuation to avoid rebound or withdrawal symptoms
Buspirone[b] (BuSpar)	10–60 mg in divided doses	GAD	Not for situational anxiety; therapeutic benefit may not be achieved for ≤1 month No risk of physical or psychological dependence Avoid in patients with severe renal or hepatic impairment

[a]All benzodiazepines are Schedule IV controlled substances.
[b]Generic formulations are available.
CR, controlled release; GAD, generalized anxiety disorder; IM, intramuscular; IV, intravenous; OCD, obsessive-compulsive disorder; PMDD, premenstrual dysphoric disorder; PTSD, posttraumatic stress disorder; XR, extended release.

cognition and is not additive with alcohol. The most common side effects are restlessness, dizziness, and headache. Recent studies suggest that buspirone may be effective as adjunctive therapy in treatment resistant depression.

5. Tricyclic antidepressants (TCAs)—These may be considered after failed trials of SSRIs, when other agents are not an option because of side effects or concerns of addiction or dependence. They are more commonly used as adjunctive therapy when the patient also has insomnia or chronic pain. Adherence is low secondary to the high incidence of intolerable side effects such as dry mouth, constipation, and urinary retention.

6. β-Blockers—These are used primarily to reduce the autonomic symptoms (rapid heart rate, flushing, sweating) associated with performance or social anxiety. The medication is usually taken only when needed ~30 minutes before an anxiety-inducing situation. Dizziness, drowsiness, and lightheadedness are the most common side effects.

7. Atypical anticonvulsants—These agents are being used frequently as adjunctive therapy to augment the activity of SSRIs in patients with refractory symptoms of anxiety. Gabapentin (Neurontin) has been shown to augment SSRI activity in the treatment of panic disorder and OCD and to reduce anxiety associated with chronic pain syndrome. Pregabalin (Lyrica) has also been used for GAD but is approved only for fibromyalgia and peripheral neuropathy. Clinical studies have also demonstrated the effectiveness of other atypical anticonvulsants such as carbamazepine, valproic acid, and lamotrigine. Doses should start low and be titrated to effective dose to minimize side effects. The most common side effects are drowsiness, dizziness, and blurred vision.

B. Psychotherapeutic Interventions

1. Behavioral therapy—This form of therapy focuses on overt behavior, with an emphasis on "how to" improve rather than "why" the problem exists. Several forms of behavioral therapy are available to assist patients in managing anxiety. The family physician's role involves explaining a behavioral procedure and prescribing homework. Time management need not suffer; 15-minute office visits sequenced about 1-2 weeks apart are usually adequate to provide therapy.

During *exposure therapy* the patient is repeatedly brought into contact with what is feared until discomfort subsides. The longer the exposure interval and the more intensive the exposure experience (massed trials) are, the better. To enhance adherence initially, often a significant other is present, or a benzodiazepine is used; as therapy proceeds, both are gradually eliminated.

Although few people are formally educated in stress management, a large repertoire of coping skills is available. **Table 57-4** offers a partial list of such strategies that can be given as a patient handout.

Table 57–4. Effective coping strategies.

Talk or write about stressful problems
Do enjoyable activities
Get enough rest and relaxation
Exercise regularly
Eat properly (beware of caffeine, chocolate, and alcohol)
Plan your time and set priorities
Accept responsibility for your role in a problem
Make expectations realistic
Get involved with others
Build in self-rewards
Utilize a sense of humor
Learn assertiveness
Attend support groups

Numerous types of relaxation training are useful in the treatment of all anxiety disorders and also have been shown to assist in anger management. Learning to relax is an inexpensive and easily accessible strategy. Reduction in the body's consumption of oxygen, blood lactate level (associated with muscle tension), metabolism, and heart and respiration rates occurs during practice. Home practice for ≥20 minutes twice each day in a quiet place produces significant effects. Commercialized relaxation tapes are available for eidetic imagery and progressive muscle relaxation.

Panic attacks can be mediated by a highly effective technique, *breathing retraining*, which involves slow, deep (diaphragmatic) breathing. Slow inhalation, holding the breath, and slow exhalation are repeated for ≥10 sequences. During slow, deep breathing the patient is told to substitute realistic thoughts ("I'm having a panic attack and I'm not in any danger") for panic-inducing thoughts ("I'm having a heart attack and I'll die soon"). This provides a sense of self-mastery and restores oxygen–carbon dioxide balance to the body. *Interoceptive exposure*, in which patients go through the symptoms of a panic attack (elevated heart rate, hot flashes, sweating, etc) in a controlled setting, can also be beneficial, by reinforcing for patients that these symptoms need not develop into a full-blown attack.

In the *worry exposure technique*, the patient is asked to do the following:

1. Identify (perhaps write down) and distinguish worrisome thoughts from pleasant thoughts.

2. Establish a 30-minute worry period at the same place and time each day.

3. Use the 30-minute period to worry about concerns and to engage in problem solving.

4. Postpone worries outside the 30-minute worry period with reminders that they can be considered during the next worry period (the patient may choose to write down new worries to avoid worrying about forgetting them).

5. During intrusions replace worries with attention to present-moment experiences, activities, or pleasant memories.

This strategy challenges dysfunctional beliefs about the uncontrollability of thoughts and the dangerous consequences of failing to worry. Delusional jealousy also can be mediated by this approach.

In *mismatch strategy*, the physician asks the patient to write a detailed account of the content of the worry (eg, exposure to a particular situation normally avoided) and then asks the patient to worry about what could happen in that situation. Finally, the patient is instructed to enter the situation and observe what really happens to assess the validity of the worry thoughts.

Finally, the family physician can ask the patient to practice alternative endings for worry sequences. Rather than rehearsing catastrophic outcomes, the patient contemplates positive scenarios in response to worry triggers.

2. Cognitive therapy—Cognitive therapy is behavioral therapy of the mind. Based on the theory that thoughts, images, and assumptions usually account for the onset and persistence of anxiety, cognitive therapy assumes that the way patients perceive and appraise events and interpret arousal-related body sensations as dangerous (anxiety sensitivity) provokes symptoms of anxiety. Patients with social phobia demonstrate overestimation of the probability of negative outcomes in social situations and they also exaggerate the costs of negative social events. Cognitive changes are the best predictors of treatment outcome for the anxiety disorders.

Achieving thought control is of central importance to mental health. Patients with OCD and GAD are especially prone to poor thought control. These patients devalue their ability to adequately deal with threats. Homework involving "self-talk" must be considered useful by the patient because alternative interpretations and explanations (*cognitive restructuring*) are always available for upsetting events; patients can assume more control of and accept more responsibility for their adaptation. Acceptance of these assumptions empowers the patient. Documented durable improvement results from cognitive restructuring (substituting rational assumptions and perspectives and transforming the meaning of events and physiologic arousal cues).

Although it is not possible to control all outside events, it is possible to control one's reaction to any event. Patients are advised that as soon as they are aware of being upset, they should pause and reflect on the following:

1. The event.
2. Thoughts about the event.
3. Associated feelings.
4. Another way to perceive the event (another meaning) that is also true, makes sense, but is not upsetting.

When time permits, patients may enter this information in a small notebook for review with the family physician at a subsequent office visit.

Halm MA. Relaxation: a self-care healing modality reduces harmful effects of anxiety. *Am J Crit Care* 2009; 18:169. [PMID: 19255107]
Mobini SR, Mackintosh S, et al. Clinical implications of cognitive bias modification for interpretative biases in social anxiety: an integrative literature review. *Cogn Ther Res*. 2013; 37(1):173.

C. Complementary and Alternative Therapies

Use of alternative therapies is more common among people with psychiatric problems and especially people with self-defined anxiety than among the rest of the population. Most alternative therapies are used without supervision. Because there are so few data on the relative effectiveness of these therapies, most people tend to try a therapist who has been recommended and, by trial and error, find a preferred therapy.

Massage therapies can be classified as energy methods, manipulative therapies, and combinations of each. Swedish massage is the most common form of massage and is usually given with oil. Movements called *effleurage* (smooth stroking) and *pétrissage* (kneading-type movements) are done up and down the back and across many tissues of the body. The Trager method, similar to many other types of massage therapy, involves gentle holding and rocking of different body parts. *Reflexology*, an energy method, could be classified as massage therapy because it involves kneading, stroking, rubbing, and other massage procedures. These procedures are centered on particular points of the feet, hands, or ears. Although few controlled studies exist utilizing massage therapy, most people report anxiety reduction benefits. There are no empiric data on the efficacy of reflexology.

Acupuncture has been demonstrated to reduce anxiety across various populations and presenting problems. However, additional double-blind, placebo-controlled studies are needed.

Research indicates the benefits of *yoga* to quality of life and improved health. Yoga, which involves body postures and *asanas* (body maneuvers), appears to exercise various tissues, organs, and organ systems and provides an avenue to address character armors, attitudes, and tensions. Specific application to stress management is widespread with generally significant positive results. As is the case with acupuncture, however, better controlled research is needed.

Herbal therapies for anxiety include kava-kava, inositol, and melatonin. Several clinical studies have demonstrated the effectiveness of short-term use of kava-kava, which has a mechanism of action similar to that of the benzodiazepines. However, long-term use or high doses are associated with development of peripheral neuropathy. The Food and Drug Administration (FDA) has issued a warning regarding the potential for kava-kava to cause hepatotoxicity, and this product has been removed from the market in several

European countries. Inositol has been shown to be effective in the treatment of panic disorder and OCD but should not be used in combination with SSRIs. Melatonin has been promoted primarily to reduce the symptoms of jet lag and sleep-cycle disturbances.

Because of the inconsistent effects shown in only small studies, valerian, St. John's wort, and passionflower are not routinely recommended, although their side effect profiles are benign. Limited data support the role of valerian in relieving anxiety and insomnia, but it has additive effects with other CNS depressants and alcohol disturbances.

Kessler RC, et al. The use of complementary and alternative therapies to treat anxiety and depression in the United States. *Am J Psychiatr* 2001; 158:289. [PMID: 11156813]
Saeed SA, et al. Herbal and dietary supplements for treatment of anxiety disorders. *Am Fam Physician*. 2007; 76:549–556. [PMID: 17853630]

D. Consultation or Referral

Attempting the previously discussed treatment recommendations during multiple 15-minute continuity office visits often renders referral unnecessary. However, referral may be necessary when symptoms recur or when tapering a medication is difficult. Referral is appropriate when the family physician is uncomfortable with an indicated therapy, when patients are potentially suicidal or are actively abusing drugs, when noncompliance is suspected, or when psychopathology is severe.

Referral of patients with OCD and PTSD is mandatory. Given the expected need to individualize treatment and provide novel treatment options, the busy family physician has neither the time nor the expertise to engage in the comprehensive interventions required.

If psychotherapy is the preferred method of managing symptoms, the specialized training of a clinical or a counseling psychologist is recommended. When psychopharmacology is warranted, the expertise of a psychiatrist is unmatched. Sound treatment is based on specific and accurate diagnosis and relies on empirically validated procedures that take into account the personality of the patient.

Table 57-5 provides several referral treatments and their indications for the effective nonpharmacologic management of anxiety disorders.

E. Management of Specific Anxiety Disorders

1. Panic disorder—Recommended treatment includes breathing retraining, cognitive restructuring, interoceptive exposure, and relaxation training. If anxiety is short-term, benzodiazepines should be used; if anxiety is chronic, paroxetine, fluvoxamine, citalopram, fluoxetine, sertraline, nefazodone, or imipramine should be used.

Although current treatments allow control of panic disorder, full recovery is questionable. Psychological treatments involve lower relapse rates, higher levels of acceptability, and lower attrition rates, and are better tolerated than many pharmacologic treatments. Exposure and deep breathing

Table 57-5. Referral interventions and indications for use.

Type of Intervention	Description	Indications
Psychotherapy Individual Group Family	Insight, empowerment, support Interactive, common interest Therapeutic environment and patient	Privacy, complicated patient Social skills, support, vicarious learning Enabling, dysfunctional family
Eye movement desensitization and reprocessing (EMDR)	Follow oscillation movement of object (pencil) thinking of trauma Mixed results	Posttraumatic stress disorder
Hypnosis	Relaxation induction; suggestions	Suggestible patient
Biofeedback	EMG, EKG, EEG monitoring of physiologic parameters to alter activity; cost is a limiting factor	Headaches, tension, blood flow, etc
Stress innoculation/anxiety management	Multifaceted, comprehensive cognitive–behavioral therapy	All anxiety disorders
Assertiveness training	Learn skills to be firm, not nasty	Dependent, unassertive, aggressive patients
Transcranial magnetic stimulation (TMS)	Noninvasive, painless method of brain stimulation via electrical current using changing magnetic fields	Applications are in their infancy

ECG, electrocardiogram; EEG, electroencephalogram; EMG, electromyogram.

are especially effective for patients with panic attacks and agoraphobia.

The percentage of patients whose panic attacks subside or disappear because of medication is generally 50–80% in acute pharmacologic trials, and this percentage rises with longer treatment. SSRIs reduced panic attack frequency to zero in 36–86% of patients and were well tolerated over long-term administration. Additionally, because of the high rate of depression comorbidity associated with panic attacks, SSRIs are the pharmacologic treatment of choice.

Benzodiazepines are best used for acute management. In most studies relapse after discontinuation of medications has been relatively high, ranging from one-third to three-fourths of patients, suggesting the need to be on the medications for at least 6 months.

2. Simple phobias—Recommended treatment includes exposure therapy, deep breathing, relaxation training, and cognitive restructuring, as well as short-term use of benzodiazepines.

3. Social phobia—Recommended treatment includes exposure therapy, cognitive restructuring, relaxation training, social skills training, and group therapy; medications that may be helpful include paroxetine, sertraline, clonazepam, and β-blockers.

When fearing negative evaluation, patients narrow their attention to social threat cues. Cognitive therapy corrects these distortions, whereas exposure therapy reduces anticipatory fear. In cognitive behavioral group settings, 81% of patients had significant improvement that was maintained 5.5 years later.

The SSRIs sertraline and paroxetine are both approved by the FDA for treatment of social anxiety disorder. β-Blockers on an as-needed basis may be helpful in patients who experience performance anxiety, even though published data supporting their benefit are limited. These agents can reduce hand tremor and tachycardia symptoms without causing cognitive impairment.

4. Obsessive-compulsive disorder (OCD)—Recommended treatment includes referral as well as exposure therapy, response prevention, cognitive restructuring, and pharmacotherapy with fluoxetine, fluvoxamine, sertraline, or clomipramine. Behavior therapy and SSRIs are primarily recommended. Homework assignments expose patients to stimuli associated with their obsessions. During *response prevention*, patients refrain from rituals (fixed behaviors that reduce anxiety) for progressively longer intervals until discomfort diminishes.

Pharmacologic options can at best reduce OCD symptoms by 50%, which may improve the patient's quality of life. Effective dosages are usually significantly higher than those required for depression or other anxiety disorders (eg, fluoxetine ≤80 mg/d). TCAs other than clomipramine do not appear to be effective in patients with OCD.

5. Posttraumatic stress disorder (PTSD)—Recommended treatment involves referral for individual or group psychotherapy, stress management, relaxation training, cognitive restructuring, and/or eye movement desensitization and reprocessing, which includes brief exposure to trauma-related images while patients visually track the therapist's rapid finger movements or receive other bilateral stimulation and cognitive interventions. Psychological treatments lead, on average, to large improvements in PTSD symptoms. Trauma-focused cognitive behavioral therapy, including focus on exposure and cognitive restructuring, has proved superior to other therapies. Some form of exposure or desensitization is essential. Patients put frightening memories into words while receiving new and incompatible information. Systematic exposure to the traumatic memory in a safe environment allows a reevaluation of and habituation to threat cues.

Although there is no established pharmacotherapy for PTSD, ~70% of patients seem to benefit from pharmacotherapy with moderate to marked effects. SSRIs appear to have the greatest efficacy of any single class of medication. Sertraline, paroxetine, and fluoxetine have been shown to produce acute improvement and decreased relapse rates in patients with PTSD. Clonazepam and buspirone may be helpful in suppressing hyperarousal symptoms. The anticonvulsant carbamazepine has been shown to decrease flashbacks, hyperarousal, and impulsivity. Carbamazepine, lithium, and β-blockers may be helpful in patients with poor impulse control.

Like OCD, PTSD is especially difficult to treat. Early intervention reduces tendencies for substance abuse, secondary gain, litigation, and malingering. Referral is mandatory.

6. Generalized anxiety disorder (GAD)—Recommended treatment includes worry exposure, thought control techniques (mismatch, cognitive restructuring), and relaxation training. Pharmacotherapy may include venlafaxine, sertraline, escitalopram, paroxetine, buspirone, and benzodiazepines.

No treatment is convincingly effective for GAD. Although cognitive behavioral therapy (CBT) appears to produce superior results, effects remain variable. Cognitive psychotherapy decreases probability overestimation (ie, overestimating the likelihood of negative events) and catastrophic thinking, and has been shown to improve sleep quality.

Nonvalidated coping strategies such as physical action, thought replacement, analysis, counterpropaganda, and talking to a friend have been used, with varying success. No one strategy is more efficient and none is rated "very efficient" by patients. Talking to a friend may be more efficient when thoughts are intense, whereas thought replacement may work well when intensity is low.

Antidepressants are often considered first-line therapy for GAD, in part because of the frequent association of GAD with depression. Although the TCAs are effective for

GAD, the SSRIs are more frequently prescribed because of a more favorable side effect profile. The SSRIs are well-demonstrated medications of choice for most anxiety disorders, notably escitalopram (Lexapro), sertraline (Zoloft), and paroxetine (Paxil). The SNRIs, venlafaxine (Effexor), and duloxetine (Cymbalta) also have demonstrated effectiveness in the treatment of GAD The atypical anticonvulsants gabapentin (Neurontin) and pregabalin (Lyrica) also have shown benefit in GAD, especially in patients with neuropathy or chronic pain syndromes. Benzodiazepines should be reserved for initial short-term overlap with the SSRIs since SSRIs have a delayed onset of effectiveness. When conspicuous worry, apprehension, irritability, and depression exist, buspirone has been especially effective and has been shown to be comparable to benzodiazepines in multiple studies of GAD.

7. Other anxiety disorders—Treatment of patients with substance-induced anxiety disorder consists in eliminating the drug of abuse, medication, or toxin exposure that is the cause of the disorder. In patients with persistent symptoms of adjustment disorder with anxious mood, referral for psychotherapy is recommended.

Culpepper L. Generalized anxiety disorder in primary care: emerging issues in management and treatment. *J Clin Psychiatr.* 2002;63:35. [PMID: 12044106]

Ehlers A, Clark DM. Post-traumatic stress disorder: the development of effective psychological treatments. *Nord J Psychiatr.* 2008;62:11.

Kapczinski F, et al. Antidepressants for generalized anxiety disorder. *Cochrane Database Syst Rev.* 2003;CD003592.

Perugi G, et al. Diagnosis and treatment of agoraphobia with panic disorder. *CNS Drugs.* 2007;21:741.

Raj BA, Sheehan DV. Social anxiety disorder. *Med Clin North Am.* 2001;85:712. [PMID: 11349481]

Shalev AY. Acute stress reactions in adults. *Biol Psychiatr.* 2002;51:532. [PMID: 11950455]

Stewart SH, Kushner MG. Introduction to the special issue on "anxiety sensitivity and addictive behaviors." *Addict Behav.* 2001;26:775. [PMID: 11768544]

Wright JH. Combined cognitive-behavior therapy and pharmacotherapy. *J Cogn Psychiatr.* 2007;21:3.

F. Special Populations

1. Children and youth—Transient fears are common in children of all ages and represent part of the normal developmental process. Normal fears need to be distinguished from the anxiety disorders of adulthood, which are more prevalent among children and adolescents than any other mental problem. Children with anxiety disorders exhibit a high rate of comorbidity, especially with other, secondary anxiety disorders.

Anxiety is often manifested among children by avoidance behavior, distorted thinking, or subjective distress. The *DSM-5* anxiety designations of childhood and adolescence include *separation anxiety disorder* (excessive anxiety concerning separation from home or from those to whom the child is attached). Separation anxiety disorder is treated by exposure to the feared event (eg, the child attends school despite discomfort). Psychotherapy is the treatment of choice.

Cognitive behavioral treatment for children with anxiety disorders is the first-line treatment recommended. Approaches similar to those described for adults are utilized, with emphasis on exposure paradigms. Response rates for children have ranged from 70% to 80%.

Targeted use of medication to lower agitation, improve energy, decrease psychotic symptoms, or improve concentration might make certain patients more accessible to psychotherapy. Despite these advantages, caution remains in effect regarding the prominent prescribing of medication for the treatment of childhood anxiety disorders. Few data are available on the impact of age on absorption, metabolism, therapeutic levels, or possible drug interactions. It is expected that to achieve the same serum levels in children compared with adults, the relative dose should be higher.

Despite this caution, FDA indications for adults with anxiety disorders are often used in children and adolescents. Approximately 50–70% of children with these disorders respond to SSRIs. Combination therapy with cognitive behavioral treatment and sertraline has been shown to be effective and safe in children when monitored closely.

Reynolds L, Wilson S, et al: Effects of psychotherapy for anxiety in children and adolescents: a meta-analytic review. *Clin Psychiatr Rev.* 2012; 32(4):251.

Silverman WK, et al. Evidence-based psychosocial treatments for phobic and anxiety disorders in children and adolescents. *J Clin Child Adolesc Psychol.* 2008;37:105. [PMID: 18444055]

Walkup JT, et al. Cognitive behavioral therapy, sertraline, or a combination in childhood anxiety. *N Engl J Med.* 2008;359(26): 2753–2766. [PMID: 18974308]

2. The elderly—Although the most common form of psychiatric condition in the elderly, anxiety disorders are still underdiagnosed. Polypharmacy is often present. Altered pharmacokinetics and pharmacodynamics in the geriatric population lead to greater sensitivity to and prolonged half-life of the medication due to decreased clearance of the drugs. Because of these drug complications, psychotherapy is attractive.

G. Patients with Related Conditions

1. Personality disorders—Personality disorders are lifelong characterologic problems that significantly complicate treatment and outcome. Poor compliance, medication abuse, interpersonal agitation, and poor insight characterize patients with personality disorders. These patients suffer more from anxiety than patients without personality disorders. Prescribing of benzodiazepines is contraindicated. (For further discussion of personality disorders, see Chapter 54.)

2. Hyperventilation—During hyperventilation excessive rate and depth of breathing produce a marked drop in carbon dioxide and blood alkalinity. These changes can be subtle. A person may slightly overbreathe for a long time. Even a yawn may trigger symptoms, accounting for the sudden nature of panic attacks during sleep. Breathing retraining is recommended.

3. Insomnia—Patients with anxiety disorders commonly have sleep problems that worsen anxiety. Sympathomimetic amines may cause sleep-onset insomnia, whereas alcohol abuse produces sleep-termination insomnia. Benzodiazepines are frequently prescribed as sedative-hypnotics. For sleep-onset insomnia, triazolam and zolpidem are rapidly acting compounds with short half-lives. For sleep maintenance, longer-acting drugs such as flurazepam and quazepam are more effective. Tolerance for the sedative effects, alteration of sleep topography, suppression of rapid eye movement (REM; dream sleep), impaired cognitive function, the occurrence of falls, and REM rebound following discontinuation are contraindications to the use of benzodiazepines in treatment of chronic insomnia.

Sleep hygiene suggestions provide an effective initial treatment option. Patients are asked to review and alter lifestyle patterns that interfere with sleep. **Table 57-6** outlines these suggestions for patient use. Adherence with recommendations and shift work are limiting factors.

Labellarte MJ, et al. The treatment of anxiety disorders in children and adolescents. *Biol Psychiatr.* 1999;46:1567. [PMID: 10599484]

Lichstein KL, et al. Relaxation and sleep compression for late-life insomnia: a placebo-controlled trial. *J Consult Clin Psychol.* 2001;69:227. [PMID: 11393600]

Sheikh JI, Cassidy EL. Treatment of anxiety disorders in the elderly: issues and strategies. *J Anxiety Disord.* 2000;14:173. [PMID: 10864384]

Table 57-6. Sleep hygiene recommendations.

Keep a sleep diary for a few weeks and monitor sleep-related activities
Establish a regular sleep/wake cycle (go to bed at about the same time and get up at about the same time)
Get regular exercise
Reduce noise
Avoid all naps
Eat dinner at a reasonable hour to allow time to digest food
Avoid excessive amounts of caffeine (chocolates, soft drinks, coffee, tea), especially before bedtime
Avoid excessive fluid intake before bed
Avoid in-bed activities such as reading, eating, or watching TV
Avoid clock watching while trying to sleep
If not asleep within 10–15 minutes after going to bed, get up:
  If you still want to lie down, do so in another room
  When sleepy, go back to bed
  If not asleep in 10–15 min, repeat these steps

▶ Prognosis

As recently as the early 1980s, it was estimated that 80% of patients with anxiety disorders would not significantly benefit from available treatment. Today the opposite is true. For the majority of patients with anxiety disorders—especially panic disorder, specific phobias, and social phobia—treatment with a combination of CBT and an SSRI carries an excellent prognosis Although these treatments show promise in the treatment of OCD, GAD, and PTSD, efficacy is more variable.

Websites

Anxiety Disorders of America: http://www.adaa.org/.
Anxiety/Panic Internet Resource: http://www.algy.com/anxiety.
Internet Mental Health: http://www.mentalhealth.com/.

Personality Disorders

58

William G. Elder, PhD

▶ General Considerations

Personality disorders (PDs) are a heterogeneous group of deeply ingrained and enduring behavioral patterns characterized by inflexible and extreme responses to a broad range of situations, manifesting in cognition (ways of perceiving and interpreting self, others, and events), affectivity (range, intensity, lability, and appropriateness of response), interpersonal functioning, and impulse control. PDs impinge on medical practice in multiple ways, including self-destructive behaviors, interpersonal disturbances, and nonadherence. Appropriate physician responses and effective treatments exist for many PDs. Correct diagnosis and proper intervention will help to improve patient outcomes. Borderline personality disorder (BPD) is an extremely debilitating disorder that can significantly interfere with the physician-patient relationship. BPD will receive extra focus in several sections of this chapter.

Significant deliberation on PDs preceded the publication of the fifth edition of the *Diagnostic and Statistical Manual* (*DSM-5*) in May 2013. *DSM-5* continues to distinguish 10 PDs clinically, while also formulating an alternative model that emphasizes core impairments in personality functioning and pathologic traits. For *Currents*, we have chosen to retain description of all 10 PDs as it seems certain that clinicians will continue to use their labels (eg, histrionic personality) for years to come. **Table 58-1** summarizes the 10 PDs.

Personality disorders are relatively common, with a prevalence of 7.6% in the general US population. Patients with PDs may seek help from family physicians for physical complaints, rather than psychiatric help. Higher rates for all types of PDs are found in medical settings. Prevalence of BPD in the general community is 1.4%.

Personality disorders have a pervasive impact because they are central to the person's identity. They are major sources of long-term disability and are associated with greatly increased mortality. Patients with PDs have fewer coping skills and during stressful situations may have greater difficulties, which are worsened by poor social competency, impulse control, and social support. Patients with BPD are frequently maltreated in the forms of sexual, physical, and emotional abuse; physical neglect; and witnessing violence. PDs are identified in 70–85% of persons identified as criminal, 60–70% of persons with alcohol dependence, and 70–90% of persons who are drug-dependent.

Borderline, schizoid, schizotypal, and dependent PDs are associated with high degrees of functional impairments and greater risk for depression and alcohol abuse. Obsessive-compulsive and narcissistic PDs may not result in appreciable degrees of impairment. Dependent PD is associated with a marked increase in healthcare utilization.

Leichsenring F, Leibing E, Kruse J, et al. Borderline personality disorder. *Lancet.* 2011; 377(9759):74–84.
Skodol AE, Bender DS, Morey LC, et al. Personality disorder types proposed for DSM-5. *J Pers Disord.* 2011; 25(2):136–169.

▶ Pathogenesis

A. Personality Disorders

Personality disorders are syndromes rather than diseases. Avoidant, dependent, and schizoid PDs appear to be heritable. Similarly, schizotypal disorder is considered to be heritable, as one end of a schizotypal-schizophrenia spectrum. Twin and adoption studies suggest a genetic predisposition for antisocial PD, as well as environmental influences, via poor parenting and role modeling. Histrionic PD may be related to indulged tendencies toward emotional expressiveness.

Borderline personality disorder may result from both constitutional and environmental factors. BPD is 5 times more common among first-degree relatives with the disorder, but to say to what degree BPD is heritable is difficult, given the reciprocity between family and child that occurs

Table 58-1. Clinical features and clusters of 10 DSM-5 personality disorders.

Cluster	Personality Disorder	Clinical Features
Cluster A: odd, eccentric	Paranoid Schizotypal Schizoid	Suspicious; overly sensitive; misinterpretations Detached; perceptual and cognitive distortions; eccentric behavior Detached; introverted, constricted affect
Cluster B: dramatic, emotional, erratic	Antisocial Borderline Histrionic Narcissistic	Manipulative; selfish, lacks empathy; explosive anger; legal problems since adolescence Dependent and demanding; unstable interpersonal relationships, self-image, and affects; impulsivity; micropsychotic symptoms Dramatic; attention seeking and emotionality; superficial, ie, vague and focused on appearances Self-important; arrogance and grandiosity; need for admiration; lacks empathy; rages
Cluster C: anxious, fearful	Avoidant Dependent Obsessive-compulsive	Anxiously detached; feels inadequate; hypersensitive to negative evaluation Clinging, submissive, and self-sacrificing; needs to be taken care of; hypersensitive to negative evaluation Preoccupied with orderliness, perfectionism, and control

during development. BPD has been attributed to highly pathologic and conflicted early interactions between parent and child. The conflict brings great ambivalence about relationships and affects ability to regulate affect. Previously BPD was attributed to child sexual abuse, but a recent meta-analysis did not support this hypothesis. It is certainly the case that traumatic childhood experiences are common in patients with BPD. As a group, patients with antisocial and borderline PDs report higher frequencies of perinatal brain injury, head trauma, and encephalitis.

B. Common Comorbid Conditions

Substance abuse disorders frequently occur comorbidly in community and clinical populations, particularly with antisocial, borderline, avoidant, and paranoid PDs. Anorexia nervosa, bulimia nervosa, and binge eating may be seen in patients who are obsessional, borderline, and avoidant, respectively. Self-injurious skin picking can be conceptualized as an impulse control disorder and has been found with significant frequency in patients with obsessive-compulsive PD and BPD. Up to 50% of patients with BPD have major depressive disorders or bipolar disorders.

APA. *Diagnostic and Statistical Manual of Mental Disorders,* 5th ed. American Psychiatric Association; 2013 (available at http://dx.doi.org/10.1176/appi.books.9780890425596.910646).

Goodman M, New AS, Triebwasser J, et al. Phenotype, endophenotype, and genotype comparisons between borderline personality disorder and major depressive disorder. *J Pers Disord.* 2010; 24(1):38–59.

Lobbestael J, Arntz A, Bernstein DP. Disentangling the relationship between different types of childhood maltreatment and personality disorders. *J Pers Disord.* 2010; 24(3):285–295.

Ruocco AC, Amirthavasagam S, Zakzanis KK. Amygdala and hippocampal volume reductions as candidate endophenotypes for borderline personality disorder: A meta-analysis of magnetic resonance imaging studies. *Psychiatr Res.* 2012;201(3):245–252.

▶ Prevention

Except for efforts to address the roots of criminal behaviors that are common in antisocial PD, there is no literature on prevention of PDs. Primary prevention could consist of better treatment of parental mental illnesses that have a negative impact on parent-child interactions and public health interventions to reduce prenatal brain insults. Both primary and secondary prevention could occur with increased interventions in family functioning and parenting skills.

▶ Clinical Findings

Personality disorders were once referred to as *character disorders.* Various descriptive labels have appeared in the literature, such as the oral-fixated character, the impulsive personality, and the introverted personality type. Each of these represents a theory of personality (psychoanalytic, developmental, and analytical, respectively). Currently, there are few points of correspondence between personality theory and diagnosis of PDs with a relatively atheoretical, categorical perspective dominating clinical practice in the United States.

A. Symptoms and Signs

1. Personality disorder—Clinical lore about PD presentations exists. Anything extreme in appearance that is not ethnically appropriate or currently fashionable suggests a PD. Examples include flamboyant jewelry, particularly in men; tattoos and piercing in older patients; steel-toed boots in men; and excessive cosmetics and large hair ribbons in women.

The patient's style of interacting with the physician can be revealing about personality difficulties. For example, the dependent patient will seek much advice and be unable to make an independent decision. The antisocial patient may be "smooth talking" or threatening. Interactions with patients with BPD can be very difficult, with the patient switching from extreme idealization to devaluation of the physician. The patient may "split" the staff, which becomes evident when some side with the patient while others are angry with the patient. **Table 58-2** describes problem behaviors associated with various PDs, as well as helpful responses and management strategies.

Physician reactions may be a sign of patient PD. Reactions such as anger, guilt, desire to punish, desire to reject, desire to please, sexual fantasies, and a sense that the physician is the "one person" capable of helping the patient are all examples of countertransference responses. Self-reflection about the encounter will help manage the strong feelings and interpersonal conflict encountered in care of PDs.

2. Borderline personality disorder—Physicians may over- or underattribute patient difficulties to BPD; therefore, it is important to be sensitive to BPD phenomena and to ascertain whether patient difficulties and symptoms represent BPD. BPD diagnostic criteria call for a pervasive pattern of instability in interpersonal relationships, self-image, and affect, and marked impulsivity beginning by early adulthood and present in a variety of contexts as indicated by at least five of the following:

1. Frantic efforts to avoid real or imagined abandonment (not including suicidal behaviors).

2. A pattern of unstable and intense interpersonal relationships characterized by alternating extremes of idealization and devaluation.

3. Identity disturbance: a markedly and persistently unstable self-image or sense of self.

4. Impulsivity in at least two areas that are potentially self-damaging (not including suicidal behaviors).

5. Recurrent suicidal behavior, gestures, threats, or self-mutilating behavior.

6. Affective instability due to a marked reactivity of mood (eg, intense episodic dysphoria, irritability, or anxiety usually lasting a few hours and only rarely more than a few days).

7. Chronic feelings of emptiness.

8. Inappropriate intense anger or difficulty controlling anger.

9. Transient, stress-related paranoid ideation or severe dissociative symptoms.

Borderline personality disorder involves subgroups of patients differing in affective, impulsive, and micropsychotic symptoms. These differences suggest different treatments, discussed later. Patients with BPD have significantly higher rates of suicidal ideation; 70–80% exhibit self-harming behavior at least once. While suicide attempts may be regarded as manipulative gestures, suicide rates are very high: 3–9.5% of patients with BPD receiving inpatient care

eventually kill themselves. Self-harm in the form of self-mutilation, such as wrist scratching, is symptomatic. Nausea and vomiting may be a primary care analog of self-mutilation in some patients, and a common chief complaint. Obtaining a history suggesting BPD may mitigate the need for extensive gastrointestinal symptom evaluations with more efficacious treatments directed to personality functioning.

B. Special Tests

No laboratory tests exist for PDs. Structured clinical interviews and personality inventories may be helpful in differentiating PDs and tracking treatment response. Interpretation by a psychologist enhances the value of the results. A consult should be considered in cases of diagnostic uncertainty.

Gross R, et al. Borderline personality disorder in primary care. *Arch Intern Med.* 2002;162:53. [PMID: 11996618]

Sansone RA, et al. Borderline personality symptomatology, experience of multiple types of trauma and health care utilization among women in a primary care setting. *J Clin Psychiatr.* 1998;59:108. [PMID: 9541152]

Skodol A, et al. Functional impairment in patients with schizotypal, borderline, avoidant, or obsessive-compulsive personality disorder. *Am J Psychiatr.* 2002;159:276. [PMID: 11823271]

► Differential Diagnosis

A. Personality Disorders

Accurate diagnosis is essential for proper response to and treatment of PDs. The following comparisons may help avoid misattribution of BPD to other PDs:

- Histrionic PD patients are dramatic and manipulative but lack the affective instability of BPD. Impulsivity, when seen, is related to attention seeking and sexual acting out.

- Dependent PD patients fear abandonment, but patients with BPD have more affective instability and impulsivity.

- Schizotypal PD patients have the micropsychotic symptoms of BPD, but are odder and lack the affective instability of BPD.

- Paranoid PD patients have volatile anger, but lack the self-destructive and abandonment issues of the BPD patient.

- Narcissistic PD patients have rages and reactive mood, but have a stable, idealized self-image in contrast to the patient with BPD, who has an unstable identity.

- Antisocial PD patients are often less impulsive than intentionally aggressive for materialistic gains. Patients with BPD act out when needy to gain support.

B. Other Mental Disorders

A PD is not diagnosed if symptoms are explained by an axis I condition or substance use. Although PDs may share impulsivity, raging, and grandiosity with bipolar disorder,

Table 58-2. Health-related problem behaviors associated with personality disorders.

Criterion	Personality Disorder				
	Paranoid	Schizotypal	Schizoid	Antisocial	Borderline
Patient's perspective	People are malevolent; situation is dangerous.	Understanding of care may be odd or near delusional.	Illness will bring too much attention and invade privacy.	Threatened if unable to feel "on top"; illness presents opportunity for crime.	Fears abandonment. Overreacts to symptoms and situation.
Problem behaviors	Fearful; misconstrues events and explanations; irrational. Argumentative.	Odd health beliefs and behaviors. Poor hygiene. Avoids care.	Unresponsive to kindness; difficult to motivate. Avoids care.	Acts out to gain control; malingering; uses staff and physicians. Superficially charming. Drug seeking.	Idealizes, then devalues care; Self-destructive acts. Splits staff.
Helpful physician responses and management strategies	Be empathic toward patient's fears, even when they seem irrational; carefully explain care plan. Provide advance information about risks. Protect patient's independence.	Communicate directly. Avoid misinterpreting patient as intentionally noncompliant; do not reject patient for oddness; honor patient's beliefs.	Manage personal frustration at feeling unappreciated; maintain a low-key approach. Appreciate patient's need for privacy.	Do not succumb to patient's anger and manipulation. Avoid punitive reactions to pa-tients. Motivate by addressing patient's self-interest. Set clear limits that interventions must be medically indicated.	Manage feelings of hopelessness about patient. Avoid getting too close emotionally. Schedule frequent periodic checkups. Tolerate periodic angry out-bursts, but set limits. Monitor for self-destructive behavior. Discuss feelings with coworkers.
Criterion	Histrionic	Narcissistic	Avoidant	Dependent	Obsessive-Compulsive
Patient's perspective	Illness results in feeling unattractive or presents an opportunity to receive attention.	Illness results in feeling inadequate or is an opportunity to receive admiration.	Illness is personal; fears exposure.	Fears abandonment. Intensifies feelings of helplessness.	Fears losing control of body and emotions. Feels shame.
Problem behaviors	Overly dramatic, attention-seeking; Excessively familiar relationship. Not objective—overemphasis on feeling states.	Demanding and entitled attitude; will overly praise or devalue care providers to maintain sense of superiority.	Missed appointments. Delay seeking care. Extremely nonassertive.	Dramatic and urgent demands for medical attention; may contribute to or prolong illness to get attention.	Unable to relinquish control to health care team. Great difficulty and anger at any change. Excessive attention to detail.
Helpful physician responses and management strategies	Avoid frustration with patient vagueness. Show respectful and professional concern for feelings, with emphasis on objective issues. Avoid excessive familiarity.	Avoid rejecting the patient for being too demanding. Avoid seeking patient's approval. Generously validate patient's concerns, with attentive but factual response to questions. Protect self-esteem of patients by giving them a role in their care.	Provide empathic response to inadequacy. Be patient with timidity. Work toward clear treatment plans—must obtain patient's view. Treat anxiety disorder.	When exhausted by patient needs, avoid hostile rejection of patient. Give reassurance and consistency. Set limits to availability—schedule regular visits. Help patient obtain outside support.	Avoid impatience. Thorough history taking and careful diagnostic workups are reassuring. Give clear and thorough explanations. Avoid control battles; treat patient as a partner; encourage self-monitoring.

they seldom have the same intensity and rate of speech or irrationality of thought that a manic episode brings. Substance use disorders differ from antisocial PD when illegal behaviors are restricted to substance use and procurement. Dissociative identity disorder, formerly known as *multiple-personality disorder*, may have a more traumatic etiology similar to BPD. Patients with obsessive-compulsive disorder recognize that their behavior and thoughts are irrational while patients with obsessive-compulsive PD are comfortable with their behavior. A diagnosis of PD does not apply when changes in behavior result from changes in brain function. For example, although personality changes are expected in dementia, a diagnosis of PD is not indicated. An axis I diagnosis "personality change due to a … [general medical condition]" is available when a change in personality characteristics is the direct physiologic consequence of a general medical condition. Because transient changes in personality are common in children and adolescents, diagnosis of a PD is not appropriate for a patient aged <18 years unless the behavioral pattern has been present for at least 1 year.

C. Cultural Considerations

Culturally related characteristics may erroneously suggest PDs. Promiscuity, suspiciousness, and recklessness have different norms in different cultures. The degree of physical or emotional closeness sought and the intensity of emotional expression also differ. Manner of dress and health beliefs may seem strange to the conventional Western physician. Evaluate the patient's degree of acculturation. Passivity, especially with one's elders, is not a sign of dependence in most recent immigrants. Constricted affect is a normal response when entering a new environment. Asking someone from the culture if the behavior is extreme can help, as can checking for significant interpersonal difficulties.

▶ Treatment

Miller (1992) has described how experienced family physicians differentially and efficiently respond to visits that can be categorized as routine, ceremony, or drama. In some cases, good application of family medicine's care principles may be beneficial psychotherapeutically. (Compare the psychotherapy of PDs described as under with the patient-centered method of family practice.) Suggestions for helping patients with PDs in a nonpsychiatric medical setting appear in Table 58-2. **Table 58-3** offers suggestions for helping patients who present with BPD.

Previously it was commonly believed that personality cannot be changed. However, increasingly specific psychopharmacologic and psychotherapeutic interventions have brought improved outcomes and some cures. The most effective treatments are multidisciplinary, combining medications, individual and group psychotherapies, and high coordination among providers. Comorbid substance dependence, violent

Table 58-3. Working with patients with BPD in medical settings.

1. Recognize the characteristics. The patient fears abandonment and increases demands on the physician. May be noncompliant, manipulative, somatasize, or "split" the healthcare team.
2. Behavior is need-driven. Demands may be overt or covert. Identify needs and motivations. Patient has little insight into problems. Externalization is symptomatic.
3. Tolerate patient's behaviors. Speaking "harshly or strictly" will activate abandonment fears and worsen the situation. Use a nonconfrontational but an educational approach.
4. A long-term plan provides stability for the patient. Follow continuity of care principles. This may be curative for the patient.
5. Titrate closeness and visit frequency. Avoid extremes of constant availability.
6. Set limits. Make clear agreements about call and office visits. Point out to patients that you are almost always involved in solving some type of problem and are unable to give full attention to their problems without an appointment. Suggest that patients schedule fairly frequent visits so that a regular time is available to discuss the problems they are experiencing.
7. Foresee problems related to abandonment fears such as when the social situation is disturbed, when the patient is referred, or when there are changes in physician or staff.
8. Use a multidisciplinary approach. Involve a highly skilled clinical psychologist or clinical social worker in the care. Encourage communication and cooperation among the care team.
9. Monitor your and the staff's reactions. Frustration and anger may be expected. Discuss the situation. Help the staff to recognize that the etiology of the frustration might originate in the patient's personality, not in the crisis of the moment. Coordinate responses to patients.
10. Set personal limits for the number of these challenging patients that you accept into your practice.

acting out toward others, or severely self-harming behaviors must be addressed first, via inpatient care.

Angstman K, Rasmussen NH. Personality disorders: review and clinical application in daily practice. *Am Fam Physician.* 2011;84(11):1253–1260.

Miller WL. Routine, ceremony, or drama: an exploratory field study of the primary care clinical encounter. *J Fam Practice.* 1992; 34:289. [PMID: 1541955]

A. Risk Management

Physicians should acknowledge the threats and challenges associated with PDs. General risk management considerations include the following:

- Having good collaboration and communication with a qualified mental health professional.
- Attention to documentation of communications and risk assessments.

- Attention to transference and countertransference issues, described earlier.
- Consultation with a colleague regarding high-risk situations.
- Careful management of termination of care, even when it is the patient's decision.
- Informed consent from the patient and, if appropriate, family members, regarding the risks inherent in the disorder and uncertainties in the treatment outcome.

B. Consultation or Referral

Consultation or referral should be considered when the following exist:

- The patient has several psychiatric diagnoses.
- The patient is experiencing depressive or anhedonic symptoms even if subthreshold (risk for suicide).
- The patient has significant problems with self-regulation.
- The patient has moderate to severe substance use disorder(s).
- The diagnosis is uncertain or the presentation is puzzling.
- Initial treatment by the family physician is ineffective.
- The physician or staff are unable to compensate for and are overwhelmed by the patient's personality problems.

Acceptance of treatment can be difficult. Symptomatically, patients with PD may externalize blame for their problems. PD behavioral patterns tend to be *egosyntonic*; that is, patients may consider their behavior reasonable, given their perception of the circumstances. Treatment may be perceived as an attempt to control the patient; referral may be experienced as devaluing or as abandonment. Thus treatment and referral suggestions should be offered with an understanding of how patients with various PDs may perceive them. Table 58-2 describes common PD patient perspectives on care.

C. Pharmacotherapy

In many cases, medications are effective only as a means to manage stress-exacerbated symptoms. For example, under stress, paranoid, schizoid, or schizotypal patients may experience delusions, distress, and hallucinations, which can be managed with antipsychotic medications. When not stressed, the odd behavior and beliefs of these patients remain unresponsive to treatment.

Some PDs may be successfully treated with medications. Avoidant PD appears to be an alternative conceptualization of social phobia. It can be treated with selective serotonin reuptake inhibitors (SSRIs) and selective serotonin and norepinephrine reuptake inhibitors (SNRIs). Patients with obsessive-compulsive PD may become less irritable and compulsive with SSRIs. Rejection sensitivity seen in patients with dependent PD may be helped by SSRIs. Medications are not helpful for patients with narcissistic, antisocial, or histrionic PDs. Consider high rates of suicide attempts and completions when selecting medications to avoid those that are especially dangerous in overdose.

Not on the basis of diagnosis per se, Soloff (2000) has proposed three symptom-specific pharmacotherapy algorithms for PDs. They are based on differential medication effects on cognitive disturbances, behavioral dyscontrol, and affective dysregulation. Soloff's first algorithm is for treatment of PDs in which cognitive perceptual symptoms are most significant (ie, patients with suspiciousness, paranoid ideation, and micropsychotic symptoms). The second algorithm is for treatment of affective dysregulation (ie, patients with a depressed, angry, anxious, labile mood). The third algorithm is for treatment of impulsive behavioral symptoms (ie, patients with impulsive aggression, binging, or self-injuring behaviors). Practice guidelines largely in accord with Soloff's symptom-based approach were published for treatment of BPD by the American Psychiatric Association (APA) in October 2001 and again recommended in 2005. Recent systemic reviews continue to support a symptom-based approach and incorporate new studies of mood-stabilizing medications. It should be noted that current recommendations are based on a small database that lacks sufficient randomized controlled trials. Therefore, each treatment should be approached as an empirical trial, with the patient as a coinvestigator. Side effects, risk/benefit ratios, conjoint medications, and patient preferences should be considered carefully. Pharmacotherapy is an adjuvant to psychotherapy; medications do not cure character and will never be a substitute for the work of a therapist. Furthermore, some medications may worsen symptoms.

Both SSRIs and SNRIs are effective with affective dysregulation seen in cluster BPDs. Tricyclic antidepressants are no more effective than SSRIs and should not be used, given their cardiotoxic effects with overdose and a possibility of paradoxical worsening of symptoms. Monoamine oxidase inhibitors (MAOIs) proved useful in treating BPD prior to the advent of SSRIs and offer a second treatment option for affective dysregulation, including rejection sensitivity. Mood stabilizers offer an additional level of treatment, especially for anger. Valproate and carbamazepine may be offered alone, while lithium should be used in conjunction with an antidepressant, although lithium is the second choice, given its serious side effects. Although patients with BPD often complain of anxiety, benzodiazepines are contraindicated, as they have been shown to cause increased impulsivity. Clonazepam, a benzodiazepine with anticonvulsant and antimanic properties, is associated with increased serotonin levels and may be useful adjunctively for anxiety, anger, and dysphoric mood.

Antipsychotics are the most researched medications for the treatment of PDs and should be the first-line treatment when cognitive perceptual symptoms are significant. Low doses should be tried first. There is no evidence that antipsychotics are helpful for PD cognitive perceptual symptoms in the long term. Antipsychotics may also be used adjuvantly with antidepressants for affective dysregulation, particularly with anger. Antipsychotics such as risperidone may exacerbate or induce manic symptoms, although they produce symptom improvement in bipolar disorder when used in conjunction with mood-stabilizing medications. When the most recent guidelines were written, there was insufficient evidence that third-generation antipsychotics (eg, risperidone or olanzapine) would be effective with cognitive perceptual symptoms in BPD, but given the side effect profiles of conventional versus third-generation antipsychotics, the newer drugs are being used increasingly, empirically. The atypical antipsychotic clozapine is effective in personality disturbances that are cognitive perceptual and impulsive but, given its risk for agranulocytosis, should be reserved until several trials of other medications have failed.

Risperidone appears to be superior to conventional antipsychotics in treatment of impulsivity and aggression, especially in BPD. However, SSRIs at low to moderately high doses should be tried first. If needed, low-dose antipsychotics may then be added to SSRIs, or used more aggressively as a last line of treatment. Mood-stabilizing medications are indicated as midlevel treatment for impulsivity. Lithium is effective, perhaps because of its impact on serotonin levels. The anticonvulsant divalproex sodium has been used to treat irritability and impulsivity in patients with BPD who have not responded to SSRI therapy, apparently independent of the presence of abnormal electroencephalographic findings. Carbamazepine is also effective as a mood stabilizer. Use of mood stabilizers requires various laboratory tests to monitor metabolic functioning. Various antipsychotic medications carry risks for extrapyramidal symptoms, tardive dyskinesia, weight gain, diabetes mellitus, extended QT intervals, and other problems.

Feurino L, Silk KR. State of the art in the pharmacologic treatment of borderline personality disorder. *Curr Psychiatr Rep.* 2011;13(1):69–75.

Oldham JM. *Guideline Watch: Practice Guideline for the Treatment of Patients with Borderline Personality Disorder.* American Psychiatric Association; 2005 (available at http://www.psychiatryonline.com/content.aspx?aid=148718; accessed Aug. 26, 2010).

Rinne T, Ingenhoven T. Phamacotherapy of severe personality disorders: a critical review. In: van Luyn B, et al., eds *Severe Personality Disorders: Everyday Issues in Clinical Practice.* Cambridge University Press; 2007.

Soloff PH. Psychopharmacology of borderline personality disorder. *Psychiatr Clin North Am.* 2000;23:169. [PMID: 10729938]

D. Psychotherapeutic Interventions

Some PDs are amenable to some forms of psychotherapy, but there is currently limited empirical support for the treatment of most PDs. Specific treatments described below may result in significant improvements over time, when compared to wait-list control or treatment as usual. Largest changes are observed in measures of self-reported distress or symptoms (eg, target complaints, level of depression). Measures assessing interpersonal problems and social functioning also show improvement, although to a smaller degree.

Treatments of <1-year duration probably represent crisis interventions or treatments of concurrent axis I disorders rather than attempts to address core PD psychopathology. Psychotherapy for borderline and narcissistic personalities tends to take significantly longer. Even with extended duration, treatment goals tend to be for functional improvement such as decreased symptom severity and decreased acting out, rather than complete remission of symptoms. Anxiety-related PDs, such as avoidant and dependent PDs, are most amenable to psychotherapy, followed by BPD, followed by schizotypal PD. Cognitive behavioral psychotherapy, which challenges irrational beliefs, may be effective with avoidant, dependent, obsessive-compulsive, narcissistic, and paranoid PDs. Because individuals with antisocial PD are manipulative and seldom take responsibility for their behavior, psychotherapy is difficult and relatively rare, unless court-ordered interventions are counted as psychotherapy, which is questionable. Furthermore, persons showing characteristic psychopathy traits (eg, lack of remorse, aggressiveness) are the least amenable to treatment.

Successful treatment of borderline and narcissistic PDs requires high levels of therapist experience. Skills in managing the therapeutic alliance and creating a stable, trusting relationship are crucial. Psychotherapy for narcissistic PDs is highly specialized wherein the patient's hypersensitivity to slights is confronted after much trust building.

Group therapy and partial hospitalization are effective for patients with schizotypal and borderline PDs. Dialectical behavior therapy (DBT) is a unique form of psychotherapy that is efficacious for BPD. In DBT, patient beliefs, contradictions, and acting out are empathically accepted. Specifically, the patient's personhood is responded to positively, and dysfunctional behaviors are responded to matter-of-factly, neither sympathizing with, nor punishing, the patient. Sessions focus on learning to solve problems, control emotions, manage anxiety, and improve interpersonal relationships. After many months of this consistent and intensive treatment, limits are set on the patient's behavior.

Besides establishing a strong therapeutic alliance, several recommendations may be useful in the treatment of all personality disorders: (1) maintain a consistent and validating treatment process, (2) build motivation and reinforce commitment to change, (3) increase self-knowledge and foster new learning experiences, (4) target cognitive structures of personality/pathology, and (5) adopt a structured approach to treatment (eg, setting appropriate interpersonal boundaries, use of therapy contract).

Bartak A, Spreeuwenberg MD, Andrea H, et al. Effectiveness of different modalities of psychotherapeutic treatment for patients with cluster C personality disorders: results of a large prospective multicentre study. *Psychother Psychosom.* 2010;79(1):20–30.

Beck AT, et al. Dysfunctional beliefs discriminate personality disorders. *Behav Res Ther.* 2001; 39:1213. [PMID: 11579990]

▶ **Prognosis**

Perhaps half of all patients with PDs never receive treatment. Several of the PDs, although pervasive in their negative effects, are perhaps not sufficiently impairing or distressing to warrant treatment. Treatment outcomes are improving for the PDs that are extremely debilitating, such as BPD.

PDs with anxiety components have good potential for improvement. Debate remains as to whether any treatment other than incarceration can be effective for individuals with antisocial PD, and with this, whether effect seen comes with age (ie, the person becomes less disruptive as age 40 is approached). Patients with BPD appear to improve by age 40, as well. Patients with BPD who are in treatment improve at a rate of 7 times their natural course.

Sanislow CA, Marcus KL, Reagan EM. Long-term outcomes in borderline psychopathology: Old assumptions, current findings, and new directions. *Curr Psychiatr Rep.* 2012; 14(1):54–61.

59

Somatic Symptom Disorder (Previously Somatoform Disorder), Factitious Disorder, & Malingering

William G. Elder, PhD

General Considerations

Somatic symptom disorder (SSD) involves unexplained physical symptoms that bring significant functional impairment. It presents one of the more common and most difficult problems in primary care. SSD is seldom "cured" and should be approached as a chronic disease. Recognition, a patient-centered approach, and specific treatments may help alleviate symptoms and distress. Factitious disorder and malingering, although not true SSD, are addressed separately in this chapter because of their similarity in the form of medically unexplained symptoms.

Somatic symptom disorder (SSD) is a new diagnostic term that replaces *somatoform disorder* in *DSM-5*, the latest version of the diagnostic manual published by the American Psychiatric Association. Use of SSD as the prevalent term will likely increase after *DSM-5* becomes widely disseminated following publication in May 2013. The diagnostic labels previously subsumed by somatoform disorders in *DSM-4* will also be subsumed by SSD in *DSM-5*. These disorders have specific courses, symptoms, complaints, and treatments, listed in Table 59-1.

Features that characterize SSD include the following:

- Physical symptoms or irrational anxiety about illness or appearance, for which biomedical findings are not consistent with a general medical condition.

- Symptoms develop with or are worsened by psychological stress, and are not intentional.

- Extensive utilization of medical care. Paradoxically, treatment and attempts to reassure patients can be counterproductive.

- Feelings of frustration on the part of the provider. Patients are often seen as "difficult patients."

Somatic expression of psychological distress can be normal, and degree of dysfunction determines whether the symptoms constitute a disorder. Furthermore, symptoms may be sufficient to suggest that the patient's condition is better described by a primary mental disorder (eg, somatic delusions) that may respond to specific therapies.

Presentations of illness without complete physical explanation have a significant impact on practice. For instance, 10% of all medical services are provided to patients with no organic disease, 26% of primary care patients meet criteria for somatic "preoccupation"; 19% of patients have medically unexplainable symptoms and 25–50% of visits involve symptoms that have no serious cause. Where true SSD is present, symptoms persist much longer and the cost of ambulatory care is 9–14 times greater than in controls. Patients with SSD undergo numerous medical examinations, diagnostic procedures, surgeries, and hospitalizations. They risk increased morbidity from these procedures, and 82% stop working at some point because of their difficulties. With appropriate recognition and treatment, costs of care may be reduced by 50%.

American Psychiatric Association. *Diagnostic and Statistical Manual of Mental Disorders*, 4th ed. (text revision). APA; 2000.

American Psychiatric Association. *Diagnostic and Statistical Manual of Mental Disorders*, 5th ed. (DSM-5 development). APA; 2013 (available at. http://www.dsm5.org/Pages/Default. aspx; last accessed March 10, 2013).

Kroenke K. Patients presenting with somatic complaints: epidemiology, psychiatric comorbidity and management. *Int J Methods Psychiatr Res.* 2003;12:34-43. [PMID: 12830308]

Voigt K, Nagel A, Meyer B, Langs G, Braukhaus C, Löwe B. Towards positive diagnostic criteria: a systematic review of somatoform disorder diagnoses and suggestions for future classification. *J Psychosom Res.* 2010; 68(5):403–414. [PMID: 20403499]

Pathogenesis

To some degree, somatic symptoms related to psychological and emotional states are common and should be considered

Table 59-1. Somatoform disorders, factitious disorder, and malingering.[a]

Disorder	Symptoms Volitional	Symptom Presentation	Type of Symptoms	Symptom Duration	Treatment Modalities
Somatic Symptom Disorder	No	Excessive concern about one or more physical complaints	Disproportionate and persistent thoughts about seriousness of symptoms High anxiety about health or symptoms Excessive time and energy devoted to symptoms	Chronic, recurring, and/or stable	Frequent visits, therapeutic relationship with provider, active listening, avoidance of excessive or invasive treatments, focus on management vs cure, consider CAM modalities
Conversion disorder	No	Onset after acute stress	Pseudoneurologic symptom or symptom complex such as stroke-like weakness, sensory loss, or pseudoseizure	Sudden onset; short duration	Reassurance that symptom will resolve over days Avoid labeling as mental illness
Pain disorder	No	Preoccupation with pain; examination out of proportion with disease or injury	Pain insufficiently explained by any organic cause; frequently associated with disability, relationship disruptions, depression, anxiety	Sudden onset; worsens with time	Focus on functionality, symptom management, and nonnarcotic therapy
Illness Anxiety Disorder also known as Hypochondriasis	No	Fearful of disease; preoccupied with symptoms; not reassured	Multiple symptoms over time; misinterpretation of normal sensations, may have unusual health and prevention behaviors	Long history, worsens after actual illness	SSRI may be beneficial, otherwise similar to somatization
Body dysmorphic disorder	No	Excessive concern about imagined defect in appearance	Specific complaints of defect (other than obesity); behaviors to hide or avoid public exposure of "defect"	Usually several years	SSRI may be beneficial, otherwise similar to somatization
Factitious disorder with physical symptoms	Yes—motivation primary gain: sick role, attention	Unexplained fever, bleeding, injuries	Nonhealing and unremitting; tend to receive multiple procedure/operations over time; falsify records	Chronic; multiple admissions; remits with confrontation	Accurate diagnosis, may remit with confrontation
Malingering	Yes—motivation secondary gain: money, disability, drugs, etc	Similar to above Protest; demand for medical help	Vague pain and/or paralysis common; belligerent with providers if need not met	Multiple episodes of same problem	Confrontation

[a]All of these disorders are more common in the young, some beginning in the teens but most commonly in the 20s–30s. Similar symptoms presenting for the first time in the elderly should prompt more extensive investigations for organic cause. True factitious disorder is rare, while the prevalence of malingering is unknown. Supportive counseling may be considered in cases of factitious disorder and malingering if the patient does not have a personality disorder that would impede care.

normal. Examples include anger experienced through jaw tightening, tension through shoulder stiffening, loss or grief through chest discomfort, disappointment or fear through a "sinking feeling in the gut," and shame through a reddening of the face, and so on. Children often feel ill when they learn that a friend is sick or when family stress is high. An example of nonpathologic fear of having a disease is "student's syndrome," perception of medical students in pathology class that every symptom they experience could represent a serious diagnosis.

Genetic factors, demonstrated in adoption studies, appear to play a role in the development of somatic sensitivities and obsessive tendencies. Traumatic experiences in the form of sexual, physical, and emotional abuse and witnessing violence are predictive of SSD. Operant reinforcements and classically conditioned associations will also play a role, both in changes in perception of physical sensations and in pain-related behaviors. In particular, some individuals are susceptible to overexperiencing sensations. This phenomenon may occur through a difference in neuron gating, in which the threshold of firing is reduced by anxiety or psychological stress. Patients with hypochondriasis can experience a cycle of symptom amplification whereby obsession about the body focuses attention on sensations, which causes anxiety, increasing sensations and further worsening obsessiveness. Other disorders, such as body dysmorphic disorder, may be related to obsessive-compulsive disorders or even a mild thought disorder.

Because families differ in how they respond to symptoms and illnesses, individual differences in health beliefs and illness-related behaviors are to be expected. Families also shape the tendency to experience, display, and magnify somatic symptoms; thus, SSD or malingering in children may be modeled or reinforced by adults. Social risk factors include single parenthood, living alone, unemployment, and marital and job difficulties.

Gender ratios and prevalence of SSD differ across cultures. In North America, somatization, conversion, and pain disorders are more frequent in women whereas hypochondriasis and body dysmorphic disorder involve men and women equally. Somatic symptoms are more prevalent among Chinese American, Asian, and South American patients. These differences are most likely due to Western/empirical explanatory models contrasted with culturally based understandings in which ancient people's associations of phenomena and symptoms still affect the beliefs and expectations of modern populations.

Disorders with somatoform characteristics specific to certain cultures include the *dhat* syndrome in India, which is a concern about semen loss, and *koro* in Southeast Asia, a preoccupation that the penis will disappear into the abdomen. A sense of having worms in the head or burning hands is sometimes reported by people in Africa and Southeast Asia. Cultures influence how emotions should be expressed and sanction religious and healing rituals that may look like conversion disorders. Thus, somatoform-type symptoms should be evaluated for appropriateness to the patient's social context. Behaviors sanctioned by the culture are typically not considered pathologic.

Dimsdale JE, Dantzer R. A biological substrate for somatoform disorders: importance of pathophysiology. *Psychosom Med.* 2007;69:850–854. [PMID: 18040093]

Winfried R, Arthur JB. Psychobiological perspectives on somatoform disorders. *Psychoneuroendocrinology.* 2005; 30(10):996–1002. [PMID: 15958280]

▶ Clinical Findings

A. Symptoms and Signs

Diagnosis of SSD involves both exclusion of general medical conditions and inclusion of somatoform features. The following features should increase suspicion of SSD:

- Unexplained symptoms that are chronic or constantly change.

- Multiple symptoms. Fainting, menstrual problems, headache, chest pain, dizziness, and palpitations are the symptoms most likely to be somatoform.

- Vague or highly personalized, idiosyncratic complaints.

- Inability of more than three physicians to make a diagnosis.

- Presence of another mental disorder, especially depressive, anxiety, or substance use disorders.

- Distrust toward the physician.

- Physician experience of frustration.

- Paradoxic worsening of symptoms with treatment.

- High utilization, including repeated visits, frequent telephone calls, multiple medications, and repeated subspecialty referrals.

- Disproportionate disability and role impairment.

B. Diagnostic Criteria

Somatic symptom disorder is a mental disorder that involves physical symptoms or irrational anxiety about illness or appearance, and for which biomedical findings are not consistent with a general medical condition. Specific diagnosis requires that the symptoms have brought unneeded medical treatment or significant impairment in social, occupational, or other important areas of functioning. SSD cannot be caused by a general medical condition or by direct effects of substances. If the disorder occurs in the presence of a general medical condition, complaints or impairment must be in excess of what would be expected from the physical findings and history. Although SSD may occur concurrently with other mental disorders, other diagnoses such as depression or anxiety may be sufficient to supersede the SSD diagnosis.

1. Somatic Symptom Disorder—Prior to DSM-5, formal diagnosis of somatization required identification (counts) of multiple symptoms from different body sites or functions. Current diagnosis focuses on the distress or disruption experienced by patients over somatic symptoms. Patients often do have multiple symptoms. Symptoms maybe specific or general (e.g., fatigue) and may sometimes represent normal bodily sensations that do not signify significant disease. Patients with this disorder have the thoughts, feelings or behaviors associated with the symptoms that are excessive, persistent, and dysfunctional.

2. Conversion disorder—This diagnosis consists solely of pseudoneurologic symptoms [ie, deficits affecting the central nervous system (CNS), voluntary motor, or sensory functions]. Psychological factors in the form of stressors or emotional conflicts are expected and precede the symptoms. Depending on the medical naiveté of the patient, symptoms are often quite implausible, not conforming to anatomic pathways or physiologic mechanisms. The symptoms, however, are not considered volitional. Symptoms may symbolically represent emotional conflicts, such as arm immobility as an expression of anger and impotence. Other clues indicating that the symptoms are pseudoneurologic include worsening in the presence of others; noninjuries despite dramatic falls; normal reflexes, muscle tone, and pupillary reactions; and striking inconsistencies on repeated examinations. Groups of symptoms also tend to not fit together physiologically. Symptoms may be experienced with a relative lack of concern (so-called *la belle indifference*), but dramatic presentations are more common. Course is an important consideration. Conversion disorder is rare before age 10 or after age 35 years. Symptoms are transient, rarely lasting beyond 2 weeks, and respond to reassurance, suggestion, and psychological support. Although primary and secondary gains may result from conversion disorder, these gains are not the motivating factor as they would be with factitious disorder or malingering.

3. Pain disorder associated with psychological factors— This disorder is the psychiatric equivalent of chronic nonmalignant pain syndrome, except that no minimum duration of symptoms is required. Psychological factors play a significant role in the pain picture, including its onset, severity, exacerbation, and maintenance. Physical pathologies are possible and frequent, but organic findings are insufficient to explain the severity of the pain. Functional deficits are common, including disability, increased use of the healthcare system, abuse of medications, and relational and vocational disruptions. Depression or anxiety may be secondary or may also be primary or comorbid, predisposing the patient to an increased experience of pain as well as a deficient ability to cope.

4. Hypochondriasis—The individual is preoccupied with fears of having a serious disease. The preoccupation may originate in an overfocus on and misinterpretation of normal physiologic sensations (eg, orthostatic dizziness), erroneous attributions about the body (eg, "aching veins"), or obsession about minor physical abnormalities. Patients are easily alarmed by contact with ill persons or media coverage of disease. Fears persist despite medical reassurance. More global symptoms may suggest a primary diagnosis of panic disorder, while more specific body-related concerns may be better explained by a diagnosis of body dysmorphic disorder. The key to this diagnosis is primary fear of disease rather than generalized worry or fear of a specific defect or disorder.

5. Body dysmorphic disorder—This disorder involves excessive preoccupation with a minor or imagined defect of one or more body parts, excluding the diagnosis of a primary eating disorder. Although many people are concerned about their appearance, the concerns and behaviors associated with this disorder are extreme, distressing, time-consuming, and debilitating. Self-consciousness is significant, and avoidance

of public exposure, hiding of defects, and nondisclosure to the physician are common. Medical, dental, and surgical treatments are sought but may only worsen preoccupations. Concern cannot focus exclusively on a false belief that one is obese, which would indicate an eating disorder. Similarly, a belief that sexual characteristics are incorrect may be better represented in a diagnosis of gender identity disorder. Transient or more generalized concerns about appearance may indicate major depressive episodes. Patients who insist that an imagined defect is real and hideous will meet the criteria for delusional disorder, somatic type.

6. Malingering, factitious disorder, and factitious disorder by proxy—These are not SSDs; symptoms are voluntary and deceptive. Deception is obtained by feigning or self-inducing symptoms or by falsifying histories or laboratory findings. Common symptoms include fever, self-mutilation, hemorrhage, and seizures. Persons connected to health professions are common perpetrators. Malingering and factitious disorder differ by whether symptom gain is primary or secondary. In malingering, symptoms are produced to gain rewards or avoid punishments (secondary gains). Factitious disorder involves production of symptoms in order to assume the sick role (primary gain). Unlike malingering, factitious disorder is considered a mental disorder principally because the need to be in the sick role is abnormal. Factitious disorder by proxy occurs when illness is caused by a caregiver, typically to meet a need for drama and to be a rescuer of the patient. Signs of factitious disorder include direct evidence, such as inconsistent laboratory or physical findings or observations (eg, injection of bacteria), as well as vague clues, such as patients who are migratory or have no visitors, are comfortable with more aggressive treatments, including extended hospitalization, or whose presentation is exaggerated and quite dramatic (Munchausen syndrome).

C. Screening and Diagnostic Measures

Keeping SSD in the differential is the key to making the correct diagnosis over time. Valid diagnostic and screening questionnaires exist, but often lack clinical utility because of the length and training required for interpretation. A directed interview with specific questions based on patient complaints is most effective for primary care providers. When doubts remain, referral to a specialist skilled in use of diagnostic questionnaires is indicated. Patients should be screened for depression.

▶ Differential Diagnosis

Diagnosis should be considered provisional until there is considerable external support. General medical conditions characterized by multiple and confusing somatic symptoms (eg, hyperparathyroidism, porphyria, multiple sclerosis, and systemic lupus erythematosus) should be considered.

Conversion disorder, in particular, is often misdiagnosed. Daum et al. (2013) have described the high specificity of weakness, sensory, and gait symptoms in determining whether conversion presentations are pseudoneurologic. Onset of multiple physical symptoms in early adulthood suggests somatization disorder but in the elderly suggests a general medical condition. Primary or secondary depression should be considered in any patient suspected of having SSD. Personality disorders are also frequently associated with SSD. It is important to determine the primary disorder in order to choose effective treatment. Clinical factors, such as context, duration of symptoms, and age of the patient, may be able to distinguish SSD from other disorders.

Daum C, et al. The value of "positive" clinical signs for weakness, sensory and gait disorders in conversion disorder: a systematic and narrative review. *J Neurol Neurosurg Psychiatr.* 2014; 85(2):180–190. [PMID: 23467417]

▶ Complications

Failure to recognize and properly treat SSD can lead to excessive diagnostic procedures and treatments, which perpetuate patient preoccupations and place the patient at risk for iatrogenic harm. Use of unidentified, unconventional, or alternative treatments by SSD patients may interact negatively with prescribed medications. Dependences on sedative, analgesic, or narcotic agents are common iatrogenic complications.

▶ Treatment

Primary care patients who present with undifferentiated symptoms are best addressed with a comprehensive approach that includes continuity of care and attention to the physician-patient relationship. "Pathologizing" makes patients feel illegitimate, in itself a major source of distress, and produces stereotypes of patients as "crocks, whiners, or difficult." Patient characteristics considered as difficult include extensive or exaggerated complaints, nonadherence with treatment recommendations, and behaviors that raise suspicion of seeking drugs. When patients are so labeled, the relevance of the patient's experience and the potential of partnership between patient and physician are both obviated. A patient-centered method, so important to family practice, becomes impossible. Even without attributions of a mental disorder, SSD presents one of the most difficult challenges in primary care. Uncertainties associated with the diagnosis, the sense that the focus is not medical and therefore the interaction is inappropriate, patient symptom amplification, and the sense that services are being overused inappropriately contribute to the perception that the patient is difficult.

A. General Recommendations

Symptoms of SSD exist on a continuum. Comprehensive, continuous, patient-centered care appropriately addresses most primary care patient presentations. The general recommendations presented in the following paragraphs apply to such an approach.

1. First visits—A therapeutic alliance should be built by a thorough history and physical examination and a review of the patient's records. The physician should show curiosity and interest in the patient's complaints and validate the patient's suffering. Psychogenic attributions should be avoided. To appear puzzled initially is a good strategy. Delivery of a diagnosis is a key treatment step with SSD. Different disorders require different types of information.

2. Management—The disorder should be treated as a chronic illness, with the focus on functioning rather than cure. Gradual change should be expected, with periods of improvement and relapse. Physicians should try to avoid excessive and/or invasive diagnostics and treatment in order to minimize iatrogenic harm. When procedures or treatments are undertaken, they should be selected only on the basis of objective evidence, not subjective complaints. When new symptoms arise, at least a limited physical examination should be performed to avoid misdiagnosis and assure the patient that his/her concerns are taken seriously. The need for unnecessary tests and procedures can be avoided by having the patient feel "known" by the physician.

3. Management when controlled drugs are involved—Berland et al. (2012) have described a comprehensive approach for managing somatoform pain disorder where patient preferences for opioids complicate treatment. They recommend a structured approach that includes a comprehensive biopsychosocial evaluation and a treatment plan that encourages patients to set and reach functional goals.

4. Patient-centered care—Feelings of illegitimacy by patients and common physician attitudes toward patients contribute to power differentials and struggles. Physicians should speak with patients as equals, listen well, ask and answer many questions, explain things understandably, and allow patients to make decisions about their care. A collaborative relationship should be developed in which the physician works together with the patient to understand and manage patient problems. The "common ground" shared by the physician and the patient should be monitored and differences discussed.

5. Office visits—Regular, brief appointments should be scheduled, thus avoiding "as-needed" medications and office visits that render medical attention contingent on symptoms. Practical time-related strategies include negotiating and setting the agenda early in the visit, paying attention to the emotional agenda, practicing active listening through appropriate reactions and follow-up questions, soliciting the patient's attributions for the problems, and communicating empathetically.

6. Psychosocial issues—Reassurance should be provided to the patient, but not before a thorough exploration of symptoms. Psychosocial questions should be interspersed with biomedical ones to explore all issues: physiologic, anatomic, social, family, and psychological. The physician should inquire about trauma and abuse. As trust builds, the patient should be encouraged to explore psychological issues that may be related to symptoms. In this way, symptoms can be linked to the patient's life and feelings. Physicians should avoid using the term *stress* too liberally, as it may be misconstrued as the cause of the patient's symptoms or an excuse for an incomplete evaluation. Eventually and subtly, patients are likely to reveal their personal issues and concerns.

7. Family involvement—With the patient's permission, family members should be invited to participate in patient visits. An occasional family conference can be valuable. Each person's opinion about the illness and treatment can be solicited, and family members can be asked how family life would differ if the patient were without symptoms. Physicians should solicit and constantly return to the patient's and family's strengths and areas of competence.

Berland E, et al. Rational use of opioids for management of chronic nonterminal pain. *Am Fam Physician*. 2012; 86(3):252–258.

B. Pharmacotherapy

Because these patients may be extremely sensitive to side effects, psychopharmacologic agents generally should not be used unless the patient has demonstrated pharmacologically responsive mental disorder such as major depression, generalized anxiety disorder, panic disorder, or obsessive-compulsive disorder. (For further discussion of these disorders, see Chapters 52–54.) Selective serotonin reuptake inhibitors (SSRIs), other nontricyclic antidepressants, and benzodiazepines are the medications most frequently used for coexisting psychiatric conditions. Treatment should be initiated at subtherapeutic doses and increased very gradually, as described in Chapters 52–54. Exceptions to this general rule are hypochondriasis and body dysmorphic disorders. They are more similar to obsessive-compulsive disorder, and patients with these disorders may benefit from slow increases to higher doses of SSRIs if side effects are tolerated. Those with extreme but transitory dysmorphic concerns may benefit from temporary treatment with an atypical antipsychotic medication.

Somashekar B, Jainer A, Wuntakal B. Psychopharmacotherapy of somatic symptoms disorders. *Int Rev Psychiatr*. 2013;25(1): 107–115. [PMID: 23383672]

C. Consultation or Referral

Involvement of a mental health clinician may be helpful in diagnosing comorbid mental conditions, offer suggestions for psychotropic medications, and engage some patients in psychotherapy. Patients, however, are unlikely to see the value of consultation or may experience referral as an accusation that their symptoms are not authentic. Pressuring the patient to accept a consultation is unlikely to be effective and may render the consultant encounter unproductive. Trust must first be established, and psychological issues must be made a legitimate subject for discussion. The idea of referral can be introduced later. When possible, it can be more effective to see the patient along with the mental health clinician so that a comprehensive approach continues to be emphasized, the patient does not feel abandoned, and worry that the patient's concerns are not taken seriously are alleviated. Extreme distress or preoccupations worsening to delusional levels may require inpatient hospitalization.

Jackson JL, Passamonti M, Kroenke K. Outcome and impact of mental disorders in primary care at 5 years. *Psychosom Med*. 2007; 69(3):270–276. [PMID: 17401055]
Schweickhardt A, et al. Differentiation of somatizing patients in primary care: why the effects of treatment are always moderate. *J Nerv Ment Dis*. 2005; 193:813. [PMID: 16319704]

D. Psychotherapeutic Interventions

Standardized group or individual cognitive behavioral therapies (CBTs) can be an effective treatment for chronic somatoform disorders, reducing somatic symptoms, distress, impairment, and medical care utilization and costs. Cognitive interventions train the patient to identify and restructure dysfunctional beliefs and assumptions about health. Behaviorally, the patient is encouraged to experiment with activities that are counter to usual habits such as avoidance, "doctor shopping," or excess seeking of reassurance. In addition, patients can learn relaxation and meditation techniques to manage symptoms of anxiety. Patients with high emotional distress respond more rapidly to psychotherapy, and patients able to at least partially attribute symptoms to psychological factors show better therapeutic outcomes than patients who firmly believe that their physical symptoms have a physical cause.

Gropalis M, et al. Specificity and modifiability of cognitive biases in hypochondriasis. *J Consult Clin Psychol*. 2013; 81(3): 558–565. [PMID: 22563641]
Rosebush PI, Mazurek MF. Treatment of conversion disorder in the 21st century: have we moved beyond the couch? *Curr Treat Options Neurol*. 2011;13(3):255–266. [PMID: 21468672]
Sharma MP, Manjula M. Behavioural and psychological management of somatic symptom disorders: an overview. *Int Rev Psychiatr*. 2013; 25(1):116–124. [PMID: 23383673]

E. Complementary and Alternative Therapies

It is to be expected that patients with somatoform symptoms often try alternative treatments such as herbal remedies, mind-body interventions, and other non-Western medical approaches. In these patients, conventional treatments appear to have failed, distrust of physicians may be high, and distress is great. Federal regulations require that label claims and instructions on herbal products and supplements address symptoms only; therefore, there are no specific herbal agents for SSD, per se. Given the plethora of symptoms that can exist in patients with SSD, it is not surprising that there are numerous alternative medications that patients may try.

Patients with pain disorder or primary or comorbid anxiety may benefit from body and mind-body interventions such as massage, movement therapies, manipulations, relaxation, guided imagery, and hypnosis. The placebo effect of various remedies may be helpful, particularly if the agents are largely inert, as bothersome side effects seen in conventional medicines may be avoided. Alternative therapies often include "nonspecific therapeutic effects" that go beyond the placebo effect and can be beneficial. Nonspecific effects include warmth and listening skills of the practitioner, empowerment that comes from legitimization of the patient's problem, and an egalitarian approach to care. Physicians may wish to recommend alternative treatments and collaborate with alternative practitioners but should also be prepared to protect the patient by cautioning against treatments that are potentially harmful, excessively expensive, or that circumvent conventional treatments that are needed for demonstrated medical conditions.

Elder WG, et al. Managing lower back pain: you may be doing too much. *J Fam Practice*. 2009; 58:180–186. [PMID: 19358795]

F. Patient Education

The American Academy of Family Physicians has developed a patient education page for somatoform disorders. The web address for the page is http://familydoctor.org/familydoctor/en/diseases-conditions/somatoform-disorders.html.

Substance Use Disorders

Robert Mallin, MD
Maribeth Porter, MD

60

General Considerations

The prevalence of alcohol and drug disorders in primary care outpatients is between 23% and 37%. Almost one third of US adults meet the criteria for a form of alcohol use disorder during some point in their lives. The cost to society of these disorders is staggering. Each year in the United States substance use disorders are associated with 100,000 deaths and costs of approximately $100 billion. The high prevalence of these disorders in primary care outpatients suggests that family physicians are confronted with these problems daily. However, these disorders rarely present overtly. Patients in denial about the connection between their substance use and the consequences caused by it frequently minimize the amount of their use, and they rarely seek assistance for their substance use problem. One study exploring the care provided for patients with alcohol dependence found that only 11% of patients received recommended care in the primary care setting. The National Institute on Alcohol Abuse and Alcoholism (NIAAA) published a physician's guide, *Helping Patients Who Drink Too Much* (http://www.niaaa.nih.gov/guide) to help improve this discrepancy of care.

The epidemiology of alcohol and drug disorders has been well studied and is most often reported from data of the National Institute of Mental Health Epidemiologic Catchment Area Program (ECA). Lifetime prevalence rates for alcohol disorders from the ECA survey data were 13.5%. For men, the lifetime prevalence was found to be 23.8%, and for women, 4.7%. The National Comorbidity Survey revealed lifetime prevalence of alcohol abuse without dependence to be 12.5% for men and 6.4% for women. For alcohol dependence, the lifetime prevalence was 20.1% in men and 8.2% in women. The ECA data yield an overall prevalence of drug use disorders of 6.2%. As with alcohol use disorders, drug use disorders occur more frequently in men (lifetime prevalence 7.7%) than in women (4.8%). Characteristics known to influence the epidemiology of substance use disorders include gender, age, race, family history, marital status, employment status, and educational status.

Boschloo L, Vogelzangs N, van den Brink W, Smit JH, et al. Alcohol use disorders and the course of depressive and anxiety disorders. *Br J Psychiatr.* 2012; 200(6):476–484.
Willenbring M, Massey S, Gardner M. (2009). Helping patients who drink too much: an evidence-based guide for primary care physicians. *Am Fam Physician.* 80(1):44-50.

Pathogenesis

The difference between abuse and dependence is an important one. With substance abuse, patients retain control of their use. This control may be affected by poor judgment and social and environmental factors, and mitigated by the consequences of the patient's use. Patients who become dependent (addicted) no longer have full control of their drug use. The brain has been "hijacked" by a substance that affects the mechanism of control over the use of that substance. This addiction is far more than physical dependence. The need to use the drug becomes as powerful as the drives of thirst and hunger. Evidence that the brains of addicted individuals are different from those of nonaddicted persons is enormous. Many of these abnormalities predate the use of the substance and are assumed to be inherited. In genetically predisposed individuals, substances of abuse cause changes in the dopaminergic mesolimbic system that result in a loss of control over substance use. These changes are mediated by several neurotransmitters: dopamine, γ-aminobutyric acid (GABA), glutamate, serotonin, and endorphins. The different classes of substances of abuse act through one or more of these neurotransmitters, ultimately affecting the level of dopamine in the mesolimbic system (otherwise known as the "reward pathway"). These changes in the brain are permanent and are the primary reason for relapse in the addicted patient trying to maintain abstinence or control of use.

▶ Prevention

Although neurobiology plays a large role in addiction, the precursors of substance abuse are also environmental and include family, school, community, and peer factors (**Table 60-1**). These multiple factors make the design of effective prevention very difficult. Primary prevention is designed to prevent the use of substances, thereby rendering abuse impossible. These programs are designed primarily for the young. Secondary prevention consists of screening programs to identify abuse early and to redirect the patient's behavior before addiction becomes overt. In tertiary prevention, the focus is on the treatment of addictive behavior in an effort to prevent the consequences of compulsive use. Prevention programs can be divided into those that address the four environmental areas of risk: family, school, peers, and community. Family physicians can support these efforts by including the following behaviors in their practice:

- Supporting efforts to strengthen parenting skills, family support, and communication.

- Providing patient and community education about drug and alcohol use, abuse, and treatment.

- Screening and assessing patients of all ages for substance use disorders in the office and hospital.

- Supporting community efforts in substance abuse prevention.

Table 60-1. Environmental risk factors for substance abuse.

Family factors
Sexual or physical abuse
Parental or sibling substance abuse
Parental approval or tacit approval of child's substance use
Disruptive family conflict
Poor communication
Poor discipline
Poor supervision
Parental rejection
School factors
Lack of involvement in school activities
Poor school climate
Norms that condone substance use
Unfair rules
School failure
Community factors
Poor community bonding
Disorganized neighborhoods
Crime
Drug use
Poverty
Low employment or unemployment
Community norms that condone substance use
Peer factors
Bonding to peer group that engages in substance use or other antisocial behaviors

- Endorsing and promoting public policy that supports prevention, early detection, and treatment of substance use disorders.

Broning S, Kumpfer K, Kruse K, et al. Selective prevention programs for children from substance-affected families: a comprehensive systematic review [rview]. *Subst Abuse Treat, Prevent Policy*. 2012;7:23

Newton NC, O'Leary-Barrett M, Conrold PJ. Adolescent substance misuse: neurobiology and evidence-based interventions. *Curr Topics Behav Neurosci*. 2013;13:685–708.

▶ Clinical Findings

A. Symptoms and Signs

The signs and symptoms of substance abuse are varied and often subtle. This is complicated by the fact that most patients fail to recognize their substance use as the cause of their problems and are often quite resistant to that interpretation. Consequently, the family physician must have a high index of suspicion, recognizing that the prevalence of substance use disorders in outpatient primary care is high. A perspective that recognizes the prevalence of these disorders will enable physicians to interpret potential clues to substance use (**Table 60-2**).

Table 60-2. Clinical clues of alcohol and drug problems.

Social history
Arrest for driving under the influence of alcohol once (75% association with alcoholism) or twice (95% association)
Loss of job or sent home from work for alcohol or drug reasons
Domestic violence
Child abuse/neglect
Family instability (divorce, separation)
Frequent, unplanned absences
Personal isolation
Problems at work or school
Mood swings and psychological problems
Medical history
History of addiction to any drug
Withdrawal syndrome
Depression
Anxiety disorder
Recurrent pancreatitis
Recurrent hepatitis
Hepatomegaly
Peripheral neuropathy
Myocardial infarction at age <30 years (cocaine)
Blood alcohol level >300 or >100 without impairment
Alcohol on breath or intoxicated at office visit
Tremor
Mild hypertension
Estrogen-mediated signs (telangectasias, spider angiomas, palmar erythema, muscle atrophy)
Gastrointestinal complaints
Sleep disturbances
Eating disorders
Sexual dysfunction

The diagnosis of substance abuse or dependence is based primarily on a careful history. However, substance-disordered patients may be deliberately less than truthful in their history, and often the patient's denial prevents the physician from seeing the connection between substance use and its consequences. Signs of sedative-hypnotic or alcohol withdrawal may be misinterpreted as an anxiety disorder. Chronic use of stimulants may present as a psychotic disorder. In fact, in the face of active substance abuse, other psychiatric diagnoses often must wait for detoxification before they can be accurately assessed.

B. Screening Measures

The diagnosis of substance use disorders is most typically begun with a screening test that identifies a user at risk. The CAGE (cut down, annoyed, guilty, and eye opener) questionnaire (**Table 60-3**) is perhaps the most widely used screening tool for the identification of patients at risk for substance use disorders. When a patient answers yes to two or more questions of the CAGE, the sensitivity is 60–90% and the specificity 40–60% for substance use disorders. Because a screening test is more predictive when applied to a population more likely to have a disease, clinical clues to substance use disorders may be useful indicators to determine whom to screen (see Table 60-2). Men aged <65 years may be classified as at-risk or heavy drinkers if they consume >4 drinks per day or >14 drinks during a week. Women of any age and men aged >65 years are also considered at-risk or heavy drinkers if they consume >3 drinks daily or 7 drinks weekly. A *drink* can be defined as a 12-oz can or bottle of beer, a 5-oz glass of wine, or 1.5 oz of distilled spirits.

Miller MM, Goplerud E, Martin J, Ziedonis DM. New systems of care for substance use disorders: treatment, finance, and technology under health care reform [review]. *Psychiatr Clin North Am.* 2012;35(2):327–356.

Table 60-3. CAGE questions adapted to include drugs.[a]

1. Have you felt you ought to cut down on your drinking or drug use?
2. Have people annoyed you by criticizing your drinking or drug use?
3. Have you felt guilty about your drinking or drug use?
4. Have you ever had a drink or used drugs first thing in the morning to steady your nerves or to get rid of a hangover or to get the day started? (**eye-opener**)

[a]Two or more yes answers indicates a need for a more in-depth assessment. Even one positive response should raise a red flag about problem drinking or drug use.
Data from Schulz JE, Parran T Jr. Principles of identification and intervention. In: Graham AW, Shultz TK, eds. *Principles of Addiction Medicine*, 2nd ed. American Society of Addiction Medicine; 1998.

C. Methods for Differentiating Abuse from Dependence

1. Diagnostic criteria—Once a patient with a substance use problem is identified, it becomes necessary to determine whether the disorder involves abuse or dependence. Substance abuse is a pattern of misuse during which the patient maintains control, whereas in substance dependence, control over use is lost. Physiologic dependence, evidenced by a withdrawal syndrome, may exist in either state. The *Diagnostic and Statistical Manual of Mental Disorders*, fifth edition (*DSM-IV-TR*; also referred to as *DSM-5*) includes the diagnostic criteria for substance abuse and dependence.

2. Withdrawal syndromes—Although, not always seen with substance abuse, physiologic dependence suggests abuse unless the patient is on long-term prescribed addictive medicines. **Table 60-4** contrasts signs and symptoms of withdrawal from alcohol and other sedative-hypnotic drugs, opiates, and cocaine and other stimulant drugs. Alcohol withdrawal may be life-threatening, if not properly treated. Opiate withdrawal is not life-threatening; neither is withdrawal

Table 60-4. Symptoms and signs of withdrawal from alcohol, opioids, and cocaine.

Substance of Abuse	Manifestations of Withdrawal
Alcohol	Autonomic hyperactivity: diaphoresis, tachycardia, elevated blood pressure Tremor Insomnia Nausea or vomiting Transient visual, tactile, or auditory hallucinations or illusions Psychomotor agitation Anxiety Generalized Seizure activity
Opioids	Mild elevation of pulse rate, respiratory rate, blood pressure, and temperature Piloerection (gooseflesh) Dysphoric mood, drug craving Lacrimation or rhinorrhea Mydriasis, yawning, diaphoresis Anorexia, abdominal cramps, vomiting, diarrhea Insomnia Weakness
Cocaine	Dysphoric mood Fatigue, malaise Vivid, unpleasant dreams Sleep disturbance Increased appetite Psychomotor retardation or agitation

from cocaine or other stimulants, although they both may be associated with morbidity and relapse to substance abuse.

In dealing with sedative-hypnotic, alcohol, or opiate withdrawal, assessment of the degree of withdrawal is important to determine appropriate use and dose of medication to reduce symptoms and, in the case of sedative hypnotic drugs or alcohol, prevent seizures and mortality. The Clinical Institute Withdrawal Assessment of Alcohol Scale, Revised (CIWA-AR) allows quantification of the signs and symptoms of withdrawal in a predictable fashion that enables clinicians to discuss the severity of withdrawal for a given patient and thus choose intervention strategies that are effective and safe. This tool is available online and can be downloaded from the American Society of Addiction Medicine (ASAM) website (http://asam.org).

D. Laboratory Findings

Biochemical markers may help support the diagnostic criteria gathered in the history, or can be used as a screening mechanism to consider patients for further evaluation (**Table 60-5**).

American Psychiatric Association. *Diagnostic and Statistical Manual of Mental Disorders*, 4th ed. (text revision). APA; 2000.
Hannuksela ML. Liisanantti MK. Nissinen AE. Savolainen MJ. Biochemical markers of alcoholism [review;98 refs. cited]. *Clin Chem Lab Med*. 2007;45(8):953–961

▶ Differential Diagnosis

Because substance abuse is a behavioral disorder, when considering a differential diagnosis, psychiatric disorders often come to mind. Indeed, there is a high comorbidity between substance use disorders and psychiatric disorders. Approximately 50% of psychiatric patients have a substance use disorder. For patients with addictions, however, the rates of psychiatric disorders are similar to those of the general population. Problems such as substance-induced mood disorders (frequently noted in alcohol, opiate, and stimulant abuse) and substance-induced psychotic disorders (most frequently associated with stimulant abuse) complicate differentiation of primary psychiatric disorders from those that are primarily substance use disorders.

Most clinicians agree that psychiatric disorders cannot be reliably assessed in patients who are currently or recently intoxicated. Thus detoxification and a period of abstinence are necessary before other psychiatric disorders may be effectively evaluated.

Other than the dilemma of determining whether a substance-induced or comorbid psychiatric disorder is present, differential diagnosis in substance abuse revolves around the issues of abuse versus dependence (see earlier discussion). The essential difference is a loss of control over use in dependence that is not present in abuse. This distinction is complicated, however, by the chronic and waxing and waning nature of substance use disorders. As a result, it is necessary to examine a patient's behavior over an extended period of time, looking for evidence of past loss of control of use that may not currently be present. In addiction, a pattern of progressively increasing loss of control usually becomes evident as the consequences of chronic substance abuse unfold.

▶ Complications

The medical complications of substance abuse are legion and profoundly affect the health of our population (**Table 60-6**). The number of deaths attributed to the abuse of substances exceeds 500,000 yearly, with tobacco use accounting for 380,000 of these deaths. (For discussion of tobacco use, see Chapter 57.) Cardiovascular disease and cancer lead this list. Alcohol causes approximately 100,000 deaths yearly and is associated with motor vehicle and other accidents, homicides, cirrhosis of the liver, and suicide. Injection drug use is responsible for the fastest growing population of HIV infection. In addition to medical complications, substance abuse causes considerable neuropsychiatric morbidity, both as a primary cause (**Table 60-7**) and by exacerbating existing psychiatric disorders.

Acute substance-induced psychosis is often indistinguishable from a primary psychotic disorder such as schizophrenia in the setting of substance abuse. Neurocognitive states such as dementia may be substance-induced and result in permanent brain damage. Depression, commonly diagnosed and treated in the primary care setting, may often be complicated by a substance-induced mood disorder. Often what appears to be treatment-resistant depression is actually

Table 60-5. Biochemical markers of substance use disorders.

Marker	Substance	Sensitivity (%)	Specificity (%)	Predictive Value (%)
Mean corpuscular volume (MCV)	Alcohol	24	96	63
γ-Glutamyltransferase (GGT)	Alcohol	42	76	61
Carbohydrate-deficient transferrin (CDT)	Alcohol	67	97	84

Table 60-6. Medical complications of substance abuse.

Drug	Medical Complication
Alcohol	Trauma
	Hypertension
	Cardiomyopathy
	Dysrhythmias
	Ischemic heart disease
	Hemorrhagic stroke
	Esophageal reflux
	Barret esophagus
	Mallory-Weiss tears
	Esophageal cancer
	Acute gastritis
	Pancreatitis
	Chronic diarrhea, malabsorption
	Alcoholic hepatitis
	Cirrhosis
	Hepatic failure
	Hepatic carcinoma
	Nasopharyngeal cancer
	Headache
	Sleep disorders
	Memory impairment
	Dementia
	Peripheral neuropathy
	Fetal alcohol syndrome
	Sexual dysfunction
	Substance-induced mood disorders
	Substance-induced psychotic disorders
	Immune dysfunction
Cocaine (other stimulants)	Chest pain
	Congestive heart failure
	Cardiac dysrhythmias
	Cardiovascular collapse
	Seizures
	Cerebrovascular accidents
	Headache
	Spontaneous pneumothorax
	Noncardiogenic pulmonary edema
	Nasal septal perforations
Injection drug use	Hepatitis C, B
	HIV infection
	Subacute endocarditis
	Soft-tissue abscesses

the result of persistent substance abuse. Withdrawal syndromes often present as episodes of anxiety, sleep disorders, mood disorders, or seizure disorders.

Seltz R, Medical and surgical complications of addiction. In: Ries RK, et al. eds. *Principles of Addiction Medicine*, 4th ed. Philadelphia: Lippincott Williams & Wilkins; 2009: 945–969.

Table 60-7. Neuropsychiatric complications of substance abuse.

Substance-induced mood disorder, depressed/elevated
Substance-induced anxiety disorder
Substance-induced psychotic disorder
Substance-induced personality change
Substance intoxication
Substance withdrawal
Delirium
Wernicke disease
Korsakoff syndrome (alcohol-induced persisting amnestic disorder)
Transient amnestic states (blackouts)
Substance-induced persisting dementia

▶ Treatment

Many substance use disorders resolve spontaneously or with brief interventions on the part of physicians or other authority figures in the workplace, legal system, family, or society. This occurs because patients with substance abuse disorders continue to maintain control over their use, and when the consequences of that use outweigh the benefits of the drug, they choose to quit. Patients with substance dependence disorders, on the other hand, have impaired control by definition. They rarely improve without assistance.

Substance use disorders can be treated successfully. Brief interventions and outpatient, inpatient, and residential treatment programs reduce morbidity and mortality associated with substance abuse and dependence. Determining the type and intensity of treatment that is best for a given patient may be difficult. ASAM has developed guidelines for clinicians to help determine the level and intensity of treatment for patients (**Table 60-8**). Once patients have been adequately assessed, treatment can begin. Detoxification, patient education, identification of defenses, overcoming denial, relapse prevention, orientation to 12-step recovery programs, and family services are the goals of substance abuse treatment.

A. Intervention

Once screening and diagnosis are complete, it is time for the physician to share the assessment with the patient. Because of the nature of substance abuse, patients rarely choose to seek help for their alcohol or drug problem until the consequences far outweigh the positive aspects of treatment. Intervention may be seen as a means of bringing these consequences to the attention of the patient. A wide range of approaches, some quite informal and others perhaps requiring careful orchestration and execution, can accomplish this task. Physicians or family members can often intervene simply by giving patients feedback about their behavior, describing the feelings that behavior generates, avoiding enabling behavior, and offering help.

Table 60-8. American Society of Addiction Medicine placement criteria.

Levels of Service

Level 0.5:	Early intervention
Level 1:	Outpatient services
Level 2:	Intensive outpatient/partial hospitalization services
Level 3:	Resident/inpatient services
Level 4:	Medically managed intensive inpatient services

Assessment Dimensions

1. Acute intoxication and/or withdrawal potential
2. Biomedical conditions and complications
3. Emotional, behavioral, or cognitive conditions and complications (eg, psychiatric conditions, psychological or emotional/behavioral complications of known or unknown origin, poor impulse control, changes in mental status, transient neuropsychiatric complications)
4. Readiness to change
5. Relapse, continued use, or continued problem potential
6. Recovery/living environment

Data from Mee-Lee D, Shulman GD, Fishman MJ, Gastfriend DR, Miller MM, eds. *The ASAM: Treatment Criteria for Addictive, Substance-Related, and Co-Occurring Conditions*, 3rd ed. Carson City, NV: The Change Companies; 2013.

The traditional intervention for alcohol or drug addiction is a formal process, best accomplished by an addictions specialist trained in this process. This approach is often effective, resulting in positive results in ~80% of cases. Although effective, the traditional, formal model of intervention is often less than ideal for the family physician. Specialist involvement and orchestration of significant relationships of the patient are sometimes difficult to achieve. In addition, if the intervention fails, it may be difficult if not impossible for the physician to continue a relationship with the patient. Another approach to consider is that of the brief intervention. This highly effective approach to intervention is based on motivational interviewing and the stages of change model (also known as the *transtheoretical model*).

1. Stages of change—Underlying the strategy of the brief intervention is the *stages of change model*, developed by Prochascka and DiClementi. In this model, behavioral change is viewed as a process that evolves over time through a series of stages: precontemplation, contemplation, preparation, action, maintenance, and termination. The individual must progress through each of these stages to reach the next one and cannot leap past one to get to another.

Individuals in the *precontemplation* stage are not planning to take any action in the foreseeable future. This is the stage most often described as denial. Patients in this stage do not perceive their behavior as problematic. In the *contemplation stage*, people perceive that they have a problem and believe that they should do something about it. Many addicted patients who do not appear to be ready for traditional treatment programs are in this stage. They recognize that they have a substance problem, believe that they should stop using the addictive substance, but seem unable to do so. In the *preparation stage*, patients have decided to change and plan to do so soon, usually within the next month. These patients are ready to enter action-oriented treatment programs. *Action* in the present context refers to the stage of change during which patients make specific changes in their behavior. In the case of addiction, abstinence is the generally agreed-on behavior that signifies action. *Maintenance* is the period after action during which the changed behavior persists and patients work toward preventing relapse. Maintenance often requires a longer sustained effort than patients anticipate, and failure to continue with maintenance behavior is a common cause of relapse. *Termination* describes the stage in which there is no temptation, and there is no risk of returning to old habits. In the case of addiction, most patients must work toward a lifetime of maintenance rather than termination. The risk of relapse is such that few truly reach this final stage for the disease of addiction.

2. Brief interventions—Presenting the diagnosis of a substance use disorder by itself may be viewed as a brief intervention. Most physicians who have worked with these patients will not be surprised to hear that as many as 70% of patients are in the precontemplation or contemplation stage when presented with the diagnosis. The resistance associated with these stages tends to force clinicians into one of two modalities—either avoiding the diagnosis or confronting and arguing with the patient. Both of these approaches are futile. One approach in presenting the diagnosis is to use the DEATH glossary, a list of pitfalls to avoid when presenting the diagnosis of addiction. On a more positive note, the SOAPE glossary (**Table 60-9**) describes suggestions to use when talking to patients about their addiction.

Even for patients in the precontemplative stage at presentation of the diagnosis, continued use of the brief intervention strategy will ultimately reduce the amount of drug use if not result in abstinence.

Brief interventions should include some of the elements of motivational interviewing. These elements include offering empathetic, objective feedback of data; meeting patient expectations; working with ambivalence; assessing barriers and strengths; reinterpreting past experience in light of current medical consequences; negotiating a follow-up plan; and providing hope.

B. Detoxification

Detoxification and treatment of withdrawal, and any medical complications, must have first priority. Alcohol and

Table 60-9. SOAPE glossary for presenting the diagnosis.

Support: Use phrases such as "we need to work together on this," "I am concerned about you and will follow up closely with you," and "As with all medical illnesses the more people you work with, the better you will feel." These words reinforce the physician–patient relationship, strengthen the collaborative model of chronic illness management, and help convince the patient that the physician will not just present the diagnosis and leave.

Optimism: Most patients have controlled their alcohol or drug use at times and may have quit for periods of time. They may expect failure. By giving a strong optimistic message such as "You can get well," "Treatment works," and "You can expect to see improvements in many areas of your life," the physican can motivate the patient.

Absolution: By describing addiction as a disease and telling patients that they are not responsible for having an illness, but that now only they can take responsibility for their recovery, the physician can lessen the burden of guilt and shame that is often a barrier to recovery.

Plan: Having a plan is important to the acceptance of the illness. Using readiness to change categories can help in designing a plan that utilizes the patient's willingness to move ahead. Indicating that abstinence is desirable, but recognizing that all patients will not be able to commit to that goal immediately can help prevent a sense of failure early in the process. Ask "What do you think you will be able to do at this point?"

Explanatory model: Understanding the patient's beliefs about addiction may be important. Many patients believe that this is a moral weakness and that they lack willpower. An explanation that willpower cannot resolve illnesses such as diabetes or alcoholism may go a long way to reassure the patient that recovery is possible.

Data from Clark WD. Alcoholism: blocks to diagnosis and treatment. *Am J Med.* 1981; 71:285.

Table 60-10. Treatment regimens for alcohol withdrawal.

Use the Clinical Institute Withdrawal Assessment of Alcohol Scale, Revised (CIWA-AR) for monitoring:
    Assess the patient using the CIWA-AR scale every 4 hours until the score is <8 for 24 hour
    For CIWA-AR >10:
        Give either chlordiazepoxide, 50–100 mg, diazepam, 10–20 mg, oxazepam, 30–60 mg, or lorazepam, 2–4 mg
    Repeat the CIWA-AR 1 hour after the dose to assess the need for further medication
Non-symptom-driven regimens:
    For patients likely to experience withdrawal, use chlordiazepoxide, 50 mg, Q6h (every 6 hours) for four doses followed by 50 mg Q8h for three doses, followed by 50 mg Q12h for two doses, and finally by 50 mg at bedtime for one dose
    Other benzodiazepines may be substituted at equivalent doses
Patients on a predetermined dosing schedule should be monitored frequently both for breakthrough withdrawal symptoms and for excessive sedation

of alcohol withdrawal. Opiate withdrawal may not be life-threatening, but the symptoms are significant enough that without supportive treatment, most patients will not remain in treatment. **Table 60-11** outlines recommendations for the treatment of opiate withdrawal. The symptoms of cocaine and other stimulant withdrawal are somewhat less predictable and much harder to improve. Despite multiple studies with many different drug classes, no medications have been shown to reliably reduce the symptoms and craving associated with cocaine withdrawal.

Manasco A, Chang S, Larriviere J, Hamm LL, Glass M. Alcohol withdrawal [review]. *South Med J.* 2012;105(11):607-612.
Praveen KT, Law F, O'Shea J, Melichar J. Opiod dependence. *Am Fam Physician.* 2012;86(6):565-566.

Table 60–11. Treatment for opioid withdrawal.

Methadone: A pure opioid agonist restricted by federal legislation to inpatient treatment or specialized outpatient drug treatment programs. Initial dosage is 15–20 mg for 2–3 days, then tapered with a 10–15% reduction in dose daily guided by patient's symptoms and clinical findings.
Clonidine: An α-adrenergic blocker, 0.2 mg Q4h to relieve symptoms of withdrawal, may be effective. Hypotension is a risk and sometimes limits the dose. It can be continued for 10–14 days and tapered by the third day by 0.2 mg daily.
Buprenorphine: This partial μ-receptor agonist can be administered sublingually in doses of 2, 4, or 8 mg Q4h for the management of opioid withdrawal symptoms.
Naltrexone/clonidine: A rapid form of opioid detoxification involves pretreatment with 0.2–0.3 mg of clonidine followed by 12.5 mg of naltrexone (a pure opioid antagonist). Naltrexone is increased to 25 mg on the second day, 50 mg on day 3, and 100 mg on day 4, with clonidine given at 0.1–0.3 mg 3 times daily.

other sedative-hypnotic drugs share the same neurobiological withdrawal process. Chronic use of this class of drugs results in downregulation of the GABA receptors throughout the central nervous system (CNS). GABA is an inhibitory neurotransmitter and is uniformly depressed during sedative-hypnotic use. Abrupt cessation of sedative-hypnotic drug use results in upregulation of GABA receptors and a relative paucity of GABA for inhibition. The result is stimulation of the autonomic nervous system (ANS) and the appearance of the signs and symptoms listed in Table 60-4. Withdrawal seizures are a common manifestation of sedative-hypnotic withdrawal, occurring in 11–33% of patients withdrawing from alcohol.

Alcohol withdrawal seizures are best treated with benzodiazepines and by addressing the withdrawal process itself. Long-term treatment of alcohol withdrawal seizures is not recommended, and phenytoin should not be used to treat seizures associated with alcohol withdrawal. The cornerstones of treatment for alcohol withdrawal syndrome are the benzodiazepines. All drugs that provide cross-tolerance with alcohol are effective in reducing the symptoms and sequelae of alcohol withdrawal, but none has the safety profile and evidence of efficacy of the benzodiazepines. **Table 60-10** summarizes recommendations in the treatment

C. Patient Education

Patients' knowledge and understanding of the nature of substance use disorders are the key to their recovery. For patients still in control of their use, education about appropriate substance use will help them to choose responsibly if they continue to use. For patients who meet the criteria for substance dependence (addiction), abstinence is the only safe recommendation. Once having made the transition to addiction, patients can never use addictive substances reliably again. The neurobiological changes in the brain are permanent, and loss of control may occur at any time when the brain is presented with an addictive substance. Loss of control can occur unpredictably; consequently, addicted patients may find that they can use the substance for a variable period of time with control, which gives them the false impression that they were never addicted in the first place or perhaps that they have been cured. Invariably, if they continue to use addictive substances, they will lose control of their use and begin to experience consequences at or above the level they did before. Understanding that the problem of addiction is a chronic disorder for which there is remission but not cure becomes essential. The question then becomes not whether, but *how* to remain abstinent.

D. Identification of Defenses and Overcoming Denial

During this phase of treatment patients typically work in a group therapy setting and are encouraged to look at the defenses that have prevented them from seeking help sooner. Denial can best be defined as the inability to see the causal relationship between drug use and its consequences. For example, a patient who believes that he drank because he lost his job may be encouraged to consider the reverse scenario: that he lost his job because he drank.

E. Relapse Prevention

Once patients are educated to the nature of their disease and have identified destructive defense mechanisms, relapse prevention becomes the primary goal. In order to help patients maintain abstinence, it is important to help them identify triggers for alcohol and drug use, develop plans to prevent opportunities to relapse, and determine new ways to deal with problems. In most treatment programs a relapse prevention plan is developed and individualized for each patient.

F. Twelve-Step Recovery Programs

It would be difficult to overstate the contribution that 12-step programs make to recovery. Despite millions of dollars in research and the efforts of a large segment of the scientific community, no treatment, medication, or psychotherapy has taken the place of the 12 steps.

Twelve-step recovery has its roots in Alcoholics Anonymous (AA), founded in 1935. Today over 200 recovery organizations use the 12 steps with some modifications for patients with substance use disorders. These programs include Al-Anon, for friends and family of alcoholics; Narcotics Anonymous (NA), for those with drug problems other than alcohol; and Cocaine Anonymous, for those with cocaine addiction. At the heart of each of these fellowships is the program of recovery outlined in the 12 steps (**Table 60-12**). AA and related 12-step programs are spiritual, not religious, in nature. No one is required to believe in anything, including God. Agnostics and atheists are welcome in AA, and are not asked to convert to any religious belief. Newcomers in AA are encouraged to attend meetings regularly (daily is wise initially), get a sponsor, and begin work on the 12 steps. A sponsor is usually someone of the same sex, who is in stable recovery and has successfully negotiated the steps. The sponsor helps guide the newcomer through the steps and provides a source of information and encouragement.

Table 60-12. The 12 Steps of Alcoholics Anonymous.

We:
1. Admitted that we were powerless over alcohol—that our lives had become unmanageable;
2. Came to believe that a power greater than ourselves could restore us to sanity;
3. Made a decision to turn our will and our lives over to the care of God as *we understood Him;*
4. Made a searching and fearless moral inventory of ourselves;
5. Admitted to ourselves, and to another human being, the exact nature of our wrongs;
6. Were entirely ready to have God remove all these defects of character;
7. Humbly asked Him to remove our shortcomings;
8. Made a list of all persons whom we had harmed, and became willing to make amends to them all;
9. Made direct amends to such people wherever possible, except when to do so would injure them or others;
10. Continued to take personal inventory and when we were wrong promptly admitted it;
11. Sought through prayer and meditation to improve our conscious contact with God as *we understand Him*, praying only for knowledge of His will for us and the power to carry that out;
12. Having had a spiritual awakening as the result of these steps, we tried to carry this message to alcoholics, and to practice these principles in all our affairs.

Note: The Twelve Steps are reprinted with permission of Alcoholics Anonymous World Services, Inc. ("AAWS") Permission to reprint the Twelve Steps does not mean that AAWS has reviewed or approved the contents of this publication, or that AAWS necessarily agrees with the views expressed herein. A.A is a program of recovery from alcoholism *only*– use of the Twelve Steps in connection with programs and activities that are patterned after A.A, but that address other problems, or in any other non-A.A context, does not imply otherwise.

Table 60-13. Limitations of 12-step groups.

AA does not solicit members; it will only reach out to people who ask for help.

AA does not keep records of membership (although some AA groups will provide phone lists for group members).

AA does not engage in research.

There is no formal control or follow-up on members by AA.

AA does not perform medical or psychiatric diagnoses. Each member needs to decide whether s/he is an addict.

AA as a whole does not provide housing, food, clothing, jobs, or money to newcomers (although individual members may do this).

AA is self-supporting through its own members' contributions; it does not accept money from outside sources.

Data from A Brief Guide to Alcoholics Anonymous. Alcoholics Anonymous World Service Inc.; 1972.

At meetings members share their experiences, relaying information about strategies for recovery. AA meetings vary in their composition and structure; consequently, if a patient feels uncomfortable at one meeting, another may be more acceptable. There are meetings for women or men only, those for young people, physicians, lawyers, and for virtually any special interest group in most large cities. There is often a great deal of confusion about what AA does and does not do. AA is not treatment. Despite the close connection that many treatment programs have with 12-step recovery fellowships, these fellowships are not affiliated with treatment centers by design. **Table 60-13** lists some of the self-described limitations of AA and other 12-step groups.

From multiple sources, it appears clear that AA and other 12-step recovery programs are among the most effective tools to combat substance disorders. Approximately 6–10% of the population has been to an AA meeting during their lives, and this number doubles for those with alcohol problems. Although 50% of those who come to AA leave, of those who stay for a year, 67% remain sober; of those who stay for 2 years, 85% remain sober; and of those who stay sober for 5 years, 90% remain sober indefinitely. Outcome studies of 8087 patients treated in 57 different inpatient and outpatient treatment programs showed that those attending AA at 1-year follow-up were 50% more likely to be abstinent than those not attending. Adolescents studied were found to be 4 times more likely to be abstinent if they attended AA/NA when compared with those who did not. Finally, in an effort to identify which groups in AA did better than others, studies of involvement in AA (defined as service work, having a sponsor, leading meetings, etc) found that those who were involved maintained abstinence better than those who just attended meetings.

Having a list of AA members willing to escort potential new members to meetings is a powerful tool for physicians to help patients transition into recovery. Generally in every AA district, there is a person identified as the chair of the Cooperation with Professional Community Committee who can help physicians identify people willing to perform this service. Al-Anon and NA have similar contacts. These contacts can often supply physicians with relevant literature to help dispel some of the myths patients may hold regarding 12-step recovery. Patients often use these myths as excuses for why AA will not work for them, and understanding this as resistance and ambivalence about entering a life of recovery is important for the physician. Family physicians are in a unique position to encourage patients to invest in 12-step recovery. Recovering persons are keenly aware of this fact, and physicians are encouraged and welcomed at open AA and other 12-step meetings to become more familiar with the way they work.

G. Pharmacotherapeutic Treatment of Addiction

Agents useful in the treatment of withdrawal were discussed earlier (see section on detoxification). The agents discussed here are used to help prevent relapse into alcohol or other drug use. These drugs attempt to influence drug use by one of several mechanisms:

1. Sensitizing the body's response to result in a negative reaction to ingesting the drug, causing an aversion reaction such as with disulfiram and alcohol.

2. Reducing the reinforcing effects of a drug, such as the use of naltrexone in alcoholism.

3. Blocking the effects of a drug by binding to the receptor site, such as naltrexone for opiates.

4. Saturating the receptor sites by agonists, such as the use of methadone in opioid maintenance therapy.

5. Unique approaches, such as the creation of an immunization to cocaine.

Drug therapy for addiction holds promise. As our understanding of the neurobiology of addiction improves, so does the chance that we can intervene at a molecular level to prevent relapse. At the current level, however, pharmacotherapy to prevent relapse must be relegated to an adjunctive position. No drug alone has provided sufficient power to prevent relapse to addictive behavior. Still, in some patients the use of appropriate medication may give them the edge necessary to move closer to recovery.

1. Pharmacotherapy for alcoholism—Disulfiram, naltrexone, possibly other opioid antagonists, selective serotonin reuptake inhibitors (SSRIs), and acamprosate are currently used in the prevention of relapse in alcoholism. Acamprosate appears to be the most promising of these medications. Although the goal of abstinence for patients addicted to alcohol cannot be met by medication alone at this time, in selected patients it may improve their chances for stable recovery.

A. Disulfiram—Disulfiram inhibits aldehyde dehydrogenase, the enzyme that catalyzes the oxidation of acetaldehyde to acetic acid. Thus, if a patient taking disulfiram ingests alcohol, the acetaldehyde levels rise. The result is referred to as the *disulfiram-ethanol reaction*. This manifests as flushing of the skin, palpitations, decreased blood pressure, nausea, vomiting, shortness of breath, blurred vision, and confusion. The reactions are usually related to the dose of both disulfiram and alcohol. This reaction can be severe, and fatalities have been reported with doses of disulfiram of >500 mg and 2 oz of alcohol. Common side effects of disulfiram include drowsiness, lethargy, peripheral neuropathy, hepatotoxicity, and hypertension.

In the United States, doses of 250–500 mg are most commonly used. Because of individual variability in the disulfiram-ethanol reaction, often these doses do not produce a sufficient reaction to deter the patient from drinking. In the United Kingdom, it is common to perform an ethanol challenge test to determine the appropriate dose to produce an aversion effect. Whether disulfiram is actually effective in preventing relapse is the subject of some debate. Most studies have failed to show a statistically significant result. On closer examination, it appears that compliance with the medication is the most important factor. In a large Veterans Administration multicenter study, a direct relationship was found between compliance with drug therapy and abstinence. In addition, the involvement of a patient's spouse in observing the patient's consumption of disulfiram results in considerable improvement in outcome. It appears that disulfiram can be a useful adjunct for patients who have a history of sudden relapse and who have a social situation in which compliance may be adequately monitored. Because of its lack of effectiveness, potential adverse effects, and compliance issues, disulfiram is not recommended for use in the primary care setting.

B. Naltrexone—Naltrexone, an opioid antagonist, has been shown to reduce drinking in animal studies and in human alcoholics. It blocks euphoric and physiological effects of opioid agonists without causing physical dependence or tolerance. Initial optimism over the potential of this discovery was tempered by several studies indicating that the effects of reducing drinking and preventing relapse diminished over time and overall failed to reduce relapse to heavy drinking. Still, the effect of naltrexone on alcohol craving is promising in that it suggests that the opioid system is involved in the craving for alcohol in alcoholism; this may open the door to the development of other opioid-active drugs that will have an impact on drinking. Studies are also showing promise with long-acting naltrexone in the form of injections or implantations as opposed to the oral route. The long-acting form has been found to be as safe and tolerable as the oral form with better patient compliance likely due to consistent blood levels of the drug.

C. Serotonergic drugs—Animal studies have consistently shown that SSRIs reduce alcohol intake in animal models. The data with respect to humans are less clear or consistent. It appears that the SSRIs reduce drinking in heavily drinking, nondepressed alcoholics, but probably only approximately 15–20% from pretreatment levels. When abstinence is the outcome studied, the results are not promising. However, the SSRIs may eventually find a place in concert with other anticraving medication. SSRIs appear to reduce drinking in a more robust fashion in alcoholics with comorbid depression.

D. Acamprosate (calcium acetylhomotaurinate)—Acamprosate has been shown to reduce craving for alcohol in alcoholics. While the overall mechanism of action is uncertain, it appears to affect both GABA and glutamine neurotransmission, both important in alcohol's effect in the brain. Unlike the effects of naltrexone, the effects of acamprosate on relapse appear to be greater and longer-lasting. Twice as many alcoholics remained abstinent in a 12-month period while taking acamprosate compared with those who took placebo. The addition of disulfiram to the regimen appears to increase the effectiveness of acamprosate. Trials have also considered combining acamprosate with naltrexone, but the combination led to a higher rate of withdrawal from the trials because of adverse effects. Acamprosate alone has a very benign side effect profile and appears to be free of any effects on mood, concentration, attention, or psychomotor performance. Diarrhea is the only side effect that reached statistical significance in a review of 24 trials. Acamprosate has been used in Europe for >20 years and was FDA-approved for use in the United States in 2004.

Overall evidence best supports the use of acamprosate and naltrexone along with counseling for the prevention of alcohol relapse. SSRIs are an option when a comorbid mood disorder is present.

Anton RF, et al. Combined pharmacotherapies and behavioral interventions for alcohol dependence: the COMBINE study: a randomized controlled trial. *JAMA*. 2006; 295:2003–2017. [PMID: 16670409]

Blondell RD. Ambulatory detoxification of patients with alcohol dependence. *Am Fam Physician*. 2005;71(3): 495–502.

Cayley WE. Effectiveness of acamprosate in the treatment of alcohol dependence. *Am Fam Physician*. 2001; 83(5), 522–524.

Donaher P, Welsh C. Managing opiod addiction with buprenorphine. *Am Fam Physician*, 2006;73(9).

Kjome KA. Long-acting injectable naltrexone for the management of patients with opioid dependence. *Subst Abuse: Res Treat*. 2011;5:1–9.

Willenbring M, Massey S, Gardner M. Helping patients who drink too much: an evidence-based guide for primary care physicians. *Am Fam Physician*. 2009; 80(1):44–50.

Williams SH. Medications for treating alcohol dependence. *Am Fam Physician*. 2005;72(9):1775–1780.

2. Pharmacotherapy for cocaine addiction—The state of the art in the pharmacologic treatment of cocaine addiction makes it difficult to recommend any medication-based treatment with any confidence. Despite great interest and much activity devoted to finding an effective pharmacologic intervention for cocaine and other stimulant addiction, none has withstood the test of rigorous study. Heterocyclic antidepressants such as desipramine, SSRIs, monoamine oxidase inhibitors, dopamine agonists such as bromocriptine, neuroleptics, anticonvulsants, and calcium channel blockers have all been tried in cocaine addiction. Variable results, often positive in animal studies, have led to attempts to treat cocaine addicts with these drugs. As each potentially effective drug is studied more rigorously, however, little in the way of positive results is found. These drugs are used to try to ameliorate the craving for cocaine or to mediate the withdrawal symptoms of anhedonia and fatigue. An attempt to use stimulants such as methylphenidate or amphetamine for cocaine dependence in a way analogous to that of methadone maintenance for opiate addiction has produced disappointing results. One of the more interesting approaches to a pharmacologic answer to cocaine addiction has been the development of a "vaccine" for cocaine. In this approach, a cocainelike hapten linked to a foreign protein produces antibodies that attach to cocaine molecules, preventing them from crossing the blood-brain barrier. This approach has had some success in animal models but has yet to be tested on humans.

3. Pharmacotherapy for opiate addiction—Agonist maintenance treatment with methadone has been the primary pharmacologic treatment for opioid treatment. The rationale for the use of methadone and its longer-acting relative, levo-α-acetylmethadol (LAAM), is to saturate the opiate receptors, thus blocking euphoria and preventing the abstinence syndrome. Methadone and LAAM treatment programs are highly regulated by the federal government; therefore, the average family physician would not be prescribing this drug but certainly might see patients who are on a maintenance program. Methadone programs and other similar programs with buprenorphine/naloxone are frequently referred to as "harm reduction programs" because the primary beneficiary of these programs is society. Reductions in crime and in the costs of active intravenous heroin abuse are clearly demonstrated as a result of these programs. The addict also benefits with a dramatic decrease in the risk of death due to addiction or contraction of HIV disease. There is social stabilization in the addict's life as well, especially when the maintenance program provides appropriate social services.

Antagonist maintenance with naltrexone was initially considered ideal, given its essentially complete blockade of opioid-reinforcing properties. Unfortunately, only 10–20% of patients remained in treatment when this approach was used. The most important use of naltrexone at this time appears to be in the management of healthcare professionals with opioid dependence. Compliance with a naltrexone regimen ensures abstinence and allows healthcare professionals to work in an environment where opioids may be accessible. Doses of 350 mg weekly divided into 3 days will provide complete protection from the effects of opioids.

Buprenorphine, a partial opioid agonist with K antagonist effects, is now being used as an alternative to methadone maintenance treatment. Dosing of this medication is problematic, with 65% of patients remaining abstinent at 16 mg/d compared with 28% abstinence at 4 mg/d. Suboxone, a combination of buprenorphine and naloxone, is another alternative that is effective for patients who do not require higher doses of methadone. Since naloxone has poor oral absorption but antagonizes opioid receptors when injected, its inclusion in suboxone make users less likely to crush and inject the drug (Donaher and Welsh 2006). Buprenorphine may decrease the use of cocaine in opioid-dependent patients. It also has less potential for diversion, making it an attractive alternative to methadone. The Drug Addiction Treatment Act of 2000 allows office-based maintenance treatment of opioid dependence by primary care physicians who have met the necessary requirements. This criterion usually includes licensure under state law, registration by the Drug Enforcement Agency, reasonable access and ability to refer patients to ancillary services if needed, and at least 8 hours of training in the management and treatment of opioid addiction from an approved association. The FDA approved the use of suboxone for treatment of opioid addiction in 2002. Treatment with suboxone has three phases, termed *induction*, *stabilization*, and *maintenance*. Therapy should start 12–24 hours after cessation of short-acting opioids or 24–48 hours after discontinuing use of long-acting opioids. Induction typically lasts 3–7 days. Day 1 consists of starting with a 4/1 mg (4 mg buprenorphine/1 mg naloxone) dose of suboxone, followed by a second dose 2 hours later if withdrawal symptoms persist. Over the next 6 days, this dose is titrated up to a maximum of 32/8 mg/d. Stabilization then begins and usually lasts 1–2 months. The goal of this stage of therapy is to find the minimal effective dose to decrease cravings, eliminate withdrawal, and minimize side effects of suboxone. Most patients require a daily dose between 12/3 mg and 24/6 mg to achieve these goals. Maintenance therapy is indefinite and focuses on monitoring for illicit drug use, minimizing cravings, and avoiding triggers to use.

Blondell RD. Ambulatory detoxification of patients with alcohol dependence. *Am Fam Physician.*, 2005; 71(3):495–502.

Cayley WE. (2011). Effectiveness of acamprosate in the treatment of alcohol dependence. *Am Fam Physician.* 2011; 83(5):522–524.

Donaher P, Welsh C. Managing opiod addiction with buprenorphine. *Am Fam Physician.* 2006; 73(9).

Litten RZ, Egli M, Heilig M, et al. Medications development to treat alcohol dependence: a vision for the next decade. *Addict Biol.* 2012;17(3):513–527.

Lobmaier PP, Kunoe N, Gossop M, Waal H. Naltrexone depot formulations for opioid and alcohol dependence: a systematic review. *CNS Neurosci Ther*. 2011;17(6):629-636.

Miotto K, Hillhouse M, Donovick R, et al. Comparison of buprenorphine treatment for opioid dependence in 3 settings. *J Addict Med*. 2012; 6(1):68-76.

Praveen KT, Law F, O'Shea J, Melichar J. Opioid dependence. *Am Fam Physician*. 2012; 86(6):565-566.

Willenbring M, Massey S, Gardner M. (2009). Helping patients who drink too much: an evidence-based guide for primary care physicians. *Am Fam Physician*. 2009;80(1):44-50.

Williams SH. (2005). Medications for treating alcohol dependence. *Am Fam Physician*. 2005;72(9):1775-1780.

Websites

Alcoholics Anonymous: (AA):aa.org.

American Society of Addiction Medicine (ASAM):asam.org.

National Institute on Alcohol Abuse and Alcoholism: niaaa.nih.gov.

National Institute on Drug Abuse (NIDA): nida.nih.gov.

Tobacco Cessation

Martin C. Mahoney, MD, PhD, FAAFP
K. Michael Cummings, PhD, MPH

▶ Smoking Behavior & Disease Risk

Cigarette smoking, which is responsible for >400,000 deaths annually, represents the single most avoidable cause of premature death in the United States today. While the prevalence of smoking in the United States has declined since the early 1960s, >40 million adults are current smokers (20% prevalence among adults), ensuring that this behavior will continue to influence rates of premature morbidity and mortality rates for decades to come. Most people begin smoking during their teenage years and struggle to quit as adults. Clinicians need to view nicotine dependence as a chronic health condition with exacerbations and remissions.

There are benefits to quitting even among those who have already experienced health problems caused by smoking. Some of the benefits of smoking cessation occur shortly after quitting, while other smoking-related risks are not moderated for months or years. An individual's disease risk depends on previous duration and intensity of smoking, the presence of preexisting illnesses, and individual susceptibility. On a population-wide basis, it is now clear that progress achieved in extending life expectancy has been due in part to successful tobacco control, especially efforts to persuade and assist smokers to quit.

Cummings KM, Mahoney MC. Strategies for smoking cessation: what is new and what works? *Expert Rev Respir Med.* 2008; 2:201–213. [PMID: 20477249]

IARC. *Tobacco Control: Reversal of Risk After Quitting Smoking.* International Agency for Research on Cancer (IARC) Handbooks of Cancer Prevention, vol 11; 2007.

US Department of Health and Human Services. *The Health Consequences of Smoking: A Report of the Surgeon General.* US Department of Health and Human Services, Centers for Disease Control and Prevention, National Center for Chronic Disease Prevention and Health Promotion, Office on Smoking and Health, 2004.

▶ Tobacco Dependence and Implications for Treatment

Most smokers report that they want to quit, and approximately 40–50% attempt to stop smoking annually. However, most quit attempts are unplanned, usually last only a few days or weeks, and are unsupported by the provision of pharmacotherapy and counseling support. Difficulty quitting is best predicted by how much one smokes on a daily basis and smoking within 30 minutes of waking up each day, both of which are measures of nicotine dependence.

Also, many smokers turn to methods with no proven efficacy to support sustained abstinence such as switching to so-called low-yield cigarettes, hypnotherapy, acupuncture, and various pharmacological therapies [eg, selective serotonin reuptake inhibitors (SSRIs), tricyclic antidepressants (TCAs), anxiolytics, benzodiazepines, β-blockers, silver acetate, mecamylamine, appetite suppressants, caffeine, ephedrine, dextrose tablets, lobeline, moclobemide) further lowering quit success and contributing to a cycle of failed quit efforts, making the prospect of stopping smoking appear hopeless to many smokers.

The vast majority (ie, 80–90% of current smokers) are addicted to nicotine, which makes it difficult or impossible for some smokers to stop smoking cigarettes. Nicotine addiction is the fundamental reason why individuals persist in using tobacco products despite knowledge of the harms caused by tobacco use. Increasing evidence suggests that nicotine addiction is a hereditary characteristic. A recent study found that those at higher genetic risk of smoking addiction were more likely to convert to daily smoking as teenagers, progress to heavy smoking as adults, and report failed quit attempts later in life. The reality is that smoking should be regarded as a chronic relapsing problem with exacerbations and remissions.

Baker TB, Piper ME, McCarthy DE, Bolt DM, Smith SS, Kim S, et al. Time to first cigarette in the morning as an index of ability to quit smoking: implications for nicotine dependence. *Nicot Tobac Res.* 2007; 9(Suppl 4):555–570. [PMC: 2933747]

Belsky DW, Moffitt TE, Baker TB, et al. Polygenic risk and the developmental progression to heavy, persistent smoking and nicotine dependence. *JAMA Psychiatr.* 2013;13:39:37. [PMID: 23536134]

National Cancer Institute. *Phenotypes and Endophenotypes: Foundations for Genetic Studies of Nicotine Use and Dependence.* Tobacco Control Monograph 20. Bethesda, MD: US Department of Health and Human Services, National Institutes of Health, National Cancer Institute. NIH Publication 09-6366; Aug. 2009.

US Department of Health and Human Services. *How Tobacco Smoke Causes Disease: The Biology and Behavioral Basis for Smoking-Attributable Disease: A Report of the Surgeon General.* Atlanta, GA: US Department of Health and Human Services, Centers for Disease Control and Prevention, National Center for Chronic Disease Prevention and Health Promotion, Office on Smoking and Health; 2010. [PMID: 21452462]

▶ Use of Brief Interventions to Promote Smoking Cessation

Smoking cessation treatment often begins with a brief intervention, in which a physician or any other healthcare provider advises smokers to quit and may recommend methods for quitting. For many smokers, the only contact with the healthcare system may be through their family physician, and office visits often provide the impetus for smokers to attempt to stop smoking.

Meta-analyses report that brief counseling interventions have significant potential to reduce smoking rates, with even minimal brief interventions conferring an estimated 30% increased likelihood of cessation.

A Cochrane review evaluating the effectiveness of brief smoking cessation advice from a physician found that advice from a physician compared with no advice (or usual care) significantly increased the odds of being smoke-free after 6 months and yielded an absolute difference of 2.5% in the rate of smoking cessation.

The Public Health Service (PHS) guidelines for treating tobacco use and dependence, last updated in 2008, continue to recommend that healthcare workers screen all patients for tobacco use and provide advice and follow-up behavioral treatments to all tobacco users. Current users are advised to quit; those who are willing to make a quit attempt are given appropriate assistance, along with arrangements for a follow-up visit. In addition, those who are identified as former smokers are given advice to prevent relapse, and persons who have never used tobacco are encouraged to remain tobacco free.

Controlled studies have found that physician involvement, especially more extensive interventions, increases quit rates. This approach has also been found to be cost-effective since tobacco cessation interventions cost ~$2500 per year of life saved, whereas mammography screening costs ~$50,000 per year of life saved.

According to a comprehensive review of the efficacy of different smoking cessation treatments, the PHS has recommended that all smokers receive counseling and support to quit preferably in combination with approved pharmacotherapy. Despite this treatment guideline, population-based surveys reveal that most tobacco users today are still not routinely receiving treatment assistance from their healthcare provider during visits. For example, a recent survey reported that tobacco counseling occurred in <25% of physician visits by tobacco users, and cessation medications were prescribed on <3% of occasions. Studies have documented that utilization of evidence-based stop smoking treatments are lowest among those who are uninsured and have the greatest need for assistance in quitting tobacco (ie, those with mental health and other substance abuse problems). Encouraging smoking cessation is now recognized as a required part of good clinical practice.

The guideline continues to emphasize use of the "5 **A**s" in clinical settings: **ask** about tobacco use, **advise** to quit, **assess** willingness to make a quit attempt, **assist** in quit attempt, and **arrange** for follow-up. The American Academy of Family Physicians has attempted to simplify this to "2 **A**"s: **ask** about tobacco use and **act** to advise smoker to quit, as well as assessing interest in quitting, assisting in organizing pharmacotherapy, and arranging for follow-up. These systematic approaches to tobacco dependence require <3 minutes to deliver with the potential to result in behavior change. Other key points from the 2008 PHS clinical guideline include the following:

- The need for all healthcare delivery systems to systematically identify and document tobacco use status and to offer treatment to every tobacco user.

- The importance of providing pharmacotherapy to all patients making a quit attempt.

- Counseling support is effective in a variety of settings (eg, individual, group, or via telephone), and effectiveness increases with treatment intensity. Counseling should address both practical issues (problem solving/skills training) and social support.

- While counseling and pharmacotherapy are each effective when used by themselves, the combination is more effective than either alone for treating tobacco dependence.

- Use of telephone quit lines should be promoted since counseling is effective with diverse populations and offers broad geographic reach.

Physician advice to stop smoking increases the likelihood that patients will try to quit and enhances the odds that those who do quit will remain off cigarettes. Long-term cessation rates approach 20% with counseling and increase to 30% when counseling is combined with pharmacotherapy.

Fiore MC, et al. *Treating Tobacco Use and Dependence: 2008 Update.* Clinical Practice Guideline, US Department of Health and Human Services, Public Health Service; May 2008 (available at http://www.surgeongeneral.gov/tobacco/treating_tobacco_use08.pdf; accessed March 31, 2013).

Lancaster T, Stead L. Physician advice for smoking cessation. *Cochrane Database Syst Rev.* 2004(4):CD000165. [PMID: 15494989]

Piper ME, et al. Assessing tobacco dependence: a guide to measure evaluation and selection. *Nicot Tobac Res.* 2006; 8:339–351. [PMID: 16801292]

▶ Pharmacotherapy

Tobacco users have a physical dependence on nicotine, in addition to various reinforced psychological and social behaviors. The two-item Heaviness of Smoking Index (HSI) represents a reliable and valid way to assess the strength of someone's nicotine dependence. Those who use tobacco more frequently every day and find a need to use tobacco first thing when they wake up in the morning are scored as more dependent. **Table 61-1** shows a strategy for identifying smokers and determining readiness to quit as well as actions to be completed at that visit.

The use of pharmacotherapy doubles the effect of any tobacco cessation intervention. A recent Cochrane review has validated the importance of providing counseling support, in addition to pharmacotherapy, among smokers attempting to quit. Studies with four or more sessions showed the greatest impact; counseling can be delivered either in person or by telephone.

The US PHS guideline on management of tobacco dependence recommends varenicline, sustained-release bupropion, and all forms of nicotine replacement (eg, resin or gum, inhaler, nasal spray, lozenges, and patch). Patients should be queried about experiences with prior use of cessation medications and asked if they are interested in a particular agent. Clinicians are encouraged to apply appropriate clinical judgment when assessing contraindications to the use of a particular agent. The use of pharmacotherapy to support smoking cessation is summarized in **Table 61-2**.

A. Nicotine Replacement Therapy (NRT)

Nicotine patches, lozenges, and resin (gum) are available over the counter (OTC), whereas nicotine nasal sprays and the nicotine inhaler systems both require prescriptions. Reduced-dose regimens of nicotine replacement might be considered for patients consuming <10 cigarettes daily or those weighing <100 lb (~45 kg). Using two forms of nicotine replacement (eg, patch plus resin or lozenges) results in higher quit rates and should be recommended if other forms of nicotine replacement have not been effective alone. Quit rates with use of NRT range between 20% and 24%; use of NRT is recommended for a minimum of 6–8 weeks; however, some patients elect to continue nicotine-containing therapy for the long term.

Nicotine medications appear to be safe for most people. Side effects of NRT mainly include local irritation (ie, mouth sores, skin rash, nasal and throat irritation) associated with the route of administration of the medication. Side effects are typically mild and transient. Studies show that only ~1 in 12 person reports discontinuing use of NRT because of side effects.

Nicotine-containing products are not associated with the occurrence of acute cardiac events. This finding is consistent with the observation that NRT is rarely able to achieve blood levels of nicotine associated with smoking. Nonetheless, NRT should be approached cautiously among patients who are within 2 weeks of an acute myocardial infarction, are known to have significant arrhythmias, and have significant or worsening symptoms of angina.

B. Bupropion (Zyban)

Sustained-release bupropion is started at a dose of 150 mg daily for 3 days before increasing to 150 mg twice daily on day 4. Treatment with bupropion begins 1–2 weeks before the anticipated quit date; its use is contraindicated among patients with a history of seizure disorders, current substance abuse, or other conditions that may lower the seizure threshold. The standard treatment course of bupropion (Zyban) in 8 weeks yields quit rates of ~30%.

C. Varenicline (Chantix)

This agent binds to $\alpha_4\beta_2$-nicotinic receptors in the central nervous system (CNS) to moderate symptoms of nicotine withdrawal, leading to reduced craving, decreased smoking satisfaction, and diminished psychological reward. Varenicline (Chantix) is started 1 week prior to the identified quit date, titrating up from a dose of 0.5 mg daily for

Table 61-1. Simplified model for addressing tobacco use and dependence: ask and act.

Ask:
  Do you smoke?
  How much do you want to quit? (1–10 scale)
  How confident are you in your ability to quit? (1–10 scale)
Act:
  Have you set a quit date?
  Provide quit advice or referral
  Provide pharmacotherapy prescription
  Arrange for follow-up

Data from http://www.askandact.org (American Academy of Family Physicians).

Table 61-2. Chart aid for use of first-line adjunctive pharmacotherapy in smoking cessation.

Stop Smoking Medication	Used in Past	Patient Would Like to Use?	Contraindications	Side Effects	Rx Given (Dose/Frequency/Number)	Other Instructions Given
Nicotine patch (7,14, or 21 mg/24 h for 4 weeks, then taper 2 weeks and 2 weeks)	Yes—Rx/OTC No	Yes No	Concurrent smoking	Local skin reaction Insomnia	7/14/21 mg patch every 24 h for 4 weeks then taper every 2 weeks	Dosing, side effects reviewed Behavioral counseling &/or quitline referral Set quit date: _____ F/U appt: _____
Nicotine gum (1—24cigs/day—2 mg gum or 25+ cigs/day—4 mg gum; max 24 pieces/day for up to 12 weeks)	Yes—Rx/OTC No	Yes No	Concurrent smoking	Mouth soreness Dyspepsia	2 mg gum 4 mg gum Max 24 pieces/day for up to 12 weeks	Dosing, side effects reviewed Behavioral counseling &/or quitline referral Set quit date: _____ F/U appt: _____
Nicotine nasal spray (8-40 doses/day for 3-6 months)	Yes—Rx No	Yes No	Concurrent smoking	Nasal irritation	_____ doses/day for 3-6 months	Dosing, side effects reviewed Behavioral counseling &/or quitline referral Set quit date: _____ F/U appt: _____
Nicotine inhaler (6-16 cartridges/day for up to 6 months)	Yes—Rx/OTC No	Yes No	Concurrent smoking	Local irritation of mouth and throat	_____ Cartridaes/day for _____ months	Dosing, side effects reviewed Behavioral counseling &/or quitline referral Set quit date: _____ F/U appt: _____
Nicotine lozenges (if first cig smoked within 30 minutes of arising—4 mg lozenge; if first cig after 30 minutes of arising—2-mg lozenge; max 5 loz/6 h or 20 loz/day for up to 12 weeks)	Yes—Rx/OTC No	Yes No	Concurrent smoking Contains phenylalanine	Mouth soreness Dyspepsia	2-mg lozenge 4-mg lozenge Maximum 20 loz/day for up to 12 weeks	Dosing, side effects reviewed Behavioral counseling &/or quitline referral Set quit date: _____ F/U appt: _____

Zyban/bupropion SR	Yes—Rx No	Yes No	History of seizures History of eating disorder Currently treated for depression Used MAO inhibitor within past 14 days	Local skin reaction Insomnia	150 mg orally every day for 3 days, then 150 mg twice a day	Dosing, side effects reviewed Quit on day #8 Behavioral counseling &/or quitline referral Set quit date: _____ F/U appt: _____
Chantix/varenidine	Yes—Rx No	Yes No	Severe renal disease	Nausea Insomnia, abnormal dreams GI symptoms	0.5 mg orally for 3 days, then 0.5 mg twice daily for 4 days, then 1.0 mg twice daily for 12 weeks	Dosing, side effects reviewed Quit on day #8 Behavioral counseling &/or quitline referral Set quit date: _____ F/U appt: _____

F/U, follow-up; GI, gastrointestinal; MAO, monoamine oxidase; OTC, over-the-counter; Rx, prescription.

3 days, to 0.5 mg twice daily for days 4–7, then to 1 mg twice daily beginning on day 8. Rates of continuous abstinence are 44%. A full treatment course of 12 weeks is recommended, and those who are abstinent at 12 weeks may continue with another 12 weeks of treatment. The most commonly encountered side effects are nausea, insomnia, and abnormal dreams; these are generally rated as mild and often resolve within several days or may be managed with a dose reduction as needed. Varenicline is minimally metabolized and is essentially excreted in the urine. There are no known drug interactions. Dose modification is necessary only with severe renal disease.

Cases of suicidal thoughts as well as aggressive and erratic behavior has been reported in some patients who have taken varenicline. There are also reports of drowsiness that affected patients' ability to drive or operate machinery. Preliminary review by the FDA suggests that many of the cases may be newly identified mental illness in persons who experienced depressed mood, suicidal thoughts, and/or changes in emotion and behavior within days to weeks of starting on varenicline.

Varenicline's role in these cases has not been established. Trying to stop smoking, with or without treatment, is associated with nicotine withdrawal symptoms, including irritability and drowsiness; symptoms of existing mental illness may worsen with cessation. Not all of the cases reported to the FDA were known to involve patients with prior mental illness, and not all patients concerned had stopped smoking.

According to information currently available, the potential benefits of varenicline greatly outweigh its risk. Clinicians are encouraged to screen for mental health issues prior to prescribing and to monitor patients for behavioral symptoms.

Clinicians should remember to support patient quit attempts by placing a follow-up call within 1–2 weeks of the quit date. Instruct patients to contact your office if they experience unusual mood swings while using this medication. Remind patients that irritability, mood swings, and drowsiness result from nicotine withdrawal. These symptoms are most common immediately after a person stops smoking and typically lessen with time. In addition, patients should be counseled to use caution when driving or operating machinery until they know how quitting smoking with varenicline may affect them.

Clinical experience with use of the pharmacotherapies for smoking cessation among pregnant women and adolescents is generally limited. Smokers with concurrent or prior depression may benefit from use of bupropion. Clinical judgment is advised regarding a comprehensive assessment of the risks and benefits associated with use of adjunctive pharmacotherapy in each of these settings.

On the basis of the observation that the number of past quit attempts is predictive of future quit attempts, clinicians should encourage smokers to continue to try to quit smoking. However, studies show that while motivation to quit is important in predicting whether someone makes a quit attempt, it does not necessarily predict ability to remain smoke-free, which is more likely to be related to the strength of someone's nicotine dependence. Clinicians play a pivotal role in not only motivating patients to make a quit attempt but also in offering evidence-based treatments to help them cope with craving and withdrawal symptoms that are the result of their nicotine addiction. Motivational interviewing can be used to enhance both level of motivation and the patient's self-efficacy to cope with the uneasy feelings that typically accompany smoking abstinence.

E-cigarettes—Electronic cigarettes (ie, e-cigarettes) are battery-powered devices that deliver nicotine in an aerosol to the user. E-cigarettes initially emerged in China in 2003 and since have become widely available. E-cigarettes heat and vaporize a solution, often flavored, containing nicotine, and many are designed to outwardly resemble traditional tobacco cigarettes and have been touted by some as a smoking cessation aid for addicted smokers. At this time the evidence supporting the efficacy of e-cigarettes as a cessation treatment for nicotine addiction is limited, although clearly smoking e-cigarettes appears to be less risky than smoking conventional cigarettes.

Borland R, Yong HH, O'Connor RJ, Hyland A, Thompson ME. The reliability and predictive validity of the Heaviness of Smoking Index and its two components: findings from the International Tobacco Control Four Country study. *Nicot Tobac Res.* 2010; 12(Suppl):S45–S50. [PMC: 3307335]

Cobb NK, Abrams DB. E-cigarette or drug-delivery device? Regulating novel nicotine products. *N Engl J Med.* 2011; 365(3):193–195. [PMID: 21774706]

Goniewicz ML, Knysak J, Gawron M, et al. Levels of selected carcinogens and toxicants in vapour from electronic cigarettes. *Tobac Control.* (published online only, March 2013; doi:10.1136/tobaccocontrol-2012-050859). [PMID: 23467656]

Gonzales D, et al. Varenicline, an alpha4beta2 nicotinic acetylcholine receptor partial agonist, vs sustained-release bupropion and placebo for smoking cessation: a randomized controlled trial. *JAMA.* 2006; 296:47–55. [PMID: 16820546]

Heatherton TF, Kozlowski LT, Frecker RC, Rickert W, Robinson J. Measuring the heaviness of smoking: using self-reported time to the first cigarette of the day and number of cigarettes smoked per day. *Addiction.* 1989; 84:791–800. [PMID 2758152]

Henningfield JE, et al. Pharmacotherapy for nicotine dependence. *CA Cancer J Clin.* 2005; 55:281. [PMID: 16166074]

Jardin BF, Carpenter MD. Predictors of quit attempts and abstinence among smokers not current interested in quitting. *Nicot Tobac Res.* 2012;14:1197–1204. [PMC: 3457712]

Jorenby DE, et al. A controlled trial of sustained-release bupropion, a nicotine patch, or both for smoking cessation. *N Engl J Med.* 1999; 340:685. [PMID: 10053177]

Mallin R. Smoking cessation: integration of behavioral and drug therapies. *Am Fam Physician.* 2002; 65:1107. [PMID: 11925087]

Polosa R, Caponnetto P, Morjaria JB, Papale G, Campagna D, Russo C. Effect of an electronic nicotine delivery device (e-cigarette) on smoking reduction and cessation: a prospective 6-month pilot study. *BMC Public Health.* 2011; 11:786. [PMC: 3203079]

Siegel MB, Tanwar KL, Wood KS. Electronic cigarettes as a smoking cessation tool: results from an online survey. *Am J Prev Med.* 2011; 40(4):472–475. [PMID: 21406283]

Stead L, Lancaster T. Behavioural interventions as adjuncts to pharmacotherapy for smoking cessation. *Cochrane Database Syst Rev.* 2012:CD009670.

Tonstad S, et al. Effect of maintenance therapy with varenicline on smoking cessation: a randomized controlled trial. *JAMA.* 2006; 296:64–71. [PMID: 16820548]

Payments for Cessation Services

Since 2005, the Centers for Medicare and Medicaid Services has provided reimbursement for smoking cessation counseling by clinicians as a preventive service provided that the patient is a Medicare beneficiary and has a disease or adverse health effect that is either caused or affected by tobacco use. Payment as a preventive service is based on two Healthcare Common Procedural Coding System (HCPCS) codes:

- G0375: Smoking and tobacco use cessation counseling visit; intermediate, >3 minutes and ≤10 minutes.
- G0376: Smoking and tobacco use cessation counseling visit; intensive, >10 minutes.

Reimbursement for tobacco cessation counseling is also available as a standard Part B Medicare benefit as CPT codes 99406 (intermediate, 3–10 minutes) and 99407 (intensive, >10 minutes), although the patient is responsible for both copayments and unmet deductible. Payment varies by region but averages approximately $13 for G0375 and $25 for G0376. Additional payment may be received according to the evaluation and management service (99201–99215, including modifier –25) provided on that same day and separately identifiable from the smoking cessation counseling. Counseling, which lasts <3 minutes, is included in the standard physician visit and is not reported separately. Medicare beneficiaries are eligible for up to four counseling sessions for each quit attempt, and up to two quit attempts are covered over a 12-month interval.

A useful resource which provides a listing HCPCS, CPT (current procedural terminology), and ICD-9 (international classification of diseases) codes related to tobacco cessation counseling can be found at the following website:

http://www.aafp.org/online/etc/medialib/aafp_org/ documents/clinical/pub_health/askact/coding.Par.0001.File. tmp/CodingList.pdf (accessed March 23, 2013).

Private health insurance plans are variable in their policies regarding reimbursement for smoking cessation counseling services. Alternative HCPCS codes include S9075 for smoking cessation treatment and S9453 for smoking cessation classes. The patient's health record should document all services provided. Medicare Part D has covered cessation FDA-approved drug therapies for eligible beneficiaries since 2006 as part of the prescription drug benefit, although OTC formulations of nicotine replacement therapies are generally excluded.

Pohlig C. Smoking cessation counseling: a practice management perspective. *Chest.* 2006; 130:1231–1233. [PMID: 17035460]

Theobald M, Jaén CR. An update on tobacco cessation reimbursement. *Fam Practice Manage.* 2006; 13:75–78. [PMID: 16736908]

Patients at the Precontemplation Stage of Quitting

For patients who are currently unwilling to make a quit attempt, clinicians should present a brief motivation intervention structured around the "5 Rs":

1. *Relevance*—make tobacco cessation personally relevant (personal medical history, family composition).
2. *Risk*—review the negative effects of quitting (include both immediate- and long-term risks).
3. *Rewards*—identify the benefits of quitting (improved sense of taste and smell, personal sense of accomplishment, money saved, and health benefits).
4. *Roadblocks*—identify perceived barriers to quitting and ways of overcoming these impediments (symptoms of withdrawal, weight gain, lack of social supports).
5. *Repetition*—repeat this intervention at all office visits.

Relapse

Although risk of relapse is greatest immediately following the quit attempt, it can occur months or even years following cessation. Because tobacco use status will be systematically determined for all patients at each visit, physicians should encourage all former tobacco users to remain abstinent and to express specific concerns or difficulties. Approaches can include reassurance, motivational counseling, extended pharmacotherapy, recommendations for exercise, or referral to supportive or behavioral therapy.

Future Approaches to Cessation

As a potent CNS modulator, nicotine stimulates various physiologic and behavioral effects through the release of various neurotransmitters. To date, therapeutic approaches to smoking cessation have tended to focus on nicotinic acetylcholine receptors, which modulate the release of dopamine and other signaling substances, via use of nicotine replacement therapy or varenicline. In contrast, the mechanism of action for bupropion is poorly understood.

At the present time no new FDA-approved therapies are anticipated to become available for the next 5–7 years. Studies examining the use of a nicotine vaccine did not yield anticipated results. Also, cannabinoid receptor agonist agents as a potential cessation therapy have been abandoned because of unacceptable side effects. Potential candidate products for cessation therapy are focusing on central nervous neurotransmitter systems involving the actions of glutamate and GABA (γ-aminobutyric acid), as well as antagonists for selective glycine receptors, and NMDA (*N*-methyl-D-aspartate) receptors.

Additional research is examining treatment matching based on smoker genotype and phenotype information, combination therapy, and modified administration schedules in an effort to enhance the efficacy of currently available pharmacotherapies.

Henningfield JE, et al. Pharmacotherapy for nicotine dependence. *CA Cancer J Clin.* 2005; 55:281. [PMID: 16166074]
Pidoplichko VI, et al. Nicotine activates and desensitizes midbrain dopamine neurons. *Nature.* 1997; 390:401–404.

► Summary

Nicotine dependence should be considered a chronic health condition with exacerbations and remissions. Identification of smokers and provision of pharmacotherapy to support a quit attempt (with nicotine replacment, bupropion, or varenicline) can increase quit rates by 1.5–3-fold compared to placebo.

Each clinical encounter should include *asking* about tobacco use and *acting* to provide office-based or off-site counseling, as well as arranging linkages to quit lines, print and Internet-based educational materials, community-based cessation classes, and access to pharmacotherapy.

Smoking cessation treatments delivered by clinicians, whether physicians or nonphysicians (eg, psychologist, nurse, dentist, or counselor), can increase abstinence. Therefore, all members of the healthcare system should be empowered to provide smoking cessation interventions. Finally, it is important to emphasize that the combination of pharmacotherapy and behavioral counseling for each smoker will help to maximize the likelihood of achieving long-term abstinence.

Interpersonal Violence

Amy Crawford-Faucher, MD, FAAFP
Lovie J. Jackson-Foster, PhD, MSW

General Considerations

Family physicians must maintain a high index of suspicion for interpersonal violence in their patients. Despite growing public awareness, community advocacy, and education about this endemic public health problem, victims of interpersonal violence may be difficult to detect in the healthcare setting. Shame, fear, self-blame, and other cultural and social factors may limit the manner and nature of presentation and disclosure to the physician. Despite these challenges, the family physician is in a unique position to make a meaningful impact and potentially intervene before violence escalates.

Interpersonal violence includes the following:

- Emotional/psychological abuse.
- Financial abuse.
- Neglect (of dependent person).
- Physical violence.
- Sexual violence.
- Stalking, bullying, or cyberbullying/electronic aggression.
- Homicide.

Those at greatest risk for violence are children, the elderly, pregnant women, persons who are physically or mentally challenged, immigrants, members of racial or cultural minorities, and sexual minorities.

Definitions

Emotional/psychological abuse includes humiliation, controlling behavior, repeated verbal assaults (name-calling), isolation (rejection, withholding attention and affection), threats, and public harassment; all of which can produce psychological trauma that reduces a person's self-worth perception, value, and sense of efficacy. Emotional/ psychological violence often coexists with chronic physical or sexual violence, but can also stand alone.

Financial abuse is when a person withholds resources such as money or transportation, or limits freedom of movement or association (eg, domination, isolation) of another person—a tactic often found in abusive relationships. Financial abuse most often involves the inappropriate transfer or use of an elder's funds for the caregiver's purposes.

Neglect is the chronic failure of a person who is responsible for the physical and emotional needs of another person to provide for those needs. This form of abuse most often occurs in family relationships and is directed at children, elders, or disabled family members. However, caregivers in other social/community settings, including child and adult daycare, schools, group homes, nursing facilities, and hospitals, may be involved in neglect of a dependent person.

Physical violence, as defined by the Centers for Disease Control and Prevention (CDC), is the "intentional use of physical force with the potential for causing death, disability, injury, or harm." This includes, but is not limited to scratching, pushing, shoving, throwing, grabbing, biting, choking, shaking, slapping, punching, or burning; or use of a weapon, and use of restraints or one's body, size, or strength against another person. In the most extreme cases, physical violence may involve *homicide*.

Sexual violence, according to the CDC, is defined as "any sexual act that is perpetrated against someone's will." Sexual violence may include a completed nonconsensual sex act (ie, rape), an attempted nonconsensual sex act, abusive sexual contact (ie, unwanted touching), and noncontact sexual abuse (eg, threatened sexual violence, exhibitionism, verbal sexual harassment). It includes the following four types:

- "**A** *completed sex act* is defined as contact between the penis and the vulva or the penis and the anus involving penetration, however slight; contact between the mouth and penis, vulva, or anus; or penetration of the anal or genital opening of another person by a hand, finger, or other object."

- "*An attempted (but not completed) sex act.*"
- "*Abusive sexual contact* is defined as intentional touching, either directly or through the clothing, of the genitalia, anus, groin, breast, inner thigh, or buttocks of any person without his or her consent, or of a person who is unable to consent or refuse."
- "*Noncontact sexual abuse* does not include physical contact of a sexual nature between the perpetrator and the victim. It includes acts such as voyeurism; intentional exposure of an individual to exhibitionism; unwanted exposure to pornography; verbal or behavioral sexual harassment; threats of sexual violence to accomplish some other end; or taking nude photographs of a sexual nature of another person without his or her consent or knowledge, or of a person who is unable to consent or refuse."

Stalking, bullying, or *cyberbullying/electronic aggression* may involve harassment, threats, or physical violence and can lead to emotional or physical injury, or death. The CDC defines *stalking* as repeatedly following a person; appearing at a person's home or place of business; making harassing phone calls or leaving objects or written, text, or internet messages; or vandalizing a person's property. *Bullying* can include spreading rumors, teasing, imposed social isolation, and influencing others to "gang up" on someone. These acts can occur in person or through increasingly popular forms such as cyberbullying or electronic aggression—using cell phones, computers, and other electronic devices or the Internet. Cyberbullying occurs through email, chat rooms, instant messaging, websites, videos or photos that may be posted on websites, or sent through cell phones.

> Centers for Disease Control and Prevention fact sheet on interpersonal violence: http://www.cdc.gov/ViolencePrevention/intimatepartnerviolence/definitions.html

▶ Epidemiology

The prevalence of abuse and neglect vary with different populations. In general, young children and pregnant women are at highest risk of death from abuse. Child maltreatment is also more prevalent among racial/ethnic minority children whose families experience the highest levels of poverty.

A. Children

In the United States in 2011, there were >675,000 reported child victims of abuse and neglect. While this rate of 9.1 victims per 1000 children has decreased slightly from 2010, it likely also significantly underestimates the true prevalence of child maltreatment. Of these reported cases

- 78.5% of victims suffered neglect.
- 17.6% suffered physical abuse.
- 9.1% suffered sexual abuse.
- 8% suffered emotional abuse.

Childhood victimization is often a precursor to adult victimization—42% of female rapes and 18% of male rapes occur at or before age 10. In 2010 approximately 1560 children died as a result of abuse or neglect; almost 80% of the deaths occurred in children aged <4 years. The victimization rate is highest for children aged <1 year. Girls are maltreated at a slightly higher rate than are boys (9.7 vs 8.7 per 1000), but maltreatment-related deaths are higher for boys than girls (2.5 vs 1.7 per 100,000). African American children experience the highest rates of maltreatment and related death, followed by American Indian/Alaska Natives. Sadly, the vast majority of perpetrators of child abuse are parents (81.2%).

Bullying is a major public health problem among school-age children. Of a nationally representative sample, 13% reported being a bully, 11% reported being a victim of bullying, and 6% reported being both a bully and a victim. Boys are more likely to participate in physical aggression, while girls are more likely to engage in verbal aggression. Adolescents who bully are more likely to have other defiant or delinquent behaviors, while victims are more likely to have depression, anxiety, and isolation. Bullying is now a major risk factor for suicide among adolescents, with higher rates of bullying-related suicides among girls and youths who are both bully and victim of bullying. The emotional and behavioral problems associated with bullies and victims can continue into adulthood with long-term negative consequences.

B. Adults

Intimate partner violence is pervasive in the United States, where approximately 24 people per minute are victimized. This amounts to <12 million women and men. Women are at increased risk of violent victimization by an intimate partner (or stranger). A 2010 CDC survey found that

- 1.3 million women were raped in the previous year.
- The lifetime risk for rape is about 1 in 5 women and 1 in 71 men.
- Severe physical assault by an intimate partner occurs in 1 in 4 women and 1 in 7 men.
- 1 in 6 women and 1 in 19 men are victims of stalking.

Women are commonly victims of multiple forms of intimate partner violence, while men are more likely to experience physical violence alone. Stemming from these experiences are a host of co-occurring physical and mental health problems such as headaches, chronic pain, sleep difficulties, fear, and other symptoms related to posttraumatic stress disorder (PTSD, eg, anxiety, flashbacks and nightmares, exaggerated startle response).

C. The Elderly

Elder abuse, like other forms of IPV, most often occurs in the context of the family. The primary perpetrators are spouses or companions or adult children or other family members who inflict physical, emotional/psychological, sexual, or financial abuse, and neglect. While the most recent estimate of elder abuse found that 14.1% of older adults in the general population experienced these forms of interpersonal violence, the US Government Accountability Office suggests that existing research underestimates the true prevalence of elder abuse. The National Center on Elder Abuse reports that older women are more likely than younger women to experience a longer period of violent victimization, to currently be in violent relationships, and to experience related health and mental health problems.

D. Persons with Disabilities

People with disabilities, including those with cognitive, hearing, vision, ambulatory, self-care, and independent-living deficits are at higher risk for all types of abuse than are those without disabilities. At 48 per 1000, the rate of violence against those with disabilities is more than twice the rate for those who do not have disabilities (19 per 1000). Additionally, the rate of victimization increases for those with multiple disabilities.

- For 2011, the average age-adjusted (for 12 years–adult) rate of violent crime against those with a single disability type was 38 per 1000.
- For 2011, the average age-adjusted (for 12 years–adult) rate of violent crime against those with multiple disability types was 61 per 1000.

Cognitively disabled individuals are at the highest risk for victimization compared to all other disabilities.

E. Lesbian, Gay, Bisexual, Transgender (LGBT) Community

The national prevalence of intimate partner violence against lesbian, gay, and bisexual men and women has not been well studied to date; the National Intimate Partner and Sexual Violence Survey (NISVS) started reporting data from 2010 and is ongoing. NISVS found that

- Bisexual women have a significantly lifetime prevalence of rape and nonrape sexual violence by any perpetrator than do lesbian or heterosexual women.
  - Rape: 13.1% of lesbian women, 46.1% of bisexual women, 17.4% heterosexual women.

  - Other sexual violence: 46.4% lesbian women, 74.9% bisexual women, 43.3% heterosexual women.
- Bisexual women have a significantly higher lifetime prevalence of rape, physical violence, or stalking by an intimate partner compared to lesbian or heterosexual women.
- While the prevalence of rape in men could not be estimated from the survey, the prevalence of nonrape sexual violence was higher for gay men (40.2%) and bisexual men (47.4%) compared to that for heterosexual men (20.8%).

Black MC, Basile KC, Breiding MJ, et al. *The National Intimate Partner and Sexual Violence Survey (NISVS): 2010 Summary Report*. Atlanta, GA: National Center for Injury Prevention and Control, Centers for Disease Control and Prevention; 2011.

CDC National Center for Injury Prevention and Control. *Child Maltreatment Facts at a Glance*. 2012.

Cooper GD, Clements PT, Holt KE. Examining childhood bullying and adolescent suicide: implications for school nurses. *J School Nurs*. 2012; 28(4):275–283.

Hamburger ME, Basile KC, Vivolo AM. *Measuring Bullying Victimization, Perpetration, and Bystander Experiences: A Compendium of assessment Tools*. Atlanta, GA: Centers for Disease Control and Prevention, National Center for Injury Prevention and Control; 2011.

Harrell E. *Crime against Persons with Disabilities, 2009-2011— Statistical Tables*. NCJ240299; Dec. 2012 (available from http://bjs.gov/index.cfm?ty=pbdetail&iid=4574).

National Center on Elder Abuse. *Fact Sheet: Domestic Violence: Older Women Can Be Victims Too*. NCEA; 2005 (available from http://www.ct.gov/agingservices/lib/agingservices/pdf/olderwomen2-columnfinal10-11-05.pdf).

US Department of Health and Human Services, Administration for Children and Families, Administration on Children, Youth and Families, Children's Bureau. *Child Maltreatment 2011*. Washington, DC: DHHS; 2012 (available from http://www.acf.hhs.gov/programs/cb/research-data-technology/statistics-research/child-maltreatment).

US Government Accountability Office. (2011). *Elder Justice: Stronger Federal Leadership Could Enhance National Response to Elder Abuse*. Washington, DC: USGAO; 2011 (available from http://www.gao.gov/products/GAO-11-208

Walters ML, Chen J, Breiding MJ. *The National Intimate Partner and Sexual Violence Survey (NISVS): 2010 Findings on Victimization by Sexual Orientation*. Atlanta, GA: National Center for Injury Prevention and Control, Centers for Disease Control and Prevention; 2013.

NATURAL HISTORY OF INTERPERSONAL VIOLENCE IN ADULTS

Interpersonal violence among known partners occurs in cycles, and similar cycles happen with elder abuse, child abuse, and sexual predatory behavior. Violence generally escalates; with each cycle the victim is exposed to additional risk.

Detection & Intervention

Refer to Chapter 42 for more detailed information about abuse in the elderly.

A. Adults

1. Identification and screening—Victims of abuse often feel ashamed, have low self-esteem, or are unable or afraid to share their circumstances readily Creating an atmosphere that promotes a welcoming, frank, and professional discussion will allow patients the opportunity to bring their concerns forward to the physician. Actively listening, making eye contact, and giving full attention to the patient may facilitate more openness and trust between providers and at-risk patients.

The US Preventive Services Task Force (USPSTF) recently published updated guidelines on screening for intimate partner violence, giving a B recommendation (high certainty that the net benefit is moderate or moderate certainty that the net benefit is moderate to substantial) for screening asymptomatic women of childbearing age. The USPSTF recognized several validated screening tools that could identify past and current abuse or risk of future abuse (**Table 62-1**). It also found adequate evidence that effective interventions reduce violence, abuse, and physical or mental harm in this population. The USPSTF continues its "I" recommendation for screening and intervention in other groups, including the elderly and vulnerable adults, because of lack of adequate studies determining risks and benefits. (The I recommendation indicates that current evidence is insufficient to assess the balance of benefits and harms of the service; that evidence is lacking, of poor quality, or conflicting, and the balance of benefits and harms cannot be determined.) The American Medical Association and American College of Obstetricians and Gynecologists recommend specific direct questioning of patients, when appropriate, in a nonthreatening manner. The policy of the American Academy of Family Physicians regarding family violence can be found at the association's website (http://www.aafp.org/x16506.xml), and advocates that family physicians be alert for risk factors as well as signs of family violence with each

Table 62-1. Screening tests for interpersonal violence with the highest levels of sensitivity and specificity per the USPSTF.

1. Hurt, Insult, Threaten, Scream (HITS)—available in English and Spanish
2. Ongoing Abuse Screen/Ongoing Violence Assessment Tool (OAS/OVAT)
3. Slapped, Threatened, and Throw (STaT)
4. Humiliation, Afraid, Rape, Kick (HARK)
5. Modified Childhood Trauma Questionnaire—Short Form (CTQ-SF)
6. Woman Abuse Screen Tool (WAST)

Table 62-2. Screening questions for interpersonal violence in adults.

1. Do you feel safe in your current relationship?
2. Do you perceive any threats to your safety on a regular basis?
3. Have you been hit or hurt by someone in the past?
4. Would you care to share any concerns you might have regarding interpersonal violence in your home or among your friends?
5. Have you ever been or are you currently concerned about harming your partner or someone close to you?
6. Would you like information about interpersonal violence or substance abuse programs in our community?

patient encounter. Much like screening for alcohol abuse or depression, low-threat questions can be incorporated to ascertain the possibility of abuse in the home situation (**Table 62-2**). The optimal frequency of screening has not been established.

The use of prompts in electronic medical records is an interesting area of development. Certain complexes, complaints, and findings could trigger a reminder for the physician to ask a question about violence in the home or workplace. Much research remains to be done to ascertain the value of such prompting, although there is some research indicating that computerized screening and interventions are acceptable to patients and result in increased discussion and disclosure of abuse and provision of services.

Moyer VA, on behalf of the US Preventive Services Task Force. Screening for intimate partner violence and abuse of elderly and vulnerable adults: US Preventive Services Task Force recommendation statement. *Ann Intern Med.* 2013; 158(6):478-486.

2. Interventions—The abusive spouse, partner, or family member often accompanies the patient to the office visit to monitor the information being shared and the manner in which experiences are being portrayed by the victim. Although it is not abnormal for a spouse or significant other to attend a physician visit, the physician should be alert to cues, including nonverbal behaviors that might signal an abusive situation. In particular, physicians should carefully evaluate situations in which someone else does all the talking for a competent and able patient. If possible, the physician should attempt to interview the patient alone. However, as an abusive individual might revert to controlling behavior in the office or become aggressive, physicians must consider the safety of their staff when confronting such individuals.

Intensive therapy is often required for both the abuser and the victim, and referrals to appropriate resources should be readily available in medical practices. Referral to an appropriate safe house in the community and information on how to obtain a personal protective order from a judge can be important for the safety of the victim, and the patient should be encouraged to take these steps, if appropriate. Domestic violence programs can help victims follow through with these initial steps. During this period, therapy for the victim is aimed at improving objective decision making, reestablishing self-esteem, reversing the cycle of self-blaming, and addressing the reality of the situation. The abuser also requires therapy. Depending on the circumstance, this may occur in the penal system or be mandated by the courts to take place in a child welfare agency. Therapy is aimed at reordering the emotional responses of the abuser and improving self-esteem. Developing a new worldview and set of behaviors is very difficult and takes a great deal of effort on the part of the therapist and the abuser.

It is critical that the family physician be supportive of the therapist and encourage the patient to continue in therapy. "Relapse" rates (ie, returning to the abusive relationship) are high; physicians should not become judgmental about such reconciliations but rather should remain supportive of victims.

B. Children

1. Identification and screening—Emergency physicians and pediatricians advocate for specific and direct questioning about childhood injuries to determine their cause. Direct questioning of parents/caregivers should be done in private to maximize value, maintain confidence, and reassure family members of the physician's intent to help, not hurt, the child or the family. This may require or be best facilitated by a multidisciplinary team trained to assess and report child abuse, neglect, or other forms of child victimization.

There are specific cues that should heighten the physician's index of suspicion regarding domestic violence and child abuse. "Red flags" should be raised when

- One partner insists on accompanying the other parent and child, and speaks for them.
- A parent is reluctant to talk with the other partner present.
- The child's history does not fit the injury or illness.
- A parent makes frequent appointments for vague, poorly defined complaints.
- A child has recurrent, medically unexplainable somatic problems [eg, failure to thrive, abdominal or genital pain or injuries, headaches, enuresis (wetting), encopresis (fecal soiling), problems eating or sleeping].
- Medical attention for injuries is sought later than would be expected.
- The family uses emergency department services more often than is usual.
- A parent attempts to hide the child's injuries with clothing.
- A parent or child has several injuries, at various stages of healing.

Additional red flags are outlined at http://childabuse. stanford.edu/screening/signs.html (accessed April 29, 2013); see also http://www.iowaepsdt.org/EPSDTNews/2000/sum00/guide.htm (accessed April 29, 2013).

Family physicians should be alert to the symptoms and signs of potential child abuse or neglect listed in **Table 62-3**.

It is also important to recognize that children may have interpersonal violence experiences other than child abuse or neglect by family members that can manifest in similar ways in terms of physical or mental health and functional impairments. These include sexual exploitation; witnessing

Table 62-3. Symptoms and signs of potential abuse and neglect in children.

Physical Abuse	Neglect	Emotional Abuse	Sexual Abuse
Burns	Malnutrition	Self-injury	Self-injury
School problems	Lack of supervision	Anger	Inappropriate sexuality for age/seductiveness
Self-destructive or suicidal behavior	Poor dental hygiene	Depression	Genital swelling, bruises, bleeding, sexually transmitted infections, yeast or urinary tract infections, pregnancy
Unexplained cuts, bruises, or welts	Inappropriate clothing	Apathy	Poor hygiene
Inappropriate fear of adults	Poor hygiene	Eating disorders	Eating disorders
Early-onset depression, alcohol or drug use	Extreme hunger	Anxiety	Sleep disorders
Bruises in the shape of objects		Anger	Excessive aggression
Injuries in uncommon locations			Fear of a particular person
Bite marks			Withdrawal
			Suicidal behavior

violence in their communities (eg, shootings, stabbings); bullying at or after school by peers, older children, or adults; and cyberbullying or electronic aggression, which is on the rise with the growth of electronic communication devices, proliferation of social media, and barriers to parental monitoring of children's access and exposure to electronic media.

2. Interventions—There is a need to strengthen the evidence base for primary care interventions addressing child maltreatment. Models of care that provide the best opportunities for prevention of child abuse and neglect in healthcare settings are those that involve a multidisciplinary team with a social worker, nurse, developmental specialist, or other staff member who can help families access resources to meet basic needs; caregivers screening for child maltreatment risk factors (eg, depression, IPV); and are brief and inexpensive. Although few interventions of this type exist and have been tested, these factors should be considered as many practices shift to a medical home or collaborative care approach. In practices that do not yet have provisions for integrated care, ensuring that all healthcare providers understand the necessity of addressing child abuse and neglect, and the mandate to report, is the bare minimum (see section on reporting later in this chapter). Family medicine practices that provide families with information on resources and opportunities to learn about healthy child development, healthy coping and stress reduction, and mental health prevention for children and caregivers may be aiding in the prevention of child abuse and neglect.

Dubowitz H, Feigelman S, Lane W, et al. Pediatric primary care to help prevent child maltreatment: The Safe Environment for Every Kid (SEEK) model. *Pediatrics*. 2009; 123:858–864.

Zuckerman B, Parker S, Kaplan-Sanoff M, et al. Healthy steps: a case study of innovation in pediatric practice. *Pediatrics*. 2004; 114(3):820–826.

C. Special Populations

Recent immigrants; ethnic and racial minorities; homeless people; people with disabilities; and lesbian, gay, bisexual, and transgendered (LGBT) persons may have additional challenges in gaining access to and communicating with their physicians. The USPSTF recognized that abuse in these populations is understudied. A wide range of social factors may contribute to underreporting of abuse in same-sex relationships. Gay, lesbian, bisexual, and transgendered patients should be questioned, as all patients are, in a safe environment and in a nonthreatening manner. For additional discussion of LGBT issues, see Chapter 66.

Followers of some religious and cultural traditions may tolerate levels of behavior that are not accepted by the mainstream culture in the United States. The norms of acceptable or expected behaviors, including the sharing of intimate family details, child-rearing practices, discussion of mental health issues, and sexuality concerns, create additional challenges for the physician to discover abusive relationships. Understanding cultural influences is key to identifying abuse in these situations. Access to an advocate who has proper training and connection with the culture can be extremely helpful. This person may also play an important role in supporting the patient's decision making when seeking appropriate interventions.

Open-ended questions about a patient's cultural norms may provide an appropriate avenue and manner for inquiry into the presence or absence of interpersonal violence in the patient's life. Lack of trust in law enforcement may be a specific challenge in poor minority communities and among the homeless. The stigma associated with interpersonal violence may inhibit reporting or seeking of assistance. Additional information can be obtained from specific resources such as the University of Michigan Program for Multicultural Health, available at http://www.med.umich.edu/multicultural/ccp/cdv.htm. A resource for the African American community is available at http://www.dvinstitute.org, and for the American Indian or Alaska Native community, is http://www.tribal-institute.org/lists/domestic.htm.

▶ Prevention

Primary prevention of interpersonal violence is critically important in addressing this problem. The effectiveness of prevention programs remains an ongoing topic of study.

Family physicians should consider a routine discussion of interpersonal violence as part of the normal health maintenance routine. This can be part of the usual discussion of safety issues, including seat belt use, gun safety, and smoke protectors. In a matter-of-fact manner, the physician can introduce the discussion of interpersonal violence in a wide variety of contexts, including well-woman care, well-child visits, routine "physicals," and other health maintenance visits.

A routine discussion of parenting techniques, referral to appropriate parenting classes, and provision of printed information have all been shown to have a positive effect on families at risk for child abuse or neglect. A plan for abuse identification, prevention, and training can be part of the individual education plan and the transition plan for children with developmental and physical disabilities.

Living situations of elderly patients should be well documented and understood, especially if the caregivers are not well known or are not part of the physician's personal practice. Information obtained and communication established during calm, uneventful times may be useful later should an incident occur.

▶ Safety Instructions for Patients

The American Bar Association provides a domestic violence safety plan on its website at http://www.abanet.org/

tips/dvsafety.html. Adult patients can be referred to this resource for updated recommendations on how to protect themselves in situations in which interpersonal violence is an imminent threat. Family physicians should also be aware of local resources and update contacts with them annually to ensure a readily available system of referral for safe houses, therapeutic care or social services, and legal intervention. Although these options vary from community to community, local resources can usually provide assistance to physicians when dealing with complicated cases.

▶ Reporting

Healthcare providers should familiarize themselves with the laws of their state regarding the required reporting of violent crimes. In general, acts of violence that involve lethal force or firearms and rape must be reported to the local police agency. Complete documentation of all encounter details—including quotations, details, and time requirements—is an important medicolegal requirement. Family physicians working in emergency departments should follow the policies and procedures of their institution in the management and reporting of such violent crimes.

The reporting of an individual's confidentially expressed intent to harm another person places the physician in a far more difficult ethical and legal position that may require legal advice. In emergencies, particularly when a patient is believed to be in danger, the patient should be told to call 911.

The reporting of child abuse to Child Protective Services is a requirement in all 50 states. Some states require reporting to the local police agency as well. It is important for physicians to know the laws in their state, as reporting requirements and processes vary. (see Child Information Gateway website, listed at end of this chapter). To aid a physician's understanding and ease any anxiety associated with reporting, physicians should learn the process for reporting in their county or state and what happens after child victimization is reported to Child Protective Services.

Elder abuse is also covered by state laws, and physicians should report in accordance with the local law at the time of the suspected abuse. In general, Adult Protective Services (APS) should be notified of suspected neglect or abuse. Other agencies that may require notification, depending on the state, include the Area Agency on Aging and the County Department of Social Services.

Ahmad M, Lachs MS. Elder abuse and neglect: what physicians can and should do. *Cleve Clin J Med.* 2002; 69:801. [PMID: 12371803]

Websites

American Bar Association Commission on Domestic Violence: http://www.abanet.org/domviol/

Child Welfare Information Gateway: http://www.childwelfare.gov/pubs/reslist/rl_dsp.cfm?rs_id=5&rate_chno=11-11172 (for state hotline numbers), http://www.childwelfare.gov/systemwide/laws_policies/state/ (for state-specific policies), and http://www.childwelfare.gov/

Combat-Related Posttraumatic Stress Disorder & Traumatic Brain Injury

Evelyn L. Lewis, MD, MA, FAAFP

Ronald J. Koshes, MD, DFAPA

POSTTRAUMATIC STRESS DISORDER

ESSENTIALS OF DIAGNOSIS

- ▶ Directly experiences the traumatic event.
- ▶ Witnesses the traumatic event in person.
- ▶ Learns that the traumatic event occurred to a close family member or close friend (where the actual or threatened death was violent or accidental)
- ▶ Experiences firsthand repeated or extreme exposure to aversive details of the traumatic event (not through media, pictures, television, or movies unless work-related)

General Considerations

In the newly released *DSM-5* (*Diagnostic and Statistical Manual of Mental Disorders*, 5th edition), posttraumatic stress disorder (PTSD) is classified as a trauma and stressor-related disorder, not a disorder primarily of anxiety alone. The criterion for the diagnosis conceptualizes trauma as the precipitating event where the person experiences, witnesses, or is confronted with an event or events that threaten death or serious injury or posed a threat to the physical integrity of self or others, and the person's response must have involved fear, helplessness, or horror. The events are beyond the realm of usual and normal human experience and include traumatic events such as war or the Holocaust; natural disasters such as earthquakes and tsunamis, hurricanes, and volcanic eruptions; and anthropogenic disasters, including factory explosions, automobile crashes, and airplane crashes. Critical to understanding the diagnosis is the idea that the cause of the illness was a traumatic event that

occurred outside of the individual and was not due to an inherent character or personality weakness of that person.

While this condition has likely existed since human beings have endured trauma, PTSD entered the medical diagnostic realm with the publication of the *Diagnostic and Statistical Manual of Mental Disorders*, third edition (*DSM-III*) in 1980. It was first brought to public attention in relation to war veterans and, depending on the name of the war, has been known by a number of different terms to include combat fatigue, gross stress reaction, post-Vietnam syndrome, shell shock, and battle fatigue. Currently, PTSD is described as a disorder of persistent reactivity in all areas of self-regulation, not just troubling memories and chronic anxiety. Distressing memories of past traumatic events and intense stress reactions to reminders of those events that occur in the person's current life continue to serve as the cornerstone of PTSD.

Essentially, the brain is a control system that regulates the body functions. Trauma forces the brain to make profound biological adaptations in how it operates. When the body is safe and working well, the brain extends its efforts to the "higher" functions that enable you to not only survive but also become a conscious individual. However, when the brain detects serious threats to body survival, traumatic stressors such as severe accidents, disasters, violence, abuse, or betrayals, the alarm system in the brain is activated and takes control of the rest of the brain's operations, putting all systems in emergency mode until the threat is overcome. In most cases, with nontraumatic threats as well as traumatic survival threats, the alarm reaction in the brain quickly subsides and resets automatically to its normal mode. However, when the brain's alarm system doesn't automatically or rapidly reset itself and alarm continues to signal danger, even though safety has been restored (ie, the person is no longer engaged in combat), the overall functioning remains in an altered state that is the chronic stress response.

Posttraumatic stress disorder and traumatic brain injury (TBI) are the largest represented diagnoses from the wars in Iraq and Afghanistan. Understanding the diagnosis and treatment of these conditions is important for healthcare providers, many of whom may not have experience with war casualties, in either civilian or military settings. Many obstacles to the timely and proper diagnosis and treatment are present in this population of veterans, including the overlap of symptoms present in both conditions as well as cultural factors in eliciting a diagnosis. Family practice physicians, both military and civilian, are likely to encounter PTSD patients in their practices, and a knowledge of military culture, traditions, and knowledge of war-related injuries and illnesses is important to master.

TRAUMATIC BRAIN INJURY (TBI)

Various forms of traumatic brain injury have been described, and all can be understood by the injury caused when the brain is moved violently within its usual protected and physiologically stable environment. TBI was first described in antiquity. It can be divided into several categories, as listed in **Table 63-1**.

Additionally, an important characteristic of TBI is the cumulative nature of the injury. In the recent wars in Iraq and Afghanistan, blast injuries played a major role in the development of TBI. Service members were exposed to blast injuries from mortars and improvised explosive device (IED) explosions, and some have sustained at many as 5–10 blasts. While some blast injuries do not result in loss of consciousness, other TBI victims experience nausea and vomiting, are dazed, and suffer other consequences of a concussion. The simplest way to understand this type of cumulative injury is to compare it to the damage produced from repetitive boxing injuries to the head.

Most cases of mild TBI improve with time, but more sophisticated testing indicates that although performance on neuropsychological testing is not abnormal, pathophysiologic and anatomic damage is created, which may result in deficits in cognitive functioning in later years. The actual mechanism of damage from the TBI is multifactorial and probably includes one of the following mechanisms:

- Focal injury
- Diffuse axonal injury
- Superimposed hypoxia or ischemia
- Diffuse microvascular injury with loss of autoregulation

These mechanisms are described in more detail in **Table 63-2**.

Treatments that have been used to date include those that ameliorate and reverse the damage caused by the mechanisms listed above (see also **Table 63-3**). Some agents are described below.

Additionally complicating the diagnosis is the sense that the individual may not believe that there is an illness or

Table 63-1. Traumatic brain injury (TBI).

Mild TBI
Impairment in sustained attention, delayed memory, and impaired ability to process multiple items of information simultaneously
Delayed symptoms: memory difficulties, concentration, fatigue, insomnia, irritability, noise sensitivity, and depression
Moderate to severe TBI
Coma
Agitation, restlessness, overreaction to stimuli, combativeness, rambling and incoherent speech, hallucinations
Confabulations, denial, environmental and temporal disorientation, misidentification, delusions, mood changes, reduplication syndrome
Anosognosia—denial of illness, specifically memory loss

Table 63-2. Anatomic and physiologic changes following traumatic brain injury.

Focal injury
Orbitofrontal and anterior temporal lobes (where brain lies next to bony edges)
Swelling contusion, or hematomas
Sequellae: attentional, memory, and behavioral abnormalities
Diffuse axonal injury
Axonal shearing may, in fact, be axonal retraction
Alterations in calcium metabolism may be delayed 12–24 hours, making early intervention critical
Hypoxia ischemia
Hippocampus and vascular border zones of brain are particularly susceptible.
Microvascular changes
Cerebrovascular autoregulation disruption related to CO_2, hypertension (catecholemines)
Endothelium-derived relaxing factor (EDRF), or nitrous oxide increasing brain blood flow
Superoxide radical formation causing microvascular constriction
Secondary tissue changes: cascade of biochemical and physiological events
Arachidonic acid metabolites such as prostaglandins, leukotrienes
Formation of oxygen free radicals
Neuropeptide changes
Calcium and magnesium alterations
Neurotransmitter changes: acetylcholine and glutamate
Lactic acid formation
Kinin formation
Leukocyte response with release of lymphokines such as interleukin-1
Oxygen free radicals
Formed normally through mitochondrial respiration
Enhanced by leukocyte activation, and arachidonic acid after trauma or ischemia
Combined with its own metabolite, hydrogen peroxide, it forms the hydroxyl radical and causes lipid peroxidation

Table 63-3. Pharmacologic interventions.

Vitamin E
Cyclooxygenase inhibitors to block prostaglandin formation
Xanthine oxidase inhibitors such as allopurinol
Iron chelators
Superoxide dismutase (50% decrease in mortality in severely head-injured patients treated with SOD)
Other free-radical scavengers such as mannitol and dimethyl sulfoxide
Steroids

injury; this impaired perception of illness is termed *anosognosia*. The deficits may be quite apparent to others in the social and occupational circle of the injured, and these other people should be routinely questioned about functioning. Writing in the *Textbook of Military Medicine*, Dr. Edwin Weinsten, a neurologist who treated World War II veterans, noted: "Caution should be exercised in sending patients with a great deal of denial back to duty or accepting their statements about their condition at face value."

His advice was prophetic and portended the difficulties that practitioners face in dealing with TBI.

Moreover, some cultural factors may impede admission of blast exposures and actual deficits in cognitive functioning. For example, service members may not want to be removed from battle for evaluation and are likely to continue serving with their units and not disrupt the unit stability during combat. Returning Veterans may be loathe to admit a disability as they try to re-adjust to family life and continued service or a civilian life. Some helpful website are listed here:

http://www.ptsd.va.gov/professional/pages/diagnostic_criteria_dsm-5.asp
www.dsm5.org
http://www.psychologytoday.com/blog/hijacked-your-brain/201306/ptsd-becomes-more-complex-in-the-dsm-5-part-1

Prevalence

The rates of PTSD after trauma or disaster have shown considerable variation. The lifetime prevalence of PTSD is 7–30%, and affects approximately 5–7.7 million American adults in any one year. For example, in instances where the trauma is more severe, where it has less meaning, where people believe that they have carried out acts of commission or omission and blame themselves for the trauma, or where they believe others have "let the side down," as in problems of friendly fire, rates are noted to be higher.

High rates of PTSD in veterans can be found regardless of which conflict is examined. In fact, as noted previously, the diagnosis of PTSD historically originates from observations of the effect of combat on soldiers. Rates of PTSD in Vietnam veterans, Persian Gulf War veterans, and Iraq War veterans are provided below.

Vietnam Veterans

Following a congressional mandate in 1983, the US government conducted the National Vietnam Veterans Readjustment Study (NVVRS) to better understand the psychological effects of participating in the Vietnam War. While approximately 15% of men and 9% of women were found to have PTSD at the time of the study, approximately 30% of men and 27% of women had PTSD at some point in their lives following Vietnam. As one might suspect, these rates were much higher than those found among non-Vietnam veterans and civilians. The rates are alarming since they indicate that at the time of the study, there were approximately 479,000 cases of PTSD and 1 million lifetime PTSD cases as a result of the Vietnam War.

Persian Gulf War

Studies examining the mental health of Persian Gulf War veterans found that rates of PTSD ranged anywhere from almost 9% to approximately 24%. Although the Persian Gulf War was brief, the rates of PTSD were higher than what was found among veterans not deployed to the Persian Gulf. In addition, veterans have reported significant numbers of physical health problems.

Iraq War and Afghanistan

Although the war in Iraq has somewhat subsided, the conflict in Afghanistan is ongoing. Therefore the full the impact on the mental and behavioral health of US soldiers is not yet known. However, the results of one study were obtained for members of four United States combat infantry units (three army and one marine) that served in Iraq and Afghanistan. The majority of soldiers were exposed to some kind of traumatic, combat-related situations, such as being attacked or ambushed (92%), seeking dead bodies (94.5%), being shot at (95%), and/or knowing someone who was seriously injured or killed (86.5%). After deployment, approximately 12.5% had PTSD, a rate greater than that found among these soldiers before deployment.

PTSD Risk

Posttraumatic stress disorder can occur in people of all ages. However, some factors more than others render a person more prone to develop PTSD after a traumatic event:

- Experiencing other types of trauma, particularly early in life
- Being female
- Experiencing intense or longlasting trauma
- Having other mental health problems, such as anxiety or depression

- Lacking a good support system of family and friends
- First-degree relatives with mental health problems, including PTSD
- First-degree relatives with depression
- Childhood neglect and physical abuse

Women are at a twofold increase risk of PTSD because they are more likely to have experienced the types of trauma that trigger the condition. This gender difference is due primarily to a women's greater vulnerability to PTSD following events that involved sexually assaultive violence. The probability of PTSD in women versus men exposed to assaultive violence was 36% versus 6%.

Risk factors for military personnel developing PTSD include combat experience, being wounded, witnessing death, serving on graves registration duty or handling human remains, being captured or tortured, being exposed to unpredictable and uncontrollable stress, and experiencing sexual harassment or assault. Higher rates of PTSD and depression are associated with longer deployments, multiple deployments, and greater time away from base camp. Car and suicide bombs, improvised explosive devices (IEDs), and rocket-propelled grenades—all elements of the recent Iraq and Afghanistan conflicts—can exacerbate the intense stress of combat.

Ethnic minorities (African Americans, Hispanics, and Native Americans) are more likely to develop the disorder than men, boys, and Caucasians, and there is some evidence that it may run in families. Some of that difference is attributed to higher rates of dissociation soon before and after the traumatic event (peritraumatic), a tendency for ethnic minorities to harbor self blame, less social support, and an increased perception of racial prejudice, as well as differences in how ethnic minorities may express distress. Roughly 30% of Vietnam veterans developed PTSD. The disorder also has been detected in as many as 10% of Gulf War (Desert Storm) veterans, ~6–11% of veterans of the Afghanistan war, and 12–20% of veterans of the Iraq war.

American Academy of Child and Adolescent Psychiatry. *Child and Adolescent Mental Health Statistics Resources for Families.* AACAP; 2007.
http://www.medicinenet.com/posttraumatic_stress_disorder.
Loo CM. *PTSD among Ethnic Minority Veterans.* National Center for PTSD; 2007.
Perilla JL, Norris FH, et al. Ethnicity, culture and disaster response: identifying and explaining ethnic differences in PTSD six months after hurricane Andrew. *J Soc Clin Psychol.* 2002;21(1):20–45.

▶ Potential Preventive Interventions

Prevention of PTSD can potentially reduce a significant burden of individual and societal suffering. Potential preventive interventions span various psychological and pharmacological domains and include emerging interventions from complementary and alternative medicine (CAM). These interventions have been used both separately and in combination with one another. Specific psychological interventions that have been studied for the prevention of adult PTSD and include the following:

- Psychological debriefing interventions
- Critical incident stress debriefing (CISD)
- Critical incident stress management (CISM)
- Psychological first aid (PFA)
- Trauma-focused cognitive behavioral therapy (CBT)
- Cognitive restructuring therapy
- Cognitive processing therapy
- Exposure-based therapies
- Coping skills therapy (including stress inoculation therapy)
- Psychoeducation
- Normalization
- Eye movement desensitization and reprocessing (EMDR).

These therapies are designed to prevent the onset of PTSD and development of trauma-related stress symptoms soon after exposure to a traumatic event.

Various neurobiological pathways have been implicated in the development of PTSD. Consequently, pharmacotherapy has been tried as a preventive intervention for PTSD. Several drugs have been studied for PTSD prevention, including propranolol, morphine, glucocorticoids, and selective serotonin reuptake inhibitors (SSRIs). These therapies are designed to prevent the onset of PTSD and development of trauma-related stress symptoms soon after exposure to a traumatic event.

Fletcher S, Creamer M, Forbes D. Preventing post traumatic stress disorder: are drugs the answer? *Austra; NZ J Psychiatr.* 2010;44(12):1064–1071. [PMID: 21080102]
http://effectivehealthcare.ahrq.gov/search-for-guides-reviews-and-reports/?pageaction=displayproduct&productID=1444#7302.
O'Donnell ML, Lau W, Tipping S, et al. Stepped early psychological intervention for posttraumatic stress disorder, other anxiety disorders, and depression following serious injury. *J Trauma Stress.* 2012;25(2):125–133. [PMID: 22522725]
Rothbaum BO, Kearns MC, Price M, et al. Early intervention may prevent the development of posttraumatic stress disorder: a randomized pilot civilian study with modified prolonged exposure. *Biol Psychiatr.* 2012;72(11):957–963. [PMID: 22766415]

▶ Clinical Findings

A. Signs and Symptoms—Posttraumatic stress disorder symptoms typically start within 3 months of a traumatic event. However, in a small number of cases, symptoms may not appear until years after the event. The symptoms of PTSD are also known to appear and disappear sporadically. They may be more plentiful or severe when life in general is more stressful, or when reminders of the event are encountered. For example, hearing a car backfire may result in reliving combat experiences, or a news report about a rape may bring back memories of the assault. There are four categories or types of PTSD symptoms:

- **Reexperiencing the events:** Memories of the traumatic event can return at any time (spontaneous memories of the traumatic event, recurrent dreams related to it, flashbacks, or other intense or prolonged psychological distress).

- **Heightened arousal:** You may be anxious, jittery, and constantly on the lookout for danger. Sudden anger or irritability is not uncommon (aggressive, reckless, or self-destructive behavior; sleep disturbances; hypervigilance or related problems).

- **Avoidance:** You attempt to avoid situations, things, or people that bring back memories of the trauma (distressing memories, thoughts, feelings, or external reminders of the event).

- **Negative alterations in thoughts and mood or feelings:** Feelings may vary from a persistent and distorted sense of blame of self or others, to estrangement from others or markedly diminished interest in activities, to an inability to remember key aspects of the event).

In addition to these symptoms, a patient must also meet the following criteria for at least a month:

- At least one recurring symptom
- At least three avoidance symptoms
- At least two hyperarousal symptoms
- Symptoms that make it complicate daily life, going to school or work, social contacts, and performing important tasks.

Even with the assistance of the descriptive symptoms listed above, the assessment of PTSD can often be difficult for practitioners to make since most patients present with complaints other than the anxiety associated with a traumatic experience. Those symptoms tend to include expression of mental conditions as disturbed body functions (somatization), depression, or substance misuse. Most studies of Iraq war veterans tend to display more of the physical symptoms as opposed to describing the associated emotional problems. Many of the cases describe individuals with PTSD who present with a history of suicide attempts, depression, and substance abuse disorders. In addition, the diagnosis of PTSD often occurs comorbidly with bipolar disorder (manic depression), eating disorders, and other anxiety disorders such as obsessive-compulsive disorder (OCD), panic disorders, social anxiety disorder, and generalized anxiety disorder.

www.dsm5.org
www.mayoclinic.com
http://www.nimh.nih.gov/health/publications/post-traumatic-stress-disorder
National Center for PTSD, US Department of Veteran Affairs, Feb. 2011: www.ptsd.va.gov.

B. Neuroanatomic Features—Through the use of brain imaging, characteristic changes in brain structure in PTSD patients have been identified. Regions typically altered in these patients include the hippocampus, amygdala, and cortical regions (anterior cingulate, insula, and orbitofrontal region). The interconnectivity of these regions forms a circuit that mediates adaptation to stress and fear conditioning. It is the change in this circuitry that has been proposed to have a direct link to the development of PTSD.

▶ Hyppocampus

As mentioned above, the hippocampus is implicated in the control of stress responses, declarative memory, and contextual aspects of fear conditioning. It is one of the most plastic regions of the brain, which is why a reduction in hippocampal volume is considered by many to be a hallmark of PTSD. Smaller hippocampal size has been demonstrated with magnetic resonance imaging (MRI) in Vietnam veterans with PTSD and associated with trauma severity and memory impairment. It is important to note that hippocampal atrophy and functional deficits exhibit considerable reversal after treatment with SSRIs, which have been demonstrated to increase neurogenic factors and neurogenesis in some preclinical studies.

▶ Amygdala

A limbic structure critical for the acquisition of fear response is the amygdala. It mediates both the stress response and emotional learning, thereby implicating its role in the pathophysiology of PTSD. Given the linkage between increased reactivity and genetic traits that moderate risk for PTSD, increased amygdala reactivity may signify a biological risk factor in the development of PTSD.

▶ Cortex

Because of its partial connections to the amygdala, the medial prefrontal cortex exhibits inhibitory control over stress responses and emotional reactivity. In PTSD patients, decreased volumes of the frontal cortex and reduction in anterior cingulate cortex (ACC) have been associated with PTSD symptom severity in some studies. Contrary to the volume loss of the hippocampus, ACC volume loss is secondary to the development of PTSD; therefore, it is not considered a preexisting risk factor.

Sherin JE, Nemeroff CB. Post-traumatic stress disorder: the neurobiological impact of psychological trauma. *Dialogues Clin Neurosci.* 2011;13(3):263–278.

C. Imaging Studies—Traumatic stress has a broad range of effects on brain function. The areas implicated in the response of the brain to stress include the amygdala, hippocampus, and prefrontal cortex. Studies of the brain in PTSD patients replicated findings in animal studies by demonstrating alterations in these brain areas. The key alterations noted included support for the hypothesis that the amygdala is hyperresponsive in PTSD while rostral and ventral portions of the medial prefrontal cortex are hyporesponsive. Although the dorsal anterior cingulate cortex and insula appear to be hyperresponsive in numerous anxiety disorders, it is also found in PTSD. In addition, the hippocampus also appears to function abnormally in PTSD, although the direction of the abnormality tends to vary depending on the methods used in the study.

In a more recent study case subjects were identified from a group of male US veterans previously deployed to Iraq or Afghanistan. There were 29 participants; 15 of the veteran case subjects met *DSM-IV* criteria and were essentially free of psychotropic drugs except for two who were receiving the antidepressant trazodone for insomnia and 14 veterans without PTSD who participated in the MRI study. When the PTSD subjects were compared to the controls, three differences were identified: (1) greater connectivity between the amygdala and brain insular cortex, (2) reduced connectivity between the amygdala and the hippocampus, and (3) reduction of the negative correlation between the amygdala and two regions of the anterior cingulate cortex. It is important to understand that in the normal control brains, there is typically a negative correlation between signaling in the amygdala and the cingulate

cortex. In the study referenced above, a reduction in the level of this typical negative correlation was noted.

Different experiential, psychophysiological, and neurobiological responses to traumatic symptom provocation in PTSD have been reported in the literature. Two subtypes of trauma response have been hypothesized, one characterized predominantly by hyperarousal and the other primarily dissociative, each one representing unique pathways to chronic stress-related psychopathology.

Hughes KC, Shin LM. Functional neuroimaging studies of post-traumatic stress disorder. *Expert Rev Neurother.* 2011;11(2): 275–285.

Sripada RK, King AP, Garfinkel SN, et al. Altered resting-state amygdala functional connectivity in men with posttraumatic stress disorder. *Jf Psychiatr Neurosci.* 2012;37(4):241–249. [PMID: 22313617]

D. Screening Tests—Screening tests or measures for PTSD vary in a number of ways. One of the most important differences is in format (**Table 63-4**).

Measures range from a 17-item self-report measure with a single rating for each item to a structured interview with detailed inquiries about each symptom and interviewer ratings regarding the validity of reports. Structured interviews vary in format as well. Some interviews have a single gatekeeping item, some have many, and in certain interviews, the ratings reflect symptom severity and/or frequency. It is important to note that the best PTSD measure really depends on what is needed. Important elements to consider when selecting a measure include the following:

- Time required to administer the measure
- Reading level of the population being sampled
- Whether it is necessary to assess symptoms related to a single traumatic event

Table 63-4. PTSD screening instruments format.

Screens for PTSD	Number of Items	Time to Admin. (minutes)	Allows Multiple Trauma	Corresponds to DSM-IV Criteria
BAI-PC	7	3	Yes	N/A
Primary care PTSD screen (PC-PTSD)	4	2	Yes	N/A
Short form of the PTSD checklist	6	2	Yes	N/A
Short screening scale for PTSD	7	3	Yes	N/A
SPAN	4	2	Yes	N/A
SPRINT	8	3	Yes	N/A
Trauma Screening Questionnaire (TSQ)	10	4	Yes	N/A
PTSD checklist (PCL)	17	5-10	Yes	Yes

or to assess symptoms related to multiple traumatic events (or to assess symptoms when the trauma history is unknown)

- Whether the measure needs to correspond to DSM criteria for PTSD
- Psychometric strengths and weaknesses of the measure
- Cost of using the measure
- Whether complexity and language of the measure is appropriate to the population being sampled

With the release of *DSM-5*, the National Center for PTSD is developing the following measures based on the following new criteria:

- Clinician-Administered PTSD Scale (CAPS), which includes new combined ratings of symptom frequency and intensity
- PTSD checklist (PCL)
- The Primary Care PTSD Screen (PC-PTSD), which will also be available in Spanish

Of particular note is the PC-PTSD. It is a four-item screen that was designed for use in primary care as well as other medical settings and is currently used to screen for PTSD in Veterans Administration (VA) veterans. The first item on the screen is an introductory sentence that cues respondents to traumatic events (**Table 63-5**).

In most circumstances the results of the PC-PTSD should be considered "positive" if a patient answers yes to any three items. Those screening positive should then be assessed with a structured interview for PTSD. The screen does not include a list of potentially traumatic events.

Prins A, Ouimette P, Kimerling R, et al. The primary care PTSD screen (PC-PTSD): development and operating characteristics. *Primary Care Psychiatr.* 2003;9:9-14 (ibid., Corrigendum. 2004; 9:151).

Table 63-5. Primary care PTSD screen (PC-PTSD).

In your lifetime, have you ever had any experience that was so frightening, horrible, or upsetting that, in the past month, you:	
Have had nightmares about it or thought about it when you did not want to?	YES/NO
Tried hard not to think about it or went out of your way to avoid situations that reminded you of it?	YES/NO
Were constantly on guard, watchful, or easily startled?	YES/NO
Felt numb or detached from others, activities, or your surroundings?	YES/NO

Data from Prins A, Ouimette P, Kimmerling R, et al. *The Primary Care PTSD Screen (PC-PTSD).* PTSD: National Center for PTSD; 2003.

Differential Diagnosis

Clinicians may have difficulty making the diagnosis of PTSD because the patient may have other disorders as well. In particular, major depression and substance abuse are common in people with PTSD. There may also be an increased risk of panic disorder agoraphobia, obsessive-compulsive disorder, social phobia, and somatization disorder. It is not clear to whether these concomitant disorders occur before or after the traumatic event and the development of PTSD.

Complications

Persons with posttraumatic stress disorder (PTSD) most often present to their primary care physician with physical symptoms rather than psychological concerns. Studies have also shown that people with PTSD are at increased risk for a number of medical conditions, such as hypertension, diabetes, cardiovascular disease, and asthma.

When there is prolonged exposure to trauma, certain persons may develop certain long-term patterns of behavior. These include difficulty in trusting others, irregular moods, impulsive behavior, shame, decreased self-esteem, and unstable relationships. Many of these traits are also seen in persons with borderline personality disorder, and people with this disorder often have histories of childhood physical and sexual abuse, which are possible causes for PTSD.

Significant interpersonal difficulties are common in persons with PTSD. Symptoms of estrangement, irritability, and anger, or associated depression, may take their toll on a person's relationships. Persons with PTSD may find it difficult to discuss their symptoms with those who did not go through the same trauma. Sometimes, guilt about surviving or about acts done in order to survive can also cause increased isolation and tension in interpersonal relationships.

Treatment

The main treatments for PTSD typically include psychological and medical interventions, which are often used in combination. Everyone is unique; therefore, any treatment intervention should be well formulated and culturally appropriate to optimize clinical and functional outcomes. Providing information about the illness usually involves teaching individuals about what PTSD is, how it impacts others, that it is caused by extraordinary stress rather than inherent personal weakness, that there is effective treatment available, and what to expect in treatment; this information helps to dispel inaccuracies and minimize any shame. This is particularly important in populations such as military personnel, who are frequently disadvantaged by the perceived and real stigma associated with seeing a mental health professional.

A. Psychotherapy—Posttraumatic stress disorder can be effectively treated with psychotherapy, and while there are several types of psychotherapies available, they all share common elements:

- Therapy should always is individualized to meet the specific concerns and needs of each unique trauma survivor.
- Trauma therapy is performed only when the patient is not currently in crisis.
- A shared plan of therapy should be developed within an atmosphere of trust and open discussion by the patient and therapist.
- One goal is to enable the survivor to gain a realistic sense of self-esteem and self-confidence in managing bad memories.
- Trauma exploration can be done in several ways, depending on the type of posttraumatic problems that a survivor is experiencing (**Table 63-6**).

Several types of effective psychotherapy are employed to treat PTSD, including

- Group psychotherapy
  - Likely the most beneficial psychotherapy method for PTSD, especially for military personnel and veterans.

This treatment is practiced in VA PTSD clinics and medical centers for military veterans.

- This peer-to-peer exchange is an ideal therapeutic setting because trauma survivors are able to risk sharing traumatic material with the safety, cohesion, and empathy provided by other survivors.
- This builds confidence and ability to trust. This allows the patient to work through trauma-related shame, guilt, rage, fear, doubt, and self-condemnation by sharing the "trauma narrative."

- Cognitive behavioral therapy
  - Most widely accepted as useful for PTSD is *cognitive behavioral psychotherapy* (CBT), which is a relatively structured psychotherapy that involves teaching specific techniques (ie, exposure and cognitive restructuring, relaxation, self-talk, and assertiveness training) within a limited number of sessions.
  - Exposure therapy targets assistance with facing the fear and gaining control of the accompanying distress. Some care is needed to avoid retraumatizing the patient.

Table 63-6. Management of different types of PTSD.

Types of PTSD	Description	Treatment
Normal stress response	Occurs when healthy adults previously exposed to a single discrete traumatic event in adulthood experience intense bad memories, emotional numbing, feelings of unreality, being cut off from relationships or body tension and distress	Group debriefing experience is helpful: (a) debriefings by describing the traumatic event; (b) progress to exploration of survivors' emotional responses to the event; (c) open discussion of symptoms precipitated by the trauma; (d) education in which responses are explained and positive ways of coping are identified
Acute stress disorder	Characterized by panic reactions, mental confusion, dissociation, severe insomnia, suspiciousness, and inability to manage even basic self-care, work, and relationship activities	Includes immediate support; removal from scene of trauma; use of medication for immediate relief of grief, anxiety, and insomnia; and brief supportive psychotherapy provided in the context of crisis intervention
Uncomplicated PTSD	Involves persistent reexperiencing of the traumatic event, avoidance of stimuli associated with the trauma, emotional numbing, and symptoms of increased arousal	May respond to group, psychodynamic cognitive behavioral, pharmacological, or combination approaches
Comorbid PTSD	Actually much more common than uncomplicated PTSD and usually associated with at least one other major psychiatric disorder such as depression, alcohol or substance abuse, panic disorder, and other anxiety disorders	Best results are achieved when both PTSD and the other disorder(s) are treated together rather than one after the other (this is especially true for PTSD and alcohol or substance abuse); treatments used for uncomplicated PTSD should also be used for these patients in addition to carefully managed treatment for the other psychiatric or addiction problems
Complex PTSD	"Disorder of extreme stress" found among those exposed to prolonged traumatic circumstances, especially during childhood, such as childhood sexual abuse; often diagnosed with borderline or antisocial personality disorder or dissociative disorders; patients exhibit behavioral difficulties, extreme emotional difficulties, and mental difficulties	Treatment often takes much longer, may progress at a much slower rate, and requires a sensitive and highly structured treatment program delivered by a team of trauma specialists

- Cognitive restructuring involves identifying irrational patterns of thought, feeling, and behavior gradually teaches the subject how to substitute new thoughts for the old and develop new emotional and behavioral patterns.

- Eye movement desensitization and reprocessing (EMDR)

  - EMDR provides an avenue for patients to view their memories of the trauma (including all of the negative thoughts, feelings, and sensations experienced at the time of the event) in an effort to change those feelings.

B. Complementary and Alternative Medicine— *Complementary and alternative medicine* (CAM) approaches to the treatment of many medical and mental health diagnoses, including PTSD, employ a range of therapies that are not or may not be considered standard to the practice of medicine. Although the research base to support the effectiveness is not complete, there is little evidence that these interventions are harmful. Nonetheless, patients who are reluctant to accept mental health labels or interventions may be more accepting of these innovative treatment approaches. Many CAM interventions are practiced in a manner that could increase social support and reduce stress for the patient and family members. These CAM interventions promote greater resilience through an increased sense of control.

The CAM modalities are typically grouped by categories reflecting their mechanism of action. However, many of the modalities cross several categories. The CAM modality categories as delineated by the National Center for Complementary and Alternative Medicine include

- **Natural products**: Include biologically based practices that include herbs, dietary supplements, vitamins, foods, and homeopathic remedies.

- **Mind-body medicine**: Seeks to harmonize mind body function to promote health and wellness. If the focus is primarily on mental activity, it will include prayer and guided imagery. If the emphasis is on the integration of mind and body, then yoga, meditation, tai chi, expressive art therapies, and breath-oriented therapies are the focus.

- **Manipulation and body-based practices (exercise and movement):** These modalities are based on manipulation of body parts or systems of the body. This includes disciplines such as chiropractic spinal and joint manipulation, osteopathic manipulation, massage therapy, reflexology, and acupuncture

- **Energy medicine**: Practices that focus on energy medicine look to balance energetic fields that surround and penetrate the human body (qi gong, reiki, and therapeutic touch).

It has been estimated that 41% of service members and veterans rely on one or more CAM treatments, a rate very similar to estimates in civilian populations. Furthermore, CAM is more often used by those who have a greater number of health symptoms, that is, comorbid conditions. In one study, more than two-thirds of service members and veterans with a history of PTSD reported using one or more CAM treatments. Because many of the CAM modalities relate to particular cultural backgrounds, physicians and allied health professionals should pay particular attention to the desires of the patient and the family.

C. Medications—Several classes of medications are employed to help improve or eliminate symptoms of posttraumatic stress disorder. They are nearly always used in conjunction with psychotherapy for PTSD, because while medications may treat some of the symptoms commonly associated with the disorder, they will not relieve a person of the flashbacks or feelings associated with the original trauma.

The selective serotonin reuptake inhibitor (SSRI) antidepressants are the most commonly prescribed class of medications for PTSD and the first class approved by the US Food and Drug Administration (FDA). They include medications such as fluoxetine, sertraline, and paroxetine. Research shows that this group of medicines tends to decrease anxiety, depression, and panic associated with PTSD in many people. These types of antidepressants may also help reduce aggression, impulsivity, and suicidal thoughts that can occur in people with PTSD. For combat-related PTSD, there is increasing evidence that prazosin can be particularly helpful. To prevent a relapse, antidepressants should be prescribed for at least a year. Many patients may need to try several types of antidepressants before finding one that meets their needs and relieves their symptoms.

The atypical antipsychotics are the most common class of medications prescribed after antidepressants. They include medications such as risperidone, olanzapine, and quetiapine. These medicines seem to be most useful in the treatment of PTSD in those who suffer from agitation, dissociation, hypervigilance, intense suspiciousness, paranoia, or brief psychotic reactions. Although less effective, the mood stabilizers like lamotrigine, tiagabine, and divalproex sodium can be helpful. Medicines that help decrease the physical symptoms associated with PTSD include drugs such as clonidine, guanfacine, and propranolol. Benzodiazepines are sometimes prescribed for certain symptoms because they provide rapid relief of anxiety. However, their usefulness is limited because of their associated dependence. There is even a small sample of data indicating that over time they can exacerbate PTSD. While other medications such as duloxetine, bupropion, and venlafaxine are sometimes used to treat PTSD, there is little research that has studied their effectiveness in treating this illness.

The current state of evidence suggests that the SSRIs remain as the treatment of first choice for most patients requiring drug therapy for PTSD. Currently there is minimal evidence to support the use of any specific SSRI. Therefore, the differences in pharmacokinetic profile, individual tolerability, and drug interaction potential should be used to guide the selection. In the event that SSRI therapy has not provided adequate benefit, or where adverse effects or drug interactions mean that SSRI treatment is unsuitable, mirtazapine or venlafaxine can be regarded as reasonable alternatives.

Benedek D, et al. *Guideline Watch: Practice Guideline for the Treatment of Patients with Acute Stress Disorder and Posttraumatic Stress Disorder.* Focus; March 2009.

Cohen H. Treatment of PTSD. *Psych Central*; 2006 (retrieved Aug. 6, 2013, from http://psychcentral.com/lib/an-overview-of-treatment-of-ptsd/000161).

http://www.healthquality.va.gov/PTSD-FULL-2010c.pdf.

National Center for Post Traumatic Stress Disorder, Treatment of PTSD http://www.ptsd.va.gov/professional/pages/overview-treatment-research.asp, last accessed March 25, 2011.

SAMHSA. *Pharmacologic Guidelines for Treating Individuals with Post-Traumatic Stress Disorder and Co-Occurring Opioid Use Disorder*; May 2012.

Ursano RJ, Bell C, Eth S, Friedman MJ, Norwood A E, Pfefferbaum B. Practice guideline for the treatment of patients with acute stress disorder and posttraumatic stress disorder [special issue]. *Am J Psychiatr.* 2004;(suppl):161.

V A/DoD Clinical Practice Guideline Working Group. *Management of Post-traumatic Stress.* Washington, DC: Veterans Health Administration, Department of Veterans Affairs and Health Affairs; Department of Defense; Office of Quality and Performance, publication 10Q-CPG/PTSD-03; Dec 2003.

Prognosis

Overall, approximately 30% of people eventually recover completely with proper treatment, and another 40% get better, even though less intense symptoms may remain.

Treatment with psychotherapy and/or medications, such as SSRIs, has been very helpful. However, the prognosis for PTSD depends primarily on the severity and length of time that a person has suffered from the disorder. The majority of patients with PTSD respond to psychotherapy. Symptom duration is variable and is affected by the proximity, duration, and intensity of the trauma, as well as comorbidity with other psychiatric disorders. The patient's subjective interpretation of the trauma also influences symptoms. In patients who are receiving treatment, the average duration of symptoms is approximately 36 months. In patients who are not receiving treatment, the average duration of symptoms rises to 64 months. More than one-third of PTSD patients never fully recover. Those who do not receive treatment may remain in a hyperaroused state and cause further damage to their brain, have difficulty maintaining a job, have difficulty developing or retaining relationships, and have a significant risk of suicide.

Both PTSD and TBI will be an ongoing challenge for healthcare providers at every venue of healthcare entry. Family practitioners will surely be involved in the diagnosis and management of these individuals. While PTSD and TBI may not be adequately diagnosed in the service member and veteran, any patient with combat experience should be considered at risk for these conditions both separately and apart. Screening for a history of blast injuries, concussions, and traumatic exposure should be part of the clinical workup of any former service member with deployment and combat experience during the Iraq and Afghanistan wars. Family practice physicians are especially likely to encounter these patients at various stages of their illness progression, and a knowledge of how combat and deployment effects illness and health is essential.

Cultural & Linguistic Competence

Kim A. Bullock, MD, FAAFP
Darci L. Graves, MPP, MA, MA

Family physicians deliver care across the lifespan from infancy to the end of life, all within increasingly diverse communities. Many of these communities face existing and persistent health and healthcare disparities. Growing diversity and persistent disparities are among several arguments for the provision of care and services, which are patient-centered as well as culturally and linguistically appropriate. This may include decisions and actions that are congruent with the patient's value systems and orientation to health and illness.

Every patient interaction is a unique cultural experience; each encounter is an opportunity to overcome the potential impediments in the exchange of information between physicians, patients, and their families. The American Academy of Family Physicians (AAFP) recognized the importance of culturally proficient and linguistically competent care in a 2008 position paper: *Principles for Improving Cultural Competency and Care to Minority and Medically-Underserved Communities*. The AAFP is not alone in its recognition of the crucial role of cross-cultural health in the effective delivery of healthcare. The list includes other influential groups such as the American Association of Medical Colleges (AAMC), Liaison Committee on Medical Education (LCME), the Center for Medicare and Medicaid Services (CMS), and national, international bodies, such as The Joint Commission, The Commonwealth Fund, and the World Health Organization (WHO).

The Institute of Medicine (IOM) produced a landmark report entitled *Crossing the Quality Chasm*, which crystallized the failures of the American medical system and asserted that the system must be changed to one that is equitable, patient-centered, safe, and effective. The following year the IOM released *Unequal Treatment, Confronting Racial and Ethnic Disparities in Health Care*, which identified cross-cultural education as a possible intervention in the reduction of healthcare disparities. The documentary

Unnatural Causes continued this narrative by examining how social determinants of health, including racism and class distinctions, created health inequalities within communities of color across the nation.

American Academy of Family Physicians. *Principles for Improving Cultural Competency and Care to Minority and Medically-Underserved Communities* (available at http://www.aafp.org/online/en/home/policy/policies/p/princculturproficcare.html).

Institute of Medicine. *Crossing the Quality Chasm: A New Health System for the 21St Century*. Committee on Quality of Health Care in America; National Academies Press; 2001.

Liaison Committee on Medical Education. *Functions and Structure of a Medical School: Standards for Accreditation of Medical Education Programs Leading to the M.D. Degree*. LCME; 2011 (retrieved from http://www.lcme.org/functions2011may.pdf).

2011 National Health Care Disparities Report (NHDR). Rockville, MD: Agency for Healthcare Research and Quality; Jan. 2012 (available at. http://www.ahrq.gov/research/findings/nhqrdr/nhdr11/index.html).

The Joint Commission. *Advancing Effective Communication, Cultural Competency, and Patient-and Family-Centered Care: A Roadmap for Hospitals*. Oakbrook Terrace, IL: The Joint Commission; 2010.

WHY CULTURALLY AND LINGUISTICALLY APPROPRIATE SERVICES ARE NECESSARY

▶ Emergent Diversity in American Communities

The changing demographics of the United States provide one of many compelling reasons for healthcare providers to consider the impact of cultural factors on health, disease, and healthcare. The population is increasingly diverse–aging, coming out, immigrating, and acculturating (**Box 64-1**). Currently, minorities represent one-third of the US population. Projections indicate that the United States

Box 64-1: Terms to be familiar with

Culturally and Linguistically Appropriate Services

Services that are respectful of and responsive to individual cultural health beliefs and practices, preferred languages, health literacy levels, and communication needs and employed by all members of an organization (regardless of size) at every point of contact.

Health Disparities

A particular type of health difference that is closely linked with social, economic, and/or environmental disadvantage. Health disparities adversely affect groups of people who have systematically experienced greater obstacles to health based on their racial or ethnic group; religion; socioeconomic status; gender; age; sexual orientation or other characteristics historically linked to discrimination or exclusion.

Health Equity

Attainment of the highest level of health for all people. Achieving health equity requires valuing everyone equally, with focused and ongoing societal efforts to address avoidable inequalities, historical and contemporary injustices, and the elimination of health and healthcare disparities.

will be a "majority-minority" nation by 2042, with the nation projected to be 54% minority in 2050 (**Box 64-2**).

Health and Healthcare Disparities

The performance of the US healthcare system reveals significant inequities across populations with missed opportunities in terms of preventing disease, disability, and morbidity and mortality indices. Disparities in health and healthcare are due to a complex interaction between many factors, from those that increase exposure to disease to those that decrease access to healthcare. The trends reveal that individuals from communities of color are in poorer health, face greater challenges in accessing care, experience significant navigation problems within the system, and receive a quality of care that is inferior to that of their nonminority peers. Individuals with limited English proficiency and low health literacy skills have also experienced lower-quality healthcare.

Box 64-2: A cautionary word about the term *minority*

The term minority is often used with little consideration for its connotations. People feel uncomfortable with this reference because of its implied status of inferiority. A clear example expressed by an Hispanic patient toward her caregivers is the following. She states, "I felt weak, small and irrelevant when they used the term to talk about me among themselves. It sounded like they were being derogatory, which made me feel more powerless than I already was...." Alternative terms have emerged in both the medical and lay literature, such as people, or communities of color, more defined country of origin delineations, or allowing patients to offer their own identification.

(Source: Paniagua FA. Assessing and Treating Culturally Diverse Clients. Sage; 2014.)

Examples of disparities include the following:

- African Americans are 3 times more likely to die from asthma than non-Hispanic whites. Asian American adults are less likely than white adults to have heart disease; they are also less likely to die from heart disease.
- Lesbians are less likely to obtain preventive services for cancer.

Health Determinants

Family physicians should factor in population health, socioeconomic status, and structural barriers, such as number and location of public health centers, pharmacies, and hospitals that may not be easily accessible. Other factors to consider include access to fresh foods, transportation, adequate housing, and recreation, which also contribute to overall health and well-being. These ecological determinants influence health and disease prevalence, but are rarely included in patient histories. Expanding the biopsychosocial model to include ecological factors provides a larger contextual model to evaluate patient's health risks, susceptibilities, and health outcomes. Asking salient questions that reflect the patient's broader living situation is a more effective approach in guiding healthcare decisions and health interventions.

Buchmueller T, Carpenter CS. Disparities in health insurance coverage, access, and outcomes for individuals in same-sex versus different-sex relationships, 2000–2007. *Am J Public Health*. 2010; 100(3):489–495.

Dilley JA, Simmons KW, Boysun MJ, et al. Demonstrating the importance and feasibility of including sexual orientation in public health surveys: health disparities in the Pacific Northwest. *Am J Public Health*. 2010;100(3):460–467.

Like RC. Educating clinicians about cultural competence and disparities in health and health care. *J Contin Educ Health Prof*. 2011;31(3):197–207.

McCarthy D, How S, Ashley-Kay F, et al. *The Commonwealth Fund: Why Not the Best? Results from the National Scorecard on US Health System Performance. The Commonwealth Fund on a High Performance Health Care System*; Oct. 2011.

Salsbury B, et al. Measuring social determinants of health inequalities: the CADH Health Equality Index. In: Hofrichter R, Bhatia R. *Tackling Health Inequalities through Public Health Practice. Theory to Action*. Oxford University Press; 2010.

Theorizing Health and Illness Causation and Establishing the Therapeutic Relationship

Health and disease are interrelated dynamic processes. Definitions of both include biomedical, social, ecological, spiritual, and psychological constructs. Illness is a socially influenced condition and must be viewed within the socially recognized reality defined by the patient. Illness causation and etiologies influence the physician-patient interaction, and a culture-centered approach to care encourages physicians to offer solace and relief from the patient's viewpoint and experiences. There is a power differential with every clinical encounter, which impacts the physician-patient alliance. Medical and psychological problems are managed within this context and require the physician to mediate this imbalance through various techniques. These include affirmations and strengths that the patient may exhibit through healthy behaviors, lifestyle choices, beneficial existential cultural beliefs, and practices that advance health.

Family medicine offers helpful strategies through supportive and intentional counseling, such as motivational interviewing, which encourages affirmations and self-reflections that are patient-directed. Other skills that empower patients include expressing empathy during the encounter and exhibiting a practice style that encompasses and appreciates diversity. Physician attributes such as eliciting the patient's goals and projecting a willingness to negotiate care options and patient preferences has been shown to increase visit satisfaction and adherence to treatment. Although time constraints create limitations on patient interactions, these activities do not add significantly to the length of the visit and do improve overall quality of care. Finally, cultural humility, a process of continual self-reflection, awareness, and growth in learning about diverse populations, change, and the relational dynamics between patients and physicians, is crucial to providing a mutually effective partnership in practice.

Explanatory Models of Health, Illness, and Care

Patient-centered care focuses on engaging patients and their families in the care management plan and healthcare decision making. Health advocacy is linked to this model of care and encourages patients to be actively involved in the design and planning of their own healthcare delivery, in addition to the larger medical system. Attributes associated with patient-centered care mirror some of the tenets of culturally competent care. They include care that is "whole-person"-focused; encourages patient empowerment and engagement; and emphasizes communication and coordination that is sensitive to the patient's linguistic level, personal preferences, cultural strengths, and values. The foundation for these principles is derived from Engel and Roman's biopsychosocial model, which maintains the patient's human dimension as the central focus to the medical encounter. Physicians are required to go beyond the traditional reductionist biomedical approach and incorporate cultural variables regarding family and community, health beliefs, and expectations in the therapeutic process.

Engel's biopsychosocial approach recognizes the complex interactions between healthcare delivery and the patient's beliefs and behaviors concerning wellness, illness, and disease. It is supported and enhanced by the clinical lessons offered by Kleinman's explanatory model, a tool for physicians to aid in providing culturally competent care. The model is elicited through open-ended questions, originally eight questions,

focused on how patients perceive their illness state, their beliefs regarding causality, and perceived forms of treatment. This information provides contextual data, which strengthens the therapeutic alliance and informs the physician regarding diagnosis and management. The advantages in using this approach have been validated through qualitative and quantitative research that enriches medical practice as well as population health. Practical applications give physicians a living illness experience associated with their patients. It also provides information about sick roles and behaviors that are linked to care in various scenarios covering social health issues, including HIV-AIDS, domestic violence, and other community ills.

Mental and Behavioral Health

Mental health can be seen as the result of the complex interactions between biological, psychological, social, and cultural factors. The influence of any of these factors can be stronger or weaker depending on the illness or disorder. Cultural and social factors can affect a patient's belief as to symptom causation and inform their reaction and reception to a diagnosis of mental illness.

Despite its prevalence in all cultures, mental health can carry with it a significant amount of shame and stigma around a diagnosis. In other cultures, acknowledging the illness can have consequences on the perception of the entire family. Cultural and religious communities have the power to demystify mental illness, while assisting and supporting individuals and their families.

Because of the complexities that exist around mental illness, numerous disparities exist and persist in culturally diverse communities. The US Surgeon General's report on mental health found the following:

- Minorities have less access to, availability of, and receive mental health services.
- Minorities in treatment often receive a poorer quality of mental healthcare.
- Minorities are underrepresented in mental health research.
- Racial and ethnic minorities collectively experience a greater disability burden from mental illness than do whites; this higher level of burden stems from minorities receiving less care and poorer quality of care, rather than from the fact that their illnesses are inherently more severe or prevalent in the community.

Application of Cultural Information and Skills in Clinical Interactions

Several tools that are available to family physicians can provide guidance in interacting with patients and incorporate cultural elements as part of the clinical assessment. Beginning with the Berlin and Fowkes' LEARN model (**Box 64-3**), others have been developed, including the BATHE, ESFT, ETHNIC, and CRASH frameworks. They provide the

Box 64-3

> **L**isten to patients' perspectives.
> **E**xplain medical views.
> **A**cknowledge similarities and differences.
> **R**ecommend a course of action.
> **N**egotiate plans.

Box 64-4: Terms to be familiar with

> **Interpretation**
> The process of understanding and analyzing a spoken or signed message and reexpressing that message faithfully, accurately, and objectively in another language, taking the cultural and social context into account.
>
> **Translation**
> The conversion of a written text into a corresponding written text in a different language.

[*Source:* Department of Health and Human Services, Office of Minority Health [HHS OMH]. (2013). National standards for culturally and linguistically appropriate services in health and health care: A blueprint for advancing and sustaining CLAS Policy and Practice. (Retrieved from http://www.thinkculturalhealth.hhs.gov).]

patient an opportunity to engage and elaborate on signs and symptoms from their cultural perspective.

Betancourt JR, Carrillo JE, Green AR. Hypertension in multicultural and minority populations: linking communication to compliance. *Curr Hypertens Rep.* 1999;1(6):482–488. [ESFT mnemonic]

Flores G, Abreu M, Pizzo-Barone C, Bachur R, Lin H. Errors of medical interpretation and their potential clinical consequences: a comparison of professional versus ad hoc versus no interpreters. *Ann Emerg Med.* 2012;60(5): 545–553.

Institute of Medicine. *Speaking of Health: Assessing Health Communication Strategies for Diverse Populations. IOM, Committee on Communication for Behavior Change in the 21st Century: Improving the Health of Diverse Populations.* IOM; 2002.

Levin SJ, Like RC, Gottlieb JE. ETHNIC: a framework for culturally competent clinical practice. *Patient Care.* 2000;9(special issue):188. [ETHNICS mnemonic]

Weiner SJ, Schwartz A, et al. Patient-centered decision making and health care outcomes. An observational study. *Ann Intern Med.* 2013;158(8).

ENGAGING IN CULTURALLY AND LINGUISTICALLY APPROPRIATE CARE

▶ Going Beyond the Clinical Interview

Fundamental to every clinical encounter is establishing a therapeutic relationship with a patient that is affirming, inclusive, and collaborative. This chapter provides information for family physicians to assist in establishing that relationship. The information presented should be viewed as a starting point along the continuum of cultural and linguistic competency. This lifelong process begins with recognizing the inherent strengths and value of human diversity. The continuum also includes the confrontation of personal and societal bias, fosters the growth of cultural awareness and sensitivity, and develops the cross-cultural knowledge and skills that will improve clinical practice.

▶ National Standards for Culturally and Linguistically Appropriate Services (CLAS) in Health and Healthcare

The National CLAS standards provide a blueprint with which to operationalize and institutionalize the concepts of cultural and linguistic competency and are intended to advance health equity, improve quality, and help eliminate healthcare disparities. The standards can assist physicians, small practices, and large hospitals plan and implement culturally and linguistically appropriate services geared toward improving care and services. Physicians need to be active members in clinics, hospitals, and medical societies in order to create culturally and linguistically competent institutions. Physicians can be powerful advocates for hiring bilingual-bicultural workers, employing trained interpreters, creating health education approaches for patients with limited English proficiency, ensuring quality translation, and engaging institutions in caring for diverse patients (**Box 64-4**). The National CLAS standards are referenced throughout the following case study to illustrate their application; however, to achieve the intended outcomes, the standards should be implemented in their entirety. The National CLAS standards and their accompanying guidance document, *A Blueprint for Advancing and Sustaining CLAS Policy and Practice,* are available through the HHS Office of Minority Health, Think Cultural Health website.

CASE 1

GT was a 42-year-old Spanish-speaking Latin American woman who presented at the family medicine center with headaches, malaise, nausea, one episode of vomiting, and weakness of one day's duration. The patient presented with several teenage children who appeared challenging to manage in the clinic. The constant interruptions made it difficult for the provider to obtain the history and conduct a physical exam. On initial presentation the patient noted that the headaches were increasingly severe and unusual because of the intensity. Previous headaches had been relieved with over-the-counter (OTC) medications. After a series of pointed questions through the use of a nurse interpreter who spoke Spanish, the patient was informed that the diagnosis was most likely the "flu," or exacerbation of stress-related tension headaches. The vital signs and examination were nonfocal, except for bradycardia of 55, and a temperature of 99.8°F. The patient presented later to the local emergency department, and did not return to the clinic because of worsening symptoms and was urgently evaluated, and stabilized for toxic exposure to the dried oleander leaves prepared for medicinal purposes. The leaves were obtained from a curandero local to the area where the patient lived.

In the current example there are several points to consider.

▶ The Importance of Effective Communication

➢ National CLAS standards 4, 5, 6, 7, 8, and 13 are just a few of the standards that can assist in providing effective communication regardless of cultural or linguistic background.

The use of a lay or ad hoc interpreter is problematic and should not be acceptable in the clinical setting (**Box 64-5**). A certified interpreter should be the standard for healthcare communications and if unavailable, other modalities, such as phone banks and/or virtual interpreter programs should be utilized. Physicians should be familiar with the different roles and types of interpreters. This includes video remote interpreting, telephonic, and in-person interpreting. It is also important for physicians to appreciate the importance of using certified interpreters who have been assessed for their language proficiency and knowledge of medical terminology. The use of interpreters includes recognizing the importance of verbal, nonverbal cues, posture, and positioning with interpreters. In addition, the value of touch as therapeutic can be helpful in solidifying the physician-patient relationship, while the interpreter remains in the background.

Effective communication is fundamental to providing healthcare to diverse patients. Care that acknowledges and supports the patient's cultural beliefs and practices (eg, folk medicine, alternative treatments) allows patients to participate in negotiating a management plan. It may also reveal questionable or even harmful responses to the illness condition, and provide a teachable moment for change. Care that includes cultural accommodations when appropriate builds trust in the professional's and patient's faith in the clinical process. Care that includes cultural negotiations and accommodations encourages patients and their families to participate in the clinical process, and builds trust in the professional relationship.

Conversational styles vary across cultures and are challenging. For optimal communication, physicians must adapt their standard interviewing techniques to match patient's communication styles. Do not assume that one methodology will be effective for interviewing and relaying clinical information. In addition, appreciation for verbal-nonverbal cues is important. Although physicians may feel comfortable with a straightforward approach with direct eye contact, patients from various backgrounds and cultures may feel intimidated and threatened by this position. They may not answer questions, chose to change the subject, or simply remain silent. Misinterpretation of delivery of information can result in problems with adherence, follow-up, and outcomes.

Physicians can learn general approaches from community experts, such as bilingual-bicultural colleagues, and make adaptations as they are attuned to people's verbal and nonverbal cues.

▶ Recognizing the Important Roles of Traditional Medicine and Traditionalist Practitioners

➢ National CLAS standards 4, 9, 11, 12, and 13 are a few of the standards that could assist in recognizing the important roles that traditional medicine and practitioners serve as forms of community support.

Recognizing folk illness beliefs and, interpretation of signs and symptoms is also linked with how patients respond to illness and disease. Culture influences help-seeking behaviors, which will be expressed in multiple ways, such as when and who is consulted first, treatment preferences, and expectations for healing. Indigenous practices and practitioners, such as herbalists, shamanists, and curanderos, may not be discussed during the family practice visit unless rapport is established and cultural sensitivity is demonstrated. Medicinal therapies may be taken alongside prescription medications, and may be substituted because of side effects, the appearance of the pills, or confusion about the regimen. Family physicians should be familiar with some commonly used botanicals and herbs, since drug toxicities can present as chief complaints. Examples include ginseng and licorice, causing hypertension; chamomile tea, leading to anaphylaxis; ephedra (ma huang), causing a wide range of cardiovascular effects; and liver enzyme induction with eucalyptus oil, sassafras, and comfrey. In this case, early signs of oleander toxicity could have been identified during the history-gathering process, instead of the premature diagnosis of "flu," viremia, or tension headache. Family physicians should sensitively ask their patients what they are taking and encourage them to bring their remedies into the office to discuss together.

A visit to the family medicine clinic or hospital may be the last resort when patients become ill. Patients

Box 64-5: From the literature

A cross-sectional error analysis was conducted to compare interpreter errors and their potential consequences in encounters with professional versus ad hoc versus no interpreters.

Emergency department (ED) visits during 30 months in the two largest pediatric EDs in Massachusetts were audiotaped and analyzed.

The resultant error rates for the three groups were as follows:
- Professional interpreter: 12%
- Ad hoc interpreter: 22%
- No interpreter: 20%

(Source: Flores G, Abreu M, Pizzo-Barone C, Bachur R, Lin H. *Ann Emerg Med.* 2012;60;5:545-553.)

may experience shame and humiliation by other family or community members if they seek care outside of normative practices or standards. Family physicians must therefore exhibit an open and nonjudgmental attitude, avoiding bias in evaluation and treatment. Family physicians should consider mobilizing additional resources and recognized community health experts in working with culturally diverse patients, especially where there may be knowledge gaps or other challenges.

▶ Utilize an Inclusive and Participatory Care Model

➤ National CLAS Standards #1, 10, 11, and 13 are a few of the standards that could assist in identifying, utilizing and maintaining an inclusive and participatory care model.

Encourage a participatory care model. Patient's and physician's information is interpreted through a cultural lens and influences the direction of the clinical questions leading to the diagnosis. Physicians who use a participatory framework allow patients to actively participate in the physician-patient exchange. Patients can offer explanatory models about their beliefs, perceptions of illness, and disease states, as well as offer information about their treatments. Patients allowed to engage and interject their health concepts and ideas will share more crucial information during the visit. The result will be a more accurate diagnosis, more appropriate management plan, and better adherence to treatment. Patient satisfaction leads to better patient follow-up, even if the diagnosis is inconclusive, or in this case, inaccurate. In this particular case, the patient most likely felt dissatisfied with the diagnostic explanation offered and sought care in the emergency department (ED) as a last resort. This was also a missed learning opportunity for the physician, since the patient did not return for follow-up care.

Aboumater H, Cooper L. Contextualizing patient-centered care to fulfill its promise of better health outcomes; beyond who, what and why. *Ann Intern Med.* 2013;158:(8):628–629.

Flores G, Abreu M, Pizzo-Barone C, Bachur R, Lin H. Errors of medical interpretation and their potential clinical consequences: a comparison of professional versus ad hoc versus no interpreters. *Ann Emerg Med.* 2012;60(5):545–553.

Havranek EP, Hanratty R, Tate C, et al. The effect of values affirmation on race-discordant patient-provider communication. *Arch Intern Med.* 2012;172(21):1662–1666.

Riekert KA, Borrelli B, Bilderback A, et al. The development of a motivational interviewing intervention to promote medication adherence among inner-city African-American adolescents with asthma. *Patient Educ Couns.* 2011;82:177–122.

US Department of Health and Human Services, Office of Minority Health. *National Standards on Culturally and Linguistically Appropriate Services in Health and Health Care* (available at https://www.thinkculturalhealth.hhs.gov/Content/clas.asp; retrieved April 24, 2013).

The quality of interpersonal care and interpersonal communications impacts all aspects of the health encounter. Research confirms that when physicians are more inclusive in their interactions, and when patients are more involved as partners, consensus around treatment is more successful with increased satisfaction with care. A participatory model of caregiving that includes a biopsychosocioecological framework has a greater impact on positive behavior change and sustaining the physician-patient relationship. This has a direct effect on outcome rating scores, and liability protection independent of diagnostic accuracy.

Providing cross-cultural care requires physicians to participate in lifelong learning both intellectually and experientially. Continuous self-reflection, evaluation, and reevaluation is required if family physicians are to remain current in their understanding of changing demographics and emerging dominant populations regionally and nationally. Self-study, participation in discussion networks, and virtual community exchanges may be an efficient strategy to engage in the learning process. This is a required educational journey if one is to partake in the universal goal to offer care that is personally meaningful and continues the ongoing search to address human sickness and healing in society.

The following sources are recommended for further information:

- American Academy of Family Physicians (AAFP). Cultural competency video: Quality *Care for Diverse Populations* (available at http://www.aafp.org/online/en/home/clinical/publichealth/culturalprof/qcdpvideos.html).

- American Board of Family Medicine: Cultural Competency Methods in Medicine Module. Five modules that qualify for Part IV recertification credit were released in fall 2010.

- American Muslim Health Professionals: http://amhp.us/

- Asian and Pacific Islander American Health Forum: http://www.apiahf.org

- Colorado Health Foundation: http://www.coloradohealth.org/

- Cross Cultural Health Care Program: www.xculture.org

- Cultural Competence Online for Medical Practice: http://www.c-comp.org

- Ethnomed: www.ethnomed.org

- Gay and Lesbian Medical Association (GLMA): www.glma.org

- HHS Health Resources and Services Agency (HRSA) toolkits, videos: http://www.hrsa.gov/culturalcompetence/index.html

- Health Resources and Services Administration (HRSA): *Effective Communication Tools for Healthcare*

Professionals (available at http://www.hrsa.gov/publichealth/healthliteracy)

- HHS Office of Minority Health, Think Cultural Health: https://www.thinkculturalhealth.hhs.gov
- Resources include
- National Standards for Culturally and Linguistically Appropriate Services in Health and Health Care.
- A Physician's Practical Guide to Culturally Competent Care (9 CME)
- National Center for Cultural Competence (NCCC): http://nccc.georgetown.edu/.
- National Coalition for LGBT Health: http://lgbthealth.webolutionary.com/.
- National Council on Interpretation in Health Care: http://www.ncihc.org/.
- National Health Law Program: http://www.healthlaw.org.
- National Hispanic Medical Association: http://www.nhmamd.org/.
- National Institutes for Health: http://www.nih.gov/clearcommunication/culturalcompetency.htm.
- National Medical Association: http://www.nmanet.org/.
- Provider's Guide to Quality and Culture: http://erc.msh.org/mainpage.cfm?file=1.0.htm&module=provider&language=english.
- Resources for Cross-Cultural Health: www.diversityrx.org.
- Society of Healthcare Professionals with Disabilities: http://www.disabilitysociety.org/.
- W. K. Kellogg Foundation: http://www.wkkf.org./
- World Education; Culture, Health and Literacy: http://www.worlded.org/us/health/docs/culture/about.html.

Health & Healthcare Disparities

Jeannette E. South-Paul, MD

Evelyn L. Lewis, MD, MA, FAAFP

BACKGROUND & DEFINITIONS

Ethnic and racial minorities manifest significantly poorer health status than their white counterparts. Health disparities are defined by the National Institutes of Health as "differences in the incidence, prevalence, mortality, and burden of diseases and other adverse health conditions that exist among specific population groups in the United States." Cardiovascular disease, cancer, and diabetes mellitus are the most commonly reported health disparities, followed by cerebrovascular diseases, unintentional injuries, and HIV/AIDS. Assessing these differences requires that a wide variety of factors, including age, gender, nationality, family of origin, religiosity, education, income, geographic location, race or ethnicity, sexual orientation, and disability, be considered.

Healthcare disparities are defined by the Institute of Medicine (IOM) as "differences in the quality of healthcare that are not due to access-related factors or clinical needs, preferences, and appropriateness of intervention." Causes of healthcare disparities most often relate to quality and include provider-patient relationships, provider bias and discrimination, and patient variables such as mistrust of the healthcare system and refusal of treatment. Although disparities in health and healthcare can be inextricably tied to one another, distinguishing between them increases our understanding of the complexity of the problem.

One of the most significant efforts to address disparities has been the introduction of the Healthy People goals every decade beginning in the late 1990s. The changes in the demographics of the US population are reflected in changes in Healthy People goals. Healthy People 2000 goals were to reduce health disparities. Healthy People 2010 goals were to eliminate those disparities. Healthy People 2020 expands these goals further to focus on achieving health equity, eliminating disparities, and improving the health of all groups. The disparities evident in the health and/or healthcare of the US population reflect inconsistencies in implementing these principles.

Approximately one-third of Americans, or >100 million persons, self-identify as belonging to a racial or ethnic minority group, 51% (154 million) are women, 12% (36 million) not living in nursing homes or other residential care facilities, had a disability, 70.5 million live in rural areas (23% of the population), while 233.5 million (77%) live in urban areas, and 4% identified themselves as lesbian, gay, bisexual, or transgender. Each of these groups experiences certain disparities in health or healthcare. (See Chapter 66 for a comprehensive discussion on the health disparities experienced by the GLBT community.) An estimated 1 in 4 Americans (almost 70 million persons) is classified as a member of one of the four major racial or ethnic minority groups: African American, Latino/Hispanic, Native American, and Asian/Pacific Islander. The US Census Bureau estimates that by the year 2050, people of color will represent 1 in 3 Americans. These populations bear a disproportionate burden of illness and disease relative to their percentage distribution in the population. Understanding the factors that contribute to inequities in health among these populations and the strategies that have resulted in improved health can inform and promote the delivery of quality healthcare.

http://healthypeople.gov/2020/about/default.aspx (accessed 6/11/2013).

Smedley BD, et al. *Unequal Treatment: Confronting Racial and Ethnic Disparities in Health Care.* Institute of Medicine, Committee on Understanding and Eliminating Racial and Ethnic Disparities in Health Care; 2002.

US Department of Health and Human Services. *Healthy People 2010: National Health Promotion and Disease Prevention Objectives;* conference ed. in 2 vols. DHHS; 2000.

Williams DR. Race, socioeconomic status, and health. The added effects of racism and discrimination. *Ann NY Acad Sci.* 1999;896. [PMID: 10681897]

HEALTHCARE DISPARITIES & THE LITERATURE

▶ Institute of Medicine Reports

In 1999, a report from the IOM entitled *Unequal Treatment: Confronting Racial and Ethnic Disparities in Health Care* was written in response to a request from Congress to the IOM to address the extent of racial and ethnic disparities in healthcare. Following review of >100 publications, the IOM study committee concluded that research findings consistently indicated that minorities were less likely than whites to receive needed services, including lifesaving procedures. The most commonly reported healthcare disparities were seen in cardiovascular disease, cancer, and diabetes. Other illnesses included cerebrovascular diseases, mental illness, and HIV/AIDS.

The IOM committee noted factors contributing to these complex healthcare disparities related to (1) minority patients' attitudes toward healthcare, preferences for and differing responses to treatment; (2) the operation of healthcare systems and regulatory environment in which they function (eg, lack of interpretation services for those with limited English proficiency, lack of resources for those with limited health literacy); and (3) factors derived from the clinical encounter. The committee suggested that provider bias, clinical uncertainty, and stereotyping or beliefs about the behavior of minorities may have a negative impact on the health outcomes of minorities. On the other side of the clinical encounter is the patient, whose reaction to the provider's biased or stereotyped behaviors may also contribute to disparities.

▶ National Healthcare Disparities Report

With a directive from the Healthcare Research and Quality Act of 1999 (Public Law 106-129) and guidance from the IOM, the Agency for Healthcare Research and Quality (AHRQ) developed and produced two reports: the *National Healthcare Disparities Report* (NHDR) and the *National Healthcare Quality Report* (NHQR). The two reports were released simultaneously in 2003 to provide a more comprehensive view of the performance of the healthcare system, its strengths, and areas that should serve as a focal point for future improvement. The performance measures underlying the two reports have been used to monitor the nation's progress toward improved healthcare delivery. Reports have been issued annually since 2003.

The Agency for Healthcare Research and Quality, March 2009 report focused on quality of care and disparities in healthcare in America overall and AHRQ's priority populations in particular. The 2008 National Healthcare Disparities Report found that although some of the biggest disparities in quality remain, progress has been made in reducing disparities in areas, such as dialysis, hospital admissions for perforated appendix, and childhood vaccinations. Most recently, the NHDR also reported that there are significant disparities in quality documented over the years where there has not been improvement, such as new AIDS cases (AHRQ 09-0002) (http://www.ahrq.gov/news/pubcat/c_quca.htm).

A summary of the 2012 NHQR and NHDR reinforces the need to consider simultaneously the quality of healthcare and disparities across populations when assessing our healthcare system. Four themes from the two reports emphasize the need to accelerate progress if we are to achieve a higher quality and more equitable healthcare in the nation in the near future: (1) healthcare quality and access are suboptimal, especially for minority and low-income groups; (2) quality is improving; access and disparities are not improving; (3) urgent attention is warranted to ensure continued improvements in quality and progress on reducing disparities with respect to certain services, geographic areas, and populations (eg, diabetes care, cancer screening, and services in southern states); and (4) progress is uneven with respect to national priorities identified in the HHS National Quality Strategy and the Disparities Action Plan.

Website

Agency for Healthcare Research and Quality, 2012. *National Healthcare Disparities Report* (available at http://www.ahrq.gov/research/findings/nhqrdr/nhqr12/nhqr12_prov.pdf; accessed 6/12/2013)

HISTORICAL FACTORS

Original American citizens of color bear a historical legacy that affects all aspects of their integration into society today. American Indians make up a fraction of today's citizens (0.7% in the 2000 census) but have significant health disparities. The prevalence of diabetes mellitus, obesity, alcoholism, and suicide is substantially greater in this population than in other US population groups. They are the one population with a health system that was established to help meet their medical needs. The availability of these services, however, is limited by distance for the many American Indians living in rural areas, and they may be completely inaccessible to those living in urban areas.

African Americans encompass several groups who came to the United States at different times. The impact of slavery on the original Africans cannot be minimized. Residual effects of this historical tragedy have been associated with discriminatory residential practices, educational disadvantages, and treatment practices in separate but unequal healthcare facilities. Later immigrants of African origin came to the United States from the West Indies, where slavery was abolished well before the Emancipation Proclamation in the United States. These differing experiences have influenced the views of Caribbean Americans and result in differences between them and African Americans who descended directly from slaves on the North American continent. The final group of immigrants from African countries chose to come to the United States in recent years both educational, economic, and political reasons. Cultural differences often exist among these three groups and include differences in customs, family roles, religious preferences, and their definition and experience of illness and disease.

Although the foundation of the United States was a union of indigenous groups and immigrants, the preceding groups along with new immigrants bear much of the burden of disease in the nation today. The number of immigrants entering the United States since the late 1990s has increased dramatically compared with the numbers seen in the previous four decades. Political crises, natural disasters, poverty, and hunger have forced population groups of significant size to leave their homes. These migrations have resulted in loss of homes and support systems, overcrowding and overexposure, decreased access to food and medical services, and contact with new infectious agents and other toxins.

IMMIGRANTS & REFUGEES

The term *immigrant* has been applied to legal and illegal (undocumented) refugees and children adopted from other countries. As of 2011, nearly 40 million immigrants were residing in the United States, accounting for 13 percent of the total population. Most immigrants reside in linguistically isolated households (those in which no one >14 years speaks English), which were identified for the first time in the 1990 census. Four percent of US households are in this category. This figure includes 30% of Asian households, 23% of Hispanic households, and 28% of all immigrant households with school-age children.

Immigrants enter the United States from many countries, but those coming from Mexico represent the largest group. Many Mexican immigrants arrive in the United States healthier than their white counterparts. However, their health deteriorates the longer they live here, possibly as a result of lifestyle changes (years of difficult labor, poverty, smoking, poor diet, and lack of attention to prevention) and a lack of health insurance. One study found that 2.6% of recent Mexican immigrants had diabetes mellitus, compared with 7.7% of Mexican immigrants who had lived in the United States for 15 years. More than two-thirds of recent Mexican immigrants and 44.8% of "long-term immigrants" have no health insurance, compared with 22.5% of Mexican-born Americans and 12.3% of US-born whites. Fewer than 10% of recent Mexican immigrants reported using emergency departments in 2000. Furthermore, more than 33% of Mexican women aged 18–64 years who were recent immigrants had not had a Pap smear in 3 years. Approximately 37% of recent Mexican immigrants visited a health clinic instead of a physician for healthcare, compared with ~15% of US-born whites.

Noncitizens are 3 times more likely than citizens to be uninsured and have more limited access to care than US-born citizens and are less likely to obtain recommended preventive services. Noncitizens are also subject to Medicaid and CHIP eligibility restrictions—specifically, being subject to a 5-year waiting period for Medicaid or CHIP coverage even when lawfully present in the United States. This group will continue to face eligibility restrictions (such as waiting periods) for health coverage options under the Affordable Care Act. Safety net providers will remain a major source of care for immigrants.

Pregnant women are of major concern because of risk for poor pregnancy outcomes. In spite of these concerns, evidence suggests that infants of Mexican immigrants have favorable birth outcomes despite their high socioeconomic risks. These favorable outcomes have been associated with a protective sociocultural orientation among this immigrant group, including a strong family unit. Yet, one-fourth of infants of immigrants in predominantly Spanish-speaking households are at high risk for serious infectious disease despite using preventive care. As these children mature beyond the neonatal period, factors predisposing to illness are large households, poor access to care, and maternal characteristics, including smoking, pregnancy complications, and employment.

Lack of understanding by healthcare providers of traditional remedies for common ailments can result in negative interactions between patients and clinicians, misdiagnosis, and poor health outcomes. In one study, healthcare providers and the population of Vietnamese immigrants for whom they cared both identified misinterpretation of patient symptoms and healthcare provider recommendations as major issues. The special problems of unemployment, depression, surviving torture, and obtaining assistance are all made more difficult for refugees living in small communities that lack sufficiently large ethnic populations to facilitate culturally sensitive provision of health care.

With the exception of Southeast Asian refugees, there are few clinical studies on the health problems of refugees after arrival in the United States. Tuberculosis, nutritional deficiencies, intestinal parasites, chronic hepatitis B infection, lack of immunization, and depression are major problems in many groups. The great variation in health and psychosocial issues, as well as cultural beliefs, among refugees requires careful attention during the medical encounter. In addition to a complete history and physical examination, tests for tuberculosis, hepatitis B surface antigen, ova and parasites, as well as hemoglobin measurement, are advised for most groups.

American Academy of Pediatrics, Committee on Community Health Services. Health care for children of immigrant families. *Pediatrics.* 1997;100:153. [PMID: 9229707]

Chen J, et al. Health expectancy by immigrant status, 1986 and 1991. *Health Rep.* 1996;8:29. [PMID: 9085119]

Mahoney FJ, et al. Continuing risk for hepatitis B virus transmission among Southeast Asian infants in Louisiana. *Pediatrics.* 1995;96:1113. [PMID: 7491231]

Power DV, Shandy D. Sudanese refugees in a Minnesota family practice clinic. *Fam Med.* 1998;30:185. [PMID: 9532440]

Stephens J, Artiga S. *Key Facts on Health Coverage for Low-Income Immigrants Today and under the Affordable Care Act.* Kaiser Commission on Medicaid and the Uninsured: Key Facts; March 2013 (available at http://kff.org/disparities-policy/factsheet/key-facts-on-health-coverage-for-low; accessed June 11, 20130).

Wallace S, Zuniga E. *Mexican Immigrants' Health Status Worsens after Living in US* (available at http://www.kaisernetwork.org/daily_reports/re-index; accessed Oct. 14, 2005).

POVERTY

A greater percentage of African Americans (53%) and Hispanics (59%) have incomes that are below 200% of the federal poverty line than non-Hispanic white Americans (25%) across their lifespans. Financial disadvantage has an impact on health in that mortality rates around the world decline with increasing social class, a concept most easily associated with access to financial resources.

Poor, minority, and uninsured children are twice as likely as other children to lack usual sources of care, nearly twice as likely to wait ≥60 minutes at their sites of care, and use only about half as many physician services after adjusting for health status. Poverty, minority status, and absence of insurance exert independent effects on access to and use of primary care. Homelessness results in poor health status and high service use among children. Homeless children were reported to experience a higher number of acute illness symptoms, including fever, ear infection, diarrhea, and asthma. Emergency department and outpatient medical visits are also higher among the homeless group.

Urban Institute and Kaiser Commission on Medicaid and the Uninsured. Key facts: race, ethnicity and medical care. In: *Analysis of March 2002 Current Population Survey.* Kaiser Family Foundation; 2003.

Weinreb L, et al. Determinants of health and service use patterns in homeless and low-income housed children. *Pediatrics.* 1998;102:554. [PMID: 9738176]

UNINSURANCE & UNDERINSURANCE

A substantial portion of the US population is medically uninsured or underinsured. A greater percentage of racial and ethnic minorities and immigrants are in this category. These numbers increase if individuals who have been without health insurance for ≥3 months in a given year are included. Underinsurance is the inability to pay out-of-pocket expenses despite having insurance and usually implies inability to use preventive services as well. The underinsured category includes unemployed persons aged 55–64 years and those not provided health insurance coverage through their employment. These individuals are not eligible for Medicare and must pay high individual health premiums when they can obtain some form of group coverage. Lack of health insurance is associated with delayed healthcare and increased mortality. Underinsurance also may result in adverse health consequences. An estimated 8 million children from diverse groups in the United States are uninsured. Substantial differences in both sources of care and utilization of medical services exist between insured and uninsured children.

In 2005, 34% of all nonelderly adult Hispanics living in the United States lacked health insurance coverage (either private or public), compared with 21% of African American, 19% of Asian/Pacific Islander, 32% of American Indians, and 13% of non-Hispanic white nonelderly citizens. Because Hispanics are more likely to be uninsured than any other ethnic group and because they are the fastest growing minority group in the United States, it is likely that the number of uninsured in the US population will steadily increase.

There are marked discrepancies in access to and utilization of medical services, including preventive services, between uninsured and insured children, although both groups have similar rates of chronic health conditions and limitations of activity (evidence of the general health of the children being seen). The 2002 Institute of Medicine report, *Unequal Treatment*, documented the widespread evidence of racial and ethnic disparities in health care. However, only 5 of the 103 published studies cited in this report addressed health disparities in children. Yet there appear to be disparities of equivalent magnitude and persistence in children as are seen in adults. Substantial gaps in insurance coverage exist among children such that 37% of Hispanic, 23% of African American, and 20% of non-Hispanic white children have no health insurance. Children of color are more likely to be insured through public programs such as Medicaid and the State Children's Health Insurance Program (SCHIP).

Children eligible for Medicaid but who remain unenrolled are often younger than 6 years of age, live in female-headed single-parent families, or are African American or Hispanic. Not only do uninsured children lack routine medical care; they also lack appropriate well-child care compared with insured children. Children who have a chronic disease, such as asthma, face difficulties of access to care and utilize substantially fewer outpatient and inpatient services.

Parents' utilization of healthcare services has a large impact on the services used by their children. Even if all children were universally insured, parental healthcare access and utilization would remain a key determinant in children's use of services. Neglecting financial access to care for adults who serve as caregivers for children may have the unintended effect of diminishing the impact of targeted health insurance programs for children.

The uninsured can manifest similar psychopathology as is seen in refugees. Rates of current psychiatric disorders (including major depression, anxiety disorders, and history of sexual trauma) are extremely high in ethnically diverse women who are receiving public medical assistance or are uninsured. These women also report behaviors that pose serious health risks, including smoking (23%) and illicit drug use (2%). Fewer than half have access to comprehensive primary medical care. Young, poor women who seek care in public-sector clinics would benefit from comprehensive medical care addressing their psychosocial needs.

In the United States, the cost of healthcare services is a major barrier to healthcare access. In addition, three-fourths of persons in the United States who have difficulty paying their medical bills have some type of health insurance. Although the affordability of healthcare among persons without health insurance has been described, few details regarding affordability among persons who are underinsured exist.

Investigators who looked at state programs offering subsidized coverage in commercial managed care organizations to low-income and previously uninsured people found no evidence of pent-up demand or an unusual level of chronic illness between people enrolled through large employer-benefit plans and previously uninsured patients. Similarly, there was little evidence of underutilization, although dissatisfaction and reported barriers to service were more frequent among nonwhite enrollees. In another study, undocumented immigrants had more complicated and serious diagnoses on admission but a lower adjusted average length of stay than native-born populations and those with permanent residency status (insured by Medicaid or of uninsured status) admitted to the same hospital.

Although generalist physicians appear to be more likely than specialists to provide care for poor adult patients, they may still perceive financial and nonfinancial barriers to caring for these patients. Nonwhite physicians were more likely to care for uninsured and Medicaid patients than were white physicians. In addition to reimbursement, nonfinancial factors played an important role in physicians' decisions not to care for Medicaid or uninsured patients. For example, perceived risks of litigation and poor reimbursement were cited by 60–90% of physicians as important in the decision not to care for Medicaid and uninsured patients.

The Affordable Care Act (ACA) is a step toward reducing disparities and to improve health and healthcare by expanding health coverage for low- and moderate-income populations. People of color and low-income individuals have more barriers to care and receive poorer quality of care. The ACA establishes a new continuum of coverage options to include an expansion of Medicaid to a national eligibility floor of 138% FPL (federal poverty level) ($26,344 for a family

of three in 2012) and the creation of new Health Benefit Exchanges with tax credits for individuals up to 400% FPL ($76,300 for a family of three in 2012). These expansions are designed to help reduce the wide variations in access to health coverage across states and increase availability of coverage for low- and middle-income populations—significantly impacting people of color who are disproportionately uninsured or low-income.

Avruch S, et al. The demographic characteristics of Medicaid-eligible uninsured children. *Am J Public Health*. 1998;88:445. [PMID: 9518979]

Beal AC. Policies to reduce racial and ethnic disparities in child health and health care. *Health Affairs*. 2004;23(5):171–179. [PMID: 15371383]

Braveman P, et al. Socioeconomic disparities in the United States: what the patterns tell us. *Am J Public Health*. 2010;100(1):186–196.

Hanson KL. Is insurance for children enough? The link between parents' and children's health care use revisited. *Inquiry*. 1998;35:294. [PMID: 9809057]

Holt JL, et al. Profile of uninsured children in the United States. *Arch Pediatr Adolesc Med*. 1995;149-398. [PMID: 7704168]

Kaiser Family Foundation. *Focus on Health Care Disparities: Key Facts*. Dec 2012 (available at http://kff.org/disparities-policy/issue-brief/health-coverage-by-race-and-ethnicity-the-potential-impact-of-the-affordable-care-act/).

Kilbreth EH et al. State-sponsored programs for the uninsured: is there adverse selection? *Inquiry* 1998;35:250. [PMID: 9809054]

Komaromy M, et al. California physicians' willingness to care for the poor. *West J Med/* 1995;162:127. [PMID: 7725684]

Miranda J, et al. Unmet mental health needs of women in public-sector gynecologic clinics. *Am J Obstet Gynecol*. 1998;178:212. [PMID: 9500476]

Smedley D, et al. *Unequal Treatment: Confronting Racial and Ethnic Disparities in Health Care*. National Academies Press; 2003.

Thamer M, et al. Health insurance coverage among foreign-born US residents: the impact of race, ethnicity, and length of residence. *Am J Publ Health*. 1997;87:96. [PMID: 9065235]

Urban Institute and Kaiser Commission on Medicaid and the Uninsured: Key facts: race, ethnicity and Medical care. In: *Health Insurance Coverage in America: March 2005 Current Population Survey*. Kaiser Family Foundation; 2005 (available at www.kaiseredu.org/tutorials/REHealthcare/player.html; accessed Oct. 25, 2009).

HOUSING & GEOGRAPHIC FACTORS

Racial residential segregation has been suggested as a fundamental cause of racial disparities in health. Although legislation exists to eliminate discrimination in housing, the degree of residential segregation remains extremely high for most African Americans in the United States. Williams and Collins (2001) argue that segregation is a primary cause of racial differences in socioeconomic status by determining access to education and employment opportunities. Furthermore, segregation creates conditions that hamper a healthy social and physical environment. Levels of racial residential segregation grew dramatically from 1860 to 1940 and have been maintained since then.

Recent research has linked racial segregation to higher cancer risk; the risk increases as the degree of segregation increases. Minorities living in highly segregated metropolitan areas are >2.5 times more likely to develop cancer from air pollutants when compared with whites. Hispanics who live in highly segregated areas are affected the most, with a risk 6.4 times that of whites. When neighborhood poverty indicators and population density are controlled, the disparities in cancer risk persist, although at lower levels.

Skinner and colleagues (2005) noted the contribution of community of residence to health disparities. The investigators suggested that African-American patients are concentrated in a small number of poorly performing hospitals. In this study, nearly 70% of African-American patients with myocardial infarctions were treated at only ~20% of regional medical centers. The majority of those with life-threatening cardiac conditions received care at smaller health care institutions that had less experience in treating these conditions. When >1 million Medicare recipients from 1997 to 2001 were examined, death rates for patients presenting with acute myocardial infarction were 19% higher at these hospitals than at facilities that saw only white patients. Because the factors contributing to health disparities are so complex, there is no one solution. However, these findings suggest that spending must be increased and quality improved at medical centers that primarily treat minorities and the poor.

Young to middle-aged residents of impoverished urban areas manifest excess mortality from several causes, both acute and chronic. African American youth in some urban areas face lower probabilities of surviving to 45 years of age than white youths nationwide surviving to 65 years of age. Minorities constitute 80% of residents of high-poverty, urban areas in the United States and >90% in the largest metropolitan areas. The lower the socioeconomic position held, the less ability the person has to gain access to information, services, or technologies that could provide protection from or modify risks.

For most Americans, housing equity is a major source of wealth. Residential segregation in such a fashion, therefore, directly influences socioeconomic status. Income predicts variation in health for both white and African Americans, but African Americans report poorer health than whites at all levels of income. People residing in disadvantaged neighborhoods have a higher incidence of heart disease than people who live in more advantaged neighborhoods. The quality of housing is also likely to be worse in highly segregated areas, and poor housing conditions adversely affect health. For example, research reveals that a lack of residential facilities and concerns about personal safety can discourage leisure-time physical exercise.

Geronimus A. To mitigate, resist, or undo: addressing structural influences on the health of urban populations. *Am J Public Health* 2000;90:867. [PMID: 10846503]

Morello-Frosch R, Jesdale BM: Separate and unequal: residential segregation and estimated cancer risks associated with ambient air toxics in U.S. metropolitan areas. *Environ Health Perspect.* 2006;114:386. [PMID: 16507462]

Skinner J, et al. Mortality after acute myocardial infarction in hospitals that disproportionately treat Black patients. *Circulation.* 2005;112:2634. [PMID: 16246963]

Williams DR, Collins C. Racial residential segregation: a fundamental cause of racial disparities in health. *Public Health Rep.* 2001;116(5):404–416. [PMID: 12042604]

MENTAL HEALTH ISSUES

Disparities in mental health services have been known to exist among diverse communities for decades. Among these disparities is a high rate of misdiagnosis, lack of linguistically competent therapists, culturally insensitive diagnostic measures, and increased exposure to abuse.

The practice of psychiatry is heavily influenced by culture. The cultural identity of patients as well as providers, their perceptions of mental illness and appropriate treatment, their background, and their current environment potentially all have an impact on the psychiatric diagnosis made, the therapy selected, and the therapeutic outcome. Mental illness has been diagnosed more frequently in African Americans and Hispanics than in non-Hispanic white Americans for >100 years. Many of the studies reporting these data have been criticized for faulty methodology, cultural bias, and suspect racial theories.

There is some evidence that appropriate research and mental healthcare delivery for these populations are influenced by factors such as poor cultural validation of the *Diagnostic and Statistical Manual of Mental Disorders*, misdiagnosis of minority patients, and the unwillingness of many psychiatrists to acknowledge culturally defined syndromes and folk-healing systems.

General mental health screening is difficult in part because assessment of psychological health in non-English-speaking populations is impeded by lack of instruments that are language- and population-specific. Patients whose first language is not English usually undergo psychiatric evaluation and treatment in English. Cultural nuances are encoded in language in ways that are often not readily conveyed in translation, even when equivalent words in the second language are used. An appropriately trained interpreter will routinely identify these nuances for the monolingual clinician. When such an interpreter is not available, these nuances can be clarified through consultation with a clinician who shares the patient's first language and culture to maximize delivery of quality healthcare.

Collins JL, et al. Ethnic and cultural factors in psychiatric diagnosis and treatment. In: *Handbook of Mental Health and Mental Disorders among Black Americans*. Greenwood Press; 1990.

Dassori AM, et al. Schizophrenia among Hispanics: epidemiology, phenomenology, course, and outcome. *Schizophr Bull*. 1995;21:303. [PMID: 7631176]

Kirmayer LJ, Groleau D. Affective disorders in cultural context. *Psychiatr Clin North Am*. 2001;24:465. [PMID: 11593857]

Lewis-Fernandez R, Kleinman A. Cultural psychiatry. Theoretical, clinical, and research issues. *Psychiatr Clin North Am*. 1995;18:433. [PMID: 8545260]

DISCRIMINATION

In addition to cost, there are significant differences in how physicians make therapeutic decisions with respect to the minority status of the patient. Women, ethnic minorities, and uninsured persons receive fewer procedures than do affluent white male patients. Furthermore, the race and sex of a patient independently influence how physicians manage acute conditions such as chest pain. For example, women and minorities are less likely to be diagnosed with angina when presenting with comparable risk factors and the same symptoms as white men.

Illegal immigrants underutilize health services, especially preventive services such as prenatal care, dental care, and immunizations due to cost, language, cultural barriers, and fear of apprehension by immigration authorities. Further complicating efforts to provide access to healthcare for this group is fear for the well-being of family members who may be undocumented, even when the patient is here legally. The increasing number of immigrants entering the United States in recent years has resulted in more legislation seeking to restrict access of various refugee and immigrant groups to public services. Legislation such as Proposition 187, passed in California in 1994, prohibits people lacking legal residency status from obtaining all but emergency medical care at any healthcare facility receiving public funds.

This legislation has encouraged further obstacles to healthcare access for countless other people residing in the United States. For example, minorities who were born in the United States find that they are pressured to produce immigration documentation to receive care. Family physicians seeking to care for immigrants and refugees must recognize and effectively deal with problems in communication, establish trust regarding immigration concerns, understand cultural mores influencing the encounter, find the resources to provide necessary services, make an accurate diagnosis, and negotiate a treatment. Unfortunately, fear of these restrictive immigration laws and socioeconomic hardships combine to delay both seeking and obtaining curative care for these populations.

Title VI of the federal Civil Rights Act states that "no person in the United States shall, on the ground of race, color, or national origin, be excluded from participation in, be denied the benefits of, or be subjected to discrimination under any program or activity receiving Federal financial assistance." Current federal mandates ensuring access to emergency medical services and new restrictions on financing of healt care for immigrants under federal programs such as Medicaid and Medicare appear to be in direct conflict. The Personal Responsibility and Work Opportunity Reconciliation Act and the Illegal Immigration Reform and Immigrant Responsibility Act specifically reaffirm federal law on delivery of emergency services without addressing the financing of that care. Unfunded mandates in an era of diminished ability to shift costs onto insured patients create a major dilemma for the institutions that provide uncompensated care. Medicaid is considered one form of insurance, although the level of reimbursement of providers has been so low that many providers will not treat patients with that coverage.

Leape LL, et al. Underuse of cardiac procedures: do women, ethnic minorities, and the uninsured fail to receive needed revascularization. *Ann Intern Med*. 1999;130:183. [PMID: 10049196]

Schulman KA, et al. The effect of race and sex on physicians' recommendations for cardiac catheterization. *N Engl J Med*. 1999;340:618. [PMID: 10029647]

LANGUAGE & LANGUAGE LITERACY

The physician-patient relationship is grounded in communication and the effective use of language. One of the first principles taught in medical school is the importance of the patient's history. Along with clinical reasoning, observations, and nonverbal cues, skillful use of language establishes the clinical interview as the clinician's most powerful tool.

The 2000 census found that more than 46 million Americans speak a language different than that of their clinician. In the United States, the primary "other language" is Spanish. Approximately 25% of Hispanics were born outside of the United States and Puerto Rico, but >77% of them note speaking Spanish as their primary language at home. Contributing to the discrepancy, the demographic profiles of the nation's healthcare providers does not mirror population trends. In California, although 32% of the population is Hispanic, only 4% of nurses, 4% of physicians, and 6% of dentists are Hispanic.

Cultural competence is not necessarily associated with language fluency. The effectiveness of communication between a clinician and a patient is influenced by the cultural exposure that fosters command of the meaning of the words and phrases. A patient and clinician who do not share a common language face more challenges to quality care than those who share this foundation of communication. Such language differences can have a negative impact on the clinical encounter. Parents, providers, hospital staff, and quality improvement professionals agree that language and cultural differences lead to communication issues that can have a pervasive, negative impact on the quality and safety of care that children receive. There is still disagreement regarding what needs to change to improve healthcare delivery in a language-discordant environment.

Linguistic competence refers to the capacity of an organization and its personnel to communicate effectively and convey information in a manner that is easily understood by diverse groups, including persons of limited English proficiency, those who have low literacy skills or are not literate, and individuals with disabilities. Linguistic competency requires organizational and provider capacity to respond effectively to the health literacy needs of populations served. The organization must have policy, structures, practices, procedures, and dedicated resources to support this capacity (**Table 65-1**). Federal standards have been established for clinical practice when language discordance is present. To maintain quality of care and adhere to the federal guidelines defined in the National Standards for Culturally and Linguistically Competent Health and Health Care (CLAS) revised and published in 2013, clinicians must provide accommodation for patients in their chosen language.

Bethell C, et al. Quality and safety of hospital care for children from Spanish-speaking families with limited English proficiency. *J Healthcare Qual/* 2006;28(3):W3-2-W3-16.

Dower C, et al. *The Practice of Medicine in California: A Profile of the Physician Workforce.* UCSF Center for the Health Professions; 2001.

Table 65-1. Linguistic resources for healthcare.

Bilingual/bicultural and multilingual/ multicultural staff
Cultural brokers
Foreign language interpretation services, including distance technologies
Sign language interpretation services, including distance technologies
TTY (teletypewriter) services
Assistive technology devices
Computer-assisted real-time translation (CART) or viable real-time transcription
Telehealth networks
Texting
Print materials in easy-to-read, low-literacy, picture and symbol formats
Materials in alternative formats (audiotape, Braille, enlarged print)
Translation services
Ethnic media in languages other than English (eg, radio, television, Internet, newspapers, periodicals, social networking sites)

Reproduced with permission from Goode TD, Jones W. National Center for Cultural Competence, Georgetown University Center for Child & Human Development, modified 2013 (available at: http://gucchd.georgetown.edu/nccc).

Duran DG, Pacheco G eds. *Quality Health Services for Hispanics: The Cultural Competency Component.* DHHS Publication 99–21. National Alliance for Hispanic Health; 2000.

Morales LS, et al. The impact of interpreters on parents' experiences with ambulatory care for their children. *Med Care Res Rev.* 2006;63(1):110–128. [PMID: 16686075]

Woloshin S, et al. Language barriers in medicine in the United States. *JAMA.* 1995;273:724. [PMID: 7853631]

Websites

National Center for Cultural Competence. *Foundations of Cultural and Linguistic Competence, Defintion of Linguistic Competence* (available at http://nccc.georgetown.edu/foundations/index.html)

National Standards for Culturally and Linguistically Appropriate Services (CLAS) in Health and Health Care, Office of Minority Health Resource Center (http://www.omhrc.gov/CLAS)

HEALTHCARE FOR THE DISABLED

Americans with disabilities are more than twice as likely to postpone needed healthcare because they cannot afford it. In addition, the National Organization on Disability has determined that people with disabilities are 4 times more likely to have special needs that are not covered by health insurance. Many nonelderly adults (46%) with disabilities note that they go without equipment and other items because of cost. More than a third (37%) postpone care because of cost, skip doses, or split pills (36%) because of medication costs, and spend less on basics such as food, heat, and other services in order to pay for healthcare (36%). Those with Medicare alone (no supplemental coverage) report the highest rates of serious cost-related problems due to gaps in Medicare's benefit package. Those receiving Medicaid fare better because of the broad scope of benefits and relatively low cost-sharing requirements of Medicaid. However, >20% of adults with disabilities on Medicaid reported that physicians would not accept their insurance—more than twice the percentage of patients having private insurance or Medicare.

Current data suggest that health disparities among people with and without disabilities are as pervasive as those recognized among ethnic minority groups. People with disabilities were included in the Healthy People plan to provide a broad look at the health of this population. Of the 467 objectives listed in Healthy People 2010, 207 subobjectives address people with disabilities. Some of the subobjectives focus on areas outside of the usual scope of healthcare or healthcare services, such as education, employment, transportation, and housing—all of which have a direct impact on wellness and quality of life.

In addition to examining the health of all citizens with disabilities, particular focus is directed to evaluating the health status of women with disabilities. Regardless of age, women with functional limitations were consistently less likely to have received a Pap test during the past 3 years than women without functional limitations.

The National Survey of SSI (supplemental security income) Children and Families (July 2001–June 2002) examined children with *disabilities* who were receiving SSI and their families. Children receiving SSI are more likely to live in a family headed by a single mother, and approximately 50% live in a household with at least one other individual reported to have had a disability. SSI support was the most important source of family income, accounting for nearly half of the income for the children's families, and earnings accounting for almost 40%.

Although the Americans with Disabilities Act was enacted in 1990 in an effort to improve access to a broad range of services, women with physical disabilities continue to receive less preventive health screening than women with none. Furthermore, women with more severe disabilities undergo less screening than those with mild or moderate severity of disability.

Adults with developmental disabilities were more likely to lead sedentary lifestyles and 7 times as likely to report inadequate emotional support, compared to adults without. Adults with physical and developmental disabilities were significantly more likely to report being in fair or poor health. Similar rates of tobacco use and overweight/obesity were reported. Adults with developmental disabilities had a similar or greater risk of having four of five chronic health conditions compared with nondisabled adults. Significant medical care utilization disparities were found for breast and cervical cancer screening as well as for oral healthcare. These women also had 40% greater odds of violence in the 5 years preceding the interview, and these women appeared to be at particular risk for severe violence.

US Surgeon General Richard H. Carmona, MD, MPH, released *The Surgeon General's Call to Action to Improve the Health and Wellness of Persons with Disabilities* on the 15th anniversary of the American with Disabilities Act in July 2005. The four goals of the *Call to Action* are to

1. Increase understanding nationwide that people with disabilities can lead long, healthy, and productive lives.

2. Increase knowledge among healthcare professionals and provide them with tools to screen, diagnose, and treat the whole person with a disability with dignity.

3. Increase awareness among people with disabilities regarding the steps they can take to develop and maintain a healthy lifestyle.

4. Increase accessible healthcare and support services to promote independence for people with disabilities.

FUTURE DIRECTIONS & CURRENT CHALLENGES

Multiple factors contribute to the persistence of health and healthcare disparities in the United States today. These factors originate from the patients, clinicians providing care, and the systems in which they must interact. Equitable, quality healthcare for all is achievable in an environment that values cultural competence. Cultural competence is necessary in multiple domains: values and attitudes; communication styles; community and consumer participation; physical environment, materials, and resources; policies and procedures; population-based clinical practice; and training and professional development. Only by assuming responsibility and accountability for this global problem at all levels of the healthcare system will there be any hope of narrowing the gap and ensuring health for all.

Brownridge DA. Partner violence against women with disabilities: prevalence, risk, and explanations. *Violence against Women*. 2006;12(9):805–822. [PMID: 16905674]

Havercamp SM. Health disparities among adults with developmental disabilities, adults with other disabilities, and adults not reporting disability in North Carolina. *Public Health Rep.* 2004;119(4):418–426. [PMID: 15219799]

Hjern A, et al. Political violence, family stress and mental health of refugee children in exile. *Scand J Soc Med.* 1998;26(1):18–25.

Hovey JD, King CA. Acculturative stress, depression and suicidal ideation among immigrant and second generation Latino adolescents. *J Am Acad Child Adolesc Psychiatr.* 1996;35:1183–1192.

Johnson BL, Coulberson SL. Environmental epidemiologic issues and minority health. *Ann Epidemiol.* 1993;3(3):175–180.

Karter AJ, et al. Ethnic disparities in diabetic complications in an insured population. *JAMA.* 2002;287:2519–2527.

Lillie-Blanton M, Laveist T. Race/ethnicity, the social environment, and health. *Soc Sci Med.* 1996;43(1):83-89.

Marmot M. Inequalities in health. *N Engl J Med.* 2001;345:134–136.

Mollica RE. Effects of war trauma on Cambodian refugee adolescents' functional health and mental health status. *J Am Acad Child Adolesc Psychiatr.* 1997;36(8):1098–1106.

Nickens HW. The role of race/ethnicity and social class in minority health status. *Health Serv Res.* 1995;30(1, Pt 2):151–162.

Pernice R, Brooks J. Refugees' and immigrants' mental health: association of demographic and post-immigration factors. *J Soc Psychol.* (US) 1996;136(4):511–519.

Smeltzer SC. Preventive health screening for breast and cervical cancer and osteoporosis in women with physical disabilities. *Fam Commun Health.* 2006;29(1 Suppl):35S–43S. [PMID: 16344635]

Stephens DL. A longitudinal study of employment and skill acquisition among individuals with developmental disabilities. *Res Dev Disabil.* 2005;26(5):469–486. [PMID: 16168884]

Caring for Lesbian, Gay, Bisexual, & Transgender Patients

66

Steven R. Wolfe, DO, MPH

OVERVIEW

▶ Who is Lesbian, Gay, Bisexual, or Transgender?

Assuming the most recent data to be correct, 5–9% of men are gay and 3–4% of women are lesbian. Kinsey's original reports put these numbers at 10% for men and 2–6% for women. A recent international review reports that ≤15% of men report same-sex sexual activity at some time during their lives. An additional small percentage of the population experiences gender identity disorder or identify as transgender. These numbers suggest that physicians will provide care for lesbian, gay, bisexual, or transgender (LGBT) patients regardless of geographic location, or the ethnic, religious, socioeconomic, or gender demographics of their practice, and perhaps without knowing.

 ESSENTIALS OF DIAGNOSIS

▶ The first step in providing high-quality healthcare to LGBT patients is a thorough and sensitive sexual history.

▶ History forms can facilitate this, if items include options relevant for LGBT patients, for example, "marital status" should include options for domestic partner.

▶ Comprehensive information about behavior is necessary as a foundation for optimal education and health screening.

Knowing which patients are LGBT is the first and most important step in providing superior care—even if patients do not self-identify as LGBT but engage in same-sex sexual encounters. Accomplish this by taking a thorough and sensitive sexual history with all new patients and any time sexual behavior may be relevant to diagnosis and management.

▶ Taking the Sexual History

The process of taking a sexual history begins with creating a safe environment. As sexual and gender-variant minorities, many LGBT people have faced discrimination and may fear sharing the details of their sexual lives with a healthcare provider. To further complicate matters, many healthcare providers may avoid discussing sexuality and sexual orientation details with patients, especially with adolescents, because often physicians do not feel they have the skills needed to address issues of sexual orientation. By providing literature in the office relevant to LGBT patients and by displaying positive, reassuring symbols (eg, a rainbow flag or equal sign), physicians can help their patients feel more at ease. History forms should include the full range of patient responses and not contain wording that ignores LGBT patients' lives; such forms could facilitate conversation about sensitive topics. Physicians can overcome their own discomfort by routinely taking sexual histories.

The goal of taking a sexual history is to identify behaviors that can affect a patient's health. Whether a man who has sex with men (MSM) self-identifies as gay or bisexual is important for understanding his social and psychological situation, but less relevant in terms of screening for and treating organic disease processes. It is worth prefacing all sexual history taking by informing the patient that the discussion will remain entirely confidential, and that the reason why each question must be answered in full, although the questions may seem too personal and invasive, is so that the physician can provide the best, most personalized care possible.

Physicians can help their patients be forthcoming about behaviors by guaranteeing privacy, excusing family members and partners from the room (after first receiving the patient's consent to do so), and being mindful of the assumptions they make about their patients. For example, married heterosexual women may have sexual encounters with women, and self-identified lesbians have often had sexual encounters with men. Not all male-to-female (MTF) transgender people are sexually active with men, or at all. Many elderly patients remain sexually active well into their senior years. Compassionate, thorough discussion of a patient's behavior can help clarify and demystify assumptions that healthcare providers make on the basis of superficial traits or stereotypes of LGBT patients. After introducing the topic, many clinicians begin the sexual history by asking, "Are you sexually active?" This question is a good starting point, but fails to address past behavior. In addition, patients may have variable definitions of what constitutes "being sexually active." These ambiguities should be addressed by carefully listening to patients' responses and following up with more specific questions.

The second question often used by practitioners is, "Are you sexually active with men, women, or both?" Asking this emphasizes behaviors are emphasized over labels, and no assumption is made about sexual orientation. Providing a list of options instead of asking patients to fill in the blanks, makes it easier to give voice to important medical information and communicates the physician's receptivity to hear any answer.

Regarding current and former partners, the distinct sexual behaviors in which the patient has participated should be elucidated. It is these behaviors (eg, penile-vaginal intercourse, receptive or insertive anal intercourse, oral-vaginal intercourse, oral-anal intercourse), and whether barrier protection was used during intercourse, that will help determine screening and other management decisions. Without asking about specific behaviors, regardless of the fact that the gender of partners may be known, therapeutic decisions will be based on potentially incorrect assumptions.

In addition, it may be useful to identify the number of current and past partners, regardless of whether those relationships were monogamous, whether barrier protection is always used (keeping in mind that condoms are often not used properly), and whether patients and their partners have a history of sexually transmitted infection. This information is useful for approximating risk of disease exposure, and may identify ongoing risk behaviors that need attention.

A physician must understand how a patient's sexual or gender identity affects her/his life at home, at work, and in the community. In addition, all patients who are sexually active with opposite sex partners, regardless of their sexual identity, should be asked whether they are interested in birth control. All LGBT patients should be screened for experiences with domestic violence or hate crime. Because the increased rates of substance abuse and dependence in some LGBT populations, the entirety of the social history should be completed, addressing the use of tobacco, alcohol, cocaine, methylenedioxymethamphetamine (MDMA; Ecstasy or Molly), methamphetamines (crystal meth), prescriptions (including opiates, benzodiazepines and stimulants), hormones, hallucinogens, marijuana, and intravenous drugs

It is only by identifying behaviors that physicians can appropriately screen, risk-stratify, effectively educate, and provide optimal care for their patients. Individuals who are members of a sexual or gender-variant minority group are often less obvious in their identity than those of other types of minority groups. Human behavior or gender expression does not always clearly align with gender norms of male and female.

For the purposes of this chapter and in the interest of simplicity, we will refer to gay men and lesbians as if they were single populations. However, this is a gross oversimplification of very complex and diverse human behavior. The LGBT population is heterogeneous, composed of individuals, couples, and families of all genders, ages, and socioeconomic, ethnic, religious, political, and geographic backgrounds. It is for this diversity that the rainbow flag was chosen as an LGBT symbol. This diversity also serves as the complex social context of patients' lives that, in turn, shapes their experience of health and disease.

Guidelines for Care of Lesbian, Gay, Bisexual, and Transgender Patients (available at http://www.glma.org/_data/n_0001/resources/live/GLMA%20guidelines%202006%20FINAL.pdf; accessed April 21, 2009).

▶ Who Is Gay? What Is Bisexual?

The complexity of human sexual behavior defies simple categorization. Sexual orientation manifests as fantasies, desires, actual behavior, and self- or other-identified labels. For example, a man could think of himself and describe himself as heterosexual, engage in sex with men and women in equal numbers, and in his sexual fantasies focus almost exclusively on male images; a simple label fails to capture the reality of his sexuality. Even when considering only sexual behaviors, differences may exist between actual versus desired, past versus present, admitted versus practiced, and consensual versus forced.

In the medical setting, asking about a patient's label (eg, "Are you gay or bisexual?") importantly assesses her/his self perception, but may fail to identify medically significant information. Many individuals who engage in same-gender, high-risk sexual behaviors do not self-identify as gay or bisexual. MSM may be at increased risk for sexually transmitted infections (STIs) compared with men who have sex with women only. Women who have sex with men and women (WSMW) may have an increased risk for STIs and substance abuse compared with either women who have sex with women (WSW) or women who have sex with men only. Differentiation would not be possible by asking a patient only if she identifies herself as lesbian, as both WSMW and WSW may identify themselves as lesbian.

Little specific literature exists describing the characteristics of bisexual men and women separate from either strictly heterosexual or homosexual persons. Research studies that include bisexual-identified individuals typically group them with homosexual patients during statistical analysis, limiting information about bisexuality as distinct from heterosexuality or homosexuality. Historically, research focusing on LGBT patients frequently suffers from definitional differences that limit cross-study comparisons, small sample size, population sampling bias, and other shortcomings. Changing societal attitudes, improved research methodology, and increased resources are improving our knowledge gaps.

▶ Homophobia, Heterosexism, & Sexual Prejudice

Homophobia is defined as an irrational fear of, aversion to, or discrimination against homosexuality or homosexuals. *Heterosexism* is the belief that heterosexuality is the natural, normal, acceptable, or superior form of sexuality. Sexual prejudice encompasses negative attitudes toward an individual because of that person's sexual orientation. In their most extreme manifestation, homophobia and sexual prejudice result in physical violence and murder. Evolving societal attitudes may diminish such threats, but homophobia and its behavioral manifestations remain a significant threat to health.

Homophobia is dangerous. One survey of physicians found that 52% observed colleagues providing substandard care to patients due to sexual orientation. In another study, 37% of young gay men reported anti-gay harassment in the previous 6 months, resulting in increased suicidal ideation and diminished self-esteem. In HIV-seropositive gay men who were otherwise healthy, HIV infection advanced more rapidly, exhibiting a dose-response relationship, in participants who concealed their homosexual identity. A study of 1067 lesbians and gay men found that feelings of victimization resulting from perceived social stigma were a significant contributor to depression. A study of 912 Hispanic men found that experiences of social discrimination were strong predictors of suicidal ideation, anxiety, and depressed mood.

Overcoming prejudices and eliminating discriminatory practices are fundamental to healthcare for all patients. Bias against LGBT individuals seems to respond more effectively to experiential interventions (eg, interaction with LGBT individuals) than to rational interventions (eg, information dissemination). In a clinical setting, physicians can communicate acceptance and support with posters showing same-sex couples, stickers depicting a rainbow flag or equals sign, and a visible nondiscrimination statement stating that equal care is provided to all patients, regardless of age, race, ethnicity, physical ability or attributes, religion, sexual identity, and gender identity.

The perceived tolerance (or intolerance) strongly influences LGBT patients' willingness to disclose sexual orientation and details of their personal lives. A patient's sexual practices affects risk for various diseases and can influence disease screening and diagnostic evaluation, so honest discussion of the patient's sexual and social life is vital to promote optimal health. A physician who fails to identify an LGBT patient's sexual orientation may not adequately counsel or diagnose a patient and may compromise delivery of quality medical care. Incorrect assumptions about patients can have similar adverse outcomes (**Table 66-1**).

Table 66-1. Pitfalls in caring for gay and lesbian patients.

Assumption	Solution
Assumption about sexual orientation: Many patients are neither exclusively heterosexual nor exclusively homosexual.	Learn to inquire about sexual orientation in a nonjudgmental manner that recognizes the range of human diversity and apply this learning to all patients.
Assumptions about sexual activity: Lesbian and gay male patients may have numerous different sexual partners, be in a monogamous relationship, be celibate, or vary in patterns of activity over time.	Take a specific, sensitive sexual history from all patients.
Assumptions about contraception: The need for contraception arises from a wish to prevent pregnancy from heterosexual intercourse, regardless of the patient's gender identity, sexual orientation, or label.	Inquire about need (rather than assuming need) or lack of need for all patients. Tailor recommendations to patient's needs.
Assumptions about marriage: Lesbians and gay men may have been, and may still be, married to persons of the opposite sex. In some states and countries, they may be married to same-gender partners and may use the terms "partner" or "husband/wife" to refer to their spouse.	Inquire about significant relationships for all patients. Use the same terminology that your patients choose.
Assumptions about parenting: Lesbian and gay male couples are often interested in and choose to bear and raise children.	Inquire about parenting wishes and choices, and be prepared to discuss options.

Using simple conversational techniques, and mastering a very manageable amount of medical information, will allow family physicians to provide superior care to LGBT patients.

Websites

Gay and Lesbian Medical Association (GLMA): http://www.glma.org.

Parents, Families, and Friends of Lesbians and Gays (PFLAG): http://www.pflag.org.

HIV/AIDS

 ESSENTIALS OF DIAGNOSIS

▶ Not all LGBT patients are at risk for HIV, but screening for HIV infection in adolescents and adults aged 15–65 years is recommended. Younger adolescents and older adults who are at increased risk should also be screened.

▶ Periodic screening (HIV blood tests) is recommended for all persons who are sexually active outside a mutually monogamous relationship.

▶ Blood tests for HIV antibodies have sensitivity and specificity of >99%. HIV viral load tests [eg, HIV polymerase chain reaction (PCR)] should not be used for HIV screening because of the high false-positive rate.

General Considerations

Any publication on LGBT health that omitted mention of HIV would be incomplete, but thorough coverage of the topic is covered in a separate chapter.

Gay men constitute the largest number of AIDS cases in the United States. Recent literature suggests increased rates of unprotected anal intercourse ("barebacking") among certain gay populations. This trend may be due in part to decreased fear of HIV in the era of highly active antiretroviral therapy (HAART). Young gay men, those who use the Internet to meet sexual partners, and those with substance abuse problems, particularly those who use crystal meth, ecstasy, and Viagra, are at greater risk. Increasingly, African American and Hispanic men are disproportionately affected. Another quickly growing HIV-positive population is African American women who have unprotected sex with African American male partners that are on the "down low" or secretly having unprotected sex with men. Increased stigma associated with homosexuality in ethnic minority communities may drive individuals at risk to hide, complicating efforts at diagnosis and treatment.

Prevention

Until an effective vaccine is available, behavioral interventions are the best means to stop the spread of HIV. Physicians should screen all patients for risk behaviors (eg, unprotected intercourse, multiple partners, concurrent sex and substance use, injection drug use) and should intervene to reduce risk and test for HIV in patients with a positive risk history, repeating testing periodically if risk behaviors continue. Pursue a "harm reduction" strategy if it is impossible to eliminate all risk (eg, stopping needle sharing until drug abuse can be stopped, keeping condoms available when sex with a new partner is possible). Since patients engaging in risky behaviors rarely will volunteer information about their risk, physicians must proactively assess each patient's risk and intervene when needed.

Postexposure prophylaxis (PEP) may be beneficial for HIV-negative individuals exposed to HIV. The data supporting antiretroviral treatment following sexual exposure are limited, extrapolated from occupational exposure data and vetted by expert guidelines recommended to initiate a 4-week regimen of PEP as soon as possible after a significant exposure to HIV. The benefit of treatment started >72 hours after exposure is limited. Combinations of antiretroviral agents similar to those used in treating HIV may be used, with similar adverse effects. PEP is not 100% effective in preventing HIV seroconversion.

Clinical Findings

Physicians should consider and test for HIV in at-risk individuals who present with routine viral infection symptoms. Patients with acute HIV infection present with symptoms that are generally indistinguishable from common viral infections, including fever (96%), adenopathy (74%), pharyngitis (70%), rash (70%), and other nonspecific symptoms (see **Table 14-2**). HIV viral load tests (eg, PCR) become positive 1–2 weeks before routine (antibody-based) HIV tests and may be useful in diagnosis (as distinct from screening).

Latent HIV infection may remain essentially asymptomatic for years. Generalized lymphadenopathy may persist for years. Its disappearance may indicate clinically significant immune system decline, marked by nonspecific symptoms such as fevers, weight loss, and diarrhea. Early immune dysfunction results in diseases such as herpes zoster or persistent vaginal candidiasis. Without effective antiretroviral treatment, almost all patients will progress to one or more AIDS-defining illnesses.

Treatment

Patients infected with HIV require a comprehensive care plan that involves skilled physicians, ancillary health services, pharmacologic therapy, and access to social and other support services. Excellent resources exist to guide physicians in the detailed management and care of patients with HIV/AIDS (see next section). The family physician's role in HIV care will be determined by the knowledge, skill, comfort level, and personal preferences of the physician, as well as the accessibility of referral physicians. Family physicians may serve primarily in case finding, by testing and referring patients found to be HIV-positive, or may assume full responsibility for comprehensive management of HIV and its complications. Current research supports all HIV-positive patients should start HAART treatment regardless of CD4 count or viral load.

SEXUALLY TRANSMITTED INFECTIONS

 ESSENTIALS OF DIAGNOSIS

▶ Many sexually active gay men are at increased risk for most STIs, requiring routine periodic screening.

▶ Suspicion or diagnosis of one STI should routinely lead to testing for concomitant HIV and syphilis.

▶ Although generally at lower risk for STIs, lesbians have a higher incidence of bacterial vaginosis than heterosexual women.

General Considerations

Human papillomavirus (HPV), likely leading to condyloma, genital warts, or epithelial dysplasia, is the most commonly transmitted STI.

Gonorrhea, chlamydia, and nonchlamydial nongonococcal urethritis (NGU) are common problems in sexually active gay men. As each of these may cause asymptomatic infection, periodic screening may be useful to detect clinically silent disease. Antibiotic resistance to *Neiseria gonorrhea* has become so ubiquitous that the only remaining first-line treatment is ceftriaxone, and fluoroquinolones are no longer recommended for treatment in MSM. Herpes simplex and syphilis most commonly cause genital ulcer disease (GUD) in heterosexual and homosexual men.

Enteritis and proctocolitis may be caused by an STI via oral-anal contact. Enterobactericiae and *Giardia lamblia* are a common cause and should be included in the differential diagnosis of enteritis and proctocolitis in MSM, as well as CMV in the HIV-positive patient. Unprotected receptive anal intercourse can lead to the tenesmus, rectal pain, and bleeding of proctitis, in which the most common pathogens are *Neisseria gonorrhoeae, Chlamydia trachomatis, Treponema pallidum,* and herpes simplex virus.

Oral stimulation of a man's penis, mistakenly thought to be a "safe" sexual practice, may be an independent risk factor for urethral and pharyngeal gonorrhea and nonchlamydial NGU; it has been implicated in HIV transmission, and has been associated with localized syphilis epidemics in gay men. Syphilis epidemics have also been associated with high-risk sexual activity among HIV-positive men.

Some researchers have shown comparable rates of STIs between lesbians and heterosexual women. Infections, including bacterial vaginosis (BV), candidiasis, herpes, gonorrhea, and human papillomavirus infections, can be contracted by lesbians. One series found a 2.5-fold increase in BV among lesbians compared to heterosexual women, often showing similar vaginal flora between female partners.

Human herpes virus type 8 (HHV8) has been shown to predispose people to Kaposi's sarcoma. Ten studies assessed the prevalence and correlates of HHV8, with most concluding that MSM have disproportionally higher HHV8 infection rates than do comparison groups.

Hepatitis C virus is a risk factor for non-Hodgkin's lymphoma and hepatocellular carcinoma. Surveillance data suggest that hepatitis B and C viral infections have increased over time in MSM, whereas it has decreased in the general population. In addition, hepatitis C is an emerging coinfection in HIV-infected MSM regardless of IVDU.

▶ Prevention

Counseling has been shown to reduce risk behaviors, and patients reporting high-risk behaviors or those diagnosed with an STI should receive or be referred for individual or group counseling. Additionally, MSM patients engaging in sex outside a mutually monogamous relationship should receive periodic STI screening, as should women having sex with men and women (see Chapter 14 for screening recommendations and other information about STIs). If not immune, gay men should be vaccinated against hepatitis A and hepatitis B.

▶ Patient Education

Patients diagnosed or suspected to have an STI should be informed of transmission methods and how to reduce infection risk. Such patients should also be informed of specific treatment, if any, as well as potential coinfection with other sexually transmissible agents. Patients should be counseled to contact sex partners; in lieu of this, the physician or health department may notify partners.

Workowski KA, Berman SM; and Centers for Disease Control and Prevention. Sexually transmitted disease treatment guidelines, 2010. *MMWR Recomm Rep.* 2010;59(RR-12):1–110.

HUMAN PAPILLOMAVIRUS INFECTION

 ESSENTIALS OF DIAGNOSIS

▶ Human papillomavirus (HPV) causes cervical cancer in all women; lesbians should be offered Papanicolaou (Pap) smear screening according to the same guidelines used for heterosexual women.

▶ HPV causes anal dysplasia and anal cancer. HIV-positive MSM should receive yearly anal Pap smears. Research is unclear as to whether HIV-negative MSM that engage in anal-receptive intercourse would benefit as well.

General Considerations

Human papillomavirus is a pervasive infection, manifesting in >100 viral types that infect various parts of the human body. Head and neck cancers can be caused by HPV, although current research shows that the risk of oral HPV infection did not differ by sexual orientation. HPV types that infect the genitalia carry varying risk for dysplasia and neoplasia. The types that cause the most visually apparent warts are usually the types with least risk for dysplasia. Conversely, the types causing clinically inapparent disease carry high dysplastic risk.

Sexual orientation and receptive anal intercourse appear to be independent correlates of condyloma and anal intraepithelial neoplasia. Interestingly, one study even showed that anal HPV was more transient in men who have sex with women (MSW) but more persistent in MSM. Most available evidence demonstrates that MSM have a higher prevalence of anal HPV infection than do comparison groups regardless of HIV status. In addition, it appears that both HIV infection and receptive anal intercourse are significant correlates of anal squamous intraepithelial lesions, and the prevalence of anal cancer was higher in MSM with HIV than in women and heterosexual men.

Prevention

Secondary prevention via Pap smear remains the cornerstone of screening. One study of lesbians revealed that 25% of respondents had not had a Pap test within the past 3 years, and 7.6% had never had a Pap test. Lesbian patients may mistakenly believe themselves to be less susceptible to cervical cancer than heterosexuals or bisexuals, even though one study showed 79% reported previous sexual intercourse with a man. Even in women reporting no prior sex with men, HPV DNA and squamous intraepithelial lesions (SILs) may be found in ≤20% of patients. Thus cervical Pap smears supplemented with HPV DNA testing should be performed routinely using the American Society of Colposcopy and

Cervical Pathology guidelines. Individuals with abnormal screening tests should receive colposcopy or anoscopy and subsequent follow-up as indicated by findings.

A gay man's risk of anal squamous cell carcinoma is equivalent to the historical risk of cervical cancer that women faced prior to the advent of Pap screening. Anal HPV DNA is very prevalent in gay men—one study detected it in 91.6% of HIV-positive and 65.9% of HIV-negative men. HIV exacerbates HPV effects, and is associated with more prevalent HPV infection and higher-grade anal intraepithelial neoplasia (AIN). Screening HIV-positive homosexual and bisexual men for AIN and anal squamous cell carcinomas with anal Pap tests offers quality-adjusted life expectancy benefits at a cost comparable with other accepted clinical preventive interventions. Because the observed increased incidence of anal cancer does not appear to be due solely to HIV infection, high-resolution anoscopy and cytologic screening of all MSM with anal condyloma and other benign noncondylomatous anal disorders is supported by current knowledge.

No consensus guidelines exist on screening for AIN and anal cancer in men who have sex with men, regardless of HIV status. Because of the ubiquitous prevalence of HPV in the HIV-positive population, baseline cytology and yearly anal cancer screening using Pap smears for all HIV-positive MSM is recommended. Current research is conflicted on the cost-effectiveness of screening all MSM using anal Pap smear, although current expert recommendations suggest screening HIV-negative MSM every 2–3 years, similar to cervical cancer screening recommendations.

Taking an anal-rectal sample for cytology (ARC) is a simple procedure. It does not require the use of an anoscope. No special preparation is needed for the patient, although the patient may be advised to refrain from receptive anal intercourse or the use of intraanal preparations before examination.

An ARC sample can be collected with the patient in the lateral recumbent position lying on one side, with the knees drawn up toward the chest. To collect an ARC sample, a tap water–moistened Dacron swab is used. The Dacron swab is inserted approximately 5–6 cm into the anal canal past the anal verge, into the rectal vault. This is done without direct visualization of the anal canal. Firm lateral pressure is applied to the swab handle as it is rotated and slowly withdrawn from the anal canal, inscribing a cone-shaped arc. Care should be taken to ensure that the transition zone is sampled. A swab or smear of the perianal skin is an unsatisfactory sample for ARC. Avoid using cotton swabs on a wooden stick because the handle may break and splinter during collection.

For liquid-based cytology, the swab is then placed in the preservative vial and agitated vigorously several times to release the cellular harvest. If liquid-based cytology is not available, the swab can be smeared onto a glass slide and then spray-fixed as per the procedure for conventional cervical

Pap smears. The lab requisition should be labeled as a rectal Pap smear.

Experimental vaccination has been shown to prevent infection with some types of HPV commonly associated with cancer development and demonstrated to prevent genital warts. A quadrivalent vaccine against HPV is licensed and recommended for both females and males aged 9–26 years. Additional discussion of HPV appears in Chapter 14.

Palefsky J. Human papillomavirus and anal neoplasia. *Curr HIV/ AIDS Rep.* 2008;5(2):78–85. [UI 18510893]
Boehmer U, et al. Cancer and men who have sex with men: a systematic review. *Lancet Oncol.* 2012; 13: e545–e553.

SUBSTANCE ABUSE

 ESSENTIALS OF DIAGNOSIS

▶ Substance use is more common in LGBT patients than in the general heterosexual population.

▶ Methamphetamine use and addiction is particularly problematic in some gay male groups.

General Considerations

Alcohol, psychoactive drug, and tobacco use appear to be more widespread in gay men and lesbians than in the general heterosexual population. Several studies suggest that lesbians and bisexual women consume more alcohol and use other psychoactive substances more than heterosexual women. A recent meta-analysis found risk ratios of 4.0 and 3.5 for alcohol and substance dependence, respectively, among WSW and WSMW as compared to WSM. Another review of tobacco use found smoking rates among adolescent and adult lesbians, gays, and bisexuals to be higher than in the general population. Methamphetamine use has reached epidemic proportions in some gay male populations, and routine history taking should include a question regarding current and past use of this drug.

Alcohol use has been associated with high-risk sexual behavior (eg, unprotected anal and oral intercourse). Gay men who have unprotected anal intercourse are more likely to have a drinking problem than gay men who do not have unprotected intercourse, and unprotected intercourse after drinking is more common with nonsteady sexual partners.

Drug use is also associated with increased high-risk sexual behaviors. Such drugs include hallucinogens, nitrate inhalants, and cocaine and other stimulants. Drug use during high-risk sex is common. However, associations between drug use and high-risk sexual behavior exist only for current

use, not past drug or alcohol use. Providing adequate treatment to patients with substance abuse problems can diminish their subsequent risk of acquiring HIV and other STIs.

In some venues, the prevalence of illicit drug use and associated high-risk sexual activity is dramatic, with use of substances such as MDMA or Ecstasy approaching 80% of the population. Men who attend "circuit parties"—a series of dances or parties held over a weekend that are attended by hundreds to thousands of gay and bisexual men—should be considered at high risk for concurrent illicit substance use and should be counseled accordingly.

Anabolic steroid use is a problem among a subset of gay men. One British study of >1000 gay men recruited from five gymnasiums found that 13.5% of the study population used anabolic steroids, and users were more likely than never users (21% vs 13%) to report engaging in unprotected anal intercourse, increasing their risk for HIV infection.

Pathogenesis

Several theories have been proposed to explain the increased substance use seen in LGBT patients. The observed behavior has been explained in various ways—a maladaptive coping strategy to deal with societal bias against homosexuality; a consequence of bars serving as a primary social gathering place for lesbians and gay men; a genetic predisposition to substance abuse linked to genes coding for same-sex attraction; a coping method for dealing with stresses such as fear of HIV infection, lack of social support, fear of discrimination in housing or employment, and rejection by family or friends on the basis of sexual orientation; or something else. Research to date has not explained causation.

Reasons for steroid use are more straightforward: to modify the patient's musculature to conform more closely to an idealized male form. Significant social pressures may drive patients to resort to steroids to achieve an idealized masculine physique, and for these patients substantial support and counseling may be required to overcome steroid abuse.

Prevention & Treatment

Prevention, clinical findings, complications, and treatment of substance abuse in LGBT populations are similar to these management considerations in heterosexual populations (see Chapter 56 for further discussion). However, modification of standard treatment approaches to reflect LGBT culture may enhance treatment effectiveness. Differences to consider with this population include the prevalence of methamphetamine use, and its association with high-risk sexual behavior among some groups of gay men; concomitant use of sildenafil (Viagra) or other treatments for erectile dysfunction; and "club drugs" (eg, MDMA or Ecstasy, amphetamines, γ-hydroxybutyrate, ketamine). Erectile dysfunction treatments, either with or without other substance use, are associated with high-risk sexual behavior.

Marshal MP et al. Sexual orientation and adolescent substance use: a meta-analysis and methodological review. *Addiction.* 2008;103(4):546–556. [PMID: 18339100]

DEPRESSION

 ESSENTIALS OF DIAGNOSIS

▸ Depression and anxiety are more prevalent in lesbians and gay men than in the general population.

▸ Suicidal ideation, attempts at suicide, and completed acts of suicide are more common in the LGB population than in their heterosexual counterparts.

▸ Suicide risk seems to be increased around the time that an individual "comes out" (reveals his or her gay or lesbian identity to others).

▸ Lack of social supports, lack of family support, and poor relationship quality are significant predictors of depression.

General Considerations

Feelings of stigmatization, internalized homophobia (the direction of society's negative attitudes toward the self), and actual experiences of discrimination or violence contribute to LGBT distress. A study of HIV-infected men, which may be relevant to all gay men, found that men who did not demonstrate traditional gender identity were more likely to have current symptoms of anxiety and depression and to have had a lifetime history of depression. Depression has also been linked to an HIV diagnoses and the AIDS epidemic.

Well-designed studies with valid sampling techniques demonstrate that suicidal ideation, attempts at suicide, and completed acts of suicide are more common in gay, lesbian, and bisexual youth than in their heterosexual counterparts. Population-based research demonstrates significantly higher rates of suicidal symptoms and suicide attempts among men who reported having same-sex partners than those who reported having exclusively opposite-sex partners. A recent meta-analysis indicates a fourfold increase in lifetime suicide attempt prevalence among gay and bisexual men as compared to heterosexual men. Other investigators demonstrate similar findings (eg, in a study of twins in which one brother reported same-sex partners after age 18 and the other did not). Suicidality has been linked to the process of "coming out," or revealing one's homosexual orientation to others. Thus, physicians caring for gay adolescents or adults disclosing their sexual orientation to others should be especially sensitive to symptoms or signs suggesting any increase in suicide risk.

One study of lesbians considered predictors of depression and looked at relationship status, relationship satisfaction, social support from friends, social support from family, "outness" (degree to which the woman publicly shared her sexual orientation), and relationship satisfaction. Lack of social support from friends, poor relationship satisfaction, and lack of perceived social support from family were significant predictors of depression.

Prevention

Well-being is enhanced during later stages of gay identity development, which suggests that facilitation of an individual's synthesis of his or her gay identity may alleviate depressive symptoms. Conversely, in HIV-positive men, concealment of homosexuality is associated with lower CD4 counts and depressive symptoms, lending further support to the idea that facilitating gay identity development may alleviate or prevent depression in some patients, and in so doing, better equip them to maintain their health.

Clinical Findings

Symptoms and signs of depression in lesbian female and gay male patients are very similar to those in heterosexual populations (see Chapter 52). Although depression is often associated with decreased sexual activity, one study of gay men revealed that 16% had heightened sexual interest while depressed. Predictors of depression in lesbians (eg, lack of social support from friends, relationship status dissatisfaction, and lack of perceived social support from family) are similar to predictors for heterosexual women.

Haas AP, et al. Suicide and suicide risk in lesbian, gay, bisexual and transgender populations: review and recommendations. *J Homosex.* 2011;10–51.

OTHER HEALTH CONCERNS

Cancer Screening

All LGBT patients require the same age- and gender-appropriate cancer screening as heterosexual and non-gender-variant patients. As discussed above, cervical cancer screening should be offered to lesbian women, and anal cancer screening to men with a history of receptive anal intercourse, particularly if they are coinfected with HIV, although there remains insufficient evidence to universally recommend the anal Pap at this time.

Since breast and ovarian cancers may be more common in nulliparous or uniparous women, it may be more common in lesbians, but well-designed, prospective studies are lacking. One study compiling survey data from almost 12,000 women found lesbians had greater prevalence rates of obesity and alcohol and tobacco use, and lower rates of parity and birth control pill use. Another study confirmed higher prevalence of nulliparity, and also found higher prevalence of other health risk factors, including high daily alcohol intake, higher body mass index, and higher prevalence of current smoking.

In transgender patients, it is important to screen according to current anatomy as well as use of hormonal therapy. For example, many male-to-female (MTF) transgender patients are at risk for both prostate and breast cancers, and female-to-male (FTM) transgender patients often require screening for breast, uterine, cervical, endometrial, and ovarian cancers. As in any patient population, tobacco and alcohol use among LGBT patients increase risk for malignancy.

Dutton L, et al. Gynecologic care of the female-to-male transgender man. *J Midwifery Women's Health.* 2008;53(4):331–337. [PMID: 18586186]

Erectile Dysfunction

Studies have demonstrated that erectile dysfunction is more common in homosexual than in heterosexual men, although overall prevalence was still <4%. Related, gay men also report higher levels of performance anxiety (eg, more likely to agree with the statement "If I feel I'm expected to respond sexually, I have difficulty getting aroused") than do heterosexual men. This was true even when men reporting erectile dysfunction were excluded from analysis. Erectile dysfunction is more common in HIV-positive homosexual men than in HIV-negative homosexual men. Declines in serum testosterone have been associated with HIV infection, suggesting one possible etiology for his difference.

Contraception & Reproductive Health

Assuming that all women of reproductive age need contraception risks alienating lesbian patients, who may consequently decline to disclose their sexual orientation. However, lesbians who are sexually active with men may be interested in obtaining contraceptives.

Lesbian patients may also be, or wish to become, mothers and so may welcome a discussion of reproductive options. Parenthood options available to lesbians and gay men include adoption, artificial insemination, surrogacy, or heterosexual intercourse. Existing evidence suggests that gay men and lesbians have parenting skills comparable to heterosexual parents. Special considerations that may arise for lesbian and gay parents include the children's awareness of lesbian and gay relationships, heterosexism, and homophobia. When compared with children of heterosexual parents, children of gay men and lesbians seem to be no different in significant variables measured, including their sexual or gender identity, personality traits, and intelligence. Despite this,

gay men and lesbians may face unjustified barriers in their attempts to become foster and adoptive parents. Issues that warrant physician awareness include parental legal rights and durable power of attorney; gestation and pregnancy; choice of surrogate, sperm, or egg donor; possible HIV risk; and routine preconception and prenatal care. Physicians caring for lesbians and gay men wishing to become parents should maintain information about appropriate referrals to facilitate this process.

TRANSGENDER PATIENTS

ESSENTIAL FEATURES

▶ Rather than assume, physicians should determine how patients wish to be addressed and understand how they conceptualize their gender.

▶ Sex reassignment in adolescence may be indicated for carefully selected patients.

▶ Sex reassignment should be managed by multispecialty teams with experience caring for this population.

Terminology

Terminology can be problematic when describing transgender individuals. *Transgender,* used as an umbrella term, can have multiple meanings—either individuals who transcend culturally defined categories of gender in some way, or individuals experiencing incongruence between their perceived and observed gender. *Transsexual* often refers to an individual who has undergone partial or complete sex reassignment surgery (SRS). Intersex individuals are born with both male and female sexual characteristics and organs, such that unambiguous assignment of male or female sex at birth is not possible. "Gender queer" is a term characterizing an individual who doesn't identify as either male of female or accept the gender binary.

The term *male-to-female* (MTF), or as the transgender community feel as the more appropriate term, "transwoman" describes individuals born with male genitalia who presents as a male regardless of hormone or surgical intervention; the reverse is true for female-to-male (FTM) individuals, or "transman." Additional ways to characterize the biological, social, psychological, and legal identity of transgender individuals have been described. The best approach to caring for an individual patient is to determine how they wish to be addressed and understand how they conceptualize their gender.

The *Diagnostic and Statistical Manual of Mental Disorders,* fifth edition (*DSM-5*) diagnosis of *gender dysphoria* communicates the emotional distress that can result from "a marked incongruence between one's experienced/ expressed gender and assigned gender. Individuals who experience the strongest feelings of dissonance between their gender identity and their physical appearance believe the quest for full hormonal and surgical sex reassignment is vital because they actually feel "trapped" in an anatomically incorrect body. Currently, transgender people include cross-dressers, female and male impersonators, transgenderists and bigender persons (identify as both man and woman), and transsexuals who have or will undergo SRS. Limited research into the etiology of gender dysphoria suggests that it may be multifactorial, including anatomic brain differences between transsexual and nontranssexual individuals, and differences in parental rearing. Regardless of etiology or classification, transgender patient needs are increasingly recognized as valid and deserving attention from healthcare educators, researchers, policymakers, and clinicians of all types.

Treatment

A multidisciplinary team experienced with transgender care may be the most critical element in providing superior care and therapy. Some patients choose partial medical or surgical treatment, finding that living with physical components of both genders best addresses the dissonance caused by their birth physiognomy. Others use extensive medical and surgical treatment to physically manifest their "internal" gender as fully as possible. Current literature on the health needs of transgender patients focuses on psychological and psychiatric evaluation and treatment, SRS, and hormonal therapy. Although common practice is to delay initiating SRS until the patient is at least 18 or 21 years of age, treatment in adolescence is well tolerated for carefully selected individuals, does not lead to postoperative regret, and may prevent psychopathology seen in individuals forced to delay therapy. Patients considering SRS should undergo psychological evaluation by a therapist experienced in working with this population.

Intensive psychological counseling, hormonal treatment, and living in the role of the desired gender for a period of ≥1 year should precede surgical treatment. Surgical treatment can involve the breasts, genitalia, and larynx. The right to such treatment, even in health systems receiving government funding, has been sanctioned by courts. Because each patient is unique, surgical approaches must be tailored to individual patients, and patients seeking SRS should be referred to teams experienced with these procedures.

Primary care is an ideal setting for transgender healthcare, given that primary care physicians are knowledgeable of and often experienced with the administration of estrogens (for menopausal care and contraception), testosterone (for androgen-deficient states such as with human immunodeficiency virus), and testosterone-blocking medications (for hirsutism and prostatic disease), and are aware of important mental and social health issues.

Hormonal treatment is often employed in both genders. Cross-sex hormonal treatment may have substantial medical side effects, so the smallest doses needed to achieve the desired result should be used. Outcome studies suggest that known complications of hormonal therapy such as galactorrhea and thromboembolic events occur, but that the incidence of complications can be held to acceptable levels with careful attention to regimens used. Extensive experience with hormonal therapies in transsexual patients indicates that hormonal therapy, particularly if transdermal formulations are used, does not cause increased morbidity or mortality; monitoring luteinizing hormone levels in MTF transsexuals may increase the benefit-to-risk ratio by limiting hormone-related bone loss.

Sutcliffe PA, et al. Evaluation of surgical procedures for sex reassignment: a systematic review. *J Plast Reconstr Aesthet Surg.* 2009;62(3):294–306; discussion 306–308. [UI: 18222742]

Websites

DSM-5: http://www.dsm5.org/Documents/Gender%20Dysphoria%20Fact%20Sheet.pdf.
Gay and Lesbian Medical Association (GLMA): http://www.glma.org.
Parents, Families, and Friends of Lesbians and Gays (PFLAG): http://www.pflag.org.
The World Professional Association for Transgender Health (WPATH): http://www.wpath.org.
Transgender Law and Policy Institute: http://www.transgenderlaw.org.

ADOLESCENTS

Lesbian and gay adolescents growing up in a loving, supportive environment develop and mature in a manner similar to their heterosexual counterparts. However, lesbian and gay adolescents may be vulnerable to parental wrath and withdrawal of support on disclosure or suspicion of their homosexual orientation. In certain instances, this can initiate a chain of events that leaves the youth homeless and vulnerable. Lacking employable skills, some homeless gay youths may resort to prostitution or "survival sex" to support themselves.

Gay youths have an increased risk for suicide compared with their heterosexual peers. In addition, population-based surveys of adolescents indicate that lesbian and gay adolescents report being physically abused ≤2 times as often as their heterosexual peers, and sexually abused ≤10 times as often as heterosexual adolescents. Despite this, homosexual adolescents are generally more similar to than different from their heterosexual peers, face many of the same challenges, and have great potential to mature into healthy and happy adults.

Physicians caring for families need to be aware of the possibility that the typical adolescent struggle to establish identity may be compounded when a teen recognizes his/her sexual orientation, particularly when this occurs in a potentially hostile environment. Physicians can play a vital role in helping adolescents—and their families—find acceptance. Parental support can dramatically reduce the adverse effects of "coming out" and the potential risk for suicide, and can increase the likelihood of healthy psychological development and maturation.

OLDER LGBT PATIENTS

Older lesbians and gay men developed and matured in a different social milieu, when society was less tolerant of homosexuality and the consequences of being gay or lesbian included even greater threats to the individual's social and family relationships, housing, and livelihood than exist today. Thus, older patients may be even less willing to disclose their homosexual orientation to physicians, and may have special healthcare needs that would go unrecognized if the physician did not take a thorough sexual history. Incorrect assumptions about geriatric patient sexuality may lead physicians to inaccurately identify risk behaviors and to implement appropriate education or screening tests. Physicians should know that many older lesbians and gay men remain sexually active, with older gay men reporting less condom use than their heterosexual counterparts.

Although not extensive, research suggests that many lesbians and gay men successfully navigate the aging process and remain connected and involved in life. In fact, the challenges that being gay presents may cause individuals to face the challenges associated with aging more successfully than their heterosexual counterparts.

Lovejoy TI, et al. Patterns and correlates of sexual activity and condom use behavior in persons 50-plus years of age living with HIV/AIDS. *AIDS Behav.* 2008;12(6):943–956. [PMID: 18389361]

McMahon E. The older homosexual: current concepts of lesbian, gay, bisexual, and transgender older Americans. *Clin Geriatr Med.* 2003;19:587. [PMID: 14567010]

FAMILY, COMMUNITY, AND MARRIAGE

One aspect of being gay or lesbian that may be overlooked in caring for a patient's medical needs is the role of family and social networks in providing support and sustenance to the LGBT patient. In this context, family often includes individuals unrelated by biological ties. A useful concept is that of "family of origin," which consists of parents, siblings, and others with whom one shares a blood relation, contrasted with "family of choice," which includes those close friendship relationships that endure over time and incorporate the same types of support and emotions often associated with idealized views of the traditional family. The family of a lesbian or gay patient, including her/his partner, is a vital part of the individual's health and can serve as a source of both stress and support, just as with heterosexual patients. Physicians caring for gay men and lesbians need to assess the resources and stressors that exist within the family, as defined by the patient.

The American Academy of Pediatrics (AAP) has come out in support of gay marriage, saying that research indicates "that there is no causal relationship between parents' sexual orientation and children's emotional, psychosocial and behavioral development." The AAP also endorses adoption and foster parenting by gays and lesbians.

Hospice & Palliative Medicine

Eva B. Reitschuler-Cross, MD
Robert M. Arnold, MD

BACKGROUND

Homes for the dying or, as they were soon to be called, *hospices,* were established in Ireland and France in the nineteenth century. However, it was not until 1967 that the first modern hospice, Saint Christopher's Hospice, was founded in London. There, Dr. Cicely Saunders, a former nurse and social worker who had earned a medical degree, helped establish the underlying philosophy of hospice and palliative medicine. She emphasized clinical excellence in pain and symptom management; care of the whole person, including physical, emotional, social, and spiritual needs; and the need for research in this newly developing field of medicine. Interdisciplinary team care became the norm, as it became clear that no one physician, nurse, social worker, or chaplain could address all the needs of the terminally ill person. Further, although the focus of care was clearly on the dying individual, the needs of the family were also addressed.

In 1982, the Congress created the Medicare Hospice Benefit (MHB), and in 1986, the benefit was made permanent. By 2007, 4700 hospice programs were providing healthcare services to the terminally ill and their families throughout the United States.

Eligibility criteria for hospice enrollment through the MHB require that patients waive traditional Medicare coverage for curative and life-prolonging care related to the terminal diagnosis and be certified by their physician and the hospice medical director as having a life expectancy of 6 months or less if the disease runs its usual course. Recertification periods within the MHB allow for reexamination of hospice eligibility. If the hospice medical director believes that the patient has a life expectancy of ≤6 months if the disease runs its usual course, the patient may be recertified as eligible for the MHB even if the patient has already been receiving the benefit for 6 months or longer.

The goal of hospice care is to relieve suffering and improve the patient's and family's quality of daily life. To achieve those goals, hospice care has come to be defined as holistic, patient-, and family-centered rather than disease-centered. Hospice provides a team composed of those trained to care for problems in a holistic manner: physician, nurse, social worker, chaplain, bereavement counselor, nursing assistant, and volunteer. The hospice team meets weekly, under the direction of the hospice medical director, to review the care plans of all patients. The hospice program is charged with providing medications for the relief of physical distress, durable medical equipment, supplies, a multidisciplinary team to provide care, and bereavement support before and after the patient's death.

Palliative medicine has developed as a medical subspecialty in the United States since the mid-1990s, bringing a "hospicelike" approach to patients with serious illnesses regardless of prognosis or their interest in pursuing life-prolonging treatments. The goals of palliative care programs are similar to those of the hospice: pain and symptom control; emotional, social, and spiritual support of patients and families; and facilitation of clear and compassionate communication regarding goals of care. Early involvement of palliative care has been shown to significantly improve symptom management, quality of life, mood, and, in one study, survival. Furthermore, palliative care has been shown to increase patient and family satisfaction and reduce costs by limiting the use of high-technology care.

Many models of palliative care are under development. There are palliative care consultation teams in hospitals, nursing homes, and outpatient clinics. The growth of palliative care consultation programs since 2004 or so has been significant and mirrors the growth of the hospice since 1974. The number of hospital-based palliative care consultation programs has increased linearly from 632 (15%) in 2000 to 1027 (25%) in 2003 and continues to grow annually. Many larger hospitals and all VA institutions have consultative palliative care services. Many hospitals have also established inpatient palliative care units.

Palliative medicine fellowships are undergoing rapid development as well. In the early 1990s, the first US palliative medicine fellowship was initiated. By June 2006, 49 programs offered 119 fellowships for advanced training. In September 2006, the American Board of Medical Specialties officially recognized the field of palliative medicine as a subspecialty.

PAIN & SYMPTOM MANAGEMENT

Optimal symptom control is an important cornerstone of palliative medicine, because uncontrolled symptoms increase patients' and caregivers' distress. Poorly controlled symptoms often detract from patients' quality of life, impair their interactions with loved ones, and limit their ability to attend to important issues at the end of life. Many studies have documented the high frequency of symptoms in patients with serious illnesses and the tendency for symptoms to increase in intensity as a disease progresses. The following discussion reviews management of some common symptoms. As with most medical problems, successful management of symptoms starts with a careful history and physical examination, with therapy directed at identifiable underlying causes.

▶ Pain

Pain can be classified physiologically as nociceptive (somatic or visceral) or neuropathic. (**Table 67-1**). Pain can occur directly from the underlying illnesses (such as tumor involvement, cytokine release, and vasculopathy), as a consequence of therapy (particularly chemotherapy, radiation therapy, and invasive procedures), or from pathologies that are not directly related to the primary disease processes. It is important to remember that pain is a subjective experience, and it is essential to respect and accept the complaint of pain as characterized by the patient. Pain is influenced by psychosocial and spiritual issues, and effective pain management requires a multidisciplinary approach.

Unlike opioids, nonsteroidal anti-inflammatory drugs (NSAIDs) and acetaminophen have an analgesic ceiling effect. The use of opioid-nonopioid combinations therefore is limited by the dose of the NSAIDs or acetaminophen. Despite this fact, NSAIDs are effective pain medication, especially for inflammatory conditions. Their use can decrease the amount of opioids required and hence decrease the incidence of opioid side effects. Unless contraindicated, all pain protocols should include a NSAID or acetaminophen.

The general principles of pain management with opioids are as follows:

1. Assess pain using a standardized pain scale: Most commonly used is a 0–10 scale, where 0 indicates no pain and 10 represents the worst pain imaginable. Numerous validated scales can be used for patients who cannot communicate–either because they are intubated, are preverbal children, or are cognitively impaired adults.

2. In opioid-naive patients, start with a short-acting opioid (such as morphine, oxycodone, or hydromorphone) to control acute, moderate to severe pain. Unless there are contraindications, morphine is the agent of choice given its low costs and variable routes of administration [oral (PO), intravenous (IV), subcutaneous (SQ), intramuscular (IM), or rectal (PR)]. Short-acting opioids can be given as frequently as the time to peak onset of action: every 60–90 minutes for oral immediate-release formulations and every 10–15 minutes for IV formulations. For severe pain, IV administration is recommended given the faster onset of action and greater ease of titration. Conversion to oral opioids can occur once the pain is controlled.

3. Determine whether the dose is adequate, and adjust accordingly: The dose should be titrated at least every 24 hours if the pain is moderate, and as often as every 4 hours if the pain is severe, particularly while using intravenous opioids. Dose increases should be made by 25–50% for moderate pain, and by 50–100% for

Table 67-1. Classification of pain.

| | Nociceptive | | Neuropathic |
	Somatic	Visceral	
Etiology	Due to tissue damage—activation of nociceptors in cutaneous and deep tissues	Due to tissue damage—activation of nociceptors resulting from stretching, distension, or inflammation of visceral organs	Due to nervous system dysfunction ± tissue damage
Description of pain	Well localized, aching, throbbing, gnawing	Poorly localized, dull, crampy, squeezy, pressure	Burning, shooting, stabbing, tingling, electriclike, numb
Examples	Bone, soft tissues, muscle pain	Small bowel or ureteral obstruction, peritoneal carcinomatosis, hepatic distension	Peripheral neuropathy, plexopathy

severe pain. There is no specific limit to opioid doses. These agents should be titrated until pain is controlled or side effects develop.

4. Further titration or rotation of opioids is achieved by first calculating the *oral morphine equivalent* (OME) of the previous 24 hours' worth of opioid use. Equianalgesic tablets for opioids are readily available (**Table 67-2**); however, these tablets often differ slightly. It is important to remember that oral and parenteral doses are not equal because of oral medicines' first-pass hepatic metabolism– for example, 1 mg of IV morphine sulfate equals 3 mg of oral morphine sulfate, and 1 mg of parenteral hydromorphone equals 4 mg of oral hydromorphone.

5. Determine the dosing schedule: Chronic pain deserves scheduled pain medication, not just as-needed dosing: 66–75% of the patient's stable 24-hour OME needs should be given as a long-acting formulation.

6. Determine the breakthrough dose. *Breakthrough pain* is defined as a transitory exacerbation of pain that occurs on top of an otherwise stable persistent pain. An adequate breakthrough dose is calculated as 10–15% of the total daily long-acting opioid, and it should be given every 3 hours as needed. Whenever possible, the same opioid agent should be used for both short- and long-acting administration [eg, sustained-release morphine 150 mg PO Q12h (by mouth every 12 hours) and immediate-release morphine 30–45 mg PO Q3h, as needed).

7. During administration of opioid therapy, the patient's renal function should be closely monitored, as toxic metabolites can accumulate with decreased kidney function, leading to alterations in mental status,

myoclonic jerks, and seizures. Opioids that are safe to use in renal failure include hydromorphone, fentanyl, and methadone.

8. Reasons for rotating to a different opioid include renal failure, side effects, and a need to change the route of administration (such as changing from oral morphine to transdermal fentanyl). When rotating to a different opioid, the dose should be reduced by 25–50% to account for incomplete cross-tolerance.

Fentanyl patches should not be used alone for acute severe pain. Because of the delayed onset of effect (12 hours) and long half-life of this formulation, which allows for titrations only every 48–72 hours, it cannot be titrated quickly for rapid pain control. If the pain is severe or unpredictable, or if opioid requirements are unknown or increasing rapidly, patient-controlled analgesia (PCA) may be indicated. With PCA infusion pumps, opioids can be infused intravenously or subcutaneously at a continuous basal rate programmed by the care provider, while the administrations of bolus doses are controlled by the patient. There is theoretically no risk of overdose since the patient will fall asleep before serious signs of overdose occur, and for this reason, the patient's family or visitors should be carefully educated to avoid pushing the PCA button on the patient's behalf.

Guidelines on management of opioid-induced side effects are as follows:

1. **Nausea/vomiting:** Opioids can cause nausea and vomiting by decreasing gastrointestinal motility. Patients usually develop a tolerance to these side effects. It may be helpful to schedule an antiemetic for a few days, then change to as-needed administration. Dopamine receptor antagonists are most effective (haloperidol 0.5–2 m Q6–12h or metoclopramide 10–40 mg Q6h).

2. **Sedation:** This is a commonly encountered side effect, although tolerance typically develops over time to this as well. Downtitration of opioids, rotation of opiates, and use of adjuvant, nonopioid pain therapies should be considered. Other sedating agents should be eliminated whenever possible. If sedation persists despite these interventions, the addition of a central nervous system (CNS) stimulant can be helpful (methylphenidate 2.5–5 mg in the morning and at noon, or modafinil 100–200 mg daily).

3. **Constipation:** This is one of the most common side effects. Since patients rarely develop tolerance, if at all, a bowel regimen must be started for most patients with initiation of opioid therapy. A bowel stimulant (senna) is the most commonly used agent. Methylnaltrexone is a peripherally acting opioid receptor antagonist that has been approved for refractory constipation in patients receiving opioid therapy. It does not reverse central analgesia.

Table 67-2. Opioid analgesic equivalences.

Opioid Agonist	Parenteral mg	Oral mg
Morphine[a]	10	30
Oxycodone		20–30
Hydromorphone	1.5	7.5
Fentanyl	0.1[b]	
Codeine	130	200
Hydrocodone		25–30
Oxymorphone	1	10

[a]The 24-hour oral morphine equivalent (OME) divided by 2 is equal to the fentanyl patch dose in micrograms per hour (eg, 24-hour OME is 100 mg, equivalent fentanyl patch dose is 50 µg/h).
[b]Equivalency of a one-time dose of intravenous fentanyl only.

4. **Delirium/confusion/hallucinations:** In this setting, opioid dose reduction, rotation to a different opioid, and initiation of neuroleptic therapy (haloperidol 0.5–1 mg BID-QID or olanzapine 2.5–5 mg daily BID should be considered).

5. **Allergic reaction:** True allergic reactions are rare. Allergylike symptoms are usually secondary to mast cell activation and subsequent histamine release.

6. **Respiratory depression:** Tolerance to the respiratory depressant effects occurs rapidly; thus, opioids can be used safely when titrated to pain control, even in patients with underlying emphysema. Naloxone administration is indicated if (a) the patient is somnolent and difficult to arouse or (b) respiratory rate is <8/min or oxygen saturation is <92% and the respiratory rate is <12/min. A dilution of 0.4 mg naloxone (one ampoule, 1 mL) in 9 mL of normal saline to yield 0.04 mg naloxone per milliliter should be prepared, with administration of this diluted nalxone in 1–2-mL increments (0.04–0.08 mg) over 1–2-minute intervals until a change in alertness is observed. Giving naloxone in this way should not cause pain to return or opioid withdrawal. Remember that the half-life of naloxone is shorter than the half-life of most opioids, so respiratory depression may recur and a naloxone drip may be needed.

A challenge in prescribing opioid pain medications is to correctly differentiate a patient in pain from a patient with a substance abuse disorder. The key lies in understanding the specific characteristics of tolerance, physical and psychological dependence, and pseudoaddiction. *Tolerance* is a state of adaption in which exposure to a drug induces changes that result in a decreased effect of the drug dose over time. *Physical dependence* is a state of adaption that is manifested by a specific withdrawal syndrome when the drug is discontinued suddenly. Most patients on chronic opioids will develop physical dependence. If the need arises for a rapid decrease in opioid dose, administering 25–50% of the stable dose can prevent withdrawal symptoms. Both tolerance and physical dependence cannot be used to differentiate between a patient in pain and a patient with a substance abuse disorder. Psychological dependence or addiction is a primary, chronic, neurobiological disease with genetic and psychosocial factors influencing its development. It is characterized by certain behaviors, including loss of control, compulsive drug use, craving, and continued use of the drug despite harm. Research suggests that opioids used to treat pain rarely lead to psychological dependence. *Pseudoaddiction* describes a patient's behavior when the pain is undertreated. Some of these behaviors, such as "clock watching" or having "excessive pain," may mimic addiction. However, a distinguishing feature of pseudoaddiction not seen in true addiction is the resolution of these behaviors when pain is effectively treated.

A. Adjuvant Pain Therapies

Patients with neuropathic pain occasionally respond to opioids alone; however, many require the addition of adjuvant pain medications. Commonly used adjuvants for neuropathic pain include tricyclic antidepressants (TCAs), serotonin and norepinephrine reuptake inhibitors (SNRIs), anticonvulsants, and antiarrhythmics. The choice of an adjuvant is usually dictated by the individual drug side effect profile, the potential for drug interactions, and the previous drug therapy. The secondary amines, nortriptyline and desipramine, are generally better tolerated than amitriptyline. The analgesic effects of TCAs occur at lower doses and usually within several days, as compared with the antidepressant effects. Data on use of selective serotonin reuptake inhibitors (SSRIs) for neuropathic pain are not convincing; however, recent studies suggest that SNRIs may be as beneficial at tricyclic agents for pain control. Of the anticonvulsants, gabapentin, pregabalin, carbamazepine, and valproic acid are commonly used for neuropathic pain. Carbamazepine and valproic acid are cost-effective but have a higher risk of drug interactions and toxicity compared with gabapentin and pregabalin. Gabapentin requires more frequent dosing, slower titration secondary to sedation, and dose adjustments for renal insufficiency. Antiarrhythmics, topical lidocaine, and oral mexiletine have also been used successfully for neuropathic pain. For adjuvant pain medications, standard initial dosing and titration guidelines should be followed, although lower-than-usual doses have been effective for pain control. In elderly patients, it is generally safer to start at low doses and titrate at a slower rate.

Corticosteroids, benzodiazepines, and anticholinergics are also used as adjuvant pain medication. Corticosteroids, by decreasing tumor-associated edema and by their anti-inflammatory effects, are useful for pain because of multiple pathologies, including bone metastasis, liver capsule distention from metastasis, and conditions in which the tumor is compressing sensitive structures. Benzodiazepines and baclofen are indicated for pain from spasticity. Anticholinergics can relieve colic due to intestinal obstruction.

In addition to drug therapy for pain control, interventions such as palliative radiation therapy for bone metastasis, nerve blockage (eg, celiac plexus block for pancreatic cancer), palliative surgical resection, or immobilization of fractures should be considered. Before undertaking such interventions, the patient's overall prognosis and the effectiveness of less invasive measures should be considered. Complementary therapies are often used in hospice and palliative care for treatment of pain and other symptoms. Some of these therapies are described in **Table 67-3**.

Table 67-3. Complementary modalities used in palliative medicine.

Therapy	Brief Description	Recommendations
Acupuncture	Stimulation of defined points on the skin using a needle, electrical current (electroacupuncture), or pressure (acupressure). These points correspond to meridians, or pathways of energy flow with the intent to correct energy imbalances and restore a normal, healthy flow of energy in the body.	1. Acupuncture may provide pain relief in terminally ill patients with cancer pain. 2. Acupuncture may provide relief from breathlessness. 3. Acupressure may reduce chemotherapy- and radiation-induced nausea and vomiting.
Aromatherapy	Therapeutic use of essential oils, which are applied to the skin or inhaled. The impact on the emotional and psychological state is mediated through the olfactory nerve and the limbic system in the brain.	1. Aromatherapy may be used in conjunction with other complementary therapies, such as massage. 2. Aromatherapy may provide reduction in anxiety.
Massage therapy	Manipulation of the muscles and soft tissues of the body for therapeutic purposes.	1. Massage might provide short-term reduction in cancer pain. 2. Massage has been shown to reduce stress and anxiety and enhance feelings of relaxation.
Hypnosis	A state of increased receptivity of suggestion and direction.	1. Hypnotherapy can enhance pain relief. 2. Hypnotherapy may reduce nausea and vomiting in patients receiving chemotherapy.
Relaxation	The use of muscular relaxation techniques to release tension. These techniques are often used in conjunction with meditation, biofeedback, and guided imagery techniques.	1. Relaxation can reduce stress and tension. 2. Relaxation techniques can improve pain control in advanced cancer patients.
Therapeutic touch	A technique performed by physical touch and/or the use of hand movements to balance any disturbances in a person's energy flow.	1. Therapeutic touch may increase hemoglobin levels. 2. Therapeutic touch may relieve anxiety and tension and reduce the effects of stress on the immune system.
Music therapy	The use of music as a therapy to influence mental, behavioral, or physiologic disorders.	1. Music therapy may assist in the reduction of pain perception. 2. Music therapy may reduce anxiety and help persons cope with grief and loss.
Support group	The use of groups and psychosocial interventions to help persons learn how to cope better with their disease.	1. Support groups can enhance the quality of life. 2. Support group therapy can improve pain management and coping skills. 3. Support group therapy can reduce anxiety and depression.

▶ Nausea & Vomiting

Nausea and vomiting entail complex physiologic processes and are triggered by activation of one of four main pathways. An understanding of these pathways may aid in choosing an effective antiemetic regimen.

1. The *chemoreceptor trigger zone* (CTZ) is located at the area postrema of the medulla. It lies outside the blood-brain barrier and is therefore able to sample emetogenic toxins, drugs, or metabolic abnormalities such as uremia or hypercalcemia. It further receives input from the gastrointestinal tract. The main receptors involved include dopamine type 2 receptors (D2), 5-hydroxy-tryptamine type 3 receptor (5-HT-3), and neurokinin type 1 receptor (NK1).

2. Pathways from the vestibular apparatus respond to vertigo and visuospatial disorientation. The main receptors involved include muscarinic acetylcholine receptors (m-Ach) and histamine type 1 receptors (H1).

3. Peripheral pathways (vagus nerve and splanchnic nerves) mediate nausea triggered by activation of visceral chemoreceptors (local toxins) and serosal mechanoreceptors (stretch of organs and capsules). The main receptors involved include H1 and m-Ach receptors. Enterochromaffine cells release 5-HT-3 when damaged by interventions such as chemotherapy or radiation therapy.

4. Cortical pathways respond to increased intracranial pressure, sensory stimuli (smell, pain), and psychogenic stimuli (anxiety, memory, conditioning).

Each of these pathways sends signals to the *vomiting center* (VC), which triggers nausea and vomiting when thresholds are reached. The main receptors involved at the VC are H1, m-Ach, and 5-HT-2.

Table 67-4. Commonly used antiemetics.

Drug	Receptor Activity/Effect	Common Indication	Dosage/Route	Side Effects
Haloperidol	D2	Opioid-induced N/V	0.5–4 mg PO or SC or IV every 6 hours (Q6h)	Extrapyramidal symptoms (EPSs), QTc prolongation
Metoclopramide	Peripheral D2	Opioid-induced N/V, delayed gastric emptying	5–20 mg PO or SC or IV before meals and at bedtime	EPS, esophageal spasm, colic in complete bowel obstruction
Prochlorperazine	D2	Opioid-induced N/V, N/V of unknown etiology	5–10 mg PO or IV Q6h or 25 mg PR Q6h	EPS and sedation
Scopolamine	Ach, H1	Vestibular dysfunction	1.5 mg transdermal patch every 3 days	Dry mouth, blurred vision, ileus, urinary retention and confusion; patch starts being effective after 24 hours
Ondansetron	5-HT-3	Chemotherapy- or radiation therapy–induced N/V	4-8 mg PO as pill or dissolvable tablet or IV Q4–8 h	Headache, fatigue, constipation
Dexamethasone	Decreases ICP	Increased intracranial pressure, capsular stretch	4–8 mg every morning or BID, PO (pill or liquid) or IV	Agitation, insomnia, hyperglycemia
Lorazepam	GABA receptor	Anticipatory N/V	0.5–2 mg PO or IV Q4–6h	Sedation, confusion, delirium
Aprepitant	NK1	Severe chemotherapy-induced N/V	125 mg PO on day 1, 80 mg PO on days 2–3	Somnolence, fatigue, may reduce warfarin levels

BID, twice per day; EPS, extrapyramidal symptom; IV, intravenous; N/V, nausea/vomiting; PO, per mouth; PR, per rectum; SC, subcutaneous.

Treatment should focus on correcting underlying causes as well as choosing antiemetics to target specific receptors and pathways involved. Commonly used antiemetics are described in **Table 67-4**. If nausea or vomiting is persistent, severe, or refractory, it is recommended to schedule regular administrations of an antiemetic agent. A second or third antiemetic targeting a different receptor may be added (scheduled dosing, or dosed as needed).

Nausea and vomiting also may be presenting symptoms of a malignant gastrointestinal obstruction. The patent should be evaluated for invasive procedures such as venting gastrostomy, intraluminal stent, or surgical diversion. With partial obstruction, the use of metoclopramide and dexamethasone along with a low-fiber diet can provide significant symptom relief for several weeks or longer. When an obstruction becomes complete, therapy is directed at decreasing intestinal motility and decreasing secretions using anticholinergics and somatostatin analogs. Metoclopramide is contraindicated in complete bowel obstruction as it increases gastrointestinal motility and leads to exacerbation of painful abdominal cramping.

▶ Dyspnea

Dyspnea, like pain, is a subjective experience, and can be present with or without hypoxia. With a broad differential existing for dyspnea, reversible causes should always be considered first. The optimal therapy is aimed at the presumed etiology. Palliative therapy can involve chemotherapy, radiotherapy, thoracentesis, pericardiocentesis, and bronchial stent placement. General measures such as providing a fan, keeping the room temperature cool, use of relaxation techniques, or using a careful trial of supplemental oxygen (for hypoxic patients) can help dyspneic patients. Available palliative drug therapies include steroids, opioids, bronchodilators, diuretics, anxiolytics, antibiotics, and anticoagulants. All these drugs can be used in combination, depending on the etiology of dyspnea.

Opioids can relieve breathlessness, although the mechanism is unclear. Opioid administration, dose, frequency, and titration are the same as for pain control. The use of nebulized morphine sulfate is not more effective than placebo. Opioids can increase exercise tolerance and reduce dyspnea in patients with chronic obstructive airways. Fear of addiction or fear of respiratory depression should not preclude a trial of opioids in this population. Starting at low doses, carefully titrating the dose to achieve symptom control, and close monitoring allow for safe and effective use.

Steroids are useful for dyspnea from bronchospasm and tumor-associated edema. Specific indications include malignant bronchial obstruction, carcinomatous lymphangitis, and superior vena cava syndrome. Dexamethasone can be started at 4 mg twice daily and subsequently reduced to the lowest effective dose. Dexamethasone is more potent and has lower mineralocorticoid activity than other steroids, resulting in less fluid retention.

Some patients with dyspnea express disturbing fears of suffocation and choking. Understandably, anxiety often coexists with chronic dyspnea. Anxiety can heighten breathlessness, making symptom control more difficult. The use of anxiolytics such as benzodiazepines and phenothiazines can help treat dyspnea associated with a high component of anxiety. Lorazepam, 0.5–1 mg, can be tried initially. If patients show benefit, long-acting diazepam or clonazepam can then be prescribed. Low-dose chlorpromazine has also shown benefit in relieving both dyspnea and anxiety.

Anorexia & Cachexia

Anorexia (poor appetite) and cachexia (involuntary weight loss regardless of caloric intake or appetite) are prevalent distressing symptoms in patients with advanced illnesses. Mechanisms of the anorexia-cachexia syndrome include an aberrant inflammatory response, generated by disease-host reactions, as well as neurohormonal dysfunction. Exacerbating factors include delayed gastric emptying, constipation, nausea, depression, mucositis, thrush, and even ill-fitting dentures.

Little effective drug therapy is available. Megestrol acetate, a progestin, has been shown to increase appetite and result in weight gain; however, weight gain is due largely to accumulation of adipose tissue and not lean muscle mass. Doses start at 160 mg/day and can be titrated to 800 mg/day if required. Side effects include thromboembolic events and adrenal insufficiency on abrupt cessation. Corticosteroids, such as dexamethasone, can be prescribed as an appetite stimulant for patients in whom side effects of long-term steroid use are of less concern. Beneficial effects tend to be limited to several weeks. Significant weight gain is not seen with corticosteroids in this population. Dexamethasone can be started at 2–4 mg daily, with titration to 16 mg daily if required. The lowest effective steroid dose should always be used. Androgens dronabinol and growth hormones have been effective for patients with AIDS-associated anorexia and cachexia.

Nutritional support, parenteral and enteral, has not been shown to prolong survival in patients with advanced cancer who are not candidates for disease-specific therapy. Exceptions include patients with head and neck cancer undergoing radiation therapy or patients with gastrointestinal dysfunction and otherwise good performance status.

Asthenia

Asthenia is well described in patients with cancer, but it also affects patients with end-stage organ dysfunction. It is one of the most disabling symptoms yet at the same time remains underrecognized and poorly treated. It is characterized by excessive physical, emotional, and cognitive fatigue that is not relieved by rest. Etiologies are often multifactorial, and treatment should be aimed at treating underlying and reversible causes, including hypoxia, anemia, electrolyte disturbances, dehydration, insomnia, or uncontrolled symptoms (such as pain, nausea, vomiting, and constipation). Unfortunately, when disease-specific therapy is not effective, asthenia is difficult to palliate. Education of the patient and family, normalization of the experience, counseling about energy conservation, mild exercise programs, light exposure therapy, and cognitive behavioral therapy can be effective. Symptomatic drug therapy includes corticosteroids (dexamethasone 2–4 mg PO once or twice daily) and psychostimulants (methylphenidate 2.5–5 mg PO once or twice daily). To lessen potential insomnia at night, these drugs should be administered early in the day.

PSYCHIATRIC DIMENSIONS IN PALLIATIVE CARE

Depression

There is a common assumption that symptoms of depression are normal or expected in patients facing life-threatening illness. This thought promotes the underdiagnosis of depression and, in turn, its undertreatment. Depressive states exist on a continuum from normal sadness that accompanies life-limiting disease to major affective disorders. It is important that clinicians differentiate among these levels of distress.

Besides a personal or family history of psychiatric illness, risk factors for depression in palliative care patients include young age, poor social support, worsening illness, high symptom burden, poor functional status, and the use of certain medications such as corticosteroids, interferon, interleukin-2, and some chemotherapeutic agents.

Diagnosing depression in physically healthy patients depends heavily on the presence of neurovegetative symptoms such as decreased appetite, loss of energy, insomnia, loss of sexual drive, and psychomotor retardation. Given that these symptoms are frequently present in patients with advanced illness, they are less reliable for diagnosing depression in this patient population. Elements of the history that can be helpful in diagnosing depression include anhedonia, feelings of hopelessness, worthlessness, helplessness, excessive guilt, and suicidal ideation. A quick and effective way to screen for depression is to ask the following two questions: "Are you feeling down, depressed or hopeless most of the time over the last 2 weeks?" and, "Have you found that little brings you pleasure or joy over the last 2 weeks?"

Treatment of depression in the palliative care population is similar to the general population. Since antidepressants take as much as 4–8 weeks to show effect, it is reasonable to start treatment with a psychostimulant in patients with a prognosis of <6 months. Effects are usually felt within 1–2 days and include improved mood, energy, appetite, and cognition. Other effective treatment options include psychotherapeutic interventions.

It is important to differentiate depression from preparatory or anticipatory grief, which is defined as the "grief that a terminally ill person has to undergo in order to prepare himself for his final separation from this world" (Elisabeth Kübler-Ross). Features include withdrawal from loved ones, rumination about the past, sadness, crying, and anxiety. In contrast to depression, mood changes are typically transient, and patients maintain the capacity for experiencing pleasure. Further, patients' self-image is typically not disturbed, and they are able to maintain hope, although the focus of their hope may shift.

Anxiety

Anxiety is a common symptom in patients facing serious illness. It is characterized by worries or fears stemming from one's perception of a threat in either the present or the future. Anxiety may be present as part of a primary psychiatric disorder, including generalized anxiety disorder, panic disorder, adjustment disorder, phobias, and acute or posttraumatic stress disorders. Anxiety may also be a secondary component of other symptoms, including pain, shortness of breath, or nausea. Furthermore, it can be a sign of drug withdrawal, including alcohol, opioids, benzodiazepines, antidepressants, and nicotine; and in addition, it can be an adverse drug reaction from medications such as corticosteroids, psychostimulants, and some antidepressants. Anxiety may have metabolic causes such as hyperthyroidism or syndromes of adrenergic or serotonergic excess. Often anxiety is also a sign of existential or psychosocial concerns about disease progression, disability, loss, dying, legacy, family, finances, and religion or spirituality.

Several formal screening tools for anxiety exist. The Edmonton Assessment Scale and the Hospital Anxiety and Depression Scale are most frequently used. Besides a thorough history and physical exam, the evaluation of a patient with anxiety should include an assessment of prior episodes of anxiety, depression, posttraumatic stress disorder (PTSD), and alcohol and drug use. It is helpful to ascertain if there are specific thoughts or situations triggering anxiety. Symptoms that can be misdiagnosed as anxiety include agitated delirium, cardiac arrhythmias, or akathisia, which is a symptom induced by dopamine receptor blocking agents such as metoclopramide or antipsychotics and manifests as an unpleasant sensation of restlessness.

The first step of treatment is active listening, with efforts to normalize the patient's experience and provide support. Pharmacologic treatment options include medications such as SSRIs (selective serotonin reuptake inhibitors) and benzodiazepines. Longer-acting benzodiazepines such as clonezepam are usually preferred, as they are less likely to cause rebound anxiety. The patient's subjective level of distress is the primary indication for the initiation of pharmacologic treatment. Nonpharmacologic treatment options include psychotherapeutic interventions such as cognitive behavioral therapy or supportive expressive therapy. The use of relaxation techniques or guided imagery is also helpful.

Delirium

Delirium is a frequently overlooked diagnosis, and it is associated with increased morbidity and mortality. It is characterized by an alteration of consciousness with a reduced ability to focus, sustain, or shift attention. Additional features are changes in cognition (such as memory deficits, language disturbances, and disorientation) and the development of perceptual disturbances. These changes are acute in onset and typically fluctuate throughout the day. Further symptoms include changes in the sleep/wake cycle, altered psychomotor activity, or delusions. A formal diagnosis of delirium also requires evidence by history, physical exam, or laboratory data that the changes in consciousness and cognition are caused by the direct physiological consequences of a medical condition.

The main differential diagnosis of delirium is dementia, which, unlike delirium, is characterized by little or no clouding in consciousness, an insidious onset, and a chronic, progressive course. Furthermore, hypoactive delirium may be mistaken for depression; conversely, early stages of hyperactive delirium may be mistaken for anxiety or extrapyramidal symptoms.

Treatment is focused on reversing or treating underlying causes, such as dehydration, infection, hypoxia, electrolyte disturbances (particularly hypercalcemia), metabolic disturbances, urinary retention, constipation, and brain metastases. The medication list should be reviewed for offending medications and drug-drug interactions. Benzodiazepines, anticholinergics, and antihistamines are often implicated in precipitating delirium and should be discontinued or decreased as much as possible. If opioids are suspected as the culprit agent, and the treatment doses cannot be reduced because of pain needs, then rotation to a different opioid at a dose reduced by 25–50% is recommended

Simple environmental measures are often underutilized and include frequent orientation (including use of clocks, calendars, caregivers, and pictures of loved ones), ample day/night indicators (well-illuminated rooms during the day and reduced noise and light at nighttime), and treatment of hearing and vision problems.

Pharmacologic interventions include the use of antipsychotics (**Table 67-5**). Haloperidol is most commonly used.

Holland J, et al. *Quick Reference for Oncology Clinicians: The Psychiatric and Psychological Dimensions of Cancer Symptom Management.* Charlottesville, VA: IPOS Press; 2006.
McPherson ML. Demystifying opioid conversion calculations. Bethesda, MD: American Society of Health-System Pharmacists; 2010.

Table 67-5. Pharmacological treatment options of delirium.

Drug	Starting Dose (mg)	Dosing Interval	Maximum 24-hour Dose (mg)	Comments
Haloperidol	0.5–1 (2 in ICU)	Every ½–1 hour for urgent symptoms, otherwise Q6–8h	20	Most commonly used; IV has less EPS than PO but PO has less QTc prolongation than IV
Olanzapine	2.5–10	Daily	20	Sedating, helpful in restoring day/sleep cycle when given at nighttime, less EPS
Quetiapine	12.5–50	Twice a day	800	At lower doses more sedating (antihistaminic) properties, antipsychotic effects at higher doses, less EPS
Risperidone	0.25–1	Twice a day or Q≤6h	6	Least sedating, caution with renal failure

Morrison RD, Meier DE. Palliative care. *N Engl J Med.* 2004;350:2582–2590.

National Institute for Health and Care Excellence. *Opioids in Palliative Care: Safe and Effective Prescribing of Strong Opioids for Pain in Palliative Care of Adults* (available at http://www.nice.org.uk/CG140; published May 2012; accessed April 14, 2003).

Oneshuk D, Hagen N, McDonald N. *Palliative Medicine: A Case-Based Manual,* 3rd ed. Oxford, UK: Oxford University Press; 2012.

Temel J, et al. Early palliative care for patients with metastatic non-small-cell lung cancer. *N Engl J Med.* 2010;363(8):733–742.

SPIRITUAL DIMENSIONS IN PALLIATIVE CARE

Palliative care physicians observe that their patients have needs that transcend physical pain, social disruptions, and psychiatric disorders. Chochinov (2006) notes, "More ubiquitous aspects of suffering—including psychological, existential, or spiritual distress—are not necessarily well understood or researched, nor do they necessarily engender a well-considered response."

The spiritual dimensions in palliative care include consideration of the patient's religious practices (eg, prayer, sacraments, and rituals) but also attend to what may be called the existential concerns of the patient. Chochinov lists these as "an overwhelming sense of hopelessness, existential or spiritual angst; loss of sense of dignity; sensing oneself a burden to others; or a waning of one's will to live and a growing desire for death." To this list can be added concerns such as the loss of a sense of meaning, a paralyzing sense of guilt and regret, broken relationships with loved ones, difficulties with one's concept of divinity or a sense of difficulty in a relationship with a personalized deity, feelings of anger, feelings of grief, and feelings of despair. Unsatisfied religious needs and unresolved existential concerns cause spiritual distress and can also result in psychiatric disorders such as depression or anxiety, as well as an increased sense of physical pain for the patient.

Recent studies have examined the importance of spirituality to physicians and to patients who are seriously or terminally ill, and whether and how physicians should address the spiritual concerns of these patients. [For a brief summary see Astrow and Sulmasy (2004).] Holmes and colleagues (2006) considered the results of some of these studies, conducted a study of their own, and came to the following conclusions: "It seems that patients tend to desire a sophisticated and somewhat controlled relationship with PCPs [primary care providers] around spirituality: They want their concerns cared about but not discussed or talked about, and they want to be prayed for but not with. These results indicate that, instead of discussing spiritual issues, PCPs may more appropriately "care" for the spiritual concerns of their patients by simply asking and listening . . . and leave the more active roles to others who have specific training in this area."

A study conducted by MacLean and colleagues (2003) concludes that patients' "desire for spiritual interaction increased with increasing severity of illness setting and decreased with referring to more-intense spiritual interactions."

Puchalski and Sandoval (2003) offer a simple assessment tool, known by its acronym, FICA, for assessing a patient's spirituality needs:

F: Faith, belief, meaning. Ask: "Do you consider yourself spiritual or religious?" "Do you have spiritual beliefs that help you cope with stress?" If the patient answers no, the physician might ask, "What gives your life meaning?"

I: Importance and influence. Ask: "What importance does your faith or belief have in your life?" "Have your beliefs influenced you in how you handle stress?" "Do you have specific beliefs that might influence your health care decisions?"

C: Community. Ask: "Are you a part of a spiritual or religious community? Is this of support to you, and how?" "Is there a group of people you really love or who are important to you?"

A: Address/action in care. Ask: "How should the health-care provider address these issues in your healthcare?" Appropriate action might involve referral to chaplains, clergy, and other spiritual care providers.

Often the presence of spiritual suffering will emerge as patients tell their stories. To attend to this suffering requires that the healthcare professional be aware of and attentive to her/his own spirituality. The decision to share personal insights, experiences, and resources must be done with sensitivity and compassion, and with respect for the patient's faith tradition and practice.

Consultation with and referral to a chaplain or other faith-based community leader is often appropriate. Professional chaplains are trained to understand and respect religious and cultural diversity and to assist patients and families in dealing with a wide variety of spiritual issues. Meador (2004) notes that "the clergy member of the team brings an interpretive, liturgical, and communal sense of spiritual care from her or his pastoral formation unique to that vocational formation."

Victor Frankl, a psychiatrist whose writings were based on his experience in a Nazi concentration camp, observed: "Man is not destroyed by suffering; he is destroyed by suffering without meaning." Palliative care therefore extends beyond the physical dimensions of suffering to attend to the spiritual suffering that may be present. A physician can attend to this dimension of healing by offering a listening ear, a word of kindness, and a referral to a professional spiritual caregiver.

Astrow AB, Sulmasy DP. Spirituality and the patient-physician relationship. *JAMA*. 2004;291(23):2884.

Chochinov H. Dying, dignity, and new horizons in palliative end-of-life care. *CA Cancer J Clin*. 2006;56(2):84–103.

Frankl VE. *Man's Search for Meaning*. Simon & Schuster; 1984.

Holmes SM, et al. Screening the soul: communication regarding spiritual concerns among primary care physicians and seriously ill patients approaching the end of life. *Am J Hosp Palliat Med*. 2006;23(1):25–33.

MacLean CD, et al. Patient preference for physician discussion and practice of spirituality. *J Gen Intern Med*. 2003;18(1):38–43.

Meador KG. Spiritual care at the end of life: What is it and who does it? *N C Med J*. 2004;65(4):226–228.

Puchalski C, Sandoval C. Spiritual care. In: O'Neill JF et al., eds. *A Clinical Guide to Supportive & Palliative Care for HIV/AIDS*. US Department of Health and Human Services, Health Resources and Services Administration; 2003 (available at http://ask.hrsa.gov/detail_materials.cfm?ProdID=2951).

COMMUNICATION SKILLS IN PALLIATIVE CARE

Physicians treating patients with serious illness encounter several difficult conversations with the patients and their families. These conversations span the entire disease course,

from the diagnosis through the disease progression, and finally, end-of-life care. Challenging aspects of these conversations include the breaking of serious news and discussions of prognosis, goals of care, and advance directives. These conversations often culminate in the emotionally challenging decision to transition from curative or life-prolonging therapies to hospice care. While easing difficult situations, effective communication also results in improved patient adjustment to illness, increased adherence to treatments, lessened pain and other physical symptoms, reduced anxiety, decreased conflict, and avoidance of ineffective, often invasive treatments.

▶ Responding to Emotions

Difficult conversations are very complex and elicit a wide range of emotions and reactions in patients and their families. These responses may include shock, withdrawal, sadness, crying, denial, fear, anger, and acceptance. During difficult conversations, clinicians tend to focus on objective, medical data; however, it is crucial to notice and respond to emotions. Understandably, difficult conversations represent a form of danger to patients. When facing danger, we usually respond with a fight-or-flight reaction, while more cognitive, analytical responses get shifted into the background. This is the reason why patients commonly report that they "did not hear anything" after their clinician conveyed serious news. The key at this point in the conversation is to slow down and respond to emotions so the "system can cool down" and patients are able to cognitively process important medical data.

Empathy is the process of recognizing and responding to emotions in others. It starts with noticing and identifying the patient's emotion; clinicians should importantly not try to fix or quiet a patient's emotion. The next step includes acknowledging the emotion. This can be done nonverbally (such as through eye contact, changes in body position, or touch) or through explicit statements. The acronym NURSE summarizes ways to respond verbally to emotions (**Table 67-6**).

Another powerful way to respond to emotions is to normalize the experience. Examples include "Anyone receiving such news would feel anxious and sad," or, "It is completely expected to feel devastated when one's life changes so dramatically."

▶ Breaking Serious News

Conversations in which serious news is delivered by the clinician to the patient and family occur not only at the time of diagnosis but also when the illness progressed to the point at which it no longer responds to therapies. The SPIKES (set up, perception, invitation, knowledge, emotion, summarize/strategy) protocol is a six-step protocol that can be used in these stressful situations:

Table 67-6. Responding to emotions: NURSE.

N	Name the emotion	"It sounds like this has been frustrating." "I can see you are feeling sad."
U	Understand the emotion	"It must be so hard to be in pain like this." "I understand that you are feeling lonely."
R	Respect (praise) the patient	"I am very impressed that you have been able to keep up with your treatments while experiencing all these side effects."
S	Support the patient	"My team and I will be here to support you." "No matter what happens next, I will be there for you."
E	Explore the emotion	"Tell me more why you are feeling frustrated." "Tell me more how this pain has been interfering with your life."

1. Set up—prepare for the conversation. Prior to the conversation, all medical data and information about possible treatment options need to be reviewed. The conversations should take place in a quiet place where everybody who is attending can sit down. Pagers and cell phones need to be silenced, and tissues should be in the patient's reach.

2. Assess the patient's perception. This step can provide an important window into the patient's perspective, especially if a clinician is meeting the patient for the first time. It may guide how much more information the patient may need. A simple way to assess a patient's understanding is to ask, "What have other doctors told you so far about your illness?" This step may not be necessary if the clinician knows the patient very well.

3. Ask for an invitation to talk about the news. This is a very valuable step, as patients in these situations can often feel out of control. Simply asking the question, "Are you ready to talk about this?" gives patients a little bit of control and signals an intent to work cooperatively. It is also important to assess how much the patient wants to know, taking into account cultural, religious, social, or personal issues.

4. Knowledge–disclose the news. Information needs to be communicated in a way that helps the patient to process and understand. It is helpful to preface serious news with a warning statement, such as "The test result came back and there is some serious news that we need to talk about" or "I am sorry to tell you that …..". Clear language without medical jargon should be used. The information needs to be provided in small, understandable amounts; details can be filled in later.

5. Respond to the patient's emotions. A wave of emotions will follow hearing the news. Ways on how to respond have been described above.

6. Summarize the conversation and discuss the strategy (treatment plan)

7. It is important to ask for questions, summarize what has been discussed, and to outline next steps. Providing information also in writing can reduce confusion and anxiety.

▶ **Discussing Prognosis**

Discussing prognosis is difficult; telling patients that they will die from their illness may feel, at its worst, like handing down a death sentence. It may often seem easier to defer these conversations and instead focus on symptoms and other care-related issues. For this reason, clinicians may have conflicting feelings about these conversations, because they understand that, although difficult and challenging, conversations that provide information about prognosis will allow the patient and family to prepare appropriately. Patients may also have contradictory wishes for their care. Most patients report that they want to be included in decision making and receive as much information as possible. However, they also want their care providers to support their wishes.

Having conversations about prognosis has been shown to impact advance care planning, particularly with regard to do-not-resuscitate orders and timely referrals to hospice. However, physicians are poor prognosticators and tend to be overly optimistic. The accuracy of prognostication improves with experience, but it worsens as the duration of the patient-physician relationship increases.

Prognostication is not commonly taught in medical school or during postgraduate training. In addition to observational data culled from patients with specific diseases, several models and scales are available to aid in forming prognoses. Some of these models are disease-specific, such as the Seattle heart failure model, a six-month-mortality calculator for patients on maintenance hemodialysis, and the Mortality Risk Index for patients with dementia. An example of a non-disease specific tool to assess prognosis is the Palliative Performance Scale (PPS, **Table 67-7**). Several studies showed correlations of PPS scores with survival in palliative care patients (including patients with different diagnoses and in different care settings).

A conversation about prognosis entails four steps: (1) negotiating the content, (2) providing information, (3) acknowledging the patient's and family's reaction to the news, and (4) checking for understanding.

Table 67-7. Palliative performance scale.

%	Ambulation	Activity Level Evidence of Disease	Self-Care	Intake	Level of Consciousness	Estimated Median Survival in Days[a]		
						A	B	C
100	Full	Normal No disease	Full	Normal	Full	N/A	N/A	108
90	Full	Normal Some disease	Full	Normal	Full			
80	Full	Normal with effort Some disease	Full	Normal or reduced	Full			
70	Reduced	Can't do normal job or work Some disease	Full	Normal or reduced	Full	145		
60	Reduced	Can't do hobbies or housework Significant disease	Occasional assistance needed	Normal or reduced	Full or confusion	29	4	
50	Mainly sit or lie	Can't do any work Extensive disease	Considerable assistance needed	Normal or reduced	Full or confusion	30	11	41
40	Mainly in bed	Can't do any work Extensive disease	Mainly assistance	Normal or reduced	Full or drowsy or confusion	18	8	
30	Bedridden	Can't do any work Extensive disease	Total care	Reduced	Full or drowsy or confusion	8	5	
20	Bedridden	Can't do any work Extensive disease	Total care	Minimal	Full or drowsy or confusion	4	2	6
10	Bedridden	Can't do any work Extensive disease	Total care	Mouth care only	Drowsy or coma	1	1	
0	Death							

[a]Key:
(A) Survival postadmission to an inpatient palliative unit, all diagnoses.
(B) Days until inpatient death following admission to an acute hospice unit, diagnoses not specified.
(C) Survival postadmission to an inpatient palliative unit, cancer patients only.

1. **Negotiating the content**: Even though most patients are interested in hearing about prognosis, not all want the same level of detail. Therefore, it is helpful to start the conversation by asking, "How much do you want to know about your prognosis?" A clinician can further explain the range of possible information provided by saying, "Some people want to hear every detail, some want to focus on the big picture, and others may rather not discuss prognosis at all. What would be best for you?" If a patient is interested in talking about prognosis, it is recommended to ask if the patient would like to hear specific statistics or rather be informed about the best, worst, and most likely case scenarios.

2. **Providing information**: The information needs to be given straightforwardly and slowly, in digestible pieces and with sufficient pauses to allow the patient to absorb it and then react and ask relevant questions. Information about time should be given in ranges, such as hours to days, days to weeks, weeks to months, or months to years.

3. **Acknowledging the patient's and family's reaction to the news:** The patient and family will most likely have an emotional reaction of some considerable intensity. Ways to respond verbally to emotions have been outlined in Table 67-6. Acknowledging the emotion can lead to a deepening of the conversation.

4. **Checking for comprehension**: Given the complexity of these conversations, patients and families may hear only the good or bad aspects. Ways to check in and ascertain what information was understood include,

"Tell me what you are taking away from this conversation," or, "Tell me what you will tell your spouse/friend about this conversation."

Clayton JM, et al. Clinical practice guidelines for communicating prognosis and end-of-life issues with adults in the advanced stages of a life-limiting illness, and their caregivers. *Med J Austral.* 2007;186(12 Suppl):S7,S79,S83–108.

Back A, Arnold R, Tulsky J. *Mastering Communication with Seriously Ill Patients—Balancing Honesty with Empathy and Hope.* Cambridge. UK: Cambridge University Press; 2009.

CARE OF THE DYING PATIENT

Family members may turn to care providers to help them understand what to expect when their loved one is dying. Patients who are very close to the end of life display a series of signs that predict the closeness of their deaths. One of the first signs is a decrease in engagement with one's surroundings and in communication. As the body is preparing to die, the patient decreases his/her oral intake. This is often the most difficult change for family members, as they may become concerned that their loved one is suffering and starving. Often it is enough to explain to them that this is part of the normal dying process. Most of the time, patients do not report being hungry or thirsty, although they may complain of a dry mouth. In this case, effective mouth care with moistened sponges and a lip balm is sufficient.

As the dying process continues, the patient will become progressively somnolent, with fewer and shorter awake periods. Sometimes the patient may become confused or restless. The clarity of hearing and vision is also often seen to decrease. Family members sometimes ask if their loved one is still able to hear them. Hearing is the last one of the five senses to be lost, and family members should be invited to continue talking to their loved one.

As oral intake decreases and metabolic changes continue, urine output will decrease and the urine will be more concentrated. When very close to death, patients may develop urinary and bowel incontinence. Other physical changes include alterations in body temperature and blood pressure, increased perspiration, and skin changes, such as mottling or a pale, yellowish pallor. Breathing changes also occur, including increased, decreased, or irregular respirations, as well as periods of apnea. As the patient is becoming weaker and more somnolent, s/he is no longer able to clear the throat or cough. Secretions begin to pool in the throat directly above the vocal cords. As air is passing by these secretions, the sound produced may be loud and rattling, often referred to as "death rattle." Family members who never have witnessed somebody dying may become concerned and wonder if the patient is "drowning." Very often, comparing the death rattle to snoring can comfort them; like snoring, this sound may be disturbing to the person

hearing it, but is not uncomfortable to the person producing it. Measures to decrease the death rattle include simply repositioning the head or the use of anticholinergic medications (see **Table 67-8**). Deep suction is not recommended, as it is uncomfortable and can lead to bleeding.

Medical care should be simplified as much as possible. Laboratory tests, radiologic procedures, and other interventions should be done only if they will result in improvement of the patient's comfort. Nonessential medications should be discontinued. Artificially provided hydration and nutrition are seldom necessary or helpful for the dying patient. Administration of parenteral fluids may result in progressive edema, lung congestion, increased oral secretions, and frequent urination with attendant discomfort and distress. Experienced hospice professionals note no increase in discomfort or suffering with the naturally occurring dehydration that accompanies the dying process. Frequently used medications to address symptoms of the dying patient are listed in Table 67-8.

Additionally, of great importance are nursing interventions, such as daily bathing, good mouth care, and application of artificial tears and lubricating ointment to the eyes, as well as comfortable positioning in the bed with pillows placed under the calves or other areas of support. Family members may be instructed in these nursing interventions and participate in the care of their loved one. This often is very meaningful and comforting to both the patient and family members.

Ellershaw J, Ward C. Care of the dying patient: the last hours or days of life. *Br Med J.* 2003;326(7379):30–34.

Karnes B. *Gone from My Sight.* Barbara Karnes Books (available at https://www.bkbooks.com/shop/gone-my-sight).

BEREAVEMENT

Grief, which is a normal reaction to loss, is the process of adjusting to a difficult reality. Both patients and families experience grief prior to and in anticipation of death; families and friends, of course, grieve after the death of a loved one. Attention to grief and bereavement is an often neglected part of excellent end-of-life care. Clinicians can play an important role in facilitating healthy grief and assessing for complicated grief.

Grieving individuals experience a variety of difficult emotional reactions, which usually occur in waves. Grief is triggered or exacerbated predictably by new losses, such as decline in functional status, as well as significant life events, including anniversaries and holidays. But grief can also worsen unpredictably by seemingly trivial events. Elisabeth Kübler-Ross first described five stages of grief—denial, anger, bargaining, depression, and acceptance—which may occur in any order and usually peak within 6 months following a loss. Somatic symptoms of grief include insomnia,

Table 67-8. Drugs used to control symptoms in the dying patient.

Symptom	Drug Class	Drug	Route	Dose
Pain	NSAID Opioid	Ketorolac Morphine	IV/SC IV/SC PO/PR	15–30 mg Q6h 4 mg Q4h 15 mg Q4h
"Death rattle"	Anticholinergic	Scopolamine Atropine Glycopyrrolate Hyoscyamine	TD IV/SC IV/SC SL	1 patch every 3 days 0.2–0.4 mg Q2h 0.2 mg Q4h 0.125–0.25 mg Q4h
Dyspnea	Opioid	Morphine	IV/SC PO/PR	4 mg Q4h 15 mg Q4h
Restlessness/anxiety	Benzodiazepine	Midazolam Lorazepam	SC IV/SC/SL	2–5 mg Q2h 0.5–1.0 mg every 4 h
Agitation/hallucinations	Antipsychotic	Haloperidol Thorazine	IV/SC IV PR	1–2 mg Q½h to effect 12.5–25 mg Q6h 25–50 mg Q6h

IV, intravenous; NSAID, nonsteroidal anti-inflammatory drug; PR, per rectum; SC, subcutaneous; SL, sublingual.

dizziness, anorexia, nausea, restlessness, generalized weakness, and shortness of breath.

The death of a loved one is likely one of the most stressful human experiences, yet most people cope without needing professional interventions. A few individuals have more pronounced symptoms and may experience a persistent, debilitating phenomenon referred to as *complicated grief* (CG). The symptoms of CG include longing for the loved one; trouble accepting the death; feeling uneasy about moving on with one's life; inability to trust others after the death; excessive bitterness or anger about the death; persistent feeling of being shocked, stunned, or numb; intense feeling of loneliness; feeling that life is empty or meaningless without the deceased; and frequent preoccupying thoughts about the deceased. These symptoms persist after 6 months, and they cause impairments in daily function. Predisposition to CG seems related to insecure attachment styles, an unstable sense of self, weak parental bonding in childhood, female gender, low perceived social support, death in an intensive care unit, and insufficient preparation for the loss (such as after an unexpected, traumatic death). Bereavement after the death of a child should always be considered CG. No interventions have been shown to prevent CG, but there is evidence from a recent meta-analysis that it is responsive to cognitive behavioral or group therapy.

Clinicians can play an important role in facilitating a healthy grieving process. They can assess patient and family risk factors for difficulties in grieving, and they can provide psychosocial resources as needed. Factors that have been associated with better bereavement outcomes include

effective symptom management and open and honest communication about the course of the illness, prognosis, and advance care planning. Timely hospice enrollment has also been shown to positively affect bereavement outcomes.

Even after a patient's death, clinicians can facilitate healthy grieving. Throughout the course of a serious illness, clinicians become an integral part in patients' and families lives. Therefore, it is a very appreciated and meaningful act of kindness to not end this relationship suddenly when a patient dies, and rather to make a condolence call, write a condolence letter, or even attend the funeral or memorial service. Screening for insomnia, hypertension, and substance abuse, as well as complicated grief and other psychiatric illnesses, is indicated.

Stroebe MS, Hansson RO, Stroebe W, Schutt H. *Handbook of Bereavement Research: Consequences, Coping, and Care.* Washington, DC: American Psychological Association; 2001.

RESOURCES

▶ **Books**

American Medical Association. *Participant's Handbook and Trainer's Guide for Education for Physicians on End-of-Life Care (EPEC)* (available at http://www.epec.net/item-products .php?type=3).
Goldman A, et al. *Oxford Textbook of Palliative Care for Children.* Oxford, UK: Oxford University Press; 2006.

Goldstein N, Morrison RS. *Evidence-Based Practice of Palliative Medicine: Expert Consult: Online and Print.* Philadelphia: Saunders-Elsevier; 2013.

Hanks G, et al. *Oxford Textbook of Palliative Medicine*, 4th ed. Oxford, UK: Oxford University Press; 2004.

Lynn J, Harrold J: *Handbook for Mortals: Guidance for People Facing Serious Illness,* 2nd ed. Oxford, UK: Oxford University Press; 2011.

Twycross R, Wilcock A, eds. *Hospice and Palliative Care Formulary, USA.* 2nd ed. Palliativedrugs.com Ltd; 2008.

Walsh D, et al. *Palliative Medicine: Expert Consult: Online and Print.* Philadelphia: Saunders-Elsevier; 2009.

▶ Journals

Journal of Pain and Symptom Management. Portenoy RK, ed. Elsevier Science Publishers, New York.

Journal of Palliative Medicine. Weissman DE, ed. Mary Ann Liebert, Inc, Larchmont, NY.

Palliative Medicine, The Research Journal of the EAPC. Geoffrey Hanks, ed. Sage Publications, London, UK.

Supportive Care in Cancer. Senn HJ, ed. Springer-Verlag, Heidelburg, Germany.

Websites

ACP-ASIM End-of-Life Care Consensus Panel: http://www.acponline.org/ethics/eolc.htm

Alliance of State Pain Initiatives (ASPI): http://aspi.wisc.edu/

AMA: Education for Physicians in End-of-Life Care: http://www.epec.net/EPEC/webpages/index.cfm

American Academy of Hospice and Palliative Medicine: http://www.aahpm.org

American Alliance of Cancer Pain Initiatives: http://www.aacpi.org

American Board of Hospice and Palliative Medicine: http://www.abhpm.org

Canter to Advance Palliative Care: http://www.capc.or

End-of-life Nursing Education Consortium: http://www.aacn.nche.edu/elnec

End-of-Life Physician Education Resource Center (EPERC): http://www.eperc.mcw.edu/

Growth House: http://www.growthhouse.org

Last Acts: http://www.lastacts.org

National Comprehensive Cancer Network guidelines for supportive care: http://www.nccn.org/professionals/physician_gls/f_guidelines.asp#supportive

National Consensus Project for Quality Palliative Care: http://www.nationalconsensusproject.org

National Hospice and Palliative Care Organization (NHPCO): http://www.nhpco.org

Supportive Care of the Dying: http://www.careofdying.org Hospice & Palliative Medicine

The Patient-Centered Medical Home

Larry S. Fields, MD

Elizabeth G. Tovar, PhD, RN, FNP-C

The 21st century began with some very exciting changes for primary care and specifically for family medicine. These changes are continuing to accelerate, heralding a bright future for the specialty. In this chapter we will discuss why a new model of primary care is essential; describe past, current, and future efforts for redesigning primary care with a focus on the patient-centered medical home (PCMH); and conclude with a discussion of how to transform both medical practices and the nation's healthcare delivery system to take full advantage of the PCMH's potential to improve the quality of, and access to, affordable care that enhances the well-being of everyone in this country.

THE NEED FOR CHANGE

The objective of any system of healthcare should be to improve the lives of the patients it serves, in terms of both the quality and the length of those lives, to create an environment in which people feel better, avoid preventable medical problems, ameliorate the effects of existing disease, and enjoy the lives they have as fully as possible.

Currently in the United States there are too many people who do not have adequate access to care, receive care that is of less than optimal quality, and obtain care that costs too much and has significant disparities in its provision (Institute of Medicine 2001). We need to do things differently because we know that there is a better way; a way that is based on solid scientific fact, which builds on the good of our current system and that is fair to all.

We must change from rewarding doing things to people, and create incentives to do things for people, from paying to do a task to paying for thinking about the task. Is a given procedure the most appropriate one for this individual at this particular time, if ever?

Institute of Medicine. *Crossing the Quality Chasm: A New Health System for the 21st Century.* National Academy Press; 2001.

HEALTH SYSTEM REFORM

▶ Past Attempts

A. Managed Care

In the early 1990s the idea of "managed care" was introduced into the United States, primarily as a way to increase profits and control costs by the insurance industry. This was popularly known as the "gatekeeper" system. Patients were required to visit a primary care provider (even though many subspecialists functioned in this role) who was approved by their insurance carrier to provide services under a particular plan as an entry point for any further access to the healthcare system. Payment was made to the physician on a capitated basis; that is, a fixed amount was paid to the physician for each member of that insurance plan who designated that individual as his or her primary care physician. The payment was the same each month regardless of whether the patient had been seen in that particular month. Additionally, a preauthorization was required for most services provided outside the physician's office. Testing and procedures done in the physician's office were rarely compensated beyond the amount of capitation. Understandably, both patients and physicians generally despised this idea.

It deprived the patient of freedom of choice, while increasing the inconvenience of obtaining a referral, test, or most any other service. Physicians were cast in the unfamiliar and uncomfortable role of being a patient adversary rather than a patient advocate. Payments were generally slow in coming and often did not come at all, making it difficult, if not impossible, for practices to maintain financial margins sufficient to maintain viability. This system was further flawed in that physicians were selected to be the "gatekeepers" solely on the condition that they have a pulse, and not by specialty or any other criterion that might indicate the physician's ability to improve quality and control cost.

B. Case Management

Next, insurance companies and other third parties tried to charge employers and other insurance providers (such as state and federal governments) to provide chronic disease management services on the theory that managing the disease, and not the whole patient (without direct contact with the patient, by the way), would somehow improve the patient's health and long-term prognosis. The only tangible results of this idea were to increase duplication of testing and increase the cost of providing insurance with no tangible benefit to anyone except the companies providing such services.

► Present & Future

A. The Patient-Centered Medical Home

The term *medical home* originated in the 1960s with the American Academy of Pediatrics (AAP), who proposed that this entity be a repository for all medical information on certain patient populations. Since that time, the meaning and application of the concept of a medical home has varied. The idea has evolved to the *patient-centered medical home* (PCMH) as the framework for transforming healthcare in the United States.

Prior to the PCMH, there had been some progress toward conceptualizing a new model of care for chronic illnesses with the goal of improving clinical outcomes. The resulting chronic care model (CCM) (see **Figure 68-1**) was developed by Wagner and his colleagues at the MacColl Institute (Wagner 1998).

At the core of the CCM was a shift in focus from a reactive approach to a proactive one, resulting in improved outcomes through productive interactions between an informed and activated patient and a prepared and proactive practice team (ICIC 2008). The model posits that to improve the current healthcare system and promote high-quality chronic illness care, the system must be reorganized to include six essential elements. These elements include a *health system* that promotes safe, high-quality care by supporting effective and patient centered *delivery system design, decision support,* and *self-management support* strategies and *clinical information systems* as well as collaboration with *the community* to mobilize community resources to meet the needs of patients (IHI 2008).

Studies that incorporated one or more elements of the CCM provided extensive evidence to support the positive effects of CCM-based interventions on both clinical processes and patient outcomes (Glasgow et al. 2001; Ouwens et al. 2005; Tsai et al. 2005; Piatt et al. 2006) and cost-effectiveness (Bodenheimer et al. 2002). Each individual element of the CCM is important and can lead to improved outcomes. While no single element appears to be more effective than the other, the more CCM elements implemented, the better the outcomes (Tsai et al. 2005).

In the year 2000, leaders in family medicine assessed the specialty's future role with the Future of Family Medicine Project (FFM), This effort, along with similar projects by the AAP and the American College of Physicians (ACP), ultimately became the second major step in development of the medical home.

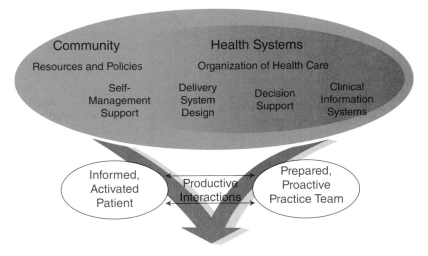

Figure 68-1. The chronic care model.

During this period much independent research, both in the United States and abroad, demonstrated that primary care was associated with higher-quality care delivered at lower cost and with increased patient satisfaction. Simultaneously, IBM, aware of this research and its own experiential data from countries with primary care–based health systems, began to search for the same value in healthcare in the United States.

In spring 2006, having become aware of the now completed FFM project and its conclusion that the country's family doctors physicians needed a "new model" of practice, representatives of IBM approached leaders of the American Academy of Family Physicians (AAFP) (Larry S. Fields, MD and Douglas Henley, MD) about collaboration on the issue.

Subsequently, the ACP and AAFP, along with IBM, convened a summit to educate and involve businesses, insurance companies, and physician groups such as the American Osteopathic Association (AOA) in the development and propagation of what came to be termed the *patient-centered medical home* (PCMH).

These groups developed and refined the principles on which the medical home would be based and formed the Patient-Centered Primary Care Collaborative (PCPCC) with headquarters in the nation's capitol to promote and disseminate the medical home idea to businesses, the public, physicians, and insurance companies as well as to federal and state governments. Currently the PCPCC has over 700 member organizations representing 333,000 primary care physicians, several Fortune 500 companies and their millions of employees, major health insurance companies, governmental agencies, other physician groups, and organizations representing patients.

The PCMH has become the most important idea for health system change since the early 1960s. It is now the accepted vehicle to finally provide quality, affordable, accessible healthcare for everyone in the United States.

American Academy of Family Physicians. *The New Model of Primary Care: Knowledge Bought Dearly*. AAFP; 2004 (available at http://www.aafp.org/online/etc/medialib/aafp_org/documents/policy/policy/primarycarepolicy.Par.0001.File.tmp/caremanagementpolicy.pdf; retrieved July 16, 2009).

Bodenheimer, T et al. Improving primary care for patients with chronic illness: the Chronic Care Model, Part 2. *JAMA*. 2002;288(15):1909–1914.

Glasgow RE, Hiss RG, Anderson RM, et al. Report of the Health Care Delivery Work Group: behavioral research related to the establishment of a chronic disease model for diabetes care. *Diabetes Care*. 2001;24(1):124–130.

Ouwens M, Wollersheim H, et al. Integrated care programmes for chronically ill patients: a review of systematic reviews. *Int J Qual Health Care*. 2005;17(2):141–146.

Piatt GA, et al. Translating the Chronic Care Model into the community. *Diabetes Care*. 2006;29(4):811–817.

Robert Graham Center. *The Patient Centered Medical Home: History, Seven Core Features, Evidence and Transformational Change*. American Academy of Family Physicians; 2007.

Tsai A, Morton S, Mangione C, Keeler E. A meta-analysis of interventions to improve chronic illness *Care Am J Manage Care*. 2005;11:478–488.

B. PCMH Evidence

Although the concept of a PCMH has been around for a while, the definition and framework are relatively new. Data demonstrating the effectiveness of PCMH care have been generated in various settings and various payment systems, including those composed of commercially insured, Medicare, Medicaid, and multipayer patient populations (PCPCC; "evidence for the PCMH" available at www.pcpcc.net). The evidence shows the PCMH's positive effect on health outcomes, patient satisfaction, processes of care, and cost effectiveness (Glasgow et al. 2001; Tsai et al. 2005; Bodenheimer et al. 2002).

Bodenheimer T, et al. Improving primary care for patients with chronic illness: the Chronic Care Model, Part 2. *JAMA*. 2002;288(15):1909–1914.

Glasgow RE, Hiss RG, Anderson RM, et al. Report of the Health Care Delivery Work Group: behavioral research related to the establishment of a chronic disease model for diabetes care. *Diabetes Care*. 2001;24(1):124–130.

Stewart E, et al. *Preliminary Answers to Policy-Relevant Questions: From the Early Analyses of the Independent Evaluation Team of the National Demonstration Project of TransforMED* (available at http://www.transformed.com/evaluatorsReports/preliminaryAnswers.cfm; retrieved July 9, 2009).

Patient Centered Primary Care Collaborative. *The Outcomes of Implementing Patient-Centered Medical Home Interventions: A Review of the Evidence on Quality, Access and Costs from Recent Prospective Evaluation Sstudies*. PCPCC; 2009. (Prepared by Kevin Grumbach, MD; Thomas Bodenheimer, MD, MPH; and Paul Grundy MD, MPH. Retrieved Aug. 20, 2010 from http://www.pcpcc.net/files/Grumbach_et-al_Evidence-of-Quality_%20101609_0.pdf).

C. PCMH Benefits

Tthe patient-centered medical home (PCMH) places patients and their interests at the center of the healthcare system. What is best for the patient is also best for the healthcare team and the system as a whole. "First, do what is right for the patient" should be the guiding principle in setting the priorities of the physician and other team members as well as the healthcare system.

The goal of the PCMH is for the patients to feel better, to have better health, to live longer and more productive lives, and to have access to less expensive services. Subspecialists can do what they are trained to do better than they do now. Hospital admissions and emergency department visits will decrease. In short, the PCMH is the only vehicle that can deliver high-quality healthcare at reasonable cost to every person in the United States.

The PCMH does not require inventing any new tests, treatments, or new specialties; it simply requires enough primary care physicians in the workforce, using the principles of the medical home, existing technology, and the best available evidence to do the "right thing" at the right time for the whole population.

Preventive services will be delivered more regularly, appropriately, and more broadly than currently. The lower the barriers to care (ie, copays) in the PCMH, the more patients will have an incentive to use its services rather than accessing the system at another, more expensive level.

The PCMH provides quality, accessible, cost-efficient healthcare that improves the health and well-being of people without depriving them of choice, riches, or independence.

ESSENTIAL ELEMENTS FOR A SUCCESSFUL PATIENT-CENTERED MEDICAL HOME

▶ Adherence to Accepted Standards & Recognition

The *patient-centered medical home* (PCMH), as defined by the National Committee for Quality Assurance (NCQA 2009), is a "healthcare setting that facilitates partnerships between individual patients, and their personal physicians, and when appropriate, the patient's family. Care is facilitated by registries, information technology, health information exchange and other means to assure that patients get the indicated care when and where they need and want it in a culturally and linguistically appropriate manner."

To describe the essential characteristics of the PCMH, the American Academy of Family Physicians, American Academy of Pediatrics, American College of Physicians, and the American Osteopathic Association (representing approximately 333,000 physicians) developed the Joint Principles of the Patient-Centered Medical Home, which are listed in **Table 68-1**.

The joint principles emphasize a patient-centered, holistic approach to patient care provided by a physician-led medical practice that should include collaboration with other disciplines such as nursing, pharmacy, nutrition, and behavioral science to meet the individual needs of the patients through integrated and/or coordinated care. No single individual can adequately meet all the needs of all the patients in a practice, thus teamwork and collaboration between disciplines in a manner that utilizes the strengths that each discipline brings to the team is essential to the success of the PCMH. The joint principles also emphasize enhanced access to care and an improved payment structure that combines enhanced fee for service as well as a per patient–per month payment or PPPM (see discussion below).

To be formally recognized as a PCMH, practices must meet a set of standards such as those established by the National Committee for Quality Assurance, URAC, The Joint Commission, or other certifying bodies that are aligned with the "Joint Principles" of the PCMH. Using this model, a practice would complete a self-assessment survey and submit documentation supporting the responses in the survey.

For practices interested in achieving PCMH status, TransforMED is an initiative of the AAFP to help practices get there by providing a framework and tools through online resources as well as direct consultation to facilitate necessary practice changes (Barclay 2006). The goal of a transformed practice is to improve quality, safety, and access while also increasing physician satisfaction [McGeeney, as cited in Barclay (2006)].

Barclay L. *AAFP Practice Redesign Initiative Aims at Transforming Primary Care* [electronic version]. Medscape Medical News; 2006 (available at http://www.medscape.com/viewarticle/529914; retrieved July 9, 2009).

National Committee for Quality Assurance. *Physician Practice Connections—Patient-Centered Medical Home*. NCQA; 2009 (available at http://www.ncqa.org/tabid/631/Default.aspx; retrieved June 17, 2009).

▶ Individual Care Coordination

"I guess you know what's happened to me since my last visit" or some variant thereof, is among the most dreaded phrases a patient can ever utter to a family physician. Dreadful because the physician immediately knows that several equally regrettable things have occurred. First, something the patient perceives as significant has taken place. Second, this event is likely to have been a nonspecific symptom (like chest pain) and involve several subspecialists, multiple tests (many of which may have been unnecessary if not redundant), and a whole lot of money. Third, and most dreadful of all, the physician has not the first clue as to what the patient is talking about.

It is clear from all available data that preventing this scenario is absolutely essential to controlling quality and cost. Regardless of whether an emergency department visit is avoided, or the number and type of tests a patient needs are more appropriately ordered, someone must be enabled to see that the care of a given individual is optimized. This function cannot be totally done in face-to-face encounters between patient and physician. Many types of "asynchronous" interactions will need to occur in order to achieve quality at acceptable cost. Delivering preventive services in the office; refilling prescriptions; educating patients about diet, exercise, and smoking cessation as well as making referrals; tracking consultations; handling abnormal test results; and a myriad of other tasks must be performed in a coordinated, well defined manner, or the game is lost.

The time and effort devoted to such asynchronous activities by all members of the healthcare team is labor-intensive and time-consuming. Properly performed, these endeavors

Table 68-1. Joint principles of the patient-centered medical home (AAFP, AAP, ACP, and AOA Consensus Panel, 2007).[a]

Personal physician	Each patient has an ongoing relationship with a personal physician trained to provide first-contact, continuous and comprehensive care.
Physician-directed medical practice	The personal physician leads a team of individuals at the practice level who collectively take responsibility for the ongoing care of patients.
Whole-person orientation	The personal physician is responsible for providing for all the patient's healthcare needs or taking responsibility for appropriately arranging care with other qualified professionals. This includes care for all stages of life, acute care, chronic care, preventive services, and end-of-life care.
Care is coordinated and/or integrated	Care is coordinated and/or integrated across all elements of the complex healthcare system (eg, subspecialty care, hospitals, home health agencies, nursing homes) and the patient's community (eg, family, public and private community-based services). Care is facilitated by registries, information technology, health information exchange, and other means to ensure that patients obtain the indicated care when and where they need and want it in a culturally and linguistically appropriate manner.
Quality and safety are hallmarks of the medical home	Practices advocate for their patients to support the attainment of optimal, patient-centered outcomes that are defined by a care planning process driven by a compassionate, robust partnership between physicians, patients, and patients' families.
	Evidence-based medicine and clinical decision support tools guide decision making. Physicians in the practice accept accountability for continuous quality improvement through voluntary engagement in performance measurement and improvement.
	Patients actively participate in decision making, and feedback is sought to ensure that patients' expectations are being met. Information technology (IT) is utilized appropriately to support optimal patient care, performance measurement, patient education, and enhanced communication.
	Practices go through a voluntary recognition process by an appropriate nongovernmental entity to demonstrate that they have the capabilities to provide patient-centered services consistent with the medical home model.
	Patients and families participate in quality improvement activities at the practice level.
Enhanced access	Enhanced access to care is available through systems such as open scheduling.
Payment	Payment appropriately recognizes the added value provided to patients who have a patient-centered medical home.

[a]The *patient-centered medical home* (PCMH) is an approach to providing comprehensive primary care for children, youth, and adults. The PCMH is a healthcare setting that facilitates partnerships between individual patients and their personal physicians, and, when appropriate, the patient's family.

will produce significant benefits to the health and well-being of individual patients, practices as a whole, and to society in general.

Care coordination is central to the success of the PCMH, as is integration of individual components of care into a unified plan and set of actions. To ensure a person's health, there must be support and incentives, which are needed for practices to add these services and assume this responsibility. The mechanism to provide such support is a monthly payment to the medical professional (usually a primary care physician) responsible for the healthcare of a given individual in the PCMH. This monthly fee is additional to any payment made to the physician for services rendered when the patient is actually seen in the PCMH, hospital, nursing home, or other venue. The monthly payment continues as

long as that patient is a member of that particular PCMH, regardless of whether the patient was seen in the PCMH in any given month. The payment must be adequate to sustain the PCMH's fiscal ability to provide the range of asynchronous services required by its patients.

Monthly payments have been called many names, including per patient–per month payment (PPPM), case management fee, disease management fee, care coordination fee, pay for reporting, pay for performance, pay for use (ie, use of a qualified electronic health record), or simply "capitation" (which it is most definitely not). Such payments are better termed "care coordination and integration fees" (CIFs), so as to better describe their purpose.

A given practice will need to meet and maintain a rigorous set of standards like those of the National Committee for

Quality Assurance (NCQA), which designates three levels that the PCMH might attain, each level having a correspondingly higher CIF.

Without the CIFs, the services mentioned above and the benefits to patients that derive from such services cannot be delivered on a consistent basis.

▶ Reduction of Barriers to Care & Disparities in Care

Reducing financial barriers to receiving care in the PCMH is vital to the functioning of a successful PCMH. Concomitant system changes to enable the attainment of these goals are integral to providing fiscally stable entities that are ubiquitous enough to allow easy access.

Next, the amount paid on a fee-for-service basis for visits to the PCMH must increase significantly. Cognitive services, which make up the majority of services rendered by the PCMH, have long been undervalued relative to payments for procedures.

Along with reasonable CIFs, enhanced payments for services delivered by the PCMH have several positive results. The stability of the PCMH is considerably improved. As noted earlier, services provided by the PCMH would be enriched and be delivered in a more consistent manner. Because of the improved economics, more medical students will be able to choose primary care careers, thereby increasing the number of medical homes and improving access to those medical homes. Evidence tells us that increased access to primary care services will reduce—and may even eliminate—disparities that currently exist in healthcare.

▶ How Do We Get There?

This question has implications for individual practices and the healthcare system as a whole. The answer is different for each. For individual practices, either large or small, the first step is the implementation of a functional *electronic medical record* (EMR) that has been certified as compliant with the standards for "meaningful use" (a governmental program supplying payments for practices implementing and appropriately using the certified EMR). Second, a thorough examination of the practice's chosen certifying body's standards for PCMH certification will provide a roadmap.

The EMR must provide functionality such as preventive care reminders, electronic prescribing, flagging of abnormal test results, performance data, referral tracking, and support for practice improvement initiatives. Written policies concerning patient access/communication and an interactive website will provide for higher levels of certification.

Changing the healthcare system to take advantage of the PCMH's benefits is well under way. There are now over 17,000 certified medical homes.

CONCLUSION

The patient-centered medical home (PCMH) is an entity designed to build on the solid scientific evidence of quality and cost-effectiveness of primary care. It does not require inventing new technologies, nor does it require creating new kinds of physicians.

The PCMH will function in any environment, and under any payment system so long as the essentials of the medical home (strict adherence to the joint principles, individual care coordination, and reduction of barriers and disparities) are not compromised.

The PCMH is the mechanism that is transforming our healthcare system to achieve quality, affordable, accessible heathcare for everyone. This is too important for partisan politics and power grabs. This is about people, our friends, our families, and our fellow citizens. This is the time to look objectively at the facts and act accordingly. This is the time, and the PCMH is the vehicle, to finally bring longer, healthier, happier, and more productive lives to all of our people.

American Academy of Family Physicians, American Academy of Pediatrics, American College of Physicians, and the American Osteopathic Association Consensus Panel (2007). *Joint Principles of the Patient-Centered Medical Home* (available at http://docs.google.com/gview?a=v&q=cache:F6_MAENFnK0J:www.medicalhomeinfo.org/joint%2520Statement.pdf+JOINT+PRINCIPLES+OF+THE+PATIENT-CENTERED+MEDICAL+HOME&hl=en&gl=us; retrieved July 16, 2009).

Bauer MS, et al. Collaborative care for bipolar disorder: Part II. Impact on clinical outcome, function, and costs. *Psychiatr Serv.* 2006;57(7):937–945.

Bray P, et al. Feasibility and effectiveness of system redesign for diabetes care management in rural areas: the eastern North Carolina experience. *Diabetes Educ.* 2005;31(5):712–718.

Chin MH, et al. Improving diabetes care in midwest community health centers with the health disparities collaborative. *Diabetes Care.* 2004;27(1):2–8.

Dwight-Johnson M, et al. Can collaborative care address the needs of low-income Latinas with comorbid depression and cancer? Results from a randomized pilot study. *Psychosomatics.* 2005;46(3):224–232.

Lozano P, et al. A Multisite randomized trial of the effects of physician education and organizational change in chronic-asthma care: health Outcomes of the Pediatric Asthma Care Patient Outcomes Research Team II Study. *Arch Pediatr Adolesc Med.* 2004;158(9):875–883.

Mangione-Smith R, et al. Measuring the effectiveness of a collaborative for quality improvement in pediatric asthma care: does implementing the Chronic Care Model improve processes and outcomes of care? *Ambulatory Pediatr.* 2005;5(2):75–82.

Montori VM, et al. The impact of planned care and a diabetes electronic management system on community-based diabetes care. *Diabetes Care.* 2002;25(11):1952–1957.

Patient Centered Primary Care Collaborative. *Patient-Centered Medical Home—Building Evidence and Momentum: Evidence on Effectiveness.* PCPCC; 2008.

Rosenthal TC. The medical home: growing evidence to support a new approach to primary care. *J Am Board Fam Med.* 2008;21(5):427–440.

Schmittdiel J, et al. Patient Assessment of Chronic Illness Care (PACIC) and improved patient-centered outcomes for chronic conditions. *J Gen Intern Med.* 2008;23(1):77–80.

Siminerio LM, et al. Implementing the chronic care model for improvements in diabetes care and education in a rural primary care practice. *Diabetes Educ.* 2005;31(2):225–234.

Stroebel RJ, et al. Adapting the chronic care model to treat chronic illness at a free medical clinic. *J Health Care Poor Underserved.* 2005;16(2):286–296.

Wang A, et al. The North Carolina experience with the Diabetes Health Disparities Collaboratives. Joint Commission. *J Qual Patient Safety.* 2004;30:396–404.

Index

Note: Page references followed by *f, t,* and *b* indicate figures, tables, and boxes respectively.